Provided as an educational resource from

The Alliance for Better Bone Health

SIXTH EDITION

GLASS' OFFICE GYNECOLOGY

Michèle G. Curtis, M.D., M.P.H.
Associate Professor
Department of Obstetrics
Gynecology and Reproductive Sciences
University of Texas Health Sciences Center Houston
Attending Physician
Lyndon Baines Johnson General Hospital
Houston, Texas

Shelley Overholt, M.D.
Family Practice Associates of McPherson, L.L.P.
Memorial Hospital of McPherson
McPherson, Kansas
Clinical Instructor
University of Kansas Medical School
Wichita, Kansas

Michael P. Hopkins, M.D., M.Ed.
Director
Department of Obstetrics and Gynecology
Aultman Hospital
Professor
Northeastern Ohio Universities College of Medicine
Canton, Ohio

LIPPINCOTT WILLIAMS & WILKINS
A Wolters Kluwer Company
Philadelphia • Baltimore • New York • London
Buenos Aires • Hong Kong • Sydney • Tokyo

Acquisitions Editor: Sonya Seigafuse
Managing Editor: Nicole Dernoski
Project Manager: Alicia Jackson
Senior Manufacturing Manager: Benjamin Rivera
Marketing Manager: Kathy Neely
Cover Designer: Vasiliky Kiethas
Production Service: TechBooks
Printer: Edwards Brothers

530 Walnut Street
Philadelphia, PA 19106 USA
LWW.com

First Edition 1976 Second Edition 1981 Third Edition 1988 Fourth Edition 1993 Fifth Edition 1998 Sixth Edition 2006

Printed in the USA

Library of Congress Cataloging-in-Publication Data

Glass' office gynecology / [edited by] Michèle G. Curtis, Shelley Overholt, Michael P. Hopkins.—6th ed.
p. ; cm.
Includes bibliographical references and index.
ISBN 13: 978-0-7817-4250-4
ISBN 10: 0-7817-4250-1
1. Gynecology. I. Glass, Robert H., 1932- . II. Curtis, Michèle G. III. Overholt, Shelley.
IV. Hopkins, Michael P. V. Title: Office gynecology.
[DNLM: 1. Genital Diseases, Female. 2. Ambulatory Care. WP 140 G549 2006]
RG103.034 2006
618.1—dc22

2005024928

10 9 8 7 6 5

To Jessica and Rachel—my sources of hope, faith, and the greatest love I have ever known.

MICHÈLE CURTIS

Thanks to my husband, Dale Ray Thiesen, for the support (and prodding when necessary) on this project.

SHELLEY OVERHOLT

To my wife, Mary Kay.

MICHAEL HOPKINS

Contents

Contributors

Jimmy D. Acklin, M.D.
Associate Professor
Department of Family and Community Health
Residency Director
AHEC Fort Smith Family Practice Residency
University of Arkansas for Medical Sciences, AHEC Fort Smith
Fort Smith, Arkansas

Tracey A. Banks, M.D.
Private Practice
North Central Women's Health Partners
Attending Physician
Medical Center of McKinney
McKinney, Texas

Kurt T. Barnhart, M.D., M.S.C.E.
Associate Professor
Departments of Ob/Gyn and Epidemiology
University of Pennsylvania
Philadelphia, Pennsylvania

Alfred E. Bent, M.D.
Associate Professor
Department of Gynecology & Obstetrics
Johns Hopkins Medicine
Chairman
Department of Gynecology
Greater Baltimore Medical Center
Baltimore, Maryland

Andrew Berchuck, M.D.
Professor
Department of Obstetrics and Gynecology/Division of Gynecologic Oncology
Duke University Medical Center
Durham, North Carolina

Abbey B. Berenson, M.D.
Professor
Department of Obstetrics and Gynecology
University of Texas Medical Branch
Galveston, Texas

Barbara M. Buttin, M.D.
Assistant Professor
Gynecologic Oncology
Department of Obstetrics and Gynecology
Northwestern University Feinberg School of Medicine
Chicago, Illinois

Mitchell D. Creinin, M.D.
Director of Gynecologic Specialties
Director of Family Planning
Department of Obstetrics, Gynecology, and Reproductive Sciences
University of Pittsburgh School of Medicine
Department of Epidemiology
Graduate School of Public Health
University of Pittsburgh
Pittsburgh, Pennsylvania

Michèle G. Curtis, M.D., M.P.H.
Associate Professor
Department of Obstetrics, Gynecology and Reproductive Sciences
University of Texas Health Sciences Center Houston
Attending Physician
Lyndon Baines Johnson General Hospital
Houston, Texas

Anthony DelConte, M.D., F.A.C.O.G.
Senior Medical Director
U.S. Clinical Development and Medical Affairs
Novartis Pharmaceuticals Corporation
East Hanover, New Jersey

Nancy L. Eriksen, M.D.
Associate Professor
Maternal Fetal Medicine
Department of Obstetrics
Gynecology and Reproductive Sciences
University of Texas Health Science Center–Houston
Houston, Texas

Andrew H. Fenton, M.D.
Assistant Professor of Surgery
Northeastern Ohio Universities College of Medicine
Department of Surgery
Akron General Medical Center
Akron, Ohio

Linda M. Frazier, M.D., M.P.H.
Professor
Department of Preventive Medicine and Public Health
Department of Obstetrics-Gynecology
University of Kansas School of Medicine–Wichita
Wichita, Kansas

Clarisa R. Gracia, M.D.
Division of Reproductive Endocrinology and Infertility
University of Pennsylvania Medical Center
Philadelphia, Pennsylvania

David A. Grainger, M.D., M.P.H.
Professor
Department of Obstetrics-Gynecology
Department of Preventive Medicine and Public Health
University of Kansas School of Medicine–Wichita
Center for Reproductive Medicine
Wichita, Kansas

Gretchen Gross, M.S.W.
Center for Health and Wellbeing
University of Vermont
Burlington, Vermont

Daniel P. Guyton, M.D.
Professor and Chair
Department of Surgery
Northeastern Ohio Universities College of Medicine
Chairman
Department of Surgery
Akron General Medical Center
Akron, Ohio

Amy E. Harrison, M.D.
Instructor
Department of Family Medicine
University of Chicago
Chicago, Illinois
Director
Women's Health Fellowship
Family Practice Residency Program, MacNeal Hospital
Berwyn, Illinois

Thomas J. Herzog, M.D.
Professor and Director
Division of Gynecologic Oncology
Department of Obstetrics and Gynecology
Columbia University College of Physicians and Surgeons
New York, New York

Lisa M. Hollier, M.D., M.P.H.
Assistant Professor
Department of Obstetrics, Gynecology, and Reproductive Sciences
University of Texas Health Sciences Center Houston
Houston, Texas

Michael P. Hopkins, M.D., M.Ed.
Director
Department of Obstetrics and Gynecology
Aultman Hospital
Professor
Northeastern Ohio Universities College of Medicine
Canton, Ohio

Justin P. Lavin, Jr., M.D.
Professor
Department of Obstetrics and Gynecology
Northeastern Ohio Universities College of Medicine
Chairman of Maternal Fetal Medicine
Children's Hospital Medical Center of Akron
Akron, Ohio

Lauren B. Marangell, M.D.
Associate Professor of Psychiatry and Behavioral Science
Department of Psychiatry
Baylor College of Medicine
Houston, Texas

James M. Martinez, M.D.
Assistant Professor
Department of Psychiatry and Behavioral Science
Baylor College of Medicine
Houston, Texas

Godwin I. Meniru, M.B.B.S., M.Med.Sci., M.F.F.P., M.R.C.O.G.
Assistant Professor of Obstetrics and Gynecology
Northeastern Ohio Universities College of Medicine
Rootstown, Ohio
Medical Director
Junaelo Institute of Reproductive Medicine
Vice Chairman
Department of Obstetrics and Gynecology
Doctor's Hospital of Stark County
Canton, Ohio

David G. Mutch, M.D.
Division of Gynecologic Oncology
Department of Obstetrics and Gynecology
Washington University School of Medicine
St. Louis, Missouri

Shelley Overholt, M.D.
Family Practice Associates of McPherson, L.L.P.
Memorial Hospital of McPherson
McPherson, Kansas
Clinical Instructor
University of Kansas Medical School
Wichita, Kansas

Wilson Sawa, M.D.
OB/Gyn Resident PGYIII
Department of Obstetrics and Gynecology
Aultman Ob/Gyn Residency Program
Aultman Health Foundation
Canton, Ohio

Vincent M.B. Silenzio, M.D., M.P.H.
Assistant Professor
Departments of Family Medicine
Community and Preventive Medicine, and Psychiatry
Univeristy of Rochester
Attending Physician
Department of Family Medicine
URMC/Highland Hospital, URMC/Strong Memorial Hospital
Rochester, New York

Monique A. Spillman, M.D., Ph.D.
Clinical Associate Faculty
Department of Obstetrics and Gynecology/
Division of Gynecologic Oncology
Duke University Medical Center
Durham, North Carolina

John F. Steege, M.D.
Chief
Division of Gynecology
Department of Obstetrics and Gynecology
The University of North Carolina at Chapel Hill
Chapel Hill, North Carolina

Meir Steiner, M.D., Ph.D., F.R.C.P.C.
Professor of Psychiatry & Behavioural Neurosciences
and Obstetrics & Gynecology
McMaster University
Director of Research
Department of Psychiatry
Director
Women's Health Concerns Clinic
St. Joseph's Healthcare, Hamilton
Ontario, Canada

John Stewart, Jr., M.D.
Department of Obstetrics and Gynecology
Akron General Medical Center
Akron, Ohio

John M. Storment, M.D.
Fertility Institute
Lafayette, Louisiana

Steven M. Strong, M.D.
Active Staff
Department of Obstetrics and Gynecology
Memorial Herman Hospital
The Woodlands, Texas

Andrea L. Zuckerman, M.D.
Assistant Professor
OB/GYN and Pediatrics
Tufts–New England Medical Center
Needham, Massachusetts

Preface

Women's health care is an ever-changing field. It relies on both quantitative and qualitative scientific advances that must be translated into clinical skills and application against the backdrop of current political, social, and global circumstances. New knowledge and technological advances explode into our daily lives with such astonishing rapidity that we are often hard-pressed to keep up with them, never mind trying to interpret them into clinical usefulness. Although scientific advances hold the promise of greater understanding, it is, at best, an incomplete understanding. The health of our patients is a reflection of more than just physiology and pathophysiology—it is a sum total of who they are (genetics), how they live (social, economic, and cultural factors), and where they live (environmental forces).

In keeping with this premise, we wanted to create a textbook that recognized that women's health care, even the gynecologic care that occurs in an office setting, involves more than a superb knowledge of scientific data and facts. For the care we render to be effective, it must incorporate the growing knowledge of how myriad forces influence and, to a large degree, determine the health of our patients.

Patients want—and have the right to ask for—feelings of understanding and connection from their health care providers. For many women, one of the primary contacts they have with the health care system is an office visit for a gynecologic condition or a well-woman exam. During these encounters, it is common for them to bring up issues that are beyond the scope of pure gynecology. This edition has been expanded to include new chapters that draw from the behavioral sciences, as well as from other disciplines, to help clinicians more fully address the variety of issues that often arise within the context of an office gynecology visit.

We are excited and pleased to bring you the sixth edition of *Glass' Office Gynecology,* and hope that you will find it informative, easy to read, and a valuable reference source in the office.

Acknowledgments

The creation of a textbook is a process that involves a large number of people. We are most appreciative of the hard work, diligence, and dedication the authors of the chapters put forth. We also want to thank several "behind the scenes" people who truly supported this endeavor and made it possible. Cathy Hoang, a former Rice University student, assisted with references and other manuscript preparation details. Our sincere thanks and gratitude also to Lauren Loder, LPN, who worked tirelessly to make sure the "nitty gritty" details of chapters were in order. Her attention to detail and rapid turnaround was essential for keeping the editors on track for project completion. Hilda Ruppal helped us locate our efforts from the last edition and facilitated our communications with several authors. Our sincere thanks to the editors at Lippincott Williams & Wilkins, who clearly understood the vagaries of life's events and the impact they have on any proposed schedule. Finally, we want to extend our sincere gratitude and appreciation to our family and friends for their love, patience, support, and understanding during this project.

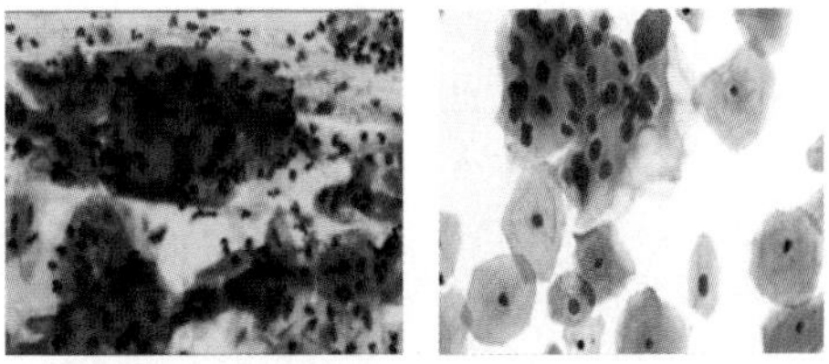

Color Plate 4.2 ● Conventional versus liquid-based cytology. (Courtesy of Matthew A. Powell, MD.)

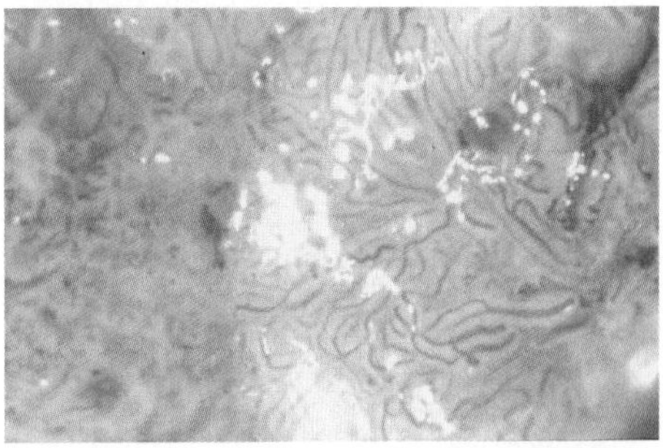

Color Plate 4.8 ● Colposcopic view of "corkscrew" (atypical) vessels. (Courtesy of Matthew A. Powell, MD.)

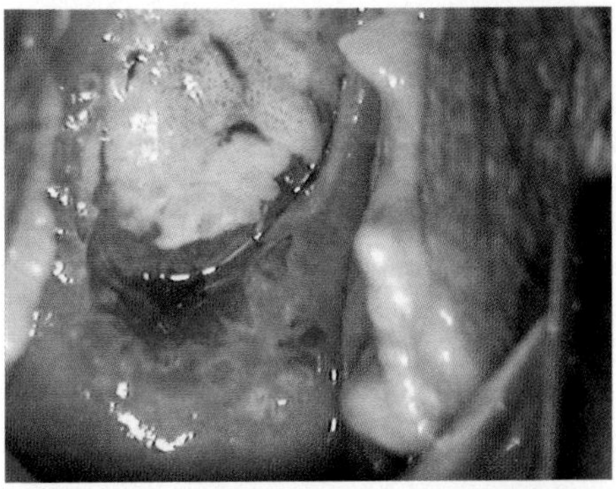

Color Plate 4.9 ● Colposcopic view of acetowhite epithelium. (Courtesy of Matthew A. Powell, MD.)

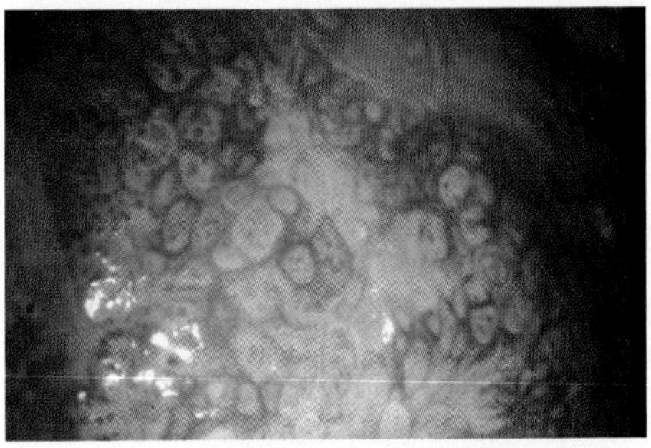

Color Plate 4.10 ● Colposcopic view of mosaicism and punctation. (Courtesy of Matthew A. Powell, MD.)

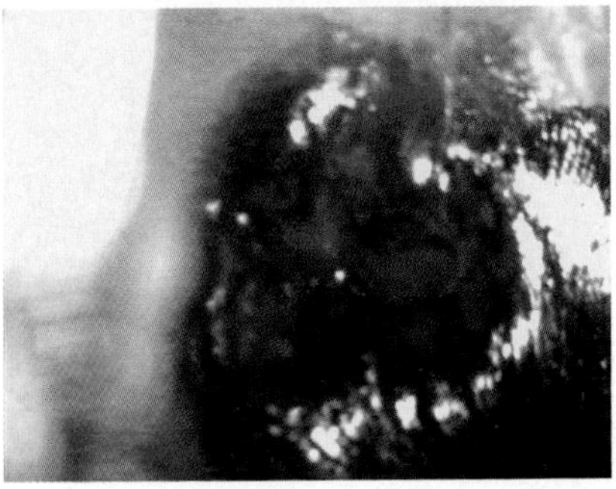

Color Plate 4.11 ● Colposcopic view of cervix with Lugol's iodine. (Courtesy of Matthew A. Powell, MD.)

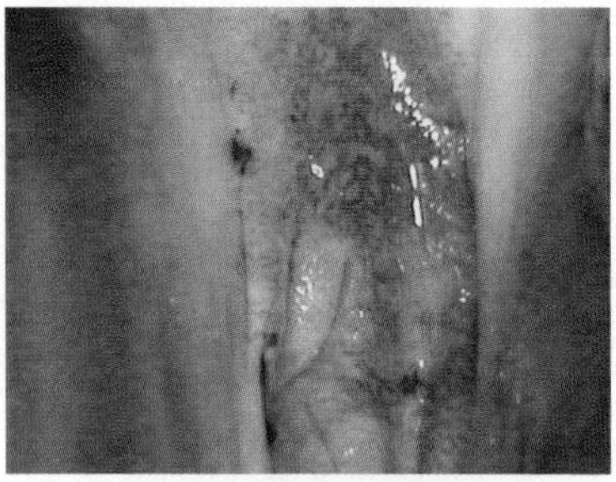

Color Plate 4.12 ● Colposcopic view of vaginal intraepithelial neoplasia. (Courtesy of Matthew A. Powell, MD.)

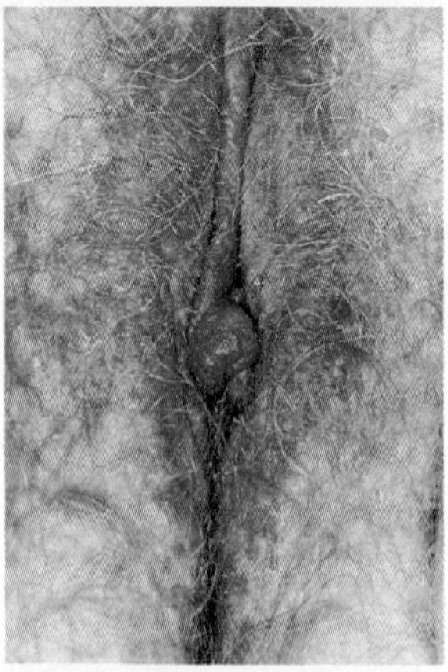

Color Plate 5.2 ● Moderate erythema in patient who complains of pruritus for 3 years. Clinical impression was eczema, and patient was advised to use hypoallergenic soap. Condition resolved. (Reprinted from Wilkinson EJ, Stone IK, eds. Atlas of Vulvar Disease. Baltimore: Williams & Wilkins, 1995:81, with permission.)

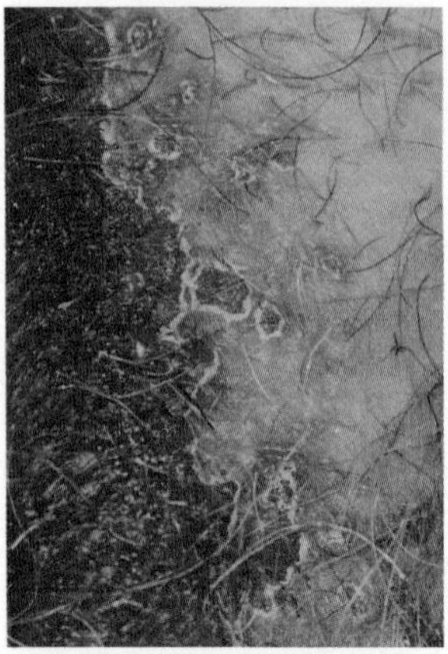

Color Plate 5.3 ● Note irregular border, erythema, and scaling of lesion. (Reprinted from Wilkinson EJ, Stone IK, eds. Atlas of Vulvar Disease. Baltimore: Williams & Wilkins, 1995:81, with permission.)

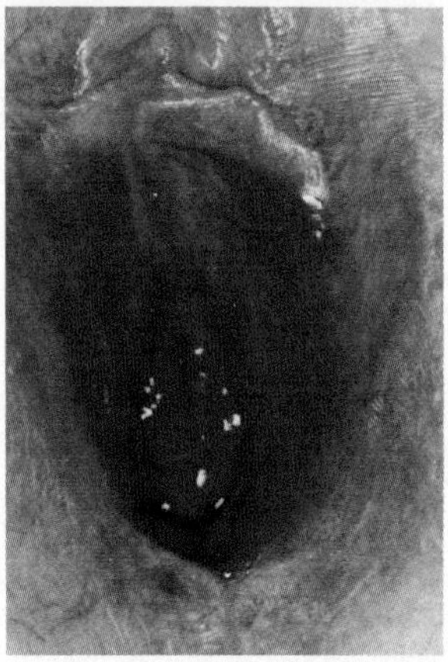

Color Plate 5.4 ● Lichen planus in a patient with dyspareunia for 8 months. Condition involved vagina and vestibule. Acute vaginal occlusion necessitated vaginal dilators (candlesticks) and topical steroids (Cort-Dome suppositories). (Reprinted from Wilkinson EJ, Stone IK, eds. Atlas of Vulvar Disease. Baltimore: Williams & Wilkins, 1995:29, with permission.)

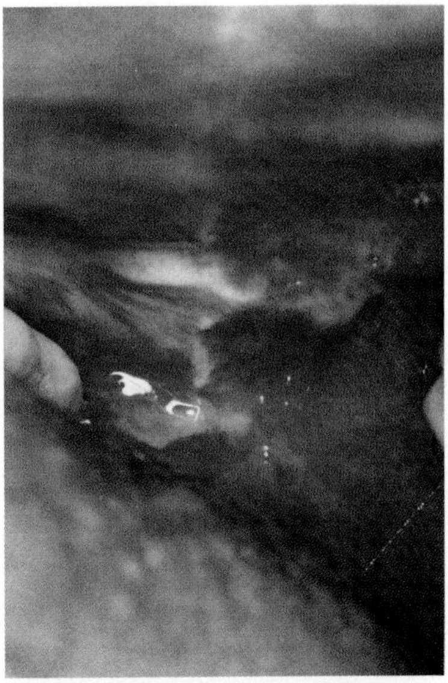

Color Plate 5.5 ● Reticular buccal mucosa lesion in a patient with vulvovaginal lichen planus. (Reprinted from Wilkinson EJ, Stone IK, eds. Atlas of Vulvar Disease. Baltimore: Williams & Wilkins, 1995:30, with permission.)

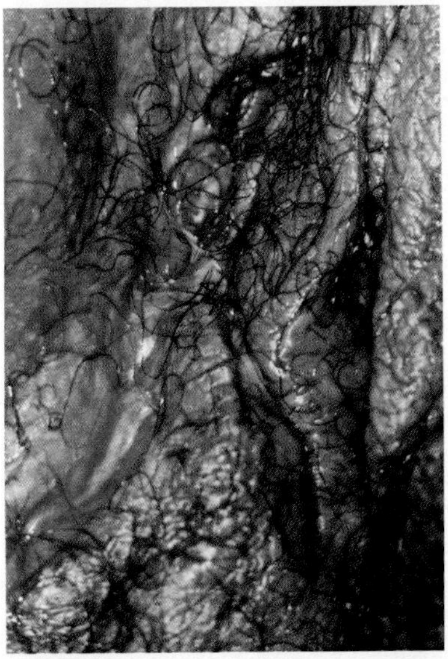

Color Plate 5.6 ● Deep vulvar ulceration in a patient with Crohn's disease of the vulva and bowel for approximately 9 years. Exacerbation of vulvar disease was unresponsive to prednisone 60 mg orally every day and metronidazole 500 mg orally three times a day. Imuran was started at 100 mg orally every day. (Reprinted from Wilkinson EJ, Stone IK, eds. Atlas of Vulvar Disease. Baltimore: Williams & Wilkins, 1995:180, with permission.)

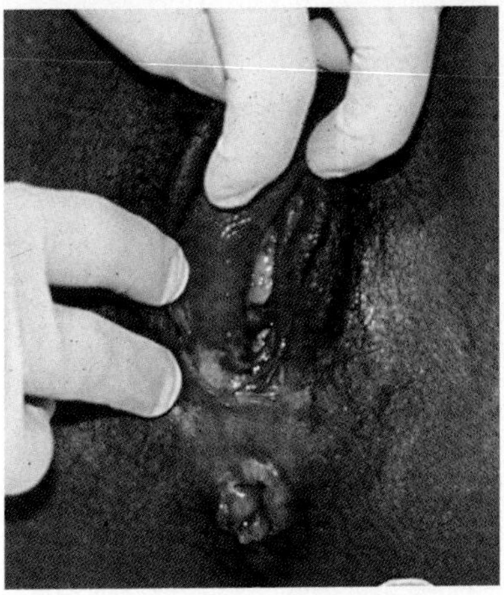

Color Plate 24.2 ● A 1-cm lesion on lower right labia minora.

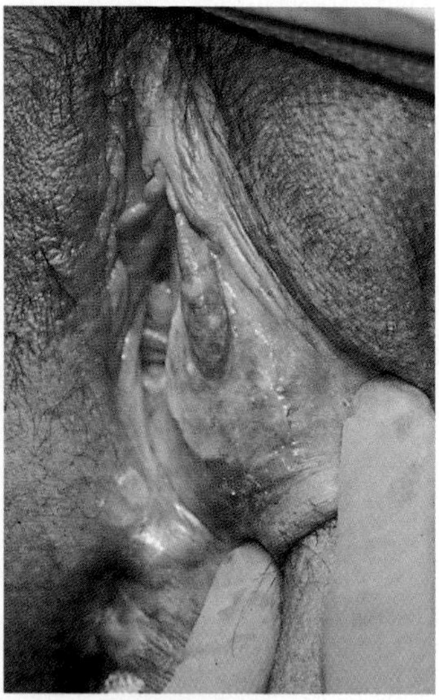

Color Plate 24.3 ● A 2 × 3 cm genital ulcer disease lesion on left vulva.

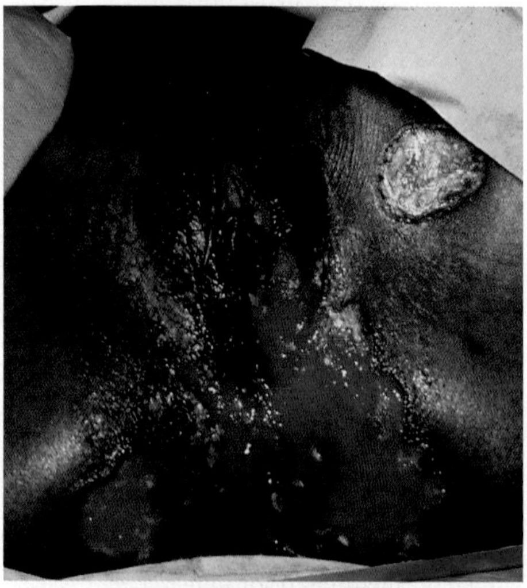

Color Plate 24.4 ● Advanced genital ulcer disease.

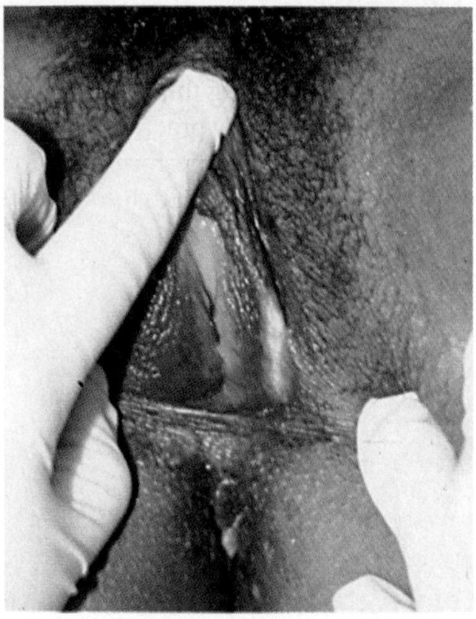

Color Plate 24.5 ● Lesion (same as in Fig. 24.2) 2 weeks after acyclovir treatment.

CHAPTER 1

Pediatric and Adolescent Gynecology

Andrea L. Zuckerman

It is not uncommon for both pediatric and adolescent patients to have gynecologic problems. Often pediatricians are not comfortable with gynecologic disorders and gynecologists are not comfortable with pediatric and adolescent patients. Therefore, these patients do not always receive the care and attention they need. Pediatric gynecologic examinations differ from adult exams in that they require more patience and different instruments. Adolescent exams can be performed similarly to adult exams, but careful preparation of the adolescent must be done prior to starting the exam, and different problems must be considered in this population.

EXAMINATION OF PEDIATRIC AND ADOLESCENT PATIENTS

All newborns should undergo a genital examination to determine whether they have normal external genitalia and a vagina present. However, patients do present at 18 years of age with vaginal agenesis, never having had an examination of their genitalia previously. If examination of the child's genitalia is performed during routine pediatric appointments, she is less likely to suffer embarrassment during her exams in her adolescent years, and congenital anomalies will be diagnosed prior to puberty.

When examining a young child, it is important to put the child at ease, and often it is helpful to distract the child during the exam. For example, allow the child to touch and look at all the instruments that will be used. The exam should be discussed with the child and her parent or guardian prior to beginning. It is helpful to look in her ears and listen to her heart, just as you would for a nongynecologic exam. This is part of the exam with which she is comfortable, and it may put her at ease. Palpation of the breasts and Tanner staging (Fig. 1.1), as well as an abdominal exam, should be performed. A child should never be forced into a gynecologic exam; postponing this part of the exam until a return visit may allow the girl to develop a relationship with a new practitioner, ultimately making the examination easier to perform. If an examination needs to be performed immediately, it may be done under anesthesia to minimize traumatization. It is important to inform the parents that an examination will not change the child's hymen unless a vaginoscope or speculum is used. If either instrument is used, the hymenal configuration may change, but this has no implications for her future health or sexuality.

A parent or guardian is usually in the room at the child's head during a gynecologic exam; this helps ease anxiety. The exam should include visualization of the external genitalia and vagina and, in some cases, a rectoabdominal exam. Different positions are used to help visualize the pediatric vagina, such as the frog-leg position or knee-to-chest position. Older children can often be placed in the lithotomy position using stirrups or by straddling the caregiver's legs. A speculum is not used in the pediatric patient unless the child is very cooperative and can tolerate the exam. If it is necessary to thoroughly examine the vagina, as in the case of undiagnosed vaginal bleeding in a young child, an exam under anesthesia should be performed with the use of a vaginoscope.

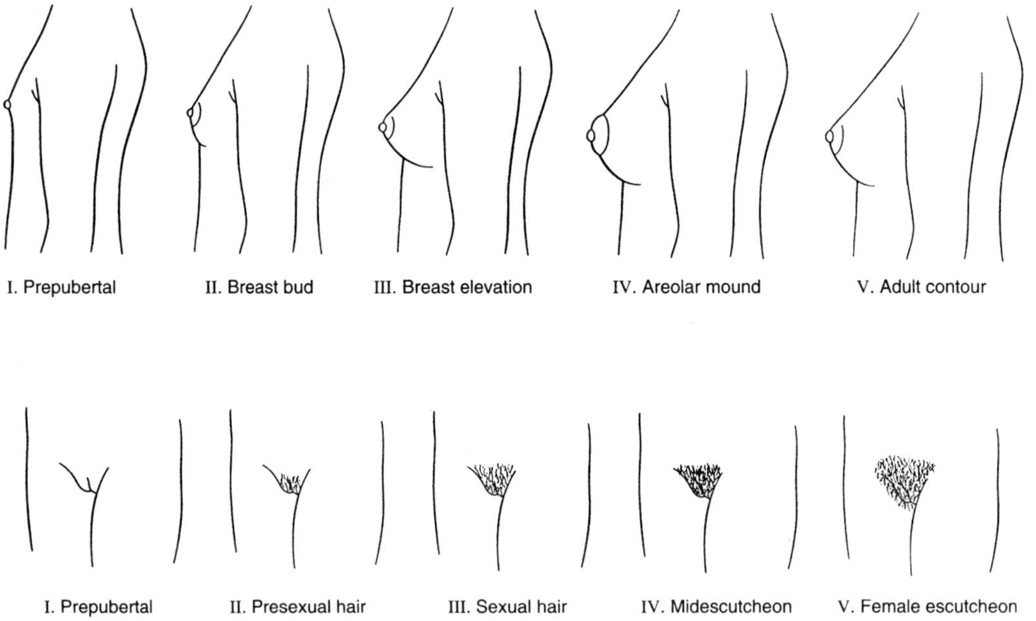

FIGURE 1.1 ● Tanner staging of thelarche and pubarche is helpful for diagnosing premature or delayed aspects of puberty. (Reprinted from Speroff L, Fritz MA. Clinical Gynecologic Endocrinology and Infertility. 7th ed. Philadelphia: Lippincott Williams & Wilkins, 2005:378–379, with permission.)

When examining the hymen and vagina in the dorsal lithotomy position, it is helpful to pull posteriorly and laterally on the labia majora of the child; in the knee-to-chest position, pull laterally and anteriorly on the labia majora. These maneuvers open the hymen and allow for better visualization of the vagina and hymen (Fig. 1.2). The knee-to-chest position is best for providing visualization of the cervix, but requires greater cooperation from the child. For those children whose hymen are redundant, making it difficult to see inside the vagina, Valsalva maneuvers are frequently helpful in opening the hymen. Use of a colposcope is helpful, if one is available, for magnification of the vulva and vagina (especially in the lithotomy position); an otoscope or ophthalmoscope can be a useful light source for the vaginal exam, especially in the knee-to-chest position.

If a vaginal infection needs to be ruled out, a culture using a moistened Calgi swab (a very small cotton swab, like those used in obtaining urethral cultures in men) should be placed in the vagina after discussion with the patient. Children respond best if they are shown the Calgi swab before the exam begins. The normal-size cotton swab used in adult women is too large and abrasive, especially when placed in a dry vagina, and is more likely to lead to hymenal changes such as clefts, strictures, or evidence of trauma.

Normal findings in the prepubertal child differ from the adolescent. Until the production of estrogen begins, the labia minora are underdeveloped, the hymen is thin, and the clitoris is small (Fig. 1.3). However, the newborn is under the influence of maternal hormones and thus may have a thickened hymen, which may last for up to 2 years after birth. Other common findings seen in the newborn female are vulvar edema, vaginal discharge and/or bleeding, and breast enlargement. About 10% of newborns will have some withdrawal bleeding. Approximately two-thirds will have a breast discharge similar to colostrum in the neonatal period. These findings are much less pronounced in premature infants, although their clitoris is relatively large. This is not a cause for concern. The effects usually resolve within the first 6 to 8 weeks of life. Neonates may present with a hymenal polyp or "tag." This is secondary to the high levels of maternal estrogen and will resolve spontaneously. If a polyp persists or the child's parents are overly concerned, resection can be performed in the operating room, but this should be combined with vaginoscopy to rule out a vaginal mass.

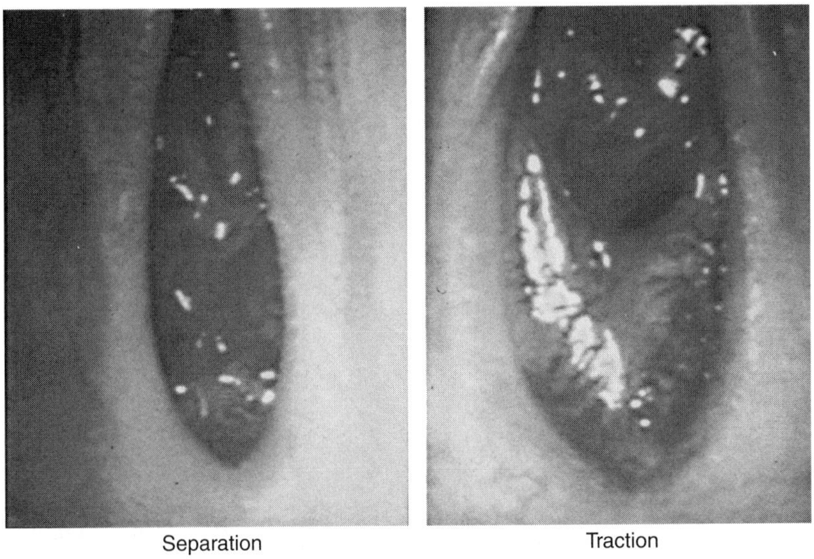

FIGURE 1.2 ● Examples of the techniques of labial separation and lateral traction for viewing the hymen of a prepubertal girl. (Reprinted from the NASPAG PediGYN Teaching Slide Set, 1996: slide 7, with permission.)

The main three normal variants of hymen configuration are annular (circumferential), crescentic, and fimbriated (folded) (Fig. 1.4A) (1). In a study by Berenson et al., all newborns examined had some hymenal tissue present, and the majority had annular hymens (1). Of note, clefts, which are splits in the rim of the hymen, are normal if present in the anterior hymenal ring. However, those found in the posterior position indicate the occurrence of trauma. This is an important finding for the evaluation of possible sexual abuse (1).

Congenital anomalies of the hymen (Fig. 1.4B) include imperforate (lacking fenestration), microperforate (with only a small opening into the vagina), cribriform (with multiple small

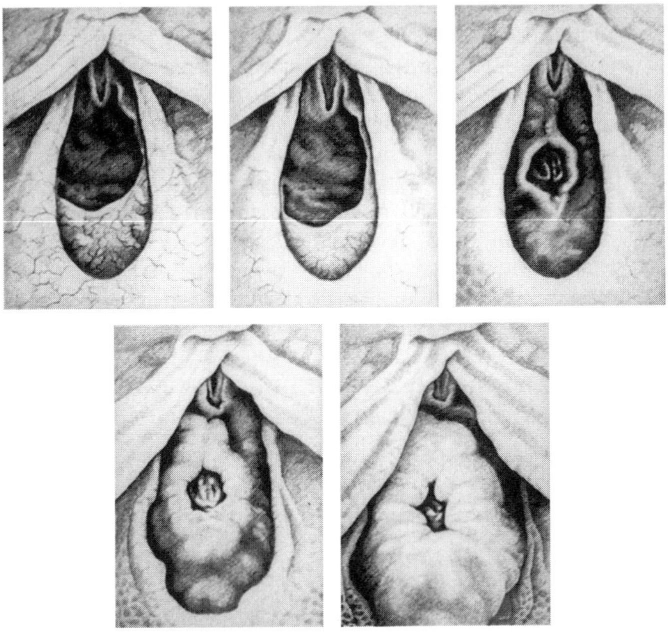

FIGURE 1.3 ● Progressive effects of estrogen on the hymen and the tissue of the vaginal vestibule, ranging from prepubertal to full sexual development. (Reprinted from the NASPAG PediGYN Teaching Slide Set, 1996: slide 6, with permission.)

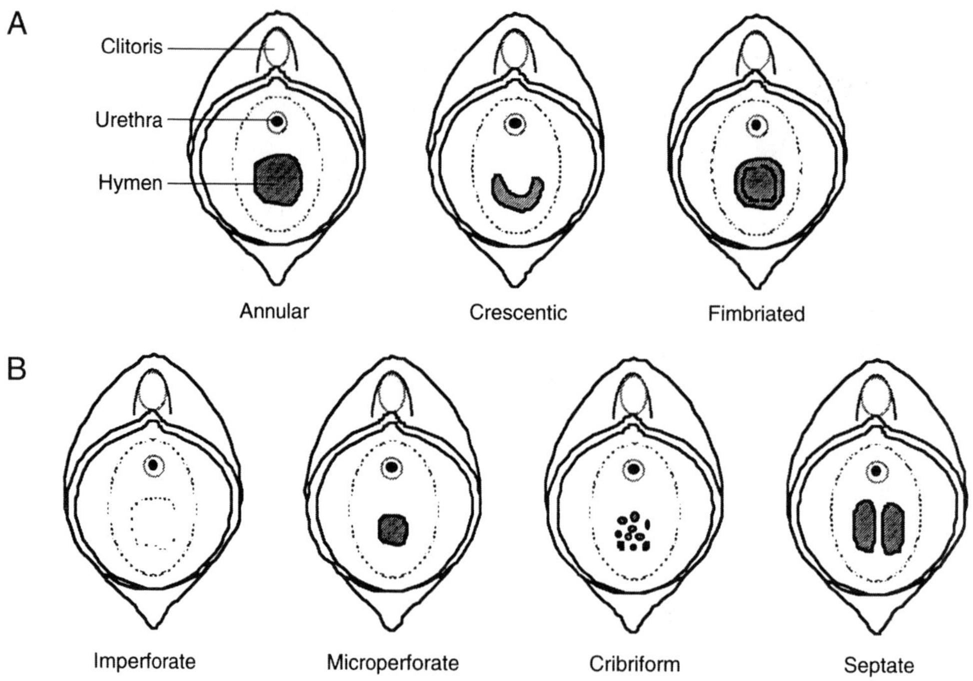

FIGURE 1.4 ● **A:** Normal variants of hymen configuration are annular (circumferential), crescentic, and fimbriated (folded). **B:** Congenital anomalies of the hymen include imperforate, microperforate, cribriform, and septate.

openings), and septate (with a soft-tissue divider forming two openings). Patients with septate hymens often present urgently with inability to remove a tampon. The septation may be ligated and cut with resultant removal of the tampon. Other congenital hymenal anomalies are managed surgically, wherein a needle-tipped cautery is used to resect the extra hymenal tissue. The procedures are quick and easily performed with mask anesthesia, but some parents prefer to wait until the child is older. Patients respond better to the surgery if performed prior to pubertal development.

Examination of the adolescent should not be rushed. A careful history with special attention to sexual activity and any gynecologic problems should be addressed. Adolescence is a time of transition that is very difficult for many patients, and they will frequently have specific concerns regarding development, sexual intercourse, and sexuality. Teens require a health care provider who will spend time with them and answer questions without the patient feeling rushed or criticized.

The exam of the adolescent should include a breast exam and Tanner staging. The pelvic exam should be discussed with the patient (with a demonstration of the speculum) prior to beginning the exam. It is helpful during the pelvic exam to ask permission for each step of the exam, giving the adolescent a sense of control. A Huffman speculum is designed to allow for easy inspection of the cervix in adolescents and is thinner than Pederson speculums; hence, it is the speculum that most patients tolerate best during their first pelvic exam (Fig. 1.5). Patients who have never been sexually active and who have a tight hymenal ring should undergo a one-finger (rather than a two-finger) bimanual exam. Occasionally, it will not be possible to do a bimanual exam; thus, a rectal examination may have to be done instead. In a prepubertal child, the size ratio of the uterine corpus compared with the cervix is 1:3, in the pubertal child it is 1:1, and in the adult woman it is 3:1.

Confidentiality

Confidentiality refers to the private and privileged nature of the health care transaction and related information. Adolescent visits to the clinician raise questions about confidentiality—physicians are often unsure under what circumstances parental consent is required. Uncertainty in this area has contributed to the underserving of patients in this population.

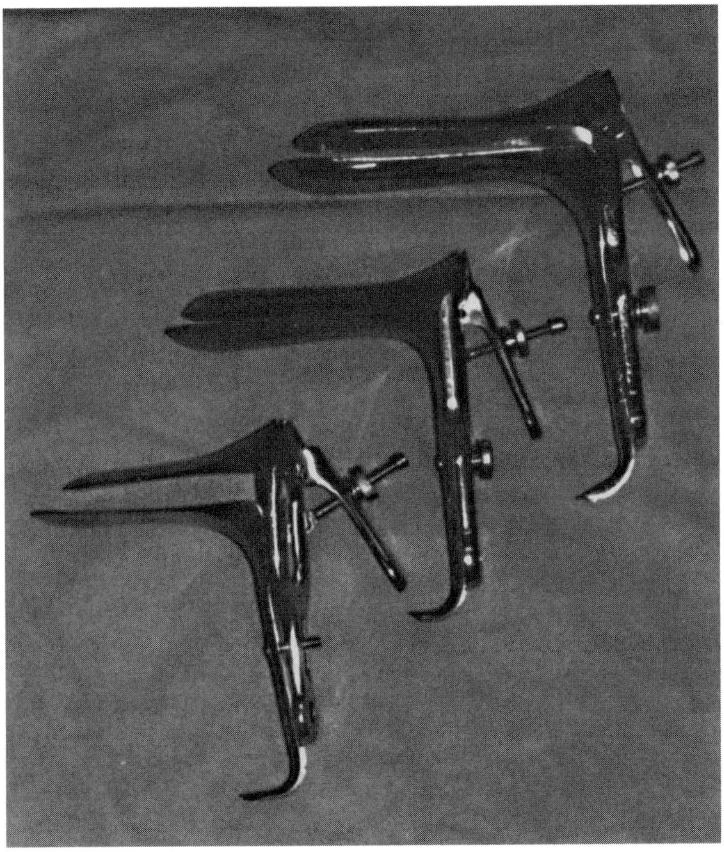

FIGURE 1.5 ● Speculums for use in the pediatric and adolescent populations are shorter and narrower. The speculum on the bottom is a Pedersen speculum. It is narrow and short. The middle speculum is a Huffman speculum. It is specially designed to fit the adolescent vagina. The speculum on top is a Graves speculum. This will cause great discomfort in the adolescent and may even be uncomfortable for the nulliparous, but nonvirginal, woman.

Every state has its own laws governing these issues. Although there are no federal laws, a person younger than the age of 18 years may consent to her own care in certain situations defined by state laws. Generally, these situations include pregnancy-related care, family planning services, sexually transmitted disease (STD) testing and treatment, emergency health care, and substance abuse treatment. Adolescents who are pregnant, parenting, married, or emancipated may consent to their own care in most states, but abortion access laws vary widely among states. An emancipated minor is a person younger than 18 years who is no longer in the custody of parents by order of a court, who is working in the armed services, and/or who is living economically independent of her parents (2). A "mature" minor is a minor who is able to consent for treatment because she can understand the risks and benefits of treatment. Although a "mature" minor is defined differently by various states, typically the law has upheld physicians' assessments of maturity and ability to consent for care (2).

An additional barrier to providing confidential care to adolescents is economics. It is more difficult to ensure confidentiality for an adolescent who wants to use her parents' insurance to cover the visit or who wants to pay cash but needs to set up a payment plan. Some private practices have offered confidential billing accounts for minor patients who want to keep charges private (3,4).

PEDIATRIC SEXUAL ABUSE

The prevalence of pediatric sexual abuse cases is difficult to ascertain. The number of cases is underreported and thus underestimates the actual number of cases. The evaluation of a child for possible sexual abuse involves a complete history by a trained sexual abuse counselor and a medical evaluation for possible sexual abuse. The medical evaluation is performed to document any pertinent findings and to rule out any infectious diseases. It is important to provide a comfortable environment for the medical evaluation and allow sufficient time for a thorough exam that is not intimidating.

A parent and clinician should view certain behavioral traits and changes as possible markers for sexual abuse. These include anxiety, sleep disturbances, social withdrawal, various vague somatic complaints, increased sex play, inappropriate sexual behavior, school problems, depression, and low self-esteem. Patients can then be screened by experts trained in sexual abuse history taking.

This chapter does not contain a complete guide to pediatric sexual abuse. Briefly, a physical examination should be performed with attention to the genital examination. Findings of sexual abuse are often subtle or absent. All infants are born with hymenal tissue (1) so the total absence of hymenal tissue is an abnormal finding. In examining the hymen, a clinician looks for clefts (V-shaped indentations on the edge of the hymenal membrane) and transections (where the indentations extend to the base). Clefts are normal in the anterior or 9 to 3 o'clock positions but are considered abnormal in the posterior or 4 to 8 o'clock positions. Suspicious findings include acute or healed lacerations of the hymen or posterior fourchette, hymenal transections to the base, and perirectal scarring. Nonspecific findings of sexual abuse include vulvar erythema, vulvovaginitis, excoriations, and increased vascular patterns. Often the exam is normal with a normal hymen even in cases of known penetration, when both the patient and the perpetrator state that penetration occurred (Table 1.1). Cultures should be obtained for gonorrhea and chlamydia, and laboratory tests for HIV, hepatitis B and C, and syphilis should be offered. The diagnosis of STDs is not common in these children; the reported incidence varies from 1 to 26%.

VULVOVAGINITIS

Vulvovaginitis, an inflammatory process involving the vagina and vulva, accounts for approximately 70% of prepubertal gynecologic complaints. The process itself may begin in either the vagina or the vulva and spread to the other site. Prepubertal girls are particularly susceptible to vulvovaginal problems for a number of reasons. Poor hygiene and lack of estrogenization of

TABLE 1.1

Documentation of Physical Findings When Sexual Abuse Is Suspected in a Child

Perineum/Labia

Document the location of lacerations, abrasions, erythema, and bruising and note any discharge.

In the vestibule, look for erythema and note any lesions around the urethra.

In the posterior fourchette, look for labial adhesions, neovascularization, and friability.

Hymen

Note the configuration (Fig 1.4A & B) and the appearance of the edges (thin and sharp, thickened, rolled, projections or notches, vascularity).

Measure the horizontal and vertical diameters, noting which position the child was in at that time.

Vagina

If visualized, comment on ridges, rugae, and discharge.

If not visualized, note why.

the vaginal epithelium are probably the two most important factors contributing to an increased susceptibility to inflammation and infection. In addition, the prepubertal labia do not cover the entire vestibule and there is a short distance from the anus to the vagina, predisposing young girls to vulvovaginitis (5).

The characteristic symptoms of vulvovaginitis include vulvar pruritus, pain, burning, vaginal discharge (mucopurulent or purulent), and dysuria. Vaginal bleeding may also be a presenting symptom, although other causes such as trauma and a foreign object need to be considered. Typical findings on physical exam may include erythema, excoriations, discharge, blood, cracks or fissures, or even lichenification if the irritation has been chronic. A rash may be present secondary to an infection (e.g., *Staphylococcus*) or dermatitis (e.g., poison ivy). The differential diagnosis of prepubertal vulvovaginitis includes infectious and noninfectious etiologies, but most commonly no specific cause can be found (Table 1.2). Cultures should be performed to rule out infectious agents. This may be done using a saline-moistened Calgi swab inserted gently through the hymenal opening. A wet prep can be done as well to look for mycotic organisms, *Trichomonas*, parasitic ova, and red and white blood cells. If bleeding is present, attempts should be made to visualize the vagina and cervix to rule out a foreign body.

TABLE 1.2

Differential Diagnosis of Prepubertal Vulvovaginitis

Infectious Causes
Respiratory Pathogens
Group A β-hemolytic streptococcus
S. pneumoniae
N. meningitides
S. aureus
H. influenzae
Enteric Pathogens
Shigella
Sexually Transmitted (some may be acquired perinatally)
N. gonorrhoeae
Chlamydia trachomatis
Herpes simplex
Human papilloma virus
Trichomonas vaginalis
Gardnerella vaginalis (questionable relationship)
Others
Candida
Enterobiasis vermicularis (pinworm)
Noninfectious Causes
Foreign body
Poor hygiene
Lichen sclerosus
Psoriasis
Seborrhea
Contact dermatitis
Persistent exposure to urine

Infectious Causes

Infectious vulvovaginitis in the prepubertal female may be due to nonsexually transmitted or sexually transmitted organisms. Respiratory and enteric organisms are most often involved, and a history may be elicited of recent respiratory infection or ear infection. Pathogens may include group A beta hemolytic streptococci, *Streptococcus pneumoniae*, *Neisseria meningitidis*, *Staphylococcus aureus*, or *Haemophilus influenzae*. Group A beta hemolytic streptococcal infection usually presents 7 to 10 days after an upper respiratory infection and may cause vaginal bleeding or a blood-tinged discharge with pronounced irritation of the vulva and perianal area. Treatment is with penicillin (Pen-Vee K, Veetids) 25 to 50 mg/kg per day divided two to four times a day (up to 125 to 250 mg four times a day) for 10 days. *Haemophilus* vaginitis may result in a greenish vaginal discharge and can be treated with amoxicillin (Amoxil, Polymox) 20 to 40 mg/kg per day divided three times a day (up to 250 to 500 mg three times a day) for 7 days. Of the enteric organisms causing vulvovaginitis, *Shigella* is the most common and may in fact cause a bloody vaginal discharge. Diarrhea is absent in most patients. The recommended treatment is trimethoprim/sulfamethoxazole (Bactrim, Septra) 40/200 per 5 mL liquid dosed at 5 mL/10 kg per dose twice a day (up to 20 mL twice a day) for 7 days. Candidal vulvovaginitis is rare in prepubertal girls, and its presence should make one suspicious for diabetes or immunosuppression. Recent antibiotic use may also rarely elicit candidal infection. Initial treatment is with an antifungal cream. Human papilloma virus (HPV) can be a cause, and it may be transmitted either neonatally or via sexual abuse (6). Pinworm (*Enterobiasis vermicularis*) may also cause vulvovaginitis; physical exam in this case may reveal anal excoriations, and symptoms include vulvar and anal pruritus. The perianal pruritus is typically worse at night. Pinworm is a common entity among children in day care and in school. Treatment is oral mebendazole (Vermox) 100 mg in a single dose to everyone in the household older than 2 years. This drug has not been extensively studied in children younger than 2 years, so the risks and benefits must be weighed. It is a category C drug for pregnancy.

In any prepubertal female with vulvovaginal symptoms, care must be taken to rule out STDs as a causal factor (including *Neisseria gonorrhea*, *Chlamydia trachomatis*, herpes simplex virus, HPV, and *Trichomonas vaginalis*) and to rule out sexual abuse, especially in children younger than the age of consent. In the prepubertal female, the primary site of an STD is the vagina, not the cervix, so a vaginal culture should be performed. *Chlamydia* may be perinatally acquired and may persist in the vagina for up to a year before being cleared by the immune system. The diagnosis of *N. gonorrhea* and *Chlamydia* should always be made by cell culture technique because the enzyme-linked immunosorbent assay test for chlamydia is often falsely positive in the prepubertal child. The findings of either *N. gonorrhea* or *C. trachomatis* should prompt evaluation for sexual abuse, and the patient should be treated to cover both organisms. For the child weighing less than 45 kg, the recommended treatment for *N. gonorrhea* is a single dose of ceftriaxone (Rocephin) intramuscularly, using 125 mg if the child weighs less than 45 kg and using 250 mg for those weighing 45 kg or more. If the child is 8 years or older, she should also receive oral doxycycline (Vibramycin, Doryx) 100 mg twice a day for 7 days to cover for *Chlamydia*. The recommended treatment for *C. trachomatis* in the child younger than 8 years is erythromycin ethyl succinate 50 mg/kg per day divided three or four times a day (up to 400 mg four times a day) for 10 days. The relationship between *Gardnerella vaginalis* (bacterial vaginosis) and sexual abuse in the pediatric patient is not clear.

Herpes simplex virus (both type I and II), HPV, and *Trichomonas* are usually sexually transmitted when seen in prepubertal girls. It is possible that the child with oral herpes infection (type I or II) may spread it to her genitalia with her hands. The possibility of abuse must, however, be explored. Genital warts can be transmitted by perinatal exposure, close physical contact, or sexual abuse. The amount of time after birth that a perinatally acquired infection may present is not known. Genital warts that appear in the first or second year of life are generally believed to represent perinatal infection. As the age of the child at diagnosis of HPV infection increases, the suspicion of abuse should also rise. More than 50% of children with anal or genital warts have a history of sexual abuse (7,8). *Trichomonas* is uncommon in prepubertal girls outside the newborn period because the organism prefers an estrogenic environment. The diagnosis is often made on a wet prep, but cultures are more sensitive. Fomites for *Trichomonas*, such as wet towels, have been demonstrated, but if the organism is found in a child, sexual abuse is extremely likely. Treatment for *Trichomonas* in the child is oral metronidazole (Flagyl) 15 mg/kg per day three times a day (up to 250 to 750 mg three times a day) for 7 to 10 days.

Cases of suspected sexual abuse should be handled by a health care team familiar with the evaluation of the prepubertal child. A careful exam should be performed (Table 1.1).

Other systemic illnesses and infections may also affect the vulva, including measles, chicken pox, Kawasaki disease, scarlet fever, and Crohn's disease, and should be considered in the differential diagnosis for vulvovaginal complaints.

Noninfectious Causes

In noninfectious cases of vulvovaginitis, a vaginal culture usually reveals normal vaginal flora, including lactobacilli, diphtheroids, *Staphylococcus epidermidis*, alpha streptococci and Gram-negative enteric organisms such as *Escherichia coli* (9). Nonspecific vulvovaginitis is most likely secondary to irritants. Poor hygiene may contribute to the etiology, and stool or toilet paper may be offending agents. The vulva can also become inflamed in response to chemical irritants such as strong soaps, perfumed or dyed toilet paper, detergents, or bubble baths. Vulvitis may be worse in obese girls or in those with urinary incontinence.

Primary vulvar diseases such as lichen sclerosus, seborrhea, psoriasis, and contact dermatitis may also cause symptoms. Rarely, congenital anomalies, such as an ectopic ureter, in which the ureter drains into the vagina, may be the underlying abnormality leading to recurrent vulvovaginitis secondary to persistent exposure to urine.

Once infectious causes have been ruled out, primary treatment of noninfectious vulvovaginitis includes removing any irritants. Improved hygiene is very important, including demonstration of proper wiping technique (from front to back only) (Fig. 1.6). Avoidance of soaps, perfumes, and strong detergent, in addition to wearing cotton underwear, avoiding tight jeans or leotards, and changing from wet bathing suits or leotards, are all important behavioral practices to recommend. Sitz baths of warm water are usually curative and soothing. Wet compresses with Burrow's solution may be helpful in cases of "weepy" vulvar lesions. Antibiotics such as amoxicillin or cephalosporin may be used in complicated or recurrent cases for 10 days (5). For persistent cases, low-dose antibiotics may need to be used for up to two months. Hydrocortisone cream 0.5 to 1.0% or triamcinolone (a midpotency topical steroid) may be used on the vulva to decrease inflammation.

Vulvovaginal complaints in adolescents follow along the lines of those seen in adults (see Chapters 5 and 10), with a few special considerations. Physiologic leukorrhea, which typically begins 6 months prior to menarche, may irritate the vulva. Yeast, bacterial vaginosis, and retained tampons are other common causes of vulvovaginitis in the adolescent. Any evaluation of an adolescent should include a history to screen for risk factors for STDs and a physical exam including pelvic exam. Counseling on the prevention of infections should be part of every visit with adolescents.

LICHEN SCLEROSUS

Lichen sclerosus is a dystrophic lesion of the vulva of unknown etiology. A classic presentation in the prepubertal female includes complaints of vulvar pruritus, irritation and dysuria, and occasional frank bleeding from persistent rubbing. Typically, the vulva appears white and atrophic. Lichen sclerosus has been described as having a "parchment paper" appearance. At times, the area may show an increase in erythema and vascular markings, although repetitive exams will show hypopigmentation in an hourglass shape involving the labial, clitoral, and perianal regions. Those lesions with pronounced vascular markings may bruise easily and produce bloody blisters that are prone to secondary infection. The diagnosis in the prepubertal child is usually made clinically and rarely requires a biopsy (Fig. 1.7).

Treatment is initially supportive, with the removal of all irritants and the use of a protective emollient (e.g., A&D ointment). A sedating antihistamine given at night may help alleviate middle-of-the-night scratching. Avoidance of straddle sports (e.g., bicycle riding) is also

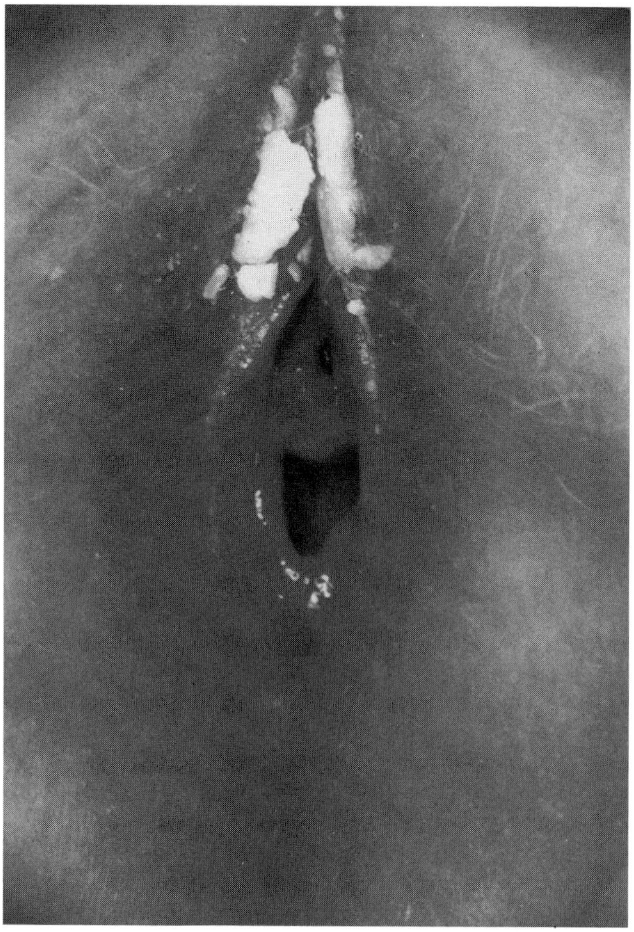

FIGURE 1.6 ● Vulvitis in a prepubertal girl. Poor perineal hygiene and external irritants (perfumed soaps, etc.) can cause this problem, which is easily treated with removal of the irritant stimulus, gentle cleansing, and thorough afterdrying. (Reprinted from the NASPAG PediGYN Teaching Slide Set, 1996: slide 43, with permission.)

beneficial. If the symptoms persist, short-term use of a topical steroid (e.g. hydrocortisone 1 or 2%) or triamcinolone acetonide (a midpotency topical steroid) can be tried. Testosterone cream (useful in postmenopausal patients) is not recommended in children because of the possibility of virilization. Laser therapy has been attempted but is no more efficacious than treatment with topical steroids (10). Lichen sclerosus resolves spontaneously or improves during puberty in more than 50% of these patients.

LABIAL ADHESIONS

Labial adhesions, complete or partial fusion of the lower labia minora, are a fairly common complaint in the prepubertal girl. The patients typically present between 6 months and 6 years of age, with most cases occurring before the age of 2 years. The etiology of labial adhesions is not known, but it is presumed that the low estrogen state is a contributing factor. In fact, labial adhesions are not seen in the neonate, probably because the maternal estrogens are still high in the newborn circulation. Inflammation of the vulvar tissue from local irritation, trauma, and infection is probably also a contributing factor to labial adhesions.

Clinically, the vagina may appear "absent" with a thin smooth membrane covering the vaginal opening (Fig. 1.8). Most patients will be asymptomatic, the problem having been discovered by a parent or on routine physical exam. Some girls have poor drainage of vaginal secretions and interference with urination, sequestration of urine, or in rare cases, acute urinary retention that requires immediate attention. Others present with recurrent urinary tract infections. Patients may complain of dysuria or recurrent vulvar or vaginal infections.

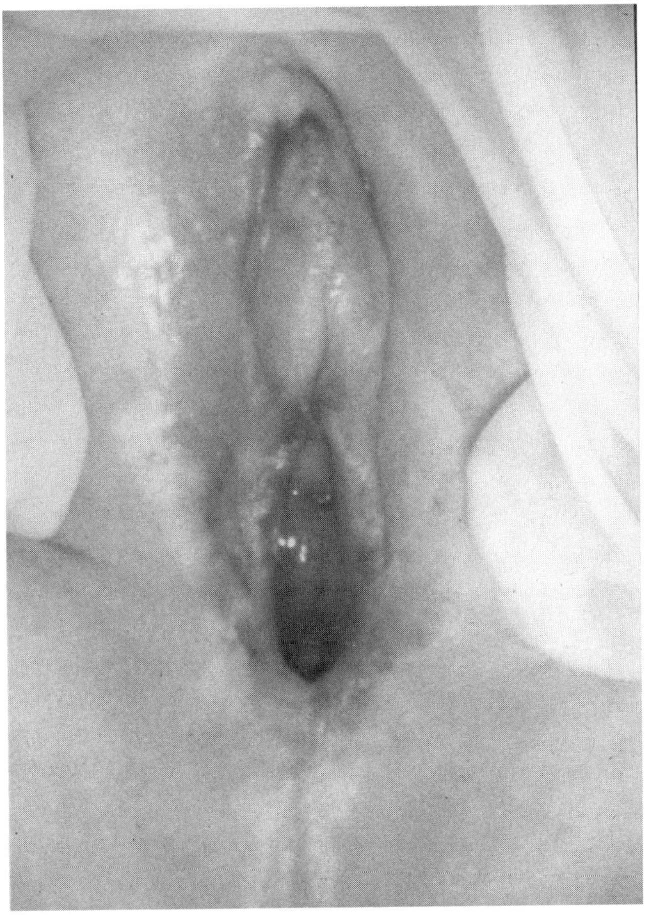

FIGURE 1.7 ● Lichen sclerosis in a 5-year-old girl. (Reprinted from the NASPAG PediGYN Teaching Slide Set, 1996: slide 101, with permission.)

Mild asymptomatic cases may simply be followed because they will resolve at puberty with the increase in systemic estrogen. If more severe, or if the parent is anxious for treatment, topical estrogen cream applied directly over the central raphe of the adhesions twice daily for 2 to 3 weeks will separate most adhesions (11). Following separation, daily use of an emollient (e.g., Desitin or A&D ointment) will keep the labia separated. Good perineal hygiene is important in these patients. In cases where medical treatment fails or acute urinary retention exists, surgical separation of adhesions is necessary. Although the adhesions separate easily, this surgery should never be done in the office without anesthesia (viscous lidocaine [Xylocaine 2%]) because it is extremely painful for the child and can lead to unnecessary psychological trauma.

PREPUBERTAL VAGINAL BLEEDING

Vaginal bleeding in childhood is a relatively rare and, for parents, alarming condition that requires immediate attention to rule out significant pathology. It may be secondary to a number of processes, including exogenous hormones, inflammation or infection, trauma, foreign body, genital tract neoplasm, or urologic pathology (Table 1.3) (12). Another possible etiology, precocious puberty, is discussed in the next section.

Exogenous Hormones

Genital bleeding in the prepubertal female may represent bleeding from the endometrium. Such bleeding may be seen as the result of estrogen withdrawal in the first few weeks of life as the maternal hormones are cleared from the newborn's circulation. No treatment is necessary, and the

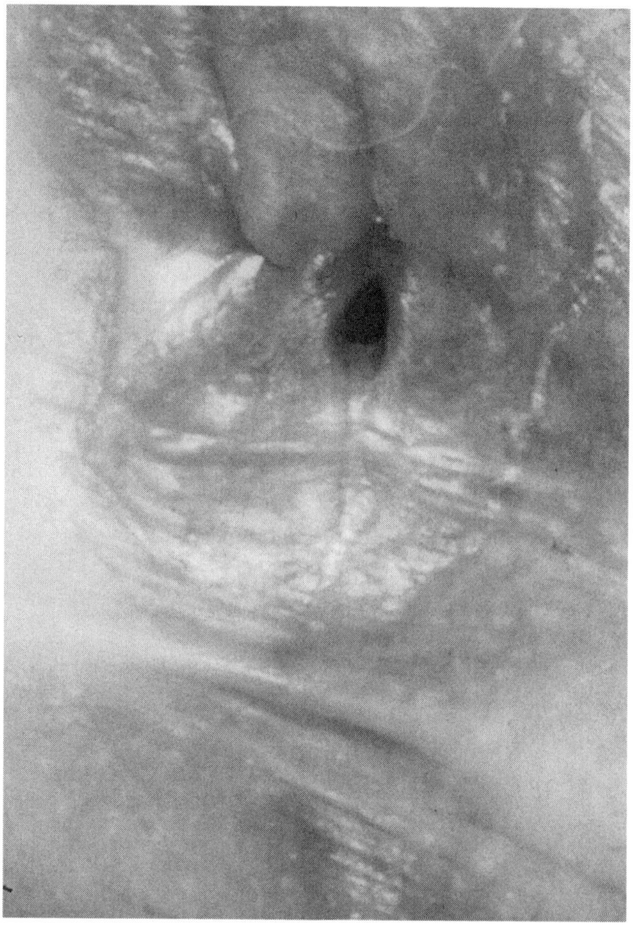

FIGURE 1.8 ● Labial adhesions in a 3-year-old girl. (Reprinted from the NASPAG PediGYN Teaching Slide Set, 1996: slide 32, with permission.)

condition is self-limiting. Iatrogenic causes, such as the use of estrogen cream for the treatment of labial adhesions, may also lead to prepubertal bleeding (13). A careful history should be taken to exclude possible ingestion of prescription hormone pills.

Isolated precocious menarche without any other signs of pubertal development is rare but has been reported. Isolated episodes of vaginal bleeding are suspected to be due to elevations in plasma estradiol as a result of transient ovarian activity and possibly due to an increased sensitivity of the endometrium to estrogens (14). In these cases, one sees normal pubertal development at

TABLE 1.3

Causes of Prepubertal Vaginal Bleeding

Exogenous hormones
Inflammation or infection
Trauma
Foreign body
Urologic pathology
Genital tract neoplasm
Precocious puberty

the appropriate age with subsequent normal fertility and attainment of expected height (15). These patients should, of course, be followed closely for any signs of true precocious puberty.

Inflammation and Infection

Some studies suggest that as many as 45% of cases of prepubertal vagina bleeding may be attributable to infection or inflammation (16). Of the specific infectious etiologies, *Shigella* has been associated with a bloody vaginal discharge and bloody diarrhea. Vaginitis caused by group A beta hemolytic *Streptococcus* often results in vaginal bleeding. Condylomata acuminatum (venereal warts) are seen in the pediatric population, most often associated with sexual abuse. These exophytic lesions, which may be vaginal or vulvar in location, may be extremely friable and present with vaginal bleeding. Lichen sclerosus and vulvovaginitis, discussed earlier in this chapter, may also have vaginal bleeding as a presenting symptom.

Trauma

Trauma may result in a vulvar hematoma and/or laceration with subsequent vaginal bleeding. Such injuries are fairly common with bike riding and other activities, especially in the summer months. Important in the evaluation of trauma is exclusion of the possibility of sexual abuse; the physician should evaluate the injury for compatibility with the patient's story. Of equal importance is determination of the extent of the injury and whether it will require an examination under anesthesia or surgical repair. In the case of an injury that is penetrating, or if hymenal injury cannot be excluded, care must be taken to ensure the peritoneal cavity was not penetrated. This may require an examination under anesthesia. Catheterization and rectal exam must be done to evaluate the integrity of the bladder and bowel. Many vulvar hematomas may be managed nonsurgically with the use of ice, observation, and serial hemoglobin measurements to ensure the hematoma is stable. Placement of a Foley catheter is often necessary in these cases because significant swelling may occur and obstruct the urethral outflow (17).

Foreign Bodies

Foreign bodies placed in the vagina by a small child are a common cause for childhood vaginal bleeding. They usually result in a foul-smelling, bloody vaginal discharge. The presentation may look suspicious for sexual abuse if changes are seen in the posterior aspect of the hymen. Usually, the child will not acknowledge or recall placing a foreign body in her vagina. The most common foreign body reported by most series is toilet paper; other common objects are pen caps, safety pins, coins, and hair pins. Most foreign bodies are not radiopaque, so x-ray studies are often not helpful (Fig. 1.9).

Management in the office using a local anesthetic and nasal speculum may be possible in some patients; however, a child should never be forced to undergo an exam. In most cases of prepubertal vaginal bleeding, examination under anesthesia with vaginoscopy should be performed to visualize the entire vaginal canal. Vaginoscopy may reveal a foreign body or simply a reactive area of the vaginal mucosa because frequently the foreign body will have been spontaneously expelled or removed by the child. Irrigation of the vagina with sterile water or saline (in the office or when examining under anesthesia) may be helpful in flushing out small foreign bodies, especially those in the lower third of the vagina. Larger objects may require use of forceps. The presence of vaginal excrescences may help differentiate vaginal bleeding due to a foreign body versus sexual abuse (18). Recurrences of vaginal foreign bodies are common, so the parents and child should be counseled regarding proper perineal hygiene.

Urologic Pathology

Disorders of the urinary tract may initially present as "vaginal bleeding." Patients with urinary tract infections and gross hematuria may present to the pediatric gynecologist with complaints of vaginal bleeding. Urethral prolapse, a complete circular eversion of the urethral mucosa, presents as a painless bleeding annular lesion above the vaginal entrance. Urethral prolapse may be seen

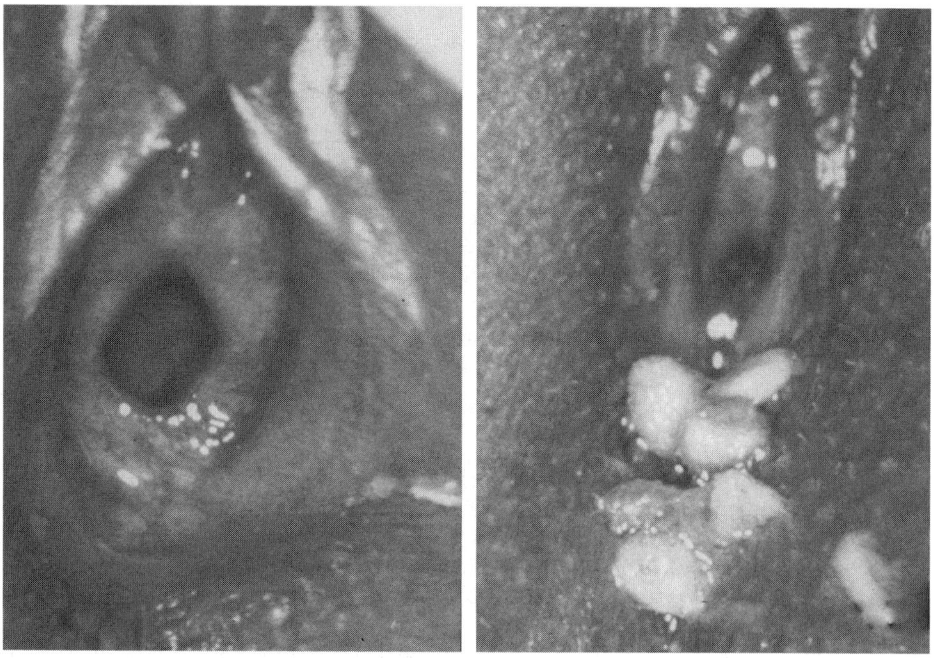

FIGURE 1.9 ● A girl with vaginal discharge and bleeding. The cause, initially unseen, is revealed to be small pieces of toilet paper. (Reprinted from the NASPAG PediGYN Teaching Slide Set, 1996: slide 40, with permission.)

secondary to trauma or medical conditions that lead to an increase in intra-abdominal pressure (e.g., constipation leading to straining). The average age of children with urethral prolapse is 5 years. Therapy consists of frequent sitz baths, estrogen cream, and, in the presence of infection, topical or oral antibiotics. With these measures, urethral prolapse will usually resolve in 4 to 6 weeks. Where possible, the underlying cause should be treated. Urethral prolapse requires surgical intervention if medical therapy fails, if the prolapsed tissue becomes necrotic, or if there is acute urinary retention. An indwelling catheter should be used for 24 hours postoperatively.

Rarer urologic abnormalities such as urethral neoplasms may also present as vaginal bleeding.

Genital Tract Neoplasms

Genital tract tumors often present with vaginal bleeding and should be completely excluded in any case of prepubertal vaginal bleeding. Vaginal polyps should be removed and examined pathologically to exclude malignancy (19). Other benign tumors of the vulva and vagina that may occur in children and adolescents include hemangiomas, simple hymenal cysts, paraurethral duct cysts, teratomas, or even benign granulomas. Hemangiomas of the capillaries usually resolve with puberty and require no intervention. Cavernous hemangiomas may bleed extensively if injured, so surgical intervention is warranted. A paraurethral duct cyst may distort the urethra, and surgical treatment is recommended. Teratomas present as midline, cystic perineal masses. They are usually benign, but because recurrence is likely, a large margin of healthy tissue is excised at the time of surgery.

Cancer of the genital tract is rare in prepubertal girls; unfortunately, these tumors often carry a poor prognosis. They are more common in girls younger than 4 years old. The most common malignant tumors of the prepubertal vagina include the embryonal rhabdomyosarcoma (more commonly known as sarcoma botryoides) and adenocarcinoma of the vagina; both may present with vaginal bleeding. Sarcoma botryoides is the most common malignancy of the lower genital tract in girls and appears as a friable polypoid tumor originating from the anterior vagina. The tumor arises in the submucosal tissues and spreads beneath the vaginal epithelium. This causes the vaginal mucosa to bulge into a series of polypoid growths. Definitive diagnosis requires a biopsy of the lesion. A combination of surgery, chemotherapy, and radiotherapy offers the best treatment success to these patients. Clear cell adenocarcinoma of the vagina, a rare malignancy, is associated with in utero exposure to diethylstilbestrol. Endodermal sinus tumor of the vagina is a rare germ cell tumor with a poor prognosis. Granulosa theca cell tumors of the ovary are the most common tumor that produces signs of precocious puberty. These may present as an abdominal mass (and abdominal pain) because the ovaries are at the pelvic brim in the prepubertal patient. Surgery consisting of a unilateral salpingo-oophorectomy is usually curative (20).

PUBERTAL ABNORMALITIES

Puberty is the development of secondary sexual characteristics and the attainment of reproductive capabilities. The changes seen during puberty are secondary to increased secretion of adrenal androgens followed by increased secretion of ovarian steroids. The regulation of these hormones is controlled by gonadotropin-releasing hormone (GnRH) secretion from the hypothalamus. GnRH is secreted in a pulsatile fashion, and this stimulates pulsatile release of luteinizing hormone (LH) and follicle-stimulating hormone (FSH) from the anterior pituitary gland.

Puberty begins with thelarche (breast development) in 85% of girls. The remainder of patients experience pubarche (pubic and axillary hair development) first (21,22). Breast development begins with a gradual increase in unopposed estrogen. Initially, estrogen levels are low, but they rise with pubertal development. At times, breast development is unilateral, although it ultimately progresses to bilateral development (23). Pubarche usually follow thelarche by about 6 months. Acceleration in the rate of growth ("growth spurt") accompanies or precedes the development of secondary sex characteristics. Often, an early hallmark of onset of accelerated growth is a sudden increase in shoe size. In early puberty, girls grow 4 to 5 cm (1.5 to 2 in) per year. This skeletal growth is initiated by very low levels of estrogen. During the growth spurt, maximal growth velocity is approximately 9 cm (3.5 in) per year and occurs in girls around age 12 years (24). By the time maximal growth velocity is reached, about 90% of final adult height has been achieved. Most girls reach maximal growth velocity 2 years after thelarche and approximately 1 year before menarche. Menarche (onset of menstruation) follows the peak of the growth spurt and occurs at a mean age of 12.8 years (25). After menarche, growth slows and usually no more than 6 cm (2.5 in) is further achieved. Puberty is complete once positive feedback of estrogen on the pituitary and hypothalamus has occurred, inducing ovulation.

The entire normal pubertal process usually occurs over a period lasting 18 months to 6 years (25). The timing of puberty appears to be largely genetic, although factors such as geographic location, health, nutrition, and psychological factors play a role (25). Pubertal abnormalities include many types of both precocious and delayed puberty, with delayed being the more common (24).

Premature Thelarche

Normal thelarche occurs between 8 and 13 years, with a mean age of 9.5 years (24), and represents the first sign of increased ovarian estradiol production (26). Premature thelarche is defined as breast development prior to 8 years of age and must be differentiated from precocious puberty (27). It may be unilateral or bilateral. Approximately 10% of patients with premature thelarche will progress to precocious puberty, whereas the remainder regress and undergo puberty at a normal time (27,28). Premature thelarche prior to 2 years of age is more common than in later childhood years, and most of these cases will regress completely and without any long-term sequelae (29,30). Bone age in these patients is equal to chronological age, and vaginal smears fail to show any estrogen effect. Surgical biopsy is *not* warranted. However, when premature thelarche occurs after 2 years of age, it more frequently persists and is often a sign of early and precocious puberty. Patients who experience persistent premature thelarche frequently have accelerated bone age (30). All patients with premature thelarche show an elevation in their FSH and LH levels (30).

The pathophysiology of premature thelarche is still unclear. It is believed to result from a transient increase in estrogen secretion (e.g., from a follicular cyst), increased sensitivity of the breast to estrogen, ingestion of estrogen via food contamination, or from activation of the hypothalamic–pituitary–ovarian axis causing increased secretion of FSH (27). Premature thelarche usually lasts 6 months to 6 years, although it may persist. It is bilateral in about half of reported cases (29). One study on premature babies with very low birth weight showed an 8.7% increased risk of premature thelarche compared with a normal population (31). This was believed to be secondary to damage to the hypothalamic–pituitary–ovarian axis.

Because the majority of precocious thelarche cases are self-limiting, treatment is not recommended (32). Patients should be followed carefully every 6 months until resolution because progression to full precocious puberty may occur.

Precocious Adrenarche and Pubarche

Adrenarche begins with the maturation of the zona reticularis of the adrenal glands leading to an increase in adrenal gland secretion of dehydroepiandrosterone (DHEA), dehydroepiandrosterone sulfate (DHEA-S), and androstenedione (21,33). This in turn stimulates pubic and axillary hair development (pubarche) and acne (21). Adrenarche occurs independent of gonadarche (maturation of the gonads and secretion of sex steroids), but they are temporally related in most cases (21,34). Gonadarche typically occurs 2 years after adrenarche.

Premature adrenarche is the secretion of adrenal androgens before age 8, and most cases occur after age 6 (33,35,36). It may be due to an adrenal enzyme deficiency or a tumor (e.g., Sertoli-Leydig cell tumor). Measurement of 17-hydroxyprogesterone will usually be adequate to exclude an adrenal enzyme deficit, specifically 21-hydroxylase deficiency. In patients with advanced bone age or circulating androgens consistent with late puberty or adulthood, an adrenocorticotropic hormone stimulation test should be performed. Precocious adrenarche does not progress into precocious puberty (21,36). Gonadotropin levels are at prepubertal levels, whereas adrenal androgen levels are at pubertal levels. Premature adrenarche may accelerate bone maturation or growth but does not lead to short adult stature (17). Typically, premature adrenarche patients reach pubic Tanner stage II and III without any breast development (33).

Premature adrenarche and pubarche are seen more commonly in certain ethnic backgrounds such as Blacks and Hispanics. Causes include precocious puberty, enzyme deficiencies such as congenital adrenal hyperplasia (CAH), heightened sensitivity to adrenal androgens, or androgen-secreting ovarian tumors (35–37).

DHEA-S, produced entirely from adrenal DHEA, is a useful marker of adrenarche (34). CAH is screened for with the dexamethasone suppression test and an 8 AM 17-hydroxyprogesterone level (35). These tests must be done in the morning because of diurnal variation.

It is recommended to follow patients every 6 to 12 months from the onset of precocious pubarche and/or adrenarche until late adolescence or early adulthood because these patients are at increased risk for menstrual irregularity, hirsutism, acne, and polycystic ovarian disorder (28). No other long-term sequelae appear to result from premature pubarche and adrenarche.

Precocious Menarche

Premature menarche is the development of cyclic vaginal bleeding without other signs of secondary sex characteristics development (38). Once other causes of prepubertal vaginal bleeding (discussed earlier in this chapter) have been excluded, this diagnosis can be made. This condition is believed to be secondary to transient estrogen production from premature follicular development, or it may result from heightened endometrial sensitivity to low estrogen levels. Estradiol levels are prepubertal, and vaginal smears fail to show estrogen effect. Adult height is not compromised in these patients, and their eventual menstrual patterns and fertility are not adversely affected.

Precocious Puberty

Precocious puberty is defined as pubertal development in girls before the age of 8, which is 2.5 SDs below the mean age of pubertal onset (24). It usually progresses from premature thelarche to menarche (as in normal puberty) because the breasts respond faster to estrogen than the endometrium (39). The incidence of precocious puberty is 1 in 5000 to 1 in 10,000 (21) and is more common in girls than boys at a ratio of 23 to 1 (24,32,37). The etiology, however, is

TABLE 1.4

Precocious Puberty Types and Causes

Central (GnRH Dependent)
Idiopathic
CNS tumors
Hydrocephaly
CNS injury secondary to trauma or infection
CNS irradiation
Neurofibromatosis
Peripheral (GnRH *Independent)*
Hormone-excreting tumor of adrenal glands or ovaries
Gonadotropin-producing tumors
Congenital adrenal hyperplasia
McCune-Albright syndrome
Severe hypothyroidism
Exogenous estrogens
Follicular cysts of the ovary

discovered more frequently in boys than in girls. In girls older than 4 years, a specific etiology for true precocious puberty is usually not found, whereas in younger girls a central nervous system (CNS) lesion is often present.

There are two main categories of precocious puberty: central (which is GnRH dependent) and peripheral (which is GnRH independent). In either case, ovulation occurs and so can pregnancy (38). Table 1.4 lists causes of central and peripheral precocious puberty, and Table 1.5 summarizes the workup of precocious puberty.

Central Precocious Puberty

Central, or true, precocious puberty is caused by activation of the hypothalamic–pituitary–ovarian axis, leading to secretion of gonadotropins and ovarian sex steroids (40). Idiopathic activation of this axis is the most common cause of central precocious puberty in girls, comprising about 80% of cases (21,32). Central precocious puberty can also be caused by tumors of the CNS (most commonly congenital hamartomas of GnRH neurons) (37), hydrocephaly, CNS injury

TABLE 1.5

Workup of Precocious Puberty

History and physical, including pelvic/rectoabdominal examination if possible
Vaginal maturation index
Lab tests: estradiol, thyroid function tests, LH, FSH
Ultrasound of abdomen/pelvis
Bone age assessment
GnRH stimulation test if ultrasound is normal. If results consistent with central causes, check head imaging to rule out lesion.

from trauma or infections, CNS irradiation, and neurofibromatosis. CNS lesions cause about 15% of central precocious puberty cases (38). When the diagnosis of true precocious puberty is made, radiographic imaging of the CNS with either computed tomography (CT) scan or magnetic resonance imaging (MRI) is done. Patients with known CNS lesions or a history of CNS irradiation and true precocious puberty should have growth hormone levels drawn in their evaluation.

Patients with central precocious puberty have a disinhibited GnRH pulse generator, leading to LH and FSH levels in the pubertal range and ratio. The LH and FSH levels may fluctuate, so multiple samples (e.g., every 30 minutes for several hours) may be necessary. A GnRH stimulation test in girls with central precocious puberty shows a pubertal response, with LH levels rising three times above baseline and elevating greater than FSH levels (39,41). The pattern of pubertal development and its chronologic progression are normal, albeit at an abnormally early age.

Peripheral Precocious Puberty

Peripheral, or pseudoprecocious, puberty is the result of the secretion of sex steroids by peripheral sources such as a hormone-secreting tumor of the adrenal gland or ovaries, gonadotropin-producing tumors, CAH, McCune-Albright syndrome (polyostotic fibrous dysplasia of the long bones, cafe au lait spots, and peripheral precocious puberty), and severe hypothyroidism (21,24,37,40). Exogenous estrogen in the form of medications, skin creams, or ingestion of estrogen-treated animal meat (particularly poultry) must be excluded. Peripheral precocious puberty can be either isosexual (same sex development) or heterosexual (masculinizing development).

Hypothyroidism may cause peripheral precocious puberty. With severe hypothyroidism, elevated FSH levels (38) and delayed bone growth are usually seen. The elevated FSH induces the formation of ovarian cysts and estrogen production. The occurrence of primary hypothyroidism and precocious puberty has also been associated with galactorrhea and pituitary enlargement. This premature puberty is reversible with thyroid hormone replacement (42).

McCune-Albright syndrome causes peripheral precocity via autonomously functioning cysts of the ovary. Diagnosis is based on the skin pigmentation changes and demonstration of bone lesions or pathologic fractures. In this condition, however, the order and progression of pubertal development does not necessarily follow the normal path (24). Vaginal bleeding is the first sign of puberty in most of these patients. Testolactone (Teslac), an androgenic agent, appears to be an effective treatment (38). Prognosis for girls with McCune-Albright syndrome is not good. Most achieve reduced adult heights secondary to premature epiphyseal closure and pathologic fractures. Most suffer menstrual irregularities and are infertile.

Follicular cysts are the most common gonadal cause of peripheral precocious puberty (24). These follicular cysts may occur spontaneously or result from benign ovarian tumors, inducing the surrounding tissue to produce estrogen. Ovarian cysts tend to be recurrent, so surgical excision is not usually helpful. Treatment with medroxyprogesterone acetate (Provera) may inhibit estrogen production and FSH release, ultimately causing cysts to regress. Testolactone, which inhibits aromatase and hence peripheral production of estrogen, may also be useful. Juvenile granulosa cell tumors are another gonadal cause; these are almost always unilateral and usually present at an early stage (24). With peripheral precocious puberty, the prolonged or repeated exposure of the CNS to estrogen may also culminate in superimposed central precocious puberty. In these cases, treatment of the peripheral cause may not be sufficient to arrest pubertal development and addition of a GnRH agonist may be required.

The evaluation of patients suspected to have precocious puberty, central or peripheral, includes a complete history with close attention to any past or current medical problems, medications ingested, family history of precocious puberty, and ethnic background. Careful questioning on the type of development, timing of development, and rapidity of progression are helpful. A complete physical examination should focus on height and weight (plotted on a growth curve), vital signs, neurologic evaluation including vision, examination of the skin (focusing on pigmentation and signs of virilization such as acne and hirsutism), thyroid, abdomen, and Tanner staging of the breasts and pubic hair (23). Some patients will allow a pelvic examination or a rectoabdominal examination. A vaginal smear for maturation index can be obtained and is helpful in quantifying the amount of estrogen present. Patients with peripheral precocious puberty do not have elevated LH and FSH levels (unless the cause is hypothyroidism). They will show a prepubertal response to a GnRH stimulation test with FSH levels remaining higher than LH levels (21). Laboratory tests should include LH, FSH, estradiol, and thyroid-stimulating hormone (TSH). Adrenal and ovarian androgen levels should be checked if signs of heterosexual development with virilization are present. An ultrasound of the abdomen and pelvis is performed to better assess the adrenals and ovaries and rule out tumor or cysts. Imaging studies of the CNS, MRI being the most sensitive (36), should be done in all patients younger than 6 years old and should be considered for patients 6 to 8 years old. A GnRH stimulation test will help differentiate central from peripheral precocious puberty. An ACTH stimulation test will help rule out adrenal causes such as CAH.

In addition to its role in bone mineral density, estrogen is important for the maturation and growth of bones during puberty. The diagnostic evaluation of precocious puberty includes a bone age to look for accelerated growth: a radiograph of the nondominant hand is compared with appropriate tables of normal bone to determine chronological ages (21). A bone age of 11 years usually corresponds with breast development, whereas a bone age of 13 years corresponds with menarche (25). Any bone age greater than 2 SDs above the mean indicates accelerated bone maturation (21). Patients with precocious puberty begin their growth spurt at a shorter height than normal and also undergo premature closure of the epiphyseal plates. Thus, the end height that these patients attain is less than if they began their growth spurt at a normal age and height (32,37,42). One-fourth to one-third of girls with untreated precocious puberty will attain adult heights less than 150 cm (5 ft) (43).

Patients with precocious puberty should undergo treatment to ensure attainment of normal adult height and to return to prepubertal status to delay the psychological and social issues incurred with puberty. Patients with untreated precocious puberty become physiologically capable of pregnancy at an earlier age (38). Often expectations are made of these children under the assumption that they are older, and this can increase their risk of sexual abuse. Treatment of peripheral precocious puberty is aimed at treating the underlying cause, as is also true when a cause of central precocious puberty can be found.

Treatment of central precocious puberty with a long-acting GnRH agonist results in arrest of pubertal development and return of estradiol levels to prepubertal levels (24,44). Pediatric patients tolerate the GnRH agonist therapy very well. Predicted adult height can be increased by 5 to 10 cm (2 to 4 in) by treatment with a slow-release GnRH agonist in a dose of 0.3 mg/kg every 4 weeks (24). A decrease in bone mass has been noted with this treatment (43–45), but preliminary studies show children undergoing treatment with a GnRH agonist will still show an increase in bone mineral density and growth consistent with rates normal for their chronological age (45). Correct dosing of the GnRH agonist can be ascertained by an abbreviated GnRH stimulation test, which should show suppressed LH and FSH levels (41). Treatment should be stopped when patients reach an appropriate age for puberty, good height prognosis is attained, or if the family desires treatment stopped. In older girls with precocious puberty, the degree of bone age advancement and rapidity of progression of the pubertal process are key issues in determining initiation, continuation, and cessation of therapy. If therapy is not initiated or if it is stopped, the amount of compromise in final adult height (based on calculated decreases in predicted adult height) must be fully addressed with the patient and her family. Once treatment is stopped, pubertal development occurs more quickly than in normal children. Menarche typically occurs just over a year after treatment is stopped (45). Women with a history of precocious puberty do not have an increased risk of developing premature menopause.

Delayed Puberty

Delayed puberty is defined as the absence of any secondary sexual characteristics by age 13, which is 2.5 SDs from the mean, or no menarche by age 15; it occurs in about 3% of children (22,24,37,46,47). It can be classified by the status of the secondary sexual characteristics. The etiology of pubertal delay may be constitutional, anatomic, or secondary to hypergonadotropic or hypogonadotropic hypogonadism (Table 1.6) (22). Patients with delayed puberty of any cause will have low estrogen levels, and bone age may be delayed to ages 11 or 12 years. If the bone

TABLE 1.6

Delayed Puberty: Types and Causes

Constitutional Eugonadism (26%)
Anatomic
Imperforate hymen
Transverse vaginal septum
Vaginal agenesis
Chronic anovulation
Polycystic ovarian disease
Hypergonadotropic Hypogonadism (43%)
Chromosomally competent
Gonadal dysgenesis
Testicular feminization (androgen insensitivity)
Swyer syndrome
Premature ovarian failure secondary to autoimmune disease, chemotherapy, irradiation
Resistant ovary syndrome
Chromosomally incompetent
Turner's syndrome (most common in this category)
Hypogonadotropic Hypogonadism (31%)
Constitutional
Congenital or acquired
CNS tumors (craniopharyngiomas, pituitary adenomas)
Infection
Trauma
Psychosocial
Illicit drug use, especially marijuana
Eating disorders
Excessive exercise
Stress
Chronic illness, including endocrinopathies
Kallman's syndrome
Isolated gonadotropin deficiency
Pituitary destruction
Delayed Puberty with Virilization
Enzyme deficiency (e.g., 21-hydroxylase deficiency)
Neoplasm
Male pseudohermaphroditism

age is more severely delayed, hypothyroidism and growth hormone deficiency should also be considered (24). Table 1.7 reviews the workup of delayed puberty.

Eugonadism

Patients categorized with eugonadism have normal gonadotropin levels but nevertheless present with pubertal delay or amenorrhea. On physical examination, patients may be found to have an anatomic cause of amenorrhea; müllerian anomalies are addressed in the following Congenital Anomalies section. If a normal vagina is found, the patient should be assessed for estrogen production to rule out chronic anovulation or polycystic ovarian syndrome. Assessment of

TABLE 1.7

Workup of Delayed Puberty

- History and physical, with attention to Tanner staging, height, weight, vital signs, and pelvic anatomy
- Assessment of estrogen status: vaginal maturation index, medroxyprogesterone challenge, bone age
- Lab tests: FSH, LH, TSH, prolactin
- If gonadotropin levels elevated, check karyotype.
  - If 46,XY, check ultrasound:
    - Normal uterus: Swyer syndrome
    - No uterus: Androgen insensitivity
  - If 46,XX, rule out other autoimmune disease (lab tests: TSH, calcium, phosphorous, ANA, consider ACTH-I stimulation test).
  - If 46,X or 45,X or mosaic of such, rule out diabetes and thyroid disease and check echocardiogram. Ensure patient's karyotype screens at least 40 cell lines to rule out a Y cell line.
- If gonadotropin levels low or normal, rule out psychosocial etiologies (anorexia nervosa, stress, excessive exercise) and congenital or acquired cerebral lesions (MRI or CT scan).
- If gonadotropin levels above normal, perform complete pituitary testing (thyroid function tests, 8 AM cortisol level, growth hormone level, GnRH stimulation test, and consider insulin tolerance test).
- Treat any underlying etiology if found. Treat patients with delayed puberty with low-dose estrogen to stimulate breast development by beginning at 0.3 mg conjugated estrogen daily and slowly increasing dose by 0.3 mg every 3 to 6 months until adequate growth of breasts (usually 9 to 18 months). Once adequate growth is achieved, add progestin therapy to cycle the patient.

estrogen levels can be accomplished in two ways. A vaginal smear may be performed by gently rolling a cotton swab on the lateral vaginal walls and then rolling the cotton swab onto a slide without overlapping the rows. Once the slide dries, it should be stained with, for example, urine sedi-stain for 1 minute before examination under a microscope. If greater than 30% of the cells seen are superficial cells, the patient has adequate estrogen production. However, if parabasal and intermediate cells predominate, the patient is hypoestrogenic. The second test for estrogen levels is the progestin challenge test. Patients are given medroxyprogesterone acetate (Provera), 10 mg daily for 12 days, and should have a normal withdrawal bleed within 1 week after stopping the progestin if they have adequate estrogen production (24).

Another cause of eugonadism with primary amenorrhea is androgen insensitivity (also called testicular feminization). In this case, patients have a 46,XY karyotype but are phenotypically female due to an androgen receptor defect. The gonads are normal testicles, usually intra-abdominal. Testosterone levels are elevated to the normal male range, patients attain tall stature, and breast development occurs because of aromatization of androgens to estrogens and a small amount of estrogen production by the testes. The breasts are abnormal because there is little actual glandular tissue, the nipples are small, and the areolae are pale in color. The quantity of patients' pubic hair ranges from normal to none, depending on whether the androgen receptor defect is complete or partial. An inguinal hernia is present in more than 50% of these patients. The labia minora are usually poorly developed, and the vagina is a short, blind pouch. A vaginal smear in these patients may be normal, but they do not have a uterus or a cervix. Because there is no dysgenesis, the gonads should be retained until after puberty to allow growth and breast development but then should be removed because they can undergo malignant transformation (24). After removal of the gonads, patients should be placed on estrogen therapy to maintain the secondary sex characteristics (24).

Patients with incomplete androgen insensitivity will exhibit signs of virilization, and removal of the gonads is done once the diagnosis is made to prevent malignant transformation. Fortunately, this variant is rare.

Congenital Anomalies

The uterus and upper two-thirds of the vagina originate from the müllerian or paramesonephric ducts (48), and congenital anomalies are found in this system in 2 to 3% of women (49). The müllerian system is closely related to the urinary system embryologically; thus, anomalies found in one system obligate a close evaluation of the other system. Both the metanephric duct (which is the embryologic origin of the ureters, kidneys, and bladder) and the paramesonephric duct originate from the mesonephric or wolffian duct (50). The müllerian ducts fuse to form the uterus and upper vagina. They also fuse with the urogenital sinus to form the vaginal plate. Initially, the vaginal plate is solid, but canalization occurs to result in a normal vagina (50).

Patients with an imperforate hymen may present as a neonate, prepubertal child, or during puberty. Bulging may be seen in the area of the hymen from a collection of mucous (a mucocolpos) in the prepubertal child or of blood (hematocolpos) in the pubertal child. Patients with hematocolpos may complain of cyclic crampy pain and the physical exam reveals normal secondary sexual characteristics. Correction is made surgically.

Hematocolpos, hematometra, and even hematoperitoneum can also result from a transverse vaginal septum, although this is much rarer than an imperforate hymen. On exam, a transverse vaginal septum will usually not bulge with Valsalva maneuvers, although an imperforate hymen will. An ultrasound will show a normal uterus and cervix, although they may be dilated with the accumulation of menstrual blood. Repair of this defect is also surgical, but it is much more complicated than that of the imperforate hymen. Care must be taken not to cause stenosis of the vagina. Postoperatively, patients often need to use vaginal dilators to prevent stricture of the vagina (48).

An adolescent with an anatomic defect may also present with complaints of cyclic crampy pain, often with progressively worsening dysmenorrhea, but with all the milestones of puberty met (48). These patients must be evaluated for a duplication of the müllerian system in which the müllerian bulbs fail to fuse. Patients may have a uterine didelphys with a longitudinal vaginal septum and a hemiobstructed vagina; these patients may complain of urinary retention and have a unilateral vaginal mass on examination. Ultrasound will reveal a pelvic mass secondary to a hematocolpos. This has at times been mistaken for a germ cell tumor. Because this anomaly is almost always associated with renal agenesis on the side of the hemiobstruction, a renal ultrasound should be performed when this diagnosis is considered. There is an increased incidence of endometriosis that usually regresses after surgical relief of the obstruction (51). MRI may be the most useful radiographic study to illustrate the exact nature of the anatomic defect(s) and help in the planning of surgical repair(s).

The two-part surgical repair of this condition first involves drainage of the hematocolpos by making an incision into the vaginal septum over the obstruction. This incision should be large enough to remain open until the second surgery is performed. The second surgery is resection of the longitudinal vaginal septum with care being given to avoid the bladder and rectum. An intraoperative hysterosalpingogram should be performed to rule out any connection between the two uterine cavities. A laparoscopy may be performed to evaluate for endometriosis (49), but in most cases, any endometriosis present resolves after adequate drainage of the hemiobstruction (52). A unicornuate uterus with a noncommunicating but functional horn may present similarly, and these patients also usually have renal agenesis (49).

The most common anatomic anomaly causing primary amenorrhea is that of müllerian agenesis or Mayer-Rokitansky-Kuster-Hauser syndrome. The incidence is approximately 1 in 5000 (53). It is second only to gonadal dysgenesis as a cause for primary amenorrhea. Often, the diagnosis is missed until the late teenage years when patients present with primary amenorrhea. Demonstration of a normal female karyotype is important to rule out some types of male pseudohermaphroditism. As discussed in the previous section, androgen insensitivity presents similarly and should be ruled out. MRI is a very useful radiologic study to aid in the diagnosis of müllerian agenesis.

Most patients with müllerian agenesis have no functioning endometrial tissue within the uterine bulbs or remnants, although a few patients will have some (50). Because the upper two-thirds of the vagina is of müllerian origin, the vagina also fails to develop. It is rare to see a normal uterus, but there have been a few reported cases of pregnancy after a connecting surgical procedure has been performed. Müllerian agenesis patients have a normal 46,XX karyotype and exhibit normal secondary sexual characteristic development and ovarian function. Urinary and renal anomalies, such as pelvic kidney and renal agenesis are common, occurring in approximately 40% of patients. Skeletal anomalies, such as scoliosis and wedge vertebrae, are also common and occur in about 12% of patients (48,50). Growth and development overall are normal.

Treatment of müllerian agenesis consists of the creation of a neovagina. This can be accomplished through the use of molds (Frank dilators) or through surgery. Patients are fitted with a dilator and shown where to place it. They then wear spandex underwear and sit on a bicycle seat, preferably a racing bike seat, to hold pressure on the mold. Patients must be cautioned to position the mold carefully so accidental dilation of the urethra does not occur. Patients should be encouraged to use the molds from 20 minutes up to 2 hours a day (to the point of modest discomfort) and to return to the office for frequent exams and refitting of the molds. An adequate vagina can be attained in a few months time. Plastic syringe covers can be used in lieu of the commercially available dilators. A more in-depth description of the use of dilators can be found in the 1971 paper by Wabrek et al. (54).

Some patients, however, prefer to undergo surgical creation of a neovagina. The most common surgical procedure is called a McIndoe (48). This procedure uses a split-thickness skin graft over a mold. A space is surgically created between the urethra and rectum, with care not to enter either. The mold is sewn in place and removed after 1 week, using cautery to remove any granulation tissue. Postoperatively, patients must use a mold to prevent scarring and stenosis of their neovagina. Operative treatment is usually reserved for patients in whom dilator usage is unacceptable or has failed, or if a well-formed uterus is present and surgery will preserve fertility.

Hypergonadotropic Hypogonadism

In evaluating patients with delayed puberty and hypogonadism, it is important to check gonadotropin levels. FSH and LH levels are secreted in a pulsatile fashion and thus levels may vary (24), but if they are found to be elevated on several occasions, the patient has hypergonadotropic hypogonadism. Hypergonadotropic hypogonadism may be divided into chromosomally competent and chromosomally incompetent categories. Patients, therefore, must have a karyotype checked (24,47).

Chromosomally Competent

Patients with hypergonadal hypogonadism can have a karyotype of either 46,XY or 46,XX. Patients with 46,XY genotype but female phenotype have either Swyer syndrome or testicular feminization (androgen insensitivity). Of the two, androgen insensitivity is more common. It is discussed in more detail earlier in the chapter (see the Eugonadism section). With Swyer syndrome, gonadal dysgenesis is present. Patients have streak gonads with a Y cell line and thus are at risk of developing gonadal malignancies (incidence more than 25%); the gonads should be removed once the patient is diagnosed. These patients have a vagina and uterus because they cannot produce müllerian-inhibiting substance, but they experience pubertal delay and need treatment with estrogen to undergo female secondary sexual characteristic development (24).

Elevated FSH and LH levels are markers for ovarian failure, whether it is prematurely or menopausally. Karyotype 46,XX patients with premature ovarian failure may present with pubertal delay or primary or secondary amenorrhea. They have normal internal and external female genitalia and may attain normal height if complete pubertal delay does not occur. Autoimmune types of thyroid disease or Addison's disease may produce concomitant premature ovarian failure, most likely due to an autoimmune response to the ovaries themselves. Other causative agents include chemotherapy, irradiation, and resistant ovary syndrome or Savage syndrome (despite high gonadotropin levels, the ovary does not respond secondary to a receptor or postreceptor defect). Evaluation includes an autoimmune workup with thyroid function tests, an 8 AM cortisol level, calcium, phosphorous, and antinuclear antibody assay (24); an adrenocorticotropic hormone stimulation test may be needed to rule out Addison's disease.

Patients with autoimmune or idiopathic premature ovarian failure may attain reproductive capabilities. There are reported cases of pregnancies in patients, so appropriate precautions should be undertaken when pregnancy is not desired, although patients should be told that the likelihood of a spontaneous pregnancy is low. These patients are candidates for donor oocyte-assisted reproduction.

Hypergonadotropic hypogonadism may be caused by previous treatment for childhood cancers. Both radiation therapy and chemotherapy may lead to premature ovarian failure. Radiation therapy will affect patients differently, depending on their age at treatment, the dose of treatment, the location of treatment, and whether they had a prophylactic oophoropexy. The younger the patient at the time of radiation, the less likely she is to suffer premature ovarian failure. This may be secondary to ovarian resistance as the ovary in a prepubertal child has less stimulation of follicles than a postpubertal patient (55). Those patients receiving 2000 to 3000 rads of abdominal or spinal radiation are less likely to have normal ovarian function after treatment. Oophoropexy is a procedure in which the ovaries are surgically tacked behind the uterus to shelter them from radiation (55). Radiation to the head can also lead to premature ovarian failure by affecting pituitary and hypothalamic function (55).

Chemotherapy may lead to premature ovarian failure via ovarian fibrosis and follicle destruction (56). Once again, the age at exposure influences the ovary's likelihood of functioning, with the prepubertal ovary showing the most resistance to chemotherapy (37,55–57). The amount of chemotherapy also affects future gonadal function (57). Some patients may initially have normal gonadal function but later develop premature ovarian failure. Postpubertal patients who receive chemotherapy and later develop amenorrhea have not been shown to regain ovarian function (57).

Patients with a history of childhood cancer and treatment should be evaluated for delayed puberty if no development has occurred by age 13 or sooner if concerns about premature ovarian failure exist. Evaluation of height, weight, and development are crucial to the evaluation. Measurement of FSH determines whether the patient has ovarian failure (FSH level more than 40 mIU/mL) or if she is hypogonadal with a low FSH. Some patients may regain ovarian function up to 5 years after chemotherapy, but it is extremely rare for this to occur beyond 5 years (55).

Chromosomally Incompetent

Of patients with hypergonadal hypogonadism, one-half will have Turner's syndrome (24). Although this is one of the more common chromosomal abnormalities among live births, most fetuses with Turner's syndrome are aborted spontaneously (58). Turner's syndrome is the most frequent cause of premature ovarian failure. The absence of an X chromosome causes premature atresia of ovarian follicles and skeletal malformations. Most of these girls have ovarian failure at birth secondary to follicular atresia that occurred in utero.

The stigmata of Turner's syndrome include short stature, webbed neck, high arched palate, low posterior hairline, and lymphedema (24). They are at risk for renal and cardiac malformations. Approximately 40 to 50% of patients will have a cardiac anomaly such as coarctation of the aorta, bicuspid aortic valve, pulmonic valve anomalies, and/or a dilated aorta. Hypertension is common in these patients, as is diabetes mellitus, obesity, and thyroid disease (24,58). Patients should be screened regularly for diabetes, thyroid disease, hypertension, and lipid abnormalities, and given periodic echocardiograms.

Turner's syndrome patients may have a single X cell line (45,X0) or may be mosaic (e.g., 45,X0/46,XX). Patients who have undergone some pubertal development are mosaic for a 46,XX cell line, whereas patients who do not undergo any pubertal development may or may not be mosaic. There are reported pregnancies in cases of mosaic Turner's syndrome. Some patients have cell lines with Y material present and hence have gonadal dysgenesis. These patients are at risk of developing virilization at puberty and gonadal tumors such as gonadoblastoma or dysgerminoma (24,58). If the gonads are left in place, approximately 15% of these patients will develop a malignancy. Thus, it is recommended to remove the gonads upon finding a Y cell line. When requesting a karyotype in patients with Turner's syndrome, one must request that at least 40 cells be examined to rule out the presence of a Y cell line.

Once a patient is diagnosed with Turner's syndrome, treatment of the pubertal delay should be undertaken. If a child is diagnosed at an early age, treatment with growth hormone can be initiated. Some studies show attainment of greater adult height when patients are treated with both recombinant growth hormone and oxandrolone (Oxandrin), an anabolic steroid (24). Untreated adults with Turner's syndrome attain a mean height of 143 cm (57 in) (58). Often, pubic hair will develop spontaneously (37). Treatment with low-dose estrogen allows breast development to occur. Patients are begun at a dose of conjugated estrogen (Premarin) 0.3 mg/day or estradiol (Estrace) 0.5 mg/day for approximately 6 months to 1 year to stimulate skeletal growth without inducing premature epiphyseal closure. The dose is then increased to 0.625 to 1.25 mg/day of Premarin or 1 to 2 mg/day of Estrace until adequate breast development occurs. Progestin therapy is then initiated for 12 to 14 days of the month to provide endometrial protection. Once through puberty, patients can be placed on a combination oral contraceptive pill for hormone replacement (24).

Hypogonadal Hypogonadism

Hypogonadal hypogonadism (pubertal delay with normal or low levels of FSH and LH) accounts for 31% of patients with pubertal delay (47). These patients do not need karyotyping unless they have an associated congenital anomaly such as Prader-Willi syndrome (mental retardation associated with loss of a region of paternal chromosome 15) (24). Constitutional delay due to hypothalamic or pituitary causes is the most frequent cause of pubertal delay in these patients (24,37,46). Congenital lesions or acquired lesions such as infection, trauma, or tumors may cause hypogonadal hypogonadism (22,46).

These patients have a delayed onset of growth spurt and delayed secondary sexual characteristic development. This may be caused by a delay in the reactivation of the GnRH pulse generator (24). Puberty is usually initiated in these patients by the time their bone age reaches 12 years, although they are chronologically older than 12 years. If the patient and her parents desire, treatment can be initiated with low-dose estrogen. Once initiated, puberty will usually progress even with discontinuation of the estrogen (24).

Patients with breast development but no menarche by age 15 must be evaluated to rule out eugonadism as discussed previously. Patients without any breast development by age 13 are hypoestrogenic; however, they may have low, normal, or elevated gonadotropins (24).

The most common types of tumors responsible for hypogonadal hypogonadism include craniopharyngiomas and pituitary adenomas. Craniopharyngiomas are tumors arising from remnants of Rathke's pouch; the capsule or tumor proper may be calcified (24,26,37). They interfere with the portal blood flow between the hypothalamus and pituitary gland. They usually become symptomatic (with signs and symptoms of increased intracranial pressure such as headache, nausea, vomiting, and visual abnormalities) between the ages of 6 and 14 years (26) and are diagnosed by head imaging studies such as CT or MRI (47). Patients often demonstrate delayed bone age, and diabetes insipidus may be present. Treatment includes surgery and radiation therapy (24,26). Some patients may present with delayed puberty as a result of the surgical resection of a cranial tumor (26).

Pituitary adenomas should be suspected when prolactin levels are elevated. These patients may present with pubertal delay or primary amenorrhea, and galactorrhea is commonly, although not always, present (37,59). If the prolactin level exceeds 100 ng/mL, imaging of the sella turcica is indicated. Head imaging studies will reveal whether the adenoma is a macroadenoma (greater than 1 cm in diameter) or a microadenoma (less than 1 cm in diameter). If a macroadenoma is present, surgical excision with postoperative irradiation may be necessary. If a microadenoma is present but the patient is asymptomatic, no treatment is indicated and follow-up imaging in 1 to 2 years is recommended. Treatment of symptomatic patients with microadenomas remains medical with bromocriptine (Parlodel). Primary hypothyroidism may also, rarely, cause hypogonadal hypogonadism. These patients often do very well in school, have short stature, and retain their deciduous teeth (26).

Complete pituitary testing should be undertaken to rule out a pituitary etiology in hypogonadal hypogonadism. This includes measurement of TSH, prolactin, LH, FSH, and 8 AM cortisol and growth hormone levels (47). Because growth hormone levels are affected by sleep, exercise, and various foods, the laboratory should be consulted prior to drawing this sample. Stimulation tests are necessary to completely evaluate pituitary gland function, including a GnRH stimulation test, wherein GnRH is given intravenously and LH and FSH levels are measured. If no rise is found in these levels, a deficiency in LH and FSH may exist. Another stimulation test involves administering thyrotropin-releasing hormone and measuring TSH and prolactin levels. An insulin tolerance test will assess the hypothalamic–pituitary–adrenal axis by inducing hypoglycemia, which should lead to secretion of growth hormone, adrenocorticotropic hormone, and prolactin (24).

Other causes of hypothalamic hypogonadism may be either reversible or permanent (24). Reversible causes include marijuana use, eating disorders, stress, and exercise. Anorexia nervosa must be considered in adolescent girls with pubertal delay or pubertal arrest (24,46,47). In severe cases of anorexia nervosa, permanent hypogonadism can be seen. Intensive exercise, such as that that can be seen in ballet dancers and gymnasts, can also lead to pubertal delay (46,47). Chronic illnesses, including chronic renal failure, severe asthma, malnutrition, gastrointestinal malabsorption, and thalassemia major, can all lead to pubertal delay (26,46).

If pituitary hormone levels are normal but the patient has pubertal delay, she is diagnosed with idiopathic hypogonadal hypogonadism or isolated GnRH deficiency (24,47). This diagnosis is often difficult to differentiate from constitutional delay of puberty. A GnRH stimulation test may be helpful in identifying the location of the deficit. If a patient has a pubertal response (LH levels rising three times above baseline and rising higher than FSH levels), the patient has a deficiency in GnRH. However, if the patient has a prepubertal response (FSH levels remain higher than LH), the patient may have pituitary deficiency. Not all patients with idiopathic hypogonadal hypogonadism, however, will respond in a prepubertal fashion to a GnRH stimulation test (47).

A rare cause of hypogonadotropic hypogonadism is Kallman's syndrome. This is an isolated deficiency of GnRH associated with intracranial anomalies and anosmia that is more common in boys than girls (24,47). Almost all patients with Kallmann's syndrome have a normal karyotype (47). Estrogen replacement therapy may be used in the initiation and sustenance of secondary sex characteristics. If pregnancy is desired, the patient will require the administration of gonadotropins or pulsatile GnRH for ovulation induction.

The treatment of patients with hypogonadal hypogonadism should focus on treating the underlying etiology whenever possible. Patients with idiopathic hypogonadal hypogonadism should be treated with GnRH given in a pulsatile fashion either subcutaneously or intravenously to initiate puberty (47). All patients with hypogonadal hypogonadism may be treated with low-dose estrogen therapy to initiate skeletal growth and breast development. Patients should initially be given unopposed estrogen in low doses to prevent premature epiphyseal closure, increasing the dose after 6 to 9 months and continuing until breast development reaches adequate size. A progestin may then be added (47).

ACUTE PELVIC PAIN

The differential diagnosis of acute abdominal pain in the adolescent is similar to that for adult women. It includes ovarian masses with torsion and cyst rupture, pelvic inflammatory disease (PID), ectopic pregnancies, and non-gynecologic causes such as appendicitis.

Ovarian Masses

Benign

Most ovarian cysts found in adolescents are benign. Functional ovarian cysts are found in 20 to 50% of cases (60), and the majority is comprised of simple follicular cysts. Although corpus luteum and theca lutein cysts may be complex cysts seen on ultrasound, they are benign. Theca lutein cysts are the least common and are usually bilateral. Corpus luteum cysts have normal endocrine function and may persist in progesterone secretion. These cysts usually spontaneously resolve in 1 to 2 months. Cysts that persist beyond this time often require surgical intervention.

Ovarian cysts in adolescents can be followed and managed conservatively. However, once a cyst reaches 10 cm, the risk of torsion markedly increases and surgery is recommended. Patients with acute abdominal pain and an ovarian cyst need to be evaluated for cyst rupture or ovarian torsion. If torsion occurs, quick progression to surgery is important to preserve ovarian tissue. Rupture of a corpus luteum cyst may result in hemoperitoneum and require surgical intervention to control the bleeding.

Malignant

Children and adolescents are at risk for developing gynecologic malignancies. The most common of these are the germ cell tumors, although the most common germ cell tumor is the benign, mature, cystic teratoma. Germ cell tumors are classified by cell types and comprise approximately 2% of ovarian tumors, although they account for 60% of ovarian tumors in the pediatric and adolescent age groups. Characteristically, these tumors grow rapidly. Patients present early with an enlarging abdominal girth, abdominal pain, and torsion. Adolescents may be found to have an adnexal mass, but in children the ovaries are intra-abdominal in location so they will present with an abdominal mass. Frequently, these tumors bleed into themselves and cause patients to present with an acute abdomen. Specific tumor markers are often elevated, including alpha-fetoprotein, beta-hCG, and lactate dehydrogenase. These tumors are aggressive but respond well to chemotherapy. Survival has markedly improved with further refinement of chemotherapy regimens (61).

There are three common types of germ cell tumors: dysgerminomas, immature teratomas, and endodermal sinus tumors. Dysgerminomas are most common in women younger than the age of 30 and are bilateral in 10 to 15% of cases (62). Dysgerminomas rarely have elevated tumor markers. Careful examination of the pathology must be undertaken to rule out a mixed germ cell tumor. Dysgerminomas are the only radiosensitive tumor, although systemic chemotherapy is now regarded as the treatment of choice, with the obvious advantage being potential preservation of fertility.

Immature teratomas resemble the mature teratoma or dermoid. However, there are immature elements, usually composed of neural tissue, within the tumor. They are most common in 10- to 20-year-old women. Usually immature teratomas are unilateral, although frequently the opposite ovary contains a mature teratoma. Postoperative chemotherapy is recommended for all patients, except those with stage 1a, grade 1 disease.

Endodermal sinus tumors, or yolk sac tumors, are the third most common malignant germ cell tumor of the ovary and often enlarge rapidly. Usually, patients present with a short history of an enlarging abdominal mass and pain (63). The tumor growth rate of endodermal sinus tumor is probably the fastest of any human malignancy; thus, endodermal sinus tumors represent a surgical and therapeutic emergency. The median age for presentation is 18 years. Frequently, patients have an elevated alpha-fetoprotein level. All patients with endodermal sinus tumors receive either adjuvant or therapeutic chemotherapy.

Rarer forms of germ cell tumors include embryonal carcinoma, choriocarcinoma, and polyembryoma. Embryonal carcinoma often occurs in the pediatric population with the median age at presentation being 14 years. Frequently, patients demonstrate isosexual (characteristic of the same sex) precocious puberty. Serum hCG and alpha-fetoprotein levels are often elevated. Choriocarcinoma can be difficult to differentiate from pregnancy-induced choriocarcinoma. Although as a pure germ cell tumor it is extremely rare, it frequently is part of a mixed germ cell tumor. Serum hCG levels are elevated in these patients. Polyembryoma is a very rare germ cell tumor and is almost exclusively part of a mixed germ cell tumor. Prognosis of the mixed germ cell tumors depends on the germ cell tumor type that has the worst prognosis. All specimens should be carefully examined by an expert in gynecologic pathology to rule out a mixed germ cell tumor (61).

Treatment of germ cell tumors should be conservative surgery (62). Even if the tumor involves both ovaries, fertility is possible with donor oocytes. Adequate staging should be performed. Postoperative chemotherapy is required in most cases except very well-differentiated stage 1 tumors.

Pelvic Inflammatory Disease

PID is an infectious process that involves the upper genital tract: the uterus, fallopian tubes, and ovaries. Teenagers account for 16 to 20% of the 1 million plus cases of PID each year in the United States. Although the overall incidence of PID seems to be stabilizing, it continues to increase in adolescents (64). Adolescents are at a three-fold greater risk for developing PID compared with women ages 25 to 29, in part because of risk-taking behavior (64–68). Risk factors include multiple sexual partners and failure to use barrier methods of contraception; it is most commonly acquired through sexual transmission.

Long-term sequelae can and do occur in this population and include tubal scarring, leading to an approximately 10% higher rate of infertility and a six- to ten-fold increase in ectopic pregnancies (69). The risk of infertility increases at all ages for increasing severity of the disease and with increasing numbers of episodes. A leading cause of maternal mortality in the United States is ectopic pregnancy, and adolescents ages 15 to 19 have the highest mortality in this group. Nongonococcal infection seems to predispose patients more to ectopic pregnancy. Thus, adolescents should be treated with antibiotics even if the diagnosis of PID is unclear. The complete discussion on PID can be found in Chapter 11. Table 11.3 reviews diagnostic criteria and considerations for PID.

PID is treated with antibiotics, either as an inpatient or outpatient. Tables 11.5 and 11.6 review inpatient and outpatient treatment regimens, respectively. In small adolescents and children, the dose of antibiotic may need to be adjusted by weight. The physician should also remember that tetracycline is not preferred in a child whose permanent teeth have not all erupted, and oral and intravenous fluoroquinolones are not approved for use in adolescents in the United States.

Compliance is often an issue in adolescents; thus, young patients with suspected PID should be hospitalized for antibiotic treatment. Other reasons patients should be admitted include uncertain diagnosis, suspected tubo-ovarian abscess, and unreliability (66). Adolescents have a higher incidence of developing tubo-ovarian abscesses compared with their adult counterparts; one study documented a 20% incidence of tubo-ovarian abscesses in adolescent girls with PID (70). Ultrasound cannot confirm or exclude simple PID, but it is helpful in diagnosing tubo-ovarian abscesses. Antibiotic therapy should be for 10 to 14 days in patients with tubo-ovarian abscesses. If improvement in symptoms and findings does not occur, surgical or CT-guided drainage can be performed.

Clinical Notes

EXAMINATION OF PEDIATRIC AND ADOLESCENT PATIENTS

- Communication, techniques, positioning, and instruments are different for the child's exam compared with an adult's exam.
- Look for congenital anomalies and deformities and signs of abuse.
- The exam may have to be done under sedation or anesthesia.
- The adolescent exam is similar to the adult exam but will involve more patient education regarding development, sexuality, and STDs.
- Confidentiality laws vary by state. Commonly, adolescents may consent to contraception, STD screening and treatment, and pregnancy care without parental consent.

PEDIATRIC SEXUAL ABUSE

- Psychosocial assessment is of key importance.
- Medical evaluation rules out any infectious diseases and documents any pertinent findings.
- Clefts and transections in the 4 to 8 o'clock position are indicative of trauma but not specific to sexual abuse.

PEDIATRIC VULVOVAGINITIS

- Can present with vulvar pruritus, pain, burning, vaginal discharge, dysuria, or vaginal bleeding.
- Infectious causes include respiratory organisms, enteric organisms, sexually transmitted organisms, yeast (rarely), viruses, and nematodes.
- Noninfectious causes are usually related to poor hygiene or chemical irritants.

LICHEN SCLEROSUS

- A dystrophic vulvar lesion of unknown etiology.
- Can present with vulvar pruritus, irritation, dysuria, or bleeding.
- Diagnosis is clinical and treatment is conservative.

LABIAL ADHESIONS

- No treatment is required unless symptomatic; if symptomatic, topical estrogen cream usually resolves it.
- Resistant or severe cases require separation in the operating room.

PREPUBERTAL VAGINAL BLEEDING

- Differential diagnosis includes exogenous hormones, inflammation and infection, trauma, foreign bodies, urologic pathology, genital tract neoplasms, and precocious puberty.

PUBERTAL ABNORMALITIES

- Premature thelarche (breast development)—usually self-limiting but follow-up required to assess for progression to full precocious puberty.
- Precocious adrenarche (elevated adrenal gland secretions) and pubarche (pubic and axillary hair development)—follow every 6 to 12 months because increased risk of menstrual irregularity, hirsutism, acne, and polycystic ovarian syndrome.
- Precocious menarche—cyclic vaginal bleeding without ovulation due to transient estrogen production; rare; diagnosis of exclusion.
- Precocious puberty (pubertal development before 8 years of age)
  - Central: usually idiopathic in girls, but can be caused by CNS tumor, hydrocephaly, CNS trauma, or neurofibromatosis; treat underlying cause; treat idiopathic with GnRH agonist.
  - Peripheral: causes include hormone-secreting tumor of adrenals or ovaries, CAH, McCune-Albright syndrome, and severe hypothyroidism; treat underlying cause.
  - Work-up: history, physical including pelvic, laboratory tests (LH, FSH, GnRH stimulation test, estradiol, TSH), ultrasound, head MRI (definitely if younger than 6 years old; consider if 6 to 8 years old), bone age studies.
- Delayed puberty
  - Absence of secondary sex characteristics by age 13 or absence of menarche by age 15.
  - Categories include eugonadism, congenital anomalies, hypergonadotropic hypogonadism (both chromosomally competent and incompetent), and hypogonadotropic hypogonadism.
  - Workup: history, physical, laboratory tests (LH, FSH, TSH, prolactin); consider stimulation testing, head imaging, karyotyping.

OVARIAN MASSES

- Benign masses are usually cysts or benign germ cell tumors. Treat conservatively unless greater than 10 cm (increased risk of torsion) or persistence more than 4 months.
- Malignant masses are usually germ cell tumors (usually dysgerminomas, immature teratomas, or endodermal sinus tumors). Treatment is surgical, usually with adjuvant chemotherapy.

PELVIC INFLAMMATORY DISEASE

- PID is more common in adolescents than adults and is more likely to be complicated by a tubo-ovarian abscess. Teens with PID are at greater risk for infertility and ectopic pregnancy than adults with PID. Always treat the adolescent with antibiotics, even if diagnosis cannot be confirmed. Consider ultrasound to rule out tubo-ovarian abscess.

REFERENCES

1. Berenson A, Heger A, Andrews S. Appearance of the hymen in newborns. Pediatrics 1991;87:458–465.
2. Diaz A, Neal WP, Nucci AT, et al. Legal and ethical issues facing adolescent health care professionals. Mt Sinai J Med 2004;71:181–185.
3. Adams KE. Mandatory parental notification: the importance of confidential health care for adolescents. J Am Med Womens Assoc 2004;59:87–90.
4. Rainey DY, Brandon DP, Krowchuk DP. Confidential billing accounts for adolescents in private practice. J Adolesc Health 2000;26:389–391.
5. Ryan K, Berkowitz R, Barbieri R. Pediatric and adolescent gynecology. In: Ryan KJ, ed. Kistner's Gynecology. 6th ed. St. Louis: Mosby, 1995:571–632.
6. Bradshaw K, Hairston L, Kass-Wolff J. Pediatric and adolescent gynecology. In: Cunningham FG, MacDonald PC, Gant NF, et al., eds. Williams Obstetrics. 20th ed. Stamford, CT: Appleton & Lange, 1997:1–14.
7. American Academy of Dermatology Task Force on Pediatric Dermatology. Genital warts and sexual abuse in children. J Am Acad Dermatol 1984;11:529–530.
8. Shelton TB, Jerkins GR, Noe HN. Condylomata acuminata in the pediatric patient. J Urol 1986;135:548–549.
9. Winter J, Good A, Simmons P. Vulvovaginitis in children—part 1. Postgrad Obstet Gynecol 1994;14:1–7.
10. Davis AJ, Goldstein DP. Treatment of pediatric lichen sclerosus with the CO_2 laser. Adolesc Pediatr Gynecol 1989;2:103–105.
11. Aribarg A. Topical oestrogen therapy for labial adhesions in children. Br J Obstet Gynaecol 1975;82:424–425.
12. Sanfilippo J, Wakim N. Bleeding and vulvovaginitis in the pediatric age group. Clin Obstet Gynecol 1987;30:653–661.
13. Hill NC, Oppenheimer LW, Morton KE. The aetiology of vaginal bleeding in children: a twenty year review. Br J Obstet Gynaecol 1989;96:467–470.
14. Blanco-Garcia M, Evain-Brion D, Roger M, et al. Isolated menses in prepubertal girls. Pediatrics 1985;76:43–47.
15. Murran D, Dewhurst J, Grant DB. Premature menarche: a follow-up study. Arch Dis Child 1983;58:142–156.
16. Imai A, Horibe S, Tamaya T. Genital bleeding in premenarcheal children. Int J Gynaecol Obstet 1995;49:41–45.
17. Pediatric gynecologic disorders. ACOG Tech Bull 1995;201:1–6.
18. Pokorny S. Long-term intravaginal presence of foreign bodies in children. J Reprod Med 1994;39:931–935.
19. Farghaly S. Gynecologic cancer in the young female: clinical presentation and management. Adolesc Pediatr Gynecol 1992;5:163–170.
20. Breen J, Bonamo J, Maxson W. Genital tract tumors in children. Symposium on Pediatric and Adolescent Gynecology. Pediatr Clin North Am 1986;28:355–366.
21. Merke DP, Cutler GB. Evaluation and management of precocious puberty. Arch Dis Child 1996;75:269–271.
22. Malasanoa TH. Sexual development of the fetus and pubertal child. Clin Obstet Gynecol 1997;40:153–167.
23. Simmons PS. Diagnostic considerations in breast disorders of children and adolescents. Pediatr Adolesc Gynecol 1992;19:91–102.
24. Layman LC, Reindollar RH. Diagnosis and treatment of pubertal disorders. Adolesc Med 1994;5:37–55.
25. Speroff L, Glass RH, Kase NG. Abnormal puberty and growth problems. In: Clinical Gynecologic Endocrinology and Infertility. 5th ed. Baltimore: Williams & Wilkins, 1994.
26. Reindollar RH, McDonough PG. Etiology and evaluation of delayed sexual development. Pediatr Clin North Am 1981;28:267–286.
27. Pasquino AM, Pucarellu I, Passeri F, et al. Progression of premature thelarche to central precocious puberty. J Pediatr 1995;126:11–14.
28. Rosenfield RL. Invited commentary: are adrenal and ovarian function normal in true precocious puberty? Eur J Endocrinol 1995;133:399–400.
29. Winter JT, Noller KL, Zimmerman D, et al. Natural history of premature thelarche in Olmsted County, Minnesota, 1940 to 1984. J Pediatr 1990;116:278–280.
30. Pasquino AM, Tebaldi L, Cioschi L, et al. Premature thelarche—a follow up study of 40 girls: natural history and endocrine findings. Arch Dis Child 1985;60:1180–1192.
31. Nelson KG. Premature thelarche in children born prematurely. J Pediatr 1983;5:756–758.
32. Brook CGD. Precocious puberty. Clin Endocrinol 1995;42:647–650.
33. Morris AH, Reiter EO, Geffner ME, et al. Absence of nonclassical congenital adrenal hyperplasia in patients with precocious adrenarche. J Clin Endocrinol Metab 1989;69:709–715.

34. Sklar CA, Kaplan SL, Grumbach MM. Evidence for dissociation between adrenarche and gonadarche: studies in patients with idiopathic precocious puberty, gonadal dysgenesis, isolated gonadotropin deficiency, and constitutionally delayed growth and adolescence. J Clin Endocrinol Metab 1980;51:548–556.
35. Siegel SF, Finegold DN, Urban MD, et al. Premature pubarche: etiological heterogeneity. J Clin Endocrinol Metab 1992;74:239–247.
36. Miller D, Emans SJ, Kohane I. Follow-up study of adolescent girls with a history of premature pubarche. J Adolesc Health 1996;18:301–305.
37. Ghali K, Rosenfield RL. Disorders of pubertal development: too early, too much, too late, or too little. Adolesc Med 1994;5:19–35.
38. Styne DM, Grumbach MM. Disorders of puberty in the male and female. In: Yen, Jaffe, eds. Reproductive Endocrinology. 3rd ed. Philadelphia: WB Saunders, 1991.
39. Borkowski AE, Cabrera JF, Leya JM. Precocious puberty without thelarche. The Female Patient 1996;21: 45–50.
40. Kornreich L, Horev G, Daneman D, et al. Central precocious puberty: evaluation by neuroimaging. Pediatr Radiol 1995;25:7–11.
41. Loughlin JS. GnRH analog treatment of precocious puberty. Semin Reprod Endocrinol 1993;11:143–153.
42. Anasti JN, Flack MR, Froehlich J, et al. A potential novel mechanism for precocious puberty in juvenile hypothyroidism. J Clin Endocrinol Metab 1995;80:276–279.
43. Murram D, Dewhurst J. Precocious puberty: a follow-up study. Arch Dis Child 1984;59:77–78.
44. Antoniazzi F, Bertoldo F, Zamboni G, et al. Bone mineral metabolism in girls with precocious puberty during gonadotropin-releasing hormone agonist treatment. Eur J Endocrinol 1995;133:421–427.
45. Oostdijk W, Rikken B, Schreuder S, et al. Final height in central precocious puberty after long-term treatment with a slow release GnRH agonist. Arch Dis Child 1996;75:292–297.
46. Albanese A, Stanhope R. Investigation of delayed puberty. Clin Endocrinol 1995;43:105–110.
47. Layman LC. Idiopathic hypogonadotropic hypogonadism: diagnosis, pathogenesis, genetics, and treatment. Adolesc Pediatr Gynecol 1991;4:111–118.
48. Meyers RL. Congenital anomalies of the vagina and their reconstruction. Clin Obstet Gynecol 1997;40:168–180.
49. Tridenti G, Bruni V, Ghiardini G, et al. Double uterus with a blind hemi-vagina and ipsilateral renal agenesis: clinical variants in three adolescent women: case reports and literature review. Adolesc Pediatr Gynecol 1995;8:201–207.
50. Griffin JE, Edwards C, Madden JD, et al. Congenital absence of the vagina. The Mayer-Rokitansky-Kuster-Hauser syndrome. Ann Intern Med 1976;85:224–236.
51. Maneschi M, Maneschi F, Incandela S. The double uterus associated with an obstructed hemivagina: clinical management. Adolesc Pediatr Gynecol 1991;4:206–210.
52. Sanfilippo JS, Waim NG, Schikler KN, et al. Endometriosis in association with uterine anomaly. Am J Obstet Gynecol 1986;154:39–43.
53. Altchek A. Pediatric and adolescent gynecology. Comp Ther 1995;21(5):235–241.
54. Wabrek AJ, Millard PR, Wilson WB Jr, et al. Creation of a neovagina by the Frank nonoperative method. Obstet Gynecol 1971;37:408.
55. Jones KP. Gynecologic issues in pediatric oncology. Clin Obstet Gynecol 1997;40:200–209.
56. Gershenson DM. Menstrual and reproductive function after treatment with combination chemotherapy for malignant ovarian germ cell tumors. J Clin Oncol 1988;6:270–275.
57. Rivkees SA, Crawford JD. The relationship of gonadal activity and chemotherapy-induced gonadal damage. JAMA 1988;259:2123–2125.
58. Saenger P. Clinical review 48: the current status of diagnosis and therapeutic intervention in Turner's syndrome. J Clin Endocrinol Metab 1993;77:297–301.
59. Badawy SZ, Marshall L, Refaie A. Primary amenorrhea-oligomenorrhea due to prolactinomas in adolescent and adult girls. Adolesc Pediatr Gynecol 1991;4:27–31.
60. Emans SJ, Goldstein DP. Ovarian masses. In: Emans SJ, ed. Pediatric and Adolescent Gynecology. 3rd ed. Boston: Little, Brown, 1990.
61. Germa JR, Perira JM, Barnadas A, et al. Sequential combination chemotherapy for malignant germ cell tumors of the ovary. Cancer 1988;61:913–918.
62. Gordon A, Lipton D, Woodruff JD. Dysgerminoma: a review of 158 cases from the Emil Novak Ovarian Tumor Registry. Obstet Gynecol 1981;58:497–504.
63. Athanikar N, Saika TK, Ramkrishan G, et al. Aggressive chemotherapy in endodermal sinus tumor. J Surg Oncol 1989;40:17–20.
64. Shafer MA, Sweet RL. Pelvic inflammatory disease in adolescent females. Pediatr Clin North Am 1989;36:513.
65. Bolan G, Burnhill MS, Catania J, et al. STD update '93: STDs in the '90s. Paper presented at: ARHP Clinical Proceedings; May 1–15, 1994.
66. Handsfield HH, Holmes KK, Berg AO, et al. The Centers for Disease Control and Prevention: sexually transmitted diseases treatment guidelines. MMWR Morb Mortal Wkly Rep 1993;42(RR-14):75–80.
67. McCormack WM. Pelvic inflammatory disease. N Engl J Med 1994;330(2):115–118.
68. Sweet RL. Pelvic inflammatory disease: prevention and treatment. Mod Med 1987;55:64–70.
69. Hillis S, Black C, Newhall J, et al. New opportunities for chlamydia prevention: applications of science to public health practice. Sex Transm Dis 1995;May-June;197–202.
70. Cromer BA, Brandstetter LA, Fischer RA, et al. Tuboovarian abscess in adolescents. Adolesc Pediatr Gynecol 1990;3:21–24.

CHAPTER 2

Care of Perimenopausal and Postmenopausal Patients

Clarisa R. Gracia and Kurt T. Barnhart

INTRODUCTION

The percentage of elderly Americans is increasing; by 2050, it is estimated that more than 20% of the population will be older than 65. In the United States, the most rapid growth is estimated to occur between 2010 and 2030, when the "baby boomers" reach 65 years of age. Because of life expectancy differences, the majority of this growing elderly population will be women (1). The average age of a woman at menopause is 51 years, and more than 90% of women are postmenopausal by 55 years of age (2). With an average life expectancy of approximately 80 years, it becomes apparent that women will spend up to one-third of their lives in the postmenopausal state. It is critical then that the changes associated with menopause be fully understood to optimize the health and well-being of this population.

The menopausal transition and ensuing menopausal state has enormous health implications for a woman. Reproductive capabilities are most obviously affected, but menopause also has a large impact on cardiovascular health, bone mass, cancer risk, and cognitive function. This chapter reviews the important changes that accompany the menopausal transition and beyond, as well as the therapies available for symptomatic relief and long-term disease prevention. This period in a woman's life should be viewed as an opportunity to promote healthy behaviors, improve the adoption of preventive measures, and increase use of screening techniques (Table 2.1).

When discussing the menopausal time period of a woman's life, there is often confusion surrounding the terminology used. In this chapter, the following commonly used terms and applicable definitions are used:

Menopausal Transition: Menopausal transition is the variations in the menstrual cycle that occur until 12 completed months of amenorrhea; these variations may be associated with an elevated follicle-stimulating hormone (FSH). This transition may also be referred to as perimenopause or climacteric and is a process that occurs over many years. There is great variability in the age of onset and duration of this period, but it appears that most women begin the transition at about age 47 (2). More recently, the Stages in Reproductive Aging Workshop (STRAW) developed a formal staging system for normal healthy women (3). This system relies on objective data, uses only reliable, inexpensive, and readily available tests, and allows women to be assigned to a specific stage.

As depicted in Figure 2.1, there are seven stages in the STRAW system: five occur prior to the final menstrual period (FMP), and two occur after the FMP. The first sign of reproductive aging is seen in the late reproductive period (stage –3) and is characterized by regular menstrual cycles with an elevated FSH. In the early menopausal transition (stage –2), women begin to experience variability in their cycle length. Late in the menopausal transition (stage –1), at least two missed cycles or 60 days of amenorrhea occur, typically with the presence of

TABLE 2.1

Recommended Screening Tests and Immunizations in Healthy Menopausal Women

Screening Test	Age and Frequency	Purpose
Pap test/pelvic exam	Yearly; if three consecutive tests are negative, then every 3 yr if low risk	Cervical cancer/ovarian cancer detection
Breast exam	Yearly by physician Monthly self-exam	Breast cancer detection
Mammogram	Every 1–2 yr after age 40; yearly after age 50	Breast cancer detection
Fecal occult blood Digital rectal exam	Yearly after age 50	Colorectal cancer detection
Flexible sigmoidoscopy	Every 3–5 yr after age 50	Colorectal cancer detection
Densitometry	Age 65 if low risk At menopause if high risk	Osteopenia/osteoporosis detection
Lipid profile	Every 2 yr after 40	Cardiovascular risk assessment
Fasting glucose	Every 3 yr after age 45	Diabetes detection
Sexually transmitted infections (STIs) and HIV testing	Yearly in high-risk patients	STIs and HIV detection
PPD skin testing	Yearly in high-risk patients	Tuberculosis detection
Immunizations		
Influenza vaccine	Yearly after age 50, or earlier if high risk	Influenza prevention
Pneumococcal vaccine	Once at age 65, or earlier if high risk	Pneumonia prevention
Tetanus-diphtheria vaccine	Every 10 yr	Tetanus and diphtheria prevention

Adapted from primary and preventive care: periodic assessments. ACOG Committee Opinion No. 292. American College of Obstetricians and Gynecologists. Obstet Gynecol 2003;102:1117–24.

Final Menstrual Period (FMP) 0

Stages:	−5	−4	−3	−2	−1	+1		+2
Terminology:	**Reproductive**			**Menopausal Transition**		**Postmenopause**		
	Early	Peak	Late	Early	Late*	Early*		Late
				Perimenopause				
Duration of Stage:	Variable			Variable		(a) 1 yr	(b) 4 yrs	Until demise
Menstrual Cycles:	Variable to regular	Regular		Variable cycle length (>*7 days different from normal*)	≥2 skipped cycles and an interval of amenorrhea (≥60 *days*)	*Amen x 12 mos*	None	
Endocrine:	Normal FSH		↑ FSH	↑ FSH		↑ FSH		

**Stages most likely to be characterized by vasomotor symptoms* ↑ = *elevated*

FIGURE 2.1 • STRAW staging system. (Reprinted from Fertil Steril 2001;76(5), with permission.)

hot flushes. Menopause is defined as having occurred after 1 full year of amenorrhea. Early postmenopause (stage +1) lasts approximately 4 years and is often associated with hot flushes. Late postmenopause (stage +2) is the final stage and is accompanied by many of the medical complications of aging. For a small percentage of women in stage +2, hot flushes may persist, although they are not usually as frequent as in earlier stages (3).

Menopause: Menopause is the permanent cessation of menses; it is considered to have occurred following 12 consecutive months of amenorrhea. By definition, menopause is a diagnosis made in retrospect. The average age of menopause is 51.3 years, according to a study of 2570 women (2). Factors associated with an earlier age of menopause include poor nutritional status, family history, vegetarianism, and living at high altitudes. Women who currently smoke appear to experience menopause 1.8 years earlier than nonsmokers. Alcoholism has also been linked to delayed menopause (4–10).

Postmenopause: Postmenopause is the remaining life period of the woman after 12 consecutive months of amenorrhea.

ENDOCRINOLOGY OF PERI- AND POSTMENOPAUSE

A woman is born with all the ovarian follicles she will ever develop; over time, these follicles become depleted. When the number of follicles drops very low, inhibin levels decrease and activin rises (11). Negative feedback from the ovary to the pituitary diminishes, resulting in rising FSH levels (12, 13). The initial elevation in FSH is first detectable only in the early follicular phase. During the menopausal transition, estradiol levels tend to be slightly elevated—not decreased—in response to the increased FSH stimulation (14, 15). Estrogen levels do not begin a major decline until a year or so before menopause (16). During perimenopause, postmenopausal levels of FSH (>20 IU/L) may be seen despite the presence of menstrual bleeding, although luteinizing hormone (LH) levels remain in the normal range. After menopause is completed, there is a 10- to 20-fold increase in FSH (>20 IU/L) and about a 3-fold increase in LH (>30 IU/L) (17). Almost all postmenopausal production of estrogen is derived from the peripheral conversion of androgens (18). Although reduced from earlier premenopausal levels, the ovary still secretes androstenedione and testosterone in the early postmenopausal years (19). In the later postmenopausal years, circulating androgens are almost all derived from the adrenal gland.

The decline in estrogen is responsible for the various physiologic effects described in the following sections.

Reproduction

For the perimenopausal women, menstrual cycle length increases and anovulation becomes more prevalent, particularly in the 2- to 8-year period prior to menopause. During this time, there is an accelerated rate of loss of ovarian follicles until the supply is finally depleted (20). Although these changes reflect increasing difficulty in achieving pregnancy, pregnancy can and does occur in perimenopausal women. Approximately 51% of pregnancies in this age group are unintended (21). Women not interested in achieving pregnancy must use contraception until definitively becoming postmenopausal.

Menstrual Cyclicity and Abnormal Bleeding

During the reproductive years, menstrual cycles occur every 21 to 35 days. In perimenopause, a reduction in progesterone production during the luteal phase is common. This reduction, coupled with increased or even normal levels of estrogen production, leads to hormonal imbalances and may be responsible for the menorrhagia some patients report during perimenopause. In early perimenopause, cycle length may shorten by 2 to 7 days secondary to a shortened follicular phase (15). The duration and amount of menstrual flow may also change during this time, although this is less predictable. In mid-late perimenopause, cycle length increases and becomes increasingly irregular. As menopause approaches, menstrual flow may become lighter, and episodes of spotting may become more prevalent (15).

Dysfunctional bleeding is common during the transition through menopause. It most often occurs as a result of the fluctuating hormonal environment and anovulation. Failure to ovulate regularly causes periods of unopposed estrogen stimulation of the endometrium. Prolonged estrogen exposure leads to proliferation, which can eventually lead to episodes of irregular and even heavy bleeding. Such unopposed estrogen stimulation also puts a woman at increased risk for hyperplasia and endometrial cancer. Evaluation of perimenopausal bleeding is important and should be aimed at excluding endometrial cancer. An office endometrial biopsy is recommended and has been shown to be more than 90% sensitive for detecting endometrial cancer (22). Alternatively, transvaginal ultrasound may be used to evaluate the endometrium; if the endometrial stripe is thicker than 4 mm, endometrial sampling is recommended (23). A D&C with hysteroscopy is recommended when an office biopsy is not possible. Persistent abnormal bleeding requires repeated evaluation. In addition, the external genitalia, vagina, and cervix should be thoroughly inspected and a Papanicolaou (or Pap) smear performed to exclude other causes of bleeding (23). For a more thorough discussion of abnormal bleeding, see Chapter 8.

Once pathology has been excluded, anovulatory bleeding may be treated hormonally. Use of a traditional postmenopausal hormone therapy regimen (estrogen with progestin) in the perimenopausal woman increases the exposure of the endometrium to excess estrogen levels in the absence of a contraceptive dose of progestin. Therefore, this approach is not recommended. Monthly progestational therapies in conjunction with an appropriate contraceptive method or a combination hormone contraceptive (e.g., oral contraceptives, the contraceptive patch, or vaginal contraceptive ring) are optimal therapies. Combined hormonal contraception preparations regulate bleeding, relieve vasomotor symptoms, and may reduce the risk of osteoporosis in women (24). The progestin intrauterine device and Depo-medroxyprogesterone acetate (MPA) have been used to control bleeding and also to provide contraception, if necessary. There is little support in the literature for cyclic MPA administration during the menopausal transition, despite its popularity (25).

Determining when it is appropriate to transition from oral contraceptives to hormone therapy is difficult. Although it has been suggested to do so based on increased FSH levels during the pill-free week, some studies show this approach is not always accurate (26, 27). Some clinicians make the change empirically when a woman reaches her early to mid-fifties.

ORGAN AND SYSTEM CHANGES IN PERI- AND POSTMENOPAUSE

Vasomotor Symptoms

Vasomotor symptoms are the most characteristic symptom of the menopausal transition and can be very troubling to women. The sudden sensation of extreme heat in the upper body, particularly the face, neck, and chest is referred to as a "hot flush" or "hot flash." It is estimated that 15 to 25% of perimenopausal women experience hot flushes (2, 28).

Oldenhave and colleagues found that hot flashes were related to the timing of the last menstrual period, and menopausal symptoms were found to be most severe in the late perimenopausal and early postmenopausal stages. These same investigators found that as vasomotor symptoms increased in severity, so did the severity of atypical complaints (e.g., tenseness, irritability, lack of self-confidence, headache, muscle or joint pain, tiredness on waking) (29). The severity and duration of hot flashes among perimenopausal women is highly variable, although they are usually more frequent and more severe at night (2).

Usually these symptoms last 1 to 2 years, but some studies show that they may persist in up to 20 to 40% of women 4 to 10 years after menopause (30, 31).

The pathophysiology of hot flashes is not fully understood. With a decline in estrogen production, the thermoregulatory center in the brain becomes unstable, leading to an acute activation of the sympathetic nervous system and vasomotor instability. Hot flashes are accompanied by an accelerated heart rate, severe peripheral vasodilation in the face and upper torso, and sweating as the internal core temperature falls (32). Vasomotor symptoms can also occur in other conditions, such as diabetes or thyroid disease, pancreatic tumors, leukemias, pheochromocytoma, carcinoid syndrome, certain drugs, neurologic disorders, and nitrites or sulfites (33).

Therapeutic Options

Estrogen therapy significantly alleviates hot flushes. In the Postmenopausal Estrogen/Progestin Intervention (PEPI) trial, all treatment combinations containing estrogen resulted in reduced severity of vasomotor symptoms, particularly in those women with more severe symptoms at baseline. The improvement was greatest at 1 year and fell thereafter (34).

There is some evidence that a combination of estrogen and androgen may alleviate symptoms in women with refractory vasomotor symptoms (30). It appears that lower doses of estrogen are required when androgens are added (35, 36). Progestins alone also appear to be an effective treatment for hot flushes. A 74% reduction in vasomotor symptoms has been demonstrated with doses of 10 to 20 mg/day of oral MPA (or 150 mg intramuscularly every 3 months), or 20 mg twice a day of oral megestrol acetate reduced symptoms in 85% of patients (37, 38).

Apart from traditional hormone replacement therapy (HRT), other medications have been used for treating hot flashes (e.g., Bellergal Retard, Veralipride, vitamin E), but these are associated with limited efficacy and/or toxicity (39–41). Transdermal clonidine (100-μg patch changed weekly) has been used but is only slightly more effective than placebo (42).

Selective serotonin reuptake inhibitors (SSRIs) have shown some promise in treating vasomotor symptoms in cancer patients unable to take estrogen (43). The mechanism of the effectiveness of SSRI remains unclear. Based on double-blinded, randomized controlled trials, it is recommended that venlafaxine (Effexor XR) therapy for hot flashes be started at a dose of 37.5 mg/day for 1 week. If the hot flashes are not adequately controlled, the dose should be increased to 75 mg/day. If no greater improvement is noted, the dose should be lowered back to 37.5 mg/day. Doses greater than 75 mg/day seem to have more toxicity but are not associated with more efficacy (44). A similar trial with fluoxetine (Prozac), 20 mg/day, also demonstrated a significant reduction in hot flashes, although its effect seemed more modest than that seen with venlafaxine (45). Another more recent trial demonstrated the efficacy of paroxetine controlled release (Paxil) at doses of 12.5 mg/day or 25 mg/day (46). Gabapentin (Neurontin) has been shown to significantly reduce hot flashes; common side effects included somnolence and dizziness. It appears to be more modest in its impact on hot flashes than SSRIs (47).

Nonmedical therapies that may alleviate symptoms include the avoidance of spicy foods, caffeine, staying in a cool environment, and wearing layers of clothing in lieu of one bulky item. Alternative therapies for hot flushing are discussed in Chapter 20.

Skin

With aging, the amount of collagen declines and thinning of the skin occurs; this results in decreased elasticity, wrinkling, and dryness. Because skin contains estrogen receptors, declining estrogen levels are believed to play a role in the atrophic changes that occur after menopause. Several studies reveal that either systemic or topical estrogen replacement can protect a woman from these changes (48–50). One observational study of 3875 postmenopausal women found that ever-users of estrogen were 30% less likely to suffer from dry and wrinkled skin than never-users (51). There is some evidence that continuous hormone therapy (HT) is associated with greater skin thickness than sequential administration (52).

Genitourinary Atrophy

At least 50% of postmenopausal women experience some form of genitourinary symptoms (53). These symptoms can significantly affect a woman's sexual, emotional, mental, and physical quality of life, resulting in social isolation and low self-esteem (54). Low circulating estrogen eventually leads to mucosal thinning and inflammation of the urethra and bladder; these changes often become apparent 2 to 5 years after the menopause (55). This results in a variety of genitourinary symptoms, including vaginitis, pruritus, dyspareunia, urethritis, frequency, urgency, dysuria, incontinence, and pelvic prolapse. Smoking appears to exacerbate genitourinary tract-related problems (56).

Vaginal dryness is associated with irritation, itching, and burning, even among women who are not sexually active. The rise in vaginal pH (>6.0) increases the likelihood of urinary tract infections, most often due to *Escherichia coli* (57).

Sexual Function

Sexuality is very important to all individuals, regardless of age. Despite the popular belief that sexuality is not a part of an elderly person's life, studies show that between 50% and 80% of older people have an interest in sex or are sexually active (58). It appears that the degree of continued sexuality activity depends on the physical condition of each partner and the strength of their relationship (59, 60). Many women are not sexually active simply because they lack a partner.

Several definite changes affecting sexual function occur with the onset of menopause. Declining estrogen levels result in decreased vaginal lubrication and genital atrophy. Intercourse may be uncomfortable and associated with the sensation of burning, irritation, and spotting. Lubricants, estrogen therapy, and regular sexual activity alleviate these symptoms (61).

It is unclear whether or to what extent the changing hormones affect libido in menopause. No *direct* correlation has ever been made between libido and androgen or estrogen levels. Libido is affected by many factors other than hormone levels. As estrogen declines after menopause, androgen production also diminishes, albeit not as dramatically. There is some evidence that hormone therapy results in improved arousal and sexual desire (62, 63). In one small trial of postmenopausal women, implants of estrogen alone or estrogen and testosterone resulted in improved sexual functioning. Data regarding the effect of oral testosterone on sexual activity, satisfaction, and orgasm are mixed (63, 64). Although not definitive, more recent studies have also supported the beneficial role of transdermal testosterone as part of HT (65, 66).

Large, randomized controlled trials examining the utility of a testosterone matrix patch for women for the treatment of sexual dysfunction during menopause are currently underway. One of the difficulties with these trials is the establishment of long-term safety for exogenous androgens in women.

Oral dehydroepiandrosterone (DHEA) and dehydroepiandrosterone-sulfate (DHEA-S) supplements are available in the United States over the counter in varying doses, but there are no national quality control standards or oversight for these products; hence, the bioavailability of DHEA-S varies by manufacturer. Results on the use of these androgens for menopausal symptoms and sexual dysfunction have been conflicting (67, 68).

Cardiovascular Disease

Cardiovascular disease (CVD) is the leading cause of death in women in the United States, and in 2000, the overall age-adjusted death rate for women was 285.8 per 100,000 for white females and 397.1 per 100,000 for black females. One in 2.4 deaths in American women is from CVD (69).

After menopause, women's risk for coronary heart disease (CHD) doubles as the atherogenic lipids reach levels greater than those in men at about age 60 years (70). The major risk factors for CHD include smoking, hypertension, diabetes, hyperlipidemia, obesity, and sedentary lifestyle. The strongest predictor of CHD in women is a low high-density lipoprotein (HDL) cholesterol (71). Diabetes and dyslipidemia have been identified as more powerful risk factors in women compared with men (72). In fact, women with diabetes lose their premenopausal estrogen advantage and are at equal risk as men of developing coronary artery disease (CAD) in their forties (73).

A low HDL cholesterol level may be a marker for the metabolic syndrome related to insulin resistance. This syndrome results partly from heredity but is strongly influenced by obesity and inactivity. The prevalence of metabolic syndrome in the United States is higher in women (40% by age 60) than men, and increases with age and increasing body mass index (74). In addition to insulin resistance and obesity, the metabolic syndrome includes three or more of the following clinical characteristics: hypertension (130/85 mm Hg or higher), triglyceride levels 150 mg/dL or higher, HDL cholesterol levels less than 50 mg/dL, a waist circumference greater than 35 inches, or a fasting glucose 110 mg/dL or higher (75). Women should be screened for hyperlipidemia through a fasting lipid profile, which should include total cholesterol, low-density lipoprotein (LDL), HDL, and triglyceride levels (Table 2.2). Levels of LDL increase by an average of 2 mg/dL per year in women between the ages of 40 and 60 years (76).

Although the goal of therapy for dyslipidemia depends in part on risk factors, the primary goal is reduction of LDL cholesterol. Statins are the first-line therapy for lowering LDL by 18 to 55%, and clinical trials have demonstrated a marked reduction in clinical cardiovascular events in women using cholesterol-lowering drugs (77). Once the LDL target is achieved, other parameters of the lipid panel must be corrected. Although a complete discussion of dyslipidemia treatment is beyond the scope of this text, the reader is referred to Table 2.2 for a summary of current recommendations on the evaluation and treatment of high blood cholesterol.

Stroke and Venous Thromboembolic Events

Stroke is the third leading cause of death in the United States. Although the incidence for stroke is about the same for men and women, at all ages, more women will die of stroke than men. Stroke rate doubles each decade after age 55 years. The most common type of stroke is atherothrombotic, accounting for 61% of all strokes. These strokes usually occur at atherosclerotic sites and lead to ischemic injury. The second most common type of stroke is cerebral embolus, accounting for 5 to 14% of all strokes (78). Risk factors for stroke include age, race, gender, and family history. A positive family history of stroke or transient ischemic attack almost doubles the risk of stroke. African Americans have the highest rates of stroke.

Venous thromboembolism (VTE) is the general term that includes deep vein thrombosis (DVT) and pulmonary embolism (PE). VTE has a yearly first-time incidence in the United States of about 100 cases per 100,000 population. The incidence varies by, and increases with, age; there are approximately 500 cases per 100,000 (0.5%) in people 80 years of age and older. Of patients with VTE, close to two-thirds have DVT alone and about one-third present with PE (79). VTE has a high recurrence rate, especially in the first few months after the initial event; the recurrence rate at 6 months is approximately 7% (79). The classic triad of risk factors for VTE is hypercoagulability, stasis, and endothelial injury. However, in 25 to 50% of patients with first-time VTE, no identifiable risk factors exist (79).

Risk factors for VTE may be general, acquired, or inherited. Known heritable mechanisms include antithrombin deficiency and protein C and protein S deficiencies. Although it is important to identify these conditions because of the heightened risk of VTE, their overall contribution to the incidence of recurrent VTE is less than 10% (80). Most activated protein C resistance is due to a mutation in the factor V gene, also known as factor V Leiden. Elevated levels of specific coagulation factors are associated with increased risk of VTE, particularly factor VIII. The exact relationship between hyperhomocysteinemia and VTE risk is not currently known (79).

Osteopenia/Osteoporosis

After approximately 30 years of age, bone mass declines gradually at a rate of approximately 0.4% per year until the menopause. With menopause, there is a dramatic and sudden increase in bone loss; bone mass losses up to 5% in trabecular bone and 1 to 1.5% of total bone mass may occur. This accelerated loss continues for about 5 years, after which it slows considerably, although age-related loss continues. It is estimated that for the first 20 years after menopause, bone loss may result in a 50% reduction in trabecular bone and a 30% reduction in cortical bone. These bone mass reductions increase the risk of fracture. The most common fractures in postmenopausal women occur in the wrist, spine, and hip (81).

In general, bone mass is higher in African American women and obese women; it is lower in Caucasian, Asian, thin, and sedentary women. Studies indicate that up to 70% of the variation in bone density is secondary to heredity (82). According to the World Health Organization (WHO), osteoporosis is defined as a bone mineral density (BMD) at least 2.5 SDs below the mean peak values in young adults, and osteopenia occurs between 1 and 2.5 SDs below the peak value (83). The longitudinal National Osteoporosis Risk Assessment (NORA) Study evaluated more than 200,000 postmenopausal women with no prior osteoporosis diagnosis. Using the WHO criteria, nearly 40% of NORA participants had low bone mass, and 7% had osteoporosis (81).

TABLE 2.2

Clinical Guidelines for Cholesterol Testing and Management

Step 1

Determine patient's LDL, total, and HDL cholesterol levels (mg/dL) after a 9- to 12-hour fast:

- LDL cholesterol—primary target of therapy
  - <100 Optimal
  - 100–129 Near or above optimal
  - 130–159 Borderline high
  - 160–189 High
  - ≥190 Very high
- Total cholesterol
  - <200 Desirable
  - 200–239 Borderline high
  - ≥240 High
- HDL cholesterol
  - ≤40 Low
  - ≥60 High

Step 2

Identify any other atherosclerotic diseases that confer high risk for coronary heart disease (CHD) events (CHD risk equivalent):

- Clinical CHD
- Symptomatic carotid artery disease
- Peripheral arterial disease
- Abdominal aortic aneurysm
- Diabetes

Step 3

Determine presence of major risk factors (other than LDL) that modify LDL goals:

- Cigarette smoking
- Hypertension (BP ≥140/90 mmHg or on antihypertensive medication)
- Low HDL cholesterol (<40 mg/dL)*
- Family history of premature CHD (CHD in male first-degree relative younger than 55 years; CHD in female first-degree relative younger than 65 years)
- Age (men older than or at 45 years of age; women older than or at 55 years of age)

*HDL cholesterol ≥60 mg/dL counts as a "negative" risk factor; its presence removes one risk factor from the total count.

Step 4

If 2+ risk factors (other than LDL) are present without CHD or CHD risk equivalent, assess 10-year (short-term) CHD risk using Framingham tables. There are three levels of 10-year risk:

- >20%—CHD risk equivalent
- 10–20%
- <10%

Step 5

Determine risk category:

- Establish LDL goal of therapy
- Determine need for therapeutic lifestyle changes (TLC)
- Determine level for drug consideration

(continued)

TABLE 2.2 (Continued)

Clinical Guidelines for Cholesterol Testing and Management

LDL Cholesterol Goals and Cut Points for Therapeutic Lifestyle Changes (TLCs) and Drug Therapy in Different Risk Categories

Risk Category	LDL Goal	LDL Level at Which to Initiate TLCs	LDL Level at Which to Consider Drug Therapy
CHD or CHD risk equivalents (10-year risk >20%)	<100 mg/dL	≥100 mg/dL	≥130 mg/dL (100–129 mg/dL: drug optional)*
2+ Risk factors (10-year risk ≤20%)	<130 mg/dL	≥130 mg/dL	10-year risk 10–20%: ≥130 mg/dL 10-year risk <10%: ≥160 mg/dL
0–1 Risk factor**	<160 mg/dL	≥160 mg/dL	≥190 mg/dL (160–189 mg/dL: LDL-lowering drug optional)

*Some authorities recommend use of LDL-lowering drugs in this category if an LDL cholesterol <100 mg/dL cannot be achieved by TLCs. Others prefer use of drugs that primarily modify triglycerides and HDL (e.g., nicotinic acid or fibrate). Clinical judgment may also call for deferring drug therapy in this subcategory.

**Almost all people with 0–1 risk factor have a 10-year risk <10%; thus, 10-year risk assessment in people with 0–1 risk factor is not necessary.

Step 6

Initiate TLC if LDL is above goal:

TLC diet

Saturated fat <7% of calories, cholesterol <200 mg/day

Consider increased viscous (soluble) fiber (10–25 g/day) and plant stanols/sterols (2 g/day) as therapeutic options to enhance LDL lowering

Weight management

Increased physical activity

Step 7

Consider adding drug therapy if LDL exceeds levels shown in Step 5 table.

Consider drug simultaneously with TLC for CHD and CHD equivalents

Consider adding drug to TLC after 3 months for other risk categories

Drugs Affecting Lipoprotein Metabolism

Drug Class	Agents and Daily Doses	Lipid/Lipoprotein Effects	Side Effects	Contraindications
HMG CoA reductase inhibitors (statins)	Lovastatin (20–80 mg), Pravastatin (20–40 mg), Simvastatin (20–80 mg), Fluvastatin (20–80 mg), Atorvastatin (10–80 mg), Cerivastatin (0.4–0.8 mg)	LDL-C ↓ 18–55% HDL-C ↑ 5–15% TG ↓ 7–30%	Myopathy Increased liver enzymes	Absolute: • Active or chronic liver disease Relative: • Concomitant use of certain drugs*
Bile acid Sequestrants	Cholestyramine (4–16 g), Colestipol (5–20 g), Colesevelam (2.6–3.8 g)	LDL-C ↓ 15–30% HDL-C ↑ 3–5% TG No change or increase	Gastrointestinal (GI) distress Constipation Decreased absorption of other drugs	Absolute: • Dysbeta-lipoproteinemia • TG >400 mg/dL Relative: • TG >200 mg/dL

TABLE 2.2 (Continued)

Clinical Guidelines for Cholesterol Testing and Management

Drug Class	Agents and Daily Doses	Lipid/Lipoprotein Effects	Side Effects	Contraindications
Nicotinic acid	Immediate-release (crystalline) nicotinic acid (1.5–3 g), extended-release nicotinic acid (Niaspan) (1–2 g), sustained-release nicotinic acid (1–2 g)	LDL-C ↓ 5–25% HDL-C ↑ 15–35% TG ↓ 20–50%	Flushing Hyperglycemia Hyperuricemia (or gout) Upper GI distress Hepatotoxicity	Absolute: • Chronic liver disease • Severe gout Relative: • Diabetes • Hyperuricemia • Peptic ulcer disease
Fibric acids	Gemfibrozil (600 mg twice a day), Fenofibrate (200 mg), Clofibrate (1000 mg twice a day)	LDL-C ↓ 5–20% (may be increased in patients with high TG) HDL-C ↑ 10–20% TG ↓ 20–50%	Dyspepsia Gallstones Myopathy	Absolute: • Severe renal disease • Severe hepatic disease

*Cyclosporine, macrolide antibiotics, various antifungal agents, and cytochrome P-450 inhibitors (fibrates and niacin should be used with appropriate caution).

Step 8

Identify metabolic syndrome and treat, if present, after 3 months of TLC Clinical Identification of the Metabolic Syndrome—Any Three of the Following:

Risk Factor	Defining Level
Abdominal obesity*	Waist circumference**
Men	>102 cm (>40 in)
Women	>88 cm (>35 in)
Triglycerides	≥150 mg/dL
HDL cholesterol	
Men	<40 mg/dL
Women	<50 mg/dL
Blood pressure	≥130/≥85 mmHg
Fasting glucose	≥110 mg/dL

*Overweight and obesity are associated with insulin resistance and the metabolic syndrome. However, the presence of abdominal obesity is more highly correlated with the metabolic risk factors than is an elevated body mass index (BMI). Therefore, the simple measure of waist circumference is recommended to identify the body weight component of the metabolic syndrome.

**Some male patients can develop multiple metabolic risk factors when the waist circumference is only marginally increased (e.g., 94–102 cm [37–39 in]). Such patients may have a strong genetic contribution to insulin resistance. They should benefit from changes in life habits, similar to men with categorical increases in waist circumference.

Treatment of the metabolic syndrome

Treat underlying causes (overweight/obesity and physical inactivity):

- Intensify weight management
- Increase physical activity

(continued)

TABLE 2.2 (Continued)

Clinical Guidelines for Cholesterol Testing and Management

Treat lipid and nonlipid risk factors if they persist despite these lifestyle therapies:
- Treat hypertension
- Use aspirin for CHD patients to reduce prothrombotic state
- Treat elevated triglycerides and/or low HDL (as shown in Step 9)

Step 9
Treat elevated triglycerides
ATP III Classification of Serum Triglycerides (mg/dL)

<150	Normal
150–199	Borderline high
200–499	High
≥500	Very high

Treatment of elevated triglycerides (≥150 mg/dl):
- Primary aim of therapy is to reach LDL goal
- Intensify weight management
- Increase physical activity
- If triglycerides are ≥200 mg/dL after LDL goal is reached, set secondary goal for non-HDL cholesterol (total – HDL) 30 mg/dL higher than LDL goal

Comparison of LDL Cholesterol and Non-HDL Cholesterol Goals for Three Risk Categories

Risk Category	LDL Goal (mg/dL)	Non-HDL Goal (mg/dL)
CHD and CHD risk equivalent (10-year risk for CHD >20%)	<100	<130
Multiple (2+) risk factors and 10-year risk ≤20%	<130	<160
0–1 Risk factor	<160	<190

If triglycerides 200–499 mg/dL after LDL goal is reached, consider adding drug if needed to reach non-HDL goal:
- Intensify therapy with LDL-lowering drug, or
- Add nicotinic acid or fibrate to further lower VLDL

If triglycerides ≥500 mg/dL, first lower triglycerides to prevent pancreatitis:
- Very low-fat diet (≤15% of calories from fat)
- Weight management and physical activity
- Fibrate or nicotinic acid
- When triglycerides <500 mg/dL, turn to LDL-lowering therapy

Treatment of low HDL cholesterol (<40 mg/dL):
- First reach LDL goal, then intensify weight management and increase physical activity.
- If triglycerides 200–499 mg/dL, achieve non-HDL goal.
- If triglycerides <200 mg/dL (isolated low HDL) in CHD or CHD equivalent, consider nicotinic acid or fibrate.

Adapted from the U.S. Department of Health and Human Services, Public Health Service, National Institutes of Health, National Heart, Lung, and Blood Institute ATP III At-A-Glance: Quick Desk Reference. NIH Publication No. 01-3305. May 2001. Available at: http://www.nhlbi.nih.gov/guidelines/cholesterol/atglance.htm. Accessed June 28, 2005.
Based on the Third Report of the Expert Panel on Detection, Evaluation, and Treatment of High Blood Cholesterol in Adults (Adult Treatment Panel or ATP III).

TABLE 2.2 (Continued)

Clinical Guidelines for Cholesterol Testing and Management

Framingham Risk Estimate Charts

Estimate of 10-Year Risk for Men

(Framingham Point Scores)

Age	Points
20–34	−9
35–39	−4
40–44	0
45–49	3
50–54	6
55–59	8
60–64	10
65–69	11
70–74	12
75–79	13

Total Cholesterol	Points Age 20–39	Age 40–49	Age 50–59	Age 60–69	Age 70–79
<160	0	0	0	0	0
160–199	4	3	2	1	0
200–239	7	5	3	1	0
240–279	9	6	4	2	1
≥280	11	8	5	3	1

	Points Age 20–39	Age 40–49	Age 50–59	Age 60–69	Age 70–79
Nonsmoker	0	0	0	0	0
Smoker	8	5	3	1	1

HDL (mg/dL)	Points
≥60	−1
50–59	0
40–49	1
<40	2

Estimate of 10-Year Risk for Women

(Framingham Point Scores)

Age	Points
20–34	−7
35–39	−3
40–44	0
45–49	3
50–54	6
55–59	8
60–64	10
65–69	12
70–74	14
75–79	16

Total Cholesterol	Points Age 20–39	Age 40–49	Age 50–59	Age 60–69	Age 70–79
<160	0	0	0	0	0
160–199	4	3	2	1	1
200–239	8	6	4	2	1
240–279	11	8	5	3	2
≥280	13	10	7	4	2

	Points Age 20–39	Age 40–49	Age 50–59	Age 60–69	Age 70–79
Nonsmoker	0	0	0	0	0
Smoker	9	7	4	2	1

HDL (mg/dL)	Points
≥60	−1
50–59	0
40–49	1
<40	2

(continued)

TABLE 2.2 (Continued)

Clinical Guidelines for Cholesterol Testing and Management

Framingham Risk Estimate Charts

Estimate of 10-Year Risk for Men

Systalic BP (mmHg)	If Untreated	If Treated
<120	0	0
120–129	0	1
130–139	1	2
140–159	1	2
≥160	2	3

Point Total	10-Year Risk %
<0	<1
0	1
1	1
2	1
3	1
4	1
5	2
6	2
7	3
8	4
9	5
10	6
11	8
12	10
13	12
14	16
15	20
16	25
≥17	≥30

10-Year risk_%

Estimate of 10-Year Risk for Women

Systalic (mmHg)	If Untreated	If Treated
<120	0	0
120–129	1	3
130–139	2	4
140–159	3	5
≥160	4	6

Point Total	10-Year Risk %
<9	<1
9	1
10	1
11	1
12	1
13	2
14	2
15	3
16	4
17	5
18	6
19	8
20	11
21	14
22	17
23	22
24	27
≥25	≥30

10-Year risk_%

Adapted from National Cholesterol Education Program. Third Report of the NCEP Expert Panel on Detection, Evaluation, and Treatment of High Blood Cholesterol in Adults (Adult Treatment Panel III) Final Report. NIG Pub. No 02-5215. Bethesda, MD: National Heart, Lung, and Blood Institute, 2002, with permission.

The risk of osteoporotic fracture depends on the bone mass at the time of menopause and the rate of bone loss following menopause (84). As a rule of thumb, for every SD drop in BMD, fracture risk increases by approximately two-fold (85). A history of osteoporotic fracture also increases the risk for future fractures. Postmenopausal women who have experienced one vertebral fracture have a 20% risk of another vertebral fracture within 1 year of the first fracture (86).

Compared with men, women have a two- to three-fold higher risk of hip fracture until age 85, when risks become equal between the genders. If hip fracture occurs, the mortality rate within the first year is 10 to 20% (87). Only 40% of hip fracture patients regain their previous level of mobility, and one-third will break the opposite hip in the future (88).

Diagnosis and Assessment

Evaluation for postmenopausal osteoporosis includes a comprehensive history and physical examination, assessment of risk factors for fractures, and BMD screening in women younger than 65 years with risk factors and in all women older than 65 years, regardless of risk factors. See Table 2.3 for a listing of known risk factors. Patients' heights should be recorded at each visit, and any changes in posture noted. In addition, caloric, calcium, and vitamin D intake need to be assessed. For those not consuming dairy products on a regular basis, the baseline calcium intake is assumed to be 500 mg/day.

Bone mass may be measured by a number of different densitometry techniques, including dual-energy x-ray absorptiometry (DXA), peripheral DXA (pDXA), single-energy x-ray absorptiometry, quantitative computed tomography, radiographic absorptiometry, and ultrasound.

DXA is currently the gold standard for assessing BMD, specifically at the lumbar spine and femoral neck. Disadvantages of DXA are that it may yield a falsely elevated BMD reading due to poor positioning, disk disease, compression fractures, scoliosis, or vascular calcifications. In the DXA results, BMD is expressed as a relationship to 2 norms: the *T* score is the number of standard deviations above or below the average BMD value for a race-matched healthy young control population, whereas the *Z* score is the number of SDs above or below the average BMD for an age-, gender-, and race-matched control population. It is the *T* score that is used for diagnosing or excluding osteopenia or osteoporosis.

pDXA units are smaller and more portable than DXA units. Measurements are generally taken at the hand, heel, and forearm sites. If osteopenia is noted on pDXA, a follow-up DXA should be performed.

Quantitative ultrasound is gaining in popularity and does not have the ionizing radiation of a DXA scan. It uses high-frequency sound waves, not radiation, to provide measurements. It gives information on bone structure and elasticity, and may be used in peripheral locations such as the heel, patella, or tibia, although the heel is the most commonly measured site. Comparisons among devices are difficult to do because of technological diversity between brands.

Bone turnover may be measured through a variety of serum or urinary markers. The markers may be classified as (a) enzymes or proteins that are secreted by osteoblasts or osteoclasts or (b) substances produced during the formation or breakdown of type I collagen, the principal protein of the bone matrix. Bone markers are often categorized as being either bone formation or bone resorption markers. Marker measurements correlate poorly with BMD. The precise clinical role for bone biomarkers in the management of osteoporosis has not been established.

If osteoporosis is diagnosed, laboratory evaluation for secondary causes should be ordered; these tests may include complete blood count (CBC), serum chemistries, urinary calcium excretion, serum thyrotropin, erythrocyte sedimentation rate, serum parathyroid hormone level, serum 25-OH vitamin D level, urinary free cortisol, and other tests for possible adrenal hypersecretion, acid-base studies, serum or urine protein electrophoresis, and, possibly, bone marrow biopsy if marrow-based diseases are suspected. More than one-third of women with osteoporosis have at least one coexisting condition that contributes to low BMD, and this must be taken into account when assessing a woman's risk for fracture.

It has been shown that a substantial proportion of women will initiate treatment and change behaviors after they have been diagnosed with either osteopenia or osteoporosis (89). Agents used for osteoporosis prevention and treatment primarily inhibit bone turnover. Such medications do not significantly increase bone mass once lost. Antiresorptive agents include estrogens, selective estrogen receptor modulators (SERMs), bisphosphonates, calcitonin, calcium, and vitamin D. Anabolic agents, such as parathyroid hormone and fluoride, promote bone formation.

Treatment of osteopenia is controversial. It is associated with a 1.8-fold increase in the risk of fracture, but not every woman with osteopenia will have progressive bone loss to osteoporosis (81). It is not unreasonable to treat osteopenia with preventive agents if the patient has one or more risk factors for osteoporosis or has documented progressive bone loss.

Postmenopausal women not taking estrogen or hormone therapy require 1200 to 1500 mg of calcium per day. Calcium supplements are best absorbed if taken in divided doses because only about 500 mg of calcium can be absorbed at a time. Calcium supplements should be taken with meals, as the acid load of the meal enhances absorption, although calcium citrate is absorbed

TABLE 2.3

Risk Factors for Osteoporosis

Nonmodifiable	Female gender	Diseases	AIDS/HIV
	First-degree relative with osteoporosis		Chronic liver or renal disease
	Caucasian or Asian		Inflammatory bowel disease
	Body mass index less than 20		Depression
	Age		Insulin-dependent diabetes
Modifiable	Low calcium intake		Chronic obstructive pulmonary disease
	Vitamin D deficiency		Cushing's disease
	Amenorrhea		Multiple myeloma
	Excessive alcohol use		Multiple sclerosis
	Smoking		Rheumatoid arthritis
	Sedentary lifestyle		Thyrotoxicosis
Drugs	Premenopausal tamoxifen		Hyperparathyroidism
	Thyroxine		Lymphoma, leukemia
	Warfarin or heparin		Eating disorders
	GnRH agonists		Pernicious anemia
	Immunosuppressives		Estrogen deficiency at early age (younger than 45)
	Anticonvulsants		
	Lithium		
	Medroxy-progesterone acetate		
	Cytotoxic agents		
	Excessive use of aluminum-based antacids		

reasonably well on an empty stomach. One cup of milk, yogurt, or calcium-fortified orange juice has about 250 to 300 mg of calcium.

For patients older than 65 years, those with chronic medical conditions, or with inadequate exposure to sunlight, 800 IU/day of vitamin D is recommended to sustain bone density and can be taken twice daily in divided doses. Although the benefits in younger women have not been clearly established, vitamin D supplementation is safe and is recommended with calcium to improve overall bone health in all women.

Lifestyle is an important component of achieving and maintaining peak bone density. To be effective, exercise must exert a load on the spine; thus, ordinary walking will not be of benefit, although brisk walking or running may benefit the hip bone mass (90). Regular walking will, however, improve cardiovascular status and decrease the risk of falling, which is associated with a lower risk of fracture (91). Smoking increases the risk of hip fracture by 40 to 45% (92). The vast majority of fractures occur after a fall; therefore, interventions that minimize the risk of falling are important preventive measures to decrease the risk of fracture.

Alzheimer's Disease

Alzheimer's disease (AD) is the most common cause of dementia. Elderly women have a higher risk of developing AD than elderly men, and although this may be because their life expectancy is longer, the age-specific incidence of AD is higher in women than in men (93, 94). The diagnosis of AD is most often based on the criteria developed by the National Institute of Neurologic and Communicative Disorders and Stroke-Alzheimer's Disease and Related Disorders Association. Using these criteria, the diagnosis is classified as definite (clinical diagnosis with histologic confirmation), probable (typical clinical syndrome without histologic confirmation), or possible (atypical clinical features but no alternative diagnosis apparent; no histologic confirmation) (95). Laboratory studies are necessary to identify causes of dementia and coexisting conditions common in the elderly (e.g., thyroid function tests and measurement of the serum vitamin B_{12} level are ordered to screen for alternative causes of dementia). In addition a CBC, as well as blood urea nitrogen, serum electrolyte, blood glucose levels, and liver function tests, should be performed. Depending on the patient's history and exam, other tests may also be indicated. Patients with dementia should have structural imaging of the brain with computed tomography or magnetic resonance imaging at least once as part of the evaluation or care (96). It is currently believed that the accumulation of beta-amyloid peptide, or A(beta) peptide, is central to the pathogenesis of AD (97). Alternative hypotheses emphasize the importance of tau proteins, heavy metals, viral infections, or vascular factors.

Treatment of AD is best provided by a health care provider with training and experience with this disease and is beyond the scope of this text.

ESTROGEN AND PROGESTIN THERAPIES

Formulations and Routes of Administration

There are a variety of estrogen preparations that may be used for therapy. Oral, transdermal, and vaginal preparations exist and are listed in Table 2.4. The choice of estrogen therapy is based on patient preference, ease of use, and differences in rate of drug release and delivery site.

There are differences in potency among various estrogens (e.g., estradiol, estriol, estrone). This is related in part to the affinity with which the estrogen binds to the nucleus; weak binding leads to more rapid clearance and is a marker for lower potency (98).

Conjugated estrogens comprise the single largest category of prescriptions for women who use estrogen therapy. There are two types of conjugated estrogens available in the United States: conjugated equine estrogens (CEE; Premarin) and synthetic conjugated estrogens (Cenestin). The two formulations differ in their compositions slightly. The conjugated estrogens in Cenestin are from plant precursors, whereas those found in Premarin are from the urine of pregnant mares. Cenestin has nine conjugated estrogenic substances in fixed concentrations similar in proportion to those found in Premarin.

Transdermal patches are designated by the amount of estradiol delivered each day. The newer matrix patches are associated with fewer skin reactions and adhere better even in high humidity. Oral estrogens are absorbed in the liver, whereas transdermal products are absorbed directly into the bloodstream. Hence, oral estrogen results in a four- to five-fold higher concentration of estrogen in the hepatic portal system compared with transdermal estrogen. Transdermal agents may result in steadier therapeutic concentrations, with less individual variability (99). Compared with oral estrogens, transdermal agents produce slightly attenuated but still significant decreases in LDL cholesterol and increases in HDL cholesterol. In contrast to oral agents, transdermal estrogens significantly lower triglyceride levels (100). In comparison to oral estrogens, transdermal agents cause fewer alterations in the levels of thrombotic and anticoagulation factors, and overall, do not disturb the balance between these factors (101). Several studies also suggest that high-sensitivity C-reactive protein levels are not elevated with transdermal estrogens as compared with oral agents (101, 102). Oral and transdermal routes of estrogen administration improve endothelial function to the same degree (103). Results from the Estrogen and Thromboembolism Risk Study suggest that oral estrogen therapy may increase the risk for venous thromboembolic events, whereas transdermal therapy does not (104).

Vaginal estrogen is often used when a prompt response of the genitourinary tissues is desired or if the patient has not gotten full relief from her vulvovaginal symptoms with oral or transdermal therapy. It is also prescribed for women who want to avoid the genitourinary atrophy associated with hypoestrogenism but do not want to use systemic therapy. Estrogens in vaginal cream may be absorbed systemically in atrophic tissue. Over 3 to 4 months, as the vaginal mucosa thickens,

TABLE 2.4

Available Hormone Therapy Preparations

Brand	Components and Strengths	Route	Recommended Starting Dose
Oral Estrogens			
Cenestin	Synthetic CE: 0.625 mg, 0.9 mg	Tablet	0.625 mg daily
Estrace	E: 0.5 mg, 1 mg, 2 mg	Tablet	0.5 mg daily
Estinyl	EE: 0.02 mg, 0.05 mg	Tablet	0.05 mg daily
Estratab, Menest	Esterified estrogens: 0.3 mg, 0.625 mg, 1.25 mg, 2.5 mg	Tablet	0.625 mg daily
Ogen	Estropipate: 0.625 mg, 1.25 mg, 2.5 mg	Tablet	0.625 mg daily
Ortho-est	Estropipate: 0.75 mg, 1.5 mg	Tablet	0.75 mg daily
Premarin	CEE: 0.3 mg, 0.625 mg, 0.9 mg, 1.25 mg, 2.5 mg	Tablet	0.625 mg daily
Transdermal Estrogens			
Alora	E: 0.05 mg/day, 0.075 mg/day, 0.1 mg/day	Patch	0.05 mg/day patch twice weekly
Climara	E: 0.025 mg/day, 0.05 mg/day, 0.075 mg/day, 0.1 mg/day	Patch	0.025 mg/day patch once weekly
Esclim	E: 0.025 mg/day, 0.0375 mg/day, 0.05 mg/day, 0.075 mg/day, 0.1 mg/day	Patch	0.025 mg/day patch twice weekly
Estraderm	E: 0.05 mg/day, 0.1 mg/day	Patch	0.05 mg/day patch twice weekly
Vivelle	E: 0.025 mg/day, 0.0375 mg/day, 0.05 mg/day, 0.075 mg/day, 0.1 mg/day	Patch	0.025 mg/day patch twice weekly
Estrogen/Testosterone Combination			
Estratest	1.25 mg esterified estrogens + 2.5 mg methyltestosterone	Tablet	Daily
Estratest HS	0.625 mg esterified estrogens + 1.25 mg methyltestosterone	Tablet	Daily
Vaginal Estrogens			
Estrace	Estradiol 0.01%	Cream	Daily, then 1–3 times/week
Estring	Estradiol 7.5 mcg/day	Ring	Change every 90 days
Premarin	CEE: 0.625 mg/g	Cream	1 g daily
Vagifem	Estradiol	Vaginal tablets	Once/day × 2 weeks, then twice/week
Combined Continuous Estrogen/Progestins			
Activella	1 mg E + 0.5 mg NE	PO tablet	Daily
FemHRT	5 mcg EE + 1 mg NE	PO tablet	Daily
Ortho-Prefest	1 mg E, 1 mg E + 0.09 mg N	PO tablet	Daily in order (alternates E × 3 days, E + N × 3 days)
Prempro	0.625 CEE + 2.5 mg MPA 0.625 CEE + 5.0 mg MPA	PO tablet	Daily

TABLE 2.4 (Continued)

Available Hormone Therapy Preparations

Brand	Components and Strengths	Route	Recommended Starting Dose
CombiPatch	0.05 mg E + 0.14 mg NE 0.05 mg E + 0.25 mg NE	Patch	Twice weekly
Combined Sequential			
Premphase	0.625 mg CEE × 14 days, then 0.625 CEE + 5 mg MPA × 14 days	PO tablet	Take daily in order
Vivelle/CombiPatch	0.05 E × 14 days, then 0.05 mg E + 0.14 mg NE OR 0.05 mg E + 0.25 mg NE × 14 days	Patch	Apply Vivelle twice weekly × 14 days, then CombiPatch twice weekly × 14 days
Oral Progestins			
Amen, Cycrin, Provera, Curretab	MPA: 2.5 mg, 5 mg, 10 mg	Tablet	5–10 mg for 12 days/month with estrogen
Prometrium	Micronized progesterone: 100 mg, 200 mg	Tablet	200 mg daily × 12 days/ month with estrogen
Aygestin	NE: 5 mg	Tablet	2.5–5 mg for at least 10 days each month
Other Progestins			
Prochieve	Micronized progesterone: 4%, 8%	Vaginal gel	1 applicator of 4% or 8% gel intravaginally every other day × 6 doses
Mirena	Levonorgestrel 20 mcg/day	Intrauterine system	Replace every 5 years

CE, conjugated estrogen; CEE, conjugated equine estrogen; E, estradiol; EE, ethinyl estradiol; N, norgestimate; MPA, medroxyprogesterone acetate; NE, norethindrone acetate.

absorption declines. One easy way to assess the adequacy of therapy is to test the pH of the lateral outer third of the vagina; if the pH is less than 4.5, treatment is adequate. Estring is a silicone ring with 2 mg of estradiol that releases 7.5 μg of estradiol daily into the vagina. It may be left in place for up to 3 months and is used to relieve the symptoms of vaginal atrophy. No endometrial changes were noted after 1 year of therapy (105). Vagifem is a 25-μg vaginal tablet placed intravaginally daily for 2 weeks and then twice weekly thereafter. A 6-month study found no change in endometrial thickness (106). Because distant target site responses have been noted with the use of vaginal estrogens (i.e., change in lipids or bone density), there are some authors that advocate endometrial surveillance after 6 to 12 months of vaginal estrogen use (107–109).

Other estrogen delivery options include estradiol gel (EstroGel, Novavax, Inc., Malvern PA) and estradiol topical emulsion (Estrasorb, Novavax, Inc., Malvern PA). EstroGel is now approved for use in the United States and is dispensed from a metered-dose pump; it delivers 1.25 g/day of gel, containing 0.75 mg/day of estradiol. It is applied once daily to the legs, thighs, or calves and is absorbed directly in to the bloodstream through the skin. It has been shown to be efficacious for the relief of menopausal symptoms (110). Estrasorb is packaged in individual pouches with 1.74 g of lotion; each gram contains 2.5 mg of estradiol, so two packs of lotion per day is the equivalent dose of a 0.05-mg patch. In this emulsion, estradiol is delivered via nanoparticle technology and not through a solvent carrier.

Although not commonly used, estradiol pellets are available in doses of 25, 50, and 75 mg for subcutaneous use twice yearly. Blood levels may exceed those achieved with oral or transdermal therapies, particularly after extended periods of use. Blood estradiol levels should be monitored in women receiving estradiol pellets. Aerodiol (oestradiol hemihydrate) is not available in the United States but is an aqueous form of estradiol administered by nasal spray. One spray in each nostril per day yields a dose of 300 μg/day, which is the equivalent of 2 mg of oral estradiol each day.

Much of the breast discomfort associated with hormone therapy is due to the progestin component of therapy. Other side effects of progestational hormones include bloating and depression. The levonorgestrel intrauterine system is an effective alternative to protect against endometrial cancer during estrogen replacement (111). Progesterone may also be administered as a vaginal gel (Prochieve 4% or 8%, Columbia Laboratories, Livingston NJ), although current studies are small, and long-term safety studies are not available (112).

Regimens of Estrogen and Progestin Administration

It is not necessary to perform an endometrial biopsy prior to initiation of hormone therapy in the absence of any signs or symptoms indicating potential endometrial pathology. Women with a uterus should receive both estrogen and progestin therapy. Combination hormone therapy may be given in either a sequential regimen or a continuous regimen. In the sequential regimen, progestins are given for 12 to 14 days each month, and progestin withdrawal bleeding occurs in 80 to 90% of women (113). In the continuous combined regimen, progestins are taken with estrogen every day.

Women without a uterus may receive estrogen therapy only, with the possible exceptions: women with a past history of endometriosis, women with the potential for residual endometrium (e.g., supracervical hysterectomy), women previously treated for endometrioid tumors of the ovary, and possibly women with a past history of adenocarcinoma of the endometrium.

The recent Women's Heart, Osteoporosis, Progestin, and Estrogen (HOPE) Study was designed to look more closely at the effects of lower doses (0.45 mg CEE and 0.3 mg CEE in combination with either 2.5 mg or 1.5 mg MPA) of hormone therapy. The goal of the HOPE Study was to determine whether lower doses of CEE alone or with MPA in a continuous regimen could relieve vasomotor symptoms and increase BMD, while yielding an acceptable safety and side effect profile. The trials found that the increase in BMD achieved with combinations using 0.45 mg of CEE were very close to those achieved with standard doses (114). For relief of vasomotor symptoms, the HOPE Study found that the lower doses of CEE are almost as effective as the standard 0.625-mg dose and that they are more effective when combined with a progestin, although the lower 1.5-mg dose of MPA was as effective as the 2.5-mg dose (115). Based on the 1-year portion of the study, the combined regimens of CEE and 1.5 mg of MPA used in this study effectively prevented the increased risk of hyperplasia associated with unopposed estrogen. The administration of unopposed 0.3 mg of CEE was demonstrated to increase the risk of endometrial cancer and this increase correlated with the duration of use (116). The HOPE trial demonstrated significant increases in HDL, decreases in LDL and total cholesterol, and modest increases of triglycerides with any of the lower doses of CEE with or without MPA (117). The trial was too small to permit any conclusions regarding the incidence of thromboembolism.

Monitoring Estrogen Levels

Monitoring estrogen levels in women on estrogenic therapies is not an easy task. Clinical assays differ in their technique and quality, and the various agents available represent a diverse array of estrogenic compounds. These variations may impede the assay's ability to adequately reflect estrogenic activity. For example, women using conjugated equine estrogens will have very low levels of estradiol detected by even highly specific assays for estradiol. Ethinyl estradiol will not be "seen" by the antibodies used in immunoassays for estradiol; hence, levels cannot be measured in women using this as hormone therapy.

Measuring hormone levels then is useful only in select populations of patients. If a woman continues to request increasing doses of estrogens for symptom relief, an assay may be able to demonstrate adequate blood levels (depending on the agent she is using). The estrogen dose may need to be tittered in women who have an inadequate bone response to therapy. FSH levels cannot be used to measure or monitor estrogen response because FSH is not regulated only by estrogen.

ADVERSE EVENTS AND SIDE EFFECTS OF HORMONE THERAPY

One of the major side effects of HT is uterine bleeding. Although bleeding tends to be somewhat predictable with sequential estrogen/progestin regimens, irregular bleeding occurs more commonly with the continuous combined estrogen/progestin combinations (113, 118). Abnormal bleeding on HT is often a manifestation of endometrial adaptation to the exogenous hormone treatment (119). In continuous combined regimens, at 6 months and 12 months, 40% and 60% of patients, respectively, will be amenorrheic (113, 120). Therefore, expectant management for 6 months may be a reasonable approach. Endometrial evaluation is recommended thereafter to exclude endometrial cancer (121).

To minimize bleeding frequency and side effects from progesterone, a 14-day course of MPA administered every 3 months was tested (122). This quarterly administration of MPA—given the first 14 days of every third calendar month—produced longer menses and a higher incidence of heavy menses and unscheduled bleeding. The study by Ettinger et al. (122) did find that this regimen is associated with endometrial hyperplasia in 1.5% of women after 1 year. In contrast to this study, a scheduled 5-year Scandinavian study using this approach had to be cancelled after 3 years because of rates of hyperplasia and one case of endometrial cancer (123). For women and clinicians who choose to use the extended cycle approach, endometrial monitoring via periodic surveillance of the endometrium or annual endometrial biopsy is necessary.

There is evidence that a higher dose of progesterone is associated with slightly less bleeding (124, 125). Others have found that continuous combined regimens with norethindrone acetate are preferable to those with MPA, with fewer patients bleeding at 6 months of therapy and a higher amenorrhea rate at 1 year (126, 127). Continued problems with recurrent bleeding may necessitate further workup and evaluation (see Chapter 8).

Gallbladder Disease

Although the epidemiologic evidence indicates that use of estrogen increases the risk of gallbladder disease, it is not an overwhelming increase. The Nurse's Health Study indicated that oral estrogens may increase the risk 1.5- to 2-fold (128). Other trials have indicated an increase in the risk of cholecystectomy in past and current users of estrogen therapy (129). The use of periodic blood tests to detect early gallbladder disease is not cost effective; waiting for clinical signs and symptoms that warrant investigation are sufficient. It has not been definitively proven that nonoral routes of administration are without adverse effects on the biliary system.

Weight Gain

As women age, there is a tendency to increase the amount of central body fat. Several studies have demonstrated that hormone therapy, whether with or without progestins, does not cause an increase in body weight (130, 131).

SPECIAL CONCERNS RELATED TO ESTROGEN AND PROGESTIN THERAPIES

Cardiovascular Disease

There is a great deal of evidence from basic science about the potential benefits of hormone therapy on cardiovascular disease. Estrogen therapy decreases LDL cholesterol, increases HDL cholesterol, and reduces lipoprotein-a. Oral estrogen increases triglyceride levels. Ovariectomized monkey model studies have demonstrated a significant reduction in atherosclerosis in monkeys treated with either estrogen alone or estrogen with progesterone (132). Both oral and transdermal estrogen is associated with vasodilation and decreased peripheral resistance (103).

Estrogen diminishes the decline in basal metabolic rate that begins at menopause and the tendency to increase central fat deposition—both of which are risk markers for cardiovascular disease (133, 134). Estrogen therapy is also associated with lower fasting insulin levels and a lower insulin response to glucose (135). An exhaustive review of the myriad of effects of hormones on cardiovascular parameters is beyond the scope of this text.

Observational studies in the literature provide support for the assertion that hormone therapy is associated with a 50% reduction in the risk of CHD (136, 137). The 20-year follow-up in the Nurse's Health Study found a 39% reduction in age-adjusted relative risk for CHD (RR = 0.61, 95% CI 0.52 to 0.71), with both 0.625 mg and 0.3 mg of conjugated equine estrogens (138).

Although there has been a fair amount of criticism over these observational studies, including the invocation of the "healthy user" effect as a large bias, several studies have been able to demonstrate that in carefully matched cohorts of women, the beneficial effect of estrogen on CVD was not due to a "healthy user" effect (139, 140).

In the final adjudication of results from the estrogen with progestin and initial results of the estrogen-only arm of the Women's Health Initiative (WHI) trial, there was no increase or decrease in the risk of CHD (141, 142).

Data regarding stroke and the use of HT have not been consistent in the epidemiologic literature (143–145). In the WHI trial, there was an increased risk of nonfatal ischemic stroke that was similar for both estrogen with progestin (RR 1.44; 95% CI 1.09 to 1.99) and estrogen-only (RR 1.39; 95% CI 1.05 to 1.84) arms of the trial. The number of cases of hemorrhagic stroke limited the power of the study to draw any conclusions regarding this type of stroke (141, 142). In another randomized controlled trial (the WEST trial), women within 90 days of an ischemic stroke or transient ischemic attack received either 1 mg of estradiol daily or placebo. After an average follow-up of 2.8 years, there was no significant difference in the risk of recurrent stroke or death between the two groups (146). On retrospective analysis, there was a significantly increased risk of stroke at 6 months in the treatment group versus placebo, but this was only based on 30 cases. The HERS trial found no difference in the risk of stroke in the treated (estrogen with progestin) group compared with placebo (145).

From the WHI and other trials, including secondary prevention trials, it is clear that hormone therapy is not an effective therapeutic intervention in established CHD (141, 142, 147, 148).

Venous Thromboembolic Events

Multiple studies have indicated that hormone therapy approximately doubles the risk of VTEs, most often in the first 2 years of therapy. A similar finding was noted in both arms of the WHI (141, 142). This risk appears to be reduced with the use of statins and low-dose aspirin, although it is not known if concurrent use of these agents will fully protect against the increased risk associated with hormone therapy (149, 150). In one French case-control study, there was a four-fold increase in the risk of VTE among users of oral estrogen but no increase in risk among transdermal users of estrogen (151).

Cognition

On average, almost all cognitive functions decline with age, but there is a large amount of variability in this decline. Many women notice increasing difficulty with recall and concentration during the menopausal transition (152). These changes are generally attributed to stress, health, and normal aging. Estrogen receptors, both alpha and beta, can be found throughout the brain, including in the cerebral cortex, forebrain, hippocampus, and cholinergic system (153–156). Several studies have demonstrated an association of HT with improved scores on verbal tests of memory and activates brain areas involved in memory, whereas other several studies have shown conflicting results (157–162). For example, a large prospective cohort study of the Rancho Bernardo retirement community failed to demonstrate any benefit from HT on cognitive tests (162). A meta-analysis of nine randomized clinical trials found that only symptomatic postmenopausal women benefit from hormonal therapy (163). It is unclear if the addition of progesterone diminishes that beneficial effect (164).

In the more recently published WHI Memory Study (WHIMS), the data reported that combination hormone therapy increased the risk of probable dementia in women 65 years of age and older and failed to prevent mild cognitive impairment in women (165). It should be noted, however, that the duration of follow-up in WHIMS was short, the average age at enrollment in WHIMS was 72.3 years, and only one combination formulation was tested. In addition, the only statistically significant finding was increased vascular dementia (not AD) in women 75 years and older and in women who had been exposed to hormone therapy for only a short term.

In a prospective trial of a fairly homogenous population in Utah, there was a reduction in the risk of AD among hormone users but only with long-term (i.e., more than 10 years) treatment (166). More research is needed to determine the effects of estrogen alone, estrogen plus progestin, and progestin alone on central nervous system function and aging.

Breast Cancer

Because the greatest risk factor for breast cancer is a woman's age, most women are diagnosed after menopause. In a more recent reanalysis of data from more than 160,000 women, the relative risk of breast cancer in current and recent users of HT (estrogen, estrogen with progestin) for more than 5 years was 1.35 compared with nonusers (95% CI 1.21 to 1.49), and the risk increased with increasing duration of use. This increase in relative risk was greatest in women with lower body weights (167). This increased relative risk amounts to two extra cases of breast cancer diagnosed by age 70 for every 1000 women using HT for 5 years. In the same study, it was also noted that current and recent users of hormone therapy had only localized disease and ever-users had less metastatic disease compared with never-users. Similar to results seen in other trials, there was no effect of family history of breast cancer (167, 168). A positive family history of breast cancer is not a contraindication to the use of hormone therapy.

A similar risk (RR 1.2 in ET users, RR 1.4 in HT users) was demonstrated in a recent large observational study and also in the estrogen-progestin arm of the WHI trial (RR 1.24, CI 1.01 to 1.54) (169). The Million Women Study was done in the United Kingdom and used data from questionnaires received from 1,084,110 women between 1996 and 2001. No increase in breast cancer risk was noted in past users, regardless of length of time since discontinuation and regardless of duration of use. It did demonstrate an increase in relative risk for breast cancer for current users (estrogen only RR 1.3, 95% CI 1.22 to 1.38, and estrogen plus progestin RR 2.00, 95% CI 1.91 to 2.09) and noted an increase in risk with increasing duration of use (170). There are many criticisms of the Million Women Study, including many differences between users and nonusers, establishment of hormone use at entry only, an average time to breast cancer diagnosis of only 1.2 years, and average time to death of only 1.7 years.

It is not clear from these and many other studies, whether the use of postmenopausal hormone therapy initiates the development of new breast cancers or if these results reflect an impact on pre-existing but undetected tumors. Interestingly, the breast cancers diagnosed in HT users tend to be less aggressive, associated with a better prognosis and decreased mortality than in women not taking HT (171–173). It has been hypothesized that this is due to increased surveillance and earlier detection, but it may also result from an effect on pre-existing tumors so they become evident at less virulent and less aggressive stages.

It is important to note that the reported increased risk of breast cancer associated with hormone therapy is smaller than that associated with other risk factors such as positive family history, obesity after menopause, and alcohol use.

Although the numbers are small and the trials were not designed to specifically compare estrogen only with estrogen plus progestin regimens, there is some evidence that combination HT increases breast cancer risk more than estrogen alone, possibly only in lean women (169, 174–176). In the more recently completed estrogen-only arm of the WHI, there was no statistically significant increase in the risk of breast cancer among women randomized to estrogen only.

Endometrial Cancer

Uterine cancer is the leading gynecologic cancer affecting women in the United States and accounts for 2% of cancer-related deaths in women (177). It has been shown that unopposed estrogen treatment in women with an intact uterus substantially increases the risk of developing endometrial cancer (178). The risk of endometrial cancer rises with higher unopposed estrogen doses, longer treatment duration, and lingers for up to 10 years after the estrogen is discontinued. The incidence can range from 20% after 1 year of unopposed therapy to up to 62% after 3 years of unopposed estrogen use (119). According to the PEPI trial, estrogen therapy increased the risk by 34%, and a more recent meta-analysis found that 10 years of unopposed estrogen increased the risk ten-fold (179, 180). The addition of either cyclic progestins for a minimum of 10 days a month or continuous progestins to estrogen eliminates this increased risk of endometrial cancer (122, 181–184). Most of the current evidence supports the use of a progestational agent for 12 to 14 days. Although estrogen-progestin therapy will not result in an increased risk in endometrial cancer, it does not preclude against the development of this disease entirely. When clinically indicated, patients on estrogen and progestin regimens should be evaluated for endometrial pathology.

Other Cancers

There is conflicting data regarding the potential risk of ovarian cancer associated with HT. Several observational studies have been conducted with variable results spanning from a slightly increased risk with more than 10 years of estrogen use to no increased risk (185–189). More recently, a cohort study of 44,271 postmenopausal women reported an increased risk of ovarian cancer in women who had used estrogen alone (RR 1.6, CI 1.2 to 2.0), especially with prolonged use. Combination HT was not associated with an elevated ovarian cancer risk in this study (190). Although the WHI concluded that combined estrogen-progestin treatment may increase the risk of ovarian cancer, the small numbers in this trial limits its statistical power to make any definitive conclusions (184).

Colorectal cancer is the third leading cause of cancer death in women and is more prevalent than cancer of the uterus or ovary (177). HT appears to be protective against colorectal cancer in postmenopausal women. This has been shown in multiple observational studies (191–196). The effect seems to be greatest for current users and is not enhanced with increasing duration of use (196). Estrogen appears to reduce the secretion and concentration of bile acids in the colon and may act directly on the colon by inhibiting the growth of human colon cancer cells (193, 197). The estrogen-progestin arm of the WHI reported a statistically significant reduced risk of colon cancer, although there were too few cases of rectal cancer to assess the impact of hormonal therapy on this disease (198). The estrogen-only arm of the WHI did not show a difference in colorectal cancer rates (142). In some studies, hormone therapy was associated with improved survival in women who had been diagnosed with colon cancer. In a study of 815 postmenopausal women diagnosed with colon cancer, Slattery and colleagues demonstrated that women who had ever used HT had a 40% lower probability of dying from colon cancer. Women who had used HT for at least 4 years had the lowest risk of dying of colon cancer (199).

Although the association between cervical cancer and HT has not been studied extensively, it appears that use of hormonal therapy does not increase the risk of cervical cancer and may be somewhat protective (200, 201).

SELECTIVE ESTROGEN RECEPTOR MODULATORS (SERMs)

Although there are benefits to hormone therapy, many women choose not to undergo this therapy because of the potential increase in the risk of breast cancer and bothersome side effects such as breast tenderness and vaginal bleeding. By exerting estrogenic effects on some tissues and antiestrogenic activities in others, SERMs may potentially provide similar benefits to hormonal therapy without some of the adverse effects. There is growing interest in developing a SERM with specific agonist activities on the bone, cardiovascular system, brain, and genitourinary system, as well as with estrogen antagonist activity in the breast and endometrium. This ideal compound has not been developed to date, but available SERMs possess some of these beneficial properties.

There are two clinically available classes of SERMs: triphenylethylenes (tamoxifen, toremifene, idoxifene, clomiphene) and benzothiophenes (raloxifene). Although beneficial effects of tamoxifen on the prevention and treatment of breast cancer have been demonstrated, its cardiovascular and skeletal effects are unclear, and there is an increased risk of venous thromboembolism, endometrial cancer, cataracts, and a worsening of vasomotor symptoms associated with its use. At this time, its use is indicated primarily for the prevention and treatment of breast cancer.

Raloxifene appears to have positive effects on the breast and bone, as well as a favorable effect on the lipoprotein profile without increasing the risk of endometrial cancer (202). However, it does not improve vasomotor or genitourinary symptoms associated with menopause and does increase the risk of venous thromboembolism approximately three-fold (203). More data are needed on the effects of raloxifene with respect to cardiovascular morbidity and mortality, as well as its effect on the central nervous system.

In view of the current evidence, raloxifene is recommended for postmenopausal women to prevent or treat osteoporosis. The recommended dose is 60 mg once daily. The most common side effects include hot flushes (particularly in younger women) and leg cramps. Women with a history of thrombosis and those who are not yet postmenopausal should not take this medication. Raloxifene should be discontinued during times of immobilization given the risk of thromboembolism.

There has been concern that SERMs may increase the risk of endometrial cancer. Indeed, early breast cancer prevention trials with tamoxifen demonstrated a more than two-fold increase in the risk of endometrial cancer in treated women, particularly in postmenopausal women (204). Postmenopausal women on tamoxifen also have a significant incidence of endometrial polyp formation (205). Although tamoxifen appears to function as an estrogen agonist on endometrial tissue, raloxifene appears to be an antagonist (206). A more recent randomized clinical trial showed no increase in endometrial thickness or proliferation in early menopausal women taking either 60 mg or 150 mg raloxifene compared with placebo (207).

Among high-risk Caucasian women, use of the SERM tamoxifen has been shown in a U.S. trial to act as a preventive agent in breast cancer development. Tamoxifen significantly reduced the incidence of invasive breast cancer by 49% and noninvasive cancer by 50% compared with placebo in women at increased risk for breast cancer (204). Raloxifene has been shown to inhibit estrogen receptor-dependent mammary tumors in vitro (208). Although not specifically designed to evaluate the effects of raloxifene on breast cancer occurrence, the MORE trial did demonstrate a reduction in new-onset breast cancer compared with placebo (203). The Study of Tamoxifen and Raloxifene (STAR), a large, multicenter randomized controlled trial is currently underway to compare these two medications in women at high risk for breast cancer development; initial results are anticipated in 2006.

ANDROGEN THERAPY

Testosterone has direct androgenic actions and is a prohormone for estradiol in the brain and other tissues. It circulates in the bloodstream highly bound to sex hormone binding globulin (SHBG); it is the level of bioavailable, free testosterone that determines whether a deficiency is present. The gold standard for measurement of free testosterone is equilibrium dialysis. A clinical or biochemical definition of androgen deficiency in women, however, does not exist. There are no studies that correlate proposed symptoms of androgen deficiency with circulating levels of androgens in women. In contrast to the abrupt decline in estradiol at menopause, testosterone levels drop gradually with age and do not change acutely across the menopausal transition (209). The change in the estrogen-to-androgen ratio associated with the menopausal transition may lead to a change in body habitus. For example, many women complain of storing fat in their midsection in lieu of their thighs or hips after menopause and mild hirsutism is present in many elderly women.

Testosterone measurement should include total testosterone, SHBG, and, when indicated, thyroid-stimulating hormone and iron studies. The testosterone level should be measured before midday, and in premenopausal women, in the middle third of the cycle. Current assays are insensitive for detecting testosterone levels at the lower-normal female range and are of little use for values that lie below this range. Values in the lower quartile of the normal range, in conjunction with clinical symptoms, may indicate testosterone insufficiency.

Many of the symptoms of androgen insufficiency are nonspecific and characteristic of other medical, psychological, and psychosocial problems; for example, decreased libido, dysphoric mood, diminished sense of well-being, and low energy may be manifest with androgen deficiency and with other problems. Because of this, alternate causes of presenting symptoms must be identified and treated before the diagnosis of androgen insufficiency is made.

Hormone therapy, either estrogen alone or in conjunction with a progesterone, should be initiated prior to any androgen therapy. Oral, but not transdermal, estrogen therapy increases SHBG concentrations and hence decreases free testosterone levels. For women who present with decreased libido after starting oral estrogen therapy, changing to a nonoral form of estrogen therapy may alleviate her symptoms.

The ideal candidate for androgen therapy is a woman who has sufficient estrogen and a physiologic reason for reduced androgen levels and for whom other causes and treatments have been considered. It is important to counsel women that no androgen therapies have been proven safe and effective in long-term trials. The only U.S. Food and Drug Administration (FDA)-approved hormonal regimen containing both estrogen and an androgen (methyltestosterone) (Estratest, Organon) is indicated for the relief of menopausal symptoms only.

Currently available androgen products include topical testosterone ointments and gels, oral methyltestosterone (MT), micronized testosterone, DHEA, intramuscular testosterone, and testosterone implants. Many of these products are compounded at the pharmacy and, as a result, lot-to-lot consistency, bioavailability, and doses are not well standardized. Topical products that are FDA approved for men, including skin patches (Androderm, Testoderm) and gels (Androgel), are not dosed for women and should not be used in women.

Oral testosterones include micronized testosterone, MT, and DHEA. Micronized testosterone is not absorbed well and is therefore not recommended. DHEA is available as a supplement and does not require a prescription. The recommended dose for women with low androgen levels is 50 mg daily, but the amount of the hormone in over-the-counter preparations varies greatly due to the lack of regulation.

Risks of androgen therapy include hirsutism, adverse lipid effects, acne, and impaired liver function. A baseline fasting lipid profile and liver function testing are recommended for women starting androgen therapy, possible with a repeat evaluation at 6 months of therapy. Other possible adverse effects include virilization, fluid retention with edema, psychological and behavioral changes, virilization of a female fetus, and exacerbation of pre-existing heart disease. As many androgens are aromatized to estrogens, it is theoretically possible that androgen therapy in women may also increase the risk of VTEs, gallbladder disease, and breast cancer.

A new transdermal testosterone patch is under development and initial trials were able to demonstrate efficacy in the treatment of diminished sexual desire, although long-term safety data is still lacking (210).

CONCLUSION

The transition to menopause marks a critical time in a woman's life. Profound but gradual changes occur that have long-term implications for the overall health, reproduction, and quality of life. The clinician should have a full understanding of these changes and the available treatments to maximize women's health and well-being.

Clinical Notes

- The menopausal transition is characterized by variable menstrual cycles and an elevated FSH.
- Menopause occurs after 12 months of amenorrhea, and postmenopause is the period from menopause until death.

- Once pathology has been excluded, irregular vaginal bleeding from anovulation in perimenopausal patients is best treated with combined oral contraceptives as long as no contraindication exists.
- HT effectively treats vasomotor symptoms, genitourinary symptoms, skin aging, and may improve sexual functioning.
- Although hormone therapy improves cardiac risk factors, more recent data indicate that it is not beneficial for the secondary prevention of CVD in postmenopausal patients.
- The long-term effect of SERMs on CVD is not yet clear.
- HT increases the risk of stroke and VTE.
- HT, bisphosphonates, and SERMs are first-line therapy for the prevention and treatment of osteoporosis in postmenopausal women.
- SERMs may be a good alternative to HT for the prevention/treatment of osteoporosis in women at risk for breast cancer; however, these medications are not effective treatment for menopausal symptoms.
- HT is associated with a small increased risk of breast cancer. These cancers appear to be less aggressive and are associated with a decreased mortality compared with cancers in women not taking HRT.
- Unopposed estrogen therapy increases the risk of endometrial cancer. However, the addition of progestin reverses this risk.
- HT should be used primarily for the treatment of menopausal symptoms and prevention or treatment of osteoporosis. Treatment should be individualized, depending on the patient's symptoms and risk factors.

REFERENCES

1. U.S. Census Bureau, Population Division, Population Projections Branch. U.S. Interim Projections by Age, Sex, Race, and Hispanic Origin. 2004. Available at: http://www.census.gov/ipc/www/usinterimproj/. Accessed June 30, 2005.
2. McKinlay SM, Brambilla DJ, Posner JG. The normal menopause transition. Maturitas 1992;14:103–115.
3. Soules MR, Sherman S, Parrott E, et al. Executive summary: Stages of Reproductive Aging Workshop (STRAW). Fertil Steril 2001;76:874–878.
4. Gonzales GF, Villena A. Age at menopause in Central Andean Peruvian women. Menopause 1997;4:32.
5. Derksen JGM, Bromann HAM, Wiegerinck MAHM, et al. The effect of hysterectomy and endometrial ablation on follicle stimulating hormone (FSH) levels up to 1 year after surgery. Maturitas 1998;29: 133–138.
6. Willett W, Stampfer MJ, Bain C, et al. Cigarette smoking, relative weight, and menopause. Am J Epidemiol 1983;117:651–658.
7. Baird DD, Tylavsky FA, Anderson JJB. Do vegetarians have earlier menopause? Proceedings of the Society of Epidemiologic Research. Am J Epidemiol 1988;19:1.
8. Torgerson DJ, Avenell A, Russell IT, et al. Factors associated with onset of menopause in women aged 45–49. Maturitas 1994;19:83–92.
9. Midgette AS, Baron JA. Cigarette smoking and the risk of natural menopause. Epidemiology 1990;1:474–480.
10. Torgerson DJ, Thomas RE, Reid DM. Mothers and daughters menopausal ages: is there a link? Eur J Obstet Gynecol Reprod Biol 1997;74:63–66.
11. Santoro N, Adel T, Skurnick JH. Decreased inhibin tone and increased activin A secretion characterize reproductive aging in women. Fertil Steril 1999;71:658–662.
12. Burger HG, Dudley EC, Hopper JL, et al. The endocrinology of the menopausal transition: a cross-sectional study of a population-based sample. J Clin Endocrinol Metab 1995;80:3537–3545.
13. Klein NA, Illingworth PJ, Groome NP, et al. Decreased inhibin B secretion in associated with the normotropic FSH rise in older, ovulatory women: a study of serum spontaneous menstrual cycles. J Clin Endocrinol Metab 1996;81:2742–2745.
14. Shideler SE, DeVane GW, Kalra PS, et al. Ovarian–pituitary hormone interactions during the perimenopause. Maturitas 1989;11:331–339.
15. Santoro N, Brown Jr, Adel T, et al. Characterization of reproductive hormonal dynamics in the perimenopause. J Clin Endocrinol Metab 1996;81:1495–1501.
16. Rannevik G, Jeppsson S, Johnell O, et al. A longitudinal study of the perimenopausal transition: altered profiles of steroid and pituitary hormones, SHBG, and bone mineral density. Maturitas 1995;21:103–113.

17. Jiroutek MR, Chen M-H, Johnston CC, et al. Changes in reproductive hormones and sex hormone-binding globulin in a group of postmenopausal women measured over 190 years. Menopause 1998;5:90–94.
18. Judd HL, Judd GE, Lucas WE, et al. Endocrine function of the postmenopausal ovary: concentration of androgens and estrogens in ovarian and peripheral vein blood. J Clin Endocrinol Metab 1974;39:1020–1024.
19. Grodin JM, Siiteri PK, McDonald PC. Source of estrogen production in postmenopausal women. J Clin Endocrinol Metab 1973;36:207–214.
20. Gougeon A, Echochard R, Thalabard JC. Age-related changes of the population of human ovarian follicles: increase in the disappearance rate of non-growing and early-growing follicles in aging women. Biol Reprod 1994;50:653–663.
21. Henshaw SK. Unintended pregnancy in the United States. Fam Plann Perspect 1998;30:24–29.
22. Stovall TG, Photopulos GJ, Poston WM, et al. Pipelle endometrial sampling in patients with known endometrial carcinoma. Obstet Gynecol 1991;77:954–956.
23. Gull B, Carlsson S, Karlsson B, et al. Transvaginal ultrasonography of the endometrium in women with postmenopausal bleeding: is it always necessary to perform an endometrial biopsy? Am J Obstet Gynecol 2000;182:509–515.
24. Kaunitz AM. Oral contraceptive use in perimenopause. Am J Obstet Gynecol 2001;185:S32–S37.
25. Lethaby A, Irving G, Cameron I. Cyclical progestogens for heavy menstrual bleeding. Cochrane Database Syst Rev 2000:CD00106.
26. Castracane VD, Gimpel T, Goldzieher JW. When is it safe to switch from oral contraceptives to hormonal replacement therapy? Contraception 1995;52:371–376.
27. Creinin MD. Laboratory criteria for menopause in women using oral contraceptives. Fertil Steril 1996; 66:101–104.
28. Dennerstein L, Smith AMA, Morse C, et al. Menopausal symptoms in Australian women. Med J Aust 1993; 159:232–236.
29. Oldenhave A, Jaszmann LJB, Haspels AA, et al. Impact of climacteric on well-being: a survey based on 5,213 women 39–60 years old. Am J Obstet Gynecol 1993;168:772–780.
30. Bachmann GA. Vasomotor flushes in menopausal women. Am J Obstet Gynecol 1999;180:S312–S316.
31. Nordin BEC, Polley KJ. Metabolic consequences of the menopause. A cross-sectional, longitudinal and intervention study of 557 normal postmenopausal women. Calcif Tissue Int 1987;41:S1–S59.
32. Freedman RR. Biomechanical, metabolic, and vascular mechanisms in menopausal hot flashes. Fertil Steril 1998;70:332–337.
33. Mohyi D, Tabassi K, Simon J. Differential diagnosis of hot flashes. Maturitas 1997;27:203–214.
34. Greendale GA, Revoussin BA, Hogan P, et al. Symptom relief and side effects of postmenopausal hormones: results from the Postmenopausal Estrogen/Progestin Interventions Trial. Obstet Gynecol 1998;92:982–988.
35. Simon JA, Klaiber E, Wiita B, et al. Double-blind comparison of two doses of estrogen and estrogen-androgen therapy in naturally postmenopausal women: neuroendocrine, psychological, and psychosomatic effects. Fertil Steril 1996;66:871.
36. Simon J, Klaiber E, Wiita B, et al. Differential effects of estrogen-androgen and estrogen-only therapy on vasomotor symptoms, gonadotropin secretion, and endogenous androgen bioavailability in postmenopausal women. Menopause 1999;6:138–146.
37. Schiff I, Tulchinsky D, Cramer D, et al. Oral medroxyprogesterone in the treatment of postmenopausal symptoms. JAMA 1980;244:1443–1445.
38. Loprinzi CL, Michalak JC, Quella SK. Megestrol acetate for the prevention of hot flashes. N Engl J Med 1994;331:347–352.
39. Bergmans MG, Merkus JM, Corbey RS, et al. Effect of Bellergal Retard on climacteric complaints: a double-blind, placebo-controlled study. Maturitas 1987;9:227–234.
40. David A, Don R, Tajchner G, et al. Veralipride: alternative anti-dopaminergic treatment of menopausal symptoms. Am J Obstet Gynecol 1988;158:1107–1115.
41. Barton DL, Loprinzi CL, Quella SK, et al. Prospective evaluation of vitamin E for hot flashes in breast cancer survivors. J Clin Oncol 1998;16:495–500.
42. Nagamani M, Kelver ME, Smith ER. Treatment of menopausal hot flushes with transdermal administration of clonidine. Am J Obstet Gynecol 1987;156:561–565.
43. Stearns V, Isaacs C, Rowland J, et al. A pilot trial of paroxetine hydrochloride in controlling hot flashes in breast cancer survivors. Ann Oncol 2000;11:17–22.
44. Loprinzi CL, Kugler JW, Sloan JA, et al. Venlafaxine in management of hot flashes in survivors of breast cancer: a randomized controlled trial. Lancet 2000;356:2059–2063.
45. Loprinzi C, Sloan J, Perez E, et al. Phase III evaluation of fluoxetine (Prozac) for treatment of hot flashes. J Clin Oncol 2002;20:1578–1583.
46. Stearns V, Beebe KL, Iyengar M, et al. Paroxetine controlled release in the treatment of menopausal hot flashes: a randomized, controlled trial. JAMA 2003;289:2827–2834.
47. Guttuso T Jr, Kurlan R, McDermott MP, et al. Gabapentin's effects on hot flashes in postmenopausal women: a randomized controlled trial. Obstet Gynecol 2003;101:337–345.
48. Callens A, Vaillant L, Lecomte P, et al. Does hormonal skin aging exist? A study of the influence of different hormone therapy regimens on the skin of postmenopausal women using noninvasive measurement techniques. Dermatology 1996;193:289–294.
49. Creidi P, Faivre B, Agache P, et al. Effect of a conjugated oestrogen (Premarin) cream on aging facial skin: a comparative study with a placebo cream. Maturitas 1994;19:211–223.

50. Maheux R, Naud F, Rioux M, et al. A randomized, double-blind, placebo-controlled study on the effect of conjugated estrogens on skin thickness. Am J Obstet Gynecol 1994;170:642–649.
51. Dunn LB, Damesyn M, Moore AA, et al. Does estrogen prevent skin aging? Arch Dermatol 1997;133:339–342.
52. Castelo-Branco C, Duran M, Gonzalez-Merlo J. Skin collagen changes related to age and hormone replacement therapy. Maturitas 1992;15:113–119.
53. Notelovitz M. Urogenital aging: solutions in clinical practice. Int J Gynaecol Obstet 1997;59(suppl 1):S35–S39.
54. McKenna SP, Whalley D, Renck-Hooper U, et al. The development of a quality of life instrument for use with postmenopausal women with urogenital atrophy in the UK and Sweden. Qual Life Res 1999;8:393–398.
55. Archer DF. Low-dose hormone therapy for postmenopausal women. Clin Obstet Gynecol 2003;46;317–324.
56. Kalogeraki A, Tamiolakis D, Relakis K, et al. Cigarette smoking and vaginal atrophy in postmenopausal women. In Vivo 1996;10:597–600.
57. Caillouette JC, Sharp CF Zimmerman GJ, et al. Vaginal pH as a marker for bacterial pathogens and menopausal status. Am J Obstet Gynecol 1997;176:1270–1275.
58. Traupmann J, Eckels E, Hatfield E. Intimacy in older women's lives. Gerontologist 1982;2:493–498.
59. Pfeiffer E, Verwoerdt A, Davis GC. Sexual behavior in middle life. Am J Psychiatry 1972;128:1262–1267.
60. Greendale GA, Hogan P, Shumaker S, et al. Sexual functioning in postmenopausal women: the Postmenopausal Estrogen/Progestin Interventions (PEPI) Trial. J Womens Health 1996;5:445.
61. Semmens JP, Tsai CC, Semmens S, et al. Effects of estrogen therapy on vaginal physiology during menopause. Obstet Gynecol 1985;66:15–18.
62. Sherwin BB. The impact of different doses of estrogen and progestin on mood and sexual behavior in postmenopausal women. J Clin Endocrinol Metab 1991;72:336–343.
63. Dow MG, Hart DM, Forrest CA. Hormonal treatments of sexual unresponsiveness in postmenopausal women: a comparative study. Br J Obstet Gynecol 1983;90:361–366.
64. Davis SR, McCoud P, Strauss BJG, et al. Testosterone enhances estradiol's effects on postmenopausal bone density and sexuality. Maturitas 1995;21:227–236.
65. Lobo RA, Rosen RC, Yang HM, et al. Comparative effects of oral esterified estrogens with and without methyltestosterone on endocrine profiles and dimensions of sexual function in postmenopausal women with hypoactive sexual desire. Fertil Steril 2003;79:1341–1352.
66. Goldstat R, Brignati E, Tran J, et al. Transdermal testosterone therapy improves well-being, mood, and sexual function in premenopausal women. Menopause 2003;10:390–398.
67. Barnhart KT, Freeman E, Grisso JA, et al. The effect of dehydroepiandrosterone supplementation to symptomatic perimenopausal women on serum endocrine profiles, lipid parameters, and health-related quality of life. J Clin Endocrinol Metab 1999;84:3896–3902.
68. Baulieu EE, Thomas G, LeGrain S, et al. Dehydroepiandrosterone (DHEA) DHEA sulfate and aging: contribution of the DHEA Age Study to a sociobiomedical issue. Proc Natl Acad Sci 2000;97:4279–4284.
69. American Heart Association (AHA). Heart Disease and Stroke Statistics—2005 Update. Dallas: AHA, 2005.
70. Matthews KA, Wing RR, Kuller LH, et al. Influence of the perimenopause on cardiovascular risk factors and symptoms of middle-aged healthy women. Arch Intern Med 1994;154:2349–2355.
71. Jacobs DR Jr, Mebane IL, Bangdiwaia SI, et al. High density lipoprotein cholesterol as a predictor of cardiovascular disease mortality in men and women: the follow-up study of the Lipid Research Clinics Prevalence Study. Am J Epidemiol 1990;131:32–47.
72. Rich-Edwards JW, Manson JE, Hennekens CH, et al. The primary prevention of coronary heart disease in women. N Engl J Med 1995;332:1758–1766.
73. Wenger N. Coronary heart disease in older women: prevention, diagnosis, management, and prognosis. Clin Geriatr 1996;4:53–66.
74. Ford ES, Giles WH, Dietz WH. Prevalence of the metabolic syndrome among US adults. Findings from the Third National Health and Nutrition Examination Survey. JAMA 2002;287:356–359.
75. Executive summary of the third report of the National Cholesterol Education Program (NCEP) expert panel on detection, evaluation, and treatment of high blood cholesterol in adults (Adult Treatment Panel III). JAMA 2001;285:2486–2497.
76. Johnson CL, Rifkind BM, Sempos CT, et al. Declining serum total cholesterol levels among US adults: the National Health and Nutrition Examination Surveys. JAMA 1993;269:3002–3008.
77. Mostaghel E, Waters D. Women do benefit from lipid lowering: latest clinical trial data. Cardiol Rev 2003;11:4–12.
78. Arnold A, Psaty B, Kuller L, et al. Incidence of cardiovascular disease in older Americans: the Cardiovascular Health Study. J Am Geriatr Soc 2005;53:211–218.
79. White RH. The epidemiology of venous thromboembolism. Circulation 2003;107(suppl 1):4–8.
80. Anderson FA Jr, Spencer FA. Risk factors for venous thromboembolism. Circulation 2003;107(suppl 1):9–16.
81. Siris E, Miller PD, Barrett-Connor E, et al. Identification and fracture outcomes of undiagnosed low bone mineral density in postmenopausal women: results from the National Osteoporosis Risk Assessment. JAMA 2001;286:2815–2822.
82. Slemenda CW, Christian JC, Williams CJ, et al. Genetic determinants of bone mass in adult women: a reevaluation of the twin model and the potential importance of gene interaction on heritability estimates. J Bone Mine Res 1991;6:561–567.
83. World Health Organization. Assessment of fracture risk and its application to screening for postmenopausal osteoporosis. Report of a WHO Study Group. World Health Organ Tech Rep Ser 1994;843:1–129.

84. Riis BJ, Hansen MA, Jensen AM, et al. Low bone mass and fast rate of bone loss at menopause: equal risk factors for future fracture: a 15 year follow-up study. Bone 1996;19:9–12.
85. Cummings SR, Black DM, Nevitt MC, et al. Bone density at various sites for prediction of hip fractures. The Study of Osteoporotic Fractures Research Group. Lancet 1993;341:72–75.
86. Lindsay R, Silverman SL, Cooper C, et al. Risk of new vertebral fracture in the year following a fracture. JAMA 2001;285:320–323.
87. Cooper C, Atkinson EJ, Jacobsen SJ, et al. Population-based study of survival after osteoporotic fractures. Am J Epidemiol 1993;137:1001–1005.
88. Koot VC, Peeters PH, de Jong JR, et al. Functional results after treatment of hip fracture: a multicentre, prospective study in 215 patients. Eur J Surg 2000;166:480–485.
89. Marci CD, Anderson WB, Viechnicki MB, et al. Bone mineral densimetry substantially influences health-related behaviors of postmenopausal women. Calcif Tissue Int 2000;66:113–118.
90. Ebrahim S, Thompson PW, Baskaran V, et al. Randomized placebo-controlled trial of brisk walking in the prevention of postmenopausal osteoporosis. Age Ageing 1997;26:253–260.
91. Feskanich D, Willett W, Colditz GA. Walking and leisure-time activity and risk of hip fracture in post-menopausal women. JAMA 2002;288:2300–2306.
92. Hopper JL, Seeman E. The bone density of female twins discordant for tobacco use. N Engl J Med 1994; 330:387–392.
93. Launer LJ, Andersen K, Dewy ME, et al. Rates and risk factors for dementia and Alzheimer's disease. Neurology 1999;1:78–84.
94. Fratiglioni L, Launer LJ, Andersen K, et al., for the Neurologic Diseases in the Elderly Research Group. Incidence of dementia and major subtypes in Europe: a collaborative study of population-based cohorts. Neurology 2000;54(suppl):S10–S15.
95. McKhann G, Drachman D, Folstein M, et al. Clinical diagnosis of Alzheimer's disease: report of the NINCDS-ADRDA Work Group under the auspices of Department of Health and Human Services Task Force on Alzheimer's Disease. Neurology 1984;34:939–944.
96. Knopman DS, DeKosky ST, Cummings JL, et al. Practice parameter: diagnosis of dementia (an evidence-based review): report of the Quality Standards Subcommittee of the American Academy of Neurology. Neurology 2001;56:1143–1153.
97. Hardy J, Selkoe DJ. The amyloid hypothesis of Alzheimer's disease: progress and problems on the road to therapeutics. Science 2002;297:353–356. [Erratum, Science 2002;297:2209].
98. Katzenellenbogen BS. Biology and receptor interactions of estriol and estriol derivatives in vitro and in vivo. J Steroid Biochem 1984;20:1033–1037.
99. Minkin MJ. Considerations in the choice of oral vs. transdermal hormone therapy. J Reprod Med 2004; 49:311–320.
100. Godsland IF. Effects of postmenopausal hormone replacement therapy on lipid, lipoprotein, and apolipoprotein (a) concentrations: analysis of studies published from 1974–2000. Fertil Steril 2001;75:898–915.
101. Vehkavaara S, Silveira A, Hakala-Ala-Pietila T, et al. Effects of oral and transdermal estrogen replacement therapy on markers of coagulation, fibrinolysis, inflammation, and serum lipids and lipoproteins in postmenopausal women. Thromb Haemost 2001;85;619–625.
102. Post MS, Thomassen MC, Van der Mooren MJ, et al. Effect of oral and transdermal estrogen replacement therapy on hemostatic variables associated with venous thrombosis: a randomized, placebo-controlled study in postmenopausal women. Arterioscler Thromb Vasc Biol 2003;23:1116–1121.
103. Zegura B, Keber I, Sebestjen M, et al. Orally and transdermally replaced estradiol improves endothelial function equally in middle-aged women after surgical menopause. Am J Obstet Gynecol 2003;188:1291–1296.
104. Scarabin PY, Oger E, Plu-Bureau G, on behalf of the Estrogen and Thromboembolism Risk Study Group. Differential association of oral and transdermal oestrogen-replacement therapy with venous thromboembolism risk. Lancet 2003;362:428–432.
105. Naessen T, Rodriguez-Macias K. Endometrial thickness and uterine diameter not affected by ultralow doses of 17 beta-estradiol in elderly women. Am J Obstet Gynecol 2002;186:944–947.
106. Dugal R, Hesla K, Sordal T, et al. Comparison of usefulness of estradiol vaginal tables and estriol vagitories for treatment of vaginal atrophy. Acta Obstet Gynecol Scand 2000;79:293–297.
107. Naessen T, Berglund L, Ulmsten U. Bone loss in elderly women prevented by ultra-low doses of parenteral 17 beta-estradiol. Am J Obstet Gynecol 1997;177:115–119.
108. Naessen T, Rodriguez-Macias K, Lithell H. Serum lipid profile improved by ultra-low doses of 17 beta-estradiol in elderly women. J Clin Endocrinol Metab 2001;86:2757–2762.
109. Speroff L, Fritz MA. Postmenopausal hormone therapy. In: Clinical Gynecologic Endocrinology and Infertility. 7th ed. Philadelphia: Lippincott Williams & Wilkins, 2005:689–779.
110. Archer DF, for the EstroGel Study Group. Percutaneous 17β-estradiol gel for the treatment of vasomotor symptoms in postmenopausal women. Menopause 2003;10:516–521.
111. Raudaskoski T, Tapanainen J, Tomas E, et al. Intrauterine 10 microg and 20 microg levonorgestrel systems in postmenopausal women receiving oral oestrogen replacement therapy: clinical, endometrial and metabolic response. Br J Obstet Gynaecol 2002;109:136–144.
112. Cicinelli E, de Ziegler D, Galantino P, et al. Twice-weekly transdermal estradiol and vaginal progesterone as continuous combined hormone replacement therapy in postmenopausal women: a 1-year prospective study. Am J Obstet Gynecol 2002;187:556–560.

113. Archer DF, Pickar JH, Bottiglioni F. Bleeding patterns in postmenopausal women taking continuous combined or sequential regimens of conjugated estrogens with medroxyprogesterone acetate. Menopause Study Group. Obstet Gynecol 1994;83:686–692.
114. Lindsay R, Gallagher JC, Kleerekoper M, et al. Effect of lower doses of conjugated equine estrogens with and without medroxyprogesterone acetate on bone in early postmenopausal women. JAMA 2002;287:2668–2676.
115. Utian WH, Shoupe D, Bachmann G, et al. Relief of vasomotor symptoms and vaginal atrophy with lower doses of conjugated equine estrogens and medroxyprogesterone acetate. Fertil Steril 2001;75:1065–1079.
116. Cushing KL, Weiss NS, Voigt LF, et al. Risk of endometrial cancer in relation to use of low-dose, unopposed estrogens. Obstet Gynecol 1998;91:35–39.
117. Lobo RA, Bush T, Carr BR, et al. Effects of lower doses of conjugated equine estrogens and medroxyprogesterone acetate on plasma lipids and lipoproteins, coagulation factors, and carbohydrate metabolism. Fertil Steril 2001;76:13–24.
118. Moore A, Noonan M. A nurse's guide to hormone replacement therapy. J Obstet Gynecol Neonatal Nurs 1996;24–31.
119. Picker JH, Archer DF, for the Menopause Study Group. Is bleeding a predictor of endometrial hyperplasia in postmenopausal women receiving hormone replacement therapy? Am J Obstet Gynecol 1997;177:1178–1183.
120. Pickar JH, Bottiglioni F, Archer DF. Amenorrhea frequency with continuous combined hormone replacement therapy: a retrospective analysis. Menopause Study Group. Climacteric 1998;1:130–136.
121. Archer DF, Lobo RA, Land HF, et al. A comparative study of transvaginal uterine ultrasound and endometrial biopsy for evaluating the endometrium of postmenopausal women taking hormone replacement therapy. Menopause 1999;6:201–208.
122. Ettinger B, Selby J, Citron J, et al. Cyclic hormone replacement therapy using quarterly progestin. Obstet Gynecol 1994;83:693–700.
123. Bjarnason K, Cerin A, Lindgren R, et al. Adverse endometrial effects during long cycle hormone replacement therapy. Maturitas 1999;32:161–170.
124. Archer DF, Dorin MH, Heine W, et al. Uterine bleeding in postmenopausal women on continuous therapy with estradiol and norethindrone acetate. Obstet Gynecol 1999;94:323–329.
125. Archer DF, Pickar JH. Hormone replacement therapy: effect of progestin dose and time since menopause on endometrial bleeding. Obstet Gynecol 2000;96:899–905.
126. Johnson JV, Davidson M, Archer D, et al. Postmenopausal uterine bleeding profiles with two forms of continuous combined hormone replacement therapy. Menopause 2002;9:16–22.
127. Simon JA, Symons J, Kempfert N, et al. Unscheduled bleeding during initiation of continuous combined hormone replacement therapy: a direct comparison of two combinations of norethindrone acetate and ethinyl estradiol to medroxyprogesterone acetate and conjugated equine estrogens. Menopause 2001;8:321–327.
128. Grodstein F, Colditz GA, Stampfer MJ. Postmenopausal hormone use and cholecystectomy in a large prospective study. Obstet Gynecol 1994;83:5–11.
129. La Vecchia C, Negri E, D'Avanzo B, et al. Oral contraceptives and noncontraceptive oestrogens in the risk of gallstone disease requiring surgery. J Epidemiol Community Health 1992;46:234–236.
130. Kritz-Silverstein D, Barrett-Connor E. Long-term postmenopausal hormone use, obesity, and fat distribution in older women. JAMA 1996;27:46–49.
131. Espeland MA, Stefanick ML, Kritz-Silverstein D, et al. Effect of postmenopausal hormone therapy on body weight and waist and hip girths. J Clin Endocrinol Metab 1997;82:1549–1556.
132. Williams JK, Anthony MS, Honore EK, et al. Regression of atherosclerosis in female monkeys. Arterioscler Thromb Vasc Biol 1995;15:827–836.
133. Tremollieres FA, Pouilles J-M, Ribot CA. Relative influence of age and menopause on total and regional body composition changes in postmenopausal women. Am J Obstet Gynecol 1996;175:1594–6000.
134. Gambacciani M, Ciaponi M, Cappagli B, et al. Body weight, body fat distribution, and hormonal replacement therapy in early postmenopausal women. J Clin Endocrinol Metab 1997;82:414–417.
135. Kanaya AM, Herrington D, Vittinghoff E, et al. Glycemic effects of postmenopausal hormone therapy: the Heart and Estrogen/progestin Replacement Study. A randomized, double-blind, placebo-controlled study. Ann Intern Med 2003;138:1–9.
136. Sullivan JM, VanderZwaag R, Lemp GH, et al. Postmenopausal estrogen use and coronary atherosclerosis. Ann Intern Med 1988;108:358–363.
137. Varas-Lorenzo C, Garcia-Rodriguez LA, Perez-Gutthann S, et al. Hormone replacement therapy and incidence of acute myocardial infarction. A population-based nested case-control study. Circulation 2000;101:2572–2578.
138. Grodstein F, Manson JE, Colditz GA, et al. A prospective, observational study of postmenopausal hormone therapy and primary prevention of cardiovascular disease. Ann Intern Med 2000;133:933–941.
139. Derby CA, Hume AL, McPhillips JB, et al. Prior and current health characteristics of postmenopausal estrogen replacement therapy users compared to nonusers. Am J Obstet Gynecol 1995;173:544–550.
140. Blumel JE, Castelo-Branco C, Roncagliolo ME, et al. Do women using hormone replacement treatment have less pre-existing cardiovascular risk. Maturitas 2001;38:315–319.
141. Manson JE, Hsia J, Honson KC, et al. for the Women's' Health Initiative Investigators. Estrogen plus progestin and the risk of coronary heart disease. N Engl J Med 2003;349:523–534.

142. The Women's Health Initiative Steering Committee. Effects of conjugated equine estrogen in postmenopausal women with hysterectomy. The Women's Health Initiative Randomized Controlled Trial. JAMA 2004;291:1701–1712.
143. Paganini-Hill A, Ross RK, Henderson BE. Postmenopausal oestrogen treatment and stroke: a prospective study. BMJ 1988;297:519–522.
144. Pedersen AT, Lidegaard O, Kreiner S, et al. Hormone replacement therapy and risk of nonfatal stroke. Lancet 1997;350:1277–1283.
145. Simon JA, Hsia J, Cauley JA, et al. for the HERS Research Group. Postmenopausal hormone therapy and risk of stroke. The Heart and Estrogen-progestin Replacement Study (HERS). Circulation 2001;103: 638–642.
146. Viscoli CM, Brass LM, Kernan WN, et al. A clinical trial of estrogen-replacement therapy after ischemic stroke. N Engl J Med 2001;345:1243–1249.
147. Hulley S, Grady D, Bush T, et al., for the Heart and Estrogen-progestin Replacement Study (HERS) Research Group. Randomized trial of estrogen plus progestin for secondary prevention of coronary heart disease in postmenopausal women. JAMA 1998;280:605–613.
148. Herrington DM, Reboussin DM, Brosnihan KB, et al. Effects of estrogen replacement on the progression of coronary-artery atherosclerosis. N Engl J Med 2000;343:522–529.
149. Herrington DM, Vittinghoff E, Lin F, et al. Statin therapy, cardiovascular events, and total mortality in the Heart and Estrogen/progestin Replacement Study (HERS). Circulation 2002;105:2962–2967.
150. Pulmonary Embolism Prevention (PEP) Trial Collaborative Group. Prevention of pulmonary embolism and deep vein thrombosis with low dose aspirin: Pulmonary Embolism Prevention (PEP) trial. Lancet 2000;355:1295–1302.
151. Scarabin PY, Oger E, Plu-Bureau G. Estrogen and Thromboembolism Risk Study Group. Differential association of oral and transdermal oestrogen-replacement therapy with venous thromboembolism risk. Lancet 2003;362:428–432.
152. Sullivan ME, Fugate Woods N. Midlife Women's attributions about perceived memory changes: observations from the Seattle Midlife Women's Health Study. J Womens Health Gend Based Med 2001;10: 351–362.
153. Shughrue PJ, Lane MV, Merchenthaler I, et al. Comparative distribution of estrogen receptor alpha and beta mRNA in the rat central nervous system. J Comp Neurol 1997;388:507–525.
154. Shughrue PJ, Scrime PJ, Merchenthaler I. Estrogen binding and estrogen receptor characterization (ER alpha and ER beta) in the cholinergic neurons of the rat basal forebrain. Neuroscience 2000;96:41–49.
155. Welland NG, Orikasa C, Hayashi S, et al. Distribution and hormone regulation of estrogen receptor immunoreactive cells in the hippocampus or male and female rats. J Comp Neurol 1997;388:603–612.
156. Luine VN, Khylchevskaya RI, McEwen BS. Effect of gonadal steroids on activities of monoamine oxidase and choline acetylase in rat brain. Brain Res 1975;86:293–306.
157. Sherwin BB. Estrogen effects on cognition in menopausal women. Neurology 1997;48:S21.
158. Rice MM, Graves AB, McCurry SM, et al. Estrogen replacement therapy and cognitive function in postmenopausal women without dementia. Am J Med 1997;103:26S.
159. Kampen DL, Sherwin BB. Estrogen use and verbal memory in healthy postmenopausal women. Obstet Gynecol 1994;83:979–983.
160. Shaywitz SE, Shaywitz BA, Puch KR, et al. Effects of estrogen on brain activation patterns in postmenopausal women during working memory tasks. JAMA 1999;281:1197–1202.
161. Resnick SM, Maki PM, Golski S, et al. Effects of estrogen replacement therapy on PET cerebral blood flow and neurophysiologic performance. Horm Behav 1998;34:171–182.
162. Barrett-Connor E, Kritz-Silverstein D. Estrogen replacement therapy and cognitive function in older women. JAMA 1993;269:2637–2641.
163. LeBlanc ES, Janowsky J, Chan BKS, et al. Hormone replacement therapy and cognition: systematic review and analysis. JAMA 2001;285:1489–1490.
164. Rice MM, Graves AB, McCurry SM, et al. Postmenopausal estrogen and estrogen-progestin use and 2-year rate of cognitive change in a cohort of older Japanese American women: the Kame Project. Arch Intern Med 2000;160:1641–1649.
165. Shumaker SA, Legault C, Rapp SR, et al., for the WHIMS Investigators. Estrogen plus progestin and the incidence of dementia and mild cognitive impairment in postmenopausal women. The Women's Health Initiative Memory Study: a randomized controlled trial. JAMA 2003;289:2651–2662.
166. Zandi PP, Carlson MC, Plassman BL, et al. Hormone replacement therapy and incidence of Alzheimer disease in older women. The Cache County Study. JAMA 2002;288:2123–2129.
167. Collaborative Group on Hormonal Factors in Breast Cancer. Breast cancer and hormone replacement therapy: collaborative reanalysis of data from 51 epidemiologic studies of 52,705 women with breast cancer and 108,411 women without breast cancer. Lancet 1997;350:1047–1059.
168. Sellers T, Mink PJ, Cerhan JR, et al. The role of hormone replacement therapy in the risk for breast cancer and total mortality in women with a family history of breast cancer. Ann Int Med 1997;127:973–980.
169. Schairer C, Lubin J, Troisi R, et al. Menopausal estrogen and estrogen-progestin replacement therapy and breast cancer risk. JAMA 2000;283:485–491.
170. Million Women Study Collaborators. Breast cancer and hormone-replacement therapy in the Million Women Study. Lancet 2003;362:419–427.
171. Collaborative Group on Hormonal Factors in Breast Cancer. Breast cancer and hormonal contraceptives: further results. Contraception 1996;54:1S–106S.

172. Gapstur SM, Morrow M, Sellers TA. Hormone replacement and the risk of breast cancer with favorable histology: results of the Iowa Women's Health Study. JAMA 1999;281:2091–2097.
173. Willis CB, Calle EE, Miracle-McMahill HL, et al. Estrogen replacement therapy and the risk of fatal breast cancer in a prospective cohort of postmenopausal women in the United States. Cancer Causes Control 1996;7:449–457.
174. Colditz GA, Rosner B, for the Nurse's Health Study Research Group. Use of estrogen plus progestin is associated with greater increase in breast cancer risk than estrogen alone. Am J Epidemiol 1998;147:64S.
175. Persson I, Weiderpass E, Bergkvist L, et al. Risks of breast and endometrial cancer after estrogen and progestin replacement. Cancer Causes Control 1999;10:253–260.
176. Ross RK, Paganini-Hill A, Wan PC, et al. Effect of hormone replacement therapy on breast cancer risk: estrogen versus estrogen plus progestin replacement therapy and breast cancer risk. JAMA 2000;283:485–491.
177. American Cancer Society (ACS). Cancer Facts and Figures—2002. Atlanta: ACS, 2002. Available at: http://www.cancer.org/docroot/STT/content/STT_1x_Cancer_Facts_Figures_2002.asp. Accessed June 28, 2005.
178. Weiss NS, Szekely DR, English DR, et al. Endometrial cancer in relation to patterns of menopausal estrogen use. JAMA 1979;242:261–264.
179. PEPI Writing Group. Effects of estrogen or estrogen/progestin regimens on heart disease risk factors in postmenopausal women: the Postmenopausal Estrogen/Progestin Interventions (PEPI) trial. JAMA 1995;273:199–208.
180. Grady D, Gebretsadik T, Kerlikowske K, et al. Hormone replacement therapy and endometrial cancer risk: a meta-analysis. Obstet Gynecol 1995;85:304–313.
181. PEPI Writing Group. Effects of hormone therapy on bone mineral density: results form the PEPI trial. JAMA 1996;276:1389–1396.
182. Voigt LF, Weiss NS, Chi J, et al. Progestogen supplementation of exogenous estrogens and the risk of endometrial cancer. Lancet 1991;338:274–277.
183. Weiderpass E, Adami H, Baron JA, et al. Risk of endometrial cancer following estrogen replacement with and without progestins. J Natl Cancer Inst 1999;91;1131–1137.
184. Anderson GL, Judd HL, Kaunitz AM, et al., for the Women's Health Initiative Investigators. Effects of estrogen plus progestin on gynecologic cancers and associated diagnostic procedures. The Women's Health Initiative Randomized Trial. JAMA 2003;290:1739–1748.
185. Hempling RE, Wong C, Piver MS, et al. Hormone replacement therapy as a risk factor for epithelial ovarian cancer: results of a case-control study. Obstet Gynecol 1997;89:1012–1016.
186. Risch HA. Estrogen replacement therapy and risk of epithelial ovarian cancer. Gynecol Oncol 1996;63:254–257.
187. Rodrigues C, Calle EE, Coates RJ, et al. Estrogen replacement therapy and fatal ovarian cancer. Am J Epidemiol 1995;141:828–835.
188. Whittemore AS, Harris R, Itnyre J, and the Collaborative Ovarian Cancer Group. Characteristics relating to ovarian cancer risk: collaborative analysis of 12 US case-control studies. II: Invasive epithelial ovarian cancers in white women. Am J Epidemiol 1992;136:1184–1203.
189. Garg PP, Kerlikowske K, Subak L, et al. Hormone replacement therapy and the risk of epithelial ovarian carcinoma: a meta-analysis. Obstet Gynecol 1998;92:472–479.
190. Lacey JV, Mink PJ, Lubin JH, et al. Menopausal hormone replacement therapy and risk of ovarian cancer. JAMA 2002;288;334–341.
191. Chute CG, Willett WC, Colditx GA, et al. A prospective study of reproductive history and exogenous estrogens on the risk of colorectal cancer in women. Epidemiology 1991;2:201–207.
192. Jacobs EJ, White E, Weiss NS. Exogenous hormones, reproductive history, and colon cancer. Cancer Causes Control 1994;5:359–366.
193. Calle EE, Miracle-McMahill ML, Thun MF, et al. Estrogen replacement therapy and risk of fatal colon cancer in a prospective cohort of postmenopausal women. J Natl Cancer Inst 1995;87:517–523.
194. Kampman E, Potter JD, Slattery ML, et al. Hormone replacement therapy, reproductive history, and colon cancer: a multicenter, case-control study in the United States. Cancer Causes Control 1997;8:146–158.
195. Troisi R, Schairer C, Chow WH, et al. A prospective study of menopausal hormones and risk of colorectal cancer (United States). Cancer Causes Control 1997;8:130.
196. Grodstein F, Martinez E, Platz EA, et al. Postmenopausal hormone use and risk for colorectal cancer and adenoma. Ann Intern Med 1998;128:705–712.
197. Prihartonon N, Palmer JR, Louik C, et al. A case-control study of the use of postmenopausal female hormone supplements in relation to the risk of large bowel cancer. Cancer Epidemiol Biomarkers Prev 2000;9:443–447.
198. Chlebowki RT, Wactawski-Wende J, Ritenbaugh C, et al. Estrogen plus progestin and colorectal cancer in postmenopausal women. N Engl J Med 2004;350:991–1004.
199. Slattery ML, Anderson K, Samowitz W. et al. Hormone replacement therapy and improved survival among postmenopausal women diagnosed with colon cancer. Cancer Causes Control 1999;5:467–473.
200. Adami HO, Persson I, Hoover R, et al. Risk of cancer in women receiving hormone replacement therapy. Int J Cancer 1989;44:833–839.
201. Parazzini F, La Vecchia C, Negri E, et al. Case-control study of oestrogen replacement therapy and risk of cervical cancer. BMJ 1997;315:85–88.
202. Delmas PD, Bjarnason NH, Mitlak BH, et al. Effects of raloxifene on bone mineral density, serum cholesterol concentrations and uterine endometrium in postmenopausal women. N Engl J Med 1997;337:1641–1647.

203. Cummings SR, Eckert S, Krueger KA, et al. The effect of raloxifene on risk of breast cancer in postmenopausal women: results from the MORE randomized trial. JAMA 1999;281:2189–2197.
204. Fisher B, Costantino JP, Wickerhan DL, et al. Tamoxifen for prevention of breast cancer: report of the National Surgical Adjuvant Breast and Bowel Project P-1 Study. J Natl Cancer Inst 1998;90:1371–1388.
205. Schwartz LB, Snyder J, Horan C, et al. The use of transvaginal ultrasound and saline infusion sonohysterography for the evaluation of asymptomatic postmenopausal breast cancer patients on tamoxifen. Ultrasound Obstet Gynecol 1998;11:48–53.
206. Anzano MA, Peer CW, Smith JM, et al. Chemoprevention of mammary carcinogenesis in the rat: combined use of raloxifene and 9-cis-retinoic acid. J Natl Cancer Inst 1996;88:123–125.
207. Goldstein SR, Scheele WH, Rajagopalan SK, et al. A 12-month comparative study of raloxifene, estrogen, and placebo on the postmenopausal endometrium. Obstet Gynecol 2000;95:95–103.
208. Short L, Glasebrook AL, Adrian MD. Distinct effects of selective estrogen receptor modulators on estrogen dependent and estrogen independent human breast cancer cell proliferation. J Bone Miner Res 1996;11 supplement 2:S482.
209. Zumoff B, Strain GW, Miller LK, et al. Twenty-four-hour mean plasma testosterone concentration declines with age in normal premenopausal women. J Clin Endocrinol Metab 1995;80:1429–1430.
210. Shifren JL, Braunstein GD, Simon JA, et al. Transdermal testosterone treatment in women with impaired sexual function after oophorectomy. N Engl J Med 2000;343:682–688.

CHAPTER 3

Lesbian, Bisexual, and Transgender Health Care

Amy E. Harrison and Vincent M. B. Silenzio

INTRODUCTION AND TERMINOLOGY

This chapter highlights the similarities and differences of caring for lesbian, bisexual, and transgendered populations compared with the heterosexual population. One area in which medical science has often lagged behind social science is in the understanding of the diverse realm of human sexual expression. The scope and content of health care for sexual minority populations in the United States has grown considerably since the beginning of the 1970s. Although precise estimates of the size and geographic distribution of these populations have been controversial and are not readily available at the community level, most office-based practitioners will provide clinical services to individuals who are members of a sexual minority (e.g., lesbian, bisexual, transgender, and intersex persons). In recognition of this fact, it is important that health care providers be able to respond to the unique needs of these populations. Unfortunately, little time is spent in medical training on lesbian, bisexual, and transgender issues; in one study, an average of 2.5 hours out of a 4-year curriculum was devoted to issues specific to homosexuality and bisexuality (1). In a survey of obstetrics/gynecology residency programs, less than 2 hours were spent for curriculum specific to lesbian health education issues (2).

In the case of sexual minorities, available language often limits our ability to comprehend the wide range and forms of psychosexual expression. This has profound political and social implications that influence the quality of health care services and access to care. For instance, the move from the term *sexual preference*, which is now considered antiquated, to *sexual orientation*, reflects a fundamental reappraisal of human sexuality. Whereas "preference" implies that these dimensions of sexual expression are completely open to free will, as a kind of acquired taste, *sexual orientation* implies a more fundamental, stable, and intrinsic component of human emotion, thought, and behavior. The following discussion of terminology is presented as an introduction for clinicians and is not intended to be exhaustive. A more comprehensive discussion can be found in other resources, including the *Healthy People 2010 Companion Document for LGBT Health* (3).

The following definitions reflect the current understanding of concepts of sexuality and sexual behavior; these definitions may—and probably will—change in the future. A summary of these terms and definitions is listed in Table 3.1. The biological concept of *sex* is that of the intrinsic phenotype of sexual anatomy. The terms *male* and *female* refer to the two distinct biological classes typically encountered. *Transsexual* refers to a change from one biologically defined sex to another. *Transsexual* individuals are in the process of, or have completed, sexual reassignment through medical intervention. Historically, individuals who are not appropriately classified as biologically or anatomically male or female have been known by terms such as hermaphrodites and currently constitute the core of the class of individuals known as *intersex* (4, 5).

Gender refers to the social and cultural classes of individuals assuming the roles, rights, and responsibilities typically assigned to the sexes. The terms *men* and *women* refer to these socially

TABLE 3.1

Definitions

Lesbian	A woman whose primary sexual and emotional partnerships are with women, or a woman who may identify as belonging to a community or subculture of similar individuals regardless of her sexual behavior. The related term *gay*, although applied exclusively to men by some, is often applied to women who have sex with women.
Bisexual	An individual who has sexual desire, attraction, or activity with members of the same or another sex or who may identify as belonging to a community or subculture of similar individuals.
Transgendered	Individuals who may have a strong sense of identification with a gender other than their original anatomic sex or the one that they have been socialized to exhibit, and who may choose to exhibit the characteristics or assume the roles and responsibilities of that gender. Transgendered individuals may identify their sexual orientation as heterosexual, gay, lesbian, bisexual, or otherwise.
Transsexual	Individuals who are in the process of or have completed sexual reassignment through medical intervention. Transsexual individuals may identify their sexual orientation as heterosexual, gay, lesbian, bisexual, or otherwise.
Intersex	Individuals born with genitalia that differ from their chromosomal makeup, caused by an endocrine (or genetic?) condition. These individuals are not appropriately classified as biologically or anatomically male or female. Formerly referred to as hermaphrodites.
Heterosexism	A term replacing *homophobia* in many instances; it refers to a societal condition in which the expectation that all individuals are heterosexual exists.
WSW	A woman who has sexual relations with women; this is inclusive of women from all racial and ethnic groups that may not readily identify or self-define themselves as lesbian or bisexual. WSW are identified across all sexual orientation identities.

Adapted from Harrison AE, Silenzio VMB. Comprehensive care of lesbian and gay patients and families. Prim Care 1996;23(1):31–46; Silenzio V. Lesbian, gay and bisexual health in cross-cultural perspective. J Gay Lesbian Med Assoc 1997;1(2):75–86, with permission.

defined classes, and these concepts are subject to widespread intercultural variation as well as intracultural variation. *Transgender* refers to partial or total assumption of another gender, which may include roles and responsibilities (5). Because transgender refers to a variety of people, including intersex newborns and heterosexual male transvestites, lumping individuals who qualify as transgender into one large group, although common, is actually misleading. *Transgendered* individuals may have a strong sense of incongruity between the gender they identify with and the gender they have been raised to exhibit and/or their anatomic sex.

Sexual orientation may be defined along three dimensions: self-identification, sexual behavior, and sexual attraction or desire. Humans may exhibit differing degrees of same- or opposite-sex sexual behavior, desire, or identity, in combinations that vary from person to person and over time (6). Hence, sexual orientation is not contingent on one's gender or sex.

The term *lesbian* has historically referred to women who have sex with other women. In more recent parlance, the term also refers to women who identify as belonging to this class of individuals, regardless of whether they are sexually active. "Lesbian" is also used in contemporary discussions to denote women whose primary emotional, romantic, and/or sexual relationships are with other women, regardless of their current or past relationships or public identity. It is also used to refer to women who partner with women (7). A list of some common slang terms used in reference to lesbians is shown in Table 3.2. The term *gay* is applied to men or women who have same-sex sexual attraction or behavior, or who may identify as belonging to a community or subculture of similar individuals. The term *heterosexual* refers to a man or woman whose predominant sexual and emotional attraction is to

TABLE 3.2

Slang Terms Commonly Used by Lesbian and Bisexual Women in North America to Self-Identify

Gay woman
Dyke
In the life
Marmacha
Two spirit
Khush
Zami
Queer

people of the opposite sex. *Heterosexism* is a worldview that regards heterosexuality as superior and repudiates homosexuality, bisexuality, and all that is not heterosexual (8–10).

Bisexual is a term referring to either women or men who have sexual desire, attraction, or sexual activity with members of the same or opposite sex. Although initially coined as an intermediate class between homosexual and heterosexual, this term has recently come to refer to a distinct, stable class of sexual orientation with which individuals may identify. Very little is known about bisexual women, so the degree to which research on lesbian women may be applied to bisexual women is also unknown. Most researchers agree that bisexual women should be viewed as a different category or subgroup of women than lesbian women (11).

A large part of the difficulty in understanding the lesbian, bisexual, gay, and transgender (LBGT) populations lies in the reality that these populations, or communities, are extraordinarily diverse. LBGT populations differ along sociodemographic lines such as ethnic, race, or cultural identities; religious preferences; residence; education; and socioeconomic status—differences that are significant for any population, not just LGBT communities. As Meyer (12) eloquently stated, LBGT persons "are also diverse in the degree to which their LGBT identities are central to their self-definition, their level of affiliation with other LGBT people, and their rejection or acceptance of societal stereotypes and prejudice." Hence, transgendered, transsexual, and intersex individuals may identify their sexual orientation as heterosexual, gay, lesbian, bisexual, or otherwise.

Sex is best viewed as a continuum (13–15). "Gender expression is also represented most accurately by a continuum . . . trying to talk about gender articulation using only the terms widely used in English today—feminine, masculine, androgynous—is as ludicrous as trying to make yourself understood in a language composed of 3 words" (16).

Although a wide range of terminology is employed to describe the sexual orientation and expression of humans, it is critical for the practicing clinician to understand that the definitions need to bend to the reality of the patients and not the other way around. This is particularly true in a multicultural society such as the United States, where various social and cultural frameworks for understanding and interpreting the meaning of same-sex phenomena coexist.

LESBIAN AND BISEXUAL PATIENTS

For the first time since its inception, the 2000 U.S. census asked directly whether an individual lived with his or her same-sex partner. The census produced the startling finding that there are more than 500,000 same-sex couples in America. Because the census data are available with respect only to individuals living with a same-sex partner (and those who would reveal this to the federal government), these 500,000 couples are most likely the tip of the iceberg regarding the true number of nonheterosexual individuals in this country. Despite the limitations and underrepresentation, every community with a population of 5,000 or more reported same-sex couples; the two communities that reported no same-sex couples were Pana, Illinois, and Renssalaer, Indiana.

It is not known how many lesbians there are in the United States, although estimates generally range from 2 to 10% of women (6, 17). The estimated percentage of American women who are lesbians varies, depending on how "lesbian" is defined. In work by Laumann et al., 3.8% of women had had at least one same-sex sexual partner since puberty, whereas 7.5% reported that they currently had feelings of desire for a female sexual partner. In the same survey, 58.7% of women reported that although they found the idea of sex with another woman to be desirable, they had never had a female sexual partner nor did they self-identify as being homosexual or bisexual (6).

Older gay men and lesbian women are estimated to make up 3 to 10% of the aging population. Connection to and activity with the lesbian community seems to improve acceptance of the aging process and satisfaction with life. Studies in older lesbian women indicate a preference for living in an intergenerational homosexual retirement community.

Not much is known about how development of sexual identity or orientation occurs and less is known about how these developments may or may not differ in the LBGT populations. Available research seems to indicate that awareness of sexual orientation occurs at an early age—around 10 years or so—and this is true for both heterosexual and lesbian subjects (18, 19). Lesbian adolescents have the same health and mental health concerns as their heterosexual peers but with the added burdens related to the stigma of homosexuality. Although lesbian adolescents come from all racial and ethnic groups, socioeconomic levels, and educational backgrounds, they are generally invisible to the larger population. Most are reluctant to share their sexual orientation or are (silently) confused by it. These adolescents may repress, deny, or attempt to change their feelings through a variety of coping mechanisms such as heterosexual activity, alcohol or drug use, pregnancy, and displacement activities (e.g., extensive involvement in extracurricular activities, sports, or school). Providers should be able to explain the difference between identity and behavior; the adolescent should also be reassured that experiencing same-sex feelings and attractions are common and do not necessarily signify homosexual identity. The development of sexual identity evolves over time and forcing "resolution" does not hasten the process. In talking with adolescents who are confused about their sexual orientation, it is important to facilitate the conversation and not force disclosure.

In the recent past, health care services specifically targeted to lesbians, bisexuals, and other sexual minorities have been heavily concentrated in major urban settings. However, the overall number and widespread geographic distribution of these patients and families requires that all practitioners be skilled in the basics of care for these populations. Access to more specialized and complex services is important, but all practitioners should be able to provide primary care for these patients.

An important distinction needs to be made between sexual identity and sexual behavior. Assessing only current or recent sexual behavior provides incomplete information to the health care provider. As Laumann et al. (6) stated: "It makes more sense to ask about specific aspects of same-sex gender behavior, practice and feeling during specific periods of an individual's life rather than a single yes-or-no question about whether a person is homosexual." For example, many women self-identify as lesbians but have sexual relationships with men or have had sex with men in the past. Surveys indicate that 75 to 80% of self-identified lesbians have had sex with men at some point (20, 21). Hence, these women's health care needs are quite similar to those of heterosexual women (e.g., contraception, sexually transmitted infection (STI) screening, cervical cancer screening).

Sexual acts or behaviors alone do not define a person's sexuality. There are many commonalities in sex practices between LGBT populations and the strictly heterosexual population. For example, approximately 25% of heterosexual males and approximately 20% of heterosexual women have ever engaged in anal intercourse. Up to 10% of heterosexual men and 9% of heterosexual women have engaged in anal intercourse in the past years, and approximately 7% of heterosexual couples engage in anal intercourse at least once a month (6).

Caring for Lesbian and Bisexual Patients

It is estimated that 6.7% of American women have engaged in same-sex sexual behavior after the age of 15 years and 3.6% have participated in same-sex sexual behavior within the last 5 years (22). Although the limited body of research on lesbian health is growing, a great deal of the studies have methodologic limitations (e.g., use of convenience samples, lack of appropriate comparison groups, inconsistencies in the way "lesbian" is defined or classified), and this makes it difficult to draw conclusions about the health status and health risks this group of women faces. Understanding both the common and the unique health risks and determinants lesbians share with heterosexual women would enhance and promote the quality of care and services lesbians receive. There are many misperceptions that exist regarding the health and health needs of lesbians (e.g., many practitioners and lesbians themselves believe they do not need cervical cytology screening or cannot contract sexually transmitted infections [STIs] such as HIV/AIDS). Yet, the cornerstones of preventive services for lesbian and bisexual women are the same as for all women (23). A more recent report by the Institute of Medicine specifically addressing lesbian health concluded that lesbians are not at "higher risk for any particular health problem simply because they have a lesbian orientation," but rather "differential risks may arise . . . because some risk or protective factors may be more common among lesbians" (11).

Because there are no identifying characteristics of lesbians and bisexual women, it is important to avoid assumptions of heterosexuality. Health care providers should use generic terms such as "partner" or "spouse" until the patient declares their sexual orientation. To encourage openness, forms should be modified to encourage a range of expression. For example, the woman in a long-term lesbian relationship may not know whether to check "single" (which she does not consider herself to be) or "married" (which she is not legally) on a standardized form. When asking about sexual behavior, use open-ended questions ("when you are sexually active, is it with men, women, or either?"). This allows the patient to define her own sexuality and lets her know that you are open to nonheterosexual sexual orientations. In addition, it avoids awkward discussions about the merits of contraceptives in a patient who may not need them. Other means to create a more supportive office environment are listed in Table 3.3. The choice to "come out" in vulnerable situations is not an easy one to make, and an encounter with a new or unknown health care provider is a situation fraught with vulnerability for all patients.

Fear of disclosure is not without cause; like the general population, health care providers have very divergent views regarding homosexuality (24, 25). When disclosure does occur, it is important that it is met by support to facilitate and promote an open dialogue with the patient.

TABLE 3.3

Steps Health Care Providers Can Take to Create a Welcoming Environment for Members of the Lesbian, Bisexual, Gay, and Transgender Population

- Display a nondiscrimination statement that includes sexual orientation.
- Use inclusive language on all intake and sexual history forms.
- Ask open-ended questions about patient's health care needs and health behaviors.
- Convey willingness to include partners in all decision-making processes if the patient desires and consents to this.
- Assure patients of the confidentiality of all discussions and written documentation.
- Provide harm reduction guidelines for HIV/sexually transmitted infections that are based on sexual behavior, not sexual identity or orientation.
- Make health resources and publications regarding LBGT populations available to patients.
- Display symbols of diversity (e.g., rainbow flags or signs designating the space as a safe one for discussing sexual orientation issues).

As with the heterosexual woman, the patient's partner should not be present during the medical interview to allow the health care provider an opportunity to inquire about domestic violence, relationship issues, or issues about monogamy.

Lesbian and bisexual women face many of the same health problems as other women. However, certain demographic trends may put these populations at higher risk for certain diseases. Lack of preventive health services is one of the major problems for this group, and there are several contributing factors to this. Because many lesbians are not covered under their partner's health insurance, these women may suffer a lack of health insurance, which impedes or precludes the utilization of screening and preventive health services. Lesbians who have had poor interactions with prior health care providers are less likely to use preventive health care resources (26, 27). In the heterosexual populations, screening exams are often done in conjunction with family planning services (contraception, prenatal care); women who do not need these services may not come in for routine screening exams (28).

Lesbian women are at higher risk for breast and gynecologic malignancies than heterosexual women; this is most likely because the lesbian population differs in their patterns of health care. They are less likely to have regular access to health care, to have had a recent mammogram, or to have had a screening well-woman exam (29). For a listing of social/behavioral factors and health concerns relevant to LGBT populations, see Table 3.4.

TABLE 3.4

Social/Behavioral Factors and Health Concerns Relevant to Lesbian, Bisexual, Gay, and Transgender Populations

Sexual Behavior	Cultural Factors	Disclosure of Sexual Orientation, Gender Identity	Prejudice and Discrimination	Concealed Sexual Activity
• Bacterial vaginosis For those women who have sex with men, other considerations include • Hepatitis A & B • Enteritis (e.g., Giardiasis, Amebiasis) • Anal cancer • HIV/AIDS • Other sexually transmitted diseases	• Body culture: eating disorders • Socialization through bars: drug, alcohol, and tobacco use • Nulliparity: breast cancer • Parenting: insemination questions, mental health concerns • Gender polarity in dominant culture: conflicts for transgender and intersex persons	• Psychological adjustment, depression, anxiety, suicide • Conflicts with family of origin, lack of social support • Physical and economic dislocation	• Provider bias, lack of sensitivity • Harassment and discrimination in medical encounters, employment, housing, child custody, etc.	• Reluctance to seek preventive care • Delayed medical treatment • Incomplete medical history (e.g., lack of disclosure of risks, sexually related complications, social factors)

Adapted from Diamant AL, Wold C, Spritzer K, et al. Health behaviors, health status and access to and use of health care: a population-based study of lesbian, bisexual, and heterosexual woman. Arch Fam Med 2000;9:1043–1051, with permission.

General Health Risks

Many of the studies on lesbian, gay, and bisexual populations have lacked population-based epidemiological methods. Most studies have been done using convenience samples of these populations, a method that is not optimally rigorous, so their results need to be interpreted in this context. Nevertheless, many studies indicate that lesbians have higher rates of tobacco and alcohol use and increased body mass indices. Studies have consistently identified lesbians as having a greater risk of alcohol abuse than heterosexual women (29–31). Based on the aforementioned risk factors, the lesbian population is at increased risk for chronic diseases linked to smoking or obesity (32).

Most studies, but not all, of lesbians show that the incidence of childhood sexual abuse is the same as it is in the heterosexual population. In a study of 523 women attending a primary health care center, women who had experienced childhood sexual abuse were more likely than women who had not to have had adult sexual experiences with women (8% versus 1%) (33). Although patterns of sexual behavior may stem, in part, from a history of childhood sexual abuse, authentic sexual identity is not formed as a result of childhood sexual abuse.

Because of cultural factors, lesbian and bisexual women (and those who are perceived to belong to one of these categories) are at higher risk of becoming victims of bias crimes. Fear of reactions when they report these crimes leads to underreporting, and many of these women may not receive appropriate medical or psychological counseling after the event—all of which may increase their risk of developing depression and posttraumatic stress disorder. Other mental health issues commonly seen in lesbian and bisexual women include high rates of depression and suicidality, especially among adolescents (34–38).

Contraception and Family Planning

Advances in reproductive technology combined with changing societal attitudes have made the 1990s the decade of the "lesbian baby boom" (39). This trend is continuing into the 21st century. Increasing numbers of lesbian women and gay men have shown the desire to become parents outside heterosexual unions. Lesbians can become parents through traditional intercourse, insemination (using fresh or frozen sperm from a known or unknown donor), use of donor oocytes and other assisted reproduction techniques, adoption, and supporting a partner through any of these methods. It is beyond the scope of this chapter to address all issues regarding childbearing in lesbians. The multitude of options that potential lesbian parents will be forced to address brings up a host of medical, social, financial, and legal issues that heterosexual couples rarely ever face. For example, use of fresh sperm leads to an increased chance of conception but may expose the patient to potential STIs, including HIV. Issues around next-of-kin and legal status with the nonbiological parent when interfacing with the health care system are major concerns.

There is no evidence that being raised in lesbian households is detrimental to the development of children in any significant respect relative to the development of children raised in heterosexual homes in otherwise comparable circumstances. Rates of homosexuality among the children of lesbian parents are similar to those of the children of heterosexual parents (40–43). The reader is referred to the excellent book *The Gay and Lesbian Parenting Handbook* for further exploration of some of these issues (39).

Because approximately three-fourths of self-identified lesbians have sex with men at some point in their lives, contraception services may be needed for some of these women. These services should be individualized, depending on the patient's situation. Being able to explore a patient's sexual practices will guide the clinician to an appropriate discussion (or omission of discussion) of contraception.

Sexually Transmitted Infections

Lesbians are generally considered to be at low risk of acquiring and transmitting STIs both within their communities and by many health care providers. In the National Lesbian Health Care Survey, less than one-fourth of the 1,925 women participating reported that they worried about contracting an STI (44). Studies have identified several STIs as transmissible through same-sex female contact, including herpes, trichomoniasis, human papillomavirus (HPV), and HIV (45–51). In a survey of 286 attendees at the Twin Cities Gay/Lesbian/Bisexual/Transgender Pride Festival, 69% of the women who consented to the interview self-identified as lesbian. Of the subgroup of women who reported only female sexual partners, 13% had a history of STI, including Chlamydia, genital warts, trichomoniasis, and pelvic inflammatory disease. In the same survey, women who self-identified as lesbian were only 27% as likely to have regular STI screening as women who self-identified as bisexual or heterosexual (21). All sexually active women, whether heterosexual, bisexual, or lesbian, should receive appropriate education and screening on STI transmission. Recommendations for use of the dental dam (a latex barrier) for oral-genital sex in women having sex with women (WSW) should be based on the individual's degree of risk.

The rate of bacterial vaginosis (BV) is consistently higher among lesbians (52, 53). In one study, 1,408 women who had ever had sex with another woman were compared with 1,423 women who had never had sex with another woman. Only 7% of the WSW had sex exclusively with women in the previous 12 months, and 12% of the overall population of WSW had never had sex with a man. BV was significantly more prevalent among WSW than controls (8% versus 5%) (52).

Debate exists over whether BV should be classified as a STI or a sexually associated infection, as it is in heterosexual women. In two studies of WSW, the incidence of BV among WSW was less than 30% but the concordance for BV infection was 72 to 95% among WSW partners (54, 55). In another study where the incidence of BV among WSW was greater than 30%, concordance was more difficult to establish (56). It might be prudent, however, to advise a patient with BV to avoid any sexual activity that would transfer her vaginal fluids to her partner's vagina until the infection is cleared and to disinfect any shared sex toys prior to use and avoid sharing sex toys until the infection is cleared.

Although less common, trichomonas may be transmitted from one woman to another through a sexual encounter. It is presumed that transmission occurs when vaginal fluids from one partner are transferred or exposed to the other partner (47). Women diagnosed with trichomonas should be advised that until the infection is cleared, she should avoid engaging in any sexual activity with her partner that might expose her partner's vagina to the patient's vaginal fluids, including the use of mutually shared sex toys.

Transmission of genital herpes simplex among WSW has been presented in the literature (57). Management is similar to that used in WSW: avoid the shared use of sex toys or physical contact with active lesions when present; inform the patient that viral shedding may occur between outbreaks; and if outbreaks are frequent, discuss prophylactic therapy.

Because HPV is linked to cervical cancer and is typically represented as a heterosexual STI, many clinicians wrongly assume LGBT women do not need a cervical cytology study. Even among women who deny ever participating in any sexual activity with men and who only engage in sex with women, HPV infection has been documented (52, 58). Patients with genital warts or recent treatments for warts should be counseled to avoid contact with the partner with the lesion or lesion sites or with any shared sex toys. The patient and her partner(s) should be informed that HPV is common in the general population, may persist or spontaneously remit, or may recur, and that some strains are associated with an increased risk for cervical neoplasia.

Patients with HIV or chronic active hepatitis B should be informed that their partner(s) should not be exposed to their menstrual blood or other sites of bleeding. A dental dam should be used for all oral-genital sex, and if this is not followed, the couple should be aware of the increased need for use of a dental dam when the infected partner is menstruating or has a genital discharge. A dental dam should also be used for all oral-anal sex. Lubricants without nonoxynol-9 and condoms should be used for all penetrative sex on either partner.

All lesbians who are involved in multiple relationships or have other well-known risk factors should be offered a hepatitis B vaccine.

Sex toys may be cleaned with household bleach diluted 1:10 with water to prevent disease transmission. Any sex toy that penetrates more than one person's vagina or anus should be covered with a new condom for each person.

TRANSGENDER, TRANSSEXUAL, AND INTERSEX CARE

Providing a safe and supportive environment for transgendered and intersex patients is a necessary prerequisite for caring for these populations. The prevalence of transsexualism, representing the end of the transgender spectrum, is relatively rare. An estimate from the Netherlands reported the prevalence of transsexualism as 1 per 11,900 males and 1 per 30,400 females (59). Competent care of transgender, transsexual, and intersex individuals and families will involve an array of medical, surgical, and behavioral health services, and is amenable to a collaborative team approach. The myriad of mental health issues facing these individuals and their families are beyond the scope of the current discussion. Ideally, medical professionals involved in transgender, transsexual, and intersex care will work closely with behavioral health professionals who are skilled and knowledgeable in this area (28).

Although homosexuality was removed from the third edition of the *Diagnostic and Statistical Manual* (DSM-III) in the 1970s, the category of Gender Identity Disorder remains in the *DSM-IV*. Gender Identity Disorder in adults and adolescents requires four diagnostic criteria: (a) a strong and persistent cross-gender identification—manifested by stated desire to be the other sex, desire to live or be treated as the other sex, or the conviction that he or she has typical feelings and reactions of the other sex; (b) persistent discomfort with his or her gender—manifested by a preoccupation with getting rid of primary and secondary sex characteristics (requests for hormones, surgery, or other procedures to simulate the other sex); (c) the disturbance is not concurrent with a physical intersex condition; and (d) the disturbance causes clinically significant distress or impairment in social, occupational, or other important areas of functioning (60).

Transsexual people may elect to undergo hormonal and surgical treatments, which may result in irreversible loss of their reproductive potential. The option of gamete banking should therefore be discussed before starting hormonal and surgical sexual reassignment treatment (61).

Treatment Protocols

General Considerations

Transgender individuals seeking medical or surgical treatments to become transsexual must meet the eligibility and readiness criteria established by the Harry Benjamin International Gender Dysphoria Association (HBIGDA) (Table 3.5). All patients must undergo a thorough evaluation by a mental health professional competent in transgender issues to establish the suitability of transsexual procedures for the individual. Ongoing collaboration between mental health and medical professionals is desirable. Whereas fundamental care to the transgender population can be successfully managed by primary care practitioners, consultation with an endocrinologist skilled in the care of transsexual or intersex individuals can be obtained to further refine the management protocol discussed here.

According to the HBIGDA criteria, individuals seeking to become transsexual must be at least 18 years of age and able to demonstrate a basic understanding of the medical and social effects (including risks and benefits) and limits of hormone therapy. They must also have either had a documented real-life experience as their desired gender for 3 months prior to beginning hormone therapy or have completed a period of psychotherapy (usually at least 3 months) with a mental health professional competent in transgender issues. Once these criteria are met, readiness for initiation of hormone therapy is assessed. The patient is considered "ready" for hormone therapy if he or she has had further consolidation of gender identity either during the real-life experience or psychotherapy, has demonstrated progress in mastering any other identified mental health issues to improve or stabilize his or her mental health, and has demonstrated an ability to take medicinal therapies (e.g., hormones) in a reliable and responsible manner (62). Medical therapy is initiated for those individuals who meet eligibility and readiness criteria. A variety of helpful patient education and informed consent materials regarding hormone treatment are available in the published literature and online. A schedule of routine care includes both initial evaluation and regular follow-up visits (63, 64).

Once an individual has met the HBIGDA criteria for readiness and eligibility, the initial history and physical exam performed prior to the initiation of medical therapy focuses on screening

TABLE 3.5

Harry Benjamin International Gender Dysphoria Association Standards of Care for Gender Identity Disorders: Eligibility and Readiness Criteria for Hormonal Therapy in Adults

Eligibility Criteria

1. 18 years of age or older
2. Knowledge of what hormones medically can and cannot do, social benefits and risks
3. *Either* documented real-life experience for at least 3 months prior to hormones *or* psychotherapy of a duration specified by the mental health professional (usually 3 months)
4. Under no circumstances should a person be provided hormones who has not fulfilled one of the criteria in item 3

Readiness Criteria

1. Further consolidation of gender identity during the real-life experience or psychotherapy
2. Progress in mastering problems leading to improving or continued stable mental health
3. Hormones likely to be taken in responsible manner

Adapted with permission from Harry Benjamin International Gender Dysphoria Association (HBIGDA). Standards of Care for Gender Identity Disorders, Sixth Version. Minneapolis: HBIGDA, 2001. Available at: http://www.hbigda.org/socv6.cfm. Accessed June 29, 2005.

for potential complications of medical therapy. The patient's past medical and family history should be reviewed for evidence of hypertension, heart disease, peripheral vascular disease, thromboembolic disorders, diabetes, obesity, hepatic dysfunction, hyperlipidemia, smoking, psychiatric disorders, alcohol or drug abuse, and hormone abuse or noncompliance. Initial physical examination should note any findings related to these issues and thoroughly document the patient's secondary sex characteristics. In-depth discussion(s) of the potential risks and benefits of medical therapy is mandatory. Baseline laboratory studies will include serum testosterone, follicle-stimulating hormone, fasting lipid panel, and hepatic function panel.

Follow-up visits should be made at 1, 2, 3, and 6 months. After 6 months, follow-up visits should occur every 6 months for patients who are on a stable medical regimen. The goal of each follow-up visit is to screen for the effectiveness and potential complications of therapy, and to adjust the medication regimen as needed. Physical and psychological developmental issues will remain complex for many individuals; therefore, ongoing clinical comanagement with a mental health professional competent in transgender issues should be encouraged. Periodic follow-up of laboratory studies is necessary; the specific studies ordered are based on the medication regimen in use.

Female-to-Male Medical Management

Female-to-male (FTM) transition is usually achieved with testosterone as a single agent (Table 3.2). Intramuscular testosterone is administered in doses ranging from 200 to 400 mg every 2 weeks. Testosterone usually cannot be administered monthly in these patients due to the unreliable serum levels of hormone after about 2 weeks post administration. Transdermal delivery of testosterone is not well established as an initial medication choice, although it may be useful in maintenance therapy (65). Once masculinization is achieved or after oophorectomy, the dose may be titrated downward by approximately one-half.

Side Effects of Testosterone Therapy

Complications of testosterone therapy include increased low-density and decreased high-density lipoprotein levels, impaired glucose tolerance, hypertension, alopecia, acne, weight gain, and fat redistribution. Mild elevations of hepatic enzyme levels may occur and hepatic neoplasms may also occur. For this reason, elevated transaminase levels should be evaluated by ultrasound to rule out structural liver disease. Endometrial hyperplasia can be induced by testosterone therapy, and hysterectomy is recommended to reduce the risk of endometrial cancer (66). Patients continue to need breast exams; Papanicolaou (or Pap) smears and evaluation for abnormal uterine bleeding remain necessary until they undergo hysterectomy. Smoking may increase the risk of coronary heart disease in individuals using testosterone (67). Common psychological effects of testosterone include increased aggressiveness, hostility, and changes in libido (68). Nearly all complications of testosterone therapy are dose related. Serum testosterone levels should be monitored and doses titrated to maintain normal male levels of circulating testosterone and suppression of endogenous estrogen production.

Male-to-Female Medical Management

Male-to-female (MTF) patients will frequently require at least two medications to achieve suppression of endogenous testosterone production and development of female secondary sexual characteristics (Table 3.3). Oral, transdermal, and intramuscular estrogen administration have all been used successfully. The specific choice of dosage and form can be individualized according to patient preferences, costs, and other factors.

Once estrogen therapy has begun, serum testosterone levels should be obtained as part of the assessment of clinical response. In addition to possible adjustments in estrogen doses, an additional antiandrogen agent can be used to further suppress endogenous hormone production and support changes in secondary sexual characteristics. The most common additional agents used off label in the United States include spironolactone, progesterone, or flutamide. The reported doses and dosing schedules of these agents vary. After sexual reassignment surgery or orchidectomy, spironolactone and progesterone as antiandrogen agents may be discontinued. However, progesterone is also believed to positively affect breast development during the first 2 years of therapy and may be discontinued after that time (64).

Side Effects of Estrogen Therapy

As for all patients on hormone therapy, it is necessary to monitor biological males taking estrogen therapy for an array of potential complications. Complications of estrogen therapy include deep venous thrombosis and the sequelae of thromboembolic disease, breast neoplasms, and elevated serum prolactin levels or prolactinoma during the first 3 years of use (69–75). Screening breast examination and mammography should be routinely monitored over time to detect the development of breast cancers. Mild elevations of hepatic enzyme levels may occur. Because this may represent hepatic neoplasms or other lesions, elevated transaminase levels should be monitored and evaluated by ultrasound to rule out structural liver disease.

The complications of estrogen therapy are dose related. Serum estrogen levels should be monitored and medications titrated to maintain normal female levels of circulating estrogen and suppression of endogenous testosterone production (68).

Intersex Care

The previously established standards of medical, surgical, and psychosocial care for intersex individuals have become increasingly controversial in more recent years, so the standards of care are also controversial at this time (28). Kipnis and Diamond (76) identified several limitations to the current clinical management of intersexuality. First, decisive distinction between male and female for these individuals is unclear and perhaps nonexistent. Second, the development of gender identity is not always alterable in these children, despite alteration of their genitalia. Third, it is not possible to confidently predict the gender—male, female, or transgendered—that an intersexed child will find comfortable in adulthood. Intersexuality, the biologically variant sexual anatomy also commonly known as hermaphroditism, disturbs the distinction between male and female persons that is so fundamental to self-identification and social status, particularly in the United States (77). For these reasons, some parents of infants with intersex conditions, as well as intersex adults, are trying to stop the practice of surgical intervention and assignment of definitive sex anatomy during infancy.

Whether to surgically alter ambiguous genitalia in infants and children is an increasingly controversial issue, which highlights the conflict between our cultural and biological definitions of gender. Although Diamond and Sigmundson (78) have published practice guidelines, clinicians are also advised to investigate other current standards of care for intersex individuals. Despite the increasing controversy surrounding surgical alteration of ambiguous genitalia in infants and children, gender assignment or reassignment of these children may continue to be the preferred approach for some time. Regardless of whether current efforts to revise this approach are successful, medical and surgical care will remain the province of interdisciplinary teams for the foreseeable future. Office-based practitioners will need to carefully individualize the approach to caring for these patients. The basic principles of medical management remain as discussed previously; however, consultation with an endocrinologist skilled in this area will be necessary in many of these cases.

CONCLUSION

Knowledge of the care of lesbian, bisexual, transgender, and intersex patients and their families is important for office-based gynecologic practitioners. Important disparities exist in the health status of these patients compared with the general population. The range of health-related needs and special considerations for these individuals and their families is becoming increasingly apparent. Whereas the knowledge base for clinicians to draw from is rapidly evolving, the overall approach to care remains fundamentally the same. Ensuring that the office setting provides a supportive and inviting atmosphere is an important first step to providing quality care services. Allowing patients to specify their own sexual and gender identities, rather than assuming or imposing them on the patient, is perhaps the simplest way to avoid confusion or miscommunication. For many patients, some specific preventive care and treatment recommendations may be individually tailored. Although the opportunities and needs for collaborative practice with other medical and mental health providers are numerous, none of the routine primary care needed by these patients is beyond the scope of the office-based gynecologic practice.

Clinical Notes

- Health care considerations regarding lesbian, bisexual, transgender, transsexual, or intersex patients are relevant for all health care providers because these individuals and their families exist in every community.
- A wide range of terminology is employed to describe the sexual orientation and expression of humans.
- It is useful to think of *sex* as a biologically defined concept, whereas *gender* represents a socially defined convention.
- Clinical and scientific terms regarding human sexual identity are useful but have their limitations. The most important consideration in caring for patients is to respect and attempt to understand their self-identification.
- Available research seems to indicate that awareness of sexual orientation occurs at an early age—around 10 years or so—and this is true for both heterosexual and non-heterosexual subjects.
- When taking a history, use nonjudgmental language and open-ended questions such as "When you are sexually active, is it with men, women, or either?"
- It is estimated that 6.7% of American women have engaged in same-sex sexual behavior after the age of 15 years and 3.6% have participated in same-sex sexual behavior within the last 5 years.
- There are many commonalities in sex practices between LBGT populations and the strictly heterosexual population.
- The cornerstones of preventive services for lesbian and bisexual women are the same as for all women.

- Lesbian women are at higher risk for breast and gynecologic malignancies than heterosexual women; this is most likely because the lesbian population differs in their patterns of health risks.
- Many studies indicate that lesbians have higher rates of tobacco and alcohol use and increased body mass indices.
- There is no evidence that being raised in lesbian households is detrimental to the development of children in any significant respect relative to the development of children raised in heterosexual homes in otherwise comparable circumstances.
- Studies have identified several STIs as transmissible through same-sex female contact, including herpes, trichomoniasis, HPV, and HIV.
- The rate of BV is higher among lesbians.
- Even among women who deny ever participating in any sexual activity with men and who only engage in sex with women, HPV infection has been documented.
- Transgender individuals seeking medical or surgical treatments to become transsexual must meet the eligibility and readiness criteria established by HBIGDA.
- The selection of medical or surgical interventions for transgendered or intersex patients must be individualized. Clinicians should understand that not all patients will opt to use all available medical or surgical therapy, and patient preferences may change over time.

REFERENCES

1. Tesar CM, Rovi SLD. Survey of curriculum on homosexuality/bisexuality in departments of family medicine. Fam Med 1998;30:283–287.
2. Amato P, Morton D. Lesbian health education: a survey of obstetrics and gynecology training programs. J Gay Lesb Med Assoc 2002;6:47–51.
3. Gay and Lesbian Medical Association and LGBT health experts. Healthy People 2010 Companion Document for Lesbian, Gay, Bisexual and Transgender (LGBT) Health. San Francisco: Gay and Lesbian Medical Association, 2001. Available at: http://www.glma.org:16080/policy/hp2010/. Accessed June 29, 2005.
4. Harrison AE, Silenzio VMB. Comprehensive care of lesbian and gay patients and families. Prim Care 1996;23(1):31–46.
5. Silenzio V. Lesbian, gay and bisexual health in cross-cultural perspective. J Gay Lesb Med Assoc 1997; 1(2):75–86.
6. Laumann EO, Gagon JH, Michael RT, et al. The Social Organization of Sexuality: Sexual Practices in the United States. Chicago: University of Chicago Press, 1994.
7. Solarz AL. Lesbian Health: Current Assessment and Directions for the Future. Washington, DC: National Academy Press, 1999.
8. Logan CR. Homophobia? No, homoprejudice. J Homosex 1996;31(3):31–53.
9. Moss D. On situating homophobia. J Am Psychoanal Assoc 1997;45(1):201–215.
10. Guindon MH, Green AG, Hanna FJ. Intolerance and psychopathology: toward a general diagnosis for racism, sexism, and homophobia. Am J Orthopsychiatry 2003;73(2):167–176.
11. Institute of Medicine. Lesbian Health: Current Assessment and Directions for the Future. Washington, DC: National Academies Press, 1999.
12. Meyer IH. Why lesbian, gay, bisexual, and transgender public health? Am J Public Health 2001;91:856–859.
13. Fausto-Sterling A. The five sexes: why male and female are not enough. Sciences (New York) 1993; March/April:20–21.
14. Fausto-Sterling A. Sexing the Body: Gender Politics and the Construction of Sexuality. New York: Basic Books, 2000.
15. Rothblatt M. The Apartheid of Sex: A Manifesto on the Freedom of Gender. New York: Crown, 1995.
16. Feinberg L. Trans health crisis: for us it's life or death. Am J Public Health 2001;91:897–900.
17. Gonsiorek JC, Weinrich JD. The definition and scope of sexual orientation. In: Gonsiorek JC, Weinrich JD, eds. Homosexuality Research Implications for Public Policy. Newbury Park, CA: Sage, 1991:1–12.
18. D'Augelli AR, Hershberger SL. Lesbian, gay and bisexual youth in community settings: personal challenges and mental health problems. Am J Commun Psychol 1993;21:421–448.
19. Pattatucci AM, Hamer DH. Development and familiarity of sexual orientation in females. Behav Genet 1995;25:407–420.
20. Diamant AL, Schuster MA, McGuigan K, et al. Lesbians' sexual history with men: implications for taking a sexual history. Arch Intern Med 1999;159(22):2730–2736.
21. Bauer GR, Welles SL. Beyond assumptions of negligible risk: sexually transmitted diseases and women who have sex with women. Am J Public Health 2001;91:1282–1286.
22. Sell RL, Wells JA, Wyrij D. The prevalence of homosexual behavior and attraction in the United States, the United Kingdom and France: results of national population-based samples. Arch Sex Behav 1995;24:235–248.

23. Mathieson CM, Bailey N, Gurevich M. Health care services for lesbian and bisexual women: some Canadian data. Health Care Women Int 2002;23(2):185–196.
24. Dardick L, Grady K. Openness between gay persons and health professionals. Ann Int Med 1980; 93:115–119.
25. Smith EM, Johnson SR, Guenther SM. Health care attitudes and experiences during gynecologic care among lesbians and bisexuals. Am J Public Health 1985;75:1085–1087.
26. Stevens PE. Lesbian health care research: a review of the literature from 1970–1990. Health Care Women Int 1992;13:91–120.
27. Dean L, Meyer IH, Robinson K, et al. Lesbian, gay, bisexual, and transgender health: findings and concerns. J Gay Lesb Med Assoc 2000;4(3):102–151.
28. Diamant AL, Wold C, Spritzer K, et al. Health behaviors, health status and access to and use of health care: a population-based study of lesbian, bisexual, and heterosexual women. Arch Fam Med 2000;9:1043–1051.
29. Abbott LJ. The use of alcohol by lesbians: a review and research agenda. Subst Use Misuse 1998;33(13): 2647–2663.
30. Skinner WF, Otis MD. Drug and alcohol use among lesbian and gay people in a southern US sample: epidemiological, comparative, and methodological findings from the Trilogy Project. J Homosex 1996;30(3):59–92.
31. Aaron DJ, Markovic N, Danielson ME, et al. Behavioral risk factors for disease and preventive health practices among lesbians. Am J Public Health 2001;91:972–975.
32. Lechner ME, Vogel ME, Garcia-Shelton LM, et al. Self-reported medical problems of adult female survivors of childhood sexual abuse. J Fam Pract 1993;36:633–638.
33. Remafedi G. Suicidality in a venue-based sample of young men who have sex with men. J Adolesc Health 2002;31(4):305–310.
34. Davidson L, Linnoila M. Report of the Secretary's Task Force on Youth Suicide, 2: Risk Factors for Youth Suicide. Washington, DC: U.S. Department of Health and Human Services; Public Health Service; Alcohol, Drug Abuse, and Mental Health Administration, 1989.
35. Savin-Williams RC. Verbal and physical abuse as stressors in the lives of lesbian, gay male, and bisexual youths: associations with school problems, running away, substance abuse, prostitution, and suicide. J Consult Clin Psychol 1994;62(2):261–269.
36. Herek GM, Gillis JR, Cogan JC. Psychological sequelae of hate-crime victimization among lesbian, gay, and bisexual adults. J Consult Clin Psychol 1999;67(6):945–951.
37. Meyer I. Minority stress and mental health in gay men. J Health Soc Behav 1995;36(March):38–56.
38. Martin A. The Lesbian and Gay Parenting Handbook: Creating and Raising Our Families. New York: Harper Perennial, 1993.
39. Golombok S, Tasker F. Donor insemination for single heterosexual and lesbian women: issues concerning the welfare of the child. Hum Reprod 1994;9:1972–1976.
40. Patterson CJ. Children of gay and lesbian parents. Child Dev 1992;63:1025–1042.
41. Tasker F, Golombok S. Adults raised as children in lesbian families. Am J Orthopsychiatry 1995;65:203–215.
42. Brewaeys A, van Ball EV. Lesbian motherhood: the impact on child development and family functioning. J Psychosom Obstet Gynaecol 1997;18:116.
43. Ryan C, Bradford J. The National Lesbian Health Care Survey: an overview. In: Granets D, Kimmel DC, eds. Psychological Perspectives on Lesbian and Gay Male Experiences. New York: Columbia University Press, 1993:541–556.
44. Johnson SR, Smith EM, Guenther SM. Comparison of gynecologic health care problems between lesbians and bisexual women: a survey of 2,345 women. J Reprod Med 1987;32:805–811.
45. Sivakumar K, De Silva AH, Roy RB. Trichomonas vaginalis infection in a lesbian. Genitourin Med 1989;65:399–400.
46. Kellock D, O'Mahoney CP. Sexually acquired metronidazole-resistant trichomoniasis in a lesbian couple. Genitourin Med 1996;72:60–61.
47. Ferris DG, Batish S, Wright TC, et al. A neglected lesbian health concern: cervical neoplasia. J Fam Pract 1996;43:581–584.
48. O'Hanlan KA, Crum CP. Human papillomavirus-associated cervical intraepithelial neoplasia following lesbian sex. Obstet Gynecol 1996;88:702–703.
49. Rich JD, Back A, Tuomala RE, et al. Transmission of human immunodeficiency virus presumed to have occurred via female homosexual contact. Clin Infect Dis 1993;17:1003–1005.
50. Troncoso AP, Romani A, Carranza CM, et al. Probable HIV transmission by female homosexual contact. Medicina 1995;55:334–336.
51. Fethers K, Marks C, Mindel A, et al. Sexually transmitted infections and risk behaviors in women who have sex with women. Sex Transm Infect 2000;76:345–349.
52. Berger BJ, Kolton S, Zenilman JM, et al. Bacterial vaginosis in lesbians: a sexually transmitted disease. Clin Infect Dis 1995;6:103–112.
53. Berger BJ, Kolton S, Zenilman JM, et al. Bacterial vaginosis in lesbians: a sexually transmitted disease. Clin Infect Dis 1995;21:1402–1405.
54. Marrazzo JM, Koutsky LA, Eschenback DA, et al. Characterization of vaginal flora and bacterial vaginosis in women who have sex with women. J Infect Dis 2002;185:1307–1313.
55. McCaffrey M, Varney P, Evans B, et al. Bacterial vaginosis in lesbians: evidence for lack of sexual transmission. Int J STD AIDS 1999;10:305–308.
56. Skinner CJ, Stokes J, Kirlew Y, et al. A case-controlled study of the sexual health needs of lesbians. Genitourin Med 1996;72:277–280.

57. Marrazzo JM, Koutsky LA, Kiviat NB, et al. Papanicolaou test screening and prevalence of genital human papillomavirus among women who have sex with women. Am J Public Health 2001;91:947–952.
58. Bakker A, van Kesteren PJ, Gooren LJ, et al. The prevalence of transsexualism in the Netherlands. Acta Psychiatr Scand 1993;87(4):237–238.
59. American Psychiatric Association. Diagnostic and Statistical Manual of Mental Disorders. Fourth Edition, Text Revision (DSM-IV-TR). Washington, DC: American Psychiatric Association, 2000.
60. De Sutter P. Gender reassignment and assisted reproduction: present and future reproductive options for transsexual people. Hum Reprod 2001;16(4):612–614.
61. Harry Benjamin International Gender Dysphoria Association (HBIGDA). Standards of Care for Gender Identity Disorders, Fifth Version. Minneapolis, MN: HBIGDA, 1998. Available at: http://www.hbigda.org/soc5.cfm. Accessed June 29, 2005.
62. Oriel K. Medical care of transsexual patients. J Gay Lesb Med Assoc 2000;4(4):185–194.
63. Boverman J, Loomis A. Cross-sex hormone treatment in transsexualism. Prim Psychiatry 2000;7(6):68–73.
64. Futterweit W. Endocrine therapy of transsexualism and potential complications of long-term treatment. Arch Sex Behav 1998;27(2):209–226.
65. Futterweit W, Deligdisch L. Histopathological effects of exogenously administered testosterone in 19 female to male transsexuals. J Clin Endocrinol Metab 1986;62:16–21.
66. Israel GE, Tarver DE. Transgender Care: Recommended Guidelines, Practical Information, and Personal Accounts. Philadelphia: Temple University Press, 1997.
67. Levy A, Crown A, Reid R. Endocrine intervention for transsexuals. Clin Endocrinol (Oxf) 2003;59(4):409–418.
68. van Kesteren PJ, Asscheman H, Megens JA, et al. Mortality and morbidity in transsexual subjects treated with cross-sex hormones. Clin Endocrinol (Oxf) 1997;47(3):337–342.
69. Ganly I, Taylor EW. Breast cancer in a trans-sexual man receiving hormone replacement therapy. Br J Surg 1995;82(3):341.
70. Pritchard TJ, Pankowsky DA, Crowe JP, et al. Breast cancer in a male-to-female transsexual. A case report. JAMA 1988;259(15):2278–2280.
71. Goh HH, Li XF, Ratnam SS. Effects of cross-gender steroid hormone treatment on prolactin concentrations in humans. Gynecol Endocrinol 1992;6(2):113–117.
72. Asscheman H, Gooren LJ, Assies J, et al. Prolactin levels and pituitary enlargement in hormone-treated male-to-female transsexuals. Clin Endocrinol (Oxf) 1988;28(6):583–588.
73. Futterweit W, Weiss RA, Fagerstrom RM. Endocrine evaluation of forty female-to-male transsexuals: increased frequency of polycystic ovarian disease in female transsexualism. Arch Sex Behav 1986;15(1):69–78.
74. Gooren LJ, Assies J, Asscheman H, et al. Estrogen-induced prolactinoma in a man. J Clin Endocrinol Metab 1988;66(2):444–446.
75. Kipnis K, Diamond M. Pediatric ethics and the surgical assignment of sex. J Clin Ethics 1998;9(4):398–410.
76. Chase C. Hermaphrodites with attitude: mapping the emergence of intersex political activism. GLQ 1998;4(2):189–211.
77. Diamond M, Sigmundson HK. Management of intersexuality. Guidelines for dealing with persons with ambiguous genitalia. Arch Pediatr Adolesc Med 1997;151(10):1046–1050.
78. Harry Benjamin International Gender Dysphoria Association (HBIGDA). Standards of Care for Gender Identity Disorders, Sixth Version. Minneapolis: HBIGDA, 2001. Available at: http://www.hbigda.org/socv6.cfm. Accessed June 29, 2005.

CHAPTER 4

Abnormal Cytology and Human Papillomavirus

Barbara M. Buttin, Thomas J. Herzog, and David G. Mutch

INTRODUCTION

Cervical cancer is the number one cause of cancer death in young women in developing countries (1). In the United States, 13,000 new diagnoses of cervical cancer are expected this year, leading to 4,100 deaths (2). With the introduction of the Papanicolaou (or Pap) smear and cytologic screening programs in the United States and other countries with universal screening programs, mortality rates from cervical cancer have decreased by 46% from 1973 to 1995 (3). Nonetheless, cervical cancer remains a major health problem in this country mostly due to nonadherence with current screening guidelines. As our understanding of the carcinogenesis of cervical cancer and its precursors continues to evolve, screening methods are being refined and guidelines revised in an attempt to improve adherence and decrease the incidence of this preventable disease. This chapter provides an overview of the human papillomavirus (HPV) as the etiologic agent of cervical dysplasia and cancer, risk factors for progression of dysplasia to invasive cancer, and the management of cervical precursor lesions, including the latest screening guidelines. The recognition and treatment of vaginal and vulvar intraepithelial neoplasia is also discussed.

HUMAN PAPILLOMAVIRUS

Epidemiology

HPV is a DNA tumor virus that is strongly associated with both cervical dysplasia and cervical cancer. Papillomaviruses can infect almost all human skin surfaces and can cause cancer in most of those sites. HPV infection of the male and female anogenital tract is sexually transmitted, and its prevalence varies depending on the population sampled and the assay used to detect it. Viral transmission only requires intimate contact between partners; it does not depend on sexual penetration or intercourse for its transmission. Asymptomatic HPV infection is detected in 10 to 20% of women of reproductive age, whereas 1 to 13% of sexually active women present with anogenital condylomata acuminata (4). The prevalence of HPV is highest among women younger than age 25 immediately after the onset of sexual activity (5). It then gradually decreases with advancing age. However, a second peak in prevalence occurs in postmenopausal women after age 55 and may be related to changes in immune and hormonal status that occur after menopause (5, 6).

Risk factors for acquiring HPV include sexual behavior, specifically frequency of sexual intercourse, number of lifetime sex partners, the male partner's number of lifetime sex partners, age, ethnicity, and smoking or living with smokers (7). Factors such as oral contraceptive use, pregnancy, and immunosuppression have been reported but are less clearly associated (4).

Most infections with HPV are transient or intermittent, with a median duration of 8 months (3, 5, 8). Ho et al. prospectively studied a cohort of 608 female college students and found that 70% had cleared their infection by 12 months and only 9% remained infected at 24 months.

TABLE 4.1

High-Risk and Low-Risk Types of Human Papillomavirus

High-risk Risk Types	Low-Risk Types
16, 18, 31, 33, 35, 39, 45, 51, 52, 55, 56, 58, 59, 66, 68	6, 11, 26, 42, 44, 54, 70, 73

In this study, persistent infection was associated with older age, infection with multiple types of HPV, and infection with a high-risk type of HPV. Most women seem to clear the virus and maintain immunity from reinfection by the viral type with which they were infected. However, prior infection with any one or multiple types of HPV has not been shown to confer immunity or protection from acquisition of another type of HPV (9).

Human Papillomavirus and Cervical Disease

HPV was first proposed as a risk factor for cervical cancer in 1974 by zur Hausen et al. (10). Since that time, it has been associated with 99.7% of all cervical cancers worldwide after more sensitive assays for its detection became available (11). In fact, many experts believe this association will eventually increase to 100% (12). For women infected with HPV, their relative risk of developing cervical cancer ranges between 20 and 70% (3, 5, 13). Even with this elevation in relative risk, the overall percentage of women infected with HPV who will develop cervical cancer is small. Factors leading to the development of persistent HPV infection and neoplastic progression are currently under investigation.

With regard to cervical dysplasia, HPV infection is associated with a 4-fold increased risk of developing atypical squamous cells of undetermined significance (ASCUS) and/or low-grade squamous intraepithelial lesions (LSIL), as well as a 13-fold risk of developing high-grade squamous intraepithelial lesions (HSIL) (14). Women with high-risk types of HPV (especially HPV-16) have an even higher risk of developing HSIL than those with low-risk types (14). Table 4.1 lists high- and low-risk types of HPV. According to a large meta-analysis of the current literature, rates of progression to/persistence of high-grade dysplasia of ASCUS, LSIL, and HSIL are about 7%, 21%, and 24%, respectively, at 24 months (15). For a further look into the progression trends of cervical dysplasia, refer to Table 4.2. It has also been established that oncogenic HPV types such as 16 and 18 progress more rapidly to HSIL (14, 16). Nonetheless, only about 1% of women infected with oncogenic HPV types actually go on to develop cervical

TABLE 4.2

Natural History of Cervical Lesions

Biopsy Result	Regress	Persist	Progress to Carcinoma in Situ	Progress to Invasion
CIN 1	57%	32%	11%	1%
CIN 2	43%	35%	22%	5%
CIN 3	32%	<56%	—	>12%

CIN, cervical intraepithelial neoplasia.

Adapted with permission from Östör AG. Natural history of cervical intraepithelial neoplasia: a critical review. Int J Gynecol Pathol 1993;12:186–192; Melnikow J, Nuovo J, Willan AR, et al. Natural history of cervical squamous intraepithelial lesions: a meta-analysis. Obstet Gynecol 1998;92:727–735.

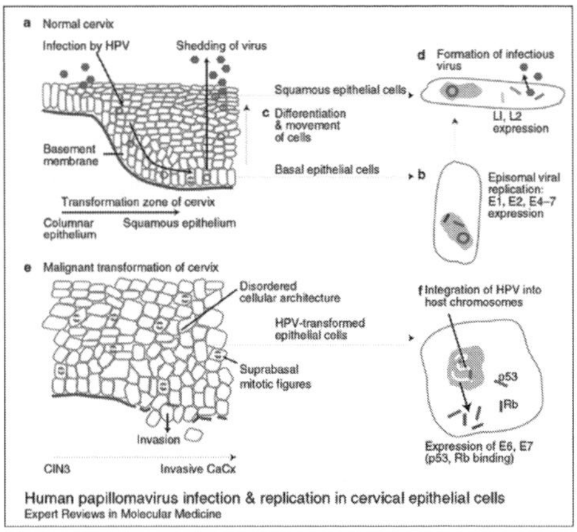

FIGURE 4.1 ● HPV-16 genome. (From Stephen Man (1998) Human cellular immune responses against human papillomaviruses in cervical neoplasia. Exp. Rev. Mol. Med. 3 July, http://www.expertreviews.org/smc/txt001smc.htm)

cancer. Therefore, current models of HPV-related carcinogenesis emphasize the role of persistent infection, immune factors, and co-carcinogens in the progression of asymptomatic infection to dysplasia and carcinoma (3).

Virology and Mechanism of Carcinogenesis

HPV is a small, nonenveloped, icosahedral double-stranded DNA virus with close to 100 subtypes identified to date. Its circular genome is about 8 kilobases in length, and only one strand is transcribed (Fig. 4.1). It contains eight open reading frames (ORFs) encoding HPV proteins. The early genes (E1 to E7) are involved in viral replication and transcription, whereas the late genes (L1, L2) encode viral capsid proteins. E6 and E7 are also associated with cellular transformation. These two ORFs show the most sequence variation, whereas L1 is the most conserved region of HPV (5). The long control region initiates replication and controls transcriptional regulation. After initial infection has occurred, the viral genome is generally present inside the nucleus of epithelial cells as an episome that can replicate. Neoplastic progression is associated with the integration of viral DNA into cellular chromosomes often involving E1 or E2. This event leads to disruption of the viral life cycle. The disruption of the E2 gene in HPV-16–positive cervical cancers has been shown to be associated with significantly shortened disease-free survival for women with cervical cancer (17).

Human Papillomavirus Testing

HPV can only infect epithelial cells and requires a specific cellular environment to replicate. Attempts at culturing HPV from tissue samples or growing the virus in tissue culture have been unsuccessful. The epithelium appears to shield the virus from the immune response, making serologic tests relatively unreliable. The diagnosis of HPV requires direct detection of viral DNA within the nucleus of an infected cell. Samples from the transformation zone of the cervix collected by cytobrush are generally a good source of infected cells.

Several assays for the detection of HPV have been developed, each with different sensitivities and specificities, depending on the method of DNA extraction from the cervical sample and the amount of DNA used. Most assays use direct hybridization techniques and nucleic acid amplification, such as the polymerase chain reaction (PCR). However, the only assays approved by the U.S. Food and Drug Administration (FDA) for HPV testing in cervical screening use Hybrid Capture (HC) assay technology and include the HC II High-Risk HPV DNA test and DNAwithPap (both by Digene, Inc., Gaithersburg, MD). The FDA initially approved the HC II High-Risk HPV DNA Test in March 2000 for testing women with abnormal Pap results to determine if they needed to be further evaluated. As such, it was approved as an adjunct for testing in the workup of abnormal cervical cytology. In March 2003, the FDA approved expanded use of the assay to allow the test to be used for screening purposes under the name DNAwithPap.

Hybrid Capture

The HC assay technology has gone through several changes and improvements. The current assay (HC II) uses a cellular sample from the cervix collected with a cytobrush and placed into a liquid cytology medium. Cellular DNA is released through lysis in solution and mixed with RNA probes specific to HPV DNA to achieve hybridization. Monoclonal antibodies that are very specific to these RNA-DNA hybrids are bound to microtiter wells and allowed to "capture" and immobilize the hybrids. The same type of antibody bound to an enzyme that gives a semiquantitative chemiluminescent signal is then incubated with the hybrids leading to the detection of the signal (3, 5, 18).

HC II comes with a low-risk probe detecting HPV types 6, 11, 42, 43, and 44 and a high-risk probe detecting HPV types 16, 18, 31, 33, 35, 39, 45, 51, 52, 56, 58, 59, and 68 (3). Specific HPV typing is therefore not possible using this assay. Overall, HC II has very good interlaboratory reproducibility and has been shown to compare favorably with PCR-based assays (18). However, cross reactivity of high-risk probes with low-risk subtypes of HPV or with subtypes not included in the assay leads to some false-positive results (17). HC II can be performed on samples collected in the manufacturer's media or by using other commercially available liquid-based cytology systems (e.g., ThinPrep by Cytyc Corp., Boxborough, MA) (3, 18).

Polymerase Chain Reaction Assays

Assays for HPV detection or typing based on PCR are currently not commercially available. These assays are the most sensitive test for HPV DNA detection, while also allowing for HPV typing by DNA sequencing of amplified PCR products or by type-specific hybridization (3, 8). Different PCR assays are widely used in HPV research; overall, PCR technology has the advantage of being applicable even on DNA extracts of poor quality, such as those derived from formalin-fixed, paraffin-embedded archival tissue. Most of these assays use one of several L1 consensus primer PCR systems, such as PGMY09/11, an improved and more sensitive version of the MY09/11 system, or the GP5+/6+ system, which has been used in several epidemiologic studies (19–21). Consensus assays use a mixture of primers to give a positive/negative result by gel electrophoresis or enzyme-linked immunoabsorbent assay, ensuring the assay covers as many HPV types as possible. The consensus product is then used for type-specific hybridization or sequencing. Alternatively, type-specific PCR can be used. Most of these assays target the highly polymorphic E6/E7 region of the HPV genome. All PCR-based assays require special equipment and training in molecular biology. They are extremely sensitive to contamination and therefore dependent on stringent techniques and appropriate controls.

Viral Load

HPV viral load has been evaluated as a tool to screen for infections at high risk for progression to cervical cancer (3, 22). In Josefsson's study, women with high amounts of HPV-16 DNA were at a 60-fold higher risk of developing cervical carcinoma in situ or invasive cancer than women who were HPV-16 negative. Although this investigational method warrants further study, it may serve as a promising test to help identify a subset of patients at high risk for persistent or progressive cervical dysplasia.

In Situ Hybridization

The technique of in situ hybridization allows for direct visualization of HPV DNA on formalin-fixed, paraffin-embedded tissue. This technique facilitates selection of the most appropriate tissue sections for further analysis (3, 5). It allows for visual distinction between episomal and integrated viral DNA within the cell nuclei. Results can be revealing but are quite technique dependent. Some amount of cross-hybridization during type-specific screening cannot be avoided.

SCREENING FOR CERVICAL CANCER PRECURSORS

Since the introduction of the Pap smear just more than 50 years ago, cytologic screening programs for cervical dysplasia have decreased the incidence of cervical cancer by almost three-fourths in the United States (23). It is estimated that 50% of women in the United States with newly diagnosed invasive cervical carcinoma have never had a Pap smear, and the other 50% occur in women who were poorly screened (had not had a Pap smear in the last 5 years), received inadequate follow-up, or were cases associated with the errors of the Pap test process (24, 25). In developing nations, however, access to and adherence with screening programs varies widely, and cervical cancer continues to be a major cause of morbidity and mortality in young women. Ongoing attempts to improve both screening modalities and accessibility with regard to early detection of cervical cancer precursors, as well as timely intervention, remain major public health goals both in this country and worldwide.

Risk factors for the development of cervical dysplasia are well known and illustrate the preventable nature of cervical cancer. They include genital HPV infection, positive HIV status, multiple sexual partners, early age at first intercourse, high parity, cigarette smoking, and low socioeconomic status.

Although long recognized as a highly effective screening test, the validity of the conventional Pap smear has been the center of controversy in the lay press, citing its high false-negative rate secondary to errors in sampling and fixation, as well as accurate and replicable interpretation (23). The conventional Pap smear has a sensitivity of approximately 50% (26). In a meta-analysis, Fahey et al. reported the sensitivity of the conventional Pap to range from 49 to 67% (27). Overall, about two-thirds of the false-negative Pap tests are related to sampling errors, and the remaining one-third are due to laboratory detection error. Although no screening test has 100% sensitivity and specificity, attempts to improve cervical cytology screening have been multifaceted. First, test quality itself is being revised with the introduction of liquid-based cytology and computerized Pap test analysis. Second, sensitivity and specificity of the Pap test are being improved with the introduction of several parallel or sequential tests such as cytology and HPV testing. Third, ongoing development of digital and spectroscopic techniques may provide physicians with valid alternatives for cervical cancer screening (28). Last, the revision and update of the 1991 Bethesda System for reporting the results of cervical cytology, as well as the development of consensus guidelines for the management of women with cervical dysplasia, are useful adjuncts to help clinicians avoid the pitfalls of ambiguous test results and multiple options for follow-up (29, 30).

Liquid-Based Cytology

Liquid-based screening systems have recently been approved by the FDA and were developed to improve the transfer of cells from the collection device to the slide, provide uniformity of the cell population in each sample, and thus decrease interpretational errors. The two systems currently available are ThinPrep and SurePath (TriPath Imaging, Inc. [formerly AutoCyte], Burlington, NC). Liquid-based cytology has been shown to result in an increased detection rate of both low- and high-grade cervical dysplasia, as well as a decrease in the ambiguous diagnosis of ASCUS (31–33). An added benefit of liquid-based cytology systems is the ability to perform "reflex" HPV testing, if desired. For this and other reasons, many health care providers have made liquid-based cytology their test system of choice despite higher cost. Figure 4.2 illustrates the differences between a conventional and a liquid-based cytology slide.

In the ThinPrep test kit, cervical specimens are collected in the usual fashion with either a broom-type device or a spatula and endocervical cytobrush, and cells are collected directly in the methanol-based fixation liquid. The sample is put through the ThinPrep processor to separate the cells from the mucous and debris. This liquid is passed through an 8-μm filter and transferred to a slide yielding a monolayer of approximately 40,000 cells. The slide is then read like a conventional Pap smear. Because the cells are fixed immediately after collection, fewer drying and fixation artifacts in cellular morphology occur, and there is diminished interference from blood or mucus. Clinical studies of the ThinPrep showed a detection rate for LSIL or worse of 9.4% compared with 8% by conventional Pap smear. The improved detection rate was higher in populations with a low risk of cervical abnormalities (65% improvement) compared with a 6% improvement in detection rate in high-risk populations (34).

The other method, SurePath, was FDA approved in 1999 under the name AutoCyte PREP. This is an automated liquid-based sample preparation system. After the cervical sample is collected, the tip of the brush is placed in an ethanol-based preservative. The PrepStain slide processor then prepares the sample by layering the cells onto a density reagent to remove blood, mucus,

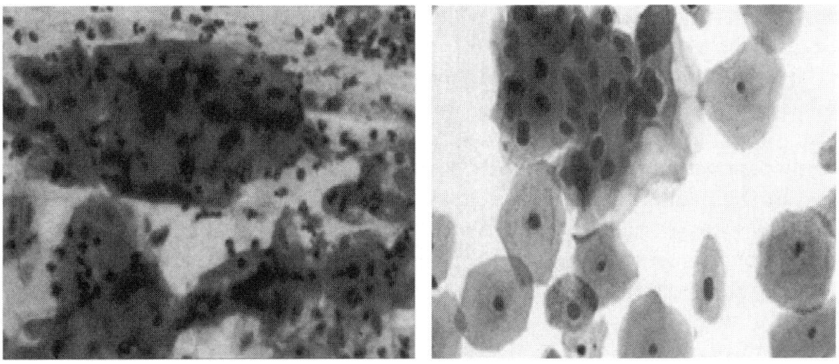

FIGURE 4.2 ● Conventional versus liquid-based cytology. (Courtesy of Matthew A. Powell, MD.)

and other debris from the sample. The remaining cells are then transferred by cytospin to a slide and stained. In a multisite trial using 58,580 SurePath slides collected prospectively and a comparison historical cohort of 58,988 conventional Pap smears, the SurePath slides had a 64.4% increase ($p < 0.00001$) in the detection of HSIL. In addition, the SurePath slides showed a detection rate for LSIL and more serious lesions of 3.4% compared with a detection rate of 1.6% for conventional slides. There was an unsatisfactory slide rate of 0.2% for SurePath slides compared with 0.5% for conventional slides (package insert).

The only concern with this type of screening method is its relatively high cost for the small return in public health benefit (24). When focusing strictly on the number of lives saved per number of screening tests, two recent cost-benefit analyses reached the same conclusion, stating that conventional Pap tests are still the most cost-effective screening method (35). A comprehensive review of the literature issued by the Agency for Healthcare Research and Quality (AHRQ) in 2001 on the subject of cervical sampling methods concluded that the current evidence is not sufficient to determine if the new technology is better than the conventional Pap smear and should replace the Pap test. In their review of the data available, they found that most of the studies of thin layer technology did not have proper control groups and that information about the sensitivity, specificity, and predictive values was scant at the time of the literature assessment (36).

In the same review, a cost analysis showed that the benefits of liquid-based cytology could be achieved well below the accepted health care cost-effectiveness threshold of $50,000 if the patients were screened every 2 years rather than yearly using the traditional Pap smear (36). In a separate cost and outcomes analysis using mathematical modeling, Montz et al. evaluated the impact of liquid-based cytology and compliance on a theoretic cohort of 100,000 women of different races, ages, and compliance levels (37). They found 32 to 33% reduction in cervical cancer incidence without compromising on cost effectiveness (37).

Neural Network Technology

Two computerized automated screening systems have been developed with the intent to minimize false-positive and false-negative results that will inevitably occur with the reliance on technologists to recognize a few abnormal cells in the midst of thousands of normal ones. AutoPap (TriPath Imaging, Inc., Burlington, NC) and the formerly available PAPNET (Neuromedical Systems, Inc., Suffern, NY) are semiautomated, neural network systems that optically scan Pap smears and use artificial intelligence to select an area on the slide with the most abnormal-appearing cells. This area is then presented to the cytotechnologist for review.

PAPNET was compared with conventional cytology as a primary screening modality in a large multicenter trial in the United Kingdom (38). Both systems were similar with regard to sensitivity (51 to 88%), but PAPNET had better specificity than conventional screening (77% versus 42%, respectively). Total screening time was also lower for PAPNET than for manual screening. However, the manufacturer of the PAPNET test, Neuromedical Systems, no longer exists, and the test is not available.

The current automated screening system, AutoPap, has demonstrated improved performance for detection of low- and high-grade dysplasia (39). It is currently FDA approved for both primary screening and for quality assurance review of normal Pap smears. The FDA more recently approved a new automated system, The ThinPrep Imaging System (Imager) (Cytyc Corp., Boxborough, MA) for commercial use. Opinions on the cost-effectiveness of this kind of technology are variable. Although their use could potentially reduce the false-negative rate generated by manual screening, many centers already have effective quality control programs in place. The exact role of this technology will have to be established by large-scale clinical trials.

Human Papillomavirus Testing as a Screening Modality

Several studies have evaluated the value of HPV testing as a screening tool for the detection of cervical dysplasia. For instance, a large-scale study from France found that HPV testing with HC II was superior to screening cytology with referral to colposcopy at a threshold of ASCUS for the detection of high-grade dysplasia (40). High-risk HPV detection with HC II had a sensitivity of 100% for the detection of high-grade dysplasia versus 85.3% with cytology/colposcopy. Wright et al. published an interesting study on 1415 previously unscreened South African women comparing self-collected vaginal swabs used for HPV testing to Pap smears, direct visual inspection of the cervix with acetic acid, cervicography, and HPV testing on a physician-obtained cervical sample (41). Self-collected specimens with HPV testing and Pap smears with colposcopy threshold of ASCUS were similarly effective for the detection of high-grade dysplasia, whereas physician-collected specimens with HPV testing were most sensitive. Although these results clearly underscore the value of HPV testing as a screening modality, they also suggest that underserved areas with little access to conventional screening programs may benefit from patient-obtained specimen collection.

Overall, the sensitivity for HPV testing as a screening modality for cervical dysplasia has been shown to be at least 10% higher than that of conventional cytology screening (84 to 100% versus 20 to 86%) (3). Its high sensitivity combined with a high negative predictive value makes a negative test a very reassuring result for patients and their health care providers. However, its positive predictive value and specificity are somewhat low, depending on the threshold used for the HC II assay. Strategies to improve this shortcoming, such as quantitative viral load measurement, are being developed.

Human Papillomavirus Testing as a Triage Modality

HPV testing in addition to liquid-based cytology has been evaluated as a triage strategy for patients with the diagnosis of "ASCUS" as it was defined in the old Bethesda System (42). The management of patients with ASCUS Pap smears has been particularly problematic because adherence with the recommended follow-up smear in 4 months tends to be poor, and many patients are lost to follow-up. This is concerning because patients with a diagnosis of ASCUS have a 5 to 17% chance of harboring high-grade dysplasia (confirmed on biopsy), and high-grade dysplasia was identified in 24 to 94% of those with ASCUS smears by colposcopically directed biopsy (30, 43–46).

To facilitate the management of patients with equivocal cytology results or low-grade lesions, the National Cancer Institute sponsored the ASCUS/LSIL Triage Study (ALTS), a large, multicenter trial comparing three management strategies for ASCUS and low-grade (LSIL) Pap smears (44, 47). The three strategies included immediate colposcopy, HPV testing with colposcopy if positive, and repeat cytology with colposcopy only for second Pap of HSIL or higher.

The ALTS compared the outcomes of three different treatment strategies for women with a Pap smear read as ASCUS. The women were randomized to either immediate colposcopy, triage by HPV DNA testing using the HC II assay, or conservative therapy with repeat cytology at 6-month intervals. Women in the HPV triage were referred for colposcopy only if they tested positive for high-risk HPV, and women in the conservative arm were referred for colposcopy only if they developed HSIL on a follow-up Pap smear. For all women, a loop electrosurgical excision procedure (LEEP) was recommended if a colposcopically directed biopsy showed cervical intraepithelial neoplasia (CIN) 2 or higher.

The data showed that 64% of the patients with CIN 2 or higher were identified initially by the immediate colposcopy referral, and 70% were detected by the HPV triage approach. Only 55% of the women with CIN 2 or higher were detected before the exit examination in the conservative treatment arm. The conservative treatment approach missed a significant number of cases, and it would probably be even worse in the noninvestigative setting where loss of follow-up rates tend to be higher. Of the three approaches, HPV triage was slightly better and cost less because only approximately 50% of the patients in this arm were eventually referred for colposcopy. This trial clearly showed that cytology with HPV testing is a viable option for triaging patients with equivocal (ASCUS) Pap tests to conservative management with follow-up at 6 to 12 months versus immediate colposcopy (48).

In the LSIL part of the ALTS trial, more than 1500 women with a community-based diagnosis of LSIL were randomized to one of the same three management protocols. Of the patients randomized to HPV DNA testing, more than 80% were positive for high-risk HPV types. This high frequency of high-risk HPV DNA, which was confirmed by PCR on a subset of the women, demonstrated that the usefulness of HPV testing for triage in women with LSIL is clearly limited (49).

Cervicography

This technique involves photography of the cervix after the application of acetic acid. The image is then magnified and projected onto a screen where expert reviewers evaluate it. Although cervicography has been proposed to increase the sensitivity of conventional screening cytology, several studies evaluated the technique and were unable to substantiate the claim (50, 51). The sensitivity was noted to be particularly poor in postmenopausal women older than 50. Cervicography is therefore not recommended as a screening alternative to cytology, although its use in certain populations and settings warrants further investigation.

Visual Inspection

Visual inspection of the cervix is done with 3 to 5% acetic acid wash followed 1 minute later by a naked-eye assessment of the cervix. This technique has been evaluated as a viable screening option in underdeveloped countries where cytology-based screening is unavailable secondary to cost and lack of infrastructure. A study from the University of Zimbabwe compared the performance of visual inspection with acetic acid and the Pap smear in the hands of midlevel providers, and established direct estimates for sensitivity, specificity, and positive and negative predictive value for the detection of high-grade dysplasia with the technique (52). These estimates are considered direct because all women testing negative or positive on screening were offered colposcopy and biopsy as indicated. In this study, visual inspection had sensitivity for HSIL positivity of 76.7%, compared with 44.3% sensitivity for cytology, although visual inspection had a lower specificity of 64.1% compared with 90.6% for cytology for the detection of high-grade dysplasia. The lower specificity has been ascribed to a high rate of sexually transmitted diseases in the population and to the limited training of some of the providers performing the screening. The most important result of the study is the high negative predictive value of this simple and inexpensive technique, thereby eliminating the need for further testing in those patients that screen negative.

In a more recent review of the literature, Gaffikin et al. found that of 15 qualifying studies, the sensitivity of visual inspection ranged between 66% and 96% and specificity between 64% and 98%. They noted that authors that compared visual inspection with cytology found that in low resource settings, the overall usefulness of visual inspection compared favorably with that of the Pap test (53).

The long-term effectiveness (i.e., reductions in the incidence of and mortality from cervical cancer) of visual inspection-based testing is not yet available because the test has not been in use long enough to yield sufficient data for these outcomes.

Speculoscopy

This method of visual inspection uses a chemiluminescent light source named Speculite (Trylon Corp., Torrance, CA) to evaluate abnormal areas on the cervix. A handheld optic device provides four to six times magnification after the application of acetic acid. Shulman compared conventional cytology with speculoscopy in a cohort of pregnant adolescents and found it to be similarly effective (54). More important, a study by Parham showed that 90.6% of women with normal cytology results but persistently abnormal speculoscopy after 6 months had biopsy-proven dysplasia that would have been missed even with repeat cytology at 6 months (55). These results strongly suggest that there may well be a role for visual techniques such as speculoscopy in improving the sensitivity of conventional cytology screening.

MANAGEMENT OF CERVICAL INTRAEPITHELIAL NEOPLASIA

In 2001, the 1991 Bethesda System for reporting cervical/vaginal cytologic diagnoses underwent an extensive re-evaluation and revision process, resulting in the new 2001 Bethesda System (29, 42). This system provides a standardized framework for laboratory reports, including both a descriptive statement and an evaluation of specimen adequacy. Alongside the new system, a set of consensus guidelines for the management of each cytologic diagnosis was developed, helping eliminate many inconsistencies and misinterpretations among the myriad of women's health care providers. The new system recommends specifying whether cells from the transformation zone are present in a cervical sample as an indication of specimen quality. The lack of transformation cells as the only criterion to classify a Pap as unsatisfactory and to require a repeat test is controversial. Some argue that there is no definitive research on the value of having endocervical cells in a Pap, whereas others note that obscuring blood and inflammatory cells are often seen on Paps done in women with invasive cervical cancer. The new Bethesda System is shown in Table 4.3.

Management of Women With Atypical Squamous Cells of Undetermined Significance

In the new Bethesda System, the category of ASCUS has been divided into ASCUS and ASC-H (atypical squamous cells, cannot exclude HSIL). All designations of atypical squamous cells (ASC) are now considered to be suggestive of dysplasia. The category of "ASCUS favor reactive" was thus eliminated, and pathologists are required to clearly state "negative for intraepithelial lesion or malignancy" for such cases. Because a significant number of patients with the old diagnosis of ASCUS were found to have high-grade dysplasia by biopsy, although only very few (less than 0.5%) were found to have invasive cancer, it was suggested that women with this equivocal Pap smear diagnosis require some form of additional workup. However, the routine recommendation of repeat cytology in 3 to 6 months, with referral to colposcopy only if abnormal on repeat screening, has not only resulted in considerable loss of patients to follow-up, but also in a delay of treatment for those harboring high-grade dysplasia.

Figure 4.3 illustrates the management algorithm for women with ASCUS. Although repeat cytology at 4 to 6 months, immediate colposcopy, or HPV testing are all viable options, each has advantages and disadvantages that should be considered carefully in the context of an individual patient's situation. The disadvantages of repeat cytology even in adherent patients are obvious because a delay in diagnosis and treatment of dysplasia is inevitable, and the false-negative rate of repeat cytology is quite high. Although the advantage of immediate colposcopy is clearly that significant pathology can be ruled out instantly, the practitioner should consider his or her colposcopic level of expertise, patient discomfort and anxiety, and that this strategy has the highest cost of the three options. Furthermore, up to 80% of patients will be overtreated with routine colposcopy for ASCUS (42, 47).

Advantages of HPV testing were outlined previously. Its negative predictive value approaches 1.0, and thus, a negative test result returns the patient to the low-risk pool with yearly cytology screening. However, a positive test result is more difficult to interpret. Between 31% and 60% of women with ASCUS will test positive for high-risk HPV types (30). It is unknown how to

TABLE 4.3

2001 Bethesda System

Specimen Adequacy
- Satisfactory for evaluation (endocervical component present/absent, comments on quality indicators)
- Unsatisfactory for evaluation

General Categorization (Optional)
- Negative for intraepithelial lesion or malignancy (see Interpretation/Results)
- Epithelial cell abnormality (see Interpretation/Results)
- Other (see Interpretation/Results)

Interpretation/Results
- Negative for intraepithelial lesion or malignancy
    - ○ Organisms
        - ← *Trichomonas vaginalis*
        - ← Fungal organisms morphologically consistent with *Candida* species
        - ← Shift in flora suggestive of bacterial vaginosis
        - ← Bacteria morphologically consistent with *Actinomyces* species
        - ← Cellular changes consistent with herpes simplex virus
    - ○ Other nonneoplastic findings (optional)
    - ○ Reactive cellular changes associated with inflammation
    - ○ Radiation
    - ○ Intrauterine contraceptive device
    - ○ Glandular cells status post hysterectomy
    - ○ Atrophy
- Epithelial cell abnormalities
    - ○ Squamous cell
        - ← Atypical squamous cells
            - Of undetermined significance
            - Cannot exclude high-grade squamous intraepithelial lesions (HSIL)
        - ← Low-grade squamous intraepithelial lesions
            - Human papillomavirus
            - Mild dysplasia
            - Cervical intraepithelial neoplasia (CIN) I
        - ← HSIL
            - Moderate and severe dysplasia
            - CIN II and III, carcinoma in situ
        - ← Squamous cell carcinoma
    - ○ Glandular cell
        - ← Atypical glandular cells (AGC), specify endocervical, endometrial, or not otherwise specified
        - ← AGC favor neoplastic, specify endocervical or not otherwise specified
        - ← Endocervical adenocarcinoma in situ
        - ← Adenocarcinoma
- Other (list not comprehensive)
    - ○ Endometrial cells in a woman at or older than 40 years of age

From Solomon D, Davey D, Kurman R, et al. The 2001 Bethesda System: terminology for reporting results of cervical cytology. JAMA 2002;287:2114–2119.
Automated review and ancillary testing (include as appropriate).
Educational notes and suggestions (optional).

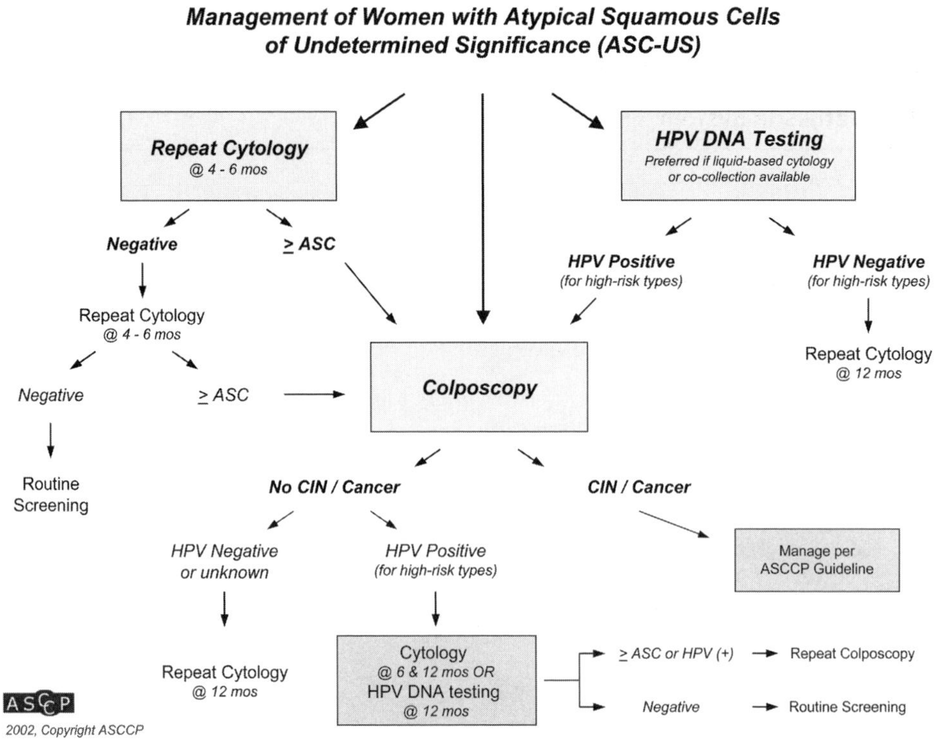

FIGURE 4.3 ● ASCUS (atypical squamous cells of undetermined significance) algorithm. (From the Journal of Lower Genital Tract Disease, Vol. 6, Issue 2; reprinted with the permission of ASCCP © American Society for Colposcopy and Cervical Pathology 2002. No copies of the algorithms may be made without the prior consent of ASCCP.)

manage those patients testing positive for high-risk HPV types that do not have evidence of dysplasia on colposcopically directed biopsy.

Liquid-based cytology with reflex HPV testing for patients with ASCUS appears to be the preferred management approach and is supported by the recent Consensus Guidelines by the American Society for Colposcopy and Cervical Pathology (ASCCP) (30). If negative, patients can be reassured and routine yearly screening resumed. If positive, patients are referred to colposcopy. If repeat cytology in 4 to 6 months is used, the patient should be referred to colposcopy if her repeat Pap smear shows at least ASCUS. Otherwise, she can be returned to yearly screening after two consecutive negative Pap smears at 4- to 6-month intervals are obtained. If immediate colposcopy is performed, those patients without evidence of dysplasia can be returned to routine yearly screening.

Atypical Squamous Cells of Uncertain Significance in Special Circumstances

Special circumstances include postmenopausal women, immunosuppressed women, and pregnant women. For postmenopausal women with a diagnosis of ASCUS on Pap smear, a short course of 8 to 12 weeks of intravaginal estrogen is recommended, provided the patient has no contraindications and shows clinical evidence of atrophy. Cytology should then be repeated 1 week after completing the treatment and again in 4 to 6 months if negative. If either the first or second repeat cytology shows at least ASCUS, the patient needs colposcopy.

All immunosuppressed women such as those infected with HIV should be referred for immediate colposcopy. The management of pregnant women with ASCUS on Pap smear should be the same as in nonpregnant women.

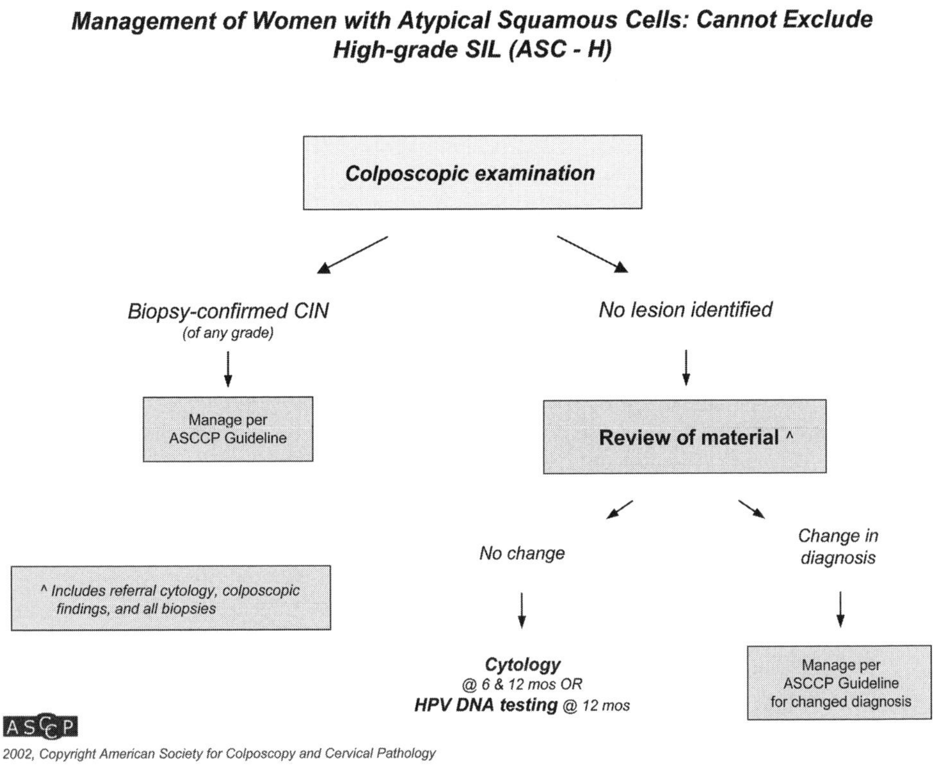

FIGURE 4.4 ● ASC-H (atypical squamous cells, cannot exclude high-grade squamous intraepithelial lesions) algorithm. (From the Journal of Lower Genital Tract Disease, Vol. 6, Issue 2; reprinted with the permission of ASCCP © American Society for Colposcopy and Cervical Pathology 2002. No copies of the algorithms may be made without the prior consent of ASCCP.)

Management of Women With Atypical Squamous Cells—Cannot Exclude High-Grade Lesions

The new diagnosis of ASC-H is believed to apply to 5 to 10% of all ASC cases (29). Women with ASC-H should be referred for immediate colposcopy as is illustrated in Figure 4.4. In cases in which no corresponding lesion can be found or when biopsies show inflammation only, a qualified pathologist should review all histologic and cytologic material on that patient and determine if correlation of cytologic and histologic findings can be established. If histologic findings explain the diagnosis of ASC-H, patients can be followed with repeat cytology at 6 or 12 months versus HPV DNA testing at 12 months. If the review changes the diagnosis to dysplasia, management of the patient needs to be adjusted accordingly. In cases that are highly suspicious for high-grade dysplasia in the absence of a lesion on colposcopy of the cervix, colposcopy of the vagina and endocervical curettage, or a diagnostic excision procedure, may be indicated.

ATYPICAL GLANDULAR CELLS

The classification of glandular cell abnormalities has undergone significant revisions in the new Bethesda System. The former diagnosis of "AGUS (atypical glandular cells of undetermined significance)" has been eliminated and atypical glandular cells (AGC) are now classified as endocervical, endometrial, or glandular cells not otherwise specified (AGC-NOS). Furthermore, AGC is classified as "favor neoplasia" or "endocervical adenocarcinoma in situ (AIS)." A diagnosis if AGC is not common, with a reported frequency between 0.13% and 2.5% (56, 57). A larger percentage (10 to 39%) of patients with AGC than those with ASCUS have been shown to have underlying high-grade lesions, including CIN II, CIN III, AIS, or invasive cancer (58, 59).

Management of Women With Atypical Glandular Cells

The management of patients with AGC is illustrated in Figure 4.5. The most common changes that result in an AGC Pap result are chronic cervicitis, endometriosis, and Arias-Stella reaction, to list a few. The differential diagnosis, however, just includes low- and high-grade CIN, AIS, adenocarcinoma of the cervix, and endometrial hyperplasia or carcinoma. The majority of patients with AGC will have underlying CIN, and the initial workup for all patients with AGC includes a colposcopy and endocervical sampling (60). Repeat cytologic testing alone is associated with lower sensitivities than colposcopy for the detection of CIN in patients with AGC (61). Therefore, all patients diagnosed with AGC-NOS or AGC favor neoplasia should be referred for immediate colposcopy, endocervical sampling, and, if the patient is older than 35 years or has unexplained vaginal bleeding, an endometrial biopsy. If these tests are negative and the initial diagnosis was AGC-NOS, the Pap should be repeated in 4- to 6-month intervals until four consecutive normal tests are obtained. However, if the diagnosis of AGC persists, referral to a specialist versus a diagnostic excision procedure is highly recommended. If the initial diagnosis was "AGC favor neoplasia" or AIS, a diagnostic excision procedure is required because the incidence of premalignant or malignant lesions in patients with this diagnosis is high. There is currently no role for HPV testing in the management of women with a cytologic diagnosis of AGC (60).

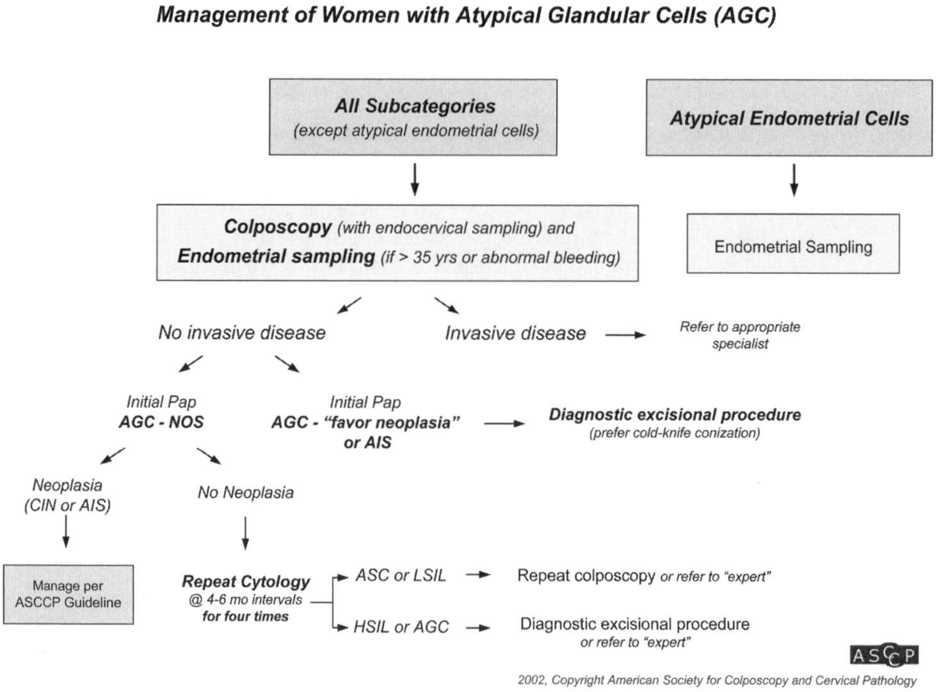

FIGURE 4.5 ● AGC (atypical glandular cells) algorithm. (From the Journal of Lower Genital Tract Disease, Vol. 6, Issue 2; reprinted with the permission of ASCCP © American Society for Colposcopy and Cervical Pathology 2002. No copies of the algorithms may be made without the prior consent of ASCCP.)

SQUAMOUS INTRAEPITHELIAL LESIONS

The new Bethesda System retains the two-tiered terminology of low- and high-grade squamous intraepithelial lesions (LSIL/HSIL). This distinction has been shown to be quite reproducible between pathologists, whereas the subdivision of cytologic HSIL into moderate and severe is more difficult to reproduce. Nonetheless, the three-tiered CIN I/II/III system also remains in use either as an alternative to the LSIL/HSIL terminology or as an additional set of descriptive terms (29).

Management of Women With Low-Grade Squamous Intraepithelial Lesions

Laboratories in the United States report the diagnosis of LSIL between 1.6% and 7.7% of the time, depending on the population served. However, 15 to 30% of women with LSIL on Pap smear will harbor CIN II or III on colposcopically directed biopsy (62, 63). Most patients with LSIL on Pap have CIN I, which tends to regress on its own. Table 4.4 summarizes the general progression of cervical lesions. Alternatively, no cervical lesion may be found colposcopically secondary to complete excision of a lesion by biopsy. The old suggestion of repeat cytology for LSIL has been largely abandoned due to high rates of loss to follow-up and the relatively high incidence of finding true pathology.

Currently, the ASCCP recommends that all women with LSIL undergo colposcopy (Fig. 4.6), except for those in "special circumstances" (see the Low-Grade Squamous Intraepithelial Lesions in Special Circumstances section). Individual treatment options should only be offered following a precise histologic diagnosis. Initial management of LSIL generally does not include any excisional or ablative procedures because these are reserved for documented dysplasia. Nor is there a role for HPV testing because its specificity was shown to be quite low (47). Rather, management depends on colposcopic findings and often can be adjusted to the individual patient's situation.

If colposcopy is satisfactory and a lesion is identified, a biopsy of the lesion should be taken and endocervical curettage is optional. If no lesion is identified on colposcopy, endocervical curettage is strongly recommended if the patient is not pregnant. Likewise, in the setting of

TABLE 4.4

Further Review of Evolution of Cervical Dysplasia

	Grade of Dysplasia		
	Within 2 yr	**Within 5 yr**	**Within 10 yr**
Progression			
Mild to moderate or worse	11.1%	20.4%	28.8%
Mild to severe or worse	2.1%	5.5%	9.9%
Moderate to severe or worse	16.3%	25.1%	32%
Regression			
Mild to first normal Pap	44.3%	74 %	87.7%
Moderate to first normal Pap	33 %	63.1%	82.9%
Mild to second normal Pap	8.7%	39.1%	62.2%
Moderate to second normal Pap	6.9%	29 %	53.7%

Adapted from Holowaty P, Miller AB, Rohan T, et al. Natural history of dysplasia of the uterine cervix. J Natl Cancer Inst 1999;91:252–258, with permission.

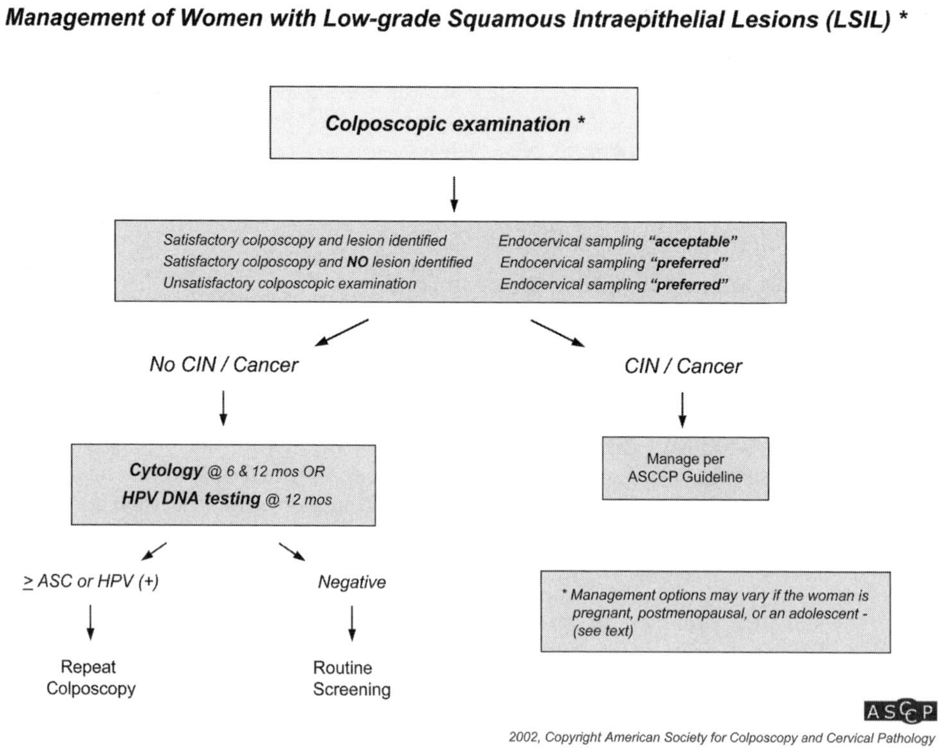

FIGURE 4.6 ● LSIL (low-grade squamous intraepithelial lesions) algorithm. (From the Journal of Lower Genital Tract Disease, Vol. 6, Issue 2; reprinted with the permission of ASCCP © American Society for Colposcopy and Cervical Pathology 2002. No copies of the algorithms may be made without the prior consent of ASCCP.)

an unsatisfactory colposcopy (i.e., if a lesion is not seen in its entirety or if the transformation zone is not entirely visible), endocervical curettage should be performed unless the patient is pregnant.

For both satisfactory and unsatisfactory colposcopic examinations where endocervical curettage and biopsy fail to detect dysplasia, several management options are available. Generally, the patient can be reassured and asked to follow-up for repeat cytology in 6 and 12 months with referral for repeat colposcopy for a Pap smear of at least ASCUS. Alternatively, HPV testing can be offered at 12 months with referral to colposcopy if positive for a high-risk type at that time. The risk of missing dysplasia in cases with satisfactory or unsatisfactory colposcopy but no identifiable lesion is unclear. Some investigators believe a fair number of such patients would be diagnosed with dysplasia on a subsequent LEEP specimen, even though several small studies on patients with LSIL and biopsy confirmed CIN I or unsatisfactory colposcopy after LSIL Pap smear demonstrated only very low rates of significant dysplasia (64). It is no longer recommended that every woman with LSIL Pap and unsatisfactory colposcopy necessarily undergo LEEP cone biopsy.

Low-Grade Squamous Intraepithelial Lesions in Special Circumstances

Postmenopausal women with LSIL Pap smears may be managed without initial colposcopy by simply repeating cytology in 4 to 6 months. If two negative repeat Pap smears are obtained, the patient may return to routine screening. If any repeat Pap smear is ASCUS or above, the patient should be referred to colposcopy. Alternatively, HPV testing at 12 months can be offered with referral to colposcopy if positive for a high-risk type. For women with clinical or cytologic evidence of atrophy in the absence of contraindications to estrogen therapy, a course of intravaginal estrogen followed by repeat Pap smear 1 week after completing therapy may be tried.

Pregnant women with LSIL Pap smear should undergo colposcopy by an experienced clinician. Biopsy of lesions is preferred if high-grade dysplasia or cancer is suspected and may also be performed for low-grade appearing lesions. In cases of unsatisfactory colposcopy in pregnancy, repeat examination is recommended in 6 to 12 weeks because chances are high that colposcopy will become satisfactory as pregnancy progresses. Endocervical curettage should not be performed on a pregnant patient. Similarly, diagnostic excisional procedures are only indicated if invasive cancer is suspected. Follow-up colposcopy and cytology should be performed no sooner than 6 weeks postpartum.

Adolescents may also be treated with repeat cytology at 6 and 12 months or undergo HPV testing at 12 months with referral to colposcopy for either ASCUS or higher or for positive high-risk HPV DNA testing after 12 months. This approach needs to be individualized depending on follow-up reliability.

Management of Women With High-Grade Squamous Intraepithelial Lesions

Women with HSIL on Pap have a 70 to 75% chance of having CIN II–III and a 1 to 2% chance of having invasive cancer (30). Thus, colposcopy with biopsies and endocervical curettage are indicated for all women with this diagnosis, except for pregnant women in whom endocervical curettage is contraindicated (Fig. 4.7). If no cervical lesion is identified, a vaginal lesion must be ruled out as the etiology of the Pap smear. If a thorough diagnostic evaluation does not reveal a lesion with biopsy-proven high-grade dysplasia, but rather no lesion is visualized or biopsy shows CIN I, a qualified and experienced pathologist should review all available cytologic and histologic material. Sometimes, a correlation can be established between findings on cytology testing and biopsy results to explain the apparent discrepancy (65–67). However, if the review

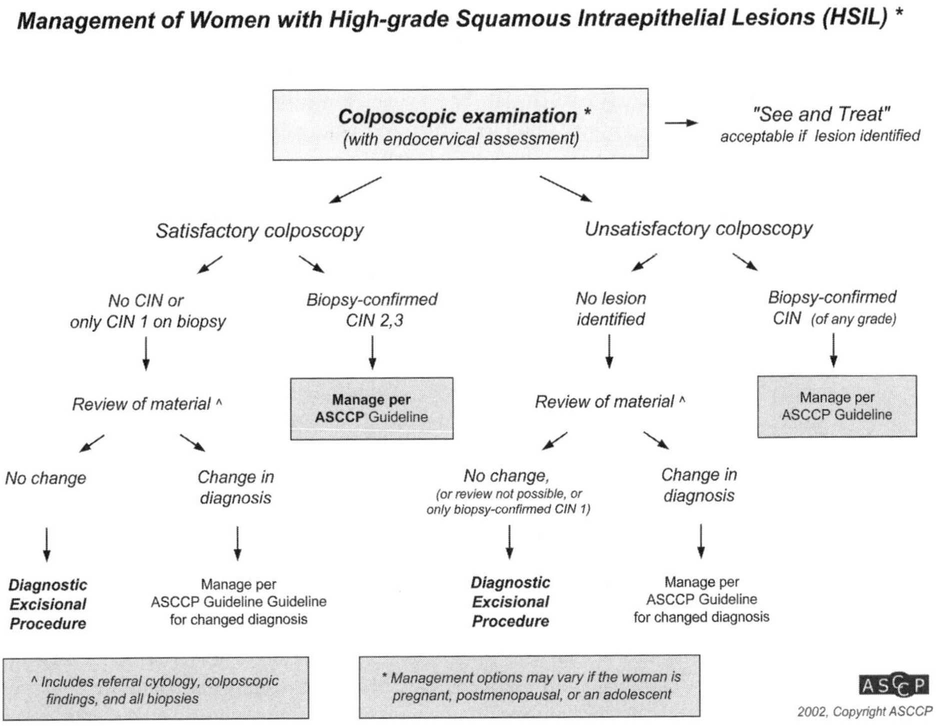

FIGURE 4.7 • HSIL (high-grade squamous intraepithelial lesions) algorithm. (From the Journal of Lower Genital Tract Disease, Vol. 6, Issue 2; reprinted with the permission of ASCCP © American Society for Colposcopy and Cervical Pathology 2002. No copies of the algorithms may be made without the prior consent of ASCCP.)

does not explain the observed discrepancy, a diagnostic excision procedure is indicated. The same management should be applied to an unsatisfactory colposcopic examination when no lesion can be identified or when biopsy shows CIN I. Ablative therapy with cryotherapy, topical concentrated trichloroacetic acid (TCA), or cold coagulation is not an option in women with HSIL on Pap to avoid the possibility of ablating an underlying malignancy.

Some practitioners question whether a cervical lesion in a pregnant patient with HSIL on Pap should necessarily be biopsied because of concerns over increased bleeding risk. Studies have shown that the risk of missing cancer in a pregnant patient far outweighs the small risk of bleeding from a biopsy site. No reports of life-threatening hemorrhage or pregnancy loss secondary to cervical biopsies have been substantiated. However, as mentioned previously, endocervical curettage is contraindicated in pregnancy.

For high-risk populations with large numbers of patients being lost to follow-up, the so-called "see and treat" strategy has been advocated as a safe and cost-effective approach to treating women with HSIL, especially in the hands of an expert colposcopist (68, 69). This strategy allows for a LEEP cone to be performed at the time of colposcopy if a suspicious lesion is identified. Older women in whom fertility preservation is not crucial may also benefit from such an approach to treatment.

Young, nulliparous women with HSIL on Pap in whom no lesion with CIN II–III can be identified may be observed with repeat colposcopy and cytology every 4 to 6 months for up to 1 year provided that endocervical curettage is negative and the patient is willing to accept the risk of missing a lesion. If HSIL persists, a diagnostic excision procedure is indicated.

DIAGNOSIS AND TREATMENT OF CERVICAL DYSPLASIA

Colposcopy

Colposcopy is the close visual inspection of the cervix, vagina, and anogenital area using magnified illumination and the application of specific solutions that highlight abnormal areas. Its main purpose is to help the clinician identify and biopsy target lesions and to rule out neoplasia. Colposcopy is indicated for any cytologic test showing ASCUS with positive HPV test or persistent ASCUS, ASC-H, AGC, LSIL, HSIL, or suspicion for invasive disease. A gross lesion on the cervix should be examined and biopsied colposcopically. Other possible indications depend on the clinical scenario and can include postcoital or unexplained bleeding, history of exposure to DES in utero, history of vulvar or vaginal neoplasia, or genital warts (condylomata acuminata).

Every time a patient presents for colposcopy, it is important to take a complete medical, surgical, and social history to elicit possible risk factors for dysplasia. The practitioner should also remember that a good visual examination of the vulva and perineum, a speculum exam of vagina and cervix, and a bimanual exam to rule out obvious pelvic pathology need to be part of every patient visit for colposcopy.

Colposcopy is performed with the patient in the dorsal lithotomy position using a standard speculum. First, a cotton swab with normal saline is applied to the cervix to clear it of mucus and debris. This application facilitates the visualization of hyperkeratosis (white epithelium seen before the application of acetic acid) and allows for biopsy of such areas. Atypical vessels can also be seen with saline alone, often in conjunction with the green filter on the colposcope. These "corkscrew"-like vessels can be the hallmark of invasive cancer (Fig. 4.8).

Second, 3% or 5% acetic acid is liberally applied to the cervix. After 30 seconds, the cervix should be carefully inspected under low power and high power. Abnormalities commonly seen include acetowhite epithelium (due to abnormal intracellular keratin and protein agglutination, as well as cellular dehydration) suggestive of both low- and high-grade dysplasia (Fig. 4.9), and vascular abnormalities such as mosaicism and punctation (Fig. 4.10). These two findings often result from the capillary proliferative effect of HPV and as an effect of tumor angiogenesis factor. Although acetowhite epithelium and mosaicism/punctation may also be seen in association with benign processes such as inflammation and normal metaplastic transformation, biopsy of such lesions is always recommended.

Third, Lugol's iodine may be applied to the cervix and/or the vaginal walls (Fig. 4.11). This solution is particularly useful when looking for a vaginal lesion because normal ectocervical and

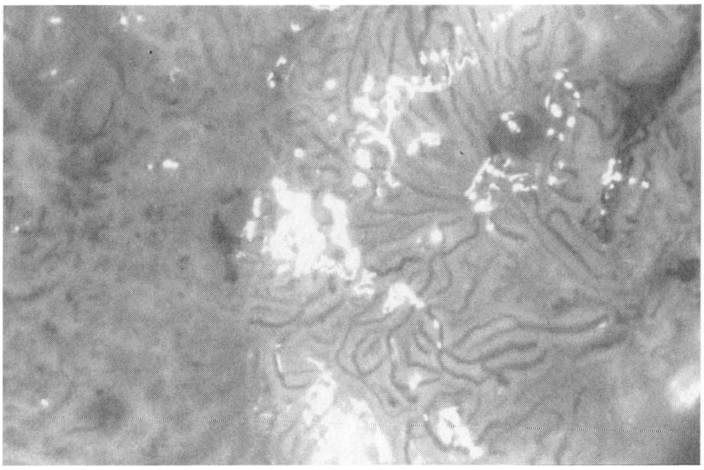

FIGURE 4.8 • Colposcopic view of "corkscrew" (atypical) vessels. (Courtesy of Matthew A. Powell, MD.)

vaginal squamous epithelium stains dark brown with its application while columnar, squamous metaplastic, or dysplastic epithelium appears light yellow. This effect is due to the presence of glycogen in normal squamous epithelium. Lugol's iodine may be helpful in detecting subtle dysplastic lesions on the cervix and in the vagina, although both a high false-negative and a high false-positive rate have been described.

Colposcopy is deemed satisfactory if the entire transformation zone is visualized because the incidence of dysplasia above this junction is minimal. Almost all cervical neoplasia arises in the transformation zone, which is defined as the area between the original squamocolumnar junction and the colposcopically visible new squamocolumnar junction. An unsatisfactory colposcopic exam either does not allow for full visualization of the new squamocolumnar junction and transformation zone or for full visualization of the extent of a lesion.

Endocervical curettage assesses the portion of the endocervical canal not visualized by colposcopy. It may help in the detection of occult lesions of the endocervix especially because both AGC and AIS are often associated with squamous CIN lesions (70). In the context of satisfactory colposcopy, the value of routine endocervical curettage is questionable. However, it is recommended for the practitioner with limited colposcopic experience and in the absence

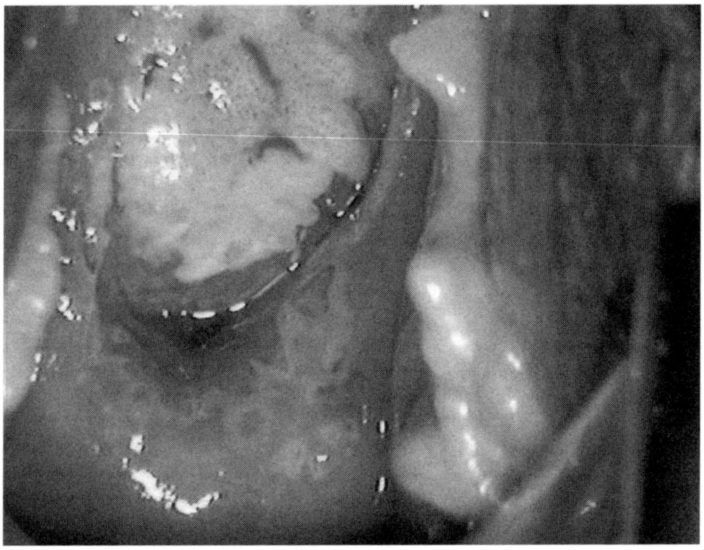

FIGURE 4.9 • Colposcopic view of acetowhite epithelium. (Courtesy of Matthew A. Powell, MD.)

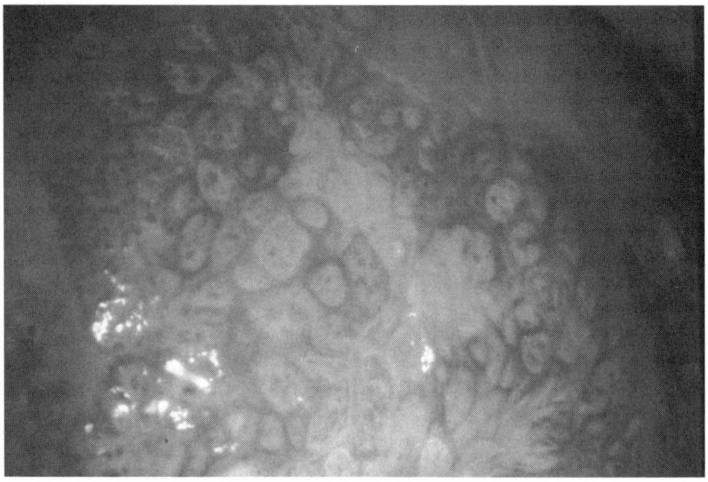

FIGURE 4.10 ● Colposcopic view of mosaicism and punctation. (Courtesy of Matthew A. Powell, MD.)

of a visible lesion. Some literature suggests that collection of an endocervical specimen with a cytobrush instead of a Kevorkian curette may be more sensitive than endocervical curettage for the detection of squamous and glandular abnormalities, although specificity is lower (71).

All colposcopic findings should be recorded on a schematic drawing labeled such that another health care provider can easily reconstruct the location and extent of all visualized lesions, their appearance, biopsy sites, and the adequacy of the exam. Photo or video documentation can also be helpful.

Ablative Treatment of Cervical Dysplasia

Ablative treatment strategies generally do not yield a histologic specimen. It is therefore extremely important to make an accurate tissue diagnosis of dysplasia and to rule out any possibility of invasive disease prior to proceeding with ablative treatment. However, reports of missed invasive cancer have been published in conjunction with all forms of ablative treatment. It has thus fallen out of favor with many physicians and has been largely replaced by LEEP.

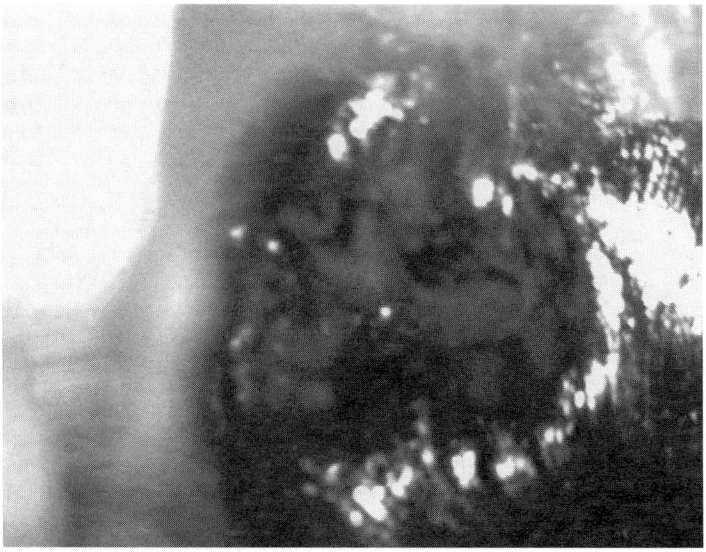

FIGURE 4.11 ● Colposcopic view of cervix with Lugol's iodine. (Courtesy of Matthew A. Powell, MD.)

Topical concentrated TCA (50 to 80%) has been used as a topical ablative treatment for dysplasia both in the cervix and in the vagina. It should be applied with colposcopic guidance. However, failure rates even after multiple applications are significant, and patients must be monitored closely for the persistence of disease.

Cold coagulation is a popular ablative treatment in Europe. Despite its name, it uses a 100°C Teflon probe that is directly applied to the cervix. Two to five applications of less than a minute each per treatment lead to destruction of the transformation zone. Reported failure rates of this method are around 7%, and the procedure is short, pain free, and relatively inexpensive.

Cryotherapy is another type of ablative treatment that is cost effective and easily performed in the outpatient setting. Similar to cold coagulation, cryotherapy is well suited for persistent biopsy confirmed low-grade lesions that are less than 3 cm in diameter and do not extend into the endocervical canal. It should not be performed if the patient has active cervicitis or is menstruating. In fact, it is preferably done during the early part of the menstrual cycle to prevent possible outlet obstruction at the time of menstruation. Cryotherapy leads to destruction of the transformation zone via cryonecrosis using the evaporation of liquid refrigerants, most commonly nitrous oxide (N_2O). Compressed N_2O is allowed to expand through a small jet producing an ice ball at the tip of a metal probe, which is brought in contact with the surface to be destroyed. Cell death results from crystallization of intracellular water at –20 to –30°C. To achieve a 5-mm depth of freezing, the probe must cover the entire transformation zone and produce a total lateral spread of freeze of 7 mm. Creasman advocates a freeze-thaw-freeze technique (3-5-3 minutes) with a repeated freeze after the tissues have visually thawed from the first freeze (72). With this technique, he observed a decrease in failure rates from 29 to 7%. Other investigators claim similar success with only one freeze. It is important to warn the patient of a watery, foul-smelling discharge after cryotherapy and to enforce pelvic rest for 4 weeks.

Carbon dioxide (CO_2) laser vaporization is still a widely used ablative treatment for dysplasia. The CO_2 laser is mounted on a colposcope and controlled via a micromanipulator that controls the beam. The surgeon can adjust spot size, power, and mode settings. The entire transformation zone must be visualized with acetic acid or Lugol's prior to initiating laser treatment. Flowers and McCall recommend the following conditions to maximize the success of the procedure: (a) destruction of the lesion to a visual depth of 5 to 7 mm ensures the treatment of glandular involvement; (b) a 5-mm visible width beyond the lesion is recommended; (c) a continuous tissue exposure mode setting should be used; and (d) if the equipment permits, high-power settings of at least 20 to 25 W or higher should be used to minimize lateral thermal damage (73). The patient can be given local anesthesia via a paracervical block. Also, use of a defocused beam and/or vasopressive injectable agents can control bleeding. If used appropriately, laser vaporization can be very effective in treating cervical dysplasia with failure rates of less than 5%.

Excisional Treatment of Cervical Dysplasia

Excisional treatment of cervical dysplasia is highly effective whether it is used to perform a cone biopsy or simply to treat a persistent low-grade lesion. It always has the advantage of producing a pathologic specimen confirming the initial diagnosis and assessing the margins of excision.

Cold-knife conization is the old standard for performing a cone biopsy. Although indications for cone biopsy have remained unchanged (Table 4.5), several other methods have been shown to be equally effective for performing a cone biopsy with adequate and interpretable margins. Some physicians still prefer cold-knife conization for certain clinical scenarios, such as AGC favor neoplasia or endocervical adenocarcinoma in situ, although operator experience for cone versus LEEP should be considered. Cold-knife conization is performed in the operating room usually under general anesthesia. After colposcopic examination, lateral sutures at 3 and 9 o'clock are placed for traction and hemostasis. The portio of the cervix is infiltrated with a vasopressive agent, and the endocervical canal is sounded to determine length and direction. The cone-shaped specimen is then excised using a scalpel after tagging it at 12 o'clock with a suture for proper orientation. Hemostasis is achieved using cautery or simple U sutures anteriorly and posteriorly. This technique avoids distortion of the remaining anatomy, which can make follow-up quite difficult. Disadvantages of cold-knife conization over other methods include higher cost

TABLE 4.5

Indications for Cone Biopsy

- Unsatisfactory colposcopy
  - Inability to see the entire transformation zone
  - Inability to see the full extent of a lesion
- Treatment of biopsy-proven high-grade dysplasia
- Suspicion for microinvasive squamous cell carcinoma
- Atypical glandular cells—favor neoplastic
- Endocervical adenocarcinoma in situ
- Two-grade discrepancy between cytologic, colposcopic, or histologic diagnosis
- Positive endocervical curettage

secondary to the need for an operating room, higher risk for bleeding and infection, and higher incidence of cervical incompetence and stenosis. Success rates in competent hands exceed 95%.

LEEP of the transformation zone is currently the preferred method for performing either a true cone biopsy (diagnostic LEEP) or a simple excision procedure (therapeutic LEEP). It has been shown in multiple studies to be equally effective as cold-knife or laser conization. Furthermore, most studies agree that difficulty in interpreting margins secondary to cautery artifact is quite rare and is easily outweighed by the many advantages of the procedure (74).

LEEP can be performed in the outpatient setting with local anesthesia via a paracervical block. Bleeding is only seen in about 2 to 5% of patients and is rarely heavy. Similarly, infection rates are quite low as compared with cold-knife conization. Cervical incompetence and stenosis are rare occurrences (less than 1% of patients), although they remain an important part of the informed consent for the procedure. Last, the equipment to perform LEEPs in the outpatient setting is relatively inexpensive, and the skills needed to perform the procedure are readily acquired.

Prior to performing a LEEP, the patient should undergo colposcopy as is required before the other excisional procedures. A plastic-coated speculum attached to suction is used that may also have vaginal sidewall retractors to achieve optimal exposure of the cervix and minimize the risk for thermal injury to the vaginal fornices. Depending on the size of the lesion, the correct size loop is chosen, and the cervix is anesthetized. It is important to ensure the patient has a grounding pad attached to her thigh. The electrosurgical generator should be set to 55 W of pure cutting or blended current. The surgeon can control the generator with the handle of the loop and excises the specimen with the loop perpendicular to the cervix either from side to side or from top to bottom. A visible margin of 2 mm should be left next to the lesion of interest, and a depth of approximately 5 to 7 mm should be achieved. Larger lesions may require more than one pass. Also, if a true cone biopsy is required, the surgeon can switch to a smaller loop and excise an additional endocervical specimen giving the two specimens combined a "top hat" configuration. Bleeding of the LEEP bed is controlled with electrocautery, and the use of a ball electrode and/or the application of Monsel's solution. Patients are placed on pelvic rest for 3 to 4 weeks after the procedure.

FUTURE DIRECTIONS: A HUMAN PAPILLOMAVIRUS VACCINE

Research on both prophylactic and therapeutic HPV vaccines is ongoing (75, 76). The important role of the immune system in modulating the response to HPV infection is illustrated by the fact that 60% of low-grade cervical dysplasia resolves on its own, as well as by the observation that immunosuppressed patients are at much higher risk for HPV infection and persistence. The E6 and E7 gene product of high-risk HPV types form the basis of proposed immunotherapy because their role in the immortalization of human keratinocytes is well known. In addition, these two proteins are ideal targets for the development of a vaccine because they have no sequence homology to human cellular proteins. Their continued expression in cervical tumors appears to be necessary for maintenance of the neoplastic state (77, 78).

Development of a prophylactic HPV vaccine would require the induction of antibody production before viral infection occurs. However, a vaccine based on crude viral extracts or inactivated virus has not been achieved thus far secondary to the inability of culturing HPV. Papillomavirus-like particles (VLPs) formed from viral major capsid proteins L1 and L2 can be synthesized with microbial or cellular expression systems (79, 80). In early trials, vaccines with HPV-16 VLPs were generally well tolerated and generated high levels of antibodies against HPV-16 (81).

In 2002, the results from a double-blind, multicenter, randomized clinical trial performed to determine whether a vaccine could prevent HPV-16 infection in women were released (82). The study included 1533 women between the ages of 16 and 23 years of age who were randomized to receive either a placebo or the vaccine at baseline, month 2, and month 6. The women in the trial had no history of abnormal Pap smears and reported less than five male sex partners in their lifetime. After a median of 17.4 months of follow-up from completed vaccination, the results showed that in the vaccine group, the incidence of persistent HPV-16 infection was 0 per 100 women at risk. The placebo group had an incidence of HPV-16 infection of 3.8 per 100 women at risk. All cases of new HPV-16 infection ($n = 41$) occurred among placebo recipients, as did all cases of cervical dysplasia. Antibody conversion occurred in 99.7% of the vaccinated women. Adverse events were similar in both groups. Although longer follow-up is needed to determine persistence of HPV-16 antibodies and rates of cervical cancer, this study is the best evidence to date that a vaccine approach to the prevention of cervical cancer can be successful.

More recent data from a mouse model has led to the hypothesis that cell-mediated immune responses may be useful in both the development of a prophylactic and a therapeutic vaccine (83). Traditionally, a therapeutic vaccine is used to fight an already existing infection. The E6 and E7 gene products are tumor-specific antigens and as such are known to be of major importance in the T-cell–mediated immune response against high-risk HPV–mediated cervical tumors. Although several studies report to have successfully generated a cytotoxic T-cell–mediated immune response in vivo against several peptides derived from HPV-16 E7, they were unable to demonstrate a clinical response in cervical cancer patients to date (84–86). Attempts to further refine this approach are currently underway.

MANAGEMENT OF VAGINAL AND VULVAR INTRAEPITHELIAL NEOPLASIA

Vaginal intraepithelial neoplasia (VAIN) is presumed to have a similar natural history as CIN, although it has been less extensively studied. It accounts for approximately 0.4% of all lower genital tract neoplasia (87). In the past when many women underwent hysterectomy as excisional treatment for high-grade dysplasia, VAIN was noted to develop in about 5% of these women postoperatively, usually at the vaginal cuff suture line. HPV and high-risk sexual behavior have been implicated in its etiology (88, 89). Thus, risk factors are presumed to be the same as for cervical dysplasia, as is explained by the "field effect" of the lower genital tract.

Similar to cervical dysplasia, VAIN is reported as VAIN I through III. The progression risk of VAIN to invasive cancer has been less well established. Only very limited series have been published reporting an overall progression risk to cancer of 9%, with 13% persistence and 78% spontaneous regression (90). Some investigators report that almost 30% of patients undergoing an excision procedure for VAIN III were found to have underlying cancer (91).

The diagnosis of VAIN is made by vaginal colposcopy (Fig. 4.12). Acetic acid should be used, and care must be taken to achieve optimal exposure of the sometimes redundant vaginal vault in its entirety. Lugol's iodine may also be helpful. VAIN can be both unifocal or multifocal with discrete or coalescent lesions. The most common reason to perform colposcopy of the vagina is a posthysterectomy Pap smear of at least ASCUS. Any suspicious-appearing lesions should be biopsied. Scarring or involution of vaginal tissue during closure of the vaginal cuff at hysterectomy can sometimes obscure the vaginal cuff area, precluding visual identification of a lesion. Therefore, in the absence of an identifiable lesion during vaginal colposcopy, it is sometimes necessary to excise a cuff scar or extensively biopsy the vaginal cuff area.

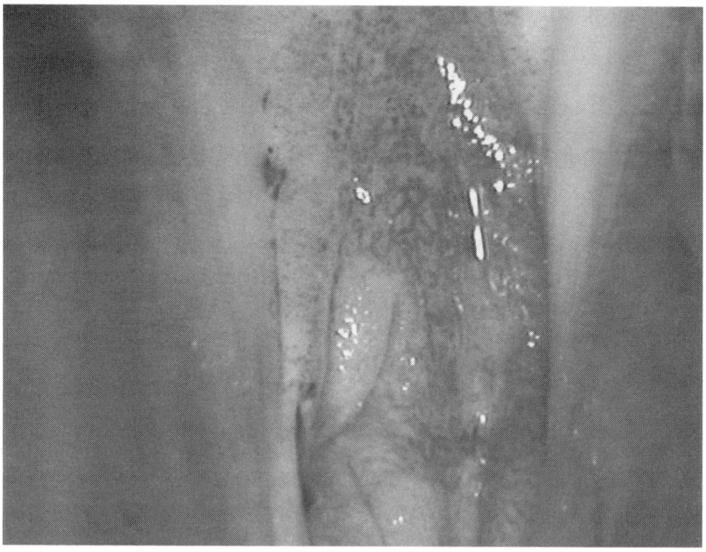

FIGURE 4.12 ● Colposcopic view of vaginal intraepithelial neoplasia. (Courtesy of Matthew A. Powell, MD.)

Treatment for VAIN can be accomplished by CO_2 laser vaporization. However, optimal depth of ablation and success rates are variable in the literature. Thus, it is recommended that an experienced clinician perform the procedure. Topical 5-fluorouracil (5-FU) cream has also been advocated as a treatment option for VAIN. Although this treatment is easy to administer, it is associated with considerable side effects and variable success rates. Some investigators report particularly high failure and recurrence rates with 5-FU alone and prefer combining this topical agent with subsequent surgical excision. Excision alone in the form of upper vaginectomy is the treatment modality with the highest reported success rates. Secondary to the risk of injury to rectum and bladder during this procedure, it should only be performed in the operating room by an experienced surgeon. Overall cure rates of 94% have been reported for patients with VAIN after a combination of surgery and ablation or 5-FU were performed (92).

Vulvar intraepithelial neoplasia (VIN) was first described by Bowen in 1912 as a precancerous dermatosis (93). It is more common in immunocompromised and postmenopausal women but can also be seen in healthy younger women. Risk factors are similar to those associated with cervical dysplasia, and HPV-16 is the most commonly associated HPV subtype. Up to 50% of patients with VIN also have CIN or VAIN (87).

Patients with VIN often present with symptoms of vulvar irritation and pruritus or a palpable and visible lesion they have noticed. Most patients, however, are asymptomatic, and disease is noted during routine gynecologic examination. Lesions are unifocal or multifocal; can appear gray, white, or reddish in color; and may be raised or flat. They can involve the labia majora and minora, the periclitoral area, and/or the perianal area. Lesions are sometimes seen extending into the vagina or involving the urethra or anus. Acetic acid of at least 5% strength should be applied for 4 to 5 minutes, but it is not always helpful in diagnosing VIN, and any suspicious-appearing lesion should be biopsied.

As is the case with both CIN and VAIN, VIN may regress spontaneously, persist or recur after treatment, or progress to invasive cancer. VIN II–III has been associated with underlying occult cancer in about 8% of cases. Progression rates of 2 to 18% have been reported; however, VIN is rarely left untreated, and most physicians would only allow for very brief periods of observation before proceeding with definite treatment (94, 95).

Treatment can be either excisional or ablative after the possibility of malignancy is ruled out. Topical treatment with 5-FU is associated with significant patient discomfort and variable success rates. It is thus rarely used for the treatment of VIN. The most common forms of treatment include both CO_2 laser ablation and wide local excision. Laser ablation is preferred for smaller lesions in non–hair-bearing regions. Its downsides include a substantial amount of postoperative pain and a fairly slow healing process, as well as the absence of a pathologic specimen. Wide local excision is preferred with localized as opposed to multifocal disease. It allows for precise excision of such lesions and the pathologic assessment of margins. A 5-mm margin of uninvolved tissue is believed by most to be adequate for VIN (87) whenever this is possible without compromising surrounding structures. For large lesions, skinning vulvectomy with the creation of skin flaps can be used, whereas for extensive multifocal disease, a combination of surgery and laser ablation is often recommended.

Clinical Notes

- HPV is associated with 99.7% of all cervical cancers.
- Ten percent to 20% of reproductive age women have asymptomatic HPV infection.
- HPV is most prevalent in women younger than 25 years of age with a second peak in prevalence after age 55.
- Risk factors: frequency of intercourse, number of lifetime sexual partners, male partner's number of lifetime sexual partners, age, ethnicity, smoking, living with smokers.
- HPV-infected women have a relative risk of 20 to 70% for developing cervical cancer, a four-fold increased risk for ASCUS/LSIL, and a 13-fold increased risk for HSIL.
- Progression to/persistence of high-grade dysplasia: ASCUS 7%, LSIL 21%, and HSIL 24% at 24 months.
- The only FDA-approved assay for HPV testing: HC II.
- Risk factors for developing cervical dysplasia: HPV infection, HIV, multiple sexual partners, early age at first intercourse, high parity, smoking, low socioeconomic status.
- Liquid-based cytology: higher detection rate of LSIL, HSIL, and ASCUS, but higher cost; can be used for reflex HPV testing with HC II.
- Sensitivity of HPV testing as screening modality for cervical dysplasia is at least 10% higher than conventional cytology screening.
- Preferred management of ASCUS Pap smears: liquid-based cytology with reflex HPV testing; yearly follow-up if negative, colposcopy if positive.
- Management of ASC-H: colposcopy, histologic correlation; if negative, vaginal colposcopy, endocervical curettage, or diagnostic excision procedure.
- Management of AGC: colposcopy, endocervical curettage, endometrial biopsy if older than 35 years of age or unexplained vaginal bleeding; AGC favor neoplasia: if no diagnosis needs diagnostic excision procedure; AGC-NOS: may repeat cytology.
- Management of LSIL: colposcopy with biopsy; endocervical curettage if no visible lesion (nonpregnant); if no diagnosis, repeat cytology in 6 to 12 months; management of persistent LSIL must be individualized.
- Management of HSIL: colposcopy, biopsy, endocervical curettage; if no diagnosis or discrepant histologic findings, search for vaginal lesion, pathologic correlation, or diagnostic excision procedure.
- Never perform ablative therapy for HSIL cytology or in the absence of histologic diagnosis, excluding occult malignancy.
- Preferred excisional procedure for therapeutic or diagnostic purposes is LEEP.

REFERENCES

1. International Agency for Research on Cancer (IARC), World Health Organization. GLOBOCAN 2000: Cancer Incidence, Mortality and Prevalence Worldwide, Version 1.0. IARC CancerBase No. 5. Lyon: IARCPress, 2001.
2. American Cancer Society (ACS). Cancer Facts & Figures 2002. Atlanta: ACS, 2002. Available at: http://www.cancer.org/docroot/STT/content/STT_1x_Cancer_Facts__ Figures_2002.asp. Accessed June 29, 2005.

3. Wright JD, Herzog TJ. Human papillomavirus: emerging trends in detection and management. Curr Womens Health Rep 2002;2:259–265.
4. Koutsky L. Epidemiology of genital human papillomavirus infection. Am J Med 1997;102:3–8.
5. Unger ER, Duarte-Franco E. Human papillomaviruses: into the new millennium. Obstet Gynecol Clin North Am 2001;28:653–666.
6. Herrero R, Hildesheim A, Bratti C, et al. Population-based study of human papillomavirus infection and cervical neoplasia in rural Costa Rica. J Natl Cancer Inst 2000;92:464–474.
7. Burk RD, Ho GY, Beardsley L, et al. Sexual behavior and partner characteristics are the predominant risk factors for genital human papillomavirus infection in young women. J Infect Dis 1996;174:679–689.
8. Ho GY, Bierman R, Beardsley L, et al. Natural history of cervicovaginal papillomavirus infection in young women. N Engl J Med 1998;338:423–428.
9. Thomas KK, Hughes JP, Kuypers JM, et al. Concurrent and sequential acquisition of different genital human papillomavirus types. J Infect Dis 2000;182:1097–1102.
10. Zur Hausen H, Meinhof W, Schreiber W, et al. Attempts to detect virus-specific DNA sequences in human tumors: nucleic acid hybridization with complementary RNA of human wart virus. Int J Cancer 1974;13:650–656.
11. Walboomers JM, Jacobs MV, Manos MM, et al. Human papillomavirus is a necessary cause of invasive cervical cancer worldwide. J Pathol 1999;189:12–19.
12. Walboomers JM, Meijer CJ. Do HPV-negative cervical carcinomas exist? J Pathol 1997;181:253–254.
13. Wallin KL, Wiklund F, Angstrom T, et al. Type-specific persistence of human papillomavirus DNA before the development of invasive cervical cancer. N Engl J Med 1999;341:1633–1638.
14. Liaw KL, Glass AG, Manos MM, et al. Detection of human papillomavirus DNA in cytologically normal women and subsequent cervical squamous intraepithelial lesions. J Natl Cancer Inst 1999;91:954–960.
15. Melnikow J, Nuovo J, Willan AR, et al. Natural history of cervical squamous intraepithelial lesions: a meta-analysis. Obstet Gynecol 1998;92:727–735.
16. Koutsky LA, Holmes KK, Critchlow CW, et al. A cohort study of the risk of cervical intraepithelial neoplasia grade 2 or 3 in relation to papillomavirus infection. N Engl J Med 1992;327:1272–1278.
17. Vernon SD, Unger ER, Miller DL, et al. Association of human papillomavirus type 16 integration in the E2 gene with poor disease-free survival from cervical cancer. Int J Cancer 1997;74:50–56.
18. Peyton CL, Schiffman M, Lorincz AT, et al. Comparison of PCR- and hybrid capture-based human papillomavirus detection systems using multiple cervical specimen collection strategies. J Clin Microbiol 1998;36:3248–3254.
19. Gravitt PE, Peyton CL, Alessi TQ, et al. Improved amplification of genital human papillomaviruses. J Clin Microbiol 2000;38:357–361.
20. Nobbenhuis MA, Walboomers JM, Helmerhorst TJ, et al. Relation of human papillomavirus status to cervical lesions and consequences for cervical-cancer screening: a prospective study. Lancet 1999;354:20–25.
21. De Roda Husman AM, Walboomers JM, van den Brule AJ, et al. The use of general primers GP5 and GP6 elongated at their 3' ends with adjacent highly conserved sequences improves human papillomavirus detection by PCR. J Gen Virol 1995;76:1057–1062.
22. Josefsson AM, Magnusson PK, Ylitalo N, et al. Viral load of human papillomavirus 16 as a determinant for development of cervical carcinoma in situ: a nested case-control study. Lancet 2000;355:2189–2193.
23. Cohn DE, Herzog TJ. Emerging trends and technologies in cervical cancer screening. Womens Oncol Rev 2001;1:11–15.
24. Sawaya GF, Grimes DA. New technologies in cervical cytology screening: a word of caution. Obstet Gynecol 1999:94:307–310.
25. NIH Consensus Statement Online 1996 April 13;14(1):1–38. Available at: http://www. consensus.nih.gov/cons/102/102_statement.htm. Accessed June 29, 2005.
26. Agency for Health Care Policy and Research (AHCPR). Evaluation of Cervical Cytology: Summary, Evidence Report/Technology Assessment: Number 5. AHCPR Publication No. 99–E010. Rockville, MD: AHCPR, 1999. Available at: http://www.ahrq.gov/clinic/epcsums/cervsumm.htm. Accessed June 29, 2005.
27. Fahey MT, Irwig L, Macaskill P. Meta-analysis of Pap test accuracy. Am J Epidemiol 1995;141:680–689.
28. Soler ME, Blumenthal PD. New technologies in cervical cancer precursor detection. Curr Opin Oncol 2000;12:460–465.
29. Solomon D, Davey D, Kurman R, et al. The 2001 Bethesda System: terminology for reporting results of cervical cytology. JAMA 2002;287:2114–2119.
30. Wright TC, Cox JT, Massad LS, et al. 2001 Consensus guidelines for the management of women with cervical cytological abnormalities. JAMA 2002;287:2120–2129.
31. Hutchinson ML, Zahniser DJ, Sherman ME, et al. Utility of liquid-based cytology for cervical carcinoma screening: results of a population-based study conducted in a region of Costa Rica with a high incidence of cervical carcinoma. Cancer 1999;87:48–55.
32. Diaz-Rosario LA, Kabawat SE. Performance of a fluid-based, thin-layer Papanicolaou smear method in the clinical setting of an independent laboratory and an outpatient screening population in New England. Arch Pathol Lab Med 1999;123:817–821.
33. Vassilakos P, Schwartz D, de Marval F, et al. Biopsy-based comparison of liquid-based, thin-layer preparations to conventional Pap smears. J Reprod Med 2000;45:11–16.
34. Lee KR, Ashfaq R, Birdsong GG, et al. Comparison of conventional Papanicolaou smears and a fluid-based, thin-layer system for cervical cancer screening. Obstet Gynecol 1997;90:278–284.

35. Brown AD, Garber AM. Cost-effectiveness of 3 methods to enhance the sensitivity of Papanicolaou testing. JAMA 1999;281:347–353.
36. Hartmann KE, Nanda K, Hall S, et al. Technologic advances for evaluation of cervical cytology: is newer better? Obstet Gynecol Surv 2001;56:765–774.
37. Montz FJ, Farber FL, Bristow RE, et al. Impact of increasing Papanicolaou test sensitivity and compliance: a modeled cost and outcomes analysis. Obstet Gynecol 2001;97:781–788.
38. PRISMATIC Project Management Team. Assessment of automated primary screening on PAPNET of cervical smears in the PRISMATIC trial. Lancet 1999;353:1381–1385.
39. Wilbur DC, Prey MU, Miller WM. Detection of high grade squamous intraepithelial lesions and tumors using the AutoPap system: results of a primary screening clinical trial. Cancer 1999;87:354–358.
40. Clavel C, Masure M, Bory JP, et al. Hybrid Capture II-based human papillomavirus detection, a sensitive test to detect in routine high-grade cervical lesions: a preliminary study on 1518 women. Br J Cancer 1999;80:1306–1311.
41. Wright TC, Denny L, Kuhn L, et al. HPV DNA testing of self-collected vaginal samples compared with cytologic screening to detect cervical cancer. JAMA 2000;283:81–86.
42. Solomon D, Schiffman M, Tarone R. The Bethesda system for reporting cervical/vaginal cytologic diagnoses. Report of the 1991 Bethesda Workshop. Am J Surg Pathol 1992;16:914–916.
43. Wright TC Jr, Lorincz A, Ferris DG, et al. Reflex human papillomavirus deoxyribonucleic acid testing in women with abnormal Papanicolaou smears. Am J Obstet Gynecol 1998;178:962–966.
44. Solomon D, Schiffman M, Tarrone R. Comparison of three management strategies for patients with atypical squamous cells of undetermined significance. J Natl Cancer Inst. 2001;93:293–299.
45. Eskridge C, Begneaud WP, Landwehr C. Cervicography combined with repeat Papanicolaou test as triage for low-grade cytologic abnormalities. Obstet Gynecol 1998;92:351–355.
46. Sherman ME, Solomon D, Schiffman M. Qualification of ASCUS: a comparison of equivocal LSIL and equivocal HSIL cervical cytology in the ASCUS LSIL Triage Study (ALTS). Am J Clin Pathol 2001;116:386–394.
47. The Atypical Squamous Cells of Undetermined Significance/Low-Grade Squamous Intraepithelial Lesions Triage Study (ALTS) Group. Human papillomavirus testing for triage of women with cytologic evidence of low-grade squamous intraepithelial lesion: baseline data from a randomized trial. J Natl Cancer Inst 2000;92:397–402.
48. National Cancer Institute, National Institutes of Health and Human Services. Results of a randomized trial on the management of cytology interpretations of atypical squamous cells of undetermined significance ASCUS–LSIL Triage Study (ALTS) Group. Am J Obstet Gynecol 2003;188:1383–1392.
49. The ASCUS–LSIL Triage Study (ALTS) Group. A randomized trial on the management of low-grade squamous intraepithelial lesion cytology interpretations. Am J Obstet Gynecol 2003;188:1393–1400.
50. Autier P, Coibion M, De Sutter P, et al. Cytology alone versus cytology and cervicography for cervical cancer screening: a randomized study. Obstet Gynecol 1999;93:353–358.
51. Schneider DL, Herrero R, Bratti C, et al. Cervicography screening for cervical cancer among 8460 women in a high-risk population. Am J Obstet Gynecol 1999;180:290–298.
52. University of Zimbabwe/JHPIEGO Cervical Cancer Project. Visual inspection with acetic acid for cervical cancer screening: test qualities in a primary-care setting. Lancet 1999;353:869–873.
53. Gaffikin L, Lauterbach M, Blumental PD. Performance of visual inspection with acetic acid for cervical cancer screening: a qualitative summary of evidence to date. Obstet Gynecol Surv 2003;58:543–550.
54. Shulman LP, Klett CC, Phillips OP. Preliminary comparison of Papanicolaou smear and speculoscopy for assessing cervical cancer precursor lesions in pregnant adolescents. J Pediatr Adolesc Gynecol 1999;12:78–82.
55. Parham GP, Andrews NR, Lee ML. Comparison of immediate and deferred colposcopy in a cervical screening program. Obstet Gynecol 2000;95:340–344.
56. Eddy GL, Ural SH, Strumpf KB, et al. Incidence of atypical glandular cells of uncertain significance in cervical cytology following introduction of the Bethesda system. Gynecol Oncol 1997;67:51–55.
57. Raab SS, Snider TE, Potts SA, et al. Atypical glandular cells of undetermined significance: diagnosis accuracy and interobserver variability using select cytologic criteria. Am J Clin Pathol 1997;107:299–307.
58. Soofer SB, Sidawy MK. Atypical glandular cells of undetermined significance: clinically significant lesions and means of patient follow-up. Cancer 2000;90:207–214.
59. Eddy GL, Strumpf KB, Wojtowycz MA, et al. Biopsy findings in five hundred thirty-one patients with atypical glandular cells of uncertain significance as defined by the Bethesda system. Am J Obstet Gynecol 1997;177:1188–1195.
60. Levine L, Lucci JA III, Dinh TV. Atypical glandular cells: new Bethesda terminology and management guidelines. Obstet Gynecol Surv 2003;58:399–406.
61. Kim TJ, Kim HS, Park CT, et al. Clinical evaluation of follow–up methods and results of atypical glandular cells of undetermined significance (AGUS) detected on cervicovaginal Pap smears. Gynecol Oncol 1999;73:292–298.
62. Jones BA, Novis DA. Follow-up of abnormal gynecologic cytology: a College of American Pathologists Q-probes study of 16,132 cases from 306 laboratories. Arch Pathol Lab Med 2000;124:665–671.
63. Lonky NM, Sadeghi M, Tsadik GW, et al. The clinical significance of the poor correlation of cervical dysplasia and cervical malignancy with referral cytologic results. Am J Obstet Gynecol 1999;181:560–566.

64. Spitzer M, Chernys AE, Shifrin A, et al. Indications for cone biopsy: pathologic correlation. Am J Obstet Gynecol 1998;178:74–79.
65. Stoler MH, Schiffman M. Interobserver reproducibility of cervical cytologic and histologic interpretations: realistic estimates from the ASCUS–LSIL Triage Study. JAMA 2001;285:1500–1505.
66. Grenko RT, Abendroth CS, Frauenhoffer EE, et al. Variance in the interpretation of cervical biopsy specimens obtained for atypical squamous cells of undetermined significance. Am J Clin Pathol 2000;114:735–740.
67. Milne DS, Wadehra V, Mennim D, et al. A prospective follow up study of women with colposcopically unconfirmed positive cervical smears. Br J Obstet Gynaecol 1999;106:38–41.
68. Holschneider CH, Felix JC, Satmary W, et al. A single-visit cervical carcinoma prevention program offered at an inner city church: a pilot project. Cancer 1999;86:2659–2667.
69. Santos C, Galdos R, Alvarez M, et al. One-session management of cervical intraepithelial neoplasia: a solution for developing countries. A prospective, randomized trial of LEEP versus laser excisional conization. Gynecol Oncol 1996;61:11–15.
70. Townsend DE, Richart RM. Diagnostic errors in colposcopy. Gynecol Oncol 1981;12:259–264.
71. Weitzman GA, Korhonen MO, Reeves KO, et al. Endocervical brush cytology. An alternative to endocervical curettage? J Reprod Med 1988;33:677–683.
72. Creasman WT, Weed JC, Curry SL, et al. Efficacy of cryosurgical treatment of severe cervical intraepithelial neoplasia. Obstet Gynecol 1973;41:501–506.
73. Flowers LC, McCall MA. Diagnosis and management of cervical intraepithelial neoplasia. Obstet Gynecol Clin North Am 2001;28:667–684.
74. Herzog TJ, Williams S, Adler LM, et al. Potential of cervical electrosurgical excision procedure for diagnosis and treatment of cervical intraepithelial neoplasia. Gynecol Oncol 1995;57:286–293.
75. Schiller JT, Lowy DR. Papillomavirus-like particle based vaccines: cervical cancer and beyond. Expert Opin Biol Ther 2001;1:571–581.
76. Murakami M, Gurski KJ, Steller MA. Human papillomavirus vaccines for cervical cancer. J Immunother 1999;22:212–218.
77. Munger K, Phelps WC, Bubb V, et al. The E6 and E7 genes of the human papillomavirus type 16 together are necessary and sufficient for transformation of primary human keratinocytes. J Virol 1989;63:4417–4421.
78. Crook T, Morgenstern JP, Crawford L, et al. Continued expression of HPV-16 E7 protein is required for maintenance of the transformed phenotype of cells co-transformed by HPV-16 plus EJ-ras. EMBO J 1989;8:513–519.
79. Zhou J, Sun XY, Stenzel DJ, et al. Expression of vaccinia recombinant HPV 16 L1 and L2 ORF proteins in epithelial cells is sufficient for assembly of HPV virion-like particles. Virology 1991;185:251–257.
80. Kirnbauer R, Hubbert NL, Wheeler CM, et al. A virus-like particle enzyme-linked immunosorbent assay detects serum antibodies in a majority of women infected with human papillomavirus type 16. J Natl Cancer Inst 1994;86:494–499.
81. Harro CD, Pang YY, Roden RB, et al. Safety and immunogenicity trial in adult volunteers of a human papillomavirus 16 L1 virus-like particle vaccine. J Natl Cancer Inst 2001;93:284–292.
82. Koutsky LA, Ault KA, Wheeler CM, et al. A controlled trial of a human papillomavirus type 16 vaccine. N Engl J Med 2002;347:1645–1651.
83. Ressing ME, Sette A, Brandt RM, et al. Human CTL epitopes encoded by human papillomavirus type 16 E6 and E7 identified through in vivo and in vitro immunogenicity studies of HLA-A*0201-binding peptides. J Immunol 1995;154:5934–5943.
84. Steller MA, Gurski KJ, Murakami M, et al. Cell-mediated immunological responses in cervical and vaginal cancer patients immunized with a lipidated epitope of human papillomavirus type 16 E7. Clin Cancer Res 1998;4:2103–2109.
85. Alexander M, Salgaller ML, Celis E, et al. Generation of tumor-specific cytolytic T lymphocytes from peripheral blood of cervical cancer patients by in vitro stimulation with a synthetic human papillomavirus type 16 E7 epitope. Am J Obstet Gynecol 1996;175:1586–1593.
86. Steller MA, Schiller JT. Human papillomavirus immunology and vaccine prospects. J Natl Cancer Inst Monogr 1996;4:145–148.
87. Cardosi RJ, Bomalaski JJ, Hoffman MS. Diagnosis and management of vulvar and vaginal intraepithelial neoplasia. Obstet Gynecol Clin North Am 2001;28:685–702.
88. Sugase M, Matsukura T. Distinct manifestations of human papillomaviruses in the vagina. Int J Cancer 1997;72:412–415.
89. Minucci D, Cinel A, Insacco E, et al. Epidemiological aspects of vaginal intraepithelial neoplasia (VAIN). Clin Exp Obstet Gynecol 1995;22:36–42.
90. Aho M, Vesterinen E, Meyer B, et al. Natural history of vaginal intraepithelial neoplasia. Cancer 1991;68:195–197.
91. Bornstein J, Kaufman RH. Combination of surgical excision and carbon dioxide laser vaporization for multifocal vulvar intraepithelial neoplasia. Am J Obstet Gynecol 1988;158:459–464.
92. Sillman FH, Fruchter RG, Chen YS, et al. Vaginal intraepithelial neoplasia: risk factors for persistence, recurrence, and invasion and its management. Am J Obstet Gynecol 1997;176:93–99.
93. Bowen JT. Precancerous dermatosis—a study of chronic atypical epithelial proliferation. J Cutan Dis Syphilology 1912;30:241–255.
94. Buscema J, Naghashfar Z, Sawada E, et al. The predominance of human papillomavirus type 16 in vulvar neoplasia. Obstet Gynecol 1988;71:601–606.
95. Crum CP, Liskow A, Petras P, et al. Vulvar intraepithelial neoplasia (severe atypia and carcinoma in situ). A clinicopathologic analysis of 41 cases. Cancer 1984;54:1429–1434.

CHAPTER 5

Benign Disorders of the Vulva and Vagina

Wilson Sawa and Michael P. Hopkins

INTRODUCTION

Benign disorders of the vulva and vagina are a common cause for visits to the primary care physician's office. Fortunately, most disorders that involve the vulva and the vagina are nonmalignant in nature. It is incumbent, however, for the examining physician to distinguish disorders that are serious and require further investigation and intervention from those that only need topical therapies. The gold standard for the management of chronic vulvar disease is a biopsy to establish a tissue diagnosis (1, 2). If there is any question regarding a lesion, biopsy must be performed.

Benign growths of the vagina are usually diagnosed at the time of the routine examination. The entire vagina should be inspected which requires rotating the speculum 90 degrees throughout the exam. A vaginal lesion can be missed if it is present beneath the blades of a speculum. Physical examination of the anogenital area is required in the patient with vulvar-based complaints. When evaluating a vulvar lesion, three features must be considered: (a) lesion type, (b) lesion location, and (c) associated systemic and laboratory findings (3). Examination of other skin sites such as the mouth, eyes, and scalp should also be done as nongenital-based disease may preset with manifestations in the vulvar or vaginal areas.

This chapter covers common benign disorders affecting the vulva and vagina. A brief discussion of premalignant conditions that affect the vulva and vagina are also presented. Information related to the vulvar or vaginal effects of STI's or HPV may be found in Chapters 11 and 4 respectively.

VULVOVAGINAL ATROPHY

Estrogen deficiency leads to thinning of the genital epithelium. The vaginal mucosa is dry, pale, and fragile (4). This may cause severe pruritus, bleeding, and dyspareunia. Conditions with relative estrogen deficiency, such as the postpartum period with breast-feeding or oral contraceptive use, can cause similar symptoms. Topical or systemic estrogen therapy will usually relieve the symptoms.

VULVAR PAIN

At the seventeenth World Congress in 2003, the International Society for the Study of Vulvovaginal Disease (ISSVD) re-established vulvodynia as the preferred term for vulvar pain occurring *in the absence of an underlying recognizable disease*. Vulvodynia is characterized by vulvar burning, stinging, soreness, rawness, or pain; the pain may be one sided or bilateral, sporadic or constant. Patients may report a swelling sensation and paresthesia. There may be periods of time when the patient is symptom free. The classification of vulvodynia is based on the site of the

TABLE 5.1

ISSVD Terminology and Classification of Vulvar Pain (2003)

A) Vulvar pain related to a specific disorder
   1. Infectious (e.g., candidiasis, herpes)
   2. Inflammatory (e.g., lichen planus, immunobullous disorders)
   3. Neoplastic (e.g., Paget's disease, squamous cell carcinoma)
   4. Neurologic (e.g., herpes neuralgia, spinal nerve compression)

B) Vulvodynia
   1. Generalized
      i. Provoked (sexual, nonsexual, or both)
      ii. Unprovoked
      iii. Mixed (provoked and unprovoked)
   2. Localized (vestibulodynia, clitorodynia, hemivulvodynia, etc.)
      i. Provoked (sexual, nonsexual, or both)
      ii. Unprovoked
      iii. Mixed (provoked and unprovoked)

ISSVD, Moyal-Barracco M, Lynch PJ 2003 ISSVD terminology and classification of vulvodynia: a historical perspective. J Reprod Med 2004;49:772–777.
Vestibulitis has been eliminated from the ISSVD terminology because the presence of inflammation, as implied by the suffix "-itis," has not been documented so far.

pain, whether it is generalized or localized, and whether it is provoked, unprovoked, or mixed (Table 5.1) (5, 6).

Several causes have been proposed for vulvodynia, including increased urinary oxalates, hormonal factors, neuropathic changes, inflammation, genetic or immune factors, and infection. The prevalence of vulvodynia is estimated to be 16% in women ages 18 to 64 years of age (7). Women seeking medical care for vulvodynia are often incorrectly diagnosed and treated several times before receiving the correct medical diagnosis.

Treatment begins with accurate diagnosis and patient education (Fig. 5.1). Pain theories, pathophysiology, and proposed treatments should be explained and discussed. Triggers to pain need to be treated as an adjunct to therapy. For example, eliminating any fungal infections is important, although their elimination alone may not cure the vulvodynia. A diagram of the pain locations is helpful to assist in assessing the pain over time.

Localized Vulvodynia

This may also be referred to as vestibulodynia, clitorodynia, or hemivulvodynia. The older terminology for vestibulodynia was vulvar vestibulitis, but this term has been eliminated from the ISSVD terminology because the presence of inflammation, as implied by the suffix "-itis," has not been documented so far.

Vestibulodynia is the most common cause of long-standing dyspareunia in premenopausal women (8). Although previously believed to be a predominantly Caucasian female disease, Harlow and Stewart reported a similar incidence among African American women (9). Women with sexual pain do not differ from controls in terms of premorbid depression, sexual abuse history, sexual behavior patterns, or sexual dysfunction (10). Even after successful treatment and resolution of the pain, sexual dysfunction may continue and complementary short-term sexual therapy may be necessary.

Vestibulodynia is characterized by dyspareunia and focal erythema (11). The etiology of vestibulodynia is unknown, although associated symptoms may last for months or years. Diagnosis is usually made by the "touch test." This involves firmly touching a cotton tip swab to

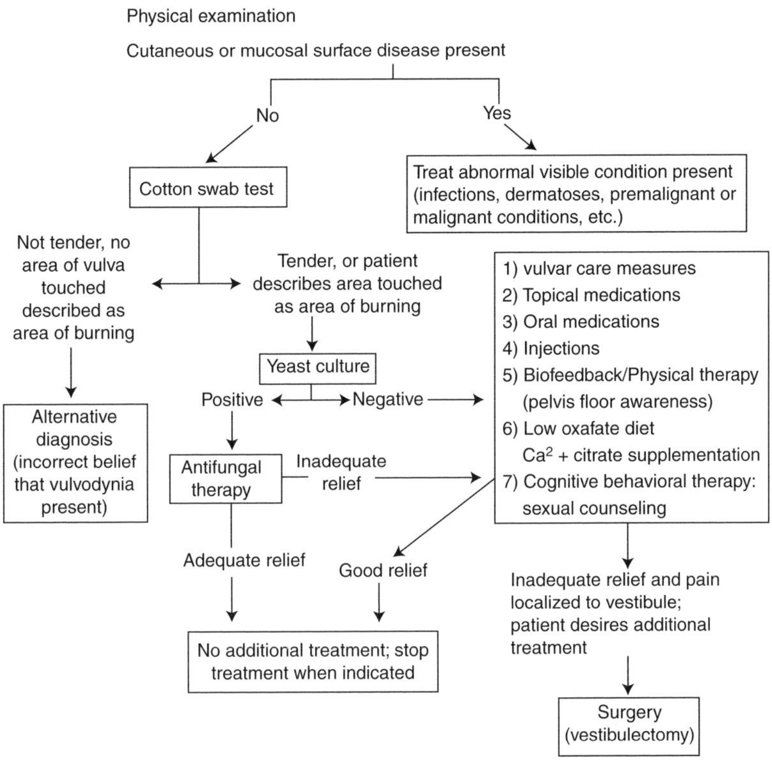

FIGURE 5.1 ● Vulvodynia algorithm. (Reprinted from Haefner HK, Collins ME, Davis GD, et al. The vulvodynia guideline. J Lower Genital Tract Dis 2005;9[1]:42, with permission.)

the labia majora, interlabial sulci, and lateral labia minora. This is followed by firmly touching the ostia of the Skene's glands and the major and minor vestibular glands. Although there is no increased sensitivity to the lateral genital structures, patients with vestibulodynia do have heightened pain sensitivity associated with touch of the gland openings.

Proposed risk factors for vestibulodynia are genital infections, especially candidiasis, and exposure to irritant agents. More recent studies hinted at a relationship between the development of superficial dyspareunia and vestibulodynia and oral contraceptive use (12, 13). In a small case-control study by Bohm-Starke et al. (14), quantitative sensory tests were performed on the vestibular mucosa; the vestibulodynia cases were using oral contraceptives, whereas the control patients were not. Testing included detection of warmth and cold thresholds and mechanical and heat pain thresholds in the anterior and posterior portion of the vestibule. Compared with controls, the authors found significantly lower mechanical pain thresholds in both areas of the vestibule in women using oral contraceptives, although the most sensitive area was the posterior vestibule. There were no significant differences in the thermotest evaluation between the two groups. Although further study is needed, the authors postulate that oral contraceptives may increase vestibular mucosal sensitivity in young women and may be a contributing factor in the development of vulvar vestibulodynia.

There is no clearly defined cure for vestibulodynia. Tricyclic antidepressants (TCAs) such as Amitriptyline (10 to 75 mg) have been used with some success in treating vestibulodynia (15). Patients should be started on 5 mg (half of a 10-mg tablet) and gradually increased so possible side effects are minimized. The dose is titrated up to 150 mg or symptom control, whichever comes first. Desipramine is also used and is less sedating; the dose schedule is the same as that of Amitriptyline.

TABLE 5.2

Topical Medications Used to Treat Vulvodynia

Topical Medication	Dosage	Side Effects[a]
5% lidocaine ointment	Apply to skin as needed; dispense 30-g tube. Do not use >20-g of ointment in a 24-h period.	Erythema or edema. Rare cases of purpura. If ointment is present on skin during intercourse, the partner may experience numbness.
EMLA cream (lidocaine 2.5% and prilocaine 2.5%; AstraZeneca Pharmaceuticals LP, Wilmington, DE	Apply to skin prn. Do not exceed 2.5 g over 20–25 cm^2 of skin surface (for example, a 5- × 5-cm area). Dispense 30-g tube.	Paleness, erythema, and swelling.
L-M-X 4, formerly ELA-Max 4% cream (lidocaine 4%; Ferndale, Ferndale, MI)	Apply to skin as needed. Dispense 30-g tube.	Erythema and edema.
L-M-X 5, formerly ELA-Max Anorectal 5% cream (lidocaine 5%); Ferndale, Ferndale, MI		
Estrogens Estrace vaginal cream (estradiol vaginal cream 0.01%); Bristol-Meyers Squibb Company, Princeton, NJ	These can be used intravaginally or topically. For treatment of vulvar and vaginal atrophy associated with the menopause, the lowest dose and regimen that will control symptoms should be chosen and medication should be discontinued as promptly as possible. Usual dosage: The usual dosage range is 2 to 4 g (marked on the applicator) daily for 1 or 2 weeks, then gradually taper. Tube contains 1.5 oz (42.5 g) with a calibrated plastic applicator for delivery of 1, 2, 3, or 4 g.	Common reactions Vaginal bleeding, spotting, breast changes, nausea, vomiting, headache, fluid retention, mood changes, weight changes, rash Serious reactions Thromboembolism, stroke, MI, breast, endometrial changes, fibroid enlargment, gallbladder disease, cholestatic jaundice, pancreatitis, asthma worsening, depression, hypertension.
Premarin vaginal cream (conjugated estrogens 0.625 mg/g); Wyeth-Ayerst Company, Philadelphia, PA	0.5 to 2 g daily, intravaginally, depending on the severity of the condition. Taper gradually to every other day, twice weekly, etc. Patients with an intact uterus should be monitored closely for signs of endometrial cancer, and appropriate diagnostic measures should be taken to rule out malignancy in the event of abnormal vaginal bleeding. Each contains net wt. 1.5 oz (42.5 g) tube with one plastic applicator calibrated in 0.5-g increments to a maximum of 2 g. Taper gradually.	

TABLE 5.2 (Continued)

Topical Medications Used to Treat Vulvodynia

Topical Medication	Dosage	Side Effects[a]
Amitriptyline 2%/baclofen 2% in water washable base (Elavil 2%/Lioresal 2% in water washable base) Elavil (AstraZeneca Pharmaceuticals LP, Wilmington, DE) Lioresal (Geigy Novartis Pharmaceuticals Corp., East Hanover, NJ)	Topical amitriptyline 2% with baclofen 2% in water washable base (WWB); squirt 0.5 mL from syringe onto finger and apply to affected area one to three times daily. Dispense 30-day supply	Common reactions (amitriptyline) Irritation, contact dermatitis, dry mouth, drowsiness, dizziness, constipation, weight gain, urinary retention, tachycardia, blurred vision, confusion Serious reactions (amitriptyline) Seizures, stroke, myocardial infarction, agranulocytosis, thrombocytopenia Common reactions (baclofen) Drowsiness, dizziness, weakness, nausea, confusion, hypotension, headache, insomnia, constipation, muscle weakness, rash, sweating, fatigue Serious reactions (baclofen) Depression, respiratory problems, ataxia, syncope, seizures, hallucinations, exacerbation of spasticity

prn, as needed; MI, myocardial infarction.
[a] Generally, the side effects of topical medications are less than when taken systemically.
Reprinted from Haefner HK, Collins ME, Davis GD, et al. The vulvodynia guideline. J Lower Genital Tract Dis 2005;9(1):43, with permission.

For women who cannot tolerate TCAs, gabapentin may be considered. Its mechanism of action is unknown. This is an anticonvulsant and is less sedating than the TCA therapies. It is started at a dose of 300 mg three times a day and may be increased up to a maximum dose of 1200 mg three times a day (16). It should not be discontinued abruptly because it can lead to withdrawal-related side effects. One advantage over TCAs is a reasonably good side effect profile; the most common being drowsiness, nausea, and dizziness.

Patients whose primary complaint is one of painful intercourse may find application of 0.2% nitroglycerin cream immediately prior to intercourse to be helpful. Headache appears to be a common side effect (17). Nightly topical 5% lidocaine has also shown promising initial results for treatment (18). Other topical medications that may be used to treat vulvodynia—both localized and generalized—are listed in Table 5.2. The current focus of therapy combines a centrally acting drug with a topical anesthetic (e.g., topical lidocaine combined with a TCA). Patients with vestibulodynia may benefit from using creams and ointments made with hypoallergenic bases such as acid mantle or Aquaphor. Some pharmacists are able to compound ointments or creams using these bases.

Antihistamines do not appear to be effective, and cromolyn has been shown to be ineffective (19). Capsaicin and imiquimod may be helpful but have irritant properties. Medium- and high-potency steroids have been reported to be helpful, but evidence of this is limited. Locally injected interferon alpha has been reported to be beneficial, but sustained improvement 1 year after therapy is variable (20). There is some evidence that biofeedback and physical therapy aimed to alleviate vulvar pain referred from ligaments and joints in the spine and pelvis provide some relief (21). There have been no controlled trials of the efficacy of a low-oxalate diet in improving symptoms.

Surgery for vestibulodynia is controversial, although it seems clear that it should be performed only when all other treatment regimens have failed, and only in carefully selected patients. Typically, about 5 mm of mucosa and underlying stroma is removed. One common long-term complication is Bartholin duct cysts, and in 5% of patients, persistent or increased vestibular tenderness occurred postoperatively. Failure rates have been reported in the 20% range, and in one study by Bornstein et al. (22), they concluded that there are two groups of patients who will not be helped by surgical intervention: women with primary pain on intercourse and women with constant pain in addition to dyspareunia. Predictors of surgical failure include primary vestibulitis, diffuse vulvar pain, urinary symptoms, and muscle hypertonicity.

Generalized Vulvodynia

Generalized vulvodynia usually affects an older patient population than localized vulvodynia. It is characterized by a chronic, burning pain and may be associated with dysuria or lower back pain. Examination reveals no abnormalities, but pain sensation disproportional to the stimulus may be noticed. Some patients have altered sensory perception (e.g., gentle pressure is felt as burning).

The etiology is unknown, although many factors have been implicated. Neuropathic pain, pudendal neuralgia, chronic reflex pain syndrome, pelvic floor abnormalities, and referred visceral pain are among suggested causes of dysesthetic vulvodynia. Contrary to previous belief, more recent studies do not support psychosexual dysfunction as a cause of vulvar dysesthesia. However, increased anxiety in patients with vulvar vestibulitis may present with lower pain thresholds. Dysesthetic vulvodynia is diagnosed after specific causes of vulvar pain have been excluded.

Therapy consists of tricyclic medications (Amitriptyline, Imipramine, or Desipramine) or Neurontin. Other oral medications that may be used to treat localized or generalized vulvodynia are listed in Table 5.3. In a small, retrospective study, rehabilitation methods through physical therapy (e.g., the Glazer method) have been shown to be effective. Other therapies include local injection of interferon-α, injection of triamcinolone, Oral gabapentin, topical estrogen, topical capsaicin, topical nitroglycerine, acupuncture, or surgical excision. There are no randomized controlled trials on the effects of any of these treatments (23–25).

VULVAR DERMATITIS

Allergens, Irritants, and Contact Dermatitis

When a patient presents with vulvar pruritus and no obvious cause can be found, an environmental or dietary etiology of contact dermatitis should be considered as a possible cause. Chemicals in deodorant soaps, bubble bath products, or perfumed feminine hygiene products can be irritating and either cause or intensify symptoms (26). Although atopic dermatitis, or eczema, may acutely present as a vesicular eruption with erythema, chronic eczema is often erythematous and scaly (Figs. 5.2 and 5.3). It is important to remember that a patient may have used an agent for months or years without any problem and then have an "allergy" develop.

Two major types of eczema occur: exogenous and endogenous. Exogenous is also known as irritant or allergic contact dermatitis, and endogenous may be referred to as atopic dermatitis. Potential irritants include almost everything. Irritant or allergic dermatitis lesions are usually seen in areas of contact with the environmental irritants or antigens. However, in atopic dermatitis other sites of the skin may be involved, such as the scalp or the ears (27, 28). Patch testing should be considered if the patient has not responded to therapy or if the diagnosis is unclear.

Treatment of contact dermatitis involves identification and elimination of the irritating agent. Compresses with 1:20 dilution of Burrow's solution may be used for 20 to 30 minutes three times a day to relieve symptoms. Other local methods include using cotton underwear washed in bland detergent, taking sitz baths (using plain tepid water twice a day), or applying a thin plain petrolatum film or zinc oxide 10 to 20% ointment after bowel movements. Use of an antidepressant such as doxepin may be considered for the treatment of pruritus. Doxepin or hydroxyzine may be particularly helpful when antihistamines do not control the symptoms.

(*text continues on page 116*)

TABLE 5.3

Oral Medications Used to Treat Vulvodynia[a]

Medication Category Medication	Dosage	Side Effects
Antidepressants Amitriptyline (Elavil; AstraZeneca Pharmaceuticals LP, Wilmington, DE)	Initial amitriptyline prescription: Amitriptyline 10 mg or 25 mg. Directions: 1 by mouth each night for 1 week; if symptoms persist, 2 by mouth each night for 1 wk; if symptoms persist, 3 by mouth each night for 1 wk; if symptoms persist, 4 by mouth nightly. Maintain nightly dose that relieves symptoms. Generally, do not exceed 100 to 150 mg nightly. Start at 10 mg in patients age 60 or older, or in patients that have not been able to tolerate higher dosages. Increase by 10 mg weekly. Often other medications should be tried in the elderly population than amitriptyline. Do not stop suddenly. Wean by 25 mg every 3 to 4 days. Discuss Interaction with alcohol (no more than one drink per day). If patient is in the reproductive age group, discuss contraception.	Common reactions (amitriptyline) Dry mouth, drowsiness, dizziness, constipation, weight gain, urinary retention, tachycardia, blurred vision, confusion Serious reactions (amitriptyline) Seizures, stroke, myocardial infarction, agranulocytosis, thrombocytopenia.
Nortriptyline (Pamelor; Novartis Pharmaceuticals Corp., East Hanover, NJ)	Same dosing as amitriptyline.	Common reactions Dry mouth, drowsiness, dizziness, constipation, urinary retention, tachycardia, blurred vision, weight gain, confusion Serious reactions Seizures, MI, stoke agranulocytosis, thrombocytopenia
Desipramine (Norpramin, Hoechst Marion Roussel for Aventis Pharmaceuticals, Bridgewater, NJ)	Same dosing as amitriptyline, except desipramine is often taken in the morning instead of the evening.	Common reactions Drowsiness, dizziness, blurred vision, dry mouth, constipation, tachycardia, urinary retention, diaphoresis, weakness, nervousness, rash, seizures, tinnitus, anxiety, confusion Serious reactions Seizures, sudden death, arrhythmias, stroke, myocardial infarction, atrioventricular block, thromobocytopenia

(*continued*)

TABLE 5.3 (Continued)

Oral Medications Used to Treat Vulvodynia[a]

Medication Category Medication	Dosage	Side Effects
Venlafaxine (Effexor XR; Wyeth Pharmaceuticals, Madison, NY) Consider this in patients that do not respond to the common tricyclic antidepressants. Often used in conjunction with an anticonvulsant.	It is started at 37.5 mg daily (in the morning) with an increase to 75 mg daily (in the morning) after 1 to 2 weeks. Can increase gradually (dose changes every 1 to 2 weeks) to a maximum dose of 150 mg daily. When stopping the medication, wean by 75 mg/week. Well tolerated in the elderly population.	Common reactions Headache, nausea, somnolence, weight loss, anorexia, constipation, anxiety, vision changes, diarrhea, dizziness, dry mouth, insomnia, weakness, sweating, hypertension Serious reactions Seizures, suicide ideation, depression
Other antidepressants are used to treat pain. These include: fluoxetine (Prozac; Eli Lilly & Co., Indianapolis, IN); sertraline (Zoloft; Pfizer Inc., New York, NY) paroxetine (Paxil; GlaxoSmithKline, Research Triangle Park, NC); citalopram (Celexa; Forest Laboratories Inc., New York, NY)		
Anticonvulsants Gabapentin (Neurontin; Pfizer Inc., New York, NY)	Gabapentin comes in 100-, 300-, 400-, 600-, and 800-mg tablets. Generally, it is started at 300 mg by mouth daily for 3 days, then 300 mg by mouth twice daily for 3 days, then 300 mg by mouth three times daily. It can be increased gradually to 3600 mg total daily. Ideally, gabapentin is given in a three times daily dosage, but if the patient is unable to comply with that, it can be given in a twice-daily dosage. However, if using higher doses, a three times daily regimen should be followed. Do not exceed 1200 mg in a dose. For the elderly population, do not exceed 2700 mg/day.	Common reactions Somnolence, dizziness, ataxia, fatigue, nystagmus, tremor, diplopia, rhinitis, blurred vision, nausea, vomiting, nervousness, dysarthria, weight gain Serious reactions Leukopenia
Carbamazepine XR (Tegretol-XR; Novartis Pharmaceuticals Corp., East Hanover, NJ)	Start at 100 mg by mouth nightly. Add 100 mg every 3 days, titrating with blood levels. Requires serial blood tests (drug level, liver function tests, and complete blood count). For pain, the general dose is 200 to 400 mg by mouth twice daily. Maximum dose is 1200 mg/day. Comes in 100-, 200-, 400-mg tablets.	Common reactions Dizziness, drowsiness, unsteadiness, incoordination, nausea/vomiting, blurred vision, nystagmus, allergic rash, confusion, elevated liver transaminases, hyponatremia, ataxia Serious reactions Hypersensitivity reactions, seizures, Arrhythmias, syncope, aplastic anemia, agranulocytosis,

TABLE 5.3 (Continued)

Oral Medications Used to Treat Vulvodynia[a]

Medication Category Medication	Dosage	Side Effects
		thrombocytopenia, leukopenia, pancytopenia, hepatitis, cholestatic jaundice, hyponatremia, water intoxication, porphyria, Steven's-Johnson syndrome, toxic epidermal necrolysis, erythema multiforme, pancreatitis
Topiramate (Topamax; Ortho Pharmaceutical Corp., Raritan, NJ)	Start at 25 mg daily to twice daily. If symptoms persist, 50 mg by mouth twice daily for 1 week; if symptoms persist, 75 mg by mouth twice daily for 1 week. If symptoms persist, 100 mg by mouth twice daily. Maintain at the doses above where symptoms are controlled. In the elderly and chronically ill, or those with renal or hepatic dysfunction, start at a lower dose and titrate more slowly.	Common reactions Asthenia, fatigue, paresthesia, tremor, ataxia, confusion, difficulty with concentration or attention, dizziness, breast pain, dysmenorrhea, diplopia, myopia, acute and secondary angle closure glaucoma, nystagmus, memory problems, nervousness, psychomotor retardation, somnolence, nausea, speech or language problems. Serious reactions Hyperthermia, oligohidrosis, anemia (rare), leukopenia (infrequent), dyspnea (rare), hepatic failure, hepatitis, pancreatitis, renal calculi, renal tubular acidosis, hyperchloremic, nonanion gap metabolic acidosis
Other medications that have been used for vulvodynia Tramadol (Ultram; Ortho Pharmaceutical Corp., Raritan, NJ)	This is a synthetic 4-phenyipiperidine analog of codeine. Studies have shown that it is effective for long-term pain management in the elderly population. 50–100 mg by mouth every 4–6 hours. Start at 25 mg by mouth in the morning then increase by 25 mg per day every 3 days to 25 mg four times daily then increase by 50 mg/day every 3 days to 50 mg four times daily, then maintenance. Do not stop suddenly. Maximum dose is 200 mg/day in the elderly population; up to 400 mg/day may be used in the general population.	Common reactions Dizziness, nausea, constipation, headache, somnolence, vomiting, pruritus, nervousness, confusion, euphoria, tremor, spasticity, emotional liability, vasodilation, visual disturbances, urinary retention, incoordination, anorexia, rash Serious reactions Seizures, respiratory depression, anaphylaxis, angioedema, bronchospasm. Stevens-Johnson syndrome, toxic epidermal necrolysis, hypotension, orthostatic serotonin syndrome, hallucinations, suicidal ideation, dependency

MI, myocardial infarction.

[a] With all of the antidepressants discussed, adequate time for a treatment trial must be given before abandoning them, as long as the side effects are tolerable.

Reprinted from Haefner HK, Collins ME, Davis GD, et al. The vulvodynia guideline. J Lower Genital Tract Dis 2005;9(1):45, with permission.

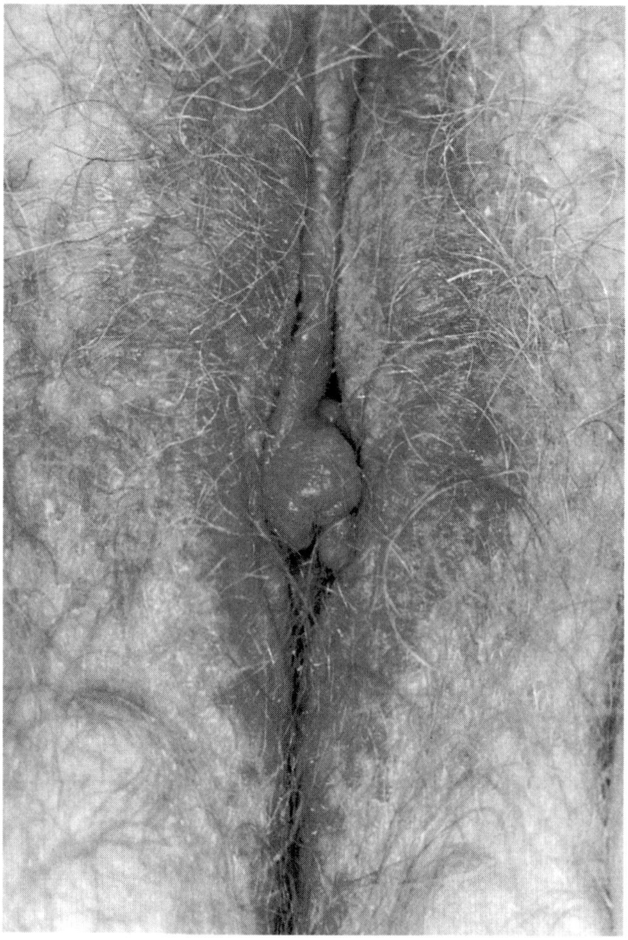

FIGURE 5.2 ● Moderate erythema in patient who complains of pruritus for 3 years. Clinical impression was eczema, and patient was advised to use hypoallergenic soap. Condition resolved. (Reprinted from Wilkinson EJ, Stone IK, eds. Atlas of Vulvar Disease. Baltimore: Williams & Wilkins, 1995:81, with permission.)

They are used primarily at nighttime because they are both sedating; the initial starting dose for doxepin is 10 mg, but this may be titrated up to 100 mg. During the day, topical doxepin may be used as an effective antipruritic agent.

Topical steroids may be used for 2 to 3 weeks to reduce inflammation and promote healing. Treatment options include triamcinolone ointment 0.1% twice a day, or halobetasol or clobetasol ointment 0.05% twice a day. Severe cases of dermatitis or vulvar dermatoses may require pulsing of ultra–high-potency corticosteroids such as clobetasol .05% for 7 to 10 days per month. Complications from long-term use of this therapy include secondary skin atrophy and rebound inflammation. For maintenance therapy, a less potent corticosteroid such as 1 to 2.5% hydrocortisone ointment is chosen, and the frequency of use is diminished. Systemic steroids, such as prednisone 0.5 to 1 mg/kg per day tapered over 14 to 21 days or subcutaneous injection of triamcinolone acetonide 10 mg/mL (3 mL) with 1% lidocaine hydrochloride (7 mL) may be necessary in cases unresponsive to topical treatment (27, 28). The newer topical treatments such as the calcineurin inhibitors tacrolimus and pimecrolimus are also helpful.

Seborrheic Dermatitis

Seborrheic dermatitis is very rare on the vulva. It usually affects the scalp, face, presternal, and intrascapular areas; it may be behind the ears. Lesions are pale to yellowish red, with greasy, nonadherent scales. Vulvar lesions are usually distributed symmetrically, and involvement of labia minora is rare. Clinically, it may be confused with psoriasis, candidiasis, tinea cruris, or

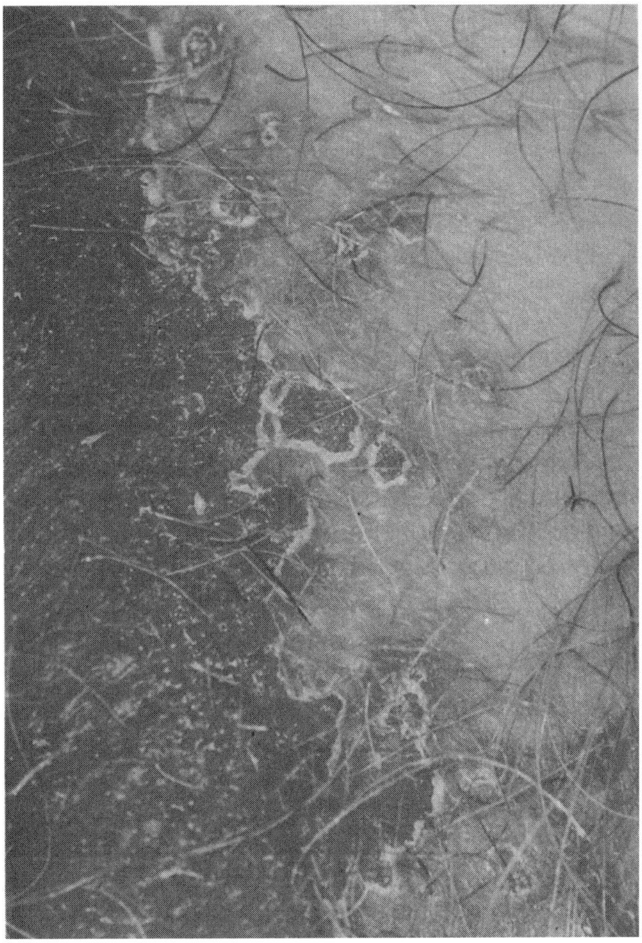

FIGURE 5.3 ● Note irregular border, erythema, and scaling of lesion. (Reprinted from Wilkinson EJ, Stone IK, eds. Atlas of Vulvar Disease. Baltimore: Williams & Wilkins, 1995:81, with permission.)

lichen simplex chronicus. The diagnosis is one of exclusion. There will often be other seborrheic dermatitis lesions in other areas of the body. If the vulva is swollen and wet, soaks with aluminum acetate may help. Initial use of a corticosteroid lotion may be followed by a corticosteroid cream as the patient is able to tolerate pressure on the vulva. Therapies used to treat seborrheic dermatitis on other body parts can also be used on vulva and include selenium sulfide, salicylic acid, and tar shampoo.

VULVAR DERMATOSES

Psoriasis

Psoriasis is a chronic papulosquamous disorder that occurs in 1 to 2% of the population. About one-third of patients with psoriasis have a family history of the disease. Psoriasis on the vulva may lack the typical silver scale and usually appears as red or reddish-yellow papules in the intertriginous areas. These often enlarge into distinct, dull-red plaques that bleed easily (4, 27). It may be mistaken on visual examination for candidiasis. Patients complain of intense pruritus.

Genital psoriasis lesions often appear on the mons and labia. A pinkening of the gluteal cleft may indicate psoriasis. Psoriasis may involve only the vulva, although other areas of the body (scalp, extensor surfaces, and trunk) are usually also affected. Psoriasis is associated with Köbner's phenomenon (i.e., the disease can flare at any site of injury, including surgical sites).

Treatment usually requires mid- to high-potency topical steroids, injectable corticosteroids, or topical tacrolimus. For ongoing therapy, the lowest possible potency topical steroid should be used because psoriasis becomes accustomed to steroid therapy. Other treatment options may include anthralin, tar, UV light, or cytotoxic agents. In some cases, it might be best if treatment is given in collaboration with a dermatologist.

Extramammary Paget's Disease

Vulvar Paget's, or extramammary Paget's, is a rare condition that often presents with itching, burning, or bleeding. A red, scaly, eczematous plaque—often described as a velvety lesion—is often noted. It may be mistaken for vulvar eczema and treated with topical steroids, but it will not respond to this therapy. It is an intraepithelial disease; hence, final diagnosis is by biopsy. In up to 26% of cases, there is a concurrent noncontiguous, underlying adenocarcinoma, and in 4% of cases, a contiguous adenocarcinoma is noted (29, 30). Because of the increased risk of a noncontiguous adenocarcinoma, if the diagnosis of vulvar Paget's is made, the workup should include colonoscopy, cystoscopy, mammogram, and colposcopy. Treatment usually includes wide local excision, but because local recurrence is high, this is a disease best managed in consultation with a gynecologic oncologist.

Acanthosis Nigricans

Acanthosis nigricans is a pigmented, raised, papillomatous lesion that will rarely involve the vulva. It can become extensive, and excision for diagnosis and cosmetic reasons may be necessary.

Intertrigo

Intertrigo can involve the vulva along the genitocrural folds. It results from chronic moisture and is typically seen beneath an abdominal pannus. An associated fungal or bacterial infection may be present. Efforts to promote dryness such as absorbent cotton garments can be helpful.

Vitiligo

Vitiligo results from a loss of melanin and produces depigmentation of the skin. Because this is a benign condition, no therapy is necessary.

LICHENOID VULVAR DERMATOSES

The more common vulvar dermatoses include "the three lichens": lichen simplex chronicus, lichen sclerosus (LS), and lichen planus (LP). Although they are discussed separately in this section, they may coexist simultaneously.

Lichen Simplex Chronicus

Lichen simplex chronicus is also known as squamous hyperplasia. It represents an end-stage disorder resulting from long-standing irritation, endogenous eczema, allergens, or infection (31). Patients often present with intractable itching and pruritus. The pruritus is often worse at night, and chronic scratching may lead to lichenification, fissures, and postinflammatory pigment changes. The vulvar surface in lichen simplex chronicus has a leathery appearance, and the cutaneous markings are quite pronounced. Treatment is removal of the infectious agents, irritants, or allergens if they are identifiable and topical application of mid- to high-potency corticosteroids. The potency of the steroid chosen depends on the degree of lichenification.

Lichen Sclerosus

LS is a common vulvar disorder; the mean age of onset is approximately 50 years, although there is a childhood variant in prepubertal girls. The etiology of LS is unknown. There is a 20% incidence of associated autoimmune disease in patients with LS. LS is characterized by thinning and whitening of the perianal and perivaginal skin, with an accompanying loss of mucocutaneous markings and skin elasticity. There is atrophy of the involved tissues and a loss of vulvar architecture, with complete flattening of the skin folds. LS may cause scarring and narrowing of the introitus. The acute phase may be red to purple in appearance and have an hourglass shape involving the vulva, perineum, and perianal area (26, 32, 33). LS does not involve the vagina. Clinical diagnosis should be confirmed by biopsy. Symptoms include intense itching, dysuria, and dyspareunia. LS may be linked to autoimmune disorders and the production of autoantibodies, particularly thyroid antibodies (34).

Randomized, prospective trials have demonstrated that high-potency steroids are more effective than testosterone therapy (35, 36). Treatment includes use of ultrapotent (class I) topical steroids, one to two times daily, for about 12 weeks. The patient should be re-examined at 4- to 6-week intervals. Maintenance therapy may be required, and this is done with weaker steroid preparations or less frequent use of potent steroids. Topical steroid use may increase the risk of dermal atrophy, rebound reactions, striae formation, hypothalamic-pituitary axis suppression, and secondary candidal or bacterial infection.

LS is a T-lymphocyte–mediated disorder. For this reason, use of a topical macrolide immunosuppressant, such as pimecrolimus or tacrolimus, has been suggested as an effective and safe therapy for LS. There are some small studies and case reports to support this treatment approach (37–39). Unlike high-potency steroids, macrolide immunosuppressants do not affect collagen synthesis, so they do not cause thinning of the dermis. Even in the pediatric population, both pimecrolimus and tacrolimus have been shown to be safe, with minimal systemic absorption even when applied to large areas of the body (40).

Although controversial, there may be an association between squamous cell carcinoma (SCC) and LS. Prospective and retrospective studies report that up to 5% of women with vulvar LS will eventually develop invasive cancer (41). If new or suspicious lesions arise in a patient previously diagnosed with LS, (repeat) biopsy is indicated. The risk of neoplasia is increased when there is histologic evidence of associated hyperplasia or cellular atypia with LS (42).

Excisional surgery with skin grafting is not curative because the disease recurs in the skin graft that is applied. Perineoplasty, however, is effective surgical management for treating the scarring and fissuring from LS (41).

Lichen Planus

Lichen planus (LP) is an inflammatory process of the mucocutaneous tissues of unknown etiology. It tends to occur in the third to sixth decades of life. It may be associated with various medications, such as diuretics or beta-blockers, as well as with autoimmune disorders and hepatitis. LP may cause significant scarring and adhesion formation in the vagina, and diffuse erosions may incur secondary bacterial infections (Fig. 5.4). Patients with LP who require surgery should have the procedure followed with aggressive steroid therapy. Like psoriasis, LP can exhibit Köbner's phenomenon (i.e., the disease can flare at any site of injury, including surgical sites).

LP presents in two ways. In the classic presentation, there are clearly demarcated, violaceous, flat-topped plaques on oral and genital membranes that are highly pruritic. On moist skin, they may appear as fine white reticulated papules. Oral lesions have a lacy appearance and occur on the posterior buccal mucosa and on the gingival surfaces (Fig. 5.5). These lesions often resolve spontaneously in 6 to 24 months.

In the erosive form, patients rarely complain of pruritus, but do note symptoms of vulvar pain, burning, soreness, dyspareunia, and dysuria. Lesions appear as brightly erythematous, superficial ulcerations that are scattered in distribution extending up into the vaginal canal. Oral lesions are demarcated areas of erythema at the gingival-dentate junction, are extremely pruritic, and may be painful. Patients may require the use of vaginal dilators to maintain vaginal patency. The premalignant potential of oral lesions should be regarded as uncertain (43).

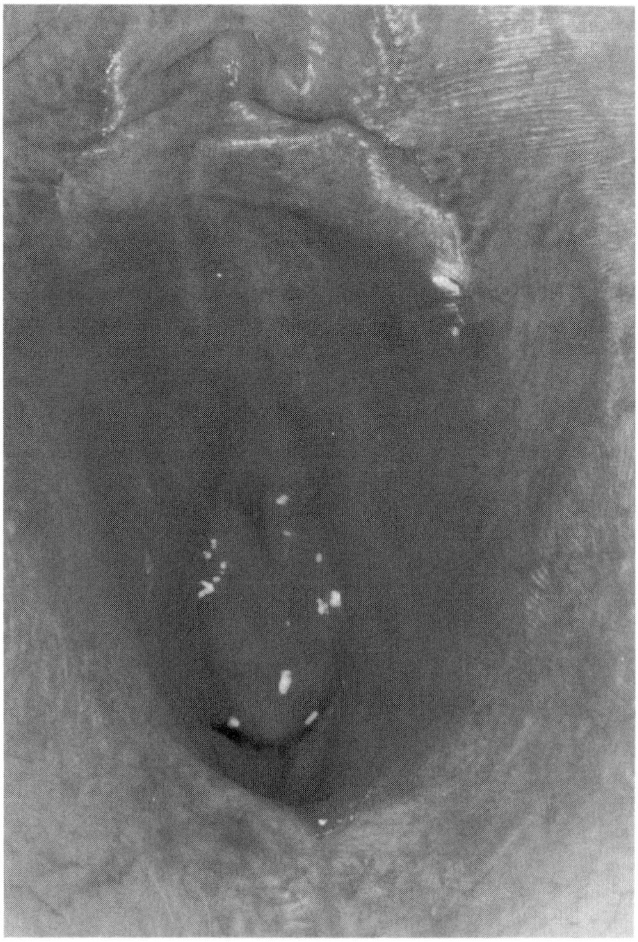

FIGURE 5.4 ● Lichen planus in a patient with dyspareunia for 8 months. Condition involved vagina and vestibule. Acute vaginal occlusion necessitated vaginal dilators (candlesticks) and topical steroids (Cort-Dome suppositories). (Reprinted from Wilkinson EJ, Stone IK, eds. Atlas of Vulvar Disease. Baltimore: Williams & Wilkins, 1995:29, with permission.)

Of the three lichens, LP is the most difficult to treat. Corticosteroids are first-line therapy, with ultrapotent ointment being used for external vulvar lesions and corticosteroid suppositories or foams used intravaginally. Although no therapy has clinically been proven effective, therapeutic options include cyclosporine, corticosteroids, psoralen plus ultraviolet A, topical or systemic retinoids, or tacrolimus. Incision or ablative therapies of the lesions are contraindicated.

Plasma Cell Vulvitis

Plasma cell vulvitis, also called Zoon's vulvitis or vulvitis circumscripta plasmacellularis, is a very rare chronic inflammatory disease of the vulva. It is usually diagnosed in postmenopausal women, although it can occur in women ages 8 to 80. Less than 50 cases have been reported in the literature. It causes red macular lesions anywhere in the vulva with pinpoint darker spots. There may also be erosions. Lesions are most often seen on the medial surface of the labia minora and periurethral mucosa. The specific cause of this condition is unknown. Patients may complain of pruritus, burning, pain, and dyspareunia. Diagnosis of plasma cell vulvitis requires histologic examination. Topical steroid creams and intralesional injections have been used with varying degrees of success (44).

There are many vulvar diseases that have similar clinical features to plasma cell vulvitis. As such, the existence of plasma cell vulvitis is questioned by some, and it has been referred to as a variant of LP (45, 46).

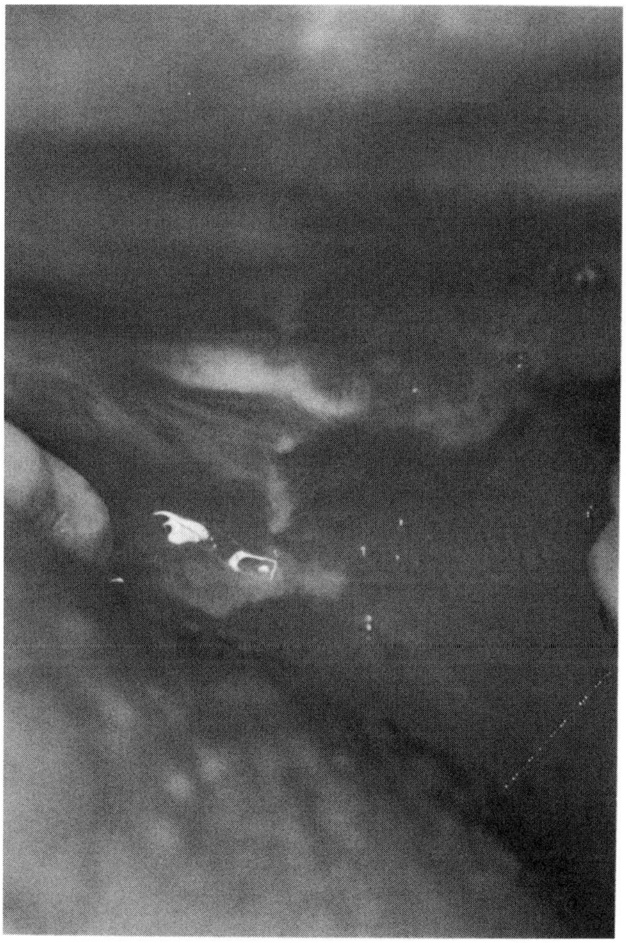

FIGURE 5.5 • Reticular buccal mucosa lesion in a patient with vulvovaginal lichen planus. (Reprinted from Wilkinson EJ, Stone IK, eds. Atlas of Vulvar Disease. Baltimore: Williams & Wilkins, 1995:30, with permission.)

INFECTIOUS CONDITIONS

Common Genital Infections

Infections are the leading cause of acute vulvar pruritus. Candidiasis, bacterial vaginosis, herpes simplex virus (HSV), human papillomavirus (HPV), and molluscum contagiosum are the most common infectious causes of vulvar itching (47). Infestation with scabies and lice are other possible causes.

Erythrasma

Erythrasma is a superficial bacterial skin infection of intertriginous sites caused by *Corynebacterium minutissimum* (short Gram-positive diphtheroid). It spreads slowly, is pruritic, has slight pink to brown macular patches, and occurs mostly in the axillary groin, pubic, or intergluteal and inframammary folds. It is common in diabetic patients and often occurs with cutaneous candida or *Taenia versicolor*. This particular rash fluoresces a coral red color under a Wood's lamp—a response caused by porphyrin production. A potassium hydroxide preparation may show negative results, but Gram's stain may show Gram-positive filamentous rods *(Corynebacterium minutissimum)*. Treatment is with erythromycin.

Hidradenitis Suppurativa

Hidradenitis suppurativa is a chronic, refractory infection of the skin and subcutaneous tissue arising from the apocrine glands. It may be found anywhere along "the milk line." It is most commonly found in women of reproductive age, and patients often have a family history of this condition. In long-standing cases, there may be multiple skin abscesses, draining subcutaneous sinus tracts, scarring, and deformity. Hidradenitis suppurativa has been associated with high morbidity, spondyloarthropathy, and carcinoma, including SCC and verrucous carcinoma, arising in lesional sites (48–50).

Examination of the vulva should determine if there is involvement of the inner aspects of the labia minora or vestibule—if there is, hidradenitis suppurativa is excluded because there are no apocrine glands at these locations and an alternative diagnosis (e.g., Crohn's disease) should be considered.

Therapeutic intervention is aimed at decreasing bacterial overgrowth, treating infection, and diminishing pain, drainage, and odor. Historically, treatment with oral antibiotics, topical clindamycin, isotretinoin, systemic and intralesional corticosteroids, and surgery have been inconsistently effective (51). Other reported interventions include methotrexate, acitretin, hormonal therapy with cyproterone acetate and ethinyl estradiol in female patients, cyclosporine, and carbon dioxide laser (51–53). Use of Infliximab (Remicade) in recalcitrant cases has been reported in the literature (54). In advanced cases, antibiotics are usually ineffective and surgical treatment is required. These patients may need referral to a specialist for long-term follow-up.

SYSTEMIC CONDITIONS ASSOCIATED WITH VULVAR OR VAGINAL MANIFESTATIONS

Crohn's Disease

Crohn's disease can affect the vulva and present as persistent, nonhealing or poorly healing ulcers (Fig. 5.6). It may also present as rectovaginal or anocutaneous fistulae. The vulvar manifestations may precede the onset of bowel disease. Systemic treatment for Crohn's is necessary (55). Consultation with a gastrointestinal or general surgeon is indicated.

Behçet's Syndrome

Behçet's syndrome is a rare and recurrent vasculitis syndrome with an unknown etiology characterized by recurrent oral and genital mucosal ulcers that may occur concurrently or separately. In addition to oral ulceration, at least two of the following signs must be present to confirm the diagnosis of Behçet's: (a) genital ulceration or scarring; (b) erythema nodosum or an acnelike rash on the arms, legs, and trunk; (c) uveitis or retinal vasculitis; and (d) a positive pathergy test (skin hypersensitivity to needle puncture) (56). Ocular involvement begins as superficial inflammation that may develop into uveitis and even blindness. When oral and genital ulcers are present, but the criteria for Behçet's disease are not met, the diagnosis is oral-genital aphthoses. Diagnosis is based on clinical symptomatology because biopsy pathologic analysis generally is nonspecific.

An ideal therapeutic regiment does not exist. Topical steroid (clobetasol propionate 0.05% ointment twice daily, with a gradual decrease to daily) is used at the initial sign or symptom of a Behçet vulvar ulcer formation. When ulcers are enlarged, however, topical steroids are not efficacious and may be irritating. In these instances, oral prednisone (60 mg/day for 1 to 2 weeks) with a slow taper (decrease by 10 mg every 1 to 2 weeks) may be tried. Recurrences are common and are unpredictable.

Neurofibromatosis

Generalized neurofibromatosis and café au lait spots (Von Recklinghausen's disease) rarely involve the vulva, but when it does, excision is required for diagnosis and is the treatment of choice for symptomatic tumors (55, 57).

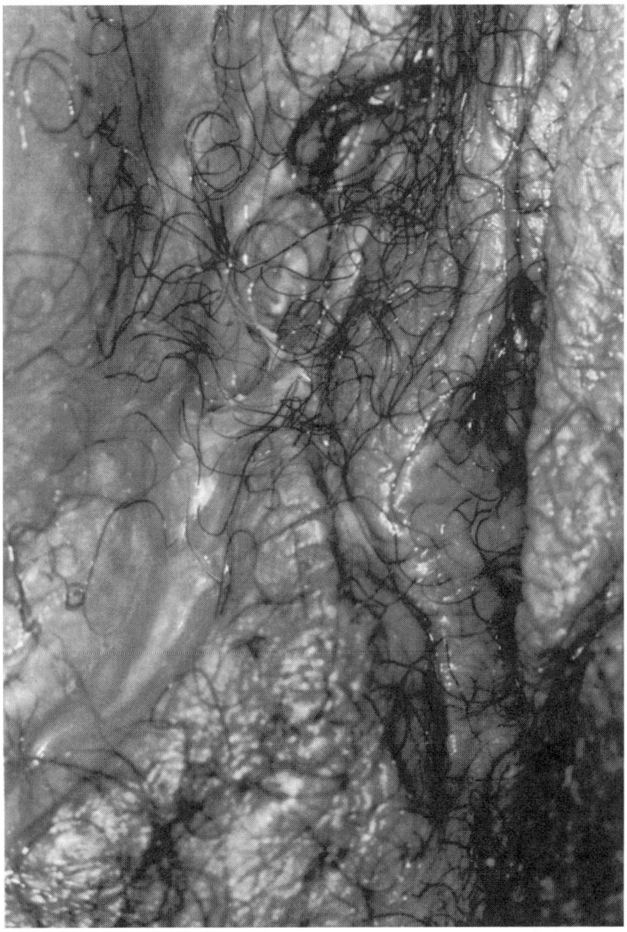

FIGURE 5.6 • Deep vulvar ulceration in a patient with Crohn's disease of the vulva and bowel for approximately 9 years. Exacerbation of vulvar disease was unresponsive to prednisone 60 mg orally every day and metronidazole 500 mg orally three times a day. Imuran was started at 100 mg orally every day. (Reprinted from Wilkinson EJ, Stone IK, eds. Atlas of Vulvar Disease. Baltimore: Williams & Wilkins, 1995:180, with permission.)

Cicatricial Pemphigoid

Cicatricial pemphigoid is an autoimmune disease that results in blistering of the mucosal surfaces and occurs mostly in older patients. Patients may present with superficial vulvovaginal ulcers, desquamative vaginitis, and conjunctivitis. Because the conjunctiva may scar somewhat extensively, the optic manifestations should be treated fairly aggressively. Diagnosis is made by biopsy of the vulvovaginal lesion(s). This should be treated in consultation with a dermatologist.

Vulvar Pyoderma Gangrenosum

Vulvar pyoderma gangrenosum (PG) is an uncommon condition that manifests as a single ulcer or multiple painful ulcers; its etiology is unknown. It is associated with systemic diseases such as inflammatory bowel disease, rheumatoid arthritis, chronic active hepatitis, and hematologic malignancies in at least 50% of patients who are affected. Ulcerations of PG may occur after trauma or injury to the skin in 30% of patients. The ulcers have a well-defined violaceous border, an overhanging ulcer edge, and necrotic tissue at the base. Conservative wound care and systemic corticosteroids are usually effective therapy.

SOLID TUMORS

Patients may discover a growth on the vulva and will often come to the office describing this as "a lump." The anxiety level in this situation is usually high because the patient presumes it is malignant. Fortunately, most of these growths are benign. The clinician, however, must be aware of the potential for malignancy. Usually, biopsy or complete removal of any growth is required. This can be performed in an elective fashion in the office or operating room, depending on the size and location of the lesion. Patients with large lesions and/or lesion(s) close to the clitoris will require anesthesia. These should be removed in the operating room.

Fibroma

Fibroma(s) of the vulva is the most common benign, solid vulvar tumor. It arises from the fibrous tissue of the vulva, tends to be pedunculated, and is small to moderate in size. Vulvar fibroma usually develops along the insertion of the round ligament into the labium majus. Microscopically, it is similar to a fibroid of the uterus. These are benign processes that should be removed because a leiomyosarcoma or sarcoma of the vulva can arise in the same area, and removal is necessary to establish the diagnosis.

Lipoma

Lipomas are the second most common benign, solid vulvar tumor. They are superficial and commonly located in the labium majus, and their risk of malignant transformation is very low. They can involve the vulva and should be locally removed. They are usually asymptomatic.

Nevi

Nevi of the vulva are very common and elective removal should be considered because of their malignant potential. If the decision is made to observe the lesion(s), digital photography is an excellent way to monitor for changes over time (3). They have a wide variety of appearances and may range in size from a few millimeters up to 2 cm. When excised, a margin of 5 to 10 mm of normal skin surrounding the nevus and the underlying dermis should be removed. This can be done at the time of an obstetric delivery or in the office with local anesthesia. Any recent changes in size, shape, color, or demonstration of friability mandate biopsy.

Mammary Tissue

Supernumerary mammary tissue can involve the vulva on one or both sides. This follows the "milk line" from the breast down to the vulva. This tissue may go unnoticed until the patient is pregnant or lactating. Simple excision is all that is necessary. Rarely do these develop malignancy.

Hidradenoma

Hidradenomas are benign tumors arising from the apocrine (sweat) glands (58). They may also originate from the interlabial eccrine glands. Hidradenomas are usually located in the interlabial sulcus, are solitary, nontender, and may have an umbilicated center. They may present as an ulcerated lesion. These tumors are found in Caucasian women 30 to 70 years of age and are rare in African American women. Treatment is with surgical excision.

Fox-Fordyce Disease

Fox-Fordyce disease presents as pruritic papules originating from apocrine glands on the mons, on the labia majora, and in the axillae. It is most commonly seen in women of color. Patients develop multiple, firm, small papules that are flesh colored to hyperpigmented. The pruritus can be severe and is provoked by physical exercise, mental stress, and emotions. It is most common in women ages 13 to 35 years. Numerous treatments, including oral contraceptives, oral antihistamines, and topical clindamycin have been tried. Topical application of tretinoin may be effective but may provoke irritation. Although topical corticosteroids may help relieve the itch, prolonged use of corticosteroids in skin folds or occluded sites carries a high risk of corticosteroid side effects. Surgical removal of the apocrine glands in recalcitrant cases has been reported to relieve symptoms of pruritus and significantly decrease the number of papules.

Syringomata

Syringomata are benign papules that are of eccrine gland origin. The typical clinical appearance of syringoma is firm, with skin-colored to brown papules on the eyelids. They may also occur on the malar area, scalp, peripheral parts of the body, and vulva. Cosmetic considerations are generally the only reason to treat syringoma. Surgical and chemical destructive treatments carry the risks of scarring, postinflammatory pigmentary changes, and recurrence.

Polyps

Fibroepithelial polyps (acrochordon) are benign growths that should be removed to ensure they are not malignant. Fibroepithelial polyps can arise from the lateral walls of the vagina or at the vaginal cuff after hysterectomy. These are benign but require excision for diagnosis.

Granular Cell Myoblastoma or Schwannoma

Granular cell myoblastoma or schwannoma of the vulva is a very rare entity. It was initially believed to be related to smooth muscle cells; however, the currently accepted theory is that granular cell tumor of the vulva is of a neurogenic origin. The vulva is involved in 5 to 15% of cases of granular cell tumor (59). Clinically, it is characterized by a slow-growing, solitary, and firm subcutaneous nodule. These are infiltrating and increase in size, which may lead to erosion through the skin surface and result in an ulcerative lesion that may be confused with cancer. This tumor can recur after excision due to benign local invasion. Malignant granular cell tumor, although rare, does not respond to radiation or chemotherapy.

Endometriosis

This may present as either a solid, cystic, or mixed lesion on the vulva or in the vagina. It is usually a secondary presentation of pelvic endometriosis. The patient may complain of cyclical, painful swelling in the vulva, as well as dyspareunia, dysmenorrhea, pelvic pain, or dysuria. Examination may reveal brown (or black) mucoid cystic lesions on the external genitalia. Systemic therapy for endometriosis will be effective for this, although excision (or destruction by electrocautery or laser) of the lesion is usually the treatment of choice.

CYSTIC LESIONS

Vaginal wall cysts are most common in the thirties and forties, and in most cases, an accurate diagnosis can be made on history and physical examination. During physical examination, the lesion should be assessed for location, mobility, tenderness, definition, and consistency. Malignancy must always be considered in the differential diagnosis.

Bartholin's Duct Cyst

The Bartholin's duct cyst is the most common cystic growth in the vulva. The majority of these are unilateral nontender cystic masses in the lateral introitus, medial to the labia minora. Ductal obstruction due to infection or thickened mucus leads to cyst formation (60). It commonly occurs in younger women, and treatment in young women is rendered only if the cyst is infected, enlarges, or is producing symptoms. The ductal cyst or the gland itself may become infected and form an abscess. The infection is usually polymicrobial, with anaerobic and aerobic vaginal bacteria isolated. An infected Bartholin's gland or ductal cyst should be treated with antimicrobials (e.g., Ceftriaxone 125 mg intramuscularly or Cefixime 400 mg orally); Clindamycin (or Flagyl) may be added to cover anaerobes. Azithromycin is added if *Chlamydia trachomatis* is present.

One of the more common management errors is premature incision and drainage. The abscess should be allowed to fully "mature" so a well-developed, walled-off structure is formed. At this point, an incision should be made on the mucosal side, where the abscess cavity is closest to the mucosa. Treatment may include simple incision and drainage, use of a Wood catheter, or marsupialization. Pain medications and warm sitz baths may be necessary until the abscess is well developed. A postmenopausal patient who develops an enlarged Bartholin gland or duct cyst should have it removed because there is an increased risk for underlying malignancy in this age group (61, 62).

Müllerian Cysts

Although Müllerian cysts may occur anywhere in the vaginal wall, they are most commonly noted in the anterolateral wall. They are the most common type of vaginal cyst and vary in size from 1 to 7 cm. The majority of these cysts are small, asymptomatic, and require no treatment.

Gartner Duct Cysts

Gartner's duct cysts arise from Wolffian remnants and occur on the lateral vaginal sidewalls. They are usually about 1 cm in diameter and are firm on palpation. Distinction between a Müllerian cyst and Gartner's duct cyst is not clinically relevant. If they enlarge, Gartner's duct cysts may be confused for a urethral diverticulum or even cystocele. Gartner's duct cysts may be associated with abnormalities of the metanephric urinary system. If the cyst is large or symptomatic, excision is indicated; otherwise, it may be followed.

Skene's Duct Cysts

A Skene's gland (paraurethral gland) cyst can occur in the suburethral area when these glands become occluded. If they become infected, Skene's duct cysts may form. These cysts are rare, but if they enlarge to greater than 2 cm, they may interfere with urination. A Skene's duct cyst must be distinguished from a urethral diverticulum. Compression of a Skene's duct cyst will not result in fluid extravasation, a finding commonly—but not uniformly—found with a urethral diverticulum.

Small Skene's cysts may also be observed. They are usually small and can be followed conservatively. If they enlarge significantly, they may require removal.

Cyst in the Canal of Nuck

A hydrocele or cyst in the canal of Nuck is a rudimentary peritoneal sac that accompanies the round ligament into the labium majus through the inguinal canal. Occlusion of the canal may lead to formation of a cyst. These cysts are usually found at the superior end of the labium or in the inguinal canal. An inguinal hernia is present in up to one-third of patients with a hydrocele of the canal of Nuck (63). Rarely, a bowel loop is also present in the canal. Drainage of the cyst fluid is not effective treatment (60). Treatment must include ligation of the peritoneal sac at the inguinal ligament or the cyst will recur.

Epidermal Inclusion Cyst

Epidermal inclusion cysts are a common disorder usually presenting as a small hard lump and contain a white sebaceous-looking material. Inclusion cysts are a result of buried epithelial tissue during episiotomy repair or other vaginal surgery (60). They are usually asymptomatic and do not require treatment unless they cause dyspareunia or pain or become infected. If infected, incision and drainage is the mainstay of therapy. Those with recurrent infections or those producing pain should be excised after the acute inflammation has subsided.

Vaginal Emphysematosa

Vaginitis emphysematosa is a rare condition characterized by gas-filled cysts in the vaginal wall. Most cases are associated with *Trichomonas vaginalis* (64). Diagnosis is made on physical examination; the cysts are usually in the upper two-thirds of the vagina and are discrete, tense, and smooth. They may make a popping sound when they are ruptured. This condition is self-limiting and does not require any specific therapy other than treatment of any underlying vaginal infections.

PREMALIGNANT CONDITIONS

Vulvar Intraepithelial Neoplasia

Vulvar dysplasia, or vulvar intraepithelial neoplasia (VIN), is reported as VIN I, II, or III (synonymous with carcinoma in situ). The incidence of VIN has increased significantly since the 1970s (65, 66). This increase has occurred mainly in women who are younger than 40 years of age and in women who smoke (65).

There are two types of VIN: simplex or differentiated and classic or bowenoid. Both are distinct entities that differ clinically and pathologically. In some instances, VIN may have mixed simplex and classic features. Although classic VIN is diagnosed more frequently than simplex VIN, the latter may play a larger role in the pathogenesis of vulvar SCC.

Most of the women who have VIN are asymptomatic. The most common presenting symptom, if it does occur, is pruritus. When examining the patient for VIN, the buttocks must be separated to allow for careful examination of the perianal area. VIN is highly variable in its gross appearance and may only be apparent with colposcopy. When using colposcopy to evaluate for VIN, it is important to remember that the vulvar area must be soaked with acetic acid for about 5 minutes. Acetowhite changes do not determine the diagnosis, rather they only serve to indicate where biopsies should be taken. A biopsy is necessary for any raised, hyperpigmented lesion. Treatment of VIN is wide local excision or laser therapy for patients with no evidence of gross or microscopic invasion. In one small nonrandomized trial, imiquimod was used in patients with VIN II/III with success (67).

Circumscribed lesions of the vulva should be treated by wide local excision. Although large comparative trials are needed, one trial showed loop electrosurgical excision procedure to be a clinically effective treatment for VIN and the most cost effective (68). Superficial but multifocal disease may be treated by "skinning vulvectomy," followed by split-thickness skin graft. Laser therapy may have a role in a clinical trial of patients expected to be at very low risk of invasion, such as patients younger than 40 years of age with multifocal disease. Patients treated for VIN should be followed with colposcopy every 3 to 4 months until they are disease free for 2 years; follow-up after that can occur every 6 months.

Classic

Classic VIN (also known as bowenoid or undifferentiated VIN or Bowen's disease) accounts for at least 90% of cases of VIN and is easy to recognize histologically. It may occur at any age, but its peak prevalence is in the third and fourth decades. These lesions are strongly HPV associated, with HPV-16 implicated in 70% of cases (69). Patients with classic VIN often have a history of condyloma acuminatum, sexually transmitted infections, current HIV-positive status, or cigarette smoking.

Classic VIN tends to be pigmented and multifocal. When excised specimens of VIN are sent to the pathologist, they must be extensively sampled and carefully examined for stromal invasion as occult areas of invasive carcinoma have been identified in 6 to 7% of patients in some series (70). Only 3 to 10% of women with classic VIN will go on to develop invasive SCC (71). Women older than 40 and those who are immunosuppressed are at the greatest risk of progression. Younger women with multifocal small papular pigmented lesions (a clinical entity referred to as bowenoid papulosis) are the most likely to experience spontaneous resolution of the lesions, particularly if they are pregnant or postpartum at the time of diagnosis (72).

Simplex

Simplex lesions are less bulky and are more subtle than those of classic VIN; they often appear as grayish white lesions with a rough surface or as a raised, thickened plaque. They account for about 2 to 10% of VIN cases. The lesions may be multifocal. Simplex or differentiated

VIN typically occurs in postmenopausal women. Histologically, it may easily be mistaken for nonspecific squamous hyperplasia or acanthosis.

Although simplex VIN accounts for only 2 to 10% of biopsy specimens with VIN, it is more likely to progress to SCC than classic VIN. Grading is applicable to classic VIN but not simplex VIN. By definition, simplex VIN is a high-grade lesion. Unlike classic VIN, simplex VIN lesions do not normally contain HPV, nor do any associated malignancies (73). VIN found in patients with LS and vulvar "dystrophy" is usually of the simplex type.

Vaginal Intraepithelial Neoplasm

Vaginal intraepithelial neoplasm (VAIN) is the terminology used to describe vaginal dysplasia. This spans the spectrum from VAIN I (mild dysplasia) to VAIN III (severe dysplasia or carcinoma in situ). Premalignant neoplasms (VAIN) are almost always asymptomatic and often detected by an abnormal Pap smear. A tissue diagnosis must be established when an abnormal cytologic smear of the vaginal cuff is obtained. Colposcopy is performed with biopsy of the most abnormal area. If there is any question of invasion, excision under anesthesia must be undertaken. VAIN is usually multifocal, and one-third to one-half of patients with VAIN have been treated for similar disorder of the cervix or vulva. VAIN can be satisfactorily treated with 5-fluorouracil (5-FU) therapy (Efudex cream), reserving local excision for those patients who fail conservative therapy. Because VAIN is usually multifocal, follow-up should occur every 3 to 4 months with colposcopy of the entire lower genital tract for 2 years, and 6 months thereafter until they have been disease free for 5 years.

CONCLUSION

Vulvovaginal disease can be a challenging and vexing problem for the clinician. Many problems can arise if an accurate diagnosis is not established. The hallmark of diagnosis should be biopsy. If there is any question whatsoever, biopsy is mandatory to rule out malignancy. Once an accurate diagnosis is established, therapies can be selectively directed to the problem. The problems can be chronic in nature, and the clinician must remember that other problems may develop over time. Thus, constant vigilance and re-examination with rebiopsy may be necessary when following these patients. Satisfactory results can usually be achieved when an accurate diagnosis is established.

Clinical Notes

- Vulvodynia is defined as vulvar pain occurring in the absence of an underlying recognizable disease. The classification of vulvodynia is based on the site of the pain, whether it is generalized or localized, and whether it is provoked, unprovoked, or mixed.
- The older terminology for vestibulodynia was vulvar vestibulitis, but this term has been eliminated from the ISSVD terminology because the presence of inflammation, as implied by the suffix "-itis" has not been documented so far.
- TCAs, such as Amitriptyline (10 to 75 mg), have been used with some success in treating vestibulodynia.
- Other treatments for vestibulodynia include gabapentin, nitroglycerin cream, lidocaine gel, steroids, and biofeedback.
- Treatment of contact dermatitis involves identification and elimination of the irritating agent. Topical steroids may be used for 2 to 3 weeks to reduce inflammation and promote healing.
- Doxepin or hydroxyzine may be particularly helpful when antihistamines do not control pruritic symptoms, although both may be sedating.

- Because of the increased risk of a noncontiguous adenocarcinoma, if the diagnosis of vulvar Paget's is made, the workup should include colonoscopy, cystoscopy, mammogram, and colposcopy.
- Lichen simplex chronicus represents an end-stage disorder resulting from long-standing irritation, endogenous eczema, allergens, or infection.
- LS does not involve the vagina.
- LP presents in two ways: classic and erosive forms; it may involve the vagina.
- LP and psoriasis can exhibit Köbner's phenomenon (i.e., the disease can flare at any site of injury, including surgical sites).
- Therapeutic intervention in hidradenitis suppurativa is aimed at decreasing bacterial overgrowth, treating infection, and diminishing pain, drainage, and odor.
- Vulvar fibroma usually develops along the insertion of the round ligament into the labium majus.
- One of the more common management errors with Bartholin's duct cysts is premature incision and drainage. The abscess should be allowed to fully "mature" so a well-developed, walled-off structure is formed.
- The incidence of VIN has increased significantly since the 1970s.
- Although classic VIN is diagnosed more frequently than simplex VIN, the latter may play a larger role in the pathogenesis of vulvar SCC.
- When using colposcopy to evaluate for VIN, it is important to remember that the vulvar area must be soaked with acetic acid for about 5 minutes. Acetowhite changes do not determine the diagnosis, rather they only serve to indicate where biopsies should be taken.
- VAIN is usually multifocal and can be satisfactorily treated with 5-FU therapy (Efudex cream), reserving local excision for those patients who fail conservative therapy.

REFERENCES

1. Taylor PT. Biopsy of lesions of the female genital tract. Surg Oncol Clin N Am 1995;4(1):121–135.
2. Kaufman RH, Gardner HL. Vulvar dystrophies. Clin Obstet Gynecol 1978;21(4):1081–1106.
3. Foster DC. Vulvar disease. Obstet Gynecol 2002;100:145–163.
4. Welsh BM, Berzins KN, Cook KA, et al. Management of common vulval conditions. MJA 2003;178:391–395.
5. Haefner HK, Collins ME, Davis GD, et al. The vulvodynia guideline. J Lower Genital Tract Dis 2005;9(1): 40–51.
6. Edwards L. Subsets of vulvodynia: overlapping characteristics. J Reprod Med 2004;49:883–887.
7. Harlow BL, Stewart EG. A population-based assessment of chronic unexplained vulvar pain: have we underestimated the prevalence of vulvodynia? J Am Med Womens Assoc 2003;58:82–88.
8. Meana M, Ninik YM, Khalife S, et al. Biopsychosocial profile of women with dyspareunia. Obstet Gynecol 1997;90:583–589.
9. Harlow BL, Stewart EG. A population-based assessment of chronic unexplained vulvar pain: have we underestimated the prevalence of vulvodynia? J Am Med Womens Assoc 2003;58:82–88.
10. Danilsson I, Sjoberg I, Wikman M. Vulvar vestibulitis: medical, psychosexual and psychosocial aspects, a case-control study. Acta Obstet Gynecol Scand 2000;79:872–878.
11. McKay M. Vulvitis and vulvovaginitis: cutaneous considerations. Am J Obstet Gynecol 1991;165:1176–1182.
12. Bouchard C, Brisson J, Forteier M, et al. Use of oral contraceptive pills and vulvar vestibulitis: a case control study. Am J Epidemiol 2002;156:254–261.
13. Berglund AL, Nigaard L, Ruander E. Vulvar pain, sexual behavior and genital infections in a young population: a pilot study. Acta Obstet Gynecol Scand 2002;8:738–742.
14. Bohm-Starke N, Johannesson U, Hilliges M, et al. Decreased mechanical pain threshold in the vestibular mucosa of women using oral contraceptives: a contributing factor in vulvar vestibulitis? J Reprod Med 2004;49:888–892.
15. Pagano R. Vulvar vestibulitis syndrome: an often unrecognized cause of dyspareunia. Aust N Z J Obstet Gynaecol 1999;39:79–83.
16. Scheinfeld N. The role of gabapentin in treating diseases with cutaneous manifestations and pain. Int J Dermatol 2003;42:491–495.
17. Walsh KE, Berman JR, Berman LA, et al. Safety and efficacy of topical nitroglycerin for treatment of vulvar pain in women with vulvodynia: a pilot study. J Gend Specif Med 2002;5:21–27.
18. Zolnoun DA, Hartmann KE, Steege JF. Overnight 5% lidocaine ointment for treatment of vulvar vestibulitis. Obstet Gynecol 2003;102:84–87.

19. Nyirjesy P, Sobel JD, Weitz MV, et al. Cromolyn cream for recalcitrant idiopathic vulvar vestibulitis: results of a placebo controlled study. Sex Transmit Infect 2001;77:53–57.
20. Marinoff SC, Turer ML, Hirsch RP, et al. Intralesional alpha interferon: cost-effective therapy for vulvar vestibulitis syndrome. J Reprod Med 1993;38:19–24.
21. Bergeron S, Binik YM, Khalife S, et al. A randomized comparison of group cognitive-behavioral therapy, surface electromyographic biofeedback, and vestibulectomy in the treatment of dyspareunia resulting form vulvar vestibulitis. Pain 2001;91:297–306.
22. Bornstein J, Goldik Z, Stolar Z, et al. Predicting the outcome of surgical treatment for vulvar vestibulitis. Obstet Gynecol 1997;89:695–698.
23. Smart OC, MacLean AB. Vulvodynia. Curr Opin Obstet Gynecol 2003;15(6):497–500.
24. Davis GD, Hutchison CV. Clinical management of vulvodynia. Clin Obstet Gynecol 1999;42(2):221–233.
25. Edwards L. New concepts in vulvodynia. Am J Obstet Gynecol 2003;189:S24–S30.
26. Friedrich EG. Vulvar dystrophy. Clin Obstet Gynecol 1985;28:178–187.
27. Foster DC. Vulvar disease. Obstet Gynecol 2002;100:145–163.
28. Margesson LJ. Contact dermatitis of the vulva. Dermatol Ther 2004;17:20–27.
29. Feuer J, Shevchuk M, Calanog A. Vulvar Paget's disease: the need to exclude an invasive lesion. Gynecol Oncol 1990;38:81–89.
30. Fanning J, Lambert HC, Hale TM, et al. Paget's disease of the vulva: prevalence of associated vulvar adenocarcinoma, invasive Paget's disease, and recurrence after surgical excision. Am J Obstet Gynecol 1999;180:24–27.
31. Virgili A, Bacilieri S, Corazza M. Managing vulvar lichen simplex chronicus. J Reprod Med 2001;46:343–346.
32. Panet-Raymond G, Girard C. Lichen sclerosus et Atrophicus. Can Med Assoc J 1972;106(12):1332–1334.
33. Ridley CM. Lichen sclerosus. Dermatol Clin 1992;10(2):309–318.
34. Meyrick-Thomas RH, Ridley CM, McGibbon DH, et al. Lichen sclerosus and autoimmunity—a study of 350 women. Br J Dermatol 1988;118:41–46.
35. Bracco Gl, Carli P, Sonni L, et al. Clinical and histologic effects of topical treatments of vulval lichen sclerosus: a critical evaluation. J Reprod Med 1993;38:37–40.
36. Bornstein J, Heifetz S, Kellner Y, et al. Clobetasol dipropionate 0.05% versus testosterone propionate 2% topical application for severe vulvar lichen sclerosus. Am J Obstet Gynecol 1998;178:80–84.
37. Goldstein AT, Marinoff SC, Christopher K. Pimecrolimus for the treatment of vulvar lichen sclerosus: a report of 4 cases. J Reprod Med 2004;49:778–780.
38. Assmann T, Becker-Wegerich P, Grewe M, et al. Tacrolimus ointment for the treatment of vulvar lichen sclerosus. J Am Acad Dermatol 2003;48:935–937.
39. Bohm M, Frieling U, Luger TA, et al. Successful treatment of anogenital lichen sclerosus with topical tacrolimus. Arch Dermatol 2003;139:922–924.
40. Gupta AK, Chow M. Pimecrolimus: a review. J Eur Acad Dermatol Venerol 2003;17:493–503.
41. Carlson JA, Ambros R, Malfetano J, et al. Vulvar lichen sclerosus and squamous cell carcinoma: a cohort, case control and investigational study with historical perspective: implications for chronic inflammation and sclerosis in the development of neoplasia. Hum Pathol 1998;29:932–948.
42. Rodke G, Friedrich EG, Wilkinson EJ. Malignant potential of mixed vulvar dystrophy (lichen sclerosus associated with squamous cell hyperplasia). J Reprod Med 1988;33:545–550.
43. van der Meij E, Schepman K, Smeele L, et al. A review of the recent literature regarding malignant transformation of oral lichen planus. Oral Surg Oral Med Oral Pathol Oral Radiol Endod 1999;88:307–310.
44. Kavanagh GM, Burton PA, Kennedy CTC. Vulvitis circumscripta plasmacellularis (Zoon's vulvitis). Br J Dermatol 1993;129:92–93.
45. Neill S. K. Reddy et al's case report on a rare case of plasma cell vulvitis (Zoon's vulvitis). J Obstet Gynecol 2002;22:230.
46. Pelisse M. The vulvo-vaginal-ginigival syndrome: a new form of erosive lichen planus. Int J Dermatol 1989; 28:381–384.
47. Weichert GE. An approach to the treatment of anogenital pruritus. Dermatol Ther 2004;17:129–133.
48. von der Werth JM, Jemec GB. Morbidity in patients with hidradenitis suppurativa. Br J Dermatol 2001; 144:809–813.
49. Leybishkis B, Fasseas P, Ryan KF, et al. Hidradenitis suppurativa and acne conglobata associated with spondyloarthropathy. Am J Med Sci 2001;321:195–197.
50. Cosman BC, O'Grady TC, Pekarske S. Verrucous carcinoma arising in hidradenitis suppurativa. Int J Colorectal Dis 2000;15:342–346.
51. Mortimer P. Management of hidradenitis suppurativa [Abstract]. Clin Exp Dermatol 2002;27:328.
52. Jemec GB. Methotrexate is of limited value in the treatment of hidradenitis suppurativa. Clin Exp Dermatol 2002;27:528–529.
53. Scheman AJ. Nodulocystic acne and hidradenitis suppurativa treated with acitretin: a case report. Cutis 2002;69:287–288.
54. Adams DR, Gordon KB, Devenyi AG, et al. Severe hidradenitis suppurativa treated with infliximab infusion. Arch Dermatol 2003;139(12):1540–1542.
55. Cormen ML, Veidengeimer MC, Coller JA, et al. Perineal wound healing after proctectomy for inflammatory bowel disease. Dis Colon Rectum 1978;21(3):155–159.
56. International Study Group for Behçet's Disease. Criteria for diagnosis of Behçet's disease (review). Lancet 1990;335:1078–1080.
57. Lewis FM, Lewis-Jones MS, Ton PG, et al. Neurofibromatosis of the vulva. Br J Dermatol 1992;127(5):540–541.

58. Virgili A, Marzola A, Corazza M. Vulvar hidradenoma papilliferum. J Reprod Med 2000;45:616–618.
59. Simone J, Schneider GT, Begneaud W, et al. Granular Cell tumor or the vulva: literature review and case report. J La State Med Soc 1996;148:539–541.
60. Eilber KS, Raz S. Benign cystic lesions of the vagina: a literature review. J Urol 2003;170:717–722.
61. Leuchter RS, Hacker NF, Voet RL, et al. Primary carcinoma of the Bartholin gland: a report of 14 cases and review of the literature. Obstet Gynecol 1982;60(3):361–368.
62. Dunn S. Adenoid cystic carcinoma of Bartholin's gland. A review of the literature and report of a patient. Acta Obstet Gynecol Scand 1995;74:78–79.
63. Block RE. Hydrocele of the canal of Nuck. A report of five cases. Obstet Gynecol 1975;45:464–466.
64. Gardner HL, Fernet P. Etiology of vaginitis emphysematosa. Am J Obstet Gynecol 1964;88:680.
65. Sturgeon SR, Brinton LA, Devesa SS, et al. In situ and invasive vulvar cancer incidence trends. Am J Obstet Gynecol 1992;166:1482–1485.
66. Iversen T, Tretli S. Intraepithelial and invasive squamous cell neoplasia of the vulva: trends in incidence, recurrence and survival rate in Norway. Obstet Gynecol 1998;91:969–972.
67. Marchitelli C, Secco G, Perrotta M, et al. Treatment of bowenoid and basaloid vulvar intraepithelial neoplasia 2/3 with imiquimod 5% cream. J Reprod Med 2004;49:876–882.
68. Vlastos AT, Levy LB, Malpica A, et al. Loop electrosurgical excision procedure in vulvar intraepithelial neoplasia treatment. J Lower Genital Tract Dis 2002;6(4):232–238.
69. Crum CP, McLachlin CM, Tate JE, et al. Pathobiology of vulvar squamous neoplasia. Curr Opin Obstet Gynecol 1997;9:63–69.
70. Rettenmaier MA, Berman ML, DiSaia PJ. Skinning vulvectomy for the treatment of multifocal vulvar intraepithelial neoplasia. Obstet Gynecol 1987;69:247–250.
71. Jones RW, Rowan DM. Vulvar intraepithelial neoplasia III: a clinical study of the outcome in 113 cases with relation to the later development of invasive vulvar carcinoma. Obstet Gynecol 1994;84:741–745.
72. Jones RW, Rowen DM. Spontaneous regression of vulvar intraepithelial neoplasia 2–3. Obstet Gynecol 2000;96:470–472.
73. Yang B, Hart WR. Vulvar intraepithelial neoplasia of the simplex (differentiated) type: a clinicopathologic study including analysis of HPV and p53 expression. Am J Surg Pathol 2000;96:470–472.

CHAPTER 6

Benign Disorders and Diseases of the Breast

Daniel P. Guyton and Andrew Fenton

INTRODUCTION

Diseases of the breast comprise a diverse clinical spectrum. The etiologies and therapies of breast diseases remain clouded by clinical inaccuracies, social myths, and continually evolving medical controversies. Fortunately, the majority of patients with breast disease in a busy clinician's practice will have one of the more common benign breast diseases and not breast cancer. From the patient's perspective, however, benign disease may be as frightening as breast cancer. The physician must recognize that fear of cancer is widespread and is often the motivating factor in seeking medical attention.

All physicians who treat women must be familiar with the clinical fundamentals of benign breast disease. This chapter discusses breast anatomy, proper history and examination skills, and benign breast disease.

CLINICAL ANATOMY

The breast is composed of fat and parenchymal tissue, which often extends well into the axilla. The amount of fat and parenchyma varies with age and parity. Breast fat increases with age, body mass, and total breast volume, although this is not absolute. It is estimated that half of women have a volume difference of 10% between the left and right breasts and up to 25% of women have a 20% difference; in these instances, the left breast is usually larger than the right (1).

The breast consists of lobes separated from each other by fascial envelopes. Within a breast lobe are 40 or more lobules, and each lobule contains 10 to 100 alveoli or acini, the basic secretory unit of the lactiferous system. Each lobe is drained by a ductal system from which a lactiferous sinus opens on the nipple. Duct-containing tissue may extend to the midline of the chest wall and well up into the axillae. In some instances, the breast tissue may extend below the costal margin or beyond the anterior border of the latissimus dorsi. This is why it is extraordinarily difficult to remove all breast tissue in a subcutaneous mastectomy.

From about the age of 35 until the onset of menopause, there is a gradual loss of lobules, and the loose connective tissue around the lobules changes into dense collagen. Around the onset of menopause and beyond, the lobules lose their characteristic shape and are replaced by a dense collagen with only a compressed remnant of epithelium. This process of lobular involution may lead to the formation of microcysts. As the woman ages, fat deposition into the breast is accelerated and connective tissue becomes less prominent. This causes the breast to change shape and also accounts for the ability of mammography to more easily detect masses in older patients (2).

The blood supply to the breast is from the axillary artery (via its thoracoacromial, lateral thoracic, and subscapular arteries) and from the subclavian artery via the internal thoracic, or internal mammary, artery. The major lymphatic drainage is through the axillary and internal mammary chains of lymph nodes. A small amount of lymph drains across to the opposite breast. Supraclavicular lymph nodes should not be palpable. Enlargement of this nodal group usually occurs with late-stage breast cancer but may also be noted in other disease processes. The skin overlying the breast is relatively thin compared with other regions of the body. It rarely exceeds 1.5 mm in thickness. Thus, patchy, irregular thickness of the skin is abnormal and may occur with tumor infiltration, infection, or other breast and/or systemic disorders.

Ectopic glandular tissue is commonly present in the axilla and this can proliferate during pregnancy and cause significant discomfort. Such proliferation will regress either with delivery or cessation of lactation. From a histologic perspective, this is normal breast tissue and is subject to both benign and malignant disorders. It should not be confused with a prominent axillary tail of Spence, a normal anatomic variant that may also enlarge during pregnancy. The axillary tail of Spence is usually continuous with the glandular tissue of the breast in contrast to ectopic axillary tissue, which may be totally discrete from the breast parenchyma.

DEVELOPMENTAL ABNORMALITIES

The premenarchal breast consists of only a few ducts; under the hormonal influences associated with puberty, lobular structures are added to the developing ductal system. In the early and midreproductive years, these are undifferentiated, budlike structures that later become replaced by more mature and less active lobules. Developmental abnormalities of the breast may be unilateral or bilateral and involve the nipple, breast or both.

Supernumerary nipples or polythelia typically occur alone, although they may occur in conjunction with accessory glandular breast tissue. Supernumerary nipples are most commonly found on the lower part of the breast, chest wall, and upper abdomen (Fig. 6.1). It is a common condition (1 to 2%), and no treatment is required unless the nipple is accompanied by active breast tissue or the patient finds it unacceptable (3).

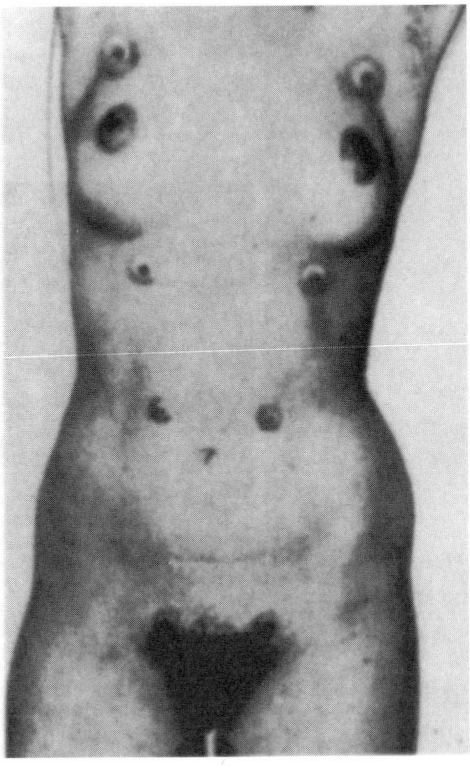

FIGURE 6.1 ● Supernumerary nipples may develop anywhere along the mammary ridge but are most common in the lower abdominal area. (Reprinted from Mitchell GW Jr, Bassett LW. The Female Breast and Its Disorders. Baltimore: Williams & Wilkins, 1990:10, with permission.)

Nipple inversion is common, and there are three primary causes: congenital, periductal inflammation, and tumor infiltration. The true incidence of nipple inversion is unknown, and problems related to it are functional (i.e., difficulty breast-feeding) or cosmetic. The nipple plays a relatively small role in the structural process of suckling; the infant's suckling makes a teat from the surrounding breast tissue and the nipple in a 3:1 ratio. For this reason, women with inverted nipples should be reassured that the contribution of the nipple to the process of breast-feeding is small and should be encouraged to simply ensure the infant has an adequate mouthful of breast tissue to form the teat (2). Supernumerary breasts, or accessory breasts, are structures that contain hormonally responsive breast tissue and may produce milk in the right circumstances. Supernumerary breast tissue is not always accompanied by a nipple and may be bothersome during pregnancy and lactation. This ectopic breast tissue is subject to all physiological processes seen in the breast and so must be adequately examined. The most common site of accessory breasts is in the axillae. Treatment is indicated only if it is bothersome to the patient or if clinical findings warrant diagnostic or therapeutic intervention.

Complete lack or absence of breast development is very rare. Genetic abnormalities such as Turner's syndrome (45 X0) or Klinefelter's syndrome (47 XXY) lead to stunting of breast development of variable degrees. Both of these chromosomal abnormalities are characterized by notable physical features involving body height and habitus, distribution of facial or body hair, and/or skeletal aberrations (4).

Amastia or lack of breast development is a rare condition and is assumed to result from failure of the milk line to develop. It is usually unilateral. Absence of a nipple, or athelia, is very rare and usually associated with absence of the breast.

Poland's syndrome is characterized by congenital absence of both breast tissue and the underlying muscle, as well as associated syndactyly. It is always unilateral, and the lack of both the pectoralis major and minor muscles serves as the distinguishing features. Partial forms of Poland's syndrome are more common than the fully manifested syndrome and often go undiagnosed when there is only breast asymmetry and partial absence of the pectoralis muscle.

Tubular breasts or "trunk breast" occur when the areola is excessively large in comparison to the rest of the breast. In extreme cases, the breast is elongated from a narrow base and has a sausage-shaped contour.

The placement of the breasts on the chest wall varies widely; in one extreme, the breasts are fused in the midline. This may cause discomfort with clothing and may be surgically remedied.

Adolescent breast hypertrophy results from stromal hyperplasia during the time of breast development. Gigantomastia represents the most extreme example of breast hypertrophy. The etiology is unknown. It is likely there is an underlying hormonal basis, although no underlying hormonal problems have been identified in these patients. When the enlargement occurs rapidly, drugs such as danazol and bromocriptine may be tried, although their efficacy and proper treatment regimens have not been fully established through clinical trials (5, 6). When medical treatment is indicated, danazol appears to be the first choice based on its safety and side effect profile. Surgery is usually deferred until 17 years of age or greater, but each case must be assessed individually.

Moderate hypertrophy is more common than gigantism but may still result in psychological and physical morbidity. Treatment is indicated when this condition is severe because of the psychological and physical morbidity associated with excessive size and weight of breasts.

Premature breast development in children usually results from estrogen stimulation of an idiopathic etiology. This should not be confused with precocious puberty in which not only breast, but also labial enlargement and pubic hair growth, are stimulated. See Chapter 1 for discussion of this pediatric problem.

PATIENT HISTORY

The first step in evaluating a woman with a suspected breast mass begins with a complete history. The length of time the mass has been present, any fluctuations in size with the menstrual cycle, and any associated pain should be solicited. For those patients with a self-detected breast mass, it is very important to review, in the patient's own words, exactly how she identified the problem. Lesions uncovered through screening mammography will often be nonpalpable and are frequently the most difficult, psychologically, for the patient to deal with.

A careful family history focuses on any relative with benign breast disease, as well as breast or ovarian cancer, especially a mother, sister, or daughter, and their approximate age at cancer diagnosis. All of this should be recorded.

The patient should be asked about any associated pain with the mass(es). Pain was once believed to be a rare symptom of invasive cancer because nerves that track pain are more sensitive to acute stretching than to slow growth. Hence, a cyst that enlarges very rapidly was believed to cause a greater sense of pain than a slowly growing tumor. However, several large series point out that pain can be a symptom of invasive cancer and has been found in 5 to 22% of patients with invasive tumors (7, 8). Thus, the presence of pain should not be used to avoid or delay further evaluation.

EXAMINATION OF THE BREASTS

Proper examination of the breast is fundamental to detecting, diagnosing, and treating breast disease. Pooled data from various studies yield an overall estimate for the sensitivity of clinical breast exam of 54% (95% CI 48.3 to 59.8) and 94% for the pooled specificity (95% CI 90.2 to 96.9) (9). A thorough breast exam requires both a visual and a physical inspection. The following sections describe a complete breast exam. The reader is also referred to Figure 6.2 for a visual display of the proper, complete breast examination.

Inspection

The initial step in the breast exam is inspection. The physician should stand in front of the patient who is seated with her arms bent and her hands on her iliac crests. The patient is asked to exert pressure on her iliac crests while the physician searches for asymmetry, dimpling, or retraction of the overlying skin, or any mass altering the contour of the breast. Retraction, when present, is usually not a subtle finding. Although most common with carcinoma, retraction may also be seen with a chronic abscess associated with periductal mastitis, a large cyst or fibroadenoma arising centrally, or fat necrosis. The color of the skin should be noted because it may be altered with infection, edema, or the classic peau d'orange of carcinoma (which is due to obstruction of the dermal lymphatics). The patient is then asked to raise her arms above her head and press her hands against each other while the physician once again visually inspects the breast. This process is repeated a third time with the patient leaning slightly forward and pushing her hands against her knees with her elbows slightly bent.

The nipple-areolar complex is inspected carefully. A physiologically inverted nipple can almost always be manually everted but a nipple retracted secondary to periductal inflammation or an underlying malignancy cannot. The presence of an encrustation or scaly covering may represent Paget's disease—carcinoma involving the nipple, and not infrequently the areola, but without an underlying palpable mass.

Palpation

Palpation of the breasts should occur with the patient in both the sitting and the supine positions. In sequence, the supraclavicular region, the breast, and the axilla should all receive careful palpation. To best examine the axilla, it is necessary to bend the arm at the elbow and slightly abduct the entire arm. This serves to open the apex of the axilla and permit accurate examination by the examiner's hand as it slides against the rib cage in search of adenopathy. It is important for the patient to relax her arm and shoulder so both are freely movable.

The breasts should be examined in the sitting position as part of the complete breast examination. The examiner supports the breast in the extended nondominant hand and lightly palpates the breast in a sequential fashion with the fingertips of the dominant hand. This exam is

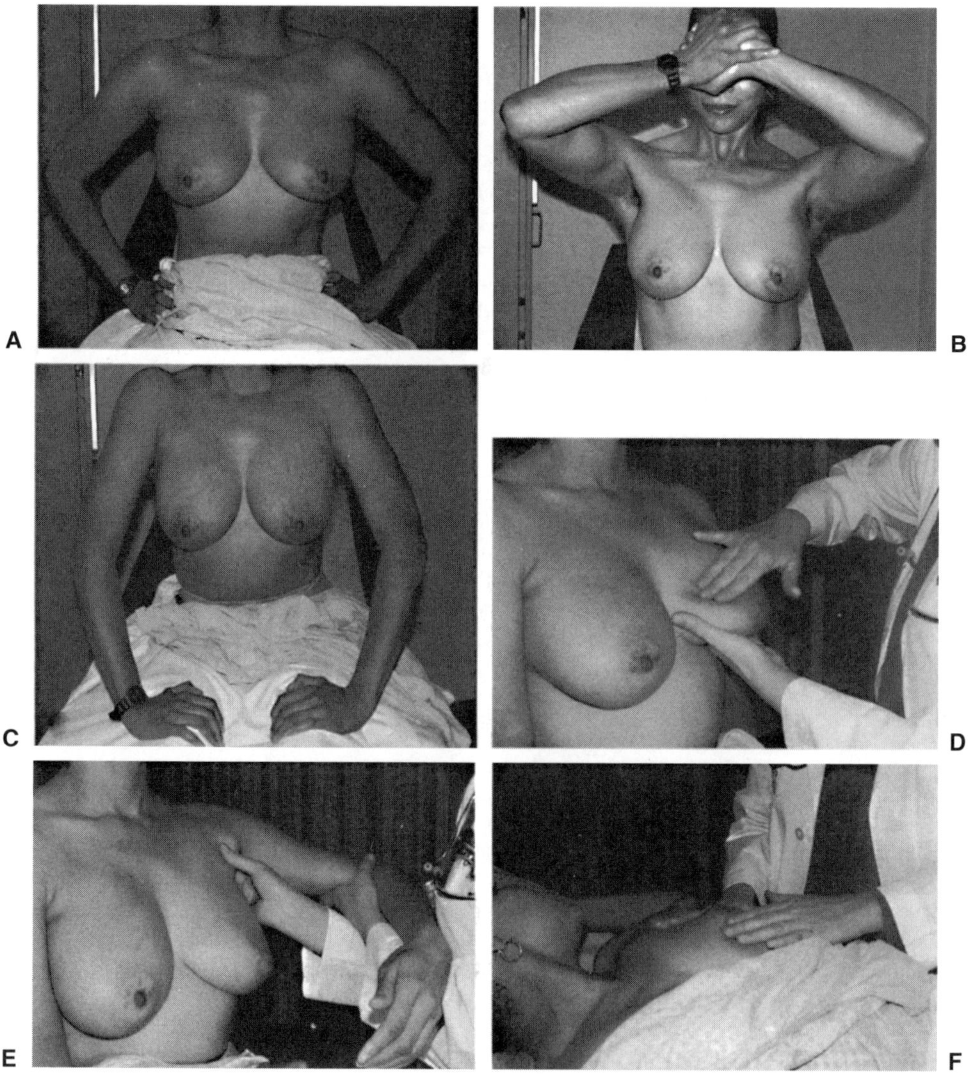

FIGURE 6.2 ● **A:** The patient places her hands on her iliac crests/hips and pushes on them. The breasts are inspected for symmetry, skin changes, dimpling, and/or retraction. **B:** The patient clasps her hands overhead and pushes her hands against each other. The breasts are inspected for symmetry, skin changes, dimpling, and/or retraction. **C:** The patient places her hands on her knees, leans forward slightly, and pushes her hands against her knees. The breasts are inspected for symmetry, skin changes, dimpling, and/or retraction. **D:** For larger breasts, palpation with one hand while the other supports the breast (in the sitting position) may reveal masses not otherwise felt on supine examination. **E:** The axilla are palpated while the ipsilateral arm is supported. To do a thorough examination, it is very important for the patient to relax the arm and shoulder as much as possible (i.e., the arm should be freely movable by the physician). **F:** The breast is inspected with the patient in the supine position with the ipsilateral arm slightly raised.

particularly helpful in women who have large, pendulous breasts. Frequently, there is a ridge of fibrous tissue occupying the inframammary fold bilaterally. This tissue is curvilinear in shape with a variable degree of thickness and represents the attachment of the breast to the underlying chest wall. This should be a symmetric finding.

Next, the patient is asked to assume a recumbent position. If the patient has reported a mass, it may be advantageous to examine the opposite breast initially to gain an appreciation for any masses that may be symmetric. Occasionally, it is helpful to have her rotate her upper body slightly to one side. This will elevate the breast, allowing exposure of the lateral chest wall. Using a small circular motion, the entire breast is examined in a systematic fashion. The ipsilateral arm is then raised with the hand placed behind the head and the breast examined again.

When a lesion is palpated, its consistency, surface characteristics, and mobility in relation to its surrounding tissue should be noted. Even among experienced clinicians, it is often difficult to distinguish between simple glandular tissue and a mass requiring biopsy. It may be useful to stand behind the patient and palpate both breasts simultaneously to more accurately determine if the mass is unilateral or bilateral and symmetric. If the patient is premenopausal, it may be helpful to reexamine her in the first half of the next menstrual cycle.

Distinction between a tense cyst and a solid mass is extremely difficult (if not impossible) by palpation alone. Both cystic and solid masses that prove histologically benign may present with a smooth, rounded surface. Mobility is a key feature to look for and evaluate because malignancies tend to be irregular and fixed to the adjacent tissue. Due to their infiltrative nature, malignancies, particularly those located at the periphery of the breast or below the nipple, will lead to retraction of the overlying tissue. Although these features are helpful palpatory findings in distinguishing a benign mass from a malignant one, they should never serve to singularly exclude biopsy.

Special Situations

Pregnancy

During the first and second trimesters of pregnancy, ductal proliferation occurs under the influence of circulating hormones. This enlargement should be symmetric, although rare instances of massive enlargement of one breast (unilateral gigantism) have been reported. Breast examination during this period of rapid growth in pregnancy may be difficult and confusing. The best safeguard is careful examination of both breasts at the time of the initial office visit, along with thorough documentation of the initial findings. A new asymmetric mass noted during the pregnancy should not be followed; it must be fully evaluated. Surgery on the breast during pregnancy is not without potential complications: damage to the ducts in late pregnancy or postpartum may lead to the formation of milk fistula. Nonetheless, breast masses noted for the first time during pregnancy must be evaluated as fully as if the patient were not pregnant.

The Equivocal Examination

Little is written on this common and frequently vexing problem; that is, what should be done for the patient with an equivocal breast examination? An equivocal examination is one where no discrete mass is evident, nothing is seen radiographically, and yet after careful palpation the physician remains uncertain. Usually, findings consist of glandular prominence. They should not be confused with a "lump" or "mass" because these require histologic diagnosis. If the patient has no genetic or social risk factors and is premenopausal, then re-examination after the next menstrual cycle should be performed. Appropriate referral should not be delayed when the area in question persists through one cycle, in a patient with recognized risk factors, or when the patient is postmenopausal (irrespective of hormone replacement) because the incidence of breast cancer increases with age. In the presence of asymmetry, prompt referral is indicated.

Breast Augmentation

Implants placed for augmentation alter the *shape* of a woman's breast but should not alter the nature of the glandular tissue. It is important to determine if any breast reduction or sculpturing was performed concomitantly because excisional surgery may lead to palpatory differences. Implants can occasionally induce the formation of a fibrous capsule, resulting in breasts that are very firm. Granulomas can also form in patients with silicone implants. These granulomas will be discrete, rock hard, and fixed to the surrounding tissue. They are often superficial and readily palpable; excisional biopsy is required for diagnosis. Needle aspiration of a breast mass in a patient with silicone-filled implants should be performed by an experienced clinician using ultrasound guidance to decrease risk of puncturing the implant, thus causing leakage and potential granuloma formation.

There is no evidence of an excess of any individual connective tissue disease or all connective tissue diseases combined, including both established and atypical or undefined connective tissue disease, among women with cosmetic silicone breast implants (10). It is not necessary to remove silicone implants unless specific problems directly attributable to the implants arise. Silicone implants are available and given their superior cosmetic effects will increase in use.

Postirradiation

The examination of the patient who has completed a course of irradiation should follow the same procedure as outlined in the previous section with one caveat. The physician must carefully examine the incision for tumor recurrence, which will present as a firm, raised lesion within or adjacent to the surgical incision. Mammography represents an important adjunct in this situation.

Palpatory changes secondary to irradiation are actually unusual, and the overall incidence of late skin changes or fibrosis is small. The treated breast may appear slightly smaller and may have a slight generalized firmness in the previous tumor bed. Subtle changes may be more difficult to detect postirradiation.

RADIOGRAPHIC EVALUATION OF THE BREAST

Screening Mammography

Until more recently, most meta-analyses of pooled trials have demonstrated screening mammography to be effective in reducing mortality from breast cancer (11, 12). Two more recent meta-analyses have created controversy around the efficacy of mammography in improving survival: the Cochrane Review and the U.S. Preventive Services Task Force (USPSTF) in 2002 (13, 14). The Cochrane Review found no reduction in breast cancer mortality by screening mammography for women of any age. One criticism of this review is the use of all-cause mortality in lieu of breast cancer mortality as an analytic end point; breast cancer mortality is only a small fraction of all-cause mortality. As such, even a large effect of screening mammography would yield only a small reduction in all-cause mortality.

In contrast, the analysis by the USPSTF showed a significant reduction in breast cancer mortality for women ages 39 to 74 years (14). After 14 years of observation, they found a significant reduction in breast cancer mortality among women ages 40 to 49 who underwent screening in comparison to those that did not. Based on these results, the USPSTF recommended that breast cancer screening for women begin at age 40. The USPSTF report included corrected data from an updated report of the Swedish trials that was not available when the Cochrane Review was done (13, 15).

The decision to use the age of 50 as the threshold for screening has been relatively arbitrary. Although the USPSTF study found a decrease in breast cancer mortality, approximately 1800 women in their forties would need to be screened for 14 years to prevent one death from breast cancer (14). Although the evidence appears to support a reduction in breast cancer mortality among women younger than age 50 who have screening mammography, whether this benefit is due to the initiation of screening before the age of 50 is unclear and still controversial. Perhaps the same benefit would be seen in women who initiate screening at age 50? Trials are currently underway to elucidate the answers to these controversies.

Until the Cochrane Review, the prevailing epidemiologic evidence supported a benefit for screening mammography in women 50 years and older. The Cochrane Review showed no substantial benefit for this age group, although the larger of the two trials included in this review was the Canadian National Breast Screening Study-2 (NBSS-2), a trial designed to test whether mammography contributed any additional breast cancer mortality benefit compared with clinical breast examination alone (16). The USPSTF report reported a 22% reduction in breast cancer mortality for women older than age 50 who underwent mammographic screening (14).

Controversy persists around the benefit of screening mammography for women age 70 and older. Part of this stems from an absence of data and competing risks of death from non–breast-related causes. It is estimated that although women older than 70 comprise only 11% of the U.S. population, they account for 35% of the new breast cancer diagnoses and 52% of the breast cancer deaths (17, 18). The two randomized, controlled trials that included women older than 65 years did suggest a benefit (15, 19). Several studies suggest, however, that screening mammography may not be indicated in women with significant comorbid illness or with a life expectancy of less than 3 to 5 years (20).

There is very little evidence about the effectiveness of breast cancer screening in specific subgroups of women at higher risk for breast cancer than the general population. While guidelines have been put forth for women with known BRCA mutations or who have a family history suggestive of hereditary breast cancer, no guidelines have been issued for screening women who are not BRCA mutation carriers but are at increased risk for breast cancer (21). A few small studies have suggested that magnetic resonance imaging (MRI) may be more effective in screening for breast cancers in high-risk women, including women with mutations in BRCA genes, than mammography (22, 23). It is unclear if this improved detection will correspond to a significant reduction in morbidity and mortality from breast cancer.

There is controversy over whether breast implants adversely impact early breast cancer detection, although one meta-analysis did not demonstrate a delay in diagnosis or decrease in survival (24). Women with implants typically require more invasive diagnostic procedures to evaluate breast lesions.

Mammography currently has a 10 to 15% false-negative rate and a 6 to 10% false-positive rate. The risk of false-positives is affected by both patient and radiologic variables (25). Performing screening mammograms in the first 2 weeks of the menstrual cycle and stopping hormone therapy 10 to 30 days before repeat mammograms may help decrease breast density and reduce mammographic abnormalities (26, 27). False-negative mammograms may be reduced with the addition of a clinical breast examination, which has been shown to detect 3 to 45% of cancers missed by screening mammography (28, 29).

When the abnormal area is indeterminate or only vaguely abnormal, a shortened interval follow-up, usually 6 months, is recommended. This is valuable for assessing any change in the radiographic appearance of the lesion. Additional views (magnified or modified compression views) may be helpful in sorting out a true mass from vague abnormalities secondary to tissue superimposition. Radiographically indeterminate lesions require histologic diagnosis in the presence of clinical suspicion or high patient anxiety. The radiographic characteristics of various benign breast disorders are reviewed in Table 6.1.

Computer-aided mammography may lead to earlier detection of mammographic abnormalities. This emerging technique uses computer screening of mammograms in an attempt to avoid human error involved in interpretation.

Microcalcifications

As utilization of screening mammography increases, an increase in the detection of microcalcifications is likely to follow suit. The significance of microcalcifications is that they may represent one of the earliest signs of detectable malignant disease, particularly ductal-type carcinoma. There may or may not be an associated mass evident. Calcifications that are solitary, scattered, or random in distribution are most likely benign. The microcalcifications of benign lesions are usually larger, rounder, fewer, and vary less in size than the microcalcifications of malignancy.

Some benign disorders such as sclerosing adenosis, fat necrosis, and apocrine metaplasia may have microcalcifications similar to those of carcinoma(s). The absolute number of calcifications does not correlate with either benign or malignant disease.

Ultrasonography

Ultrasound, easily done in the office, is most commonly employed to help identify palpable cystic and solid masses. It may also help characterize masses seen on mammography and identify lesions that are palpable on exam but not visible on mammography. Because no compression of the surrounding breast tissue is required, it is a nearly painless procedure. Ultrasound is an important adjunct for evaluating palpable masses in younger women whose breasts are dense

TABLE 6.1

Radiographic Findings in Benign Breast Disorders

Benign Breast Disorders	Mammographic Characteristics
Cysts	Frequently multiple Smooth, sharp border May have thin radiolucent halo
Intramammary lymph node	Upper outer quadrant, near chest wall Usually less than 1 cm Kidney bean shaped with smooth outline May be partially replaced by fat
Mole	Well circumscribed
Fibroadenoma	Sometimes multiple Lobulated but with a small margin May have thin radiolucent halo If hyalinized, may have coarse calcifications
Surgical scar	May have radial spiculations if recent Follow-up mammogram will show decreasing size/prominence
Lipoma	May be difficult to detect on mammography
Sclerosing adenosis	The most common benign disorder that mimics malignancy on mammogram, it falls in the spectrum of breast changes in fibrocystic breast disease May appear as ill-defined, mottled, or nodular process May appear as homogenous soft-tissue density with indistinct margins
Breast abscess	May appear similar to inflammatory carcinoma (primarily diagnosed on aspiration or biopsy)
Traumatic fat necrosis	Variable mammographic features May be confused with carcinoma

and fibrous. The sensitivity and specificity of ultrasound are too low, however, to allow for its use as a screening tool for malignancy.

Breast tissue is very heterogenous, so abnormalities near the surface of the breast may be distorted or missed in the near fields of the transducer. To adequately perform breast ultrasound, a fluid offset must be located between the breast and the transducer. A water-filled plastic bag or commercially available offset pad is used if the transducer does not have a built-in fluid offset. For breast imaging, the transducer should be 5 MHz or greater, and the depth of focus should not exceed 2 cm.

Ultrasound is ideal for evaluation and follow-up of patients with multiple breast cysts. It can detect breast cysts as small as 2 mm. The most reliable diagnostic feature of a cyst in ultrasound is an anechoic interior. With compression, cysts usually flatten. Simple cysts demonstrate a clear, fluid-filled space between the anterior and posterior wall. These are almost always benign. Complex cysts appear with echogenic structures between the anterior and posterior border and may be septated. Failure to visualize a palpable mass on ultrasound does not preclude the need for continued evaluation and workup.

Ultrasound-guided biopsy or aspiration may be performed on solid and cystic lesions (30, 31). In skilled hands, this is technically simple, straightforward, and associated with a high degree of accuracy.

Magnetic Resonance Imaging

MRI using gadolinium contrast is a newer radiographic tool. The label accumulates around tissue composed of a high degree of vascularity, such as that seen with invasive cancer. There have been reports on the utility of MRI in identifying cancers when a suspicious lesion is seen only on one view of the mammography or when mammography findings are equivocal in patients who have had breast conservation therapy for previous breast cancer (32). Although cysts may be reliably detected by MRI, ultrasonography is less expensive and more accessible. Presently, MRI has no role in screening, but it can be helpful in equivocal situations where the traditional modalities are confounded by extensive fibrocystic changes or dense breast tissue. MRI may also be useful for follow-up of the irradiated breast due to skin and soft-tissue thickening.

Stereotactic-Guided Biopsy

Stereotactic-guided biopsy uses specialized mammography-like equipment and computer software. A single-view mammogram is taken from two opposing angles, and a computer then calculates the x-, y- and z-axes, thus determining the exact location of the lesion in the breast. Digitalized equipment now permits near real-time visualization of the biopsy procedure. It may be used for all types of mammographic abnormalities, including masses and calcifications. It may be used on women with breast implants.

The patient's ability to maintain the needed position for the biopsy, the breast size and thickness, or the location of the abnormality in the breast may impose limitations on the utility of stereotactic biopsy. In instances where the mass may not be visualized by ultrasound or stereotactic imaging, MRI or computed tomography may be used for guidance in performing a breast biopsy.

FINE NEEDLE ASPIRATION OF A MASS

Fine needle aspiration (FNA) is a technique for obtaining tissue from a solid lesion for cytologic evaluation. It can be diagnostic when malignant cells are recovered and therapeutic when employed to aspirate a cyst. Its usefulness is limited by the need for a skilled cytopathologist, a high rate of insufficient samples, and an inability to differentiate between in situ and invasive carcinoma. It is usually contraindicated in the presence of breast implants or in women taking anticoagulants.

For accuracy, the mass must be discrete and not simply glandular parenchyma of the breast. After preparation of the skin with alcohol, the mass is aspirated using a 20- or 22-gauge syringe (Fig. 6.3). Aspiration is not begun until the mass is entered, and four or five passes in a very short time period are necessary for an adequate specimen. If a long time is taken in obtaining the biopsy, the specimen will be contaminated with blood or blood clots. Frank blood will obscure the cellular pattern so the procedure should be repeated. It is usually possible to tell when the needle has entered the mass because of differences in its consistency compared with the surrounding tissue. The aspirated contents are then deposited on a glass slide, smeared, and fixed immediately using a commercially available fixative, such as that used for a Papanicolaou smear.

Several points regarding the interpretation of FNA material bear emphasis. With any patient, the decision to perform this aspiration should not be regarded as an end point in the evaluation of a discrete mass. Rather, it represents only an initial component of the entire evaluative process. Grant et al. (33) showed that FNA has a false-negative rate of 6%, no false-positive results, and an accuracy of 94%. The false-negative rate reported in the literature is 1 to 35% (34). Clinicians should view a negative report as nondiagnostic. The actual false-positive rate depends highly on the skill levels of both the clinician and the cytopathologist. Both a small tumor size and an aspirate containing a sparse number of cells may lead to diagnostic difficulties (35).

Complications from FNA are relatively few with the most frequent being hematoma formation. If this occurs, it will be readily apparent and should be treated with gentle direct compression until expansion of the underlying tissue is no longer noted. If mammography is performed soon after a hematoma, the original mass may be obscured; therefore, mammography should be

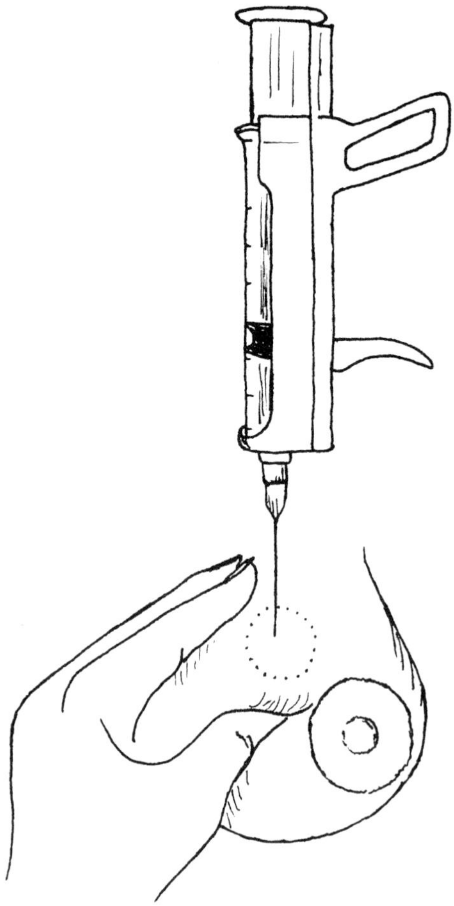

FIGURE 6.3 ● Fine needle aspiration (FNA) technique. The needle is placed in the mass and withdrawn at different angles and different areas at the mass at least five times. This should be done in a minimum of time to avoid contamination of the specimen. Suction must be maintained throughout the biopsy process but is discontinued with the entry of biopsy material into the needle hub. The needle is then withdrawn, the syringe removed, and 5 to 10 cc of air drawn into the syringe. The needle is reattached and the air used to place the cytologic specimen onto the slide. If adequate material is not obtained, repeat the aspiration by entering a separate track.

performed before attempting aspiration or no less than 2 weeks after the aspiration. A more unusual complication with FNA is pneumothorax. This is more prone to occur when the lesion lies in close proximity to the chest wall or the patient is very thin, but the risk can be diminished by manipulating the mass over a rib when possible. Infection following FNA is extremely rare.

EVALUATION OF NIPPLE DISCHARGE

Nipple discharge may present in women of all age groups and is the third most common breast complaint after breast pain and lumps. In taking the history and performing the exam, several things should be noted: nature of the discharge, factors that elicit the discharge (spontaneous or requiring pressure), relation to menses, presence or absence of a mass, unilateral or bilateral, and single or multiple ducts involved. The physician should also ask about conditions of overstimulation of the nipple. These might include tight clothes, inadequate support while exercising, and constant examination of the breasts for discharge (Table 6.2). Most nipple discharge is secondary to a benign etiology; only 2 to 25% of patients with an initial complaint of nipple discharge have breast cancer (36, 37).

One approach to evaluating nipple discharge is to classify it as physiologic or nonphysiologic. Physiologic discharge usually occurs only with breast stimulation, is bilateral, involves multiple ducts, and is nonbloody and often milky in appearance. Nonphysiologic nipple discharge is often spontaneous, unilateral, involves a single duct, and may be any color or have blood present.

TABLE 6.2

Causes of Nipple Discharge

Idiopathic

Physiologic
Lactation, pregnancy, postlactation, mechanical stimulation, hyperprolactinemia

Drug Induced
Antihypertensives, opiates, antipsychotic, phenothiazines, antipsychotics, antidepressants, selective serotonin reuptake inhibitors, synthetic hormones, antimigraine agents, anticonvulsants, benzodiazepines, sedatives, hypnotics, histamine antagonists

Breast Lesions
Intraductal papilloma, ductal ectasia, carcinoma, breast abscess

Central Nervous System Lesions
Pituitary stalk disorders such as aneurysm, empty sella syndrome, pseudotumor cerebri, pituitary adenoma or other tumors; hypothalamic disorders; head trauma

Medical Conditions
Primary hypothyroidism, chronic renal failure, multiple sclerosis, acromegaly, sarcoidosis, Schüller-Christian disease, Cushing's disease, hepatic cirrhosis

Chest Wall Lesions
Thoracotomy, herpes zoster

Physiologic discharge is usually the result of an endocrinologic or pharmacologic effect. Nipple discharge due to oral contraceptives is usually from multiple ducts, is usually more evident just prior to menses, and resolves upon stopping the medication. Endocrinologic disturbances that produce physiologic discharge either directly increase prolactin secretion or impair the inhibition of prolactin secretion. Physiologic nipple discharge may also be idiopathic. A small amount of fluid can be elicited with the application of manual pressure to the ducts of the nipple in up to 67% of premenopausal women (38). In postpartum women, galactorrhea may be present for a year or two after pregnancy, even if the woman is not breast-feeding (39).

Nonphysiologic discharge is often caused by local pathology and may be due to the following lesions (of most common to least common): papillomas and papillomatosis, duct ectasia and nonlactational infections, fibrocystic breast changes, ductal carcinoma in situ, and invasive cancer (40).

The most common cause of nonphysiologic discharge is an intraductal papilloma, a benign lesion involving the ductal system in proximity to the nipple. In about half of the women with papillomas, the discharge is bloody; in the other half, it is serous (41). With nonphysiologic discharge, a mass may or may not be present. The involved duct(s) should be identified. This is usually accomplished by exerting pressure at different sites around the nipple at the margin of the areola. Cytologic examination of the discharge should be done, bearing in mind that a negative result does not rule out cancer (42, 43).

A multicolored, sticky, or cheesy discharge is most often due to mammary duct ectasia or nonlactational infections.

Advancing age is associated with an increased risk of cancer in patients presenting with nipple discharge; in the study by Selzer et al. (44), 32% of patient older than age 60 presenting with nonphysiologic nipple discharge were found to have an underlying malignancy.

Examination of the breast should help determine whether the discharge is unilateral or bilateral, whether it arises from a single duct or multiple ducts, and whether it is associated with any underlying mass or lymphadenopathy. Occult blood in a discharge may be identified using a reagent paper and developer (e.g., Hemoccult or Hemostix). The utility of sending nipple discharge for cytology is controversial; although the sensitivity is low (35 to 67%), the specificity is high (up to 99%) (45). Obtaining nipple discharge for cytology is done by holding a glass slide at the opening of the duct, expressing the discharge, and moving the slide directly across the fluid on the surface of the nipple. Because the discharge contains more cells in the last drops of secretions, several (i.e., four to six) slides should be obtained. Occasionally, neither the physician nor the patient is able to replicate the discharge and a return office visit is required. Application of a small amount of benzoin to the nipple to temporarily block the duct drainage for 48 hours prior to the office visit is said to be an effective aid in the identification of discharge.

If the discharge appears to be physiologic, a workup for endocrinologic causes should be started. Initial tests include a pregnancy test, thyroid function tests, and serum prolactin level. If the history or physical is suggestive for acromegaly, Cushing's, renal, or liver disease, tests to evaluate for these diseases should be ordered. Diagnostic breast imaging is not likely to be helpful in the case of physiologic nipple discharge. Women ages 40 and older or at high risk for breast cancer should consider having a screening mammography, if appropriate.

If an underlying endocrinologic disorder is found as the cause of the physiologic discharge, it should be treated appropriately. Medications found to be the etiology should be stopped if possible; if the patient must continue on them, she should be reassured. If the etiology for physiologic discharge is not found, the patient may be reassured and advised that frequent breast manipulation and nipple stimulation may exacerbate her symptoms.

In cases of nonphysiologic breast discharge, women should undergo breast imaging with either ultrasonography or mammography. Which imaging modality is chosen depends on the age of the patient and whether they are pregnant. Women with an obvious breast infection should have the infection treated and resolved prior to breast imaging; if the infection does not resolve in a timely fashion, the patient should proceed to breast imaging.

Galactography involves cannulation of the affected ducts and injection of a water-soluble contrast agent into the duct. A specialized mammographic technique is then used to visualize the injected duct system. The role of galactography in evaluating nonphysiologic nipple discharge is controversial. Although there are galactographic patterns that indicate the possible need for surgery, a normal galactogram does not obviate the need for surgery (46). Galactography is able to identify abnormalities or lesions of the ductal system, but it cannot distinguish between benign and malignant intraductal tumors.

Ductal lavage can be used for risk stratification of high-risk women or to evaluate pathologic nipple discharge in conjunction with the traditional modalities of physical exam, mammography, and ductography. The fluid-producing milk duct is cannulated with a fine microcatheter using local anesthesia. The duct is then lavaged with sterile saline, and the fluid collected and placed in cell preservative and analyzed cytologically. A large numbers of cells can be collected with this technique, and they are examined for possible atypia or malignant changes. The information from lavage may be useful in helping a woman decide if a risk reduction strategy, such as Tamoxifen therapy, is indicated.

Evaluation and treatment of a nonphysiologic discharge often requires surgical consultation. Women with biopsy-proven ectasia as the cause of the nonphysiologic discharge should be referred for surgery only if the discharge is bothersome or if it interferes with their quality of life.

BENIGN CONDITIONS

For a list of possible causes of benign breast masses, see Table 6.3.

Cysts

Cysts are very common, and it is estimated that 7 to 10% of all women will develop a symptomatic breast cyst during their reproductive life. The incidence of breast cysts peaks among women ages 40 to 50 years. Most breast cysts are simply aberrations of normal lobular involution. The etiologic agents responsible for breast cyst formation are unknown. Breast cysts vary widely in size; larger cysts often present as an individual occurrence, although they are likely to be accompanied by multiple, bilateral cysts that are nonpalpable. The fluid contained in a cyst may range in color from light brown to almost black. A small increase in fluid volume in the cyst

TABLE 6.3

Possible Causes of Benign Breast Masses

Normal breast tissue
Normal or cyclical nodularity
Prominent fat lobule
Solid lesions
Duct papillomas
Fibroadenoma
Sclerosing adenosis
Stromal fibrosis
Phyllodes tumor
Lipoma
Cystic lesions
Simple
Complex
Galactocele
Sebaceous cyst
Trauma
Hematoma
Fat necrosis
Infections or Inflammation
Abscess
Mastitis
Foreign body granuloma
Tuberculosis
Hidradenitis suppurativa

has a disproportionate effect on the intracystic pressure. Hence, a previously undetected cyst may suddenly appear and be associated with pain or discomfort over a period of days. Cysts may reach such large size that they actually result in asymmetry on inspection of the breasts. Fifty-five percent of cysts are found in the left breast and 45% in the right; two-thirds of breast cysts occur in the upper outer quadrant, with the second most common location being the upper inner quadrant (2). Palpable cysts will usually be smooth, rounded, and relatively mobile, but occasionally they may blend into the underlying tissue due to associated fibrosis. They often create a "shotty" consistency in the breast. Some cysts will be exceptionally firm and nontender; in this situation, it is very difficult to distinguish cystic from solid lesions on the basis of physical examination alone. In these instances, an ultrasound is useful in distinguishing between cystic and solid lesions.

Breast cysts may be managed by ultrasound, aspiration, and inspection of the cystic fluid. Mammographic imaging is not necessarily required in the evaluate of breast cysts, although some believe screening mammography is indicated for women older than age 35 who present with breast cysts (2). Breast cysts can be classified as simple or complex, or single or clustered, based on ultrasound imaging results. A limitation of ultrasound is its inability to detect very small (less than 5 mm) lesions. Radiographically simple cysts (free from any septation) may be aspirated if palpable, or they may be observed. Aspiration is often performed in the case of a palpable cyst so as not to interfere with breast examination by either the patient or the physician. Upon aspiration, fluid that is clear yellow, straw colored, green, or brown (typical features of benign cystic fluid) can be discarded. Complex cysts should be aspirated for cytology or excision to provide definitive diagnosis.

Although a blood-tinged aspirate may result from a traumatic aspiration, this type of fluid requires cytologic evaluation. If there are no malignant cells, diagnostic mammography and targeted ultrasonography should be performed to assess for cyst resolution and to exclude other worrisome features. With successful aspiration of a breast cyst, the dominant mass should disappear, and a clinical breast exam should be repeated in 4 to 6 weeks. Recurrence of the mass should prompt evaluation with diagnostic mammography and ultrasonography to exclude any associated malignancy. If a mass is found after successful cyst aspiration, excisional biopsy is required because a small carcinoma may have occluded the duct, leading to cyst formation. Other indications for cyst excision are early recurrence (less than 6 weeks after complete aspiration) and recurrence of the same cyst after two aspirations. Recurrence may be indicative of persistent ductal obstruction. Changes in size, appearance, or consistency of a known breast cyst requires immediate follow-up (47).

A galactocele is an uncommon cyst that forms after a period of lactation; the cyst is filled with a milky material. The patient usually notes a painless swelling in her breast that occurs anywhere from a few weeks to a few months after she has stopped lactating. The mass is smooth and mobile and feels very much like the more common breast cyst. Cure can often be achieved with a single aspiration (the fluid withdrawn will appear milky), and the mass disappears completely. Galactoceles may be found anywhere in the breast, although they tend to occur more commonly near the areola.

Fibroadenomas

Fibroadenomas are the most common benign breast tumors, occurring most frequently in young women. Classically, a fibroadenoma presents as a firm, discrete solid mass detected by the patient. They are more common in the left breast and are predominantly found in the upper outer quadrant (48). These are generally painless, and the median age at diagnosis is 30 years, although they may also be identified in teenage girls. Because of the widespread use of oral contraceptives in younger women, it is difficult to determine conclusively if there is any relationship between their use and the development of fibroadenomas. Many will regress spontaneously, and evidence supports the observation of breast masses cytologically diagnosed as fibroadenomas (49).

Fibroadenomas usually decrease in size in the later reproductive years. They may eventually calcify and form a characteristic "popcorn" pattern of microcalcifications on mammogram. This may occur when a large fibroadenoma degenerates. Coarse microcalcifications seen with fibroadenomas on mammography are different from the coarse microcalcifications associated with ductal carcinoma.

On occasion, there is a rapid growth of a fibroadenoma, and it is referred to as a "giant" fibroadenoma; this designation is on the basis of physical size alone (usually greater than 5 cm). These giant fibroadenomas tend to have a bimodal distribution at the extremes of reproductive life, although they are slightly more common among adolescents than menopausal women (48). On examination of the mass, the surface feels smooth and is occasionally lobulated. These are not infiltrative lesions, so they are typically highly mobile. They are firm, discrete, and nontender masses, and usually measure 1 to 5 cm in diameter, although they can grow to be quite large (the giant fibroadenoma). Multiple lesions occur in one or both breasts in as many as 10 to 15% of patients. The use of cyclosporine for more than 1 year increases the risk of multiple fibroadenomas (50).

Histologically, fibroadenomas demonstrate an increased cellularity with large numbers of regularly shaped epithelial cells. The fibrous stroma is of low cellularity and regular cytology. They are considered proliferative lesions in the Page/Dupont classification system (51). In a more recent review of the relationship between fibroadenoma and breast cancer, Dupont et al. found no increased risk for a patient with a simple fibroadenoma and no family history of breast cancer. Patients with a complex hyperplasia and family history of breast cancer had an increase in the relative risk of breast cancer by three- to four-fold (52). The incidence of carcinoma arising in association with a fibroadenoma is quite low, with less than 200 cases having been reported in the medical literature (53). Ductal carcinoma may occur in association with a fibroadenoma rather than from within it and may either directly infiltrate the fibroadenoma or grow along the duct into the epithelial clefts of the fibroadenoma. Either way, treatment should be decided by the malignancy and not be influenced by the presence of the fibroadenoma.

Lesions in which the stroma shows markedly increased cellularity and atypia are termed phyllodes tumor. Hence, the diagnosis of a phyllodes tumor is based not on size but on histologic criteria. Phyllodes tumor is macroscopically and histologically distinct from a giant fibroadenoma. It is unclear if phyllodes tumors arise de novo or if they develop from a fibroadenoma. Phyllodes tumors grow rapidly and are not fixed to the adjacent breast tissue like malignancies. They feel softer than fibroadenomas, and the skin overlying them may have large, dilated veins or even ulcerations from pressure of the tumor on the skin. Phyllodes tumors tend to behave in a benign manner, although they more frequently recur, particularly if the excision margin was close to the tumor. Rarely, a phyllodes tumor will undergo malignant transformation (54). In women younger than the age of 20, phyllodes tumors may be treated by enucleation; management in older patients is not so clear. In one of the largest series reported, Haagensen (41) recommends wide local excision as the primary approach to treatment. The four generally accepted indications for removal of a fibroadenoma are:

- Inability to differentiate between benign and malignant processes
- Recent enlargement or increase in size on serial examinations
- Periareolar location
- Patient concern

Fat Necrosis

Fat necrosis is a pathologic and clinical term descriptive of lesions that, on palpation, may readily be confused with malignancy. A careful history may disclose a traumatic incident preceding the examination by several weeks to months. In instances where an associated traumatic event is clear, the patient may have noticed a painful hematoma that slowly resolved. Lack of a recalled traumatic event does not, however, preclude the diagnosis. Only about 50% of patients are able to recall a history of trauma or injury to the breast. It is common to see fat necrosis after radiation therapy and/or segmental resection of the breast.

There are two forms of fat necrosis: one that mimics cancer and another that simulates simple cysts that may be accompanied by a dull, aching pain (2). The former type of fat necrosis is more common in the elderly, and the mass is usually discrete, fixed to the underlying breast tissue, and may be very hard. This lesion will occasionally lead to retraction of the overlying skin that is indistinguishable from that seen with carcinoma; mammographic findings can also resemble those of carcinoma. Ultrasound appearances of these lesions may be quite variable. With the latter form of fat necrosis, palpation will reveal one or more cystic areas that may be tender to palpation. Aspiration typically produces an oily fluid and is curative.

If the history is clear and the mass follows a well-documented trauma, a short period of observation may be indicated to await resolution. The clinical dilemma that arises is the presence of such a mass without any external evidence of trauma. FNA may yield a small amount of fluid with an oily consistency. If the mass does not appreciably decrease in size, excisional biopsy is usually required to rule out malignancy. Histologic examination shows only the presence of chronic inflammation with a predominance of lymphocytes. This lesion is not associated with an increased risk of breast cancer.

Lipoma

Lipomas may be found in the breast and clinically are smooth, slightly lobulated, and mobile. It is important to distinguish a lipoma from a variant of carcinoma—the pseudolipoma that is produced when carcinomatous infiltrates cause a shortening of Cooper's ligaments. This causes intervening fat lobules to become compressed and to take on the lobulated form typical of lipoma. On mammography and ultrasonography, the lesions are circumscribed and translucent, and are seen compressing surrounding tissues. If there is any doubt about the diagnosis, excision is indicated.

Sclerosing Adenosis

Sclerosing adenosis may present as a firm, ill-defined fibrotic mass that may be mistaken for cancer. It is nodular and circumscribed in contrast to the stellate pattern of cancer. Localized pain may or may not be present and may be worse premenstrually. Pressure often increases the pain, and patients may complain of an inability to sleep well secondary to the pain (55). Mammographically, it may mimic invasive cancer, and excisional biopsy is required to differentiate this lesion from invasive cancer. Histologically, it may prove difficult for pathologists to differentiate this lesion from invasive cancer, particularly on frozen section specimens. Diagnosis may be easier if the tumor is viewed on a low-power view rather than attempting to assess cytology on a high-power view.

Fibrocystic Disease

Historically, the clinical diagnosis "fibrocystic disease" or "mammary dysplasia" was given to women who had prominent areas of glandular tissue ("lumpy breasts") but who had no histologic evaluation performed. This term is often applied to explain normal physiologic changes that may be painful or uncomfortable and that are associated with cyclic production of estrogen and progesterone in the premenopausal woman. It is common among women 30 to 50 years of age and is rare in the postmenopausal woman.

"Fibrocystic disease" is a diagnosis that should be used only when a biopsy has been done that demonstrates either characteristic proliferative or nonproliferative changes. If no biopsy has been done, the diagnosis should not be applied to the patient's condition.

Lactational Breast Infection and Abscesses

Lactational breast abscesses occur in the postpartum period and result from a progression of mastitis. Eighty-five percent of lactational breast abscesses occur during the first month after delivery (56). The other time period associated with an increased risk for developing lactational abscess is when the mother is attempting to wean the child from the breast. The patient usually develops an acutely painful, red, and swollen breast. The infection is believed to arise from a mechanical obstruction of a duct, leading quickly to infection by a skin organism, commonly *Staphylococcus aureus*. The infection should be treated immediately with antibiotics (oxacillin or dicloxacillin), and drainage of the breast through either breast-feeding or pumping should continue. Although the bacteria are present in the milk, they do not harm the infant; hence, breast-feeding can and should be continued.

If the lesion progresses and forms a localized mass with signs of infection, an abscess is present that must be drained, with concurrent antibiotic coverage to prevent systemic infection. Drainage may use an open technique or be done via repeated aspirations (57). After an abscess has been drained, suckling from that breast may be difficult, although the mother may continue to feed on the unaffected side. The breast with the surgical site should continue to be drained through either manual expression or with a pump until breast-feeding is resumed.

Nonlactational Breast Abscess

Nonlactational breast abscesses tend to occur in older women and fall into two groups: subareolar or peripheral abscesses. The microbiologic profile of nonlactational abscess is much more variable than for lactational abscesses. Subareolar abscess is most commonly seen in reproductive age women and is due to the duct ectasia/periductal mastitis complex, which covers a number of different processes that may exist alone or in combination. These processes include ectasia (duct dilation), periductal mastitis, and periductal fibrosis. Cigarette smoking significantly increases the risk of severe inflammatory complications with this disease entity (58). The patient often complains of a sudden onset of tenderness, erythema, induration, and a breast mass (59). If the abscess is not treated, it may burst spontaneously, which may be followed by clinical relief from any pain or discomfort, but a persistent sinus will remain and the abscess will eventually recur, usually at the same site. If a subareolar abscess is to be treated conservatively (i.e., with antibiotics alone), a prolonged course of therapy (4 to 6 weeks) is recommended to prevent recurrence (60). Some authors recommend treatment for 6 to 8 weeks in patients without obvious sinus or fistula formation in conjunction with multiple aspirations, concluding that incision and drainage may lead to fistula formation (61, 62). If a fistula or draining sinus is present, treatment is prolonged antibiotic therapy with surgical fistulectomy performed anywhere from 3 to 10 days after initiation of antibiotics (62).

Peripheral abscesses are less common than the subareolar abscess. They typically present in the postmenopausal woman as either a recent-onset condition or a chronic condition with no underlying pathology (59). The pathogenesis of these abscesses is uncertain. *S. aureus* is commonly cultured from aspirate obtained from the mass. Management with simple drainage either with or without antibiotics is usually effective therapy. Similar abscesses may be seen in patients with diabetes or who are on steroids, although in these instances the bacteria are usually less pathogenic (63).

Patients with breast infections should be followed closely in the first 2 weeks of antibiotic therapy. Re-evaluation for response should first occur within 72 hours of initiating therapy. If response is adequate, they should be seen approximately 1 week later and then every 2 to 3 weeks until the infection is resolved. Palpable abscesses may take 2 to 3 months to resolve completely. Radiographic imaging should be ordered 2 to 3 weeks after all symptoms have resolved to ensure there is no underlying or residual tissue abnormality. Some authors recommend follow-up every 3 months for the next 6 months after the infection has resolved to ensure there is no recurrence (61, 62).

Patients who appear septic should be admitted to the hospital for intravenous antibiotic therapy (e.g., ampicillin/sulbactam 1.5 mg every 6 hours) and possible abscess drainage. If the abscess is large (i.e., larger than 3 cm), prompt surgical intervention is warranted, followed by several days of intravenous antibiotics and a prolonged course of oral antibiotics. Smaller abscesses may often be treated with oral antibiotics with a wide spectrum of activity on an outpatient basis. Possible regimens include clindamycin 300 mg every 6 hours or amoxicillin/clavulanate 875/125 mg every 12 hours. Patients with penicillin allergies may be treated with a combination of cephalexin 500 mg four times a day or, alternatively, with erythromycin 500 mg twice daily and metronidazole 500 mg three times a day (62).

Breast Abscesses in Immunocompromised Patients

Abscesses found in immunocompromised patients tend to contain unusual organisms and may progress to overwhelming sepsis rapidly. In patients with HIV/AIDS, tuberculosis is commonly seen as the causative agent of a breast abscess, and in some instances, may be the first manifestation of HIV positivity (64). Hence, the bacteriologic evaluation of nonlactational abscesses should encompass a wide variety of organisms.

Nonbacterial Infections

Two common conditions can mimic bacterial infections: hidradenitis suppurativa and superficial Candida infection. Hidradenitis may lead to chronic infection of the breasts, draining abscesses, and fistula formation. Treatment depends on the stage of the disease. In early stages, in which there is no evidence of scarring or sinus tract formation, treatment regimens may include use of topical clindamycin (1% lotion twice daily for 3 months), cyproterone acetate and ethinyl estradiol (65).

Candidiasis may mimic cellulites or be complicated by secondary cellulites. Typically, the skin in the inframammary fold appears quite erythematous and may be "weeping." Examinations of scrapings taken from the area will usually demonstrate hyphae and budding yeast. Treatment is with a topical antifungal agent, and the patient is instructed to keep the area clean and dry. If there is an accompanying cellulites that is moderate in nature, treatment may include an antibiotic with antistaphylococcal activity.

Mastodynia

Mastodynia, or the broader term mastalgia, describes the complaint of breast pain. It is a common entity with an estimated 40 to 60% of women experiencing breast pain (66). Although patients are often concerned that the pain is a symptom of an underlying cancer, most causes of mastalgia are benign. Studies show that only 2% of patients presenting with breast pain alone had an underlying cancer (66, 67). Although this incidence is low, it is still higher than in the general screening population, so cancer must be excluded in the evaluation of mastodynia.

Mastodynia is often difficult to treat, and many health care providers view it as a condition that occurs more frequently in women who are depressed or anxious. Many studies have been done to evaluate the relationship between mastalgia and affective disorders, but the results are very inconsistent (68, 69).

Mastodynia may be divided into two categories: cyclical and noncyclical. Studies show the severity of the pain and its impact on the quality of life are the same for both categories (70). Cyclical pain is more common and accounts for the majority of mastodynia cases; it is usually relieved with the onset of menstruation or menopause. It is classically described as a heavy, dull ache that is usually bilateral and most pronounced in the upper outer quadrants of the breast (70).

Noncyclical breast pain is present throughout the menstrual cycle or occurs intermittently and irregularly. This pain is often described as sharp, burning, and localized. Patients may be able to demonstrate a pathway of the pain pattern. Although the severity of the pain is variable, it does seem to be related to the size of the area affected (70). It is occasionally of such degree that the patient is unable to lie on her stomach to sleep, and any type of external pressure accentuates her discomfort.

When seeing and evaluating the patient for the first time, it is important to determine if the breast pain is cyclical or noncyclical (Fig. 6.4). Although the cause of cyclical mastalgia is believed to be endocrinologic, the specific pathways and mechanisms remain unknown. Extramammary causes of the pain must be excluded. There are several validated questionnaires to help evaluate the impact of the pain on the patient's quality of life (e.g., the McGill Modified Questionnaire). See Appendix 1 for a copy of the breast pain questionnaire (70).

A breast pain diary kept for 2 months gives a much better assessment of mastalgia than relying on patient recall in the office. The patient should include a daily measure of the pain severity and the patient's menstrual cycle (if applicable) (71). Pain severity is best evaluated with a visual analog pain scale; with this system, pain is rated from 0 to 10, with 10 being the most severe. The diary should also note the use of any self-prescribed efforts by the patient to alleviate the pain (e.g., the use of pain relievers) and any improvements in breast pain.

The treatment plan must first recognize the patient's pain. Reassurance and support are essential measures. A search for underlying pathologies that may mimic the syndrome of myalgia such as muscular strain or blunt trauma should be undertaken. Regardless of the cyclicity or noncyclicity of the pain, diagnostic imaging studies must be ordered where appropriate. Mammography may be indicated to any nonpalpable causes, such as a cyst deep within the glandular structures or, rarely, a malignancy. For younger patients with dense breast tissue, ultrasound may be the imaging study of choice.

Most breast pain will resolve with reassurance, lifestyle changes, and over-the-counter medications. If these measures fail and the pain significantly interferes with the patient's daily activities, prescription therapies may be of value. Noncyclical breast pain is more difficult to treat than cyclical and has a higher associated failure rate with both lifestyle changes and over-the-counter medications, as well as with prescriptive modalities. Treatments for mastalgia that were recommended in the past but that have not been proven more effective than placebo include vitamin B6, vitamin E, and diuretics (72–74).

Lifestyle changes to be recommended for patients with mastalgia include purchase of a well-fitting bra after being measured by a knowledgeable fitter; tapering of caffeine intake to avoid caffeine withdrawal headaches, with the ultimate goal being caffeine cessation (although studies have been mixed on this issue, it is a low-cost intervention to try); a low-fat diet; and relaxation therapy and hypnosis. Over-the-counter remedies include nonsteroidal anti-inflammatory drugs and evening primrose oil. Evening primrose oil contains gammalinolenic acid, a deficiency of

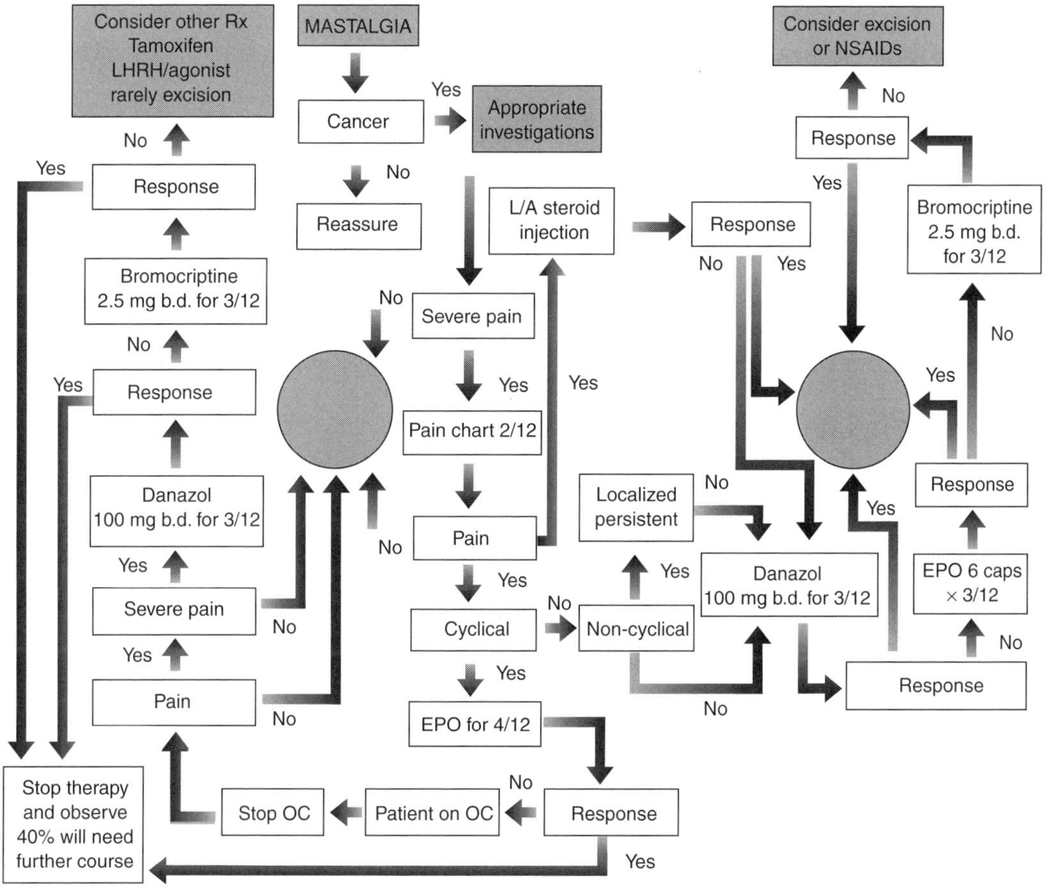

FIGURE 6.4 ● Flowchart of the management of mastalgia (Reprinted from Hughes LE, Mansel RE. Breast anatomy and physiology. In: Hughes LE, Mansel RE, Webster DJ, eds. Benign Disorders and Diseases of the Breast: Concepts and Clinical Management. 2nd ed. Philadelphia: WB Saunders, 2000:114, with permission.)

which may make breast tissue more sensitive to the normal premenstrual elevation of prolactin. Some authors believe evening primrose oil should be used as first-line therapy in mild to moderate cases of mastalgia (2). A controlled trial using 1.5 g orally twice a day demonstrated an improvement in both cyclical and noncyclical pain (75). However, not all studies have found the same salutary effect (76). It may take 3 to 4 months to see an effect from the primrose oil. Possible side effects include nausea, stool softening, and flatulence.

When conservative measures fail and the pain is severe, a variety of prescription medications may be tried in the treatment of mastalgia. These include danazol, tamoxifen, bromocriptine, medroxyprogesterone acetate, goserelin, or topical diclofenac. With the exception of topical diclofenac, all are contraindicated in pregnancy. If they provide relief of symptoms, therapy should be continued for 3 to 6 months. Studies done in Europe indicate that only 15% of patients require pharmaceutical therapy for their mastalgia (75). Failure of one form of pharmaceutical therapy does not predict failure with another type of agent.

Danazol is much more effective in treating cyclical breast pain than noncyclical breast pain; response rates in cyclical breast pain patients range from 70 to 79% (75, 77). It suppresses gonadotropin synthesis, which ultimately generates an antiestrogen, antiprogestogen, and androgenic hormonal environment. Drawbacks to danazol include the high incidence of side effects (up to 30% of patients), and the relapse rate may be as high as 70%—a much higher rate than that seen with tamoxifen. Some authors believe the introduction of a low-dose regimen will sufficiently lower the incidence of side effects to warrant the use of danazol as first-line therapy in cases of moderate to severe mastalgia. The regimen they use is a starting dose of 200 mg daily, followed by a maintenance dose of 100 mg every other day. With this regimen, the drop-out rate is lowered to 10% (2, 78). Common side effects include weight gain acne, headaches, and irregular menses. Serious complications such as intracranial hypertension, pancreatitis, and Stevens-Johnson syndrome have also been reported (72, 79). Patients using danazol must be receiving and practicing adequate contraception techniques.

Tamoxifen has long been used for the treatment of mastalgia. It decreases the availability of estrogen by elevating levels of sex hormone binding globulin. In one study, response rates for cyclical and noncyclical breast pain were 98% and 56%, respectively, with a daily dose of 10 mg (80). Relapse rates range from 25 to 48% upon discontinuation of tamoxifen therapy (81, 82). In a large trial, the frequency of the dose was reduced to days 15 to 25 of the cycle for a period of 3 months, and doses of 10 mg and 20 mg were compared with no placebo controls. There was no advantage to the higher dose and a higher incidence of side effects (83). Current recommendations are to use 10 mg per day for 3 months and to repeat for relapse, if necessary (2). Caution must be exercised in using tamoxifen long term due to the higher risks of thromboembolic events, stroke, and uterine cancer (84). For this reason, some authors recommend using tamoxifen only in cases of resistant and recurrent cases of mastalgia (2). Care must be taken that patients using tamoxifen are using adequate contraception techniques.

Bromocriptine is a prolactin inhibitor and is most effective for cyclical mastalgia, although in one trial drop-out rates were up to 30% because of side effects such as nausea, dizziness, vomiting, and headaches (85). The severity of side effects can be reduced by introducing the drug incrementally and avoiding doses higher than 2.5 mg twice daily. One recommended regimen is to start therapy at 1.25 mg at night with food for 3 days. This is increased to 2.5 mg at night with food for days 4 to 7. Next, a 1.25-mg dose is introduced in the morning with food and the 2.5-mg dose at night with food is maintained for days 8 to 11. From the twelfth day onward, the regimen is 2.5 mg in the morning and 2.5 mg at night, both times with food (2). A clinical response may take up to 3 months after initiation of therapy, and this may last for 3 to 6 months after discontinuation of the drug.

Depo-medroxyprogesterone acetate (Depo-Provera), an injectable form of contraception, is another pharmacologic agent used in the treatment of mastalgia. It is believed to exert its effect by inhibiting ovarian steroidogenesis, decreasing synthesis of estrogen receptors, and enhancing estrogen degradation. Side effects include irregular menses, weight gain, and depression. Serious side effects include bone density loss.

Goserelin is a luteinizing hormone-releasing agonist that inhibits gonadotropin release and ovarian steroidogenesis. It is given subcutaneously (3.6 mg) monthly and is associated with an 81% response rate in mastalgia (86). Because it induces an artificial menopause, side effects are similar to the symptoms of menopause, including decreased bone density.

Topical diclofenac gel contains 3% diclofenac and is available in the United States. In one prospective, randomized, controlled trial, a 50-mg dose used three times daily for 6 months significantly improved both cyclical and noncyclical pain symptoms. In this trial, 47% cyclical and 50% of noncyclical mastalgia patients reported no pain at 6 months (87).

Although mastalgia is not commonly seen in menopausal women, it does occur. In these instances, nonbreast causes must be excluded (e.g., biliary pain or musculoskeletal referred pain). Because older women have a higher incidence of breast cancer, radiologic examination, in conjunction with physical exam, may need to be undertaken to evaluate focal, chronic pain. The use of hormone therapy may cause breast pain in some older patients; cessation of therapy may lead to resolution of the mastalgia.

CONCLUSION

Although much focus and attention is given to the issue of breast cancer, the majority of diseases of the breast are, fortunately, benign conditions. Patients presenting with breast complaints are always concerned about cancer, and although it is of paramount importance to ensure cancer is not the cause of their condition, it is of equal significance that health care providers be familiar with the many benign conditions of the breast to accurately diagnose and adequately treat them.

Clinical Notes

- It is estimated that half of women have a volume difference of 10% between the left and right breasts and up to 25% of women have a 20% difference; in these instances, the left breast is usually larger than the right.
- Any new mass should be evaluated, regardless of pregnancy state.
- There is no evidence of an excess of any individual connective tissue disease or all connective tissue diseases combined, including both established and atypical or undefined connective tissue disease, among women with cosmetic silicone breast implants.
- Mammography should never serve to replace further evaluation of a breast mass with histologic examination.
- Ultrasound is helpful to distinguish between solid and cystic masses.
- FNA is helpful when positive. Negative results are to be viewed as nondiagnostic.
- Physiologic nipple discharge usually occurs only with breast stimulation, is bilateral, involves multiple ducts, and is nonbloody and often milky in appearance. Nonphysiologic nipple discharge is often spontaneous, unilateral, involves a single duct, and may be any color or have blood present.
- The most common cause of nonphysiologic discharge is an intraductal papilloma, a benign lesion involving the ductal system in proximity to the nipple.
- It is estimated that 7 to 10% of all women will develop a symptomatic breast cyst during their reproductive life. The incidence of breast cysts peaks among women ages 40 to 50 years.
- Fibroadenomas are the most common benign breast tumors, are more common in the left breast, and are predominantly found in the upper outer quadrant.
- Fibroadenomas should be removed in the event of recent enlargement, patient concern, periareolar location, or when they are unable to be distinguished from a malignant process.
- There are two forms of fat necrosis: one that mimics cancer and another that simulates simple cysts that may be accompanied by a dull, aching pain.
- Eighty-five percent of lactational breast abscesses occur during the first month after delivery.
- Nonlactational breast abscesses tend to occur in older women and tend to fall into two groups: subareolar or peripheral.
- Mastodynia may be divided into two categories: cyclical and noncyclical. Studies show that the severity of the pain and its impact on quality of life is the same for both categories. Noncyclical breast pan is more difficult to treat.

APPENDIX 6.1

Breast Pain Questionnaire

Name: Ethnicity (optional): Birthdate:

Have you ever been diagnosed with breast cancer? _____Yes _____No

Postmenopausal?_____Yes _____No

1. Have you experienced breast pain within the **last three months**? _____Yes _____No
   If yes, please continue to fill out the rest of this survey.
2. **What does your breast pain feel like?**
   Please check one of the four categories (none, mild, moderate, or severe) for each descriptor.

	None	Mild	Moderate	Severe
Throbbing				
Shooting				
Stabbing				
Sharp				
Cramping				
Gnawing				
Hot-Burning				
Aching				
Heavy				
Tender				
Splitting				
Tiring-Exhausting				
Sickening				
Fearful				
Punishing-Cruel				

3. What is the **amount** of your overall breast pain? Write a number between 0 and 10, where 0 means no pain and 10 the worst possible pain.
4. Which word below best describes the **amount** of your overall breast pain? Check one.
   _____ Mild
   _____ Discomforting
   _____ Distressing
   _____ Horrible
   _____ Excruciating

5. How does your breast pain change in time?
   A. Which word or words would you use to describe the **pattern** of your breast pain?

_____ Continuous	_____ Rhythmic	_____ Brief
_____ Steady	_____ Periodic	_____ Momentary
_____ Constant	_____ Intermittent	_____ Transient

   B. What kind of things **relieve** your breast pain?
   C. What kind of things **increase** your breast pain?
6. Is your breast pain related to your **menstrual cycle**?_____ Yes _____ No
   If yes:
   Which day is your breast pain the **worst**? Write a number between 0 and 28 where 28 indicates menstruation.
   How long does your breast pain usually last? Write a number between 0 and 28 where 28 indicates menstruation.
7. How **often** does your breast pain occur? Check one.
   _____ Every hour _____ Every day _____ Every week _____ Every month
8. How **long** have you had your breast pain? ___ Number of years ___ Number of months
9. **Where**, exactly, does the pain occur? Please shade painful areas.

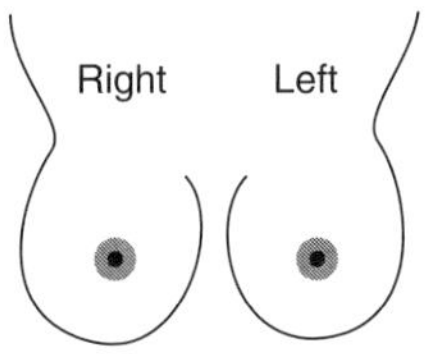

10. Has your breast pain affected your **work** schedule? _____ Yes _____ No
11. Has your breast pain affected your **sleep** pattern? _____ Yes _____ No
12. Has your breast pain affected your **sexual** activity? _____ Yes _____ No
13. Do you take **medications** to relieve your breast pain?_____ Yes _____ No
    If yes, write the type of medications and doses that you take.
14. Do you have **other pains** besides breast pain? _____Yes _____ No
    If yes, write where.
    How often?
    Does it coincide with your breast pain? _____Yes _____ No
    Do you take any medications to relieve this pain? _____Yes _____ No
    If yes, write the type of medications and doses that you take.
15. If you have any comments regarding your breast pain that was not covered above please write them here:

Reprinted with permission from Breast Pain Questionnaire. Pain & Qualia Lab, Northwestern University, Department of Physiology, Chicago, IL. Available at: www.apkarianlab.northwestern.edu/breast.html. Accessed June 30, 2005.

REFERENCES

1. Loughry CW, Shefer DB, Price TE, et al. Breast volume measurement in 598 women using biostereometric analysis. Ann Plastic Surg 1989;22:380–385.
2. Hughes LE, Mansel RE. Breast anatomy and physiology. In: Hughes LE, Mansel RE, Webster DJ, eds. Benign Disorders and Diseases of the Breast: Concepts and Clinical Management. 2nd ed. Philadelphia: WB Saunders, 2000:7–20.
3. Lewis EJ, Crutchfield CE. Accessory nipples and associated conditions. Pediatr Dermatol 1997;14:333–334.
4. Keller-Wood M, Bland KI. Breast physiology in normal, lactating and diseased states in the breast. In: Bland KI, Copeland EM, eds. The Breast: Comprehensive Management of Benign and Malignant Diseases. 1st ed. Philadelphia: WB Saunders, 1991:36–45.
5. Taylor PJ. Successful treatment of D-penicillamine induced breast gigantism with danazol. BMJ 1981; 282:362–363.
6. Hedberg K, Karlsson K, Lindstedt A. Gigantomastia during pregnancy: effect of a dopamine agonist. Am J Obstet Gynecol 1979;133:928–931.
7. Pierce PE, Hughes LE, Mansel RE, et al. Clinical syndromes of mastalgia. Cancer 1976;2:670–673.
8. River, L, Silverstein I, Grant J, et al. Carcinoma of the breast: the diagnostic significance of pain. Am J Surg 1951;82:733–735.
9. Barton MB, Harris R, Fletcher SW. Does this patient have breast cancer? The screening clinical breast examination: should it be done? How? JAMA 1999;282:1270–1280.
10. Lipworth L, Tarone R, McLaughlin JK. Silicone breast implants and connective tissue disease: an updated review of the epidemiologic evidence. Ann Plast Surg 2004;52(6):598–601.
11. Glasziou P, Irwig L. The quality and interpretation of mammographic screening trials for women ages 40–49. J Natl Cancer Inst Monogr 1997;22:73–77.
12. Glasziou PP. Meta-analysis adjusting for compliance: the example of screening for breast cancer. J Clin Epidemiol 1992;45:1251–1256.
13. Olsen O, Gotzsche PC. Cochrane Review on screening for breast cancer with mammography. Lancet 2001;358:1340–1342.
14. Humphrey LL, Helfand M, Chan BK, et al. Breast cancer screening: a summary of the evidence for the U.S. Preventive Services Task Force. Ann Intern Med 2002;5:347–360.
15. Nystrom L, Anderrson I, Bjurstam N, et al. Long-term effects of mammography screening: updated overview of the Swedish randomized trials. Lancet 2002;359:909–919.
16. Miller AB, To T, Baines CJ, et al. The Canadian National Breast Screening Study–2: 13-year results of a randomized trial in women aged 50–59 years. J Natl Cancer Inst 2000;92:1490–1499.
17. Population Projections Program, Population Division, U.S. Census Bureau. Projections of the Total Resident Population by 5-Year Age Groups, and Sex with Special Age Categories: Middle Series, 2006 to 2010. Available at: http://www.census.gov/population/projections/nation/summary/np-t3-c.txt. Accessed June 30, 2005.
18. American Cancer Society (ACS). Breast Cancer Facts & Figures, 2001–2002. Atlanta: ACS, 2001:1. Available at: http://www.cancer.org/downloads/STT/BrCaFF2001.pdf. Accessed June 30, 2005.
19. Tabar L, Fagerberg G, Chen HH, et al. Efficacy of breast cancer screening by age: new results form the Swedish Two-county Trial. Cancer 1995;75:2507–2517.
20. Walter LC, Eng C, Covinsky KE. Screening mammography for frail older women: what are the burdens? J Gen Intern Med 2001;16:779–784.
21. Burke W, Daly M, Garber J, et al. Recommendations of follow-up care of individuals with an inherited predisposition to cancer: II. BRCA1 and BRCA2. JAMA 1997;277:997–1003
22. Stoutjesdijk MJ, Boetes C, Jager GJ, et al. Magnetic resonance imaging and mammography in women with a hereditary risk of breast cancer. J Natl Cancer Inst 2001;93:1095–1102.
23. Warner E, Plewes DB, Shumak RS, et al. Comparison of breast magnetic resonance imaging, mammography, and ultrasound for surveillance of women at high risk for hereditary breast cancer. J Clin Oncol 2001;19:3524–3531.
24. Nass SJ, Henderson IC, Lashof JC, eds. Mammography and Beyond: Developing Technologies for the Early Detection of Breast Cancer. Washington, DC: National Academy Press, 2001:1–165.
25. Elmore JG, Bargon MB, Moceri VM, et al. Ten-year risk of false positive screening mammograms and clinical breast examinations. N Engl J Med 1998;338:1089–1096.
26. White E, Velentas P, Mandelson MT, et al. Variation in mammographic breast density by time in menstrual cycle among women aged 40–49 years. J Natl Cancer Inst 1998;90:906–910.
27. Harvey JA, Pinkerton JV, Herman CR. Short-term cessation of hormone replacement therapy and improvement of mammographic specificity. J Natl Cancer Inst 1997;89:1623–1625.
28. Roberts MM, Alexander FE, Anderson TJ, et al. Edinburgh trial of screening for breast cancer: mortality at seven years. Lancet 1990;335:241–246.
29. Burns PE, May C, Gutter Z, et al. Relative accuracy of clinical examination and mammography in a breast clinic in Alberta. J Can Assoc Radiol 1978;29:22–27.
30. Jokich PM, Monticciolo DL, Adler HT. Breast ultrasonography. Radiol Clin North Am 1992;30:993–1009.
31. Meyer JE, Christian RE, Frenna TH, et al. Image guided aspiration of solitary occult breast "cysts". Arch Surg 1992;127:433–435.
32. Orel SG, Schnall MD. MR imaging of the breast for the detection, diagnosis, and staging of breast cancer. Radiology 2001;220:13–30.

33. Grant CS, Goellner JR, Welch JS, et al. Fine-needle aspiration of the breast. Mayo Clin Proc 1986;61:377–381.
34. Layfield LJ, Glasgow BJ, Cramer H. Fine-needle aspiration in the management of breast masses. Pathol Annu 1989;24(part 2):23–62.
35. O'Malley F, Casey TT, Winfried AC, et al. Clinical correlates of false negative fine needle aspiration of the breast in a consecutive survey of 1005 patients. Surg Gynecol Obstet 1993;176:360–364.
36. Hou MF, Huang TJ, Liu GC. The diagnostic value of galactography in patients with nipple discharge. Clin Imaging 2001;25:75–81.
37. Ambrogetti D, Berni D, Catarzi S, et al. The role of ductal galactography in the differential diagnosis of breast carcinoma. Radiol Med (Torino) 1996;91:198–201.
38. Wyner EL, Hill P, Laakso K, et al. Breast secretion in Finnish women. Cancer 1981;47:1444–1450.
39. Firorica JV. Nipple discharge. Obstet Gynecol Clin North Am 1994;21:453–460.
40. Varkey AB. Nipple discharge. In: Ganschow PS, Norlock FE, Jacobs EA, et al., eds. Breast Health and Common Breast Problems: A Practical Approach. Philadelphia: American College of Physicians, 2004:225–241.
41. Haagensen CD. Diseases of the Breast. 3rd ed. Philadelphia: WB Saunders, 1986.
42. Tabar L, Dean PB, Penteck Z. Galactography: the diagnostic procedure of choice for nipple discharge. Radiology 1983;149:31–38.
43. Philip J, Narris WG. The role of ductography in the management of patients with nipple discharge. Br J Clin Pract 1984;38:293–297.
44. Selzer MH, Perloff LJ, Kelley RI, et al. Significance of age in patients with nipple discharge. Surg Gynecol Obstet 1970;131:519–522.
45. Dunn JM, Lucarotti ME, Wood SJ. Exfoliative cytology in the diagnosis of breast disease. Br J Surg 1995;82:789–791.
46. Dinkel HP, Gassel AM, Muller T, et al. Galactography and exfoliative cytology in women with abnormal nipple discharge. Obstet Gynecol 2001;97:625–629.
47. Pruthi S. Detection and evaluation of a palpable breast mass. Mayo Clin Proc 2001;76(6):641–648.
48. Foster ME, Garrahan N, Williams S. Fibroadenoma of the breast—a clinical and pathological study. J R Coll Surg Edinb 1988;36:16–19.
49. Cant PJ, Madden MV, Coleman MG, et al. Non-operative management of breast masses diagnosed as fibroadenoma. Br J Surg 1995;82:792–794.
50. Baildam AD, Higgins RM, Hulrey E, et al. Cyclosporin A and multiple fibroadenomas of the breast. Br J Surg 1996;83:1755–1757.
51. Page DL, Dupont WE. Anatomic indicators (histologic and cytologic) of increased breast cancer risk. Breast Cancer Res Treat 1993;28:157–166.
52. Dupont WD, Page DL, Parl FF, et al. Long term risk of breast cancer in women with fibroadenoma. N Engl J Med 1994;331:10–15.
53. Fukuda M, Nagao K, Nishimura R, et al. Carcinoma arising in fibroadenoma of the breast: a case report and review of the literature. Jpn J Surg 1989;19:5993–5596.
54. Moffat CJC, Pinder SE, Dixon AR, et al. Phyllodes tumour of the breast. A clinico-pathological review of 32 cases. Histopathology 1995;27:205–218.
55. Preece PE. Sclerosing adenosis. World J Surg 1989;13:721–725.
56. Newton M, Newton NR. Breast abscess. A result of lactation failure. Surg Gynecol Obstet 1950;91:651–655.
57. O'Hara RJ, Dexter SPL, Fox JN. Conservative management of infective mastitis and breast abscesses after ultrasonographic assessment. Br J Surg 1996;83:1413–1414.
58. Bundred NJ, Dover MS, Aluwihari N, et al. Smoking and periductal mastitis. BMJ 1993;307:772–773.
59. Maier WP, Au FC, Tang C. Nonlactational breast infection. Am J Surg 1994;60:247–250.
60. Giamarellou H, Soulis M, Antoniadou A, et al. Periareolar nonpuerperal breast infection: treatment of 38 cases. Clin Infect Dis 1994;18:73–76.
61. Jacobs EA, Collins KL. Breast infections. In: Ganschow PS, Norlock FE, Jacobs EA, et al, eds. Breast Health and Common Breast Problems: A Practical Approach. Philadelphia: American College of Physicians, 2004:241–251.
62. Dixon JM. Breast infection. BMJ 1994;309:946–949.
63. Surani S, Chandna H, Weistein RA. Breast abscess: coagulase negative staphylococcus as a sole pathogen. Clin Infect Dis 1993;17:701–704.
64. Hartstein M, Leaf HL. Tuberculosis of the breast as a presenting manifestation of AIDS. Clin Infect Dis 1992;15:692–693.
65. Mortimer PS, Lunniss PJ. Hidradenitis suppurativa. J R Soc Med 2000;93:420–422.
66. Barton MB, Elmore JC, Fletcher SW. Breast symptoms among women enrolled in a health maintenance organization: frequency, evaluation, and outcome. Ann Intern Med 1999;130:651–657.
67. Kerin M, O'Hanlon DM, Khalid AA, et al. Mammographic assessment of the symptomatic nonsuspicious breast. Am J Surg 1997;173:181–184.
68. Colegrave S, Holcombe C, Salmon P. Psychological characteristics of women presenting with breast pain. J Psychosom Res 2001;50:303–307.
69. Preece PE, Mansel RE, Hughes LE. Mastalgia: psychoneurosis or organic disease? BMJ 1978;1:29–30.
70. Khan SA, Apkarian AV. The characteristics of cyclical and non-cyclical mastalgia: a prospective study using the modified McGill Pain Questionnaire. Breast Cancer Res 1998;60:102.
71. Tavaf-Motamen H, Ader DN, Browne MW, et al. Clinical evaluation of mastalgia. Arch Surg 1998;133:211–214.
72. Pye JK, Mansel RE, Hughes LE. Clinical experience of drug treatments for mastalgia. Lancet 1985;2:373–377.

73. Meyer RC, Sommers DK, Reitz CJ, et al. Vitamin E and benign breast disease. Surgery 1990;107:549–551.
74. Preece PE, Richards AR, Owen GM, et al. Mastalgia and total body water. BMJ 1975;4:498–500.
75. Gateley CA, Miers M, Mansell RE, et al. Drug treatments for mastalgia: 17 years experience in the Cardiff mastalgia clinic. J R Soc Med 1992;85:12–15.
76. Blommers J, de Lange-de Klerk ESM, Kuik DJ, et al. Evening primrose oil and fish oil for severe chronic mastalgia: a randomized double-blind, controlled trial. Am J Obstet Gynecol 2002;187:1389–1394.
77. O'Brien PM, Abukhalil IE. Randomized controlled trial of the management of premenopausal syndrome and premenstrual mastalgia using luteal phase-only danazol. Am J Obstet Gynecol 1999;180:18–23.
78. Mansel RE, Wisbey JR, Hughes LE. Controlled trial of the antigonadotrophin danazol in painful nodular benign breast disease. Lancet 1982;i:928–931.
79. Kontostolis E, Stefanidis K, Navrozoglou I, et al. comparison of tamoxifen with danazol for treatment of cyclical mastalgia. Gynecol Endocrinol 1997;11:393–397.
80. Fentiman IS, Caleffi M, Brame K, et al. Double blind controlled trial of tamoxifen therapy for mastalgia. Lancet 1986;i:287–288.
81. Fentiman IS, Caleffi M, Hamed H, et al. dosage and duration of tamoxifen treatment for mastalgia: a controlled trial. Br J Surg 1988;75:845–846.
82. Messinis IE, Lolis D. Treatment of premenstrual mastalgia with tamoxifen. Acta Obstet Gynecol Scand 1988;67:307–309.
83. GEMB Group. Tamoxifen therapy for cyclical mastalgia. Dose randomised trial. Breast 1997;5:212–213.
84. Braithwaite RS, Chlebowski RT, Lau J, et al. Meta-analysis of vascular and neoplastic events associated with tamoxifen. J Gen Intern Med 2003;18(11):937–947.
85. Mansel RE, Dogliotti L. European multicenter trial of bromocriptine in cyclical mastalgia. Lancet 1990;335:190–193.
86. Hamed H, Calefi M, Chaudary MA, et al. LHRH analogue for treatment of recurrent and refractory mastalgia. Ann R Coll Surg Engl 1990;72:221–224.
87. Colak T, Ipek T, Kanik A, et al. Efficacy of topical nonsteroidal anti-inflammatory drugs in mastalgia treatment. J Am Coll Surg 2003;196:525–530.

CHAPTER 7

Premenstrual Syndromes

Meir Steiner

INTRODUCTION

Epidemiologic surveys have estimated that as many as 75% of women of reproductive age experience some symptoms attributable to the premenstrual phase of the menstrual cycle (1). More than 100 physical and psychological symptoms have been reported (2); however, most women are able to manage these symptoms through lifestyle changes and conservative therapies. This phenomenon is often classified by the generic term *premenstrual syndrome (PMS)*, and most often refers to any combination of symptoms that appears during the week prior to menstruation and that resolves within a week of onset of menses (3). Conversely, 3 to 8% of women of reproductive age report premenstrual symptoms of irritability, tension, dysphoria, and lability of mood, which seriously interfere with their lifestyle and relationships (4–11). So disruptive is the latter that a series of research diagnostic criteria for what is now labeled premenstrual dysphoric disorder (PMDD) have been developed and published in the 4th edition of the *Diagnostic and Statistical Manual of Mental Disorders* (*DSM-IV*) (Table 7.1) (12). Women who are found to meet the diagnostic criteria of PMDD do not usually respond to conservative and conventional interventions, and they often seek the expertise of a health professional (13).

ETIOLOGY

The etiology of PMS, and specifically of PMDD, is still largely unknown. Attempts have been made to explain the phenomena in terms of biology, psychology, or psychosocial factors, but most of these explanations have failed to be confirmed by laboratory and treatment-based studies.

As is true for all female-specific mood disorders, the role of female sex hormones in PMDD has been considered of central importance. To date, however, studies attempting to attribute the disorder to an excess of estrogen, a deficit of progesterone, a withdrawal of estrogen, or changes in estrogen-to-progesterone ratio have been unable to find specific differences between women with PMDD and those without the disorder (14). Treatment studies have suggested that progesterone and progestogens may actually provoke rather than ameliorate the cyclical symptom changes of PMDD (15). The hypothesis that ovarian cyclicity is important in the etiology of PMDD is, nevertheless, supported by research. Efforts to suppress ovulation with estradiol patches and cyclical oral norethisterone, use of gonadotrophin-releasing hormone (GnRH) agonists, or bilateral oophorectomy resulted in the disappearance of premenstrual mood disturbances and physical symptoms (16–18).

The current consensus seems to be that normal ovarian function (rather than hormone imbalance) is the cyclical trigger for PMDD-related biochemical events within the central nervous system and other target tissues. A psychoneuroendocrine mechanism triggered by the normal endocrine events of the ovarian cycle seems the most plausible explanation (19). This viewpoint is attractive in that it encourages investigation of the neuroendocrine-modulated central

TABLE 7.1

Summary of Premenstrual Dysphoric Disorder *DSM-IV* Criteria

A. Symptoms must occur during the week before menses and remit a few days after onset of menses. Five of the following symptoms must be present and include at least one from numbers 1, 2, 3, or 4.
   1. Depressed mood or dysphoria
   2. Anxiety or tension
   3. Affective lability
   4. Irritability
   5. Decreased interest in usual activities
   6. Concentration difficulties
   7. Marked lack of energy
   8. Marked change in appetite, overeating, or food cravings
   9. Hypersomnia or insomnia
   10. Feeling overwhelmed
   11. Other physical symptoms (breast tenderness, bloating)

B. Symptoms must interfere with work, school, usual activities, or relationships

C. Symptoms must not merely be an exacerbation of another disorder (major mental disorder, personality disorder, or general medical condition)

D. Criteria A, B, and C must be confirmed by prospective daily ratings for at least two cycles

Adapted from American Psychiatric Association. Diagnostic and Statistical Manual of Mental Disorder, 4th ed. Washington, DC: American Psychiatric Association, 1994:717–718.

neurotransmitters and the role of hypothalamic-pituitary-gonadal (HPG) axis in PMDD. Data regarding the hypothalamic-pituitary-adrenal (HPA) axis function in women with PMS are conflicting. Overall, no differences between PMS patients and controls have been observed, but more recently there is some indication that despite the ubiquity of affective symptoms in PMS, HPA axis function in PMS is distinctly different from that seen in major depression. Women with PMS fail to show the normal increase in HPA axis response to exercise and also seem to have a blunted adrenal sensitivity (20). They also appear to have an abnormal response to normal levels of progesterone (21), including physical evidence for an abnormal brain response to progesterone (22).

Of all the neurotransmitters studied to date, increasing evidence suggests that serotonin may be important in the pathogenesis of PMDD (23–27). PMDD also shares many of the features of other mood and anxiety disorders linked to serotonergic dysfunction (28–31). In addition, reduction in brain serotonin neurotransmission is believed to lead to poor impulse control, depressed mood, irritability, and increased carbohydrate craving—all mood and behavioral symptoms associated with PMDD (32).

Reciprocity between fluctuations in ovarian steroids and serotonergic function has been established in animals showing that estrogen and progesterone influence central serotonergic neuronal activity. In the hypothalamus, estrogen induces a diurnal fluctuation in serotonin (33), whereas progesterone increases the turnover rate of serotonin (34).

More recently, several studies concluded that serotonin function may also be altered in women with PMDD. Some studies used models of neuronal function (e.g., whole blood serotonin levels, platelet uptake of serotonin, platelet tritiated imipramine [Tofranil] binding) and found altered serotonin function during all phases of the menstrual cycle (23, 35–38). Other studies that used challenge tests (with L-tryptophan, fenfluramine [Pondimin], and buspirone [BuSpar]) suggested abnormal serotonin function in symptomatic women but differed in their findings as to whether the response to serotonin is blunted or heightened (25, 39–42). These studies imply, at least in part, a possible change in 5-hydroxytryptamine (serotonin) ($5HT_{1A}$) receptor sensitivity in women with PMDD.

The current consensus is that women with PMDD may be behaviorally or biochemically subsensitive or supersensitive to biological challenges of the serotonergic system (43, 44). It is not yet clear whether these women present with a trait or state marker of PMDD.

RISK FACTORS

Epidemiologic surveys from around the world continue to demonstrate convincingly that, for adult women, the lifetime prevalence of mood disorders is substantially higher than it is among men. Most studies confirm that the ratio of affected women to men is approximately 2:1, and this ratio is maintained across ethnic groups (45). The higher incidence of depression among women is primarily seen beginning at puberty and is less marked in the years after menopause (46). The relationship between PMDD and other psychiatric disorders is complicated by the observation that a high proportion of women presenting with PMDD have a history of previous episodes of mood disorders and that women with an ongoing mood disorder report premenstrual magnification of symptoms, as well as an emergence of new symptoms (29, 31, 47–53). Likewise, several family studies have identified a concordance in rates of premenstrual tension between first-degree female family members (54–56).

Women with PMS/PMDD also report more stressful life events (57), and more women with PMDD have histories of abuse (either sexual or physical) when compared with controls (58, 59).

PRESENTATION AND DIAGNOSIS

To aid in the study of menstrual cycle disorders, each menstrual cycle is characterized as containing two prominent phases: the follicular phase occurs after the onset of menses, and the luteal phase refers to the premenstrual interval. The temporal relationship between fluctuations in psychopathology and different phases of the menstrual cycle are well documented. It is therefore essential to ascertain whether the presenting premenstrual symptomatology is unique to the luteal phase or whether it is a worsening of an ongoing, persistent physical or psychiatric disorder.

Unfortunately, investigators have yet to reach consensus on how to best define the follicular and luteal phases of the menstrual cycle. Some investigators use set days, and others use cycle-adjusted days; other combinations also exist (Fig. 7.1). Although researchers are still defining

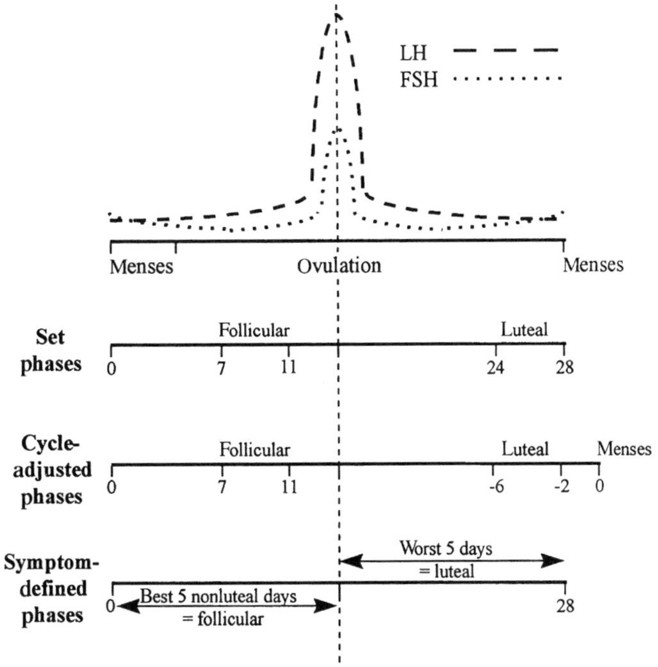

FIGURE 7.1 ● The follicular and luteal phases can be defined in various ways for research purposes. The cycle-adjusted phases illustrated in the middle graph seem most appropriate to clinical settings. LH, luteinizing hormone; FSH, follicle-stimulating hormone.

Baseline weight on Day 1 _________ lbs. or kg.
(circle one)

Day of Menstrual Cycle	1	2	3	4	5	6	7	8	9	10	11	12	13	14	15	16	17	18	19	20	21	22	23	24	25	26	27	28	29	30	31	32	33	34	35
Bleeding																																			
Month: Date:																																			
SYMPTOMS																																			
Irritable																																			
Fatigue																																			
Inward anger																																			
Labile mood (crying)																																			
Depressed																																			
Restless																																			
Anxious																																			
Insomnia																																			
Lack of control																																			
Edema or rings tight																																			
Breast tenderness																																			
Abdominal bloating																																			
Bowels: const. (c) loose (l)																																			
Appetite: up ▲ down ▼																																			
Sex drive: up ▲ down ▼																																			
Chills (C)/sweats (S)																																			
Headaches																																			
Crave: sweets, salt																																			
Feel unattractive																																			
Guilty																																			
Unreasonable behavior																																			
Low self-image																																			
Nausea																																			
Menstrual cramps																																			
LIFESTYLE IMPACT																																			
Aggressive towards others: Physically																																			
Aggressive towards others: Verbally																																			
Wish to be alone																																			
Neglect housework																																			
Time off work																																			
Disorganized, distractible																																			
Accident prone/clumsy																																			
Uneasy about driving																																			
Suicidal thoughts																																			
Stayed at home																																			
Increased use of alcohol																																			
LIFE EVENTS																																			
Negative experience																																			
Positive experience																																			
Social activities																																			
Vigorous exercise																																			
MEDICATIONS																																			

FIGURE 7.2 ● The Premenstrual Record of Impact and Severity of Menstruation. Instructions for completing this calendar are provided in Table 7.2. (Reprinted from Reid RL. Premenstrual syndrome. Curr Probl Obstet Gynecol Fertil 1985;8:1–57, with permission.)

the temporal boundaries of the follicular and luteal phases (60), a definition of the follicular phase as days 7 through 11 after onset of bleeding and the luteal phase as 6 days before bleeding through 2 days before bleeding seems most appropriate in clinical settings.

Another challenge in the delineation of premenstrual disorders is that most women report varying combinations of the most troubling symptoms. Some investigators attempted to divide

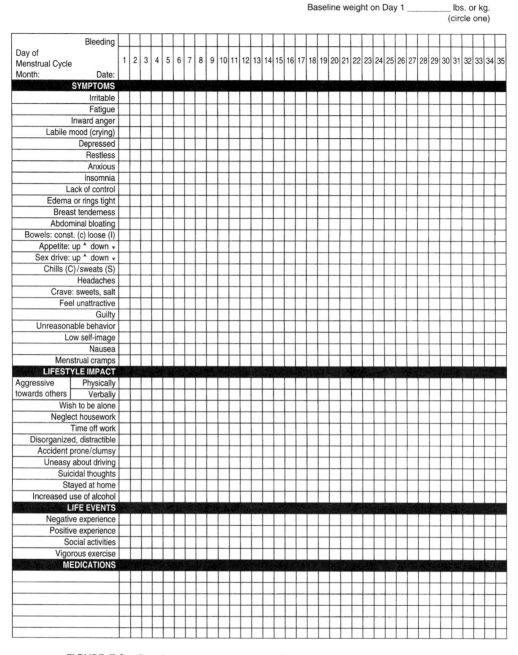

TABLE 7.2

Instructions for Completing the Premenstrual Record of Impact and Severity of Menstruation Calendar

Prepare the calendar on the first day of menstruation. Considering the first day of bleeding as day 1 of your menstrual cycle, enter the corresponding calendar date for each day in the space provided. Each evening, at about the same time, complete the calendar column for that day as described here:

• Bleeding:	Indicate if you have had bleeding by shading/filling in the box above that day's date; for spotting, use an "X".
• Symptoms:	If you do not experience any symptoms, leave the corresponding box blank. If present, indicate the severity by entering a number from 1 (mild) to 7 (severe).
• Lifestyle impact:	If the listed phrase applies to you that day, enter an "X".
• Life events:	If you experienced one of these events that day, enter an "X".
	Experiences: For positive (happy) or negative (sad/disappointing) experiences unrelated to your symptoms, specify the nature of the events on the back of the form.
	Social activities: This implies such events as a special dinner, show, or party, etc., involving family or friends.
	Vigorous exercise: This implies participation in a sporting event or exercise program lasting more than 30 minutes.
• Medication:	In the bottom five rows, list medication used, if any, and indicate days when medication was taken by entering an "X".

From RL. Premenstrual syndrome. Curr Probl Obstet Gynecol Fertil 1985;8:1–57, with permission.

the most prominent symptoms into physical and psychological domains; however, a complete separation is not possible. Measurement tools developed for depression and other mood disorders have not performed well in the diagnosis of PMS (61). A review by Budeiri et al. (2) identified at least 65 instruments developed specifically to measure various combinations of premenstrual symptoms. Generally, if an instrument has been tested for reliability and validity in this population, it is appropriate for both facilitating diagnosis and assessing treatment outcomes. There has yet to be consensus as to which instruments are most appropriate for diagnosis and measurement of treatment efficacy (2, 62), so most investigators use at least two or three of these instruments in their clinical trials.

Women presenting with premenstrual complaints should be instructed to chart their symptoms daily over the course of several menstrual cycles to measure symptom change within each cycle. The current emphasis is on prospective self-report instruments, which are easy to administer and score without jeopardizing validity. The Daily Record of Severity of Problems (DRSP) assesses 20 symptoms associated with PMDD and specifically measures functional impairment in work and social realms (63). The Premenstrual Record of Impact and Severity of Menstruation (PRISM) (64) and the Calendar of Premenstrual Experiences (COPE) (65) are detailed one-page calendars that have also been validated and used in clinical trials. Figure 7.2 is a copy of the PRISM calendar, and Table 7.2 provides the instructions for completing it. These calendars allow respondents to rate a variety of physical and psychological symptoms, indicate negative and positive life events, record concurrent medications, and track menstrual bleeding and cycle length.

The lack of objective diagnostic tests for PMS or PMDD mandates taking a complete history of symptoms when one of these diagnoses is suspected. In addition to a history of the premenstrual symptoms, this interview should also include a complete review of physical systems (with particular attention to gynecologic and endocrinologic symptoms) and medical disorders, as well as a psychiatric history and a detailed review of family history looking for mental illness. Because the symptoms of anemia and thyroid disease often mirror those of PMS or PMDD, the patient should undergo laboratory studies if there is any hint of an underlying medical cause for the symptoms. In addition, women who are suspected to meet criteria for PMDD should be assessed by their physicians at least once during each cycle phase to ensure the patient subjectively endorses phase-appropriate mood symptoms that support their daily charting (minimal or no symptoms during follicular phase, lifestyle-impairing symptoms during the luteal phase).

The *DSM-IV* multiaxial classification system includes five axes, each of a different domain of information that may help the clinician in the comprehensive and systematic evaluation of the patient (12). It draws attention to the various major mental disorders (axis I) and personality disorders (axis II), to general medical conditions (axis III), and to psychosocial and environmental factors (axis IV), and provides a global assessment of functioning (axis V). In using the *DSM-IV* criteria for PMDD (Table 7.1), a certain familiarity with the multiaxial system is assumed. Thus, for PMDD, criterion C is crucial in excluding any current axis I, II, or III illness or episode. The other essential features of the *DSM-IV* PMDD criteria are the cyclicity of symptoms and the emphasis on core mood symptoms (criterion A), the requirement that the symptoms must interfere markedly with lifestyle (criterion B), and most important, the requirement that the disorder must be confirmed prospectively by daily ratings for at least two menstrual cycles (criterion D). Prospective daily rating of symptoms is now the only acceptable means of confirming a provisional *DSM-IV* diagnosis of PMDD.

The PRISM, COPE, DSR, and DRSP calendars contain the core symptoms and most of the additional symptoms considered for the *DSM-IV* diagnosis of PMDD. In using one of the daily calendars, the clinician must identify *a priori* the patient's chief complaints and the symptoms to be followed throughout treatment. Daily symptoms are rated by the patient using scales that range from none (for a score of 0) to severe (for a score of 7 on the PRISM, 3 on the COPE). Scores for the symptoms of interest are added for the 5 follicular days and the 5 luteal days, and these total phase scores are then compared.

Investigators have typically followed a diagnostic severity criterion that is applied in addition to the criteria listed for PMDD in the *DSM-IV*. Conventionally, an increase in symptom scores (worsening) of at least 30% from follicular to luteal phase scores within a single cycle is required to meet PMDD criteria (66). For inclusion of subjects in clinical trials, within-cycle worsening of at least 50% has been suggested (67). The within-cycle percent change is calculated by subtracting the follicular score from the luteal score, dividing by the luteal score, and multiplying by 100:

$$[(\text{luteal score} - \text{follicular score}) \div (\text{luteal score})] \times 100\% \qquad (7.1)$$

Thus, a patient presenting with a mean follicular score of 20 and a luteal score of 50 would demonstrate a within-cycle symptom increase of 60%. A change of this proportion demonstrates the cyclicity of symptomatology and is typical of women who meet criteria for PMDD (68).

On completion of the two-cycle prospective diagnostic assessment phase, women may qualify for one of the following diagnostic categories. Applying these criteria to women who seek help for premenstrual complaints will facilitate the clinician in planning management interventions.

Premenstrual Dysphoric Disorder

Women who receive this diagnosis meet criteria for PMDD only. They have no other concurrent psychiatric disorder or unstable medical condition but may have a history of a past psychiatric disorder. They have charted symptoms daily for two cycles, and their chief complaints include one of the four core symptoms and at least 5 of the 11 total symptoms (Table 7.1). Their symptoms have occurred with most menstrual cycles during the past year and have interfered with social or occupational roles. Their symptoms demonstrate clear worsening premenstrually and remit within a few days after the onset of the follicular phase. In addition, worsening between the follicular and luteal phases must be at least 30%.

Premenstrual Syndrome

Women who receive this diagnosis do not meet all *DSM-IV* criteria for PMDD but do demonstrate symptom exacerbation premenstrually. Symptoms may include mild psychological discomfort and feelings of bloating and weight gain, breast tenderness, swelling of hands and feet, various aches and pains, poor concentration, sleep disturbance, and change in appetite. Only one of these symptoms is required for this diagnosis, although the symptoms must be restricted to the luteal phase of the menstrual cycle, reach a peak shortly before menstruation, and cease with the menstrual flow or soon after (3).

Premenstrual Magnification/Exacerbation

Women who receive this diagnosis may meet criteria for PMS or PMDD but are in the process of being assessed for, or have already been diagnosed with, a current major psychiatric disorder or an unstable medical condition (53, 68). Medical disorders that are commonly exacerbated during the luteal phase include migraine headaches, allergies, asthma, seizures, and genital herpes. Psychiatric conditions that can be magnified include depression, anxiety, panic, bulimia, substance abuse, mania, and psychosis (69).

Other Psychiatric Diagnosis Only

These women do not demonstrate premenstrual symptoms that meet criteria for PMDD but do meet *DSM-IV* criteria for another psychiatric disorder. Women meeting criteria for intermittent depressive disorder or cyclothymia may fall into this category, where the cyclical nature of their symptoms does not necessarily match the phases of their menstrual cycle.

No Diagnosis

In these women, the diagnosis of PMS or PMDD cannot be made and medical, gynecologic, and psychiatric screening is negative. These women experience disruptive symptoms that tend to occur throughout the cycle. It is often difficult to delineate the exact problem. Careful examination of the entire diary, especially the follicular phase, and discussion with the patient may show low-grade psychiatric or medical problems. These include situational, vocational, or marital stress, mild dysthymia, generalized anxiety disorder, personality disorders, irritable bowel syndrome, chronic fatigue syndrome, headache, fibromyalgia or other pain syndromes, and sleep disorders.

TREATMENT

Women who present with premenstrual magnification of a major psychiatric disorder, personality disorder, or general medical disorder should be treated for the primary disorder at the discretion of the supervising clinician. Referral to an appropriate specialist is often indicated for newly diagnosed disorders.

A wide range of therapeutic interventions have been tested in the treatment of premenstrual symptoms, from lifestyle changes to advanced hormonal treatment.

Conservative Therapies

It is prudent to start all women with premenstrual symptoms on a program of lifestyle changes (Table 7.3). For women who do not meet criteria for PMS, PMDD, or other physical or psychological disorders, management without pharmacologic interventions should be encouraged. Unfortunately, there have been few randomized controlled trials to determine the efficacy of these more conservative interventions. There is some evidence, however, to support that these patients may best respond to individual or group psychotherapy in combination with lifestyle changes (70, 71). Recommended dietary changes (especially during the luteal phase) should include the reduction or cessation of tobacco, chocolate, caffeine, and alcohol consumption. Some women report improvement with small, frequent, complex carbohydrate meals with vitamin and mineral supplements. Patients should be encouraged to decrease sodium in their diets when edema or

TABLE 7.3

Conservative Treatment Modalities for Premenstrual Symptoms

Charting of Symptoms Daily

Diet

Reduce or eliminate (especially in the luteal phase) salt, chocolate, caffeine, and alcohol

Small frequent complex carbohydrate meals

Vitamins and minerals in moderation

Moderate, Regular Aerobic Exercise

Stress Reduction

Stress management course and/or counseling if necessary

Relaxation course or audio tape

Assertiveness course and/or marital counseling if necessary

Self-Help Books, Groups if Available

fluid retention occurs and, if possible, to reduce weight to within 20% of ideal weight. Regular exercise is important and particularly effective when combined with the regular practice of stress management techniques. Patients should also be taught to review their own monthly diaries and identify triggers for symptom exacerbation.

Evidence-Based Low-Risk Therapies

Women who meet criteria for PMS should be encouraged to practice the lifestyle changes described previously, but they may also respond to some of the tested conservative therapies (Table 7.4).

Vitamin B_6 has demonstrated mild to moderate efficacy in relieving PMS symptoms in clinical trials, using a wide range of dosing strategies from 50 to 500 mg daily (72). Because of reports of sensory neuropathy, dosing in clinical practice should not exceed 150 mg daily, given during the last 2 weeks of each cycle.

Calcium (1200 to 1600 mg daily) demonstrated significant improvement in overall symptoms scores from baseline compared with placebo (73, 74). No untoward side effects were reported with this dose.

TABLE 7.4

Evidence-Based Low-Risk Treatment Options for Premenstrual Symptoms

	Dosage
Vitamin B_6	50–150 mg daily
Calcium	1200–1600 mg daily
Magnesium	360 mg daily for the 14 days prior to menses
Optivite	Up to 6 tablets daily
Vitamin E	400 IU daily
Spironolactone	100 mg daily from day 12 until the first day of the next menstrual cycle for bloating
Bromocriptine	1.25–7.5 mg daily during luteal phase for premenstrual mastodynia

Oral magnesium (360 mg daily) from the fifteenth day of the menstrual cycle to the onset of menstrual flow significantly improved premenstrual pain and negative affect in one randomized controlled trial (75).

Optivite (Otimox Corp., Torrance, CA) is a vitamin/mineral supplement. In one clinical trial, subjects were randomized to 6 or 12 tablets daily of the supplement or placebo for three menstrual cycles and demonstrated significant treatment effects in physical symptoms and depression (76). No unusual side effects were reported. Up to six Optivite tablets daily during the luteal phase of the menstrual cycle may relieve symptoms.

Vitamin E (alpha-tocopherol) was administered in a randomized trial to women with benign breast disease who scored the severity of their premenstrual symptoms before and after 2 months of vitamin E therapy (150, 300, or 600 IU per day versus placebo) (77). Significant improvements in physical symptoms and depression were demonstrated by all three treatment groups compared with placebo. Vitamin E therapy can safely begin at 400 IU daily.

Evening primrose oil (gamma-linolenic acid) has not demonstrated efficacy superior to placebo in several randomized controlled trials and should not be recommended as treatment for PMS or PMDD (78).

Naproxen sodium (Anaprox, Aleve) improved pain and premenstrual behavior changes in one randomized trial when taken 7 days premenstrually (79) and menstrual migraine specifically in another randomized trial when it was taken daily (80).

Mefenamic acid (Ponstel) was superior to placebo for improving physical and mood symptoms in one randomized controlled trial (81); however, the use of this medication should be limited (7 to 10 days) because of gastric side effects.

Spironolactone (100 mg daily) from day 12 of the menstrual cycle until the first day of the next menstrual cycle significantly reduced bloating compared with placebo in one randomized controlled trial (82). The potential for diuretic abuse and hyperkalemia (and thus contraindication of potassium supplements) necessitates the use of this drug for severe symptoms only.

Bromocriptine (at least 5 mg daily) has demonstrated significant improvement in premenstrual mastodynia (83) but has not demonstrated efficacy with the mood symptoms associated with the premenstruum. Randomized controlled trial evidence suggests that a dosing range of 1.25 to 7.5 mg daily during the luteal phase of the menstrual cycle is appropriate for clinical use.

Women who continue to experience severe premenstrual symptoms after the commencement of lifestyle changes and the previous conservative therapies may be considered for the pharmacologic treatment regimens indicated for PMDD.

Pharmacotherapies

Therapeutic interventions for women who meet criteria for PMDD but fail conservative therapies are available. These range from treatment of the most troublesome symptoms with psychotropic medications (Table 7.5) to hormonal therapy to eliminate ovulation.

Listed as follows is a summary of the randomized controlled trial evidence for the most common therapies used to treat PMDD. It is important to note that only studies that used prospective diagnostic criteria that could meet *DSM-IV* PMDD classification have been cited.

Psychotropic Medications

Serotonin reuptake inhibitors have proven to be very successful in the treatment of PMDD symptoms. Of the selective serotonin reuptake inhibitors (SSRIs), fluoxetine (Prozac) 20 mg daily has been proven superior to placebo in several randomized trials (67, 84–89). One of these trials used a higher dose, 60 mg daily, but the improvement demonstrated by this group did not differ from the 20-mg group, and the side effect profile was significantly higher at the 60-mg dose (67). Sertraline (Zoloft) 50 to 150 mg daily (90), paroxetine (Paxil) 10 to 30 mg daily (91), citalopram (Celexa) 10 to 30 mg daily (92), and the selective serotonin and norepinephrine reuptake inhibitor (SNRI) venlafaxine (Effexor) 50 to 150 mg daily (93, 94) have also demonstrated efficacy in randomized controlled trials in the treatment of PMDD. More recent studies have demonstrated the efficacy of intermittent serotonin reuptake inhibitor

TABLE 7.5

Psychotropic Medications for Premenstrual Dysphoric Disorder and Premenstrual Syndrome Refractory to Conservative Treatment

	Dosage
First-Line Treatment: Antidepressants	
Luteal phase only or continuous	
Citalopram	10–30 mg daily
Clomipramine	25–75 mg nightly
Fluoxetine	20 mg daily
Paroxetine	10–30 mg daily
Sertraline	50–150 mg daily
Venlafaxine	25–75 mg twice a day[a]
Second-Line Treatment: Anxiolytics	
Luteal phase only	
Alprazolam	0.25–2 mg three to four times daily (max 5 mg daily)
Buspirone	10–15 mg twice a day

[a]An extended-release preparation is also available—venlafaxine-XR 75–150 mg daily.

dosing during the last 2 weeks of the menstrual cycle (95–97). The tricyclic antidepressant (but primarily serotonin reuptake inhibitor) clomipramine (Anafranil) has also been proven superior to placebo in two randomized controlled trials. One study used 25 to 75 mg daily (98) and the other the same dose range for only the luteal phase of each menstrual cycle (99). Thus, the serotonin reuptake inhibitors to date have demonstrated their effectiveness in significantly improving the psychological and physical symptoms of PMDD compared with placebo, with only mild, mostly tolerable side effects. The side effect profile is similar among agents in the class, the most troublesome include headache, nausea/gastrointestinal upset, sleep disturbance/insomnia, tremulousness, sweating, dry mouth, and anorgasmia. These side effects can usually be managed through dosing changes, the use of intermittent versus daily dosing schedules, or by switching to other serotonin reuptake inhibitor compounds.

Anxiolytics have been tested for the treatment of PMDD because of its mood disorder component. Alprazolam (Xanax) has successfully alleviated the symptoms of PMDD in several (100–103), but not all (104), randomized controlled trials. The risk of dependence and concerns regarding withdrawal prompted investigators to test the efficacy of alprazolam versus placebo when administered in the luteal phase only. Patient-modified dosing was allowed, and efficacious dosing ranged from 0.25 to 5 mg daily from 6 to 14 days before menstruation. One study also allowed women who demonstrated mild follicular symptoms to take this medication as needed during the follicular phase of the cycle (102). Sedation and drowsiness were the two most frequently identified side effects of this treatment. Significant improvements in mood and physical symptoms were reported for the positive studies. The 5-HT_{1A} receptor partial antagonist buspirone (BuSpar) has also demonstrated efficacy in one randomized controlled trial when administered with a mean daily dose of 25 mg for the 12 days prior to menstruation (105).

Hormonal Therapies

GnRH agonists can reversibly suppress the menstrual cycle, and this is often referred to as medical ovariectomy or medical menopause. GnRH agonists have proven to be very successful in clinical trials (16, 17). Unfortunately, the long-term (more than 6 months cumulative) use of

GnRH agonists has been inhibited by the occurrence of side effects that mimic menopause, and the potential for hypoestrogenism and osteoporosis. The "add-back" of estrogen and progesterone to goserelin (Zoladex) (106) or leuprolide (Lupron) (21) has led to the reappearance of mood and anxiety symptoms. Because it has been shown that women with severe PMS and PMDD have an abnormal response to normal hormonal fluctuation (21), it is not surprising that the addition of hormones led to the induction of mood and anxiety symptoms, in turn reducing the benefit of the hormone replacement therapy.

More recently, a trial of women receiving leuprolide with added tibolone (a compound with some estrogenic activity) versus added placebo reported equal efficacy for premenstrual symptoms and fewer hot flushes (18).

Estradiol treatment can suppress ovulation and thus has been proven effective in reducing the symptoms of PMDD, although adjunct progestogen therapy is necessary to prevent endometrial hyperplasia. Luteal phase-only administration of conjugated estrogen (Premarin) was ineffective in one randomized controlled trial (107); however, transdermal estradiol (Climara, Estraderm, Vivelle) or estradiol implants combined with luteal phase norethisterone, medroxyprogesterone (Premarin), or dydrogesterone improved physical and mood symptoms in three randomized controlled trials (108–110). Transdermal estradiol (100- to 200-μg patches) applied twice weekly with low-dose progestogen daily from days 17 to 26 of each cycle is appropriate for clinical use.

Danazol (Danocrine), a synthetic androgen, alleviates symptoms of PMS when administered at 200 to 400 mg daily (111). A more recent study reported that luteal phase–only danazol was not effective for general premenstrual symptoms but was highly effective for the relief of premenstrual mastalgia (112). Although danazol has been proven to be superior to placebo in several randomized controlled trials (111,113–115), the adverse effect profile of this treatment is considerable and may be the result of both its androgenic activity and antiestrogen properties. Tested doses include 100 to 400 mg daily, and both mood and physical symptoms improved significantly when compared with placebo. The most prominent side effect at doses over 200 mg was altered menstrual cycle length, but at higher doses, women can get acne, bloating, depression, and permanent lowering of the voice. One study of women with PMS found that intermittent danazol, 200 mg given daily from the onset of symptoms to the onset of menses, significantly improved mood symptoms and bloating compared with placebo (116). Clinical dosing at 200 to 400 mg daily during symptoms is appropriate.

Progesterone has been shown to be no more effective than placebo in treating PMS or PMDD symptoms in the majority of trials and should not be used as a primary treatment for these disorders (103, 117–125). Despite this mounting evidence demonstrating their lack of efficacy, progestogens, including progesterone, are the most widely prescribed treatment for PMS in the United Kingdom (126).

Oral contraceptives suppress ovulation while maintaining menstruation with periodic steroid withdrawal. The one randomized controlled trial that tested oral contraceptives for premenstrual symptoms was a negative study (127) that supported the conclusions of other less rigorous studies. Overall, the current consensus is that oral contraceptives do not influence premenstrual mood in most women (128). A more recent initial report on the effectiveness of a new unique oral contraceptive containing a combination of drospirenone (with spironolactone-like activity) and estradiol (Yasmin) has renewed the interest in this type of intervention for women with PMDD (129).

To date, no one pharmacologic intervention has proven to be effective for all women with PMDD. Serotonin reuptake inhibitors continue to prove efficacious in women with PMDD who have failed conservative treatment and are currently the first treatment of choice. Alprazolam and buspirone have demonstrated efficacy in the reduction of psychological symptoms in randomized controlled trials, but side effects and dependence concerns with the benzodiazepines limit their efficacy.

The last line of treatment for women with PMDD who do not report efficacy with the symptom-modifying drugs are the GnRH agonists. Due to the potential long-term side effects of this treatment, low-dose estrogen-progesterone add-back should be considered but is likely to affect efficacy. Estradiol and danazol may also be effective, and gynecologic interventions such as surgery may need to be considered (130, 131).

ASSESSMENT OF TREATMENT EFFICACY

Patients should be assessed every 2 weeks (i.e., during both the follicular phase and the luteal phase) within the first month of commencing any therapy, and they should be instructed to continue to chart symptoms daily for at least two to three additional cycles. Dosing strategies vary, but most recent investigations demonstrated the efficacy of most therapeutic drugs at low doses. If efficacy has not been attained after several dose increases, alternative treatment options should be considered. There is increasing evidence that treatment effect is seen relatively quickly in this population. Therefore, if there is no change in symptomatology, an alternate therapy should be considered within two to three menstrual cycles. Continued symptom charting using a daily calendar will help track efficacy, symptom response to dosing changes, symptoms on termination of therapy, and side effects. For example, women who report headaches or nausea as side effects are often surprised to see that they rated these symptoms just as severe prior to commencing therapy.

Investigators have yet to reach a consensus on how to define efficacy. Clinically, the easiest way to define efficacy is by the reduction of luteal symptoms so the luteal symptoms remit significantly or the within-cycle percent change (see Eq. [1]) is less than 30%.

What has become obvious is that the intervention alone cannot predict efficacy, and more consideration is now being given to past psychiatric history and to family psychiatric history, especially of mood disorders in the families of women with PMDD.

Clinical Notes

ETIOLOGY

- The etiology of PMS and PMDD is still largely unknown.
- The current consensus seems to be that normal ovarian function (rather than hormone imbalance) is the cyclical trigger for PMDD-related biochemical events within the central nervous system and other target tissues.
- Evidence suggests that serotonin may be the predominant neurotransmitter involved.

PREVALENCE

- Epidemiologic surveys have estimated that as many as 75% of women with regular menstrual cycles experience some symptoms of PMS. The majority of these women do not require medical or psychiatric interventions.
- PMDD, however, is much less common, affecting only 3 to 8% of women in this age group. It is much more severe, specifically exerting a much greater psychological toll.

PRESENTATION AND DIAGNOSIS

- *DSM-IV* lists criteria for PMDD (Table 7.1). Women who do not meet these criteria may be categorized with PMS, premenstrual magnification (of a psychiatric or medical condition), other psychiatric diagnosis only, or no diagnosis.

TREATMENT

- Conservative treatment is used for all patients, including those with premenstrual complaints but no diagnosis.
- Low-risk/evidence-based modalities, including vitamins, minerals, and nonsteroidal anti-inflammatories, are used for women with PMS or PMDD.
- Psychotropics such as serotonin reuptake-inhibiting antidepressants or anxiolytics may be useful for women with PMDD or PMS refractory to conservative treatment.

- Hormonal therapies should be reserved for refractory PMDD patients because of the adverse effects associated with "medical menopause."
- Neither progesterone alone nor combination oral contraceptives are efficacious in treating PMDD or PMS.

ASSESSMENT OF EFFICACY

- Patients should continue charting their symptoms. If on pharmacologic therapy, the physician should evaluate them during both the follicular phase and the luteal phase of at least one cycle.

REFERENCES

1. Johnson SR. The epidemiology and social impact of premenstrual symptoms. Clin Obstet Gynecol 1987;30:367–376.
2. Budeiri DJ, Li Wan Po A, Dornan JC. Clinical trials of treatments of premenstrual syndrome: entry criteria and scales for measuring treatment outcomes. Br J Obstet Gynaecol 1994;101:689–695.
3. World Health Organization (WHO). Mental, Behavioral and Developmental Disorders. Tenth Revision of the International Classification of Diseases (ICD-10). Geneva: WHO, 1992.
4. Andersch B, Wendestam C, Hahn L, et al. Premenstrual complaints. Prevalence of premenstrual symptoms in a Swedish urban population. J Psychosom Obstet Gynaecol 1986;5:39–49.
5. Johnson SR, McChesney C, Bean JA. Epidemiology of premenstrual symptoms in a nonclinical sample. I. Prevalence, natural history and helpseeking behaviour. J Reprod Med 1988;33:340–346.
6. Ramcharan S, Love EJ, Fick GH, et al. The epidemiology of premenstrual symptoms in a population based sample of 2650 urban women. J Clin Epidemiol 1992;45:377–392.
7. Sveindottir H, Backstrom T. Prevalence of menstrual cycle symptom cyclicity and premenstrual dysphoric disorder in a random sample of women using and not using oral contraceptives. Acta Obstet Gynecol Scand 2000;79:405–413.
8. Angst J, Sellaro R, Merikangas MR, et al. The epidemiology of perimenstrual psychological symptoms. Acta Psychiatr Scand 2001;104:110–116.
9. Wittchen HU, Becker E, Lieb R, et al. Prevalence, incidence and stability of premenstrual dysphoric disorder in the community. Psychol Med 2002;32:119–132.
10. Cohen LS, Soares CN, Otto MW, et al. Prevalence and predictors of premenstrual dysphoric disorder (PMDD) in older premenopausal women. The Harvard Study of Mood and Cycles. J Affect Disord 2002;70:125–132.
11. Steiner M, Macdougall M, Brown E. The Premenstrual Symptoms Screening Tool (PSST) for clinicians. Arch Women Ment Health 2003;6:203–209.
12. American Psychiatric Association. Diagnostic and Statistical Manual of Mental Disorders. 4th ed. Washington, DC: American Psychiatric Association, 1994:715–718.
13. Halbreich U, Borenstein J, Pearlstein T, et al. The prevalence, impairment, impact, and burden of premenstrual dysphoric disorder (PMS/PMDD). Psychoneuroendocrinology 2003;28:1–23.
14. Roca CA, Schmidt PJ, Bloch M, et al. Implications of endocrine studies of premenstrual syndrome. Psychiatr Ann 1996;26:576–580.
15. Hammarback S, Backstrom T, Holst J, et al. Cyclical mood changes as in the premenstrual tension syndrome during sequential estrogenprogestogen postmenopausal replacement therapy. Acta Obstet Gynecol Scand 1985;64:393–397.
16. Johnson SR. Premenstrual syndrome therapy. Clin Obstet Gynecol 1998;41:405–421.
17. Pearlstein T, Steiner M. Non-antidepressant treatment of premenstrual syndrome. J Clin Psychiatry 2000;61:22–27.
18. Di Carlo C, Palomba S, Tommaselli GA, et al. Use of leuprolide acetate plus tibolone in the treatment of severe premenstrual syndrome. Fertil Steril 2001;75:380–384.
19. Rubinow DR, Schmidt PJ. The treatment of premenstrual syndrome—forward into the past. N Engl J Med 1995;332:1574–1575.
20. Roca CA, Schmidt PJ, Altemus M, et al. Differential menstrual cycle regulation of hypothalamic-pituitary-adrenal axis in women with premenstrual syndrome and controls. J Clin Endocrinol Metab 2003;88:3057–3063.
21. Schmidt PJ, Nieman LK, Danaceau MA, et al. Differential behavioral effects of gonadal steroids in women with and in those without premenstrual syndrome. N Engl J Med 1998;338:209–216.
22. Smith MJ, Adams LF, Schmidt PJ, et al. Abnormal luteal phase excitability of the motor cortex in women with premenstrual syndrome. Biol Psychiatry 2003;54:757–762.
23. Rojansky N, Halbreich U, Zander K, et al. Imipramine receptor binding and serotonin uptake in platelets of women with premenstrual changes. Gynecol Obstet Invest 1991;31:146–152.
24. Rapkin AJ. The role of serotonin in premenstrual syndrome. Clin Obstet Gynecol 1992;35:629–636.
25. Yatham LN. Is $5HT_{1A}$ receptor subsensitivity a trait marker for late luteal phase dysphoric disorder? A pilot study. Can J Psychiatry 1993;38:662–664.
26. Steiner M, Lepage P, Dunn EJ. Serotonin and gender specific psychiatric disorders. Int J Psychol Clin Prac 1997;1:3–13.

27. Steiner M, Dunn E, Born L. Hormones and mood: from menarche to menopause and beyond. J Affect Disord 2003;74:67–83.
28. Pearlstein TB, Frank E, RiveraTovar A, et al. Prevalence of axis I and axis II disorders in women with late luteal phase dysphoric disorder. J Affect Disord 1990;20:129–134.
29. Endicott J. The menstrual cycle and mood disorders. J Affect Disord 1993;29:193–200.
30. Wurtman JJ. Depression and weight gain: the serotonin connection. J Affect Disord 1993;29:183–192.
31. Bailey JW, Cohen LS. Prevalence of mood and anxiety disorders in women who seek treatment for premenstrual syndrome. J Womens Health Gend Based Med 1999;8:1181–1184.
32. Meltzer HY. Serotonergic dysfunction in depression. Br J Psychiatry 1989;155:25–31.
33. Cohen IR, Wise PM. Effects of estradiol on the diurnal rhythm of serotonin activity in microdissected brain areas of ovariectomized rats. Endocrinology 1988;122:2619–2625.
34. Ladisich W. Influence of progesterone on serotonin metabolism: a possible causal factor for mood changes. Psychoneuroendocrinology 1977;2:257–266.
35. Taylor DL, Mathew RH, Ho BT, et al. Serotonin levels and platelet uptake during premenstrual tension. Neuropsychobiology 1984;12:16–18.
36. Rapkin AJ, Edelmuth E, Chang LC, et al. Whole blood serotonin in premenstrual syndrome. Obstet Gynecol 1987;70:533–537.
37. Ashby CR Jr, Carr LA, Cook CL, et al. Alteration of platelet serotonergic mechanisms and monoamine oxidase activity on premenstrual syndrome. Biol Psychiatry 1988;24:225–233.
38. Steege JF, Stout AL, Knight DL, et al. Reduced platelet tritium-labeled imipramine binding sites in women with premenstrual syndrome. Am J Obstet Gynecol 1992;167:168–172.
39. Bancroft J, Cook A, Davidson D, et al. Blunting of neuroendocrine responses to infusion of L-tryptophan in women with perimenstrual mood change. Psychol Med 1991;21:305–312.
40. Bancroft J, Cook A. The neuroendocrine response to d-fenfluramine in women with premenstrual depression. J Affect Disord 1995;36:57–64.
41. FitzGerald M, Malone KM, Li A, et al. Blunted serotonin response to fenfluramine challenge in premenstrual dysphoric disorder. Am J Psychiatry 1997;154:556–558.
42. Steiner M, Yatham LN, Coote M, et al. Serotonergic dysfunction in women with pure premenstrual dysphoric disorder: is the fenfluramine challenge test still relevant? Psychiatry Res 1999;87:107–115.
43. Halbreich U, Tworek H. Altered serotonergic activity in women with dysphoric premenstrual syndromes. Int J Psychiatry Med 1993;23:1–27.
44. Leibenluft E, Fiero PL, Rubinow DR. Effects of the menstrual cycle on dependent variables in mood disorder research. Arch Gen Psychiatry 1994;51:761–781. [Erratum Arch Gen Psychiatry 1995;52:144.]
45. Weissman MM, Olfson M. Depression in women: implications for health care research. Science 1995;269: 799–801.
46. Weissman MM, Bruce ML, Leaf PJ, et al. Affective disorders. In: Robins LN, Regiers DA, eds. Psychiatric Disorders in America. New York: Free Press, 1991:53–80.
47. Harrison WM, Endicott J, Nee J, et al. Characteristics of women seeking treatment for premenstrual syndrome. Psychosomatics 1989;30:405–411.
48. Graze KK, Nee J, Endicott J. Premenstrual depression predicts future major depressive disorder. Acta Psychiatr Scand 1990;81:201–205.
49. Fava M, Pedrazzi F, Guaraldi GP, et al. Comorbid anxiety and depression among patients with late luteal phase dysphoric disorder. J Anxiety Disord 1992;6:325–335.
50. McLeod DR, Hoehn–Saric R, Foster GV, et al. The influence of premenstrual syndrome on ratings of anxiety in women with generalized anxiety disorder. Acta Psychiatr Scand 1993;88:248–251.
51. Bancroft J, Rennie D, Warner P. Vulnerability to perimenstrual mood change: the relevance of a past history of depressive disorder. Psychosom Med 1994;56:225–231.
52. Kaspi SP, Otto MW, Pollack MH, et al. Premenstrual exacerbation of symptoms in women with panic disorder. J Anxiety Disord 1994;8:131–138.
53. Miller MN, Miller BE. Premenstrual exacerbations of mood disorders. Psychopharmacol Bull 2001;35:135–149.
54. Kendler KS, Silberg JL, Neale MC, et al. Genetic and environmental factors in the aetiology of menstrual, premenstrual and neurotic symptoms: a population based twin study. Psychol Med 1992;22:85–100.
55. Condon JT. The premenstrual syndrome: a twin study. Br J Psychiatry 1993;162:481–486.
56. Treloar SA, Heath AC, Martin NG. Genetic and environmental influences on premenstrual symptoms in an Australian twin sample. Psychol Med 2002;32:25–38.
57. Fontana AM, Palfai TG. Psychosocial factors in premenstrual dysphoria: stressors, appraisal, and coping processes. J Psychosom Res 1994;38:557–567.
58. Girdler SS, Sherwood A, Hinderliter AL, et al. Biological correlates of abuse in women with premenstrual dysphoric disorder and healthy controls. Psychosom Med 2003;65:849–856.
59. Wittchen HU, Perkonigg A, Pfister H. Trauma and PTSD—an overlooked pathogenic pathway for premenstrual dysphoric disorder. Arch Women Ment Health 2003;6:293–297.
60. Schnurr PP, Hurt SW, Stout AL. Consequences of methodological decisions in the diagnosis of late luteal phase dysphoric disorder. In: Gold JH, Severino SK, eds. Premenstrual Dysphorias: Myths and Realities. Washington, DC: American Psychiatric Press, 1994:715–718.
61. Haskett RF, Steiner M, Osmun JN, et al. Severe premenstrual tension: delineation of the syndrome. Biol Psychiatry 1980;15:121–139.

62. Haywood A, Slade P, King H. Assessing the assessment measures for menstrual cycle symptoms: a guide for researchers and clinicians. J Psychosom Res 2002;52:223–237.
63. Endicott J, Harrison W. Daily Record of Severity of Problems. 1992. Available from Dr. Endicott, New York State Psychiatric Institute, Biometrics Unit, 722 West 168th Street, New York, NY 10032.
64. Reid RL. Premenstrual syndrome. Curr Probl Obstet Gynecol Fertil 1985;8:1–57.
65. Mortola JF, Girton L, Beck L, et al. Diagnosis of premenstrual syndrome by a simple, prospective, and reliable instrument: the calendar of premenstrual experiences. Obstet Gynecol 1990;76:302–307.
66. National Institute of Mental Health (NIMH). NIMH Premenstrual Syndrome Workshop Guidelines. Rockville, MD: NIMH, April 14–15, 1983.
67. Steiner M, Steinberg S, Stewart D, et al. Fluoxetine in the treatment of premenstrual dysphoria. N Engl J Med 1995;332:1529–1534.
68. Steiner M, Wilkins A. Diagnosis and assessment of premenstrual dysphoria. Psychiatry Ann 1996;26:571–575.
69. Pearlstein TB. Hormones and depression: what are the facts about premenstrual syndrome, menopause and hormone replacement therapy. Am J Obstet Gynecol 1995;173:646–653.
70. Morse C, Dennerstein L, Farrell E, et al. A comparison of hormone therapy, coping skills training and relaxation for the relief of premenstrual syndrome. J Behav Med 1991;14:469–489.
71. Christensen AP, Oei TP. The efficacy of cognitive behaviour therapy in treating premenstrual dysphoric changes. J Affect Disord 1995;33:57–63.
72. Wyatt KM, Dimmock PW, Jones PW, et al. Efficacy of vitamin B-6 in the treatment of premenstrual syndrome: systematic review. BMJ 1999;318:1375–1381.
73. Thys-Jacobs S, Starkey P, Bernstein D, et al. Calcium carbonate and the premenstrual syndrome: effects on premenstrual and menstrual symptoms. Am J Obstet Gynecol 1998;179:444–452.
74. Ward MW, Holimon TD. Calcium treatment for premenstrual syndrome. Ann Pharmacother 1999;33:1356–1358.
75. Facchinetti F, Borrella P, Sances G, et al. Oral magnesium successfully relieves premenstrual mood changes. Obstet Gynecol 1991;78:177–181.
76. London RS, Bradley L, Chiamori NY. Effect of a nutritional supplement on premenstrual symptomatology in women with premenstrual syndrome: a double-blind longitudinal study. J Am Coll Nutr 1991;10:494–499.
77. London RS, Murphy L, Kitlowski KE, et al. Efficacy of alpha-tocopherol in the treatment of the premenstrual syndrome. J Reprod Med 1987;32:400–404.
78. Budeiri DJ, Li Wan Po A, Dornan JC. Is evening primrose oil of value in the treatment of premenstrual syndrome? Control Clin Trials 1996;17:60–68.
79. Facchinetti F, Fioroni L, Sances G, et al. Naproxen sodium in the treatment of premenstrual symptoms: a placebo controlled study. Gynecol Obstet Invest 1989;28:205–208.
80. Sances G, Martignoni E, Fioroni L, et al. Naproxen sodium in menstrual migraine prophylaxis: a double-blind placebo controlled study. Headache 1990;30:705–709.
81. Mira M, McNeil D, Fraser IS, et al. Mefenamic acid in the treatment of premenstrual syndrome. Obstet Gynecol 1986;68:395–398.
82. Vellacott ID, Shroff NE, Pearce MY, et al. A double blind, placebo controlled evaluation of spironolactone in the premenstrual syndrome. Curr Med Res Opin 1987;10:450–456.
83. Andersch B. Bromocriptine and premenstrual symptoms: a survey of double blind trials. Obstet Gynecol Surv 1983;38:643–646.
84. Stone AB, Pearlstein TB, Brown WA. Fluoxetine in the treatment of late luteal phase dysphoric disorder. J Clin Psychiatry 1991;52:290–293.
85. Wood SH, Mortola JF, Chan YF, et al. Treatment of premenstrual syndrome with fluoxetine: a double-blind, placebo-controlled crossover study. Obstet Gynecol 1992;80:339–344.
86. Menkes DB, Taghavi E, Mason PA, et al. Fluoxetine's spectrum of action in premenstrual syndrome. Int Clin Psychopharmacol 1993;8:95–102.
87. Su TP, Schmidt PJ, Danaceau MA, et al. Fluoxetine in the treatment of premenstrual dysphoria. Neuropsychopharmacology 1997;16:346–356.
88. Steiner M, Romano SJ, Babcock S, et al. The efficacy of fluoxetine in improving physical symptoms associated with premenstrual dysphoric disorder. Br J Obstet Gynaecol 2001;108:462–468.
89. Steiner M, Brown E, Trzepacz P, et al. Fluoxetine improved functional work capacity in women with premenstrual dysphoric disorder. Arch Women Ment Health 2003;6:71–77.
90. Yonkers KA, Halbreich U, Freeman E, et al. Symptomatic improvement of premenstrual dysphoric disorder with sertraline treatment. A randomized controlled trial. Sertraline Premenstrual Dysphoric Collaborative Study Group. JAMA 1997;278:983–988.
91. Eriksson E, Hedberg MA, Andersch B, et al. The serotonin reuptake inhibitor paroxetine is superior to the noradrenaline reuptake inhibitor maprotiline in the treatment of premenstrual syndrome. Neuropsychopharmacology 1995;12:167–176.
92. Wikander I, Sundbald C, Andersch B, et al. Citalopram in premenstrual dysphoria: is intermittent treatment during luteal phases more effective than continuous medication throughout the menstrual cycle? J Clin Psychopharmacol 1998;18:390–398.
93. Freeman EW, Rickels K, Yonkers KA, et al. Venlafaxine in the treatment of premenstrual dysphoric disorder. Obstet Gynecol 2001;98:737–744.

94. Hsiao MC, Liu CY. Effective open label treatment of premenstrual dysphoric disorder with venlafaxine. Psychiatry Clin Neurosci 2003;57:317–321.
95. Steiner M, Korzekwa M, Lamont J, et al. Intermittent fluoxetine dosing in the treatment of women with premenstrual dysphoria. Psychopharmacol Bull 1997;33:771–774.
96. Cohen LS, Miner C, Brown EW, et al. Premenstrual daily fluoxetine for premenstrual dysphoric disorder: a placebo-controlled, clinical trial using computerized diaries. Obstet Gynecol 2002;100:435–444.
97. Halbreich U, Bergeron R, Yonkers KA, et al. Efficacy of intermittent, luteal phase sertraline treatment of premenstrual dysphoric disorder. Obstet Gynecol 2002;100:1219–1229.
98. Sundblad C, Modigh K, Andersch B, et al. Clomipramine effectively reduces premenstrual irritability and dysphoria: a placebo controlled trial. Acta Psychiatr Scand 1992;85:39–47.
99. Sundblad C, Hedberg MA, Eriksson E. Clomipramine administered during the luteal phase reduces the symptoms of premenstrual syndrome. Neuropsychopharmacology 1993;9:133–145.
100. Smith S, Rinehart JS, Ruddock VE, et al. Treatment of premenstrual syndrome with alprazolam: results of a double-blind, placebo-controlled, randomized crossover clinical trial. Obstet Gynecol 1987;70:37–43.
101. Harrison WM, Endicott J, Nee J. Treatment of premenstrual dysphoria with alprazolam. Arch Gen Psychiatry 1990;47:270–275.
102. Berger CP, Presser B. Alprazolam in the treatment of two subsamples of patients with late luteal phase dysphoric disorder: a double-blind, placebo-controlled crossover study. Obstet Gynecol 1994;84:379–385.
103. Freeman EW, Rickels K, Sondheimer SJ, et al. A double-blind trial of oral progesterone, alprazolam, and placebo in the treatment of severe premenstrual syndrome. JAMA 1995;274:51–57.
104. Schmidt PJ, Grover GN, Rubinow DR. Alprazolam in the treatment of premenstrual syndrome: a double-blind, placebo-controlled trial. Arch Gen Psychiatry 1993;50:467–473.
105. Rickels K, Freeman E, Sondheimer S. Buspirone in the treatment of premenstrual syndrome [Letter]. Lancet 1989;1:777.
106. Leather AT, Studd JW, Watson NR, et al. The treatment of severe premenstrual syndrome with goserelin with and without 'add-back' estrogen therapy: a placebo-controlled study. Gynecol Endocrinol 1999;13:48–55.
107. Dhar V, Murphy BE. Double-blind randomized crossover trial of luteal phase estrogens (Premarin) in the premenstrual syndrome (PMS). Psychoneuroendocrinology 1990;15:489–493.
108. Magos AL, Brincat M, Studd JW. Treatment of the premenstrual syndrome by subcutaneous estradiol implants and cyclical oral norethisterone: placebo controlled study. BMJ 1986;292:1629–1633.
109. Watson NR, Studd JW, Savvas M, et al. Treatment of severe premenstrual syndrome with estradiol patches and cyclical oral norethisterone. Lancet 1989;2:730–732.
110. Smith RN, Studd JW, Zamblera D, et al. A randomized comparison over 8 months of 100 micrograms and 200 micrograms twice weekly doses of transdermal oestradiol in the treatment of severe premenstrual syndrome. Br J Obstet Gynaecol 1995;102:475–484.
111. Hahn PM, VanVugt DA, Reid RL. A randomized, placebo-controlled crossover trial of danazol for the treatment of premenstrual syndrome. Psychoneuroendocrinology 1995;20:193–209.
112. O'Brien PM, Abukhalil IE. Randomized controlled trial of the management of premenstrual syndrome and premenstrual mastalgia using luteal phase-only danazol. Am J Obstet Gynecol 1999;180:18–23.
113. Watts JF, Butt WR, Logan Edwards R. A clinical trial using danazol for the treatment of premenstrual tension. Br J Obstet Gynaecol 1987;94:30–34.
114. Halbreich U, Rojansky N, Palter S. Elimination of ovulation and menstrual cyclicity (with danazol) improves dysphoric premenstrual syndromes. Fertil Steril 1991;56:1066–1069.
115. Deeny M, Hawthorn R, McKay Hart D. Low dose danazol in the treatment of premenstrual syndrome. Postgrad Med J 1991;67:450–454.
116. Sarno AP Jr, Miller EJ Jr, Lundblad EG. Premenstrual syndrome: beneficial effects of periodic, low-dose danazol. Obstet Gynecol 1987;70:33–36.
117. Sampson GA. Premenstrual syndrome: a double-blind placebo controlled trial of progesterone and placebo. Br J Psychiatry 1979;135:209–215.
118. Dennerstein L, Spencer-Gardner C, Gotts G, et al. Progesterone and the premenstrual syndrome: a double-blind, cross-over trial. BMJ 1985;290:1617–1621.
119. Maddocks S, Hahn P, Moller F, et al. A double-blind placebo-controlled trial of progesterone vaginal suppositories in the treatment of premenstrual syndrome. Am J Obstet Gynecol 1986;154:573–581.
120. Dennerstein L, Morse C, Gotts G, et al. Treatment of premenstrual syndrome: a double-blind trial of dydrogesterone. J Affect Disord 1986;11:199–205.
121. Rapkin A, Chang LH, Reading AE. Premenstrual syndrome: a double blind placebo controlled study of treatment with progesterone vaginal suppositories. J Obstet Gynecol 1987;7:217–220.
122. Freeman E, Rickels K, Sondheimer SJ, et al. Ineffectiveness of progesterone suppository treatment for premenstrual syndrome. JAMA 1990;264:349–353.
123. West CP. Inhibition of ovulation with oral progestins—effectiveness in premenstrual syndrome. Eur J Obstet Gynecol Reprod Biol 1990;34:119–128.
124. Kirkham C, Hahn PM, VanVugt DA, et al. A randomized, double-blind, placebo-controlled, cross-over trial to assess the side effects of medroxyprogesterone acetate in hormone replacement therapy. Obstet Gynecol 1991;78:93–97.
125. Chan AF, Mortola JF, Wood SH, et al. Persistence of premenstrual syndrome during low-dose administration of the progesterone agonist RU 486. Obstet Gynecol 1994;84:1001–1005.
126. Wyatt KM, Dimmock PW, Frischer M, et al. Prescribing patterns in premenstrual syndrome. BMC Womens Health 2002;2:4.

127. Graham CA, Sherwin BB. A prospective treatment study of premenstrual symptoms using a triphasic oral contraceptive. J Psychosom Res 1992;36:257–266.
128. Joffe H, Cohen LS, Harlow BL. Impact of oral contraceptive pill use on premenstrual mood: predictors of improvement and deterioration. Am J Obstet Gynecol 2003;189:1523–1530.
129. Freeman EW. Evaluation of a unique oral contraceptive (Yasmin) in the management of premenstrual dysphoric disorder. Eur J Contracept Reprod Health Care 2002;7:27–34.
130. Casper RF, Hearn MT. The effect of hysterectomy and bilateral oophorectomy in women with severe premenstrual syndrome. Am J Obstet Gynecol 1990;162:105–109.
131. Casson P, Hahn PM, Van Vugt DA, et al. Lasting response to ovariectomy in severe intractable premenstrual syndrome. Am J Obstet Gynecol 1990;162:99–105.

CHAPTER 8

Abnormal Uterine Bleeding

Godwin I. Meniru and Michael P. Hopkins

INTRODUCTION

More than 10 million women in the United States suffer from abnormal uterine bleeding, and it is estimated that one-third of all outpatient gynecologic visits annually are for abnormal uterine bleeding (1, 2). For some of these women, abnormal uterine bleeding constitutes a serious health risk due to the resulting anemia and general debility. In other cases, it could be the symptom of a serious illness such as endometrial cancer, leukemia, or a coagulation disorder. Even in the most innocuous cases, abnormal bleeding patterns constitute a nuisance and impinge on a woman's social, sexual, psychological, and occupational functioning due to unpredictable or heavy bleeding.

Successful management of abnormal uterine bleeding can often be achieved on an outpatient basis using an informed and efficient approach. This chapter provides background information on the problem of abnormal uterine bleeding and considers various management options. Age-specific information is provided in relevant sections. Abnormal uterine bleeding shares a similar presentation with vaginal and other extrauterine genital tract lesions that cause bleeding. Therefore, these lesions are mentioned briefly in this discussion.

PHYSIOLOGY OF MENSES

Ovarian Cycle

At cyclic intervals, cohorts of primordial follicles commence further development in the ovaries and become responsive to follicle-stimulating hormone (FSH). This hormone serves to propel some of the follicles into the pool from which the Graafian follicle is selected. All other follicles eventually stop developing and become atretic. Estrogen is produced by FSH-responsive follicles and exerts a negative feedback inhibition of the hypothalamic output of gonadotropin-releasing hormone (GnRH) and the pituitary production of FSH and luteinizing hormone (LH) for most of the cycle. However, during a brief period close to the midcycle, high estrogen levels cause a sudden large output of FSH and LH. The surge in LH induces final maturation of the Graafian follicle and serves to trigger ovulation. Following ovulation, the collapsed follicle, which is now referred to as the *corpus luteum*, commences progesterone synthesis for approximately 10 days.

Menstrual Cycle

The endometrium consists of three layers: the superficial layer (stratum compactum), middle or functional layer (stratum spongiosum), and deep layer (stratum basalis). The deep, or basal, layer is supplied by basal arteries and serves mainly as a source of cellular and intercellular material from which the endometrium is regenerated following each menstrual period. The middle, or functional, layer forms the bulk of the endometrium at the height of endometrial development, from midcycle to onset of menstrual periods. It is supplied by spiral arteries that arise from the basal arteries. Unlike the basal arteries, the spiral arteries are hormone sensitive. Spiral arteries also supply the stratum compactum, which consists mainly of epithelial cells that line the endometrium and the terminal portions of the endometrial glands.

Cyclical changes in the morphology and function of the endometrium occur in tandem with the ovarian cycle. Estrogen that is produced by developing ovarian follicles stimulates the proliferation of endometrial glands, stroma, and epithelium. There is also development of the spiral arteries, which are uncoiled in the early proliferative phase. Following ovulation, progesterone induces luteal (secretory) changes in the endometrium, including edema of the stroma with increased convolution of the endometrial glands and intense coiling of the spiral arteries.

Prostaglandins (PGs) are synthesized by the endometrial stromal cells and within the walls of the spiral arterioles, which also contain PG receptors. Cyclo-oxygenase (COX) is an enzyme that is found in the endometrium and converts arachidonic acid into PGs. There is a substantial increase in the endometrial tissue levels of the prostaglandin $PGF_{2\alpha}$, which is a powerful vasoconstrictor. Although the tissue levels of PGE_2 also increase, a high $PGF_{2\alpha}$:PGE_2 ratio is maintained. Other PGs produced in the endometrium include thromboxane (thromboxane A_2; a vasoconstrictor) and prostacyclin (PGI_2; a vasodilator).

If implantation fails to occur, the corpus luteum undergoes involution and production of progesterone ceases. This leads to a series of complex chemical and biological activities in the endometrium that result in shrinkage of the endometrium, intense vasoconstriction of the spiral arteries, and ischemia of the endometrium. Eventually, breaks occur in the endometrial vessels, leading to bleeding within the endometrium and subsequent sloughing of the middle and superficial layers of the endometrium. Uterine contractions are caused by the prostaglandins $PGF_{2\alpha}$ and $PGE_{2\alpha}$. Hemostasis is achieved during menstruation by a combination of vasoconstriction; myometrial spasms; production of thrombin, which induces fibrin deposition; platelet activation; and other changes, including regeneration of the surface epithelium of the endometrium. In patients with menorrhagia, the prostaglandins $PGE_{2\alpha}$ and PGI_2 (both vasodilators) predominate over the vasoconstrictive prostaglandins $PGF_{2\alpha}$ and thromboxane A_2.

Normal Cycle Parameters

Irregular menstrual cycles are common in the first few years following menarche. However, most women ovulate regularly and menstrual periods become regular by 5 to 7 years after menarche. At this time, the normal menstrual cycle length is conventionally accepted as ranging between 24 and 35 days (average 28 days), with menstrual bleeding occurring from 3 to 7 days (average 4 days) and an average menstrual loss of 35 mL (range 20 to 80 mL) (3). Any bleeding pattern that falls outside this range is regarded as abnormal.

Definitions

Abnormal uterine bleeding is described in various ways, and specific terminology has traditionally been used to characterize particular bleeding patterns. The terminology is sometimes used inappropriately, and proposals for using only descriptions of the specific abnormal bleeding pattern have been suggested but not universally adopted. The definitions shown in Table 8.1 are still prevalent in clinical notes and the medical literature.

Prevalence

Menstrual disturbances are one of the primary reasons a woman seeks gynecologic care; it is estimated that 9 to 30% of the women of reproductive age suffer from menorrhagia (4, 5). Of the 600,000 hysterectomies performed each year in the United States, about 20% will be done for dysfunctional uterine bleeding (DUB; bleeding without an identifiable anatomic etiology, even on histologic examination) (6–8).

Etiology

Many local and systemic factors have been causally linked with the etiology of abnormal uterine bleeding (Table 8.2). These are described briefly in the following sections. Other causes of genital tract bleeding not secondary to abnormal uterine bleeding are shown in Table 8.3. These

TABLE 8.1

Classification of Abnormal Uterine Bleeding

Menorrhagia: heavy bleeding; loss of more than 80 mL of blood and/or increased duration of flow (>7 days) at regular intervals
Metrorrhagia: bleeding at irregular intervals or bleeding between menstrual periods
Menometrorrhagia: increased loss or duration of bleeding occurring at irregular intervals
Polymenorrhea: menstrual bleeding occurring at less than 21-day intervals
Oligomenorrhea: menstrual cycle length of more than 35 days
Amenorrhea: lack of menstrual periods for more than 6 months
Intermenstrual bleeding: bleeding between two regular menstrual periods
Postmenopausal bleeding: bleeding occurring after more than 1 year of reaching menopause

conditions may present with vaginal bleeding that mimics that of abnormal uterine bleeding, and differentiation of the true source(s) depends on a thorough history, clinical evaluation, and workup.

Uterine Disease

Leiomyomas are the most common benign tumors of the uterus and are found clinically in 20 to 30% of women older than 30 years of age. They are found in up to three-fourths of hysterectomy specimens when they are looked for systematically (9). They are largely asymptomatic but may cause abnormal uterine bleeding, pain, pelvic pressure, and, occasionally, infertility. Abnormal bleeding may be in the form of menorrhagia, but with submucous leiomyomas, irregular bleeding patterns may arise from the endometrium that overlies the tumor.

TABLE 8.2

Etiology of Abnormal Uterine Bleeding

Uterine disease
- Leiomyoma
- Adenomyosis
- Polyps
- Cancer
- Endometritis
- Endometrial hyperplasia

Medications
- Psychotropic drugs
- Combined oral contraceptives
- Progestins
- Dilantin
- Intrauterine contraceptive devices
- Tamoxifen

Coagulation disorders
- von Willebrand's disease
- Thrombocytopenia
- Leukemia
- Autoimmune disease
- Anticoagulant therapy

Systemic disease
- Obesity
- Liver failure

Endocrine
- Anovulation
- Hyperprolactinemia
- Thyroid dysfunction
- Estrogen-producing tumors
- Adrenal dysfunction
- Ovarian failure

TABLE 8.3

Other Causes of Genital Tract Bleeding

Pregnancy complications	Pelvic pathology
• Miscarriage	• Oophoritis
• Ectopic pregnancy	• Pelvic inflammatory disease
• Gestational trophoblastic disease	• Endometriosis
Cervical pathology	• Fallopian tube cancer
• Infection	• Pyosalpinx
• Cancer	Vulva
• Polyps	• Lacerations
• Hemangioma	• Cancer
Vaginal lesions	• Vulvitis
• Vaginitis	• Other lesions
• Cancer	Miscellaneous
• Foreign body	• Congenital anomalies
Puerperal complications	• Hemorrhoids
• Retained products of conception	• Hematuria
• Endomyometritis	

Adenomyosis can be found in 20 to 30% of women of all ages and consists of islands of endometrial glands and stroma located within the myometrium; the frequency of adenomyosis appears to be greater in patients with leiomyomata than those without leiomyomata (10). It has been suggested that a common pathogenetic mechanism is shared between leiomyomata and adenomyosis because both occur in the myometrium and both are associated with polymorphism of estrogen receptor alpha (11). Current theories of the pathogenesis of adenomyosis suggest that the disease arises from a downward growth of endometrial tissue from the stratum basalis of the endometrium. Between 80 and 90% of adenomyosis cases occur in parous patients, which suggests that the trauma of childbirth creates an initial breach in tissue barriers existing between the endometrium and the myometrium. Puerperal endometritis may also serve as a factor in causing this break (12). The statistical correlation found between adenomyosis and prior dilatation and curettage adds further credence to the hypothesis that a trauma initially induces the breach in the endometrium-myometrium barrier (12, 13). Adenomyosis and endometriosis probably represent entirely different and distinct disorders. Endometriosis is found in only 6 to 20% of all women with adenomyosis of the uterus (14). Adenomyosis is asymptomatic in a large proportion of patients (19 to 35%) but can present with severe dysmenorrhea, dyspareunia, chronic pelvic pain, and menorrhagia (15). In patients for whom the only existing pelvic pathology is adenomyosis, 40 to 50% will report menorrhagia, 15 to 30% note dysmenorrhea, and 20% will complain of both symptoms (16, 17)

Endometrial polyps are outgrowths from the endometrial surface consisting of endometrial glands, stroma, and blood vessels. These are most commonly found in women between 40 and 50 years of age, and the prevalence of polyps in the general population is estimated to be 24% (18). Endometrial polyps can cause irregular, prolonged, and/or heavy bleeding. Although the majority of these polyps are benign, malignant transformation can occur in a small number of cases. More recent studies have found carcinoma in 1.5 to 3.2% of endometrial polyps studied (19, 20).

Endometrial cancer is the most common gynecologic malignancy in women in the United States, and an estimated 40,320 cases of uterine cancer are expected to be diagnosed in 2004 (21). Incidence rates of uterine cancer increased from 1988 to 1998, but leveled off after that through the year 2000 (21). It is a disease that affects mostly postmenopausal women and usually presents with irregular bleeding. Although the peak incidence is in women in their 50s and early 60s, the likelihood that endometrial cancer is the cause of postmenopausal bleeding increases with the age of the woman.

Endometrial malignancy usually occurs in the postmenopausal period, but 20 to 25% of cases occur in premenopausal women, and 3 to 5% are diagnosed in women younger than the age of 40 (22). It is estimated that almost 5% of incident endometrial cancers in women ages 20 to 54 years may be attributed to a family history of endometrial cancer, and 2% may be attributable to a family history of colorectal cancer (23). Risk factors for developing endometrial cancer include obesity, delayed menopause, unopposed estrogen therapy, chronic use of tamoxifen, polycystic ovary syndrome (PCOS), nulliparity, and estrogen-producing ovarian tumors.

Endometrial hyperplasia usually results from unopposed estrogenic stimulation and is classified as simple, complex, or atypical based on histologic features. These histologic groupings also exhibit varying premalignant potential with the least risk of progression to endometrial cancer being noted in simple hyperplasia. Atypical endometrial hyperplasia has the highest risk of malignant transformation; 11 of 48 patients reported by Kurman et al. progressed to endometrial adenocarcinoma. Women with atypical hyperplasia have a 23% risk of endometrial carcinoma over the next decade (24). Because of the frequent association between atypical hyperplasia and endometrial carcinoma, clinicians must be concerned that there is an undetected, concomitant carcinoma when endometrial biopsy (EMB) results demonstrate atypical hyperplasia. In a retrospective analysis of 44 women who underwent hysterectomy within 10 weeks of uterine sampling exhibiting atypical hyperplasia, 19 (43%) demonstrated coexistent endometrial carcinoma. Among these patients, 17 (89%) had myometrial invasion, including 7 patients (37%) with deep invasion (FIGO stage IC or higher) (25). In another study of endometrial hyperplasia, 12 of 24 hysterectomy specimens with known atypical endometrial hyperplasia on preoperative biopsy had concomitant endometrial carcinoma, and 75% of these patients were stage IB or greater (26).

Coagulation Disorders

Coagulation disorders are a significant cause of abnormal uterine bleeding, especially in younger females. The more severe the abnormal uterine bleeding is, the greater the chance of finding an underlying problem. The most common hematologic cause of abnormal uterine bleeding is von Willebrand's disease, a heterogeneous bleeding disorder with several recognized subtypes.

Another coagulation disorder that may present as abnormal uterine bleeding is thrombocytopenia. This is caused by a host of diseases, including leukemia, idiopathic thrombocytopenic purpura, aplastic anemia, and hypersplenism. It can also result from chemotherapy. Glanzmann's thrombasthenia is a rare disease in which there is a platelet aggregation dysfunction. Other coagulation disorders that have been found in women with menorrhagia include factors V, X and XI deficiency (27, 28). Menorrhagia can occur right from menarche (29). The incidence of bleeding disorders has ranged from 5 to 20% of adolescents who have abnormal uterine bleeding that is severe enough to require hospitalization (30, 31). Frequently, other clinical features of coagulation defects may be present, such as a history of easy bruising or prolonged bleeding from cuts, petechial hemorrhages, and epistaxis. Patients with von Willebrand's disease often have a history of heavy menstrual loss right from the onset of their menarche. However, absence of such a history does not exclude the possibility of the disease because an acquired form of von Willebrand's disease can occur in patients with systemic lupus erythematosus who produce anti–von Willebrand factor antibody (32).

Systemic Disease

Systemic diseases can be associated with abnormal uterine bleeding. Women with liver or renal disease may have an impairment of estrogen metabolism, leading to prolonged (unopposed) estrogen stimulation of the endometrium, endometrial hyperplasia, and menometrorrhagia. Liver disease may impair liver synthesis of clotting factors (e.g., fibrinogen) and is associated with hypothrombinemia—all of which exacerbates the bleeding tendency. Similar coagulopathies may be found in patients with liver transplant.

In adipose tissue, androstenedione is converted to estrone; in obese patients, the amount of estrone produced may be quite large. These high levels of estrone cause anovulation by feedback inhibition of the pituitary output of gonadotropins. The high estrone levels also stimulate hyperplastic endometrial growth, which is unopposed because of the lack of progesterone due to anovulation.

Endocrine Causes

Both hyperprolactinemia and hypothyroidism cause anovulation and subsequent amenorrhea. This amenorrheic state is associated with prolonged periods of unopposed estrogen action on the endometrium, and in some patients, may lead to irregular heavy bleeding. Menstrual irregularities are associated with both hypothyroidism (23.4% of cases) and hyperthyroidism (21.5% of cases) (33, 34).

Late-onset adrenal hyperplasia, Cushing's syndrome, and Addison's disease can cause abnormal uterine bleeding as a result of anovulation.

Estrogen-producing ovarian tumors such as granulosa cell tumor and thecoma frequently cause endometrial hyperplasia, amenorrhea, and/or menometrorrhagia (35, 36). Up to 5% of patients with granulosa cell tumors have a coexisting endometrial cancer most likely resulting from the unopposed estrogenic endometrial stimulation (36). Irregular vaginal bleeding may be experienced by some patients with impending ovarian failure for a variable length of time before amenorrhea eventually supervenes.

Medications

There are specific medications associated with menorrhagia and a few are listed in Table 8.4. Psychotropic drugs such as antidepressants and antipsychotics may interfere with both stimulatory and inhibitory nervous impulses that control hypothalamic function resulting in anovulation and abnormal uterine bleeding.

The pattern of abnormal bleeding that occurs as a result of the use of hormonal preparations such as oral contraceptive pills and progestin-only contraception (minipill, injectables, and implants) depends on the dose and timing. Initial bleeding patterns may be in the form of breakthrough bleeding, which is irregular and possibly heavy. However, with continued use of the medication amenorrhea may result, but irregular bleeding can also occur in the long term from endometrial atrophy. Not completing the full monthly course of oral contraceptives (OCs) or skipping tablets can also cause abnormal bleeding patterns. Copper-bearing intrauterine contraceptive devices (IUCDs) increase the amount of blood loss up to two-fold and the duration of menstrual loss an average of 1 day; progestin-releasing IUCDs reduce mean menstrual blood loss to about 5 mL, compared with a normal mean loss of 35 mL (37, 38).

TABLE 8.4

Medications Associated With Onset of Menorrhagia

Corticosteroids
Digoxin
Propranolol
Tricyclic antidepressants
Phenothiazines
Butyrophenones
Major tranquilizers
Monoamine oxidase inhibitors

Tamoxifen is an estrogen agonist and antagonist, but the estrogenic effect is believed to be what causes endometrial hyperplasia (atypical) on prolonged use (39, 40).

The use of anabolic steroids by female athletes may lead to amenorrhea or irregular bleeding due to the androgenic effects of the steroids. Aspirin and other prostaglandin synthetase inhibitors irreversibly inhibit platelet function, thereby being a potential cause of abnormal uterine bleeding. Heparin and warfarin also interfere with clotting mechanisms and have been implicated in cases of abnormal uterine bleeding (41).

Dysfunctional Uterine Bleeding

Abnormal uterine bleeding in the absence of an organic cause (Tables 8.2 and 8.3) is commonly classified as dysfunctional uterine bleeding (DUB). As such, DUB is a diagnosis of exclusion that can only be made with a reasonable degree of certainty after a comprehensive evaluation of the patient. There is controversy, however, about the true meaning of DUB and the ovulatory status of the patient. Although many reports consider only anovulatory patients in the definition of DUB, others identify two subclasses—namely anovulatory and ovulatory varieties of DUB. Those who accept only anovulation in their definition of DUB may use the term *essential menorrhagia* to classify patients presenting with DUB in the presence of ovulatory cycles (42). For purposes of clarity, the term *DUB* is not used in this chapter. Rather, the phrase *anovulatory uterine bleeding* is used to describe patients with ovulatory dysfunction who have abnormal uterine bleeding in the absence of an identifiable local genital tract lesion or an obvious systemic disease.

Anovulatory Uterine Bleeding

Absence of ovulation in a woman with normal or high estrogen levels means that the progesterone-driven maturational and luteal changes normally found in the endometrium in the second half of the menstrual period are lacking. This leads to continued proliferative changes in the endometrium, which subsequently becomes hyperplastic in a significant proportion of cases. More important, there is asynchronous endometrial growth with poor stromal development and increasing tissue fragility.

At the biochemical level, there is a general increase in the endometrial tissue levels of PGE_2 but a relative deficiency of $PGF_{2\alpha}$ leading to a reduced $PGF_{2\alpha}$:PGE_2 ratio. This reversal of the $PGF_{2\alpha}$:PGE_2 ratio correlates with an increase in the amount of menstrual blood loss (43). There is also an increase in the PGI_2 levels and decrease in the TXA_2 content of the endometrium. Several other alterations in the absolute and relative tissue levels of PGs and their precursors have been documented in the literature (44).

These altered relationships in PG levels favor vasodilation, relaxation of the myometrial muscle fibers, impairment of platelet function, and other hemostatic mechanisms consequently increasing endometrial blood loss. The end result of all these changes is an absence of uniform sloughing of the stratum compactum and spongiosum that normally takes place at the time of menstrual bleeding. Instead, there is patchy desquamation and re-epithelization of the endometrium that further prolongs irregular bleeding patterns.

The incidence of anovulatory uterine bleeding shows two peaks in the life of a woman: during adolescence and at the perimenopausal period. At both times, the frequency and regularity of ovulation is suboptimal. However, there are many other causes of anovulation that are not related to these reproductive milestones, and these may manifest at any time during the reproductive life of the woman (Table 8.5).

Ovulatory Abnormal Uterine Bleeding (Essential Menorrhagia)

Patients with ovulatory abnormal uterine bleeding are relatively small in proportion compared with patients with anovulatory uterine bleeding. Ovulatory abnormal uterine bleeding presents as regular cyclic bleeding that is usually quite heavy. Causes to consider include anatomic factors (e.g., myomas, polyps, or adenomyosis), hematologic disorders (e.g., von Willebrand's disease in adolescents), or undetected pregnancy. Ovulatory abnormal uterine bleeding without any anatomic, organic, or systemic cause is not common, although in some cases there seems to be a derangement in the relative proportion of PGs in the endometrium and increased fibrinolysis (45, 46).

TABLE 8.5

Causes of Anovulatory Bleeding

Hypothalamic dysfunction from excessive weight loss, exercise, and stress
Obesity
Hyperprolactinemia
Hypothalamic-pituitary "immaturity" of adolescence
Lactation
Menopausal transition
Thyroid disorders, especially hypothyroidism
Polycystic ovary syndrome
Late-onset adrenal hyperplasia
Ovarian tumors
Adrenal steroid excess, including congenital or acquired adrenal hyperplasia
Medications
Discontinuation of oral contraceptives
Granulosa cell tumors

Etiology of Abnormal Uterine Bleeding in Various Reproductive Age Groups

Childhood (Younger Than 10 Years)

Withdrawal of in utero estrogen support of the newborn female endometrium after delivery may cause transient vaginal bleeding. Common causes of vaginal bleeding in childhood include foreign objects, vaginitis, or trauma (47). The finding of genital trauma should initiate an investigation of the child's domestic circumstances for evidence of abuse or rape. Appearance of secondary sex characteristics in a child with vaginal bleeding may indicate the presence of an ovarian tumor or may be due to precocious puberty (48). (This issue is discussed in more detail in Chapter 1.)

Adolescence (12 to18 Years)

Anovulation is the most common cause of abnormal uterine bleeding in this age range. This is because it may take 2 to 3 years for regular ovulatory bleeding to be established after menarche; if irregular periods continue beyond this time frame, further evaluation is needed (49). Much still remains unknown about pathophysiologic mechanisms because not all anovulatory postmenarchal females have abnormal uterine bleeding patterns.

The second most common etiology for abnormal uterine bleeding among adolescents, but the most important to consider, is a coagulation disorder (50). In one study, a hematologic abnormality that caused bleeding diathesis and acute menorrhagia was diagnosed in 7 of 25 patients (28%). There were four cases of immune thrombocytopenic purpura, two cases of von Willebrand's disease, and one case of acute promyelocytic leukemia (51).

Disorders of platelet number or function can also present as abnormal uterine bleeding. Examples include idiopathic thrombocytopenic purpura, leukemia, aplastic anemia, hypersplenism, and thrombocytopenia or platelet dysfunction secondary to medications. Women with coagulopathies frequently have marked blood loss with menses. Fraser et al. reported that the average blood loss in women with various coagulopathies is 400 mL per menses (52).

Congenital reproductive organ/tract malformations or malfunctions may manifest at this stage, including premature ovarian failure from gonadal dysgenesis.

Reproductive Age (19 to 39 Years)

Pregnancy-associated complications are a common source of abnormal uterine bleeding in this age group, and a pregnancy test must be performed at the outset of evaluation of any reproductively capable woman who presents with abnormal uterine bleeding. The most common endocrinopathy to be considered is PCOS (defined as oligo- or anovulation in combination with hyperandrogenism), which affects 5 to 7% of all reproductive age women (53–55).

Fibroids are benign tumors of the uterus, arising from smooth muscle, which occur in 30% of women. They can result in symptoms such as pain, infertility, and abnormal bleeding; alternatively, they may be entirely asymptomatic. One-third of fibroids will cause abnormal bleeding, usually in the fourth or fifth decades of life. The fibroids that are commonly related to significant menorrhagia are located in the submucous position. The reason the myoma in this position causes heavier bleeding is not entirely clear. One theory is that submucous myomas increase the surface area of the endometrium, which results in an abnormal venous pattern, with stasis and a change in venous drainage. This disruption of the vascular supply to the endometrium results in abnormal bleeding.

Endometrial hyperplasia is the proliferation of endometrial glands of irregular size and shape, with crowding of the glands and an increase in the gland-to-stroma ratio. This process may occur in response to unopposed estrogen stimulation. Endometrial hyperplasia can be divided into two groups: those with atypia and those without atypia. Hyperplasia with atypia refers to the presence of atypical cells lining the glands, showing a loss of polarity, prominent nucleoli, and enlarged pleomorphic nuclei. Hyperplasia with atypia has a tendency to recur following treatment and a higher chance of developing into endometrial adenocarcinoma (56). Less than 2% of women diagnosed with hyperplasia without atypia will progress to adenocarcinoma, but 23% of women having hyperplasia with atypia will develop adenocarcinoma (24).

Late Reproductive Age (40 to 45 Years)

Perimenopausal women have an increased incidence of anovulatory uterine bleeding as ovarian oocyte stores are depleted. As estrogen production is maintained and actually increased by the higher levels of FSH, there is an increase in the incidence of endometrial hyperplasia. There is also an increasing problem with pelvic and genital tract tumors. A worsening of the symptoms of pre-existing uterine pathology, such as leiomyoma and adenomyosis, may occur at this age. Endometrial polyps are also another common finding in this age group.

Women ages 40 to 44 years have a significantly higher hysterectomy rate compared with any other age group. In the United States, from 1994 to 1999, 52% of all hysterectomies were performed among women younger than 44 years of age (6).

Menopausal Transition and Postmenopause (Older Than 45 Years)

Although changes in menstrual patterns and flow are a normal part of the menopausal transition, it is abnormal for a patient to report heavier than usual bleeding, prolonged bleeding, periods occurring more frequently than every 3 weeks, intermenstrual bleeding, or bleeding after intercourse (57). For perimenopausal women, anovulatory bleeding is common, and it continues until final cessation of menstrual periods. This anovulatory bleeding is associated with a higher incidence of endometrial hyperplasia and possible adenocarcinoma secondary to the long-standing activity of unopposed estrogen.

There are more than 41,000 new cases of endometrial carcinoma each year; the median age at diagnosis is 63 (21). Postmenopausal bleeding must be considered endometrial carcinoma until proven otherwise. Risk factors for endometrial carcinoma are obesity, nulliparity, late menopause, hypertension, and diabetes. Women with prolonged exposure to unopposed estrogen are at increased risk of developing adenocarcinoma. This may occur through exogenous administration, such as hormone replacement of estrogen without a progestin, or through prolonged anovulation.

Up to 80% of postmenopausal women with bleeding may have endometrial pathology such as polyps, hyperplasia, and submucous leiomyomas (58). Bleeding in late menopause may be due to endometrial atrophy, but this diagnosis can only be accepted after the most painstaking search for endometrial cancer and other lesions.

Clinical and Laboratory Evaluation of Patients

The diagnosis of abnormal uterine bleeding can be straightforward if a cause is immediately apparent. Often, a careful search for all possible etiologies, especially age-specific problems, is required. Therefore, the utilization of the traditional sequence of history taking, physical examination, laboratory testing, and advanced diagnostic procedures will optimize the identification of causative pathology. The role of history taking cannot be overemphasized because this could help identify the etiology or at least exclude a significant number of possibilities from being considered further. Likewise, a careful examination may clinch the diagnosis or help eliminate more differential diagnoses.

Clinical History

Summary demographic data including age, gravidity, and parity are obtained, followed by an enquiry into the nature and duration of the abnormal bleeding. For many of the causes of abnormal bleeding, the history of the onset of menorrhagia will be highly suggestive of the diagnosis (Table 8.6). Other required information include the last (normal) menstrual period; cyclicity of the bleeding; amount of blood loss as deduced by several parameters, such as number of pads or tampons used and their extent of saturation with menstrual lochia; bleeding in clots, staining of clothing or bedding; and the duration of the bleeding. If available, a menstrual diary can be very useful. The presence of provoking factors such as sexual intercourse is ascertained together with other associated symptoms such as dysmenorrhea, dyspareunia, abnormal vaginal discharge, and pelvic pressure. Regular cyclical bleeding; "ovulation" pain (mittelschmerz); and premenstrual symptoms such as a feeling of bloating, edema, breast tenderness, pelvic congestion, and mood changes, if present, suggest ovulatory cycles.

Further questioning is carried out while keeping in mind the etiologic factors discussed in previous sections (Tables 8.2 and 8.3). Thus, information on the timing and outcome of the most recent pregnancy is required, as is data regarding any significant previous or current illnesses, history of uterine leiomyoma, and other genital tract disorders. Knowledge of previous medical and/or surgical treatments will provide further insight into the nature and cause of the bleeding, as well as prevent repetition of already conducted investigations and the application of treatment that was ineffective in the past.

The patient is asked about her use of preventive health care services, specifically regular cervical cytology (Papanicolaou) smears. An assessment of past and current medications is done. The review of symptoms should inquire about other etiologically suggestive symptoms, such as fever, dizziness, urinary symptoms, rectal symptoms, easy bruising of the skin, prolonged bleeding from cuts and abrasions, and frequent bleeding from the gum after tooth brushing or dental surgery. The review of symptoms should be very thorough (i.e., it should include

TABLE 8.6

Onset of Menorrhagia in Relationship to Diagnosis

Onset of Menorrhagia	Probable Diagnosis
Immediately after menarche, or in late 40s or 50s	Physiologic (anovulation; perimenopause transition)
Since onset of medication or soon after start of medication	Medication induced
With weight gain or symptoms of hyperandrogenism	Anovulation
Either gradual increase over months or sudden and noncyclic	Fibroid; hyperplasia; carcinoma
Occurring with increasing disability from systemic disease	Chronic disease

questions regarding dry skin, lethargy, environmental temperature intolerance, constipation, hair loss, visual defects, headache, unprovoked milk discharge from the nipples, excessive body hair, greasy skin, acne, hot flashes, and vaginal dryness).

The family and social history is reviewed for clues to familial diseases and behavioral traits such as bleeding disorders, use of recreational drugs, smoking, occupation, chemicals in the workplace, and spousal relationships. Stress of domestic or occupational origin and evidence of eating disorders may be uncovered by careful questioning.

Quantifying Vaginal Blood Loss

In a normal menstrual cycle, 30 to 40 mL of blood is lost, and 90% of women lose less than 80 mL during a cycle. Anemia typically develops at losses of 60 mL or greater per cycle (59). The menstrual effluent is not composed entirely of blood. Fraser and colleagues determined the percentage contribution of blood to total menstrual discharge and found that the mean contribution from whole blood was 36% (range 1.6 to 81%), whereas the remainder of menstrual discharge consisted of endometrial fluid (60). The blood–fluid ratio changes with the use of different contraceptive methods (e.g., the blood–fluid ratio decreases with OC pills and increases with the use of an intrauterine device). This variation in composition of menstrual discharge contributes to the difficulty in estimating amount of menstrual bleeding.

It is important to quantify the amount of blood loss accurately, but studies demonstrate that underestimates or overestimates are commonly made regarding the amount of menstrual blood loss (61). An alkaline hematin method has been described for the laboratory quantification of menstrual blood loss (62, 63). Attempts have been made to quantify the menstrual loss in ambulatory settings by counting the number of pads or tampons used and assessing the degree of soaking. Using this method, utilization of 10 to 15 pads or tampons in each menstrual period is regarded as being normal. However, different brands of sanitary pads and tampons have varying absorptive potential, making it difficult to use this general rule for individual patients. Moreover, the frequency of pad changing may reflect more on the individual's habits than on the extent of soaking.

Another scoring system uses a pictorial blood loss assessment chart (PBAC) with which the patient visually assesses the amount of staining on their pad or tampon and matches it to a corresponding picture. More than 80 mL blood loss per cycle is equivalent to a score higher than 100 (64, 65). The PBAC method is criticized as being quasi-objective and overly influenced by the nonblood component of the menstrual flow. In one more recent study, the authors noted that the PBAC score did not accurately diagnose menorrhagia (66). However, in another study comparing total blood volume (using alkaline hematin measurements) in sanitary products with total menstrual fluid volume (by weighing used pads and tampons and converting grams into milliliters), there was a strong correlation between total menstrual fluid and actual menstrual blood loss (67). The finding of anemia or low ferritin stores in a patient complaining of heavy vaginal bleeding provides supporting evidence of excessive uterine bleeding.

Physical Examination

A preliminary impression of the patient's clinical state is determined at the time of history taking. The vital signs in an acutely bleeding patient with significant blood loss may indicate hypovolemia by the presence of a rapid thready pulse and hypotension. However, these are not usually present in a woman with chronic or recurrent mild to moderate vaginal bleeding, although she may be pallid from anemia. Height and weight are measured to calculate the body mass index. A general physical examination is performed to identify any signs of disorders that may be responsible for the abnormal bleeding, for example, hirsutism in a patient with PCOS.

Petechiae and ecchymoses are sought for by inspecting the conjunctiva and other parts of the body. The thyroid gland is palpated for diffuse enlargement or nodules. The nipples are squeezed gently with the fingers to check for expressible galactorrhea, although this sign can be a normal finding in parous women. Abdominal examination is carried out to detect any masses, tenderness, or ascites. A detailed pelvic examination is performed. The vulva, vagina, and cervix are inspected for lesions (e.g., signs of infection, trauma, and tumor), followed by the sampling of cervical secretions with microbiological swabs for gonorrhea and chlamydia screening tests.

TABLE 8.7

Initial Laboratory Tests for Evaluation of Abnormal Uterine Bleeding

Pregnancy test
Complete blood count (including hemoglobin concentration and platelet count); other indices within the full blood count may more accurately assess iron state
Tests for coagulopathies such as von Willebrand's disease should only be undertaken when specifically indicated by the history
Thyroid function test (thyroxine-stimulating hormone and thyroxine)
Papanicolaou smear
Screening for sexually transmitted diseases

A Papanicolaou smear is also performed at this time if the patient has not had one within the previous 12 months. A bimanual pelvic examination is then carried out for assessment of uterine size and shape, as well as presence of adnexal masses and/or tenderness. Careful inspection of the anus may occasionally reveal a fissure-in-ano. After a change of gloves to avoid contamination of the stool specimen with blood from the vagina, a rectal examination is performed to detect any palpable rectal masses, hemorrhoids, and tenderness. A stool sample should be tested for occult blood.

Laboratory Investigations

The first investigation to be performed in a woman capable of reproduction is a pregnancy test. Other preliminary tests include a complete blood count, thyroid test, and other tests as suggested by the clinical picture (Table 8.7). Additional testing depends on the information derived from the clinical evaluation of the patient and differential diagnoses (Table 8.8).

TABLE 8.8

Additional Laboratory Tests as Indicated for Evaluation of Abnormal Uterine Bleeding

Androgen assay (testosterone and dehydroepiandrosterone sulfate)
17-Hydroxyprogesterone
Prolactin
24-Hour urinary free cortisol
Ristocetin cofactor assay
Liver function test (aspartate aminotransferase, alanine transferase, alkaline phosphatase, bilirubin, and prothrombin time)
Purified protein derivative skin test
Luteinizing hormone
Follicle-stimulating hormone
Progesterone
Renal function test (serum electrolytes, urea, and creatinine)
Ferritin
Glucose tolerance test

Advanced Diagnostic Techniques

Ultrasonography

Transabdominal ultrasound scanning permits complete evaluation of the uterus and other reproductive tract organs, and can be used to rule out pelvic masses such as ovarian tumors and uterine leiomyoma. If smaller pelvic masses are suspected or suggested on other imaging modalities, transvaginal ultrasonography (TVUS) is ideally suited for their evaluation, particularly if the mass is closer to the vagina than the anterior abdominal wall. For optimal imaging using TVUS, the pelvic mass should be within 6 cm of the transducer in the vagina and not more than 8 to 9 cm away. Pelvic ultrasonography should be performed in the early follicular phase in premenopausal women just after conclusion of the menstrual period when the endometrium is thinnest.

Ultrasonography is useful for the diagnosis of ovarian tumors and uterine leiomyoma, and measurement of endometrial thickness. During the reproductive years, there is a wide range of fluctuations in endometrial thickness (4 to 8 mm in the proliferative phase and 8 to 14 mm in the secretory phase), so it is best to schedule TVUS for these women right after the menses (i.e., on cycle days 4 to 6). Additional evaluation with saline infusion sonography (SIS) (also referred to as hysterosonography and sonohysterography), EMB, and/or hysteroscopy may be required to confirm the clinical impression.

TVUS is very helpful in evaluating women with postmenopausal bleeding. Because postmenopausal hormone therapy may cause endometrial proliferation, TVUS is less specific in women using hormone replacement therapy. It is of minimal use in premenopausal women because specific cut-off levels or morphologic features do not accurately denote the presence or absence of endometrial hyperplasia or cancer (68). Endometrial cancer is found in less than 0.5% of postmenopausal women with endometrial thickness of less than 5 mm. If the cut-off point is reduced to 4 mm, virtually all women with complex hyperplasia, atypical hyperplasia, and endometrial cancer will be identified (69, 70). Postmenopausal bleeding in the presence of an endometrial thickness of more than 4 to 5 mm should be evaluated further. Other pathology found in women with increased endometrial thickness includes submucosal leiomyoma, endometrial hyperplasia, and polyps.

To improve the detection of endometrial cancer, the texture of the endometrium should also be examined. A heterogenous appearance of the endometrium is an indication for further evaluation using other modalities. Bleeding from an atrophic endometrium is suggested by the finding of an endometrial thickness of less than 4 mm.

Ultrasonography may not always distinguish between an endometrial polyp, adenomyosis, and submucosal leiomyoma. Endometrial tissue debris and blood clots present in the uterine cavity may not exhibit any characteristic sonographic features. The exact spatial relationships between endometrial polyps or submucosal leiomyoma and the endometrial cavity may not be readily obvious during conventional ultrasonography, although the use of SIS should help discriminate between these pathologies. In one direct comparison of unenhanced vaginal ultrasonography and SIS in premenopausal women with abnormal uterine bleeding, the use of SIS increased specificity from 21 to 95% (71, 72).

Saline Infusion Sonohysterography

This imaging technique involves the instillation of fluid into the uterine cavity with simultaneous TVUS being performed. It allows for examination of the contours of the uterine cavity and is useful in identifying pathology such as endometrial polyps, submucosal leiomyoma, and intrauterine adhesions (Fig. 8.1). It is also used for further evaluation of any suspicious findings in the endometrium noted during conventional pelvic ultrasonography. When TVUS is followed with SIS, the extent of the myometrial portion of submucosal leiomyoma can be mapped more accurately than what can be done with the hysteroscope. The findings may influence the decision to perform hysteroscopic resection of the leiomyoma or transabdominal myomectomy. In well-selected patients, SIS is a cheaper and more optimal alternative than hysteroscopy, but it does not obviate the need for hysteroscopy in all cases.

Saline infusion sonohysterography is ideally carried out in the early proliferative phase of the menstrual cycle. Normal saline, lactated Ringer's solution, or glycine is used for distension of the uterine cavity. The patient should void before the procedure. Conventional ultrasonography, preferably TVUS, is performed followed by the insertion of a vaginal speculum to expose the

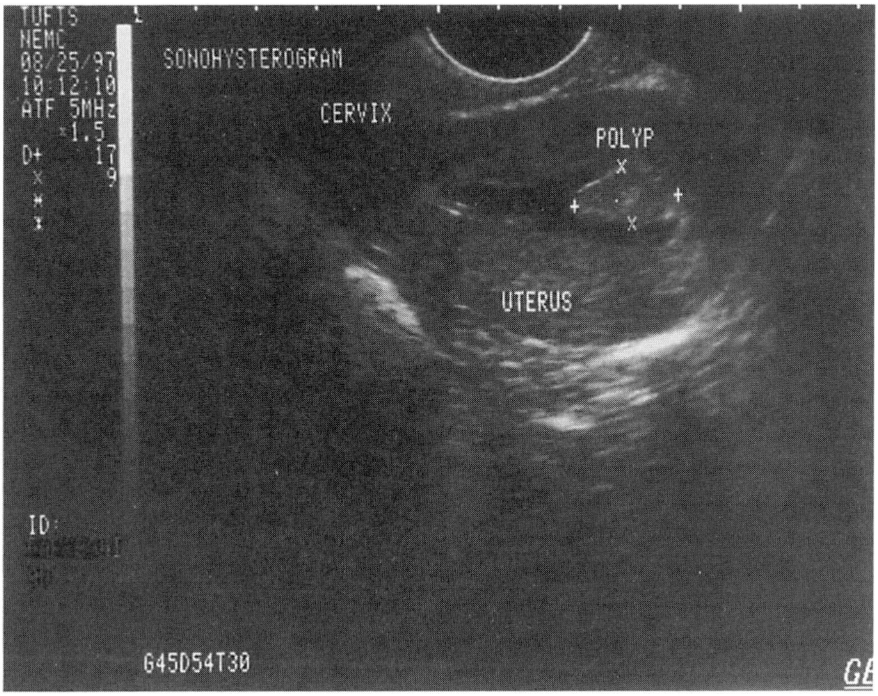

FIGURE 8.1 • Sonohysterogram depicting a submucosal polyp.

cervix. The cervix and visible parts of the vaginal wall are cleansed with an antiseptic solution. Various disposable catheter systems have been developed for instillation of fluid into the uterine cavity. The catheter is filled with fluid prior to introduction into the cervix to expel all air and to prevent the injection of air bubbles into the uterine cavity. It is then slowly introduced into the uterine cavity. When introducing the catheter, touching the fundus of the uterus with the tip of the catheter should be avoided if possible because this can cause pain and/or produce a vasovagal response. The speculum is removed, followed by the introduction of the vaginal ultrasound transducer into the vagina. The midline echo of the endometrium is brought into focus on the monitor. Fluid is then gradually injected into the uterine cavity while slowly moving the transducer in a systematic manner to allow for a full examination of the uterine cavity.

Saline infusion sonohysterography is well tolerated by patients, although uterine cramps may be stimulated by the presence of the catheter in the uterine cavity and during the fluid instillation. Administration of a nonsteroidal anti-inflammatory drug (NSAID) 1 to 2 hours prior to the procedure may reduce the severity of the cramps. Occasionally, especially in grand multiparous patients, a hysterosalpingogram balloon catheter must be used to prevent leakage of the saline through the cervical os and to allow adequate distention of the uterine cavity. The inflation of the balloon will cause a moderate degree of discomfort.

Complications associated with SIS include uterine perforation with the flexible catheter (although this is extremely rare), bleeding, and infection. Although the risk of infection is rare and has been reported to be less than 1%, it is important to consider prophylactic antibiotics for patients having a history of pelvic inflammatory disease and those who require systemic bacterial endocarditis prophylaxis (73). A vasovagal reaction is possible but is extremely rare (i.e., less than 0.3%) (74). If this occurs, intravenous administration of atropine will quickly reverse the reaction, but resuscitation equipment should be readily available in the procedure room in case it is needed.

SIS is not readily accomplished in all patients. If the volume of the uterine cavity is large (e.g., an enlarged uterus secondary to leiomyoma), the cavity may not be distended adequately with the usual volumes of fluid. This renders visualization of the uterine cavity difficult or impossible.

Introduction of the catheter may be impossible due to cervical stenosis, and although gentle cervical dilatation may be tried, it may be very painful. Other technical difficulties may be experienced with this procedure, including poor visualization of the endometrial cavity due to extreme uterine retroversion or anteversion or the presence of air bubbles in the uterine cavity (75). Saline infusion sonohysterography may lead to an erroneous diagnosis of endometrial polyps when actually the observed "polyp" is a blood clot or redundant endometrium.

SIS is as effective as hysteroscopy with curettage in detecting a number of uterine conditions, including polyps, myomas, and adhesions. SIS is usually associated with less pain compared with hysteroscopy (76).

Endometrial Sampling

Screening for endometrial hyperplasia and adenocarcinoma remains the most common reason for carrying out endometrial sampling in women with abnormal uterine bleeding. Different criteria have been used to determine who should have this procedure performed, and these criteria usually relate to the patient's age, as well as to the nature and duration of the abnormal bleeding (77). Because of the increased risk for hyperplasia and endometrial cancer in perimenopausal and menopausal women, endometrial sampling is advised in the presence of unexplained vaginal bleeding. There is a significant and increasing trend in the incidence of endometrial hyperplasia and adenocarcinoma in these women that makes EMB prudent. The incidence of endometrial cancer is much less in younger women, and endometrial sampling is usually reserved for obese adolescents with a long history of anovulatory bleeding (78).

Endometrial sampling is a convenient and relatively easy procedure that can be performed in an office setting. Two approaches to endometrial sampling are possible: sampling for cytologic examination or sampling for tissue diagnosis. The use of endometrial cytologic sampling is no more accurate than blind biopsy for benign or malignant lesions, and it requires a skilled pathologist for interpretation; due to these factors, it is not commonly recommended or used (79).

Endometrial tissue sampling is accomplished by the use of devices that collect strips or pieces of endometrium by scraping or suction (Table 8.7). Some of these devices are disposable (e.g., Pipelle catheter, Accurette, Z-sampler, Tis-u-Trap), whereas others are reusable (e.g., Vabra aspirator, Randall curette, Novak curette). Although some devices, such as the Pipelle, may sample a relatively small proportion of the endometrial surface (4.5 to 15%), in comparison to others such as the Vabra aspirator, the Pipelle catheter is less expensive, easier to use, and as reliable at diagnosis (80–82). Other studies have shown that the Novak and Pipelle have equivalent sensitivity, and the Pipelle incurs less pain for the patient (83, 84).

There are some caveats to bear in mind with the Pipelle catheter. Up to 70% of biopsy samples are nondiagnostic, and there is a 4 to 10% chance that cervical stenosis may either complicate or preclude its use (80). With the Pipelle, the detection of endometrial cancer depends on the location and total surface area of the tumor. Endometrial carcinoma that involves less than 5% of the cavity or is located near tubal ostia may be missed. Clinically, these caveats mean that if a patient's symptoms persist, further evaluation is needed, even if the biopsy is normal.

The basic technique for endometrial sampling is broadly similar for most devices, and many clinicians advise patients to ingest an oral NSAID about 1 hour prior to the biopsy. Other anesthetic techniques may also be used and include intrauterine lidocaine, paracervical block, topical cervical gels or creams, and others (85). The procedure begins with a speculum examination of the vagina. It may be necessary to apply a single-tooth vulsellum forceps on the anterior lip of the cervix and apply slight traction to stabilize the cervix and straighten out the angle between the cervical canal and uterine cavity. Insertion of a metal uterine sound is not always necessary in women having EMB. If the biopsy device itself is graduated in centimeters, this can be used to measure the depth of the uterine cavity. The endometrial tissue sampling device is gradually introduced into the uterine cavity and used to obtain endometrial tissue using appropriate techniques.

Although infrequent, endometrial sampling is associated with complications such as uterine perforation, vasovagal reaction, hemorrhage, genital tract or pelvic infection, or pain and severe cramping either during or after the procedure. EMB is contraindicated in pregnant women, as well as in patients with active cervicitis, known endometritis, current pelvic infection, coagulation disorders, or known cervical cancer.

Diagnostic D&C has largely been replaced by in-office EMB secondary to lower cost and anesthetic risk. D&C is also associated with higher complication rates, such as hemorrhage, infection, and perforation. D&C is associated with an incidence of uterine perforation of 0.63%, compared with an associated perforation rate with EMB of 0.1 to 0.2% (86, 87). Prophylaxis for bacterial endocarditis is not required for EMB (88).

Office Hysteroscopy

Evaluation of abnormal uterine bleeding is by far the most common indication for hysteroscopy. In combination with curettage, hysteroscopy is highly accurate and clinically useful in diagnosing endometrial cancer in women with abnormal uterine bleeding; it is also moderately useful in diagnosing benign endometrial disease (89). Hysteroscopy with directed biopsy of suspicious endometrial lesions has sensitivity rates of 97 to 98% (90, 91).

Although it is commonly performed under general anesthesia in the hospital, hysteroscopy may be done in the office setting. Concern about pain is one of the major reasons patients or clinicians choose not to perform office hysteroscopy, but the literature suggests that outpatient hysteroscopy without anesthesia is a well-tolerated procedure, with an average pain score around 4 on a 10-cm visual analog scale (92, 93).

Various forms of anesthesia can be used with office hysteroscopy, such as paracervical blocks or intravenous administration of short-acting narcotic analgesics (e.g., alfentanil) and/or sedatives (e.g., propofol). A combination of these techniques can also be used. There have been reports on the efficacy of local anesthetic gel instillation into the cervical canal and uterine cavity prior to instrumentation.

Rigid, flexible, and contact hysteroscopes have been used, but the former type is currently most commonly used for the evaluation of abnormal uterine bleeding and for operative hysteroscopy. Furthermore, the diameter of hysteroscopes has decreased to the point (3 mm) where cervical dilatation with dilators is not necessary for many patients. Carbon dioxide and normal saline are the usual distension media for outpatient hysteroscopy. The hysteroscope is inserted into the uterine cavity under direct vision with the distension medium flowing and a systematic search of the endometrial cavity is conducted. Landmarks such as the tubal ostia and uterine fundus are used to guide the examination.

Therapeutic use of hysteroscopy can also be used in the office setting for removal of small endometrial polyps and IUCDs. Careful patient selection will minimize the likelihood of complications that cannot be managed effectively in an office setting. It is safer to carry out hysteroscopic resection of significant endometrial pathology within hospital operating facilities.

The risk of complications arising during hysteroscopy is less than 3% (94). Uterine perforation is the most common complication reported in most hysteroscopic reviews, although, depending on the distending medium, fluid overload is another possible complication. The risk of fluid and electrolyte disturbance is minimal given the small volumes of physiologic saline that are normally used for diagnostic hysteroscopy (95). Hysteroscopy using carbon dioxide infusion is associated with a risk of carbon dioxide embolism. In one large study, the risk of subclinical embolic events was 0.51% and 0.03% for severe events (95, 96). Even though intravasation of carbon dioxide probably occurs more often than is realized, absorption of the gas in the bloodstream is rapid secondary to the lipid solubility of carbon dioxide. As a result, when CO_2 is used and intravasation occurs, the gas bubbles rarely reach the heart.

Magnetic Resonance Imaging

The use of magnetic resonance imaging (MRI) for the evaluation of women with abnormal uterine bleeding is a relatively recent innovation. It reliably localizes pelvic pathology, allows for estimation of the size of lesions, and differentiates uterine anatomy. It is not an invasive procedure and is better at distinguishing uterine leiomyomas from adenomyosis when compared with TVUS, SIS, and hysteroscopy (75, 97). MRI permits complete localization of uterine leiomyoma, giving the surgeon the opportunity to decide preoperatively the best technique and surgical approach to use.

MRI is not cost effective in all cases, however, and is not superior to SIS or hysteroscopy in excluding abnormalities in the uterine cavity, such as endometrial polyps (97). As such, its use should be reserved for distinguishing between leiomyoma and adenomyosis, localizing lesions, or evaluating the uterine corpus or other pelvic anatomy.

Medical Treatment

Emergency Medical Treatment

A patient with vaginal bleeding that is severe enough to decrease the hemoglobin (or hematocrit) and/or render her hemodynamically unstable should receive emergency medical treatment. Such treatment consists of intravenous crystalloid and/or colloid fluid infusion, possible blood transfusion, and administration of estrogen and other medications. However, surgical treatment such as D&C or tamponade with a pediatric Foley catheter balloon may be required in resistant cases. While conducting a rapid general physical examination, the clinical history is obtained followed by pelvic examination. A pregnancy test is mandatory in all women capable of reproduction.

In the absence of an organic cause or a medical history that contraindicates estrogen treatment, the following regimen is commonly used to stop the vaginal bleeding. Nausea and vomiting are common side effects that are associated with aggressive estrogen administration. Therefore, pretreatment or concomitant administration of antiemetics will prevent or reduce the severity of the symptoms.

Acute menorrhagia that does not warrant immediate surgical intervention should be treated with high-dose estrogens. Although the specific mechanism of action by which this works is unclear, it is known that high-dose estrogen increases the level of fibrinogen and factors V and IX, and promotes aggregation of platelets (98, 99). Intravenous administration of high-dose conjugated estrogen is as efficacious as oral intake of high-dose estrogen. Intravenously, the dose is conjugated equine estrogens (CEE) 25 mg every 4 hours for 24 to 48 hours. The oral regimen may be given as CEE 2.5 to 5 mg every 6 hours or estradiol 2 mg every 4 hours for 24 to 48 hours; it is then given as a single daily dose for 7 to 10 days. If the patient does not respond to one to two doses of estrogen with a significant decline in blood loss or they are not hemodynamically stable, a D&C should be performed (100, 101). Once the bleeding is under control, efforts to maintain or induce amenorrhea are warranted. This may be done with a variety of agents, including hormone therapy, oral combination contraceptives, cyclic progesterone, or a progesterone/progestogen-releasing IUCD.

A progestin needs to be started at the same time as the high-dose estrogen and should be continued for approximately 10 days. After this, the patient should experience a withdrawal bleed. This bleeding may be heavy but is rarely prolonged. After 5 days of withdrawal bleeding, the patient then uses an agent or regimen for the next three to six cycles to regulate the frequency or flow of her cycles.

Nonemergency Medical Management

Some commonly used regimens to treat menorrhagia are provided in Table 8.9. These regimens address various levels of bleeding severity, including mild to moderate bleeding, persistent bleeding that is unresponsive to medical therapy, and severe bleeding that requires immediate hospitalization.

Iron

In treating women with excessive uterine bleeding and laboratory evidence of anemia, iron therapy is considered to be a standard approach or adjuvant. If menstrual losses exceed 60 mL per month, iron-deficiency anemia may result. For most women, the primary symptom of anemia is fatigue. In some cases, daily administration of 60 to 180 mg of iron is the only treatment necessary for abnormal uterine bleeding.

Prostaglandin Synthetase Inhibitors

Several NSAIDs inhibit cyclo-oxygenase, decrease the amount of uterine blood loss in patients with abnormal uterine bleeding, and have the added advantage of relieving dysmenorrhea. Although the exact mechanism for this reduction in blood loss is unknown, it is theorized that NSAIDs preferentially decrease the endometrial content of vasodilator PGs such as PGE_2 and PGI_2 (101). Medication usually starts from the first day of the bleeding and continues for 3 to

TABLE 8.9

Commonly Used Regimens to Treat Menorrhagia

	Bleeding Severity		
	Mild to Moderate	**Persistent and Unresponsive to Medical Therapy**	**Severe, Requiring Hospitalization**
Treatment and dose or regimen	NSAIDs • Naproxen, 375 mg orally twice a day • Meclofenamate sodium, 100 mg orally three times a day Start first day of bleeding and continue for 3–5 days or until bleeding is less. Oral contraceptives Various estrogen and progesterone types and dosages: Mild—1 pill day Moderate—1 pill three times a day for 1 week, then 1 pill a day for 3 months Progestin or progesterone agent • Medroxyprogesterone acetate 5–10 mg orally for 10–14 days monthly • Depo-Provera: 1 injection 150 mg daily every 3 months • Progesterone-releasing IUCD Androgens • Danazol 100–400 mg four times a day Iron 60–180 mg/day Antifibrinolytics • Tranexamic acid is given 1 g q6h for first 4 days of cycle (not available in United States)	Surgical—D&C Endometrial ablation Hysterectomy	High-dose estrogen in conjunction with a progestin • Conjugated equine estrogens (CEE) 25 mg intravenously q4h for 24–48 hours • CEE 2.5–5 mg orally q6h or estradiol 2 mg orally q4h for 24–48 hours • Continue progestin for 7–10 days D&C Hysterectomy

5 days or until the bleeding greatly decreases. A 50% reduction of menstrual blood loss has been documented in the literature (102), but other studies have demonstrated less dramatic diminution of blood loss (20 to 24% reduction) (103, 104). NSAIDs shown to be effective in the treatment of menorrhagia include ibuprofen, indomethacin, diclofenac, flurbiprofen, mefenamic acid, naproxen, and naproxen sodium (105). NSAIDs are less effective than either tranexamic acid or danazol. Although studies are limited, there is no significant difference in efficacy between NSAIDs and other medical treatments such as oral luteal progestogen, ethamsylate, combination OCs, or progesterone-releasing IUCDs (106).

Antifibrinolytics

The use of antifibrinolytic agents such as tranexamic acid (Cyklokapron) for the treatment of menorrhagia is based on the belief that heavy menstrual bleeding may be due to an overactive endometrial fibrinolytic system. Tranexamic acid is an inhibitor of plasminogen activation, and studies have shown its use to be associated with a decrease in the amount of menstrual blood loss by an average of 110 mL per cycle (107). Although not approved for use in the United States, tranexamic acid is administered at a dose of 1 g every 6 hours for the first 4 days of the menstrual cycle. Tranexamic acid carries a theoretical risk for thromboembolic event, but this has not been supported by the experience in Europe, where this drug has been used extensively. One retrospective study of a large group of women at increased risk for thromboembolic disease found no association between the use of tranexamic acid and thromboembolic events in this population (108).

Studies comparing tranexamic acid with COX inhibitors showed a 45 to 55% reduction in menstrual flow for women receiving tranexamic acid; the COX inhibitors led to decreases of only 20 to 24%, and use of progestins during the luteal phase actually led to a 20% increase in menstrual blood loss (103, 104, 109). In a more recent Cochrane Review, antifibrinolytic therapy was found to cause a greater reduction in objective measurements of heavy menstrual bleeding when compared with placebo or other medical therapies (NSAIDS, oral luteal phase progestogens, and ethamsylate), without any significant increase in side effects (107).

Progestins

Progestins such as medroxyprogesterone acetate and norethindrone have been used in the management of abnormal uterine bleeding, as well as for the prevention and treatment of endometrial hyperplasia. Progestins are more useful in women who are anovulatory but have adequate endogenous estrogen production. The cyclical use of progestins in such instances will induce regular withdrawal bleeding, pending the restoration of normal ovulatory activity. Treatment in each cycle lasts for a period of 10 to 12 days, depending on the dose used before stopping administration to induce a withdrawal bleed. The use of cyclical progestin treatment in women with ovulatory abnormal uterine bleeding may not immediately decrease the menstrual blood loss. In fact, a study demonstrated a 20% increase in the amount of blood loss when norethindrone was administered to such a group of women with menorrhagia (103). It is only with prolonged cyclical use of progestins that the volume of menstrual loss eventually decreases.

For women with anovulatory abnormal uterine bleeding, cyclic progestins offer a therapeutic option as a means of regularly inducing withdrawal menses. The cyclic use of norethindrone has been shown in several studies to restore regular and predictable menses in more than 50% of women with anovulatory bleeding (110).

For women with ovulatory cycles, the use of cyclic progestogens offered no advantage over other medical therapies such as danazol, tranexamic acid, NSAIDs, and the intrauterine system (IUS) in the treatment of menorrhagia (111). Progestogen therapy for 21 days of the cycle results in a significant reduction in menstrual blood loss, although women find the treatment less acceptable than intrauterine levonorgestrel. In addition, progestogen therapy from day 5 to 26 of the menstrual cycle was significantly less effective at reducing menstrual blood loss than the progesterone-releasing IUS (111). Continuous progestin-only use often leads to amenorrhea as a result of endometrial atrophy.

This property is exploited when progestin-impregnated IUCDs, such as the levonorgestrel intrauterine system (LNG IUS) (Mirena), are used for the treatment of abnormal (excessive) uterine bleeding. Women with an LNG IUS are more satisfied and willing to continue with treatment than women treated with 21 days of norethisterone each month, but they experience more side effects, such as intermenstrual bleeding and breast tenderness (112). One study demonstrated that there were no statistically significant differences between IUS and hysterectomy for the outcomes of quality of life and psychological well-being (113). There are no data available from randomized controlled trials comparing progesterone-releasing intrauterine systems to either placebo or other commonly used medical therapies for heavy menstrual bleeding.

Progestin IUCDs have been shown to reduce the amount of blood loss over time by 79 to 94% (114, 115). Further benefits derived from this treatment modality include a decreased recourse to operative treatments such as hysterectomy (116). Two studies documented that 64 to 82% of patients who had the progestin IUCD inserted for temporary control of their abnormal uterine bleeding pending hysterectomy declined proceeding with the hysterectomy (117, 118). The benefits of this treatment are experienced in both ovulatory and anovulatory abnormal uterine bleeding.

Intrauterine progestin therapy can be used for heavy menstrual bleeding associated with uterine fibroids, but there is some evidence that expulsion rates may be increased in the presence of submucous fibroids (119).

Menorrhagia due to endometrial hyperplasia without atypia can be treated with progestins. In a study where patients were cycled with 10 mg of medroxyprogesterone acetate (Provera) or a similar progestin for 14 days per month, regression of hyperplasia was noted in 80% of patients, and 92% of these patients had reverted to a normal endometrium by 12 months of therapy. No endometrial carcinomas were noted in this group after a mean 7-year follow-up therapy (56). Atypical hyperplasia can be treated successfully with progestins, but the clinician and the patient must understand that there is a significantly increased risk of progression to carcinoma, and there is a higher incidence of resistance to regression to benign endometrium (56). Because of these risks, postmenopausal women with cytologic atypia should be strongly encouraged to undergo hysterectomy. Premenopausal women with atypical hyperplasia who choose to proceed with high-dose progestin treatment must be followed closely with EMB every 3 to 6 months. Commonly used progestin regimens for this situation include medroxyprogesterone acetate (Provera) 10 to 30 mg four times a day, or megestrol (Megace) 40 to 160 mg four times a day. Progestin concentration should be adjusted based on endometrial histology.

Combined Use of Estrogens and Progestins

The use of combined OCs is a popular method of menstrual cycle control, especially in patients who are not immediately desirous of pregnancy. Again, both ovulatory and anovulatory abnormal uterine bleeding are controlled with these medications. OCs suppress ovulation in ovulatory patients and reduce the variability in estrogen levels found in anovulatory patients. The withdrawal bleeding is regular, and eventually, thinning of the endometrium occurs with prolonged usage. A combined OC that contains 30 or 35 μg of ethinyl estradiol is sufficient for the treatment of abnormal uterine bleeding.

For treatment of an acute episode of abnormal uterine bleeding, a typical regimen is one combined OC pill two to four times a day for 5 to 7 days; the bleeding will usually stop on days 2 to 4 of treatment. After these 5 to 7 days, the dosing is tapered over the next 7 days until she is taking one pill per day. At this point, a new pill pack is begun and taken in the usual manner. Variations of how to taper the doses over the next 7 days have been described. Another regimen advocates thc use of one OC tablet, three times a day, for 7 days, a withdrawal bleed for 5 days, and then standard pill cycles for 2 months (49). Studies that demonstrate superiority of one dosing or tapering regimen over others, as well as studies comparing the efficacy of various estrogen doses for the treatment of acute, moderate menorrhagia, are lacking.

If use of an OC is not possible, a regimen using hormone therapy may be initiated. Oral administration of 2.5 mg of CEE is given every 6 hours in conjunction with medroxyprogesterone acetate (MPA) 10 mg/day for 5 to 7 days. After this, the 2.5 mg CEE is taken daily with 5 to 10 mg/day MPA for the next 3 weeks. A withdrawal bleed is allowed to occur, and therapy to regulate the flow is initiated.

Androgens

Danazol is the main androgenic compound that has been used for the treatment of abnormal uterine bleeding. It is a synthetic androgen derived from 17α-ethinyl testosterone and has multiple mechanisms of action, both antiestrogenic and antiprogestational. These actions include suppression of ovulation, reduction of ovarian 17 beta estradiol production, and a direct action on endometrial estrogen receptors. Higher doses of 200 to 400 mg/day are more effective than lower doses (e.g., 100 mg/day) in reducing menstrual bleeding in women with ovulatory abnormal uterine bleeding (120). Reversible amenorrhea can also result from the treatment (121). However, androgenic side effects such as permanent voice changes limit its use, and conception following incomplete ovarian suppression is possible, especially in patients who are on lower doses of danazol.

Gonadotropin-Releasing Hormone Agonists and Antagonists

Patients with ovulatory or anovulatory abnormal uterine bleeding or bleeding in association with leiomyoma or adenomyosis may benefit from the use of gonadotrophin-releasing hormone agonists (GnRHa). These agonists produce reversible suppression of pituitary output of FSH and LH, leading to hypoestrogenemia, amenorrhea, and decrease in uterine and leiomyoma volume.

The practical use of GnRHa in these patients is to induce amenorrhea in women with heavy bleeding due to leiomyomas. This allows a return of the hemoglobin concentration back to normal levels before embarking on surgical treatment or radiologic intervention. Reduction in the size of uterine leiomyoma may make it possible for vaginal hysterectomy to be performed in situations where abdominal hysterectomy would have been necessitated by a larger uterine size prior to GnRHa administration (122). One drawback to the use of GnRHa in treating symptomatic fibroids is that within 6 months of treatment completion, the uterus returns to pretreatment size and symptoms recur (123).

In perimenopausal women with biopsy-proven absence of endometrial pathology, the use of GnRHa may serve to prevent further bleeding from myomas until natural menopause supervenes. Treatment with GnRHa is conventionally carried out for no longer than 6 months due to concerns about causing significant bone loss. However, concomitant use of low doses of estrogen and progestin can allow the administration of GnRHa to be continued for longer periods. Resumption of endogenous estrogen production following cessation of GnRHa administration often leads to tumor regrowth, with the uterus and leiomyoma returning to previous dimensions.

There is also interest in the use of GnRH antagonists such as cetrorelix acetate for injection (Cetrotide, Serono, Inc., Rockland, MA) and ganirelix acetate (Antagon, Organon, West Orange, NJ) in the management of excess bleeding in the perimenopausal woman. GnRH antagonists act by the mechanism of competitive receptor binding, which leads to an immediate arrest of gonadotropin secretion. They also do not display the "flare-up" effect commonly seen with GnRHa. Because they do not downregulate receptors, gonadal function will resume almost immediately after the cessation of treatment with the antagonist. Uterine myomas treated with antagonists showed effective reduction in size (124, 125).

Antiprogestational Agents

Mifepristone (RU-486) may be useful in the presurgical setting for similar purposes as GnRHa—increased preoperative hemoglobin and improved surgical approaches. The effect of mifepristone is believed to be mediated through its well-known antiprogestational action. It has been observed that daily low-dose (5 to 10 mg/day) mifepristone can induce a 48 to 49% reduction in the size of fibroid tumors; the tumor(s) with up to 65% of women also having accompanying amenorrhea (126). Mifepristone treatment has demonstrated a consistent reduction in leiomyoma size and a positive effect on leiomyoma symptoms, including menorrhagia, dysmenorrhea, and pelvic pressure (126).

Mifepristone induces ovarian acyclicity, but follicular levels of estrogen are maintained. One potential side effect of concern that may result from this is endometrial hyperplasia. Two studies thus far have demonstrated an increase in endometrial hyperplasia in women treated for 6 months with mifepristone. On histologic examination, the endometrial tissue showed an estrogen effect on glandular and stromal morphology combined with a minimal progesterone effect on the epithelium. In neither study was there noted to be complex hyperplastic changes or cytologic atypia (126, 127).

Clinical Notes

- More than 10 million women in the United States suffer from abnormal uterine bleeding.
- Normal menstrual function is denoted by regular periods occurring every 24 to 35 days, with a blood loss of 20 to 80 mL that takes place over 3 to 7 days in each cycle.
- Anemia typically develops at losses of 60 mL or greater per cycle.
- In patients with menorrhagia, the prostaglandins $PGE_{2\alpha}$ and PGI_2 (both vasodilators) predominate over the vasoconstrictive prostaglandins $PGF_{2\alpha}$ and thromboxane A_2.

- Of the 600,000 hysterectomies performed each year in the United States, about 20% will be done for dysfunctional uterine bleeding.
- Leiomyomas are the most common benign tumors of the uterus and are found clinically in 20 to 30% of women older than 30 years of age.
- Adenomyosis can be found in 20 to 30% of women of all ages; the frequency of adenomyosis appears to be greater in patients with leiomyomata.
- The prevalence of polyps in the general population is estimated to be 24%.
- Endometrial malignancy usually occurs in the postmenopausal period, but 20 to 25% of cases occur in premenopausal women, and 3 to 5% are diagnosed in women younger than the age of 40.
- Almost 5% of incident endometrial cancers in women ages 20 to 54 years may be attributed to a family history of endometrial cancer, and 2% may be attributable to a family history of colorectal cancer.
- Women with atypical hyperplasia have a 23% risk of endometrial carcinoma over the next decade.
- Anovulatory bleeding is the most common cause of abnormal bleeding in adolescents.
- The incidence of bleeding disorders has ranged from 5 to 20% of adolescents who have abnormal uterine bleeding that is severe enough to require hospitalization.
- The average blood loss in women with various coagulopathies is 400 mL per menses.
- In the United States, from 1994 to 1999, 52% of all hysterectomies were performed among women younger than 44 years of age.
- Twenty-three percent of women having hyperplasia with atypia will develop adenocarcinoma; less than 2% without atypia will progress to cancer.
- Endometrial cancer is found in less than 0.5% of postmenopausal women with endometrial thickness of less than 5 mm.
- In the treatment of menorrhagia, there is no significant efficacy difference between NSAIDs and other medical treatments such as oral luteal progestogen, ethamsylate, combination OCs, or progesterone-releasing IUCDs.
- For women with ovulatory cycles and menorrhagia, cyclic progestogens offer no advantage over other medical therapies (e.g., danazol, tranexamic acid, NSAIDs, progesterone-releasing IUCDs).
- Sixty-four to 82% of patients who had the progestin IUCD inserted for temporary control of abnormal uterine bleeding pending hysterectomy declined proceeding with the hysterectomy.
- Menorrhagia due to endometrial hyperplasia without atypia can be treated with progestins.
- Atypical hyperplasia can be treated successfully with progestins, but there is a significantly increased risk of progression to carcinoma and a higher incidence of resistance to regression to benign endometrium.
- Mifepristone induces ovarian acyclicity, but follicular levels of estrogen are maintained.

REFERENCES

1. Cooper JM. Contemporary management of abnormal uterine bleeding. Preface. Obstet Gynecol Clin North Am 2000;27:xi–xiii.
2. Awwad JT, Toth TL, Schiff I. Abnormal uterine bleeding in the perimenopause. Int J Fertil 1993;38:261–269.
3. Chimbira TH, Anderson ABM, Naish C, et al. Reduction of menstrual blood loss by danazol in unexplained menorrhagia: lack of effect of placebo. Br J Obstet Gynaecol 1980;87:1152–1158.
4. Snowden R, Christian B. Patterns and Perceptions of Menstruation—A World Health Organization International Study. London: Croom Helm, 1983.
5. Rosenfeld J. Treatment of menorrhagia due to dysfunctional uterine bleeding. Am Fam Physician 1996;53:165–172.
6. Keshavarz H, Hillis SD, Kieke BA, et al. Hysterectomy surveillance—United States, 1994–1999. MMWR Surveill Summ 2002;51(SS05):1–8. Available at: http://www.cdc.gov/mmwr/preview/mmwrhtml/ss5105a1.htm. Accessed on July 11, 2005.
7. Clarke A, Black N, Rowe P, et al. Indications for and outcome of total abdominal hysterectomy for benign disease: a prospective cohort study. Br J Obstet Gynaecol 1995;102:611–620.

8. Carlson KJ, Nichols DH, Schiff I. Indications for hysterectomy. N Engl J Med 1993;83:792–796.
9. Cramer SF, Patel A. The frequency of uterine leiomyomas. Am J Clin Pathol 1990;94:435–438.
10. Yin H, Mittal K. Incidental findings in uterine prolapse specimen: frequency and implications. Int J Gynecol Pathol 2004;23(1):26–28.
11. Kitawaki J, Obayashi H, Ishihara H, et al. Oestrogen receptor-alpha gene polymorphism is associated with endometriosis, adenomyosis and leiomyomata. Hum Reprod 2001;1:51–55.
12. Siegler AM, Camilien L. Adenomyosis. J Reprod Med 1994;39:841–853.
13. Parazzini F, Vercellini P, Panazza S, et al. Risk factors for adenomyosis. Hum Reprod 1997;12:1275–1279.
14. Azziz R. Adenomyosis: current perspectives. Obstet Gynecol Clin North Am 1989;16:221–235.
15. Lee NC, Dicker RC, Reuben GI. Confirmation of the preoperative diagnosis for hysterectomy. Am J Obstet Gynecol 1984;150:283.
16. Molitor JJ. Adenomyosis: a clinical and pathological appraisal. Am J Obstet Gynecol 1971;110:275.
17. Nikkanen V, Punnonen R. Clinical significance of adenomyosis. Ann Chir Gynaecol 1980;69:278.
18. Kurman RJ, Mazur MT. Benign diseases of the endometrium. In: Kurman RJ, ed. Blaustein's Pathology of the Female Genital Tract. New York: Springer-Verlag, 1994:394.
19. Anastasiadis PG, Koutlaki NG, Skaphida PG, et al. Endometrial polyps: prevalence, detection, and malignant potential in women with abnormal uterine bleeding. Eur J Gynaecol Oncol 2000;21:180–183.
20. Bakour S, Khan KS, Gupta JK. The risk of premalignant and malignant pathology in endometrial polyps. Acta Obstet Gynecol Scand 2000;70:317–330.
21. American Cancer Society (ACS). Cancer Facts & Figures 2004. Atlanta: ACS, 2004. Available at: http://www.cancer.org/docroot/STT/content/STT_1x_Cancer_Facts__Figures_2004.asp. Accessed July 11, 2005.
22. Duska LR, Garrett A, Rueda BR, et al. Endometrial cancer in women 40 years old and younger. Gynecol Oncol 2001;83:388–393.
23. Gruber SB, Thompson WD. A population-based study of endometrial cancer and familial risk in younger women. Cancer Epidemiol Biomarkers Prev 1996;5:411–417.
24. Kurman RJ, Kaminski PF, Norris HJ. The behavior of endometrial hyperplasia: a long-term study of "untreated" hyperplasia in 170 patients. Cancer 1985;56:403–412.
25. Janicek MF, Rosenhein NB. Invasive endometrial cancer in uteri resected for atypical endometrial hyperplasia. Gynecol Oncol 1994;52:373–378.
26. Widra EA, Dunton CJ, McHugh M, et al. Endometrial hyperplasia and the risk of carcinoma. Int J Gynecol Cancer 1995;5:233–235.
27. Bennett K, Daley ML, Pike C. Factor V deficiency and menstruation: a gynecologic challenge. Obstet Gynecol 1997;89:839–840.
28. Kadir RA, Economides DL, Sabin CA, et al. Frequency of inherited bleeding disorders in women with menorrhagia. Lancet 1998;351:485–489.
29. Ellis MH, Beyth Y. Abnormal vaginal bleeding in adolescence as the presenting symptom of a bleeding diathesis. J Pediatr Adolesc Gynecol 1999;12:127–131.
30. Claessens EA, Cowell CL. Acute adolescent menorrhagia. Am J Obstet Gynecol 1981;139:277–280.
31. Falcone T, Desjardins C, Bourque J, et al. Dysfunctional uterine bleeding in adolescents. J Reprod Med 1994;39:761–764.
32. Soff GA, Green D. Autoantibody to von Willebrand factor in systemic lupus erythematosus. J Lab Clin Med 1993;121:424–430.
33. Krassas GE. Thyroid disease and female reproduction. Fertil Steril 2000;74:1063–1070.
34. Krassas GE, Pontikides N, Kaltas T, et al. Menstrual disturbances in thyrotoxicosis. Clin Endocrinol 1994;40:641–644.
35. Evans AT, Gaffey TA, Malkasian GD Jr, et al. Clinicopathologic review of 118 granulosa and 82 theca cell tumors. Obstet Gynecol 1980;55:231.
36. Stenwig JT, Hazekamp JT, Beecham JB. Granulosa cell tumors of the ovary. A clinicopathological study of 118 cases with long-term follow-up. Gynecol Oncol 1979;7:136.
37. Milsom I, Andersson K, Jonasson K, et al. The influence of the Gyne-T380SIUD on menstrual blood loss and iron status. Contraception 1995;52:175–179.
38. Andersson JK, Rybo G. Levonorgestrel-releasing intrauterine device in the treatment of menorrhagia. Br J Obstet Gynaecol 1990;97:690–694.
39. Ismail SM. Pathology of endometrium treated with tamoxifen. J Clin Pathol 1994;47:827–833.
40. Mignotte H, Lasset C, Bonadona V, et al. Iatrogenic risk of endometrial carcinoma after treatment for breast cancer in a large French case-control study. Federation Nationale des Centres de Lutte Contre le Cancer (FNCLCC). Int J Cancer 1998;76:325–330.
41. van Eijkeren MA, Christiaens GCML, Haspels AA, et al. Measured menstrual blood loss in women with a bleeding disorder or using oral anticoagulant therapy. Am J Obstet Gynecol 1990;162:1261–1263.
42. Munro MG. Dysfunctional uterine bleeding: advances in diagnosis and treatment. Curr Opin Obstet Gynecol 2001;13(5):475–489.
43. Smith SK, Abel MH, Kelly RW, et al. The synthesis of prostaglandins from persistent proliferative endometrium. J Clin Endocrinol Metab 1982;55:284–289.
44. Ylikorkala O. Prostaglandin synthesis inhibitors in menorrhagia, intrauterine contraceptive device-induced side effects and endometriosis. Pharmacol Toxicol 1994;75(suppl 2):86–88.
45. Smith SK, Abel MH, Kelly RW. Prostaglandin synthesis in the endometrium of women with ovular dysfunctional uterine bleeding. Br J Obstet Gynaecol 1981;88:434–442.

46. Gleeson N, Devitt M, Sheppard BL, et al. Endometrial fibrinolytic enzymes in women with normal menstruation and dysfunctional uterine bleeding. Br J Obstet Gynaecol 1993;100:768–771.
47. Zitsman JL, Cirincione E, Margossian H. Vaginal bleeding in an infant secondary to sliding inguinal hernia. Obstet Gynecol 1997;89:840–842.
48. Imai A, Horibe S, Tamaya T. Genital bleeding in premenarcheal children. Int J Gynecol Obstet 1995;49:41–45.
49. Schwayder JM. Pathophysiology of abnormal uterine bleeding. Obstet Gynecol Clin North Am 2000;27:219–234.
50. Kanbur NO, Derman O, Kutluk T, et al. Coagulation disorders as the cause of menorrhagia in adolescents. Int J Adolesc Med Health 2004;16(2):183–185.
51. Oral E, Cagdas A, Gezer A, et al. Hematological abnormalities in adolescent menorrhagia. Arch Gynecol Obstet 2002;266(2):72–74.
52. Fraser IS, McCarron G, Markham R, et al. Measured menstrual blood loss in women with menorrhagia associated with pelvic disease or coagulation disorder. Obstet Gynecol 1986;68:630.
53. Knochenhauer ES, Key TJ, Kahsar-Miller M, et al. Prevalence of the polycystic ovary syndrome in unselected black and white women of the southeastern United States: a prospective study. J Clin Endocrinol Metab 1998;83:3078–3082.
54. Diamanti-Kandarakis E, Kouli CR, Bergiele AT, et al. A survey of the polycystic ovary syndrome in the Greek island of Lesbos: hormonal and metabolic profile. J Clin Endocrinol Metab 1999;84:4006–4011.
55. Asuncion M, Calvo RM, San Millan JL, et al. A prospective study of the prevalence of the polycystic ovary syndrome in unselected Caucasian women from Spain. J Clin Endocrinol Metab 2000;85:2434–2438.
56. Ferenczy A, Gelfand M. The biologic significance of cytologic atypia in progestogen-treated endometrial hyperplasia. Am J Obstet Gynecol 1990;160:126–131.
57. Seltzer VL, Benjamin F, Deutsch S. Perimenopausal bleeding patterns and pathologic findings. J Am Med Womens Assoc 1990;45:132–134.
58. Townsend DE, Fields G, McCausland A, et al. Diagnostic and operative hysteroscopy in the management of persistent postmenopausal bleeding. Obstet Gynecol 1993;82:419–421.
59. Hallberg L, Hogdahl A, Nilsson L, et al. Menstrual blood loss—a population study. Acta Obstet Gynecol Scand 1966;45:320.
60. Fraser IS, McCarron G, Markham R, et al. Blood and total fluid content of menstrual discharge. Obstet Gynecol 1985;65:194.
61. Fraser IS, McCarron G, Markham RA. A preliminary study of factors influencing perception of menstrual blood loss volume. Am J Obstet Gynecol 1984;149:788–793.
62. Hallberg L, Nilsson L. Determination of menstrual blood loss. Scand J Clin Lab Invest 1964;16:244–248.
63. van Eijkeren MA, Scholten PC, Christiaens GMCL, et al. The alkaline hematin method for measuring menstrual blood loss—a modification and its clinical use in menorrhagia. Eur J Obstet Gynecol Reprod Biol 1986;22:345–351.
64. Higham JM, O'Brien PM, Shaw RW. Assessment of menstrual blood loss using a pictorial chart. Br J Obstet Gynaecol 1990;97:734–739.
65. Janssen CA, Scholten PC, Heintz AP. A simple visual assessment technique to discriminate between menorrhagia and normal blood loss. Obstet Gynecol 1995;977–982.
66. Reid PC, Coker A, Coltart R. Assessment of menstrual blood loss using a pictorial chart: a validation study. Br J Obstet Gynaecol 2000;107:320–322.
67. Fraser IS, Warner P, Marantos PA. Estimating menstrual blood loss in women with normal and excessive menstrual fluid volume. Obstet Gynecol 2001;98:806–814.
68. Farquar C, Ekeroma A, Furness S, et al. A systemic review of transvaginal ultrasonography, sonohysterography and hysteroscopy for the investigation of abnormal uterine bleeding in premenopausal women. Acta Obstet Gynecol Scand 2003;82:493–504.
69. Gupta JK, Chien PF, Voit D, et al. Ultrasonographic endometrial thickness for diagnosing endometrial pathology in women with postmenopausal bleeding: a meta-analysis. Acta Obstet Gynecol Scand 2002;81:799–816.
70. Gull B, Karlsson B, Milsom I, et al. Can ultrasound replace dilation and curettage? A longitudinal evaluation of post-menopausal bleeding and transvaginal sonographic measurement of the endometrium as predictors of endometrial cancer. Am J Obstet Gynecol 2003;188:401–408.
71. Bronz L, Suter T, Rusca T. The value of transvaginal sonography with and without saline instillation in the diagnosis of uterine pathology in pre- and postmenopausal women with abnormal bleeding or suspect sonographic findings. Ultrasound Obstet Gynecol 1997;9:53–58.
72. de Vries LD, Dijkhuizen FP, Mol BW, et al. Comparison of transvaginal sonography, saline infusion, sonography, and hysteroscopy in premenopausal women with abnormal uterine bleeding. J Clin Ultrasound 2000;79:55–58.
73. Bonnamy L, Marret H, Perrotin F, et al. Sonohysterography: a prospective survey of results and complications in 81 patients. Eur J Obstet Gynecol Reprod Biol 2002;102:42.
74. Goldstein SR. Saline infusion sonohysterography. Clin Obstet Gynecol 1996;39(1):248–258.
75. Bradley LD, Falcone T, Magen AB. Radiographic imaging techniques for the diagnosis of abnormal bleeding. Obstet Gynecol Clin North Am 2000;27:245–276.
76. de Kroon CD, et al. Saline contrast hysterosonography in abnormal uterine bleeding: a systematic review and meta-analysis. Br J Obstet Gynaecol 2003;110:938.
77. Crum CP, Hornstein MD, Nucci MR, et al. Hertig and beyond: a systematic and practical approach to the endometrial biopsy. Adv Anat Pathol 2003;10(6):301–318.

78. American College of Obstetricians and Gynecologists (ACOG). Management of anovulatory bleeding. ACOG Practice Bulletin, No. 14, March 2000.
79. Mencaglia L, Valle RF, Perino A, et al. Endometrial cancer and its precursors: early detection and treatment. Int J Gynecol Obstet 1990;31:107–116.
80. Guido RS, Kanbour-Shakir A, Rulin MC, et al. Pipelle endometrial sampling: sensitivity in the detection of endometrial lesions. Cancer J Reprod Med 1995;40:553–555.
81. Rodriguez GC, Yaqub N, King ME. A comparison of the Pipelle device and the Vabra aspirator as measured by endometrial denudation in hysterectomy specimens: the Pipelle device samples significantly less of the endometrial surface than the Vabra aspirator. Am J Obstet Gynecol 1993;168:55–59.
82. Eddowes HA. Pipelle: a more acceptable technique for outpatient endometrial biopsy. Br J Obstet Gynecol 1990;97:961–962.
83. Silver MM, Miles P, Rosa C. Comparison of Novak and Pipelle endometrial biopsy instruments. Obstet Gynecol 1991;78:828–830.
84. Stovall TG, Ling FW, Morgan PL. A prospective, randomized comparison of the Pipelle endometrial sampling device with the Novak curette. Am J Obstet Gynecol 1991;165:1287–1289.
85. Leclair C. Anesthesia for office endometrial procedures: a review of the literature. Curr Womens Health Rep 2002;2(6):429–433.
86. McElin TW, Bird CC, Reeves BD, et al. Diagnostic dilation and curettage. Obstet Gynecol 1974;17:205.
87. Kaunitz AM, Masciello A, Ostrowski M. Comparison of endometrial biopsy with the endometrial Pipelle and Vabra aspirator. J Reprod Med 1988;33:427.
88. Dajani AS, Taubert KA, Wilson W, et al. Prevention of bacterial endocarditis: recommendations by the American Heart Association. JAMA 1997;277:22.
89. Clark TJ, Voit D, Gupta JK, et al. Accuracy of hysteroscopy in the diagnosis of endometrial cancer and hyperplasia: a systematic quantitative review. JAMA 2002;288(13):1610–1621.
90. Larson DM, Johnson KK, Broste SK, et al. Comparison of D&C and office endometrial biopsy in predicting final histopathologic grade in endometrial cancer. Obstet Gynecol 1995;86:38–42.
91. Van den Bosch T, Vandendal A, Van Schoubroeck D, et al. Combining vaginal ultrasonography and office endometrial sampling in the diagnosis of endometrial disease in postmenopausal women. Obstet Gynecol 1995;85:349–352.
92. De Iaco P, Marabini A, Stefanetti M. Acceptability and pain of outpatient hysteroscopy. J Am Assoc Gynecol Laparosc 2000;7:71–75.
93. Finikiotis G. Outpatient hysteroscopy: pain assessment by visual analogue scale. Aust N Z J Obstet Gynecol 1990;30:89–90.
94. Propst AM, Liberman RF, Harlow BL, et al. Complications of hysteroscopic surgery: predicting patients at risk. Obstet Gynecol 2000;96:517–520.
95. Serden SP. Diagnostic hysteroscopy to evaluate the cause of abnormal uterine bleeding. Obstet Gynecol Clin North Am 2000;27:277–286.
96. Bradner P, Neis KJ, Ehmer C. The etiology, frequency, and prevention of gas embolism during CO_2 hysteroscopy. J Am Assoc Gynecol Laparosc 1999;6:421–428.
97. Dueholm M, Lundorf E, Hansen ES, et al. Evaluation of the uterine cavity with magnetic resonance imaging, transvaginal sonography, hysterosonographic examination, and diagnostic hysteroscopy. Fertil Steril 2001;76:350–357.
98. Bar J, Tepper R, Fuchs J, et al. The effect of estrogen replacement therapy on platelet aggregation and adenosine triphosphate release in postmenopausal women. Obstet Gynecol 1993;81:261–264.
99. Zreik TG, Odunsi K, Cass I, et al. A case of fatal pulmonary embolism associated with the use of intravenous estrogen therapy. Fertil Steril 1999;71:373–375.
100. DeVore GR, Owens O, Kase N. Use of intravenous Premarin in the treatment of dysfunctional uterine bleeding—a double-blind randomized control study. Obstet Gynecol 1982;59:285–291.
101. Munro MG. Medical management of abnormal uterine bleeding. Obstet Gynecol Clin North Am 2000;27:287–304.
102. Vargyas JM, Campeau JD, Mishell DA. Treatment of menorrhagia with meclofenamate sodium. Am J Obstet Gynecol 1987;157:944–950.
103. Preston JT, Cameron IT, Adams EJ, et al. Comparative study of tranexamic acid and norethisterone in the treatment of ovulatory menorrhagia. Br J Obstet Gynaecol 1995;102:401–406.
104. Bonnar J, Sheppard BL. Treatment of menorrhagia during menstruation: randomised controlled trial of ethamsylate, mefenamic acid, and tranexamic acid. BMJ 1996;313:579–582.
105. Munro MG. Abnormal uterine bleeding in the reproductive years. Part II—medical management. J Am Assoc Gynecol Laparosc 2000;7:19–32.
106. Lethaby A, Augood C, Duckitt K. Nonsteroidal Anti-Inflammatory Drugs for Heavy Menstrual Bleeding (Cochrane Review). The Cochrane Library, Issue 3. Chichester, UK: Wiley, 2004.
107. Lethaby A, Farquar C, Cooke I. Antifibrinolytics for heavy menstrual bleeding. Cochrane Database Syst Rev 2000;4:CD000249.
108. Lindoff C, Rybo G, Astedt B. Treatment with tranexamic acid during pregnancy, and the risk of thrombo-embolic complications. Thromb Haemost 1993;70:238–240.
109. Andersch B, Milsom I, Rybo G. An objective evaluation of flurbiprofen and tranexamic acid in the treatment of idiopathic menorrhagia. Acta Obstet Gynecol Scand 1988;67:645–648.
110. Fraser IS. Treatment of ovulatory and anovulatory dysfunctional uterine bleeding with oral progestogens. Aust N Z J Obstet Gynaecol 1990;30:352–356.

111. Lethaby A, Irvine G, Cameron I. Cyclical Progestogens for Heavy Menstrual Bleeding (Cochrane Review). The Cochrane Library, Issue 3. Chichester, UK: Wiley, 2004.
112. Lethaby AE, Cooke I, Rees M. Progesterone/Progestogen Releasing Intrauterine Systems for Heavy Menstrual Bleeding (Cochrane Review). The Cochrane Library, Issue 3. Chichester, UK: Wiley, 2004.
113. Hurskainen R, Teperi J, Rissanen P, et al. Quality of life and cost-effectiveness of levonorgestrel-releasing intrauterine system versus hysterectomy for treatment of menorrhagia: a randomized trial. Lancet 2001;357:273–277.
114. Irvine GA, Campbell-Brown MB, Lumsden MA, et al. Randomised comparative trial of the levonorgestrel intrauterine system and norethisterone for treatment of idiopathic menorrhagia. Br J Obstet Gynaecol 1988;105:592–598.
115. Crosignani PG, Vercellini P, Mosconi P, et al. Levonorgestrel-releasing intrauterine device versus hysteroscopic endometrial resection in the treatment of dysfunctional uterine bleeding. Obstet Gynecol 1997;90:257–263.
116. Istre O, Trolle B. Treatment of menorrhagia with the levonorgestrel system versus endometrial resection. Fertil Steril 2001;76:304–309.
117. Barrington JW, Bowen-Simpkins P. The levonorgestrel intrauterine system in the management of menorrhagia. Br J Obstet Gynaecol 1997;104:614–616.
118. Lahteenmaki P, Haukkamaa M, Puolakka J, et al. Open randomised study of use of levonorgestrel releasing intrauterine system as alternative to hysterectomy. BMJ 1998;316:1122–1126.
119. Ikomi A, Pepra EF. Efficacy of the levonorgestrel intrauterine system in treating menorrhagia: actualities and ambiguities. J Fam Plan Reprod Health Care 2002;28:99–100.
120. Higham JM, Shaw RW. A comparative study of danazol, a regimen of decreasing doses of danazol, and norethindrone in the treatment of objectively proven unexplained menorrhagia. Am J Obstet Gynecol 1993;169:1134–1139.
121. Irvine GA, Cameron IT. Medical management of dysfunctional uterine bleeding. Bailliere's Clin Obstet Gynecol 1999;13:189–202.
122. Lethaby A, Vollenhoven B, Sowter M. Pre-operative GnRH analogue therapy before hysterectomy or myomectomy for uterine fibroids. Cochrane Database Syst Rev 2001;2:CD000547.
123. Matta WH, Shaw RW, Nye M. Long-term follow-up of patients with uterine fibroids after treatment with the LHRH agonist buserelin. Br J Obstet Gynaecol 1989;96:200–206.
124. Gonzalez-Barcena D, Ochoa EP, et al. Treatment of uterine leiomyomas with luteinizing hormone releasing hormone antagonist Cetrorelix. Hum Reprod 1997;12:2028–2035.
125. Felberbaum RE, Ludwig M, Diedrich K. Medical treatment of uterine fibroids with the LHRH antagonist: Cetrorelix. Contracept Fertil Sex 1999;27:701–709.
126. Eisinger SH, Meldrum S, Fiscella K, et al. Low-dose mifepristone for uterine leiomyomata. Obstet Gynecol 2003;101:243–250.
127. Murphy AA, Kettel LM, Morales AJ, et al. Endometrial effects of long-term low-dose administration of RU486. Fertil Steril 1995;63:761–766.

CHAPTER 9

Hirsutism

Steven M. Strong

INTRODUCTION

Hirsutism describes the presence of male pattern hair growth in a woman. Excess facial and body hair is caused by the action of androgens on androgen-sensitive hair follicles. This socially distressing complaint is commonly encountered by all practitioners who care for women. The presentation may vary in degree, distribution, and chronicity. A thorough history and physical examination, supplemented in select cases with hormonal evaluations, distinguishes between the more commonly benign and rarely sinister underlying causes. The use of oral contraceptives (OCs) has been the cornerstone of treatment in most cases, and several new medications have more recently been evaluated.

PHYSIOLOGY OF HIRSUTISM

Androgen Production and Metabolism

The main circulating androgens in women are androstenedione, dehydroepiandrosterone (DHEA), dehydroepiandrosterone sulfate (DHEA-S), testosterone, and α-dihydrotestosterone (DHT). Among these, only testosterone and DHT have androgenic activity at the target cell.

Androstenedione is produced by both the zona reticularis of the adrenal gland and in the ovary, approximately 1 mg/day from each source. About 5% of androstenedione is converted in peripheral tissues to testosterone. DHEA is produced mainly in the adrenal, with smaller amounts from the ovary, and is peripherally converted in lesser quantities to testosterone. DHEA-S arises entirely from the adrenal gland.

The normal female produces about 0.3 mg/day of testosterone. One-third to one-half of testosterone is secreted directly from the ovary, and the remainder is converted peripherally from androstenedione and DHEA so approximately two-thirds of the total daily testosterone production is accounted for by the ovaries. In most hirsute women, the ovary is the major source of excess testosterone, due to both increased direct secretion and increased production of androstenedione for peripheral conversion (1).

Only about 1% of circulating testosterone is free, with 80 to 85% tightly bound to sex hormone binding globulin (SHBG), and the remainder weakly bound to albumin. The free and albumin-bound fractions are biologically active. Hepatic synthesis of SHBG increases in response to estrogens and decreases in response to androgens, obesity, corticosteroids, and acromegaly. Most hirsute women have significantly decreased levels of SHBG. Consequently, there is a substantial increase in bioavailable testosterone.

In hair follicles and other target tissues, testosterone is converted by 5α-reductase to DHT, a biologically more potent androgen. The production of DHT depends on the amount of circulating testosterone, the amount directly secreted and that peripherally converted from androstenedione and DHEA, and the 5α-reductase activity in the target tissue (2). DHT is metabolized to 3-androstenediol, which is then conjugated to 3-androstenediol glucuronide. Testosterone is metabolized to the 17-ketosteroids, androsterone and etiocholanolone, which are excreted in the urine.

Hair Growth

The pilosebaceous unit consists of a hair canal, sebaceous glands, a dermal papilla, and an arrector pili muscle. Hair growth occurs during the anagen phase when there is a proliferation of epidermal cells in contact with the dermal papilla, causing elongation and keratinization of the hair column. This is followed by involution of the matrix cells, or the catagen phase. A resting period, the telogen phase, follows, and the existing hair is shed at the initiation of the next anagen phase. Hair length is determined by the length of the anagen phase, and the occasional appearance of shedding corresponds to increased synchrony of the individual hair follicles.

There are three different types of hair. Lanugo is the lightly pigmented, short, thin, loosely attached hair that covers the fetus. Vellus hair is soft, lightly pigmented hair that covers the body during the prepubertal years. Thick, coarse, and highly pigmented terminal hair occurs only on the scalp and eyebrows before puberty. At adrenarche, pubic and axillary hair transforms from vellus to terminal hair in response to adrenal androgens. Hirsutism, an increase in male pattern hair growth, is caused by a transformation from vellus to terminal hair in the androgen-dependent follicles of the face, chest, lower abdomen, lower back, medial thighs, and pubic area. The amount of terminal hair growth, and thus the severity of the hirsutism, depends on the degree of androgen increase, the 5α-reductase activity in the pilosebaceous unit, and the density of hair follicles. Follicle density and 5α-reductase activity are genetically determined and vary significantly between ethnic groups.

DISORDERS ASSOCIATED WITH HIRSUTISM

Hirsutism may result from an increase in circulating androgens of ovarian, adrenal, or exogenous origin or from an increase in target hair follicle sensitivity to normal levels of androgen due to excess 5α-reductase activity. In addition to hirsutism, excess androgens may result in acne, oily skin, increased libido, and alopecia. Virilization describes the effects of pronounced hyperandrogenism with extreme hirsutism, clitoromegaly, deepening of the voice, and increased muscle mass. Hyperandrogenic chronic anovulation and idiopathic hirsutism account for most cases, although care must be taken to exclude more sinister causes (Table 9.1).

TABLE 9.1

Etiologies of Hirsutism and Virilization

Ovarian	Hyperandrogenic chronic anovulation
	Androgen-producing tumors
	Stromal hyperthecosis
	Luteoma of pregnancy/hyperreactio luteinalis
Skin	Idiopathic
Adrenal	Late-onset 21-hydroxylase deficiency
	Cushing's syndrome
	Androgen-producing tumors
Exogenous	Drugs

Hyperandrogenic Chronic Anovulation

Chronic anovulation with hyperandrogenism affects 5 to 10% of women in developed countries and accounts for more than one-third of all cases of anovulation. Stein and Leventhal (3) first described a syndrome of obesity, oligomenorrhea, hirsutism, and enlarged polycystic ovaries in 1935. As the complex hormonal alterations that give rise to this syndrome have been elucidated, many authors proposed that the term *hyperandrogenic chronic anovulation* replace the traditional polycystic ovary syndrome (PCO). Indeed, several authors showed that only 70 to 80% of women with menstrual irregularity and elevated androgens, and as many as 25% of normal women, have sonographically confirmed polycystic ovaries (4, 5). In addition, although obesity in conjunction with PCO is common, it is not always present for anovulation and hirsutism to occur. The change in terminology to hyperandrogenic chronic anovulation is also supported in the most recent American College of Obstetricians and Gynecologists (ACOG) technical bulletin (6).

Patients with hyperandrogenic chronic anovulation often present with a gradual onset of symptoms of androgen excess and menstrual irregularity that usually begin perimenarcheally, although sometimes they may follow a period of weight gain. If these women began OCs shortly after menarche, they may report the onset of symptoms on discontinuation of the pill. Acne and mild to moderate hirsutism are common, but the occasional woman will exhibit severe hirsutism and alopecia. Anovulation usually presents as oligomenorrhea but varies from amenorrhea to metrorrhagia.

Although the precise initiating factor is not clear, several interrelated endocrinologic abnormalities have been described. A tonically elevated level of luteinizing hormone (LH) exists, resulting from either an increased pulsatility of gonadotropin-releasing hormone (GnRH) or heightened sensitivity of the anterior pituitary to normal GnRH levels (7). The tonic elevation of LH increases the production of testosterone and androstenedione in ovarian theca cells. Some of this testosterone and androstenedione is converted to estrone peripherally, resulting in an increase in estrogen levels. This elevation of circulating androgens inhibits production of SHBG in the liver, resulting in increased amounts of bioavailable, non–SHBG-bound testosterone. The decreased SHBG also results in an increase in bioavailable estradiol. This inhibits follicle-stimulating hormone (FSH) release from the pituitary and may even increase the pulsatility of GnRH (contributing to tonically elevated LH levels). FSH depression results in decreased aromatase activity in the granulosa cells, so little of the excess androgen is converted to estradiol and most is released into the circulation. Persistently low FSH levels allow the recruitment of multiple early follicles, but a dominant follicle is not permitted to mature, thus giving rise to anovulation and polycystic ovaries.

Although patients with hyperandrogenic chronic anovulation suffer from symptoms of androgen excess, it is important to realize they are also exposed to tonically elevated levels of estrogen. As mentioned previously, estrogen levels are increased in two ways in hyperandrogenic chronic anovulation: the decrease in SHBG results in increased amounts of bioavailable estrogen, and conversion of testosterone and androstenedione peripherally results in increased levels of estrone. This chronic exposure to relatively unopposed levels of estrogen increases the risk of endometrial hyperplasia and/or endometrial carcinoma in these patients.

Insulin resistance is common in women with hyperandrogenic anovulation and has even been shown in anovulatory adolescents (8). Elevated serum insulin levels may manifest as acanthosis nigricans, a velvety gray-brown skin discoloration, usually at the neck, axilla, and groin. Several more recent reports addressed the link between hyperandrogenism and insulin resistance (9). The action of insulinlike growth factor 1 (IGF-1) at its receptor augments LH-induced androgen production. Because of the homology between insulin and IGF-1, insulin also acts on the IGF-1 receptor to increase androgen synthesis. In addition, insulin decreases granulosa cell production of IGF-1-binding protein (resulting in increased free IGF-1) and directly inhibits hepatic SHBG production. Researchers demonstrated a decrease in circulating androgens when serum insulin levels were decreased with diazoxide (Hyperstat), metformin (Glucophage), or troglitazone (Rezulin) (10–12). Although one study found that suppressing androgen levels with a GnRH analog partially reversed insulin resistance in nonobese patients with PCO, others have been unable to confirm that hyperandrogenemia contributes to insulin resistance (13).

Obesity, affecting 50 to 80% of women with hyperandrogenic anovulation, contributes to the endocrinologic alterations in several ways (14). Increased android obesity worsens insulin resistance (15). Obesity is also associated with a decrease in SHBG and an increase in peripheral conversion of androgens to estrone (16).

In addition to hirsutism and menstrual irregularity, women with hyperandrogenic anovulation are subject to serious long-term health risks. Chronic unopposed estrogen can lead to endometrial hyperplasia and adenocarcinoma (17). A higher incidence of hypertension and diabetes has been noted in women treated for PCO (18). More recent studies addressed the association between increased cardiovascular risk and hyperandrogenism. Both elevated androgens and insulin resistance correlate with decreased high-density lipoprotein, increased triglycerides, and increased very low-density lipoprotein. These alterations confer a higher risk of coronary artery disease (19–21). Current evidence suggests that insulin resistance is the more important modifier of cardiovascular risk and that hyperandrogenism plays a smaller role or may only be a marker for hyperinsulinemia (22).

Variation in the severity of hirsutism depends on the increase in bioavailable testosterone, on follicle density, and on the level of 5α-reductase activity in the skin. A study of Japanese women diagnosed with PCO revealed levels of circulating androgens, SHBG, and serum insulin similar to those in Caucasian women with PCO, but hirsutism was uncommon in the Japanese women (23). Analysis of androgen levels in oligo-ovulatory women in the United States without hirsutism has shown that 19% have elevations in free testosterone and that the testosterone level correlated with the degree of menstrual irregularity (24). It remains to be determined whether these women are subject to similar long-term sequelae. For a graphic display of these interrelated endocrinologic processes, see Figure 9.1.

Idiopathic Hirsutism

More than one-third of women with hirsutism ovulate regularly. Because serum androgen levels in these women are most often normal, this has been called idiopathic hirsutism. Seen in certain ethnic groups and within certain families, hirsutism is gradual in onset and menses are regular. Increased 5α-reductase activity causing a local increase in DHT has been demonstrated in the

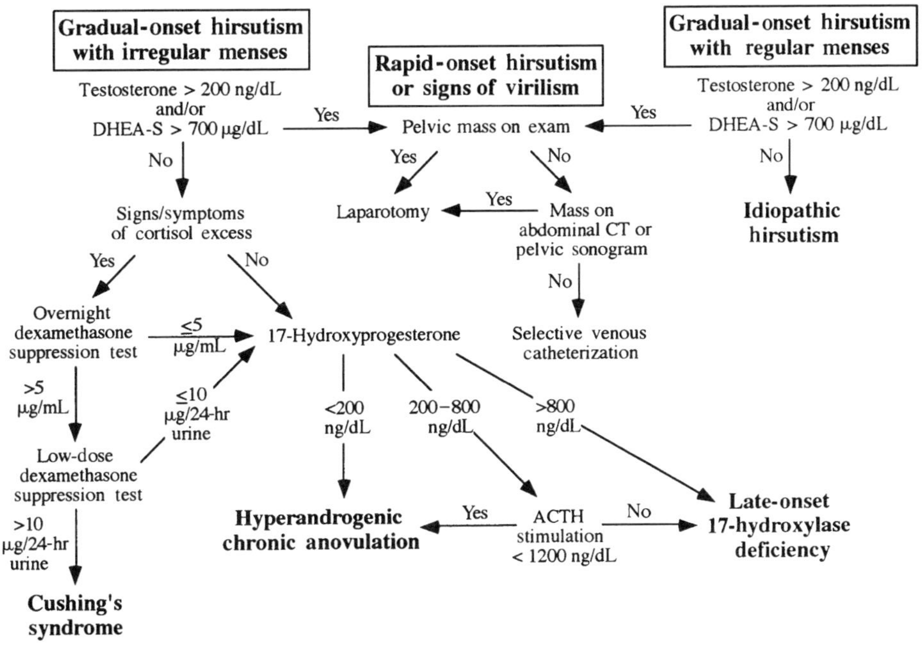

FIGURE 9.1 • Evaluation of hirsutism. ACTH, corticotropin; CT, computed tomography; DHEA-S, dehydroepiandrosterone-sulfate.

skin of these women (25). This entity should therefore be considered one of enhanced peripheral conversion of testosterone to DHT.

Because DHT is metabolized rapidly to androstenediol glucuronide, many authors attempted to measure 5α-reductase activity by measuring androstenediol glucuronide (26). Assessment of the clinical utility of this measurement is mixed (27). Androstenediol precursors arise primarily from the adrenal gland, and most glucuronidation occurs in the liver (28). Use of the 5α-reductase inhibitor finasteride has resulted in a decrease in serum androstenediol glucuronide along with a reduction in hirsutism (29–32).

Late-Onset 21-Hydroxylase Deficiency

Congenital adrenal hyperplasia is an inherited disorder of cortisol synthesis usually caused by a defect in the 21-hydroxylase enzyme and less commonly by defects in the 11-hydroxylase or 3-hydroxysteroid dehydrogenase enzymes. In the classic form, ambiguous genitalia and virilism occur in affected females. This is due to an accumulation of the 21-hydroxylase substrate 17-hydroxyprogesterone (17-OHP) that is converted to androstenedione and DHEA. A deficiency in aldosterone results in salt wasting in 75% of cases. The incidence of classic congenital adrenal hyperplasia is 1 in 1400 births.

A milder enzymatic defect results in a delay of symptoms until after puberty and so has been referred to as nonclassic congenital adrenal hyperplasia, late-onset congenital adrenal hyperplasia, or late-onset 21-hydroxylase deficiency (LOHD). The overall frequency is 0.1 to 1%, although it has been found in 3 to 9% of hirsute women. Affected women present nearly identically to those with hyperandrogenic chronic anovulation, with gradually worsening hirsutism and menstrual irregularity beginning in the perimenarcheal time period. Nearly all women with LOHD have oligomenorrhea or amenorrhea (33). Hirsutism varies from mild to severe, but virilization is rare. Although earlier reports stated that these patients are often tall in childhood and short in adulthood, as seen in those afflicted with the classic form of the disease, larger series have shown that short stature is uncommon (34).

Mutations at the gene locus for 21-hydroxylase on chromosome 6 may result in an enzyme with minimal or no activity (the severe allele) or partial activity (the mild allele). Homozygotes for the severe allele suffer from classic congenital adrenal hyperplasia. Homozygotes for the mild allele or compound heterozygotes with one mild and one severe allele manifest LOHD. Women with cryptic adrenal hyperplasia, a carrier state with one mild or one severe allele, have no symptoms and are discovered only by DNA or biochemical analysis.

Patients may be screened for LOHD by measuring serum 17-OHP levels. The 17-OHP level must be drawn in the morning because of variation in response to the diurnal pattern of corticotropin (ACTH). If the level of 17-OHP is greater than 800 ng/dL, LOHD is present. If the level is less than 200 ng/dL, an enzyme defect does not account for the presence of hirsutism. If the level is less than 800 ng/dL but greater than 200 ng/dL, an ACTH stimulation test should be performed. For this test, basal serum levels of 17-OHP are drawn in the morning and 1 hour after an infusion of 25 μg of synthetic ACTH. A level of 17-OHP greater than 1200 ng/dL in response to ACTH establishes a diagnosis of LOHD.

There is disagreement regarding the need to screen for LOHD. Treatment of LOHD depends on the patient's desires and concerns. For women most bothered by hirsutism, antiandrogens (e.g., spironolactone [Aldactone] or cyproterone [Androcur or Cyprostat]) are superior to glucocorticoids for therapy. For women desiring pregnancy, clomiphene is superior to glucocorticoids for the induction of ovulation, although many women do have resumption of ovulatory cycles and arrest of hirsutism when treated with dexamethasone 0.5 mg nightly. Women with LOHD who become pregnant may choose to undergo genetic counseling and testing for paternal carrier status so antenatal glucocorticoid therapy can be initiated for female fetuses at risk for classic 21-hydroxylase deficiency.

Cushing's Syndrome

Cushing's syndrome is a persistent increase in cortisol secretion. Cortisol excess may result from pituitary ACTH production (Cushing's disease), ectopic ACTH production by tumors, cortisol-secreting adrenal tumors, or, rarely, cortisol-secreting ovarian tumors. Women are affected five times as frequently as men, and the mean age at onset is 33 years. Findings include central obesity with moon facies, a dorsal cervical fat pad (buffalo hump), striae, ecchymoses, muscle weakness, hypertension, osteoporosis, and glucose intolerance. Of hirsute women, only those with other signs or symptoms suggestive of cortisol excess should be screened for Cushing's syndrome.

An overnight dexamethasone suppression test should be performed initially. A single dose of 1 mg dexamethasone is taken at bedtime, and plasma cortisol is measured at 8 AM. A value less than 5 μg/dL excludes Cushing's syndrome. Obese patients have false-positive rates as high as 13%. If the level is above 5 μg/dL, a low-dose suppression test is performed in which 0.5 mg of dexamethasone is given every 4 hours for 2 days. Failure to suppress the 24-hour urinary free cortisol below 10 μg on the second day establishes the diagnosis of Cushing's syndrome but does not determine the precise etiology.

Androgen-Producing Tumors

Androgen-secreting tumors as a cause of hirsutism or virilism are extremely rare. Suspicion should be aroused when signs of severe hirsutism or virilization rapidly progress over the course of several months.

Although Sertoli-Leydig and hilus cell tumors account for less than 1% of ovarian neoplasms, they are the only ovarian tumors that frequently produce excess testosterone. One-third of Sertoli-Leydig and three-fourths of hilus cell tumors produce very high levels of testosterone, resulting in virilization. The patient usually notes the onset of oligomenorrhea followed by amenorrhea, acne, and hirsutism within a few months. This rapidly progresses to temporal balding, deepening of the voice, clitoromegaly, and breast atrophy. Sertoli-Leydig cell tumors occur most often in women younger than 30 years of age. They are usually unilateral well-differentiated tumors, and 85% are palpable by the time symptoms are produced. Hilus cell tumors are almost always benign, usually occur after menopause, and are not palpable.

Adrenal cortical carcinoma has an incidence of about 1 in 1 million. Five percent of women with adrenal carcinoma have hirsutism. Benign adrenal adenomas may cause hirsutism, although this is rare. Functioning tumors may produce signs and symptoms relating to excess production of androgens, mineralocorticoids, and/or glucocorticoids. About half of women with adrenal tumors producing hirsutism also manifest Cushing's syndrome.

A testosterone level of 200 ng/dL has traditionally been used as a threshold for further evaluation of a possible ovarian or adrenal neoplasm. A DHEA-S level of greater than 700 μg/dL has been used as a marker for adrenal tumors. However, case series have been reported in which several patients with adrenal cortical carcinoma had levels of testosterone and DHEA-S that were elevated but fell below these cutoffs (35). Therefore, the presence of severe and rapidly progressing virilism, along with any increase in androgen levels, should dictate a search for ovarian or adrenal tumors, regardless of the absolute DHEA-S or testosterone levels.

When an androgen-producing neoplasm is suspected, a pelvic examination, pelvic sonogram, and computed tomography (CT) of the adrenals are the most important diagnostic procedures needed. Dexamethasone suppression has been used to establish adrenal versus ovarian origin and distinguish tumor from nontumor. However, this test is nether as sensitive nor as specific as radiologic imaging. Because selective catheterization of adrenal and ovarian veins is technically difficult, it should be reserved for those patients in which the presence of a tumor is strongly suspected but in which radiologic studies are negative.

Ovarian Stromal Hyperthecosis

Ovarian stromal hyperthecosis is an uncommon benign disorder in which the ovaries produce large amounts of testosterone. The ovaries are bilaterally enlarged, and nests of luteinized theca cells are seen on microscopic examination.

Menstrual irregularity is observed first, followed by gradually increasing hirsutism. Signs of hirsutism progress gradually, as in hyperandrogenic chronic anovulation, but when left untreated may result in more severe masculinization with temporal balding, deepening of the voice, and clitoromegaly. Signs and symptoms may appear early in life or may not appear until after the menopause. Although the severe virilization and testosterone elevation (often higher than 200 ng/dL) can mimic an androgen-producing tumor, symptoms usually progress much more slowly than those from neoplastic causes.

The diagnosis should be suspected in the presence of severe hirsutism, elevated testosterone levels, and enlarged ovaries. It is confirmed by histopathologic examination. Treatment has usually been bilateral oophorectomy, but there has been more recent success with GnRH agonists (36). It must be stressed that a response to GnRH agonists should not be used to exclude a diagnosis of tumor because testosterone production by some Sertoli-Leydig cell tumors may be suppressed by these medications (37).

Pregnancy-Related Conditions

Two rare conditions specific to pregnancy can result in hirsutism or virilism. Luteoma of pregnancy, a solid ovarian enlargement that produces large amounts of testosterone, results from an exaggeration of the normal luteinization reaction of the ovary. Hyperreactio luteinalis is a benign cystic enlargement of the ovary associated with high levels of human chorionic gonadotropin. These lesions regress postpartum but may recur in subsequent pregnancies. Although virilization of a female fetus has been reported, androgen levels in the umbilical cord are usually normal because of the high capacity of the placenta to convert androgens to estrogen (38).

Drugs

Several medications are associated with androgenic side effects. Oral and parenteral testosterone, alone or in combination with estrogen, has been used in postmenopausal and oophorectomized women to increase libido (39). Danazol (Danocrine) is sometimes used in the treatment of endometriosis and mastodynia. Systemic absorption of topical testosterone in the treatment of lichen sclerosus can cause elevated testosterone levels, and a few case reports documented severe virilization as a result (40). Various anabolic steroids bring about masculinization in addition to other serious health risks. Although some of the progestin components of OC pills are 19-nortestosterone derivatives and retain some androgenic activity, the very low doses in current formulations are unlikely to cause hirsutism. Hypertrichosis, an increase in nonandrogendependent hair, can be seen with cyclosporin (Sandimmune, Neoral), diazoxide (Hyperstat), minoxidil (Loniten), and phenytoin (Dilantin).

EVALUATION OF THE PATIENT WITH HIRSUTISM

The etiology of hirsutism in most cases may be determined with a careful history and physical examination. A concerned, sympathetic approach is important because hirsutism can greatly affect a woman's sense of femininity, attractiveness, and social acceptance. Because treatment must be undertaken for many months before results appear, a trusting relationship is necessary for the patient to persist in therapy.

The duration and extent of hirsutism are critical in distinguishing common benign causes, usually with early onset and gradual progression, from rare sinister causes, usually with rapid progression of severe hirsutism over several months. The presence of other symptoms of androgen excess, acne, or alopecia should be elicited. If cosmetic measures such as shaving, plucking, or use of depilatories are practiced, noting the frequency of use aids in assessing severity and measuring treatment effectiveness. A menstrual history establishes the likelihood of ovulation. A thorough medication history can exclude iatrogenic causes. A family history may reveal a familial pattern of hirsutism or point to the possibility of hydroxylase deficiency. A review of symptoms is important to look for evidence of cortisol excess.

The location and degree of hair growth should be noted at the physical examination and carefully recorded. Several scoring systems have been created to grade hirsutism. The system by Ferriman and Gallwey (41) assesses hair in each of nine androgensensitive body areas on a scale of 0 to 4 with total scores above 8 or 10 defining clinically significant hirsutism

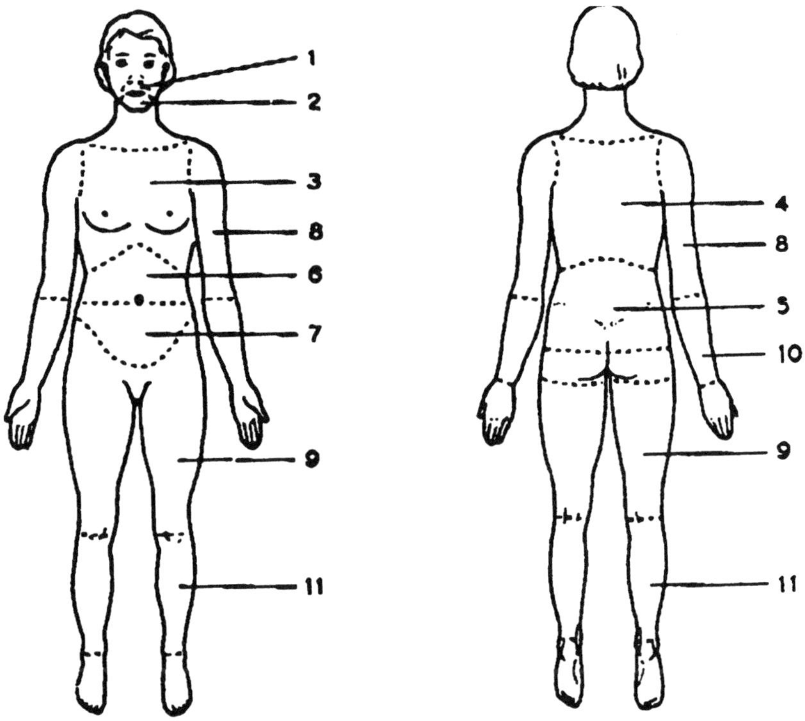

FIGURE 9.2 ● Demarcation of 11 sites used for numerically grading amount of hair growth—anterior and posterior views. (Reprinted with permission from Ferriman D, Gallwey J. Clinical assessment of body hair growth in women. J Clin Endocrinol Metab 1961;21: 1440–1447. © The Endocrine Society.)

(Fig. 9.2 and Table 9.2). An alternative is the Lorenzo method (42), in which hair growth is graded on the chin and anterior neck, upper lip, chest, abdomen, thighs, and forearms. Signs of virilization, including breast atrophy and clitoromegaly, often indicate an androgen-producing neoplasm. An adnexal or abdominal mass suggests an ovarian or adrenal tumor. Acanthosis nigricans should raise the suspicion of insulin resistance. Signs of cortisol excess warrant testing for Cushing's syndrome.

After the initial history and physical examination, further evaluation is guided by dividing hirsute women into three categories: those with a gradual onset of hirsutism and regular menses, those with a gradual onset of hirsutism and irregular menses, and those with a rapid onset of hirsutism or signs of virilism.

Gradual-Onset Hirsutism and Regular Menses

The gradual onset of mild to moderate hirsutism with regular menses supports a diagnosis of idiopathic hirsutism with increased peripheral conversion of testosterone to DHT. Although a neoplastic cause is extraordinarily unlikely, serum levels of testosterone and DHEA-S may be assessed for reassurance. For a summary of evaluative treatment plans for these categories, see Figure 9.3.

Gradual-Onset Hirsutism and Irregular Menses

A woman with long-standing hirsutism and irregular menses likely has hyperandrogenic chronic anovulation. Serum testosterone and DHEA-S are useful in ruling out ovarian or adrenal tumors. The serum testosterone level may be mildly elevated or even normal. However, the decrease in

TABLE 9.2

Definition of Hair Gradings at 11 Sites[a]

Site	Grade	Definition
Upper lip	1	Few hairs at outer margin
	2	Small moustache at outer margin
	3	Moustache extending halfway from outer margin
	4	Moustache extending to midline
Chin	1	Few scattered hairs
	2	Scattered hairs with small concentration
	3 and 4	Complete cover, light and heavy
Chest	1	Circumareolar hairs
	2	With midline hair in addition
	3	Fusion of these areas, with three-quarters cover
	4	Complete cover
Upper back	1	Few scattered hairs
	2	Rather more, still scattered
	3 and 4	Complete cover, light and heavy
Lower back	1	Sacral tuft of hair
	2	With some lateral extension
	3	Three-quarters cover
	4	Complete cover
Upper abdomen	1	Few midline hairs
	2	Rather more, still midline
	3 and 4	Half and full cover
Lower abdomen	1	Few midline hairs
	2	Midline streak of hair
	3	Midline band of hair
	4	Inverted V-shaped growth
Arm	1	Sparse growth affecting not more than one quarter of limb surface
	2	More than this; cover still incomplete
	3 and 4	Complete cover, light and heavy
Forearm	1, 2, 3, 4	Complete cover of dorsal surface: 2 grades of light and 2 of heavy growth
Thigh	1, 2, 3, 4	As for arm
Leg	1, 2, 3, 4	As for arm

Reprinted with permission from Ferriman D, Gallwey J. Clinical assessment of body hair growth in women. J Clin Endocrinol Metab 1961;21:1440–1447. © The Endocrine Society.

[a] Grade 0 at all sites indicates absence of terminal hair.

SHBG in hirsute women greatly increases the amount of bioavailable testosterone. Measurement of the free or non–SHBG-bound testosterone level is unnecessary because the presence of hirsutism alone is evidence that an excess in biologically active testosterone exists. Although the LH level is typically elevated, the normal range for LH is broad and the LH:FSH ratio is highly variable so neither the LH level itself nor the LH:FSH ratio adds useful information (7). A morning 17-OHP level should be drawn to screen for LOHD because its presentation is often similar to that of hyperandrogenic chronic anovulation.

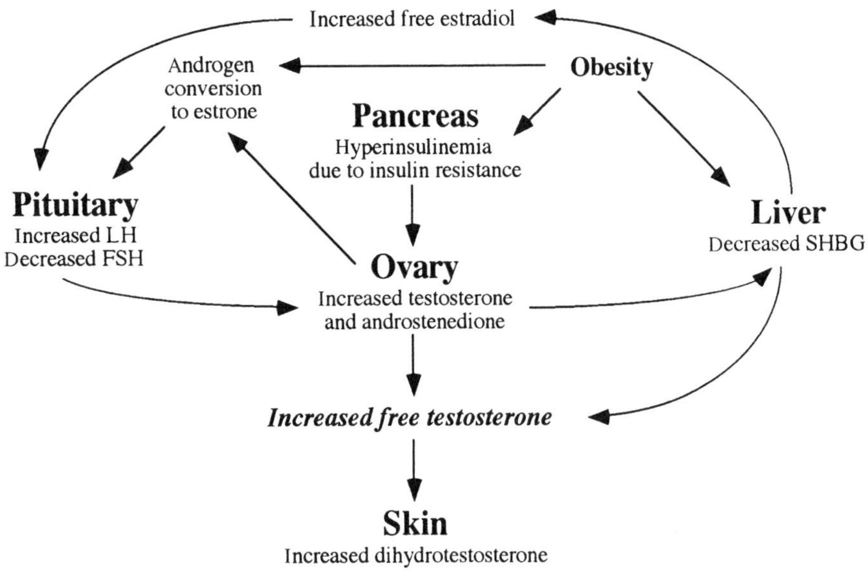

FIGURE 9.3 ● Hormonal and biochemical interactions in hyperandrogenic chronic anovulation. FSH, follicle-stimulating hormone; LH, luteinizing hormone; SHBG, sex hormone binding globulin.

Anovulation is evaluated with a thyroid-stimulating hormone and prolactin level. If amenorrhea is present, a progestin challenge is added. With long-standing anovulation, an endometrial biopsy should be performed to rule out endometrial hyperplasia or carcinoma from unopposed estrogen stimulation. The association of hyperandrogenic chronic anovulation and lipid abnormalities warrants a lipid profile. Because insulin resistance plays a significant role in the pathogenesis of hyperandrogenism, glucose tolerance should be evaluated, especially if acanthosis nigricans is found.

Rapid-Onset Hirsutism or Virilism

The rapid progression of severe hirsutism or virilism over several months suggests an androgen-producing tumor. Androgen levels are usually very high but may be only slightly elevated. In about half of all cases of adrenal tumors, patients exhibit features of Cushing's syndrome. Most androgen-producing ovarian tumors are palpable on pelvic examination. If a tumor is suspected, a pelvic sonogram and an abdominal CT should be obtained. Suppression and stimulation testing have little value in distinguishing an ovarian from an adrenal source (43). When there is a marked elevation in androgen level and the radiologic studies fail to localize a source, selective venous catheterization may be performed.

TREATMENT OF HIRSUTISM AND ASSOCIATED ANDROGENIC DISORDERS

The treatment of uncommon causes of hirsutism is usually straightforward. Androgenic medications should be discontinued. Hyperreactio luteinalis and luteoma resolve postpartum so expectant management and cosmetic measures are used. Ovarian tumors require surgical removal, most often a total abdominal hysterectomy and bilateral salpingo-oophorectomy, although a unilateral adnexectomy may be performed for a unilateral well-differentiated Sertoli-Leydig tumor in a woman who wants to preserve fertility. Adrenal tumors are removed operatively. Bilateral salpingo-oophorectomy has traditionally been performed for ovarian stromal hyperthecosis. Although successful treatment of stromal hyperthecosis with a GnRH analog has recently been reported in four postmenopausal women, further follow-up is needed to assess long-term efficacy (36).

TABLE 9.3

Treatment of Hyperandrogenism

Weight loss
Medications
Combination oral contraceptives
Progesterone
Gonadotrophin-releasing hormone analogs
Spironolactone
Drospirenone
Cyproterone acetate
Ketoconazole
Flutamide
Finasteride
Glucocorticoids
Eflornithine
Metformin
Cosmesis
Shaving
Plucking
Depilatories
Electrolysis
Laser

In most remaining cases of hirsutism, treatment involves suppressing ovarian or adrenal androgen production and blocking androgen action at the skin, either by competitively inhibiting androgen receptors or by inhibiting 5α-reductase.

Hyperandrogenic Chronic Anovulation

Table 9.3 is a summary of the multiple modalities of treatment for hyperandrogenic symptoms.

Weight Loss

Weight loss is an essential, although often underemphasized, element in treating patients with hyperandrogenic chronic anovulation who are obese. Obesity decreases serum SHBG levels and enhances insulin resistance, thereby increasing both total androgen production and the free fraction of testosterone.

Several studies demonstrated a rise in SHBG, a decrease in total and free testosterone, an improvement in Ferriman-Gallwey score, and a decrease in serum insulin in response to weight reduction (44, 45). In addition, the resumption of ovulation has been observed with regular menses and successful pregnancies (46). Although many therapies are effective in treating hirsutism, only weight loss has been proven beneficial in modifying the associated insulin resistance, hypertension, and lipid abnormalities. Advice on regular exercise and a sensible diet should be given.

Combination Oral Contraceptives

In hirsute women not currently desiring pregnancy, combined estrogen–progestin OC pills are inexpensive, easy to administer, and effective in reducing excess hair growth.

OCs act through several mechanisms to decrease the amount of bioavailable androgens and ameliorate hirsutism and acne. OCs suppress ovarian androgen production by suppressing LH, although the LH suppression is highly variable and the LH:FSH ratio is not affected. OCs increase SHBG levels, which results in decreased amounts of circulating free testosterone. Some studies found a greater rise in SHBG with OCs containing desogestrel or norgestimate (47, 48).

Because of the length of the hair growth cycle, an observable decrease in hair growth requires at least 6 months of treatment. The addition of an antiandrogen improves the response, but prolonged treatment is still necessary. Acne usually responds more rapidly. Randomized trials of low-dose combination OCs with different progestin components do not show consistent differences between various formulations. Although only one OC preparation has been U.S. Food and Drug Administration approved for a marketing claim of acne improvement, all low-dose combination OCs cause a similar decrease in free testosterone levels, which is the presumed mechanism for the improvment in acne (49, 50). Low-dose OCs are as effective as higher-dose preparations. Multiphasic OCs are as effective as monophasic OCs. Those with low-dose levonorgestrel, which is known to cause acne at high doses, are equally beneficial in treating hirsutism. Newer OCs with desogestrel and norgestimate are often recommended because of their lower androgenic activity and because they are associated with a greater increase in SHBG. However, no studies have yet documented a clinical advantage for these third-generation OCs in the treatment of hirsutism.

Additional benefits of OCs include regulation of menses and a decreased risk of both endometrial hyperplasia and cancer. In chronically anovulatory women in whom OCs are contraindicated or unacceptable, periodic withdrawal bleeding should be induced with progestin to decrease these risks.

Gonadotropin-Releasing Hormone Agonists

GnRH agonists suppress pituitary gonadotropin secretion, resulting in decreased ovarian androgen production, and hence are effective in decreasing hirsutism. Gonadotropin suppression also causes a hypoestrogenic state that results in menopausal symptoms and decreased bone density. Estrogen, usually in the form of OCs, is often added to avoid bone demineralization and ameliorate symptoms.

A more recent randomized trial comparing the combination of an OC and a GnRH agonist with either agent alone found that the GnRH agonist alone resulted in a greater reduction in Ferriman-Gallwey score at 6 months and an unacceptable decrease in bone density. The GnRH agonist-OC combination resulted in a greater score reduction than the OC alone at 3 months, but at 6 months the decrease in Ferriman-Gallwey score was equivalent, indicating a more rapid initial response with the combination, but overall equal efficacy (51). Others confirmed similar efficacy between the OC-GnRH agonist combination and OCs alone (52).

Because GnRH agonists are very expensive and their use in conjunction with OCs appears to add little additional long-term benefit, most women should be treated with an OC alone. Bisphosphonates have been shown to preserve bone density when given with a GnRH agonist so the combination of alendronate (Fosamax) and a GnRH agonist might be used where a contraindication to estrogen exists (53).

Spironolactone

Spironolactone (Aldactone) is a synthetic steroidal aldosterone antagonist used as a potassium-sparing diuretic in the treatment of hypertension. Its antiandrogenic action is three-fold: (a) it competitively binds the DHT receptor, (b) it decreases androgen production by inhibiting cytochrome P450, and (c) it inhibits 5α-reductase activity. Of these mechanisms, competitive inhibition at the DHT receptor appears most important. In addition, spironolactone has weak progestational activity.

Spironolactone is administered in doses of 25 to 100 mg twice daily. Clinical improvement usually requires 6 months of treatment. Results have been noted as early as 3 months with the higher dose (200 mg/day), but side effects are also increased (54). Side effects are mild and include diuresis and fatigue. Significant hyperkalemia in patients without renal disease does not occur. Because of its progestational activity, irregular menses are common, with a 25% frequency seen with 100 mg/day and a frequency greater than 50% seen at 200 mg/day (55). There is a theoretic risk of feminization of a male fetus; therefore, contraception is necessary.

The use of an OC with spironolactone regulates menses, further suppresses androgen production, and provides contraception. Studies with the OC-spironolactone combination demonstrate greater reductions in the Ferriman-Gallwey score than those with spironolactone alone, but the two regimens have not been compared in a single study (32, 56, 57). Daily OC use with spironolactone, 50 mg twice daily, has similar efficacy to the use of cyproterone, 50 mg/day, with ethinyl estradiol (57, 58).

Impressive efficacy, low-risk profile, and low cost make spironolactone, in conjunction with an OC, a good choice for women with hyperandrogenic chronic anovulation.

Drospirenone

Drospirenone is a synthetic progestogen used in the new OC Yasmin. Unlike progestogens contained in other OCs available in the United States, drospirenone exhibits antiandrogenic activity. Animal studies have found drospirenone to be about one-third as antiandrogenic as cyproterone acetate (59). Although Yasmin is a well-tolerated, effective contraceptive with the theoretic advantage of an antiandrogenic progestin, there have not yet been any studies showing Yasmin to be more effective than other OCs in alleviating hirsutism.

Cyproterone

Cyproterone acetate is a steroidal progestogen derived from 17-OHP. It is not approved for use in the United States but is marketed in other countries as a component of the contraceptives "Diane" (2 mg cyproterone acetate and 50 μg ethinylestradiol) and "Dianette" (2 mg cyproterone acetate and 35 μg ethinyl estradiol). It decreases androgen production by suppressing LH secretion and competitively inhibits testosterone and DHT at their intracellular receptors.

A higher dose of cyproterone is commonly used for the treatment of hirsutism. Because of its progestational activity and long half-life, it is administered with oral ethinyl estradiol in a reversed sequential regimen, 50 to 100 mg of cyproterone on days 5 to 14, with 35 μg ethinyl estradiol on days 5 to 25. Significant improvement in hirsutism has been noted within 3 months with this high-dose regimen. Although some studies found that a 2-mg dose yields results similar to higher doses at 12 months, a faster initial response with the higher doses has been documented (60, 61).

Side effects include weight gain, edema, diminished libido, headache, nausea, fatigue, and mood swings (61). Overall, however, it is well tolerated. Rare cases of hepatotoxicity have been reported in women taking cyproterone, but a causal relationship has not been established.

Ketoconazole

Ketoconazole (Nizoral) is an imidazole derivative active as an antifungal. It suppresses both adrenal and ovarian synthesis of androgens by inhibiting the 17,20-desmolase, 17-hydroxylase, and 11β-hydroxylase enzymes. Improvement may be seen in patients who complete at least 6 months of 400 mg/day therapy (62). There is a very high rate of discontinuation, however, because of frequent side effects such as headache, nausea, fatigue, and loss of scalp hair (63). Serious hepatotoxicity has also been reported. Because of poor tolerability and risk of hepatotoxicity, ketoconazole should not be used long term or as a first-line agent.

Flutamide

Flutamide (Eulexin) is a nonsteroidal antiandrogen used in the treatment of prostatic cancer. It acts primarily by competitive inhibition at the DHT receptor. Although the affinity of flutamide for the DHT receptor is much less than that of spironolactone, its lack of progestational or mineralocorticoid activity allows it to be given in much higher doses. It also suppresses adrenal androgen production by inhibiting 17,20-desmolase. At a dose of 125 mg two or three times a day, flutamide is equally as effective as spironolactone (64). Minor side effects include dry skin and increased appetite. Drug-induced hepatitis has occurred in 0.5% of men receiving flutamide and has been reported in one woman being treated for hirsutism (65, 66). Because of the risk of drug-induced hepatitis and its high cost, flutamide is not recommended for the initial treatment of hirsutism.

Cimetidine

Cimetidine (Tagamet) blocks the type 2 histamine receptor and is prescribed for peptic ulcer and gastroesophageal reflux. Because of its weak affinity for the androgen receptors, it has been investigated as a treatment for hirsutism. Results have been disappointing, with minimal clinical effect at doses up to 1200 mg/day (67). It is not recommended for the treatment of hirsutism.

Finasteride

Finasteride has also been used in the treatment of prostatic cancer (Proscar) and male-pattern baldness (Propecia). A 5α-reductase inhibitor, it blocks peripheral conversion of testosterone to DHT. A dose of 5 mg/day results in a reduction in Ferriman-Gallwey score, along with a lowering of serum DHT and androstenediol glucuronide (29–32). Clinical efficacy is similar to spironolactone (32). Doses of up to 400 mg/day have been given in men without significant side effects. Because of potential teratogenic effects, reliable contraception is necessary.

Finasteride may be the drug of choice for hirsutism in the future with its lack of side effects and good clinical response. However, the medication is costly, and further experience is needed to ensure safety.

Glucocorticoids

Prednisone, 5 to 7.5 mg/day, or dexamethasone, 0.5 mg/day, suppresses adrenal androgen production. Glucocorticoids are often used as the first-line therapy for LOHD. Its efficacy in treating hirsutism in patients with hyperandrogenic chronic anovulation with an ovarian origin is inferior to that of OCs or spironolactone. The fact that the ovary is the major source of excess androgen in these patients probably accounts for the poor response. Weight gain and depression are frequent side effects, and its use may exacerbate insulin resistance.

Eflornithine

Topical eflornithine (Vaniqa) is a specific, irreversible inhibitor of ornithine decarboxylase. Applied twice daily as a 13.9% cream, eflornithine reduces hair growth significantly compared with placebo (47% versus 15% reduction in hair length). Clinically, 58% of eflornithine and 34% of placebo recipients had some improvement in facial hirsutism, and 32% versus 8% were successfully treated, experiencing at least marked improvement (68). Systemic absorption is minimal, and side effects are limited to mild, local discomfort.

Cosmetic Measures

There are several widely used methods for the temporary removal of unwanted hair. Depilatory creams remove hair by dissolving disuffide bonds. These creams sometimes cause skin irritation and allergic dermatitis. Shaving does not stimulate hair growth but does result in stubble, which gives the appearance of thicker, coarser hair. In addition, shaving may further threaten a woman's sense of femininity and gender identity. Waxing is effective but may be time consuming and expensive. Electrolysis involves permanent hair removal by destruction of the dermal papilla with electric current.

Laser is rapidly coming into widespread use as an effective tool in hair removal. Several types of laser, now found in many plastic surgeons' and dermatologists' offices, provide safe and permanent removal of unwanted hair (69, 70). Intense marketing has helped increase use, but high cost limits its availability to many women.

Attempts at permanent hair removal without addressing the underlying hyperandrogenism are often in vain because new terminal hairs continue to be formed. Electrolysis and laser are most useful after several months of medical therapy when there is no new terminal hair growth.

Metformin

Metformin (Glucophage) is used in the treatment of type II diabetes mellitus, acting to increase insulin sensitivity at the cellular level. Because hyperinsulinemia resulting from insulin resistance exacerbates hyperandrogenism and ovulatory dysfunction in hyperandrogenic chronic anovulation, insulin-sensitizing agents such as metformin would be expected to aid in treatment. In fact, metformin has been shown to restore normal menses and decrease body mass index in women with PCO (71, 72). There is more recent evidence that metformin directly reduces androgen production in human theca cells (73, 74). In the most recent ACOG practice bulletin on the management of infertility caused by ovulatory dysfunction, the use of metformin is recommended only as an adjunct for PCO patients that do not ovulate with clomiphene alone (75). Usual dosing is 500 mg three times a day; it should not be used in women with liver dysfunction.

Idiopathic Hirsutism

Although the underlying biological mechanism in idiopathic hirsutism is different from that of hyperandrogenic chronic anovulation, the treatment is similar. The use of OCs decrease hirsutism by reducing circulating androgens to subnormal levels so less testosterone is available for conversion to DHT. Antiandrogens have proven effective in treating idiopathic hirsutism (56). Spironolactone is a prudent choice and may be combined with an OC to enhance efficacy, avoid irregular uterine bleeding, and provide contraception. Finasteride has been shown to be effective in idiopathic hirsutism and may prove especially useful because it specifically addresses the apparent etiology of this disorder by inhibiting 5α-reductase.

Late-Onset 21-Hydroxylase Deficiency

Women with LOHD may be treated with dexamethasone, 0.5 mg/day, or prednisone, 5 mg/day. Glucocorticoid therapy suppresses ACTH-induced adrenal androgen production, and has resulted in a decrease in hirsutism and a resumption of ovulatory cycles in some women. However, peripheral androgen blockade with cyproterone or spironolactone has been shown to be more effective than adrenal suppression (76).

EVALUATION OF TREATMENT

Treatment efficacy is best evaluated clinically. Useful measures include a reduction in the Ferriman-Gallwey score or a reduction in the amount of time spent in temporary hair removal. Subjective improvement may be noted in serial photographs. The amount of reduction in serum androgen levels does not correlate well with the magnitude of clinical improvement assessed by Ferriman-Gallwey score (29, 68). Therefore, measurement of serum androgens is usually not helpful.

Clinical Notes

- Hirsutism is male-pattern hair growth in a woman. It results from the stimulation of hair follicles by excess androgens and may occur on the face, chest, lower abdomen, lower back, medial thighs, and pubic area.
- Androgens are produced in the ovary and adrenal glands. Testosterone, produced in the ovary and through peripheral conversion of androstenedione and DHEA, is converted in the skin to DHT, which stimulates terminal hair growth. In addition to hirsutism, acne and alopecia are often signs of hyperandrogenism.
- Women with a gradual onset of hirsutism and regular menses likely have idiopathic hirsutism that results from an increase in the conversion of testosterone to DHT by 5α-reductase.
- Women with a gradual onset of hirsutism and irregular menses likely have hyperandrogenic chronic anovulation (also known as PCO) in which the ovary produces excess androgens in response to tonically elevated LH.
- About 5% of women with a gradual onset of hirsutism and irregular menses have LOHD (also known as late-onset congenital adrenal hyperplasia) in which excess androgens are produced in the adrenal because of a defect in the enzyme 21-hydroxylase.
- Androgen-producing ovarian or adrenal tumors are rare and usually present with the rapid onset of severe hirsutism or signs of masculinization. Other uncommon causes of hirsutism

include Cushing's syndrome, androgenic medications, ovarian stromal hyperthecosis, and luteoma or hyperreactio luteinalis of pregnancy.

- Studies for evaluation include testosterone and DHEA-S to rule out ovarian or adrenal tumors. In women with irregular menses, anovulation should be evaluated with thyroid-stimulating hormone and prolactin levels. A morning 17-OHP should be drawn to rule out LOHD. Radiologic imaging, an abdominal CT, and a pelvic sonogram should be performed when the serum androgen levels are very high, or there is a rapid progression of severe hirsutism.
- A combination of an OC to suppress ovarian androgen production and the antiandrogen spironolactone results in clinical improvement in about 6 months in most women with hyperandrogenic chronic anovulation or idiopathic hirsutism.

REFERENCES

1. Chang R. Ovarian steroid secretion in polycystic ovarian disease. Semin Reprod Endocrinol 1984;2:244–248.
2. Rittmaster RS. Clinical relevance of testosterone and dihydrotestosterone metabolism in women. Am J Med 1995;98(suppl):17S–21S.
3. Stein I, Leventhal M. Amenorrhea associated with bilateral polycystic ovaries. Am J Obstet Gynecol 1935; 29:181–191.
4. Farquhar C, Birdsall M, Manning P, et al. The prevalence of polycystic ovaries on ultrasound scanning in a population of randomly selected women. Aust N Z J Obstet Gynaecol 1994;34:67–72.
5. Polson D, Wadsworth J, Adams J, et al. Polycystic ovaries: a common finding in normal women. Lancet 1988; 1:870–872.
6. Hyperandrogenic chronic anovulation. ACOG Tech Bull 1995;202:1–7.
7. Taylor A, McCourt B, Martin K, et al. Determinants of abnormal gonadotropin secretion in clinically defined women with polycystic ovary syndrome. J Clin Enclocrinol Metab 1997;82:2248–2256.
8. Apter D, Butzow T, Laughlin G, et al. Metabolic features of polycystic ovary syndrome are found in adolescent girls with hyperandrogenism. J Clin Endocrinol Metab 1995;80:2966–2973.
9. Nestler J. Role of hyperinsulinemia in the pathogenesis of the polycystic ovary syndrome, and its clinical implications. Semin Reprod Enclocrinol 1997;15:111–122.
10. Nestler J, Barlascini C, Matt D, et al. Suppression of serum insulin by diazoxide reduces serum testosterone levels in obese women with polycystic ovary syndrome. Metabolism 1989;68:1027–1032.
11. Velazquez E, Mendoza S, Hamer T, et al. Metformin therapy in polycystic ovary syndrome reduces hyperinsulinemia, insulin resistance, hyperandrogenemia, and systolic blood pressure, while facilitating normal menses and pregnancy. Metabolism 1994;43:647–654.
12. Ehrmann D, Schneider D, Sobel B, et al. Troglitazone improves defects in insulin action, insulin secretion, ovarian steroidogenesis, and fibrinolysis in women with polycystic ovary syndrome. J Clin Endocrinol Metab 1997;82:2108–2116.
13. Moghetti P, Tosi F, Castello R, et al. The insulin resistance in women with hyperandrogenism is partially reversed by antiandrogen treatment: evidence that androgens impair insulin action in women. J Clin Endocrinol Metab 1996;81:952–960.
14. Douchi T, Ijuin H, Nakamura S, et al. Body fat distribution in women with polycystic ovary syndrome. Obstet Gynecol 1995;86:516–519.
15. Ferranini E, Natali A, Bell P, et al. Insulin resistance and hypersecretion in obesity. J Clin Invest 1997;100: 1166–1173.
16. Bernasconi D, del Monte P, Meozzi M, et al. The impact of obesity on hormonal parameters in hirsute and non-hirsute women. Metabolism 1996;45:72–75.
17. Coulam C, Annegers J, Kranz J. Chronic anovulation syndrome and associated neoplasms. Obstet Gynecol 1983;61:403–407.
18. Dahlgren E, Johansson S, Lindstedt G. Women with polycystic ovary syndrome wedge resected in 1956–1965: a long term followup focusing on natural history and circulating hormones. Fertil Steril 1992;57:505–513.
19. Castelo-Branco C, Casals E, de Osaba M, et al. Plasma lipids, lipoproteins and apolipoproteins in hirsute women. Acta Obstet Gynecol Scand 1996;75:261–265.
20. Wild R, Painter P, Coulson P, et al. Lipoprotein lipid concentrations and cardiovascular risk in women with polycystic ovary syndrome. J Clin Endocrinol Metab 1985;61:946–951.
21. Wild R. Obesity, lipids, cardiovascular risk, and androgen excess. Am J Med 1995;98(suppl):27S–32S.
22. Wild R, Alaupovic P, Givens J. Lipoprotein abnormalities in hirsute women: the association with insulin resistance. Am J Obstet Gynecol 1992;166:1191–1197.
23. Carmina E, Koyama T, Chang L, et al. Does ethnicity influence the prevalence of adrenal hyperandrogenism and insulin resistance in polycystic ovary syndrome. Am J Obstet Gynecol 1992;167:1807–1812.
24. Allen S, Potter H, Azziz R. Prevalence of hyperandrogenernia among non-hirsute oligo-ovulatory women. Fertil Steril 1997;67:569–572.
25. Mauvaisjarvis P. Regulation of androgen receptors and 5α-reductase in the skin of normal and hirsute women. Clin Enclocrinol Metab 1986;15:307–317.

26. Kirschner M, Samojlik E, Szmal E. Clinical usefulness of plasma androstanectiol glucuronicle measurements in women with idiopathic hirsutism. J Clin Endocrinol Metab 1987;65:597–601.
27. Khoury M, Baracat E, Pardini D, et al. Serum levels of androstenediol glucuronicle, total testosterone, and free testosterone in hirsute women. Fertil Steril 1994;62:76–80.
28. Rittmaster R. Androgen conjugates: physiology and clinical significance. Endocrinol Rev 1993;14:121–132.
29. Fruzzetti F, de Lorenzo D, Parrini D, et al. Effects of finasteride, a 5α-reductase inhibitor, on circulating androgens and gonadotropin secretion in hirsute womcn, J Clin Endocrinol Metab 1994;79:831–835.
30. Moghetti P, Castello R, Magnani C, et al. Clinical and hormonal effects of the 5α-reductase inhibitor finasteride in idiopathic hirsutism. J Clin Endocrinol Metab 1994;79:1115–1121.
31. Tolino A, Petrone A, Sarnacchiaro F, et al. Finasteride in the treatment of hirsutism: new therapeutic perspectives. Fertil Steril 1996;66:61–65.
32. Wong I, Morris R, Chang L, et al. A prospective randomized trial comparing finasteride spironolactone in the treatment of hirsute women. J Clin Endocrinol Metab 1995;80:233–238.
33. Panitsa-Faflia C, Batrinos M. Late-onset congenital adrenal hyperplasia. Ann N Y Acad Sci 1997;816:230–234.
34. Baskin H. Screening for late-onset congenital adrenal hyperplasia in hirsutism or amenorrhea. Arch Intern Med 1987;147:847–848.
35. Derksen J, Nagasser S, Meinders A, et al. Identification of virilizing adrenal tumors in hirsute women. N Engl J Med 1994;331:968–973.
36. Barth JH, Jenkins M, Belchetz PE. Ovarian hyperthecosis, diabetes and hirsuties in postmenopausal women. Clin Endocrinol (Oxf) 1997;46:123–128.
37. Pascale M, Pugeat M, Roberts M, et al. Androgen suppressive effect of GnRH agonist in ovarian hyperthecosis and virilizing tumours. Clin Endocrinol 1994;41:571–576.
38. Cohen D, Daughaday W, Weldon V. Fetal and maternal virilization associated with pregnancy. Am J Dis Child 1982;136:353–356.
39. Urman B, Pride S, Yuen B. Elevated serum testosterone, hirsutism, and virilism associated with combined androgen–estrogen hormone replacement therapy. Obstet Gvnecol 1991;77:595–985.
40. Joura E, Zeisler H, Bancher-Todesca D, et al. Short-term effects of topical testosterone in vulvar lichen sclerosus. Obstet Gynecol 1997;89:297–299.
41. Ferriman D, Gallwey J. Clinical assessment of body hair growth in women. J Clin Endocrinol Metab 1961; 21:1440–1447.
42. Lorenzo E. Familial study of hirsutism. J Clin Endocrinol Metab 1970;31:556–564.
43. Moltz L, Schwartz U. Gonadal and adrenal androgen secretion in hirsute females. Clin Endocrinol Metab 1986;15:229–245.
44. Pasquali R, Antenucci D, Casimirri F, et al. Clinical and hormonal characteristics of obese amenorrheic hyperandrogenic women before and after weight loss. J Clin Endocrinol Metab 1989;68:173–179.
45. Crave J, Fimbel S, Lejeune H, et al. Effects of diet and metformin administration on sex hormone-binding globulin, androgens and insulin in hirsute and obese women. J Clin Endocrinol Metab 1995;80:2057–2062.
46. Guzick D, Wing R, Smith D, et al. Endocrinologic consequences of weight loss in obese hyperandrogenic women. Fertil Steril 1994;61:598–604.
47. Breitkopf DM, Rosen MP, Young SL, et al. Efficacy of second versus third generation oral contraceptives in the treatment of hirsutism. Contraception 2003;67:349–353.
48. Odlind V, Milsom I, Persson I, et al. Can changes in sex hormone binding globulin predict the risk of venous thromboembolism with combined oral contraceptive pills? Acta Obstet Gynecol Scand 2002;81:482–490.
49. Thorneycroft IH, Stanczyk FZ, Bradshaw KD, et al. Effect of low-dose oral contraceptives on androgenic markers and acne. Contraception 1999;60:255–262.
50. Koulianos GT. Treatment of acne with oral contraceptives: criteria for pill selection. Cutis 2000;66:281–286.
51. Carr B, Breslau N, Givens C, et al. Oral contraceptive pills, gonadotropin-releasing hormone agonists, or use in combination for the treatment of hirsutism: a clinical research center study. J Clin Endocrinol Metab 1995;80:1169–1178.
52. Vegelli W, Testa G, Maggioni P, et al. An open randomized comparative study of an oral contraceptive containing ethinyl estradiol and cyproterone acetate with and without the GnRH analogue goserelin in the long-term treatment of hirsutism. Gynecol Obstet Invest 1996;41:260–268.
53. Mukherjee T, Barad D, Turk R, et al. A randomized, placebo controlled study on the effect of cyclic etidronate therapy on the bone mineral density changes associated with six months of gonadotropin-releasing hormone agonist treatment. Am J Obstet Gynecol 1996;175:105–109.
54. Lobo R, Shoupe D, Serafini P, et al. The effects of two doses on spironolactone on serum androgens and anagen hair in hirsute women. Fertil Steril 1985;43:200–205.
55. Helfer E, Miller J, Rose L. Side-effects of spironolactone therapy in the hirsute woman. J Clin Endocrinol Metab 1988;66:208–211.
56. Barth J, Cherry C, Wojnarowska F, et al. Spironolactone is an effective and well tolerated systemic antiandrogen therapy for hirsute women. J Clin Endocrinol Metab 1995;80:2966–2973.
57. Erenus M, Yucelten D, Gurbuz O, et al. Comparison of spironolactone-oral contraceptive versus cyproterone acetate-estrogen regimens in the treatment of hirsutism. Fertil Steril 1996;66:216–219.
58. O'Brien P, Cooper M, Murray P, et al. Comparison of sequential cyproterone acetate/estrogen versus spironolactone oral contraceptive in the treatment of hirsutism. J Clin Endocrinol Metab 1991;72:1008–1013.
59. Muhn P, Krattenmacher R, Beier S, et al. Drospirenone: a novel progestogen with antimineralocorticoid and antiandrogenic activity. Contraception 1995;51:99–110.

60. Barth J, Cherry C. Cyproterone acetate for severe hirsutism: results of a double-blind dose-ranging study. Clin Endocrinol 1991;35:510.
61. Belisle S, Love F. Clinical efficacy and safety of cyproterone acetate in severe hirsutism: results of a multicentered Canadian study. Fertil Steril 1986;46:1015–1020.
62. Martikainen H, Heikkinenj, Ruokonen A, et al. Hormonal and clinical effects of ketoconazole in hirsute women. J Clin Endocrinol Metab 1988;66:987–991.
63. Venturoli S, Fabbri R, Prato L, et al. Ketoconazole therapy for women with acne and/or hirsutism. J Clin Endocrinol Metab l990;71:335–339.
64. Erenus M, Gurbuz O, Durmusoglu F, et al. Comparison of the efficacy of spironolactone versus flutamide in the treatment of hirsutism. Fertil Steril 1994;61:613–616.
65. Wysowski D, Fourcroy J. Flutamide toxicity. J Urol 1996;155:209–212.
66. Wallace C, Lalor E, Chik C. Hepatotoxicity complicating flutamide treatment of hirsutism. Ann Intern Med 1993;119:1150.
67. Golditch I, Price V. Treatment of hirsutism with cimetidine. Obstet Gynecol 1990;75:911–913.
68. Balfour JA, McClellan K. Topical eflornithine. Am J Clin Dermatol 2001;2:197–201.
69. DiBernardo B, Perez J, Usal H, et al. Laser hair removal: where are we now? Plast Reconstr Surg 1999;104: 247–257.
70. Lanigan SW. Management of unwanted hair in females. Clin Exp Dermatol 2001;26:644–647.
71. Glueck CJ, Wang P, Fontaine R, et al. Metformin to restore normal menses in oligo-amenorrheic teenage girls with polycystic ovary syndrome. J Adolesc Health 2001;29:160–169.
72. Velazquez E, Acosta A, Mendoza S. Menstrual cyclicity after metformin therapy in polycystic ovary syndrome. Obstet Gynecol 1997;90:392–395.
73. Attia G, Rainey W, Carr B. Metformin directly inhibits androgen production in human theca cells. Fertil Steril 2001;76:517–524.
74. Management of infertility caused by ovulatory dysfunction. ACOG Tech Bull 2002;34.
75. Kocak M, Caliskan E, Simsir C, et al. Metformin therapy improves ovulatory rates, cervical scores, and pregnancy rates in clomiphene citrate-resistant women with polycystic ovary syndrome. Fertil Steril 2002;77:101–106.
76. Carmina E, Lobo R. Peripheral androgen blockade versus glandular androgen suppression in the treatment of hirsutism. Obstet Gynecol 1991;78:845–849.

CHAPTER 10

Vulvovaginitis

Tracey A. Banks and Michèle G. Curtis

INTRODUCTION

Vulvovaginitis, or vaginal discharge, is one of the top reasons for a woman to visit her obstetrician/gynecologist (1). Although this diagnosis is commonplace, misdiagnosis can occur and lead to ineffective treatment unless the physician pays careful attention to specific criteria.

The three most frequently diagnosed infectious causes of vaginitis are bacterial vaginosis (BV), vulvovaginal candidiasis (VVC), and trichomoniasis. Other less common etiologies include atrophic vaginitis, the vulvovaginogingival syndrome, and contact vaginitis. This chapter discusses the evaluation and treatment of these various vulvovaginitis entities.

NORMAL VAGINAL FLORA AND DISCHARGE

The vagina is an ecosystem in which the vaginal epithelium serves as the habitat for microbial flora, composed primarily of Gram-negative, Gram-positive, anaerobic, and facultatively anaerobic species (2). The predominant normal vaginal flora consists of facultative *Lactobacillus* species. These are long, Gram-positive rods that exert protective effects in the vagina by producing hydrogen peroxide, bacteriocins, and/or a lower pH that inhibits the colonization or overgrowth of potential pathogens. Physiologic or normal discharge is usually clear or white, viscous, and pools in the fornices of the vagina. It contains sloughed vaginal and cervical epithelial cells, mucoid endocervical secretions, and bacteria. The pH of normal vaginal secretions in women of childbearing age is between 3.8 and 4.5. Minimal odor may be present. Normal vaginal discharge does not cause symptoms of burning or itching.

The phase of the menstrual cycle influences the quantity of normal discharge. During the follicular phase, there is a steady increase in vaginal liquid discharge, up to the point of ovulation. In the luteal phase, after ovulation, the discharge becomes more viscous and thick. Diet, medications, or over-the-counter (OTC) dietary supplements may affect the odor of the normal vaginal discharge. There may be excessive, but normal, vaginal discharge from cervical mucorrhea if there is a large cervical ectropion. In this case, no therapy is indicated, but if it is too bothersome to the patient, cryotherapy or CO_2 laser has been used and is occasionally helpful.

MECHANISM OF INFECTION

For the most part, there is remarkable stability of the vaginal endogenous flora even in the face of aggressive douching and short-term parenteral antibiotics. Estrogen and pH exert a strong influence on this stability. A complex interaction exists between the vaginal epithelium and both the endogenous and exogenous floras. A change in the existing conditions of the vaginal tissue may alter the flora in terms of numbers and species. Thus, in some cases, the benign normal vaginal flora can become pathologic and assume a different relationship to the host.

DIAGNOSIS

The evaluation of women with vaginal symptoms requires a directed history, a physical examination, and in-office laboratory testing in all cases (Table 10.1). Symptoms alone are insufficient as a basis for diagnosis and treatment plans. Common contributing factors to the misdiagnosis of vaginitis include the following:

- Patient self-diagnoses and treatment
- Diagnosis made via phone
- Office visit does not include pelvic examination
- Inadequate examination of vulva and vestibule during the exam
- Proper laboratory tests not performed
- Use of "shotgun" therapy
- Overprescription of topical steroids
- Papanicolaou (or Pap) results used as diagnostic tool
- Possibility of topical therapy exacerbating the symptoms not considered (3)

With the current availability of OTC antifungal agents many women self-diagnose and treat. The accuracy of these self-diagnoses is notoriously poor. One study performed to assess the accuracy of patient self-diagnosis found that of 54 women who believed they had VVC, only 59% actually had the condition. The accuracy of self-diagnosis rose to 82% in women who had a prior history of VVC (4). Although it is estimated that there are cost savings of nearly $64

TABLE 10.1

Diagnostic Features of Vulvovaginitis

Feature	Normal	Bacterial Vaginosis	Candidal Vaginitis	Trichomonas Vaginitis
Symptoms	None or physiologic discharge	Thin, malodorous, white/gray discharge	Pruritus, white thick or watery discharge, vulva soreness	Profuse, offensive discharge, dyspareunia
Discharge	White or clear, variable minimal to no odor	Moderate, adherent, white to gray, homogenous	White, scant to moderate, varying from milky to cottage cheese-like	Profuse, yellowish, homogenous, frothy
Exam	Normal	No inflammation	Introital, vaginal, and vulvar erythema; exfoliations from scratching	Erythema and swelling of vulvar and vaginal wall; "strawberry" cervix
pH of vaginal fluid	<4.5	>4.5	<4.5	5–6.0
Amine (whiff) test	Negative	Positive	Negative	Occasionally positive
Saline microscopy	Normal epithelial cells and lactobacilli (long rods)	Clue cells, absence of leukocytes, decreased lactobacilli	Normal flora	Increased leukocytes, motile trichomonads, no clue cells or abnormal flora
10% KOH microscopy	Negative	Negative	Hyphae and budding yeast	Negative

million for self-treatment of VVC, whether this cost is offset, and to what extent, due to the misuse of OTC antifungal products is not known (5).

History

Vaginal discharge is the most common complaint in women with vaginitis. A thorough history should note the color, consistency, and volume of the vaginal discharge, as well as the presence or absence of odor. It should include the onset, type, duration, and extent of symptoms. Other symptoms such as itching, vulvar pain, abdominal pain, and/or dysuria should also be noted. Information regarding sexual history, previous sexually transmitted infections (STIs), contraceptive methods, and dyspareunia is contributory. A list of current medications, including OTC drugs, is included in the history. Often disregarded, but equally important, are the patient's concern or opinion about the diagnosis, remedies the patient has already tried, and finally, the patient's response to past treatments.

Physical Exam

The physical exam should be deferred if vaginal creams were used in the last 72 hours because they may obscure the diagnosis. The vulvar and vaginal vestibules, including the vaginal introitus, are inspected and palpated for any erythema, swelling, lesions, or tenderness. Vaginal speculum examinations, with only water as a lubricant, are mandatory for the diagnosis and treatment of vulvovaginitis. Inspect the vaginal walls carefully for any evidence of vaginal ulcers secondary to improper tampon use, or prolonged use of diaphragms or a pessary. Scrutinize the cervix for lesions, friability, or purulent material that may indicate cervicitis. The color, amount, texture, and odor of the vaginal and/or cervical discharge are noted. A bimanual examination is necessary to assess the size and tenderness of the uterus and adnexa.

Office Analysis

Simple office analysis provides the backbone for diagnosing the etiology of vulvovaginitis. This assessment includes the following tests:

1. pH of vaginal secretions—A drop of vaginal discharge is placed on litmus paper, and color change is noted. The normal vaginal pH is 3.5 to 4.0.
2. Amine (whiff) test—A positive test constitutes a "fishy" odor after 10% potassium hydroxide is added to vaginal secretions on the speculum or glass slide. This odor is caused by volatilization of amines in the discharge.
3. Microscopy (wet mount)—Small amounts of vaginal discharge are placed on a plain unfrosted slide and mixed with one to two drops of normal saline at one end and one to two drops of 10% potassium hydroxide (KOH) at the other. The specimens are then covered with coverslips, and the specimen is examined microscopically.

Examination of the normal saline preparation includes assessment of the background flora: a normal finding includes lactobacilli with long rods, whereas an abnormal result may reveal a predominance of short rods, cocci, and curved motile rods. A search for the presence of white blood cells, trichomonads, and/or clue cells (squamous epithelial cells studded with bacteria causing obscured borders) is also made. The KOH preparation is examined for the presence of hyphae or budding yeast. Misdiagnosis occurs when slides are not systematically examined and carefully scrutinized for each type of vaginitis. Mixed infections can and do occur (6). An accurate diagnosis is subject to many variables. Despite this, the aforementioned laboratory tests, coupled with a thorough history and careful physical examination, will provide an immediate and reliable clinical diagnosis in the majority of cases.

It is important that each aforementioned test be performed in the diagnostic workup for vulvovaginitis. Even when microscopy is done by skilled clinicians in a research setting, the sensitivity of diagnosis is only about 50% for VVC and 50 to 70% for trichomoniasis (7, 8). For this reason, use of other diagnostic evaluations such as cultures for *Trichomonas vaginalis* (TV) and *Candida* species, using modified Diamond media in addition to Sabouraud's or Nickerson's agar (for *Candida* species) may be required if the diagnosis is suspected but not confirmed on microscopy or is unsupported with pH testing. Gram's stain of vaginal secretions may be employed to diagnose BV and Candidal vulvovaginitis. However, because nonmotile trichomonads are difficult to distinguish from leukocytes, the Gram's stain is not useful in diagnosing this entity. If clinically indicated, urinalysis, pregnancy testing, or serum and/or cervical testing for concomitant sexually transmitted diseases, such as syphilis, HIV, gonorrhea, or chlamydia, is performed.

If a microscope is not available, hydrogen peroxide may be able to differentiate yeast and BV infections from those caused by trichomonas or desquamative inflammatory vaginitis. If the vaginal secretions contain white blood cells, the mixture of hydrogen peroxide and vaginal discharge produces foaming bubbles. Leukocytes are present in cases of vulvovaginitis due to trichomonas or in the vulvovaginogingival syndrome. In cases of vulvovaginitis caused by yeast or BV, there are no white blood cells in the vaginal secretions; thus, the mixture of vaginal secretions and hydrogen peroxide does not produce a foamy response. This information, in addition to the results of pH testing and the whiff test, may guide the clinician's diagnosis and therapy. The problem with this method is that the results are unreliable in the presence of a mixed infection.

During the episode of vulvovaginitis, and until treatment is completed, intercourse is either avoided, or condoms are used. It is important to keep the external genitalia dry and to avoid perfumed feminine hygiene products. The patient may find it efficacious to wear loose-fitting clothing, and use all cotton undergarments.

BACTERIAL VAGINOSIS

BV is the most common vaginal infection among reproductive age women, accounting for 40 to 50% of all cases of vaginitis (9). It has had many names in the past, including nonspecific vaginitis, *Haemophilus vaginalis* vaginitis, *Corynebacterium vaginale* vaginitis,and *Gardnerella vaginalis* vaginitis (10). The confusion over its name parallels the confusion over the disease entity itself. It is not considered an STI because it has been diagnosed in virginal women, but it is sexually associated. Initially believed to be a benign condition, more recent investigations have demonstrated that BV is associated with a variety of upper genital tract infections and complications. These include pelvic inflammatory disease (PID), postcesarean endometritis, posthysterectomy pelvic infection, chorioamnionitis, premature rupture of membranes, and preterm labor and delivery (11).

Epidemiology

BV is a common disorder that occurs among 35 to 64% of women attending sexually transmitted disease clinics, 15 to 20% of pregnant women, and 10 to 26% of women attending gynecologic clinics (12). Typically, BV affects women of reproductive age, indicating a possible role of sex hormones in its pathogenesis, but it may occur in prepubertal and menopausal women infrequently. Some women develop symptoms on a cyclical basis. There has been an association between BV and intrauterine devices, although the exact mechanism by which the intrauterine device increases the risk of BV is unknown (13). Oral contraceptives might have a protective effect on the development by promoting lactobacilli-predominant vaginal flora. This disease can also occur in women who have had a hysterectomy.

PATHOGENESIS

BV is a polymicrobial condition where there is a decrease in vaginal acidity and the concentration of lactobacilli. There is also a 100-fold or more increase in the concentrations of other organisms. These organisms include *G. vaginalis*, which is isolated from 45 to 99% of women with BV, *Mycoplasma hominis, Prevotella, Bacteroides, Peptostreptococcus* species, *Ureaplasma urealyticum,* and other anaerobic flora. The triggering mechanism that causes a decrease in lactobacilli concentration and an overgrowth of anaerobic and facultatively anaerobic organisms is not known. One hypothesis is that loss of the hydrogen-producing lactobacilli allows the overgrowth to occur; a second hypothesis believes the loss of lactobacilli is secondary to the overgrowth of the other bacteria.

Clinical Manifestations

Women often complain of a thin increased vaginal discharge present at the introitus. The discharge may be sticky and have a disagreeable or fishy odor. This odor is more noticeable after unprotected sexual intercourse because the basic pH of seminal fluid causes a volatilization of amines and the production of a strong odor. Mild to moderate itching may also occur with the vaginal discharge. These symptoms, however, might be absent in approximately half of the women with BV (9). On exam, a thin grayish-white homogeneous discharge that adheres to the vaginal wall may be noted.

In some cases of BV due predominately to *Gardnerella*, gas-filled cystic structures on the vaginal walls or cervix are seen. This is vaginitis emphysematosa and will clear with treatment of the BV. Vaginitis emphysematosa may also be seen with infections due to trichomonas.

Diagnosis

Using Amsel's critieria, BV is clinically diagnosed by the presence of three of the four following criteria (13):

1. A thin or even milky, homogenous adherent discharge.
2. A vaginal pH greater than 4.5. (This is one of most sensitive tests for the diagnosis of BV; sample only vaginal side walls and avoid cervical os or posterior fornix to avoid contamination with cervical secretions, which are more alkaline than normal vaginal fluid. Menstrual blood or semen will also falsely elevate vaginal pH levels.)
3. The presence of clue cells (squamous epithelial cells covered with bacterial rods or cocci, giving them a granular border) in the vaginal fluid on light microscopy. Normal cells may be misdiagnosed as clue cells; the key to distinguishing them is to look closely at the cellular borders. On clue cells, the borders will appear stippled or rough. Also, when looking for clue cells in the wet mount, notice the background bacteria. If there are not a lot of lactobacilli, the possibility of BV is raised. Although polymorphonuclear leukocytes are not associated with BV, their presence could be a sign of a mixed infection or cervicitis.
4. Positive whiff test as demonstrated by a fishy odor, indicating presence of amines. This is tested for by adding 10% KOH to a vaginal fluid specimen and smelling it. Presence of the amine odor is the least sensitive of the clinical tests because of its fleeting nature and the variation in olfactory sensitivity among clinicians; however, it is the most specific of the clinical criteria.

The presence of clue cells—vaginal epithelial cells with bacteria densely adherent to them and obscuring their borders—is the single most reliable predictor of BV (14). Failure to do a wet-mount preparation examination in a woman with BV misses the opportunity to potentially identify the coexistence of a sexually transmitted or sexually associated disease. BV is a noninflammatory disease. The presence of a significant number of white blood cells on microscopy should alert the clinician to at least a 20% probability of another sexually transmitted disease (15). To accurately diagnose BV, at least 20% of the epithelial cells seen on the wet mount should be clue cells (16). Interpretation of these signs can be difficult. Vaginal pH is highly sensitive but not specific; it is influenced by blood, douching, and recent intercourse.

Clue cells and changes in bacterial flora may be detected on the Pap smear. These are normally an incidental finding and have limited diagnostic significance in comparison with other methods. Gram's stains are another means of diagnosing BV that can be done in the office setting. A criteria for interpreting Gram's stains was devised by Spiegal et al. (17). BV was diagnosed if the number of *Gardnerella* morphotypes and other bacteria (cocci, fusiforms, and curved rods) were increased, and if there were fewer than five *Lactobacillus* morphotypes (large Gram-positive rods) per oil immersion field. Using these criteria, the Gram's stain has a sensitivity of 93% and a specificity of 70% for diagnosing BV (17). In one study, the sensitivity and specificity of the Gram's stain compared with the Amsel criteria were 89 and 83%, respectively. Based on this study, if the Gram's stain was considered the criterion standard for the diagnosis of BV, the sensitivity and specificity of the Amsel criteria were 70 and 94%, respectively (18).

Vaginal culture, which has a high degree of sensitivity, is not practical for diagnosing BV because these organisms are members of the normal flora. Unless clinical signs are present, the incidental finding of *G. vaginalis* in a vaginal culture is not used to diagnose BV.

The Affirm VP_{III} (Becton Dickinson Microbiology Systems, Sparks, MD) is a semiautomated system for detection of ribosomal RNA (rRNA) from the agents of vaginitis/vaginosis. Three separate probes are used, one for *G. vaginalis* as a marker organism for BV, one for *T. vaginalis*, and one for *Candida* species. A specific DNA capture probe for each organism, plus positive and negative control beads, are included on each test card. The presence of any blue color indicates a positive test. Affirm is equivalent to the microscopic exam for clue cells, a common method of diagnosis in a doctor's office setting. When compared with diagnosis of BV by Gram's stain, the specificity of Affirm is lower, a finding that may reflect improved accuracy of diagnosis when the patients are examined for the presence of multiple clinical criteria (13). Some authors recommend that Affirm be used in conjunction with the pH and amine test for diagnosis of BV to increase the specificity and positive predictive value (19).

The FemExam (Litmus Concepts, Santa Clara, CA) and Amines TestCard were developed to detect two of the four Amsel clinical criteria, namely vaginal fluid pH greater than 4.7 and the amines responsible for the "fishy odor" of BV. The FemExam kit consists of two plastic cards: card 1 is for rapid assessment of vaginal fluid pH and the presence of trimethylamine, and card 2 is for measuring proline iminopeptidase activity of *G. vaginalis*. A single vaginal swab is applied to the pH test spot on the FemExam card and then to the amine test spot. The development of plus signs in both spots is interpreted as a positive test. This test provides an assessment of clinical markers of BV, similar to conventional Amsel clinical criteria. The FemExam test compared favorably with conventional clinical diagnosis. In one more recent study, use of both FemExam cards 1 and 2 (with two of three tests positive) yielded higher sensitivity (91%) but lower specificity (62%) than use of FemExam card 1 alone (sensitivity, 71%; specificity, 73%) and FemExam card 2 alone (sensitivity, 70%; specificity, 81%) (20).

Other commercially available tests have been produced that rely on detecting biochemical changes (e.g., BVBLUE, which detects sialidase activity; the PAP test, which detects proline aminopeptidase; and elevated pH, FemExam, which detects elevated pH and trimethylamine). Another assay uses a semiquantitative polymerase chain reaction (PCR) to detect high concentrations of *G. vaginalis* as a marker of BV (21).

Sequelae

BV is a risk factor for nonobstetric infections, including postpartum endometritis, cuff cellulitis, postabortal and spontaneous PID, and nonpuerperal breast abscess (22, 23).

Several researchers have established a correlation between abnormal bacterial flora of the genital tract and upper genital tract infections. BV may contribute significantly to the development of these upper tract infections (9). Almost 67% of the time, the anaerobes and facultative bacteria responsible for BV are recovered from the upper genital tracts of women with PID. These studies provide strong evidence for the important role that anaerobic bacteria play in the etiology and pathogenesis of acute PID.

The development of postoperative infection depends on a complex interaction between host defense mechanisms and the bacterial inoculum. Most postoperative pelvic infections involve an ascending route of bacterial spread from the vagina and the cervix. Similarities between the bacteria associated with BV and those of postpartum and postsurgical infections suggest that BV may play a role in the origin of these infections (24). Preliminary data suggest that BV increases the risk of postoperative infections in both the postpartum and the postsurgical settings. However, few prospective studies are able to confirm this suspicion. If this is true, it may be prudent to consider treatment of BV (symptomatic or asymptomatic) before performing surgical or invasive procedures.

BV is also related to complications such as preterm delivery, amnionitis, postcesarean endometritis, and postdelivery pelvic infection (25–28). One hypothesis is that the bacterial products of BV-associated flora, including phospholipase A2, mucinase, endotoxin, and sialidase, have the potential to provoke premature labor (29–32). In one review of the obstetric and gynecologic sequelae of BV, nine studies were noted to have linked BV or BV-associated flora with preterm birth and/or low birth weight, the odds ratios ranged from 1.4 to 6.9. Six additional studies showed an association of BV with chorioamnionitis and amniotic fluid infection (odds ratios, 1.5 to 6.8). BV-associated flora have been recovered from the placenta, chorioamnion, and amniotic fluid of patients with clinical disease (22).

In the investigation by Ralph et al., the effect of BV on conception and first trimester miscarriage was evaluated in women undergoing in vitro fertilization. Although there was no association of BV with the rate of conception, there was a two-fold risk of miscarriage in the women who had BV immediately before egg collection (33).

At present, however, the evidence does not support screening all obstetric or gynecology patients for BV or treating women who are asymptomatic (34).

Treatment

When treating BV (Table 10.2), it is interesting to note that BV seems to actually protect against genital yeast infection by producing amines (35). Hence, studies have shown that 20 to 30% of women may develop vulvovaginal candidiasis after treatment of BV (36, 37).

Systemic Therapy

A multitude of antimicrobial agents has been used for the treatment of BV, including sulfa vaginal creams, ampicillin, and doxycycline. Metronidazole is currently the treatment of choice with reported cure rates of 72 to 100% (38). Metronidazole is inactive against facultative lactobacilli; therefore, it helps the recolonization of this organism, and thus, the restoration of the normal flora after successful therapy. Various treatment regimens with metronidazole exist. The two most common dosages are 500 mg orally, twice a day for 5 to 7 days, and 2 g as a single dose. The single 2-g dose should be considered in patients where nonadherence is a significant concern. The 7-day course achieves higher cure rates in comparison with the single 2-g dose. The single-dose regimen increases compliance, causes fewer side effects, and incurs a lower cost. These factors may render its clinical effectiveness equal to that of the 7-day regimen, but there are no firm data to support this argument.

TABLE 10.2

Treatment Options for Bacterial Vaginosis for Nonpregnant Women

Drug	Formulation
Recommended Therapy (all with equal efficacy)	
Oral Metronidazole (Flagyl, Protostat)	500 mg twice a day for 5–7 days
Metronidazole vaginal gel (0.75%)	One applicatorful intravaginally for 5 days
Clindamycin cream (2%)	One applicatorful intravaginally for 7 days
Alternative Therapies (less efficacious than those above)	
Oral Metronidazole	2-g single dose
Oral clindamycin	300 mg twice a day for 7 days
Clindamycin vaginal ovules	Intravaginally for 3 days

From Centers for Disease Control and Prevention. Sexually transmitted diseases treatment guidelines, 2002. MMWR Morb Mortal Wkly Rep 2002;51(RR6):42–44.

The common side effects of metronidazole are nausea, vomiting, anorexia, metallic taste in the mouth, secondary yeast infections, headache, dizziness, and darkening of the urine. Skin rashes are less common. The patient should not drink alcoholic beverages while taking metronidazole because it may produce a disulfiramlike effect. Metronidazole should be used with caution in patients with central nervous system diseases or blood dyscrasias.

Oral clindamycin has a significant cure rate against anaerobic bacteria and *G. vaginalis*. A dose of 300 mg twice a day for 7 days produced a 94% cure rate that is comparable to metronidazole (39). It is particularly useful in pregnancy, metronidazole treatment failure, and where patients cannot tolerate metronidazole. Adverse reactions include gastrointestinal complaints (nausea, loose stool), and on rare occasions, skin rash. It is safe to use in pregnancy, regardless of trimester.

Intravaginal Therapy

Local therapy provides high medication levels at the site of the infection and should reduce systemic side effects. Bistoletti et al. examined the effectiveness of the 500-mg intravaginal metronidazole tablets at bedtime for 7 days versus oral metronidazole and demonstrated similar efficacies—resolution of BV among 79% of women using intravaginal medication and 74% of women who were randomized to receive oral metronidazole (40). Hanson et al. compared metronidazole vaginal gel with oral metronidazole and again demonstrated equivalent efficacies for the two treatments (41). BV was eliminated by 1 week post-treatment among 83% (36 of 43) of women randomized to metronidazole vaginal gel and 85.1% (40 of 47) of women randomized to oral metronidazole. Metronidazole vaginal gel 0.75% (MetroGel-Vaginal) is an effective alternative to oral metronidazole (42). The currently recommended dosage is one applicatorful (5 g) intravaginally, twice a day, for 5 days.

Clindamycin (Cleocin) is another vaginal preparation found to be effective in limited clinical trials. The currently recommended regimen is clindamycin cream 2%, one applicatorful (5 g), intravaginally, at bedtime for 7 days. This regimen appears to be safe and well tolerated in nonpregnant women. Patients using this treatment regimen should be advised that this cream has an oil base and may weaken certain barrier contraceptives (e.g., condoms or diaphragms).

Other treatments for BV used in the past have included ampicillin, amoxicillin and clavulanate potassium, ofloxacin, erythromycin, triple sulfa cream, and vaginal acidification. These treatments are less effective than either oral or vaginal preparations of metronidazole or clindamycin and are not recommended (43–46).

Probiotics

Probiotics are live micro-organisms or microbial mixtures administered to improve the patient's microbial balance; they have been used in the gastrointestinal (GI) tract and the vagina (47). Currently available probiotics are considered nonpathogenic, but if the patient is severely debilitated or immunosuppressed, even benign microorganisms can be infective. In comparison, a "biotherapeutic agent" is considered a microbe having specific therapeutic activity against a specific disease (e.g., the oral administration of *Saccharomyces boulardii* to treat recurrent *Clostridium difficile*-associated disease) (48, 49). Although many studies of probiotics for vaginal infections have been reported, most lack a rigorous design. Nevertheless, an effective probiotic that could prevent vaginitis or help break the cycle of recurrence would be extremely helpful. For example, a probiotic could be taken whenever a woman uses an antimicrobial to decrease the risk of subsequent Candidal vulvovaginitis. Similarly, there could be an important role for probiotics in decreasing the frequency of recurrence associated with BV. Most probiotic preparations for vaginal use include one or more *Lactobacillus* species.

Lactobacillus protects the vagina from colonization by pathogens by two main mechanisms: blocking their attachment to the vaginal epithelium and producing substances that inhibit their multiplication. The same *Lactobacillus* strain can show different blocking and inhibiting activity against different pathogens. To date, only a small number of systematic clinical trials with well-characterized strains have been conducted, and there are few conclusive results. The main indications for probiotic *Lactobacillus* use in urogenital tract infections would include recurrent urinary tract infection in healthy pre- and postmenopausal women, and postinfection prophylaxis to re-establish the vaginal flora and prevent future episodes, BV, and recurrent vaginal candidiasis.

The species of *Lactobacillus* believed to be the most important in maintaining a healthy vaginal environment is *Lactobacillus crispatus*. More recently, a capsule containing *L. crispatus* has been developed for use in humans to promote and/or increase vaginal colonization by H_2O_2-producing lactobacilli. In a pilot study involving nine women ages 18 to 40 years, vaginal colonization by *L. crispatus* CTV-05 was evaluated at 1 to 3 days and 6 to 8 days following insertion of one capsule intravaginally twice a day for 3 days. *L. crispatus* CTV-05 was detected in five of nine women at the first follow-up and six of nine women at the second follow-up (50). In another study at two centers, vaginal capsules containing *L. crispatus* were used in conjunction with a single 2-g dose of metronidazole (51). Preliminary data showed that the majority of women with recurrent BV were successfully recolonized with *L. crispatus* and were significantly less likely to have a recurrence compared with women who received placebo. However, in women using the capsules who did not have recolonization of the vagina, there was an increase in the rates of BV recurrence compared with women treated with placebo. The study authors believed this was due to exogenous materials in the capsules that were unrelated to lactobacilli and facilitated overgrowth of undesirable organisms (51).

Asymptomatic Patients

Approximately 50% of women with microbiologic findings suggestive of BV are asymptomatic. Studies suggest that spontaneous resolution of laboratory-proven BV occurs in the majority of asymptomatic women (52). Currently, treatment of asymptomatic patients is not recommended. It has been recommended that patients with BV scheduled to undergo endometrial biopsy, hysteroscopy, hysterosalpingography, intrauterine device insertion, or hysterectomy receive a full course of therapy before the procedure. Although BV has been associated with premature rupture of membranes, preterm labor, chorioamnionitis, and postpartum endometritis, routine treatment of asymptomatic pregnant patients has not been recommended or accepted universally.

Sexual Partners

The role of sexual transmission of micro-organisms in BV is controversial. Randomized, double-blinded studies show no improvement in cure rates when sexual partners were also treated (53, 54).Therefore, the data indicate no benefit in treating the sexual partners of women with BV. However, some clinicians favor doing so in women who have intractable or recurrent disease.

Pregnant Women

Currently, the Centers for Disease Control and Prevention (CDC) guidelines state that evaluation for BV may be conducted at the first prenatal visit for asymptomatic patients who are at high risk for preterm labor (e.g., those who have a history of a previous preterm delivery) (60). Some specialists prefer using systemic therapy to treat possible subclinical upper genital tract infections among women at low risk for preterm delivery (i.e., those who have no history of delivering an infant before term). Existing data do not support the use of topical agents during pregnancy. Evidence from three trials suggests an increase in adverse events (e.g., prematurity, neonatal infections), particularly in newborns, after use of clindamycin cream (31, 55, 56). Multiple studies and meta-analyses have not demonstrated a consistent association between metronidazole use during pregnancy and teratogenic or mutagenic effects in newborns (57–59). Recommended treatment regimes for pregnant women with symptomatic BV are metronidazole 250 mg orally three times a day for 7 days or clindamycin 300 mg orally twice a day for 7 days. Current evidence does not support routine testing for BV in pregnancy (60).

Recurrent BV

Although there is no universally accepted definition of recurrent BV, one commonly used criteria is three or more confirmed attacks per year. Lack of cure may represent refractory disease, not recurrent episodes. Recurrence rates will vary according to the population being studied. Strategies to address recurrent BV have been described in the literature, but none have been tested in large-scale clinical trials, so data to recommend one approach over the other(s) are lacking. Empirically, one option is to prescribe the same regimen previously tried for longer durations of time. Another approach is to switch to another treatment regimen. Other techniques include the use of combination therapy or even treating the sexual partner. Use of condoms as barrier protection has also been recommended. Acidification of the vagina exogenously has been used in the past but has been demonstrated to be ineffective.

In an ongoing study to examine the efficacy of suppressive therapy with metronidazole gel, women are initially treated with 10 days of therapy with metronidazole gel, followed by a maintenance regimen of twice-weekly metronidazole gel. In an initial pilot study, this approach did demonstrate a significant reduction in cases of recurrent BV when compared with placebo, but the results seemed to disappear after the regimen was discontinued (61).

VULVOVAGINAL CANDIDIASIS

Epidemiology

Yeast infections of the vagina and vulva are among the most common gynecologic conditions affecting women (62, 63). Approximately 75% of women will have at least one episode of Candidal vulvovaginitis during their reproductive years, with 40 to 50% of these women experiencing two or more attacks (64). Fortunately, fewer than 5% of women suffer recurrent vulvovaginal candidiasis (RVVC). There is a sexual association with this condition, but it is not considered an STI.

Pathogenesis

Among the 150 species of *Candida*, only about a dozen, including *Candida albicans, Candida tropicalis, Candida parapsilosis, Candida glabrata, Candida krusei, Candida guilliermondii, Candida rugosa, Candida lipolytica, Candida lusitaniae, Candida briglis*, and *Candida kefyr*, may infect humans. Colonization rates of *Candida* in the vagina have varied from one-tenth to one-third of all healthy women of reproductive age (65–67).

Twenty-five to 40% of women who have positive vaginal cultures for *Candida* are asymptomatic. In asymptomatic carriers, usually less than ten colony-forming units of *Candida* are observed on agar culture plates. At least 90% of all strains isolated from the vagina belong to *C. albicans* (68). This suggests a colonization of *Candida* species (similar to that of many BV-associated organisms) in low numbers that may increase when faced with an altered vaginal environment. Thus, asymptomatic colonization may progress to symptomatic Candidal vulvovaginitis when changes occur in the host vaginal environment. The natural vaginal flora, predominated by lactobacilli, provides a colonization-resistant mechanism to prevent *Candida* germination and superficial mucosal invasion. Approximately 85 to 90% of yeast isolates from the vagina are *C. albicans* strains. *C. albicans* tends to show greater ability to adhere in higher numbers to vaginal epithelial cells than do non-albicans species, such as *C. tropicalis, C. krusei*, and *C. parapsilosis* (69). Both VVC and RVVC are often caused by *C. albicans*, although non-albicans species, which are generally less susceptible to commonly used antifungals to treat nonrecurrent VVC, can be found as the causative agent (63). *C. dubliniensis* is a variant of *C. albicans* (70). *Saccharomyces cerevisiae* is another isolate found in vaginitis cases (71). Typing of *Candida* strains by rDNA restriction fragment-length polymorphism may be used for evaluation of recolonization versus reinfection (72).

Predisposing Factors

It is believed that the higher levels of female sex hormones in reproductive-age women increases their susceptibility to *Candida* infections. Estrogen does enhance the adherence of yeast organisms to vaginal mucosa cells. Vaginal *Candida* colonization and genital *Candida* infections are more common in pregnant than in nonpregnant women (73).

Data regarding the relationship between oral contraceptive use and VVC or RVVC are conflicting (74–77). Claims of an association between barrier contraceptive methods and spermicides and candidosis are also inconsistent (75, 78, 79). There seems to be compelling evidence that intrauterine contraceptive device (IUCD) use may be associated with RVVC recurrences in susceptible women (80). Thus, women with RVVC should be recommended to use oral hormonal contraceptive methods and/or condoms rather than an IUCD.

The oral cavity of the male partner is believed to be a source of reinfection for RVVC (77). In one study, receptive oral sex twice or more in the previous 2 weeks was closely associated with symptomatic, culture-proven VVC (66). An increase in the detectable vaginal colonization rate between 10% and 30% has been observed in women given broad-spectrum antibiotics (76). Although frequently discussed when counseling patients, the actual role of clothing in RVVC is still controversial. It is commonly believed that pantyhose and tight pants trap moisture near the crotch, creating an environment for yeast to multiply. Although one study did demonstrate an association between tight-fitting clothing and RVC attacks, in a retrospective case-control study of American university students, the wearing of tight clothing, pantyhose, or synthetic underwear was not associated with candidiasis (66, 81).

Clinical Manifestations

The most common symptom is vulvar pruritus, which occurs in virtually all symptomatic patients and is usually more severe at night. Patients may also complain of a burning sensation after urination. This is intensified in the presence of excoriation from scratching or extensive maceration of the vulva. Vaginal discharge is typically white and cottage cheese-like in consistency, but may vary from watery to homogeneously thick. Other symptoms include vaginal irritation, soreness, burning, dyspareunia, and external dysuria. Odor is rarely present and not offensive. The symptoms are usually exacerbated in the week preceding the onset of menses. There is some relief after the onset of menstrual flow.

Physical examination of the labia and vulva often reveals erythema and swelling with discrete pustulopapular peripheral lesions. A spectrum of manifestations occurs. At one end, there is an exudative syndrome of copious discharge and white plaques on the vaginal walls. At the other end of the spectrum, there is minimal discharge and severe erythema with extensive vulvar involvement (82). Women may develop allergic reactions to *Candida*, which may occur in women after vaginal deposition of ejaculates containing IgE antibodies produced by a male sexual consort sensitized against *Candida* allergens. This can cause severe local reactions in the woman (83–85). Male counterparts of women with VVC may experience a transient rash, erythema and pruritus, or a burning sensation of the penis that occurs minutes or hours after unprotected intercourse.

Diagnosis

The value of signs and symptoms are limited in diagnosing RVVC; accurate diagnosis rests on the use of laboratory tests designed to detect the presence of *Candida* organisms (86–88). Clinically, the diagnosis is made by identifying the presence of hyphae or budding yeast in vaginal secretions mixed with 10% potassium hydroxide preparation. Microscopic examination of a saline preparation of vaginal secretions to exclude the presence of clue cells or trichomonads is also necessary. Large numbers of leukocytes are invariably absent, and if present, suggest a mixed infection. The vaginal pH is normal (4.0 to 4.5), and one in excess of 4.7 indicates BV, trichomoniasis, or a mixed infection. The Pap smear is unreliable as a diagnostic test for Candidal vulvovaginitis. As with cultures, the presence of yeast on a Pap may represent colonization, not infection.

Some argue for more aggressive use of culture in making this diagnosis. Abbott found that only 23 of 71 patients (32.4%) had culture confirmation of a previously positive wet-mount–derived diagnosis of candidiasis (89). On occasion, a woman with symptoms suggestive of a Candidal vaginitis will have no yeast forms seen on microscopic examination but will have a positive culture for *Candida*. Hence, some researchers argue that the wider use of culture would improve outpatient gynecology care (90). Some yeast species, such as *T. glabrata*, may not have typical hyphae or spores, and may be difficult to identify on microscopy. The commonly accepted culture technique has used Sabouraud dextrose agar (usually containing cycloheximide to inhibit overgrowth of unrelated mold species) and is done using samples collected from the posterior vaginal fornix (91). Cultures are also necessary to perform susceptibility testing to antifungal agents.

There is no reliable serologic technique for the diagnosis of symptomatic Candidal vaginitis. A latex agglutination slide technique, using polyclonal antibodies, is available commercially. Its sensitivity is moderately good, but this test provides no advantage over the standard microscopic examination (92).

PCR probes that can detect *Candida* DNA directly in clinical samples have been developed, but are still only available for investigation purposes (93). PCR testing is unable to distinguish between asymptomatic carriers and those suffering from a true Candidal tissue invasion.

The differential diagnosis of VVC may include lichen sclerosis, vestibulitis, vulval dermatitis, vulvodynia, lactobacillosis, and cytolytic vaginosis (a condition due to an overgrowth of lactobacilli in the vagina) (94, 95). In lactobacillosis, extremely elongated lactobacilli are seen in stained smears. The vaginal epithelial cells are not lysed in contrast to cytolytic vaginosis. In cytologic vaginosis, a massive multiplication of lactobacilli can be seen. Latex allergy may also be considered as a differential diagnosis of RVVC.

Recurrent Candidal Vulvovaginitis

Approximately 5% of the women who have experienced one or more attacks of VVC during their lifetime will develop RVVC (76). For unknown reasons, RVVC has increased in recent decades. In contrast to isolated episodes, RVVC represents a management problem, which can be disabling for affected women. RVVC is defined as four or more mycologically proven, symptomatic episodes within a 12-month period, with the exclusion of other pathogens (96). It is often difficult to differentiate between reinfection and relapse in genital *Candida* infections.

Up to one-third of patients with chronic fungal vaginitis may have a non-albicans species present. Fungal cultures may aid in confirming the diagnosis and selecting appropriate therapy. Most patients will have chronic or recurrent episodes of fungal vaginitis despite the absence of underlying medical illnesses or predisposing factors. Risk factors include exogenous hormone therapy, positive HIV serology, repeated courses of broad-spectrum antibiotics, tight-fitting clothing, and local hypersensitivity to the *Candida* antigen. Poor glycemic control in diabetic patients triggers RVVC attacks (97). Diets leading to obesity are known to increase risk of *Candida* skin infections, but have not been proven to predispose RVVC. Although an association between RVVC and frequent intercourse has been shown, it is likely that sexual activity plays a relatively minor role in the pathogenesis of RVVC (98). Chemotherapy, radiation, and corticosteroid therapy are known to increase the risk of RVVC. Unfortunately, in most women with recurrent or chronic Candidal vulvovaginitis, no underlying or predisposing factor(s) can be identified.

Theories to explain the pathogeneses of recurrent Candidal vulvovaginitis include reinfection from exogenous sources such as sexual partners, oral-genital sex, the intestinal reservoir, or vaginal relapse. Vaginal relapse hypothesizes that recurrent infections are due to the same infecting organism declining in numbers only to subsequently increase again and result in a recurrence.

Women who suffer from recurrent Candidal vulvovaginitis may experience physical and psychological sequelae. Symptoms of chronic dyspareunia may cause sexual and marital relations to suffer. These patients need support, counseling, and reassurance that virtually all cases of recurrent Candidal vulvovaginitis can be controlled.

Treatment

Locally applied azole therapies (imidazoles and azoles) are recommended for uncomplicated VVC cases and are successful in at least 80% of cases, whereas therapy of RVVC cases is less successful (Table 10.3). Antifungal drugs used for treatment of RVVC (and VVC) have the disadvantage of being fungistatic and not fungicidal in action (99). Antifungal agents are available topically as creams, lotions, vaginal tablets, and suppositories. There is no evidence

TABLE 10.3

Treatment Options for Candidal Vulvovaginitis

Drug	Formulation	Rx
Acute Cases		
Miconazole, 200-mg suppository (Monistat-3)	1 suppository intravaginally at bedtime for 3 nights	No
2% vaginal cream (Monistat 7)	1 applicatorful intravaginally at bedtime for 7 nights	No
100-mg vaginal tablet (Monistat)	1 vaginal tablet intravaginally at bedtime for 7 nights	No
Clotrimazole (Gyne-Lotrimin, Mycelex G), 100-mg vaginal tablet	1 tablet intravaginally at bedtime for 7 nights	No
(1% vaginal cream)	1 applicatorful intravaginally at bedtime for 7 nights	No
(Mycelex) 500-mg vaginal tablet	1 tablet intravaginally one time	No
Butoconazole (Femstat), 2% cream	1 applicatorful intravaginally at bedtime for 3 nights	No
Terconazole (Terazol 3), 80-mg suppository or 0.8% vaginal cream	1 suppository or 1 applicatorful intravaginally at bedtime for 3 nights	Yes
(Terazol 7) 0.4% vaginal cream	1 applicatorful intravaginally at bedtime for 7 days	Yes
Ticonazole (Vagistat), 6.5% ointment	1 applicatorful intravaginally at bedtime one time	No
Ketoconazole (Nizoral), 400 mg	1 tablet daily for 5 days	Yes
Fluconazole (Diflucan), 150 mg	1 tablet orally one time	Yes
Itraconazole (Sporanox), 200 mg	1 tablet orally daily for 3 days	Yes
400 mg	1 tablet one time	Yes
Prophylactic Regimens		
Ketoconazole, 100 mg	1 tablet daily for 6–12 months	Yes
Clotrimazole, 500 mg	1 tablet vaginally weekly or monthly for 6–12 months	No
Fluconazole, 150 mg	1 tablet orally each month for 6–12 months	Yes
Resistant Cases		
Any of the above drugs at dosage levels used for 7-day regimens for a 14- to 21-day course		
Boric acid, 600-mg capsule	600-mg capsule daily intravaginally for 14 days (requires suppository formulation by pharmacist)	Yes
Gentian violet	Apply to vagina, once or twice for 1 week	Yes

to suggest that the vehicle influences efficacy. The patient's preference should guide the choice of therapeutic vehicles. Extensive vulvar inflammation dictates local vulvar applications of cream.

Low-potency corticosteroids or nonsteroid anti-inflammatory drugs may be used concurrently with antifungal therapy to obtain a more rapid relief of local symptoms. Sitz baths with sodium bicarbonate may also help relieve itching.

The correlation between a vaginal *Candida* infection and the use of OTC antifungal medications is very poor. In one study of women who had self-diagnosed vulvovaginal candidiasis, only 37.4% of the women correctly self-diagnosed (100). In another study, 95 women who had self-diagnosed vulvovaginal candidiasis and had purchased OTC antifungal medication were evaluated (101). Of these 95 women, only 33.7% correctly self-diagnosed, and another 20% had concurrent infection in addition to *Candida*. A prior diagnosis of vulvovaginal candidiasis did not enhance the probability of making a correct diagnosis nor did reading the package insert. Of the women, 51% required a physician-prescribed medication to effect termination of symptomatology.

Topical Agents

The various imidazole and triazole vaginal preparations are broad-spectrum antimycotics, and have superior efficacy compared with polyene preparations (Nystatin). The efficacy and dosing regimens of the various azole derivatives are all comparable. Terconazole, a triazole, is more effective against the non-albicans species than the imidazoles and is equally as effective against *C. albicans*. There is a major trend toward shorter courses and single-dose regimens. These have demonstrated effectiveness in several clinical trials. These trials, however, did not include patients with severe and more intractable infections. This has led some authors to advocate single-dose therapy in patients with infrequent episodes of mild to moderate severity (82). Side effects may include local irritation or discomfort.

Probiotic treatment of Candidal vulvovaginitis holds promise, but more data from well-designed trials of defined products are needed for an objective assessment.

Oral Agents

Oral ketoconazole (400 mg daily for 5 days), itraconazole (200 mg daily for 3 days or 400 mg for 1 day), and fluconazole (150 mg for 1 day) are also often used as therapeutic agents in genital *Candida* infection, particularly when local therapy of RVVC has failed (102, 103). Only fluconazole (Diflucan) has U.S. Food and Drug Administration approval for this indication. Fluconazole was initially believed to have the advantage of eradicating or suppressing an intestinal reservoir of *Candida* and thus would be more protective against recurrences than local antifungal therapy in RVVC cases; however, this assumption has not been proven. Compared with conventional topical therapy, oral therapy demonstrates equal, if not slightly superior, efficacy. Most women, given the choice, prefer oral therapy, although it is more expensive.

The potential side effects of oral therapy are important to remember. Ketoconazole incurs GI upset up to 10% of the time, and rarely, anaphylaxis. The major concern is the risk of hepatotoxicity, which occurs in 1 of 10,000 to 15,000 women treated. Similar side effects are less frequent with itraconazole and fluconazole.

Interactions may occur with oral contraceptives and itraconazole, fluconazole, and ketoconazole. There are a number of reported interactions between ketoconazole and fluconazole with other drugs. Their use should be avoided, or the dose corrected, if they are to be used concomitantly with midazolam, cyclosporin, phenytoin, glipizide, methylprednisolone, prednisone, triazolam, warfarin, and zidovudine. Heart failure may occur if cisapride is given in combination with fluconazole. More recent reports indicate that itraconazole (Sporanox) may cause heart failure in patients with cardiac disorders.

Recurrent Vulvovaginal Candidiasis

Treatment of RVVC generally involves a longer course of antimycotic therapy than that usually recommended for VVC, regardless of the route of administration. Conventional 5- and 7-day therapy should be increased to 10 to 14 days to achieve both clinical remission and mycologic culture-negative status. Immediately after the current episode is effectively treated, a maintenance regimen is indicated. Several possible regimens may be considered, including 100 mg ketoconazole daily for 6 months, 50 to 100 mg itraconazole daily for 6 months, and 100 mg fluconazole once weekly for 6 months. In another regimen, 500-mg clotrimazole vaginal suppositories are administered once weekly. Maintenance therapy should last at least for 6 months. During maintenance therapy, 90% of patients are protected from symptomatic recurrences (104). A small percentage of women may require maintenance azole regimens for several years. Several studies have not demonstrated any resistance problem in *C. albicans* strains isolated from RVVC cases treated even for long periods with azole drugs (105–108).

Boric acid, 600 mg administered vaginally once daily in a gelatin capsule, has been shown to be effective in clinically resistant RVVC cases. Others recommend only 300 mg and thereby demonstrated a lower rate of mucosal irritation (109). Therapy is continued until cultures are negative (usually within 10 to 14 days). Maintenance therapy with boric acid in RVVC cases is used in some settings. The recommended maintenance regimen is use of the drug on alternate days and then twice weekly.

Some women attempt to cure RVVC by vaginal douching with natrium tetraborate (Borax). Others may use tampons with tea tree oil, although this frequently causes severe allergic reactions (110, 111). Concurrent treatment of the sexual partners of women with RVVC has generally not been reported to have any influence on the attack rate of RVVC (112, 113). A lower recurrence rate of RVVC was, however, found in women whose male partners were treated for harboring yeasts in their oral cavity, in the penile coronal sulcus, or in seminal fluid as compared with RVVC women without a colonized male partner (75).

The current knowledge of the role of dietary habits in the pathogenesis of RVVC is not sufficient to make dietary recommendations to patients with this condition.

Pregnancy

The incidence of Candidal vulvovaginitis during pregnancy is 2- to 20-fold higher than that in nonpregnant women. The altered hormonal milieu of pregnancy makes reinfection more common and definitive cure more difficult. Most topical antifungal agents are effective, especially when prescribed for longer periods of 1 to 2 weeks. Nevertheless, single-dose therapy with clotrimazole also has been efficacious in pregnant women. Vaginal antifungal therapy is safe in pregnancy, and there is minimal systemic absorption. Oral antifungal agents are not recommended for use during pregnancy. Because oral triazoles (and possibly ketoconazole) are excreted in breast milk, these drugs should not be used in women who are breast-feeding.

TRICHOMONAS VAGINALIS

Epidemiology

Trichomonas vaginalis (TV) is one of most common STIs in the United States, with an estimated 5 million new cases per year (compared with 3 million cases of Chlamydia and 650,000 cases of GC) (114). It is not a sexually reportable disease, which reflects a misconception that it is not an STI of great significance. This is a misconception in light of the fact that, in women, TV may play a role in preterm labor, the development of cervical neoplasia, postoperative infections, and perhaps atypical PID and infertility. In addition, infection with TV is known to increase the transmission or acquisition of HIV during intercourse. TV can also cause significant morbidity in men. It is a common cause of nongonococcal urethritis, chronic prostatitis, and a probable factor in male infertility secondary to decreases in sperm viability and motility (115–117). Epidemiologic studies show increasing prevalence of TV with age (20 to 45 years) in comparison to gonorrhea and Chlamydia, whose peak occurrence is between 15 and 24 years. These differences may be due to longer duration of infectiousness or variations in the host–parasite relationship. For example, a high vaginal pH predisposes to infection with TV, whereas a high estrogen level seems to be protective (118).

The normally acidic environment in the vagina discourages the growth of trichomonas. Menstruation, semen, or the presence of other pathogens that render the vaginal fluid more basic will favor the growth of these protozoans. Other known risk factors for trichomonas infection include multiple sexual partners, black race, previous history of sexually transmitted diseases, coexistent infection with *Neisseria gonorrhea*, and nonuse of either barrier or hormonal contraceptives.

Pathogenesis

Trichomonas is predominately sexually transmitted. The etiologic agent, *T. vaginalis*, is a flagellated anaerobic protozoan. Transmission appears to be higher from men to women, as 70% of men have disease within 48 hours of exposure, compared with 80 to 100% of exposed women (119–121). Perinatal transmission occasionally occurs and is detected in about 5% of newborn girls born to infected mothers. This is the only documented nonvenereal transmission, and the infection was confined to the genital tract. Although there are no prolonged evaluations on infant carriage, it is presumed that the infection clears in these female infants as the effects of the maternal hormonal milieu dissipates (122). Although trichomonas will survive for short periods on moist objects or exposed bodily fluids, there are no documented cases of transmission by indirect or fomite exposure.

Clinical Manifestations

Trichomonas infection ranges from a asymptomatic carrier state to severe acute inflammatory disease. Up to 50% of women are asymptomatic, but when symptoms and signs do occur they include vaginal discharge, vulvovaginitis, and dysuria (123). Up to 90% of men infected with TV are asymptomatic (120). In some studies, one-third of asymptomatic infected women became symptomatic within 6 months (123). The incubation period of symptomatic trichomonal infection, although controversial, ranges from 3 to 28 days.

The most common complaint is vaginal discharge, described as malodorous by 10% of patients. Other symptoms include vulvar irritation, dyspareunia, dysuria, and/or pruritus. These symptoms can be severe. Lower abdominal pain may also be present, but its presence should raise the possibility of concomitant salpingitis. Symptoms tend to appear or worsen during or immediately after menstruation, or during pregnancy.

On examination, excessive vaginal discharge is present in 50 to 75% of patients. The classically described frothy or bubbly, yellow-green discharge is present in less than one-half of these patients. The discharge is gray in 75% of patients. Vulvar finding may be absent, or, in severe cases, diffuse vulvar erythema may be evident. Vulvar and vaginal erythema and edema is typical. In less than 10% of women, capillary dilatation and punctate hemorrhages of the cervix will result in the characteristic "strawberry cervix." There should be no mucopurulent endocervical discharge unless *Chlamydia trachomatis* or *Neisseria gonorrhoeae* is also present.

Diagnosis

Clinical signs and symptoms of trichomoniasis are neither sensitive nor specific enough to be used alone for diagnosis (124). Signs and symptoms of trichomoniasis often overlap with those of BV, and trichomoniasis is often associated with concurrent BV. It is believed that *T. vaginalis* may alter the normal vaginal flora and contribute to the development of BV (125, 126).

Positive demonstration of the organism is required, and wet mount is most commonly relied on for diagnosis. When motile trichomonads are seen, a wet mount has a high degree of specificity (greater than 95%). The teardrop-shaped parasite is slightly larger than a leukocyte and is mobile. If the slide is too cold, the solution too hypertonic, or too many leukocytes are surrounding the organisms in solution, the parasite may not be very mobile and may be rounder in shape.

In their study of 65 wet-mount preparations found to be positive for *T. vaginalis*, Kingston et al. concluded that the positive identification of TV in wet-mount preparations is most strongly influenced by time (127). In samples where motile trichomonads were immediately identified after sampling, 20% became negative within 10 minutes of the initial reading (127).

Using the current diagnostic standard of wet-mount microscopy, some authors believe trichomonal infections are significantly underdiagnosed (128). Diagnosis based on wet mount results in lower prevalence rates than diagnosis based on culture results (118). Culture in Diamond's medium will identify up to 95% of infections and requires as few as 300 to 500 trichomonads per milliliter of inoculum to demonstrate growth (129). Compared with culture sensitivity, wet-mount sensitivity ranges from 45 to 60% (130).

The disadvantages of relying on culture to make the diagnosis include the delay in results, not having culture media easily available, expense (compared with wet mount), and the possibility that organisms may die in transit.

There is a commercially available DNA-based test called the Affirm VP system (Becton Dickinson) that uses synthetic probes for the detection of *T. vaginalis*, *G. vaginalis*, and *Candida* species from a single vaginal swab (129). This kit has a sensitivity of 92% and specificity of 98% compared with wet mount. Compared with culture, the DNA-based kit has a sensitivity of 92% and a 99% specificity (package insert, Affirm VP III).

PCR-based tests will yield even higher detection rates but as yet are only available in the research setting, due to technical complexity and cost.

With TV, the vaginal pH is almost always greater than 5. Gram's stains are of little value because of their inability to differentiate trichomonas from leukocytes. The Pap smear lacks adequate sensitivity and does not offer advantage over saline preparation microscopy.

TABLE 10.4

Therapeutic Options for Trichomonas Vaginitis

Drug	Formulation
Standard Treatment	
Metronidazole (Flagyl, Protostat), 500 mg	2 g (4 tablets) orally in a single dose
500 mg (should also treat partner)	500 mg orally twice a day for 7 days
Persistent or Recurrent Cases	
Metronidazole	500 mg orally twice a day for 14 days or repeat 2 g orally
Clotrimazole (Gyne-Lotrimin, Mycelex-G), 100-mg tablet	1 tablet vaginally at bedtime for 7 nights
Adjunctive Therapy	
Povidone-iodine suppositories (Betadine)	1 suppository intravaginally twice a day for 14–28 days
Metronidazole gel (MetroGel)	5 g intravaginally twice a day for 5 days
Pregnancy	
Metronidazole	2 g orally one time after first trimester
Clotrimazole, 100-mg tablet	1 tablet intravaginally at bedtime for 7 nights
Lactation	
Metronidazole	2 g orally one time, with discontinuation of breast-feeding for 24 hours

Treatment

Systemic metronidazole and other 5-nitromidazoles (tinidazole, ornidazole, and secnidazole) have been considered part of the standard treatment regimen for trichomoniasis for more than three decades (Table 10.4). Only metronidazole is available in the United States; its cure rates are higher than 90% when given as either a 7-day regimen (500 mg twice a day) or a single 2-g dose (129). Common side effects of treatment include nausea, vomiting, GI upset, and a metallic taste in the mouth. Patients should be instructed to avoid alcohol ingestion while undergoing treatment. Systemic therapy is required to fully treat this infection because organisms may be present in the urinary tract system and in the genital tract. Treatment consists of the following options:

1. 2 g of metronidazole as a single oral dose
2. 250 mg of metronidazole orally three times a day for 7 days
3. 500 mg twice a day for 7 days (131)

Disadvantages to the prolonged dosages include decreased compliance, greater vaginal flora disruption, and a longer period of alcohol abstinence. Intrauterine devices may be left in place except in patients with severe (upper reproductive tract) infections. Patients on medications that activate the liver enzymes, such as phenobarbital or Dilantin, may require either higher doses or longer periods of therapy to effect a cure.

Metronidazole-resistant strains of *T. vaginalis* have been reported; this has also been demonstrated with high doses of metronidazole in the United States. The CDC currently estimates that 2.5 to 5% of *T. vaginalis* isolates demonstrate some resistance to metronidazole, and there is speculation that metronidazole resistance is rising (132, 133).

In cases of resistance, some practitioners augment a high daily oral dose (1 to 2 g) with the use of topical intravaginal agents to increase the concentrations in the vaginal fluids. Such regimens include 0.75% metronidazole gel, or a 500-mg gelatin capsule of metronidazole, placed in the vagina twice a day. For those patients unable to tolerate the oral preparation because of vomiting, intravenous administration of 2 to 4 g daily is an option. In rare cases of metronidazole allergy, an intravenous incremental dosing protocol has been used with good results (134).

There are reports in the literature, including some from the United States, of successfully treating metronidazole-resistant trichomoniasis with tinidazole (135–138). In one report, 24 women who had previously failed high doses of metronidazole (in some cases, more than 20 g of metronidazole) demonstrated a 92% cure rate with the use of high-dose tinidazole (2 to 3 g orally four times a day, plus 1 to 1.5 g intravaginally four times a day) for 14 days (135). Tinidazole was well tolerated at these high doses and appears to have a lower incidence and severity of side effects compared with metronidazole. It is currently under development in the United States.

For those patients who cannot take oral therapy, vaginal treatments with either Metronidazole or Vagisec Plus are therapeutic options, although complete eradication of the organism is not usually achieved. Topical clotrimazole intravaginally for 7 days has variable low cure rates. Other options of vinegar douches, hypertonic (20%) saline douches, sitz baths, and povidone-iodine douches or suppositories offer questionable benefit.

Because trichomoniasis is an STI, sexual partners should be treated concurrently. When this is done, cure rates approach 100%, and recurrence rates are reduced (139–141).

Sequelae of Untreated or Undertreated *Trichomonas Vaginalis*

TV is an important factor in infertility in both men and women. Trichomonads attach easily to mucosal surfaces and may serve as vectors in the spread of other organisms. In women with acute salpingitis, trichomonads have been found in the abdominal cavity (142). In the study by Grodstein et al. (143), women with *T. vaginalis* infection had a 1.9-fold increased risk of tubal infertility compared with controls. For women with two to four episodes of trichomoniasis, the risk increased even higher (OR 2.5), and for women with more than four episodes, the infertility risk increased 6-fold.

Infection with TV increases both the susceptibility of an HIV-negative sexual partner and the infectivity of HIV-positive individuals (144). In a 2-year prospective study, using multivariate analysis of risk factors, infection with trichomoniasis was independently associated with seroconversion from HIV negative to HIV positive with an odds ratio of 1.9 (145).

Several studies demonstrate that TV may be an important risk factor for cervical neoplasia (146, 147).

Pregnancy

TV is associated with adverse pregnancy outcomes such as premature rupture of the membranes (PROM), pre-term delivery (PTD), and low-birth-weight infants (148, 149). The data are limited on whether treatment of TV during pregnancy reduces the incidence of these adverse events.

Use of metronidazole in the first trimester requires caution. Studies suggest that infection with *T. vaginalis* is associated with premature delivery, low birth weight, and postpartum endometritis (121). However, the role of trichomonas in contributing to adverse pregnancy outcome(s) remains controversial. Although some reports found an association between *T. vaginalis* and prematurity, there is little evidence that the micro-organism ascends into the uterus or placenta, or to the neonate.

A single 2-g oral dose is best for lactating women. Breast-feeding should be discontinued for 24 hours after treatment.

Recurrence

When initial therapy is unsuccessful, the most common reasons are noncompliance and reinfection. If single-dose therapy is ineffective, a repeated 2-g dose is given to both the patient and her sexual contacts. This is successful in 85% of cases (131). Other possibilities to consider include misdiagnosis or infection with multiple sexually transmitted diseases. If compliance is assured and sexual partners have been treated, continued infection is most likely due to resistance.

(MUCOPURULENT) CERVICITIS

Clinically, cervicitis is often suspected if endocervical bleeding is easily induced or if a mucopurulent endocervical exudate is present on examination. In the research setting, cervicitis is defined as an increased number of polymorphonuclear (PMN) leukocytes per field on endocervical Gram's stain (e.g., greater than or equal to 10 or greater than or equal to 30 PMNs at 1000 magnification) (150, 151). The association between mucopurulent cervicitis and cervical infection with *C. trachomatis* and *N. gonorrhoeae* is well established (152, 153). The CDC recommends testing for both of these organisms if mucopurulent cervicitis is present. To a lesser extent, cervicitis may be caused by herpes simplex virus (HSV); in as many as one-half of all cases, however, the etiology is unknown. Some of these "unknown etiology" cases may be due to false negatives with Chlamydia testing, although this is unlikely with nucleic acid amplification testing. A small fraction may be due to oral contraceptive pill use because the oral contraceptive may initiate inflammatory changes in the cervix, and finally, there is the possibility of chronic cervicitis where there are copious secretions from the cervix, but microscopic examination shows predominately lymphocytes and monocytes, not PMNs, which indicates the discharge is not mucopurulent.

Marrazzo et al. (154) demonstrated that the signs of cervicitis should be interpreted in the context of age. Their study found that cervical signs suggesting chlamydial or gonococcal infection had higher positive predictive value in younger women. In their analysis of 6230 new visits to a sexually transmitted disease clinic, approximately one in three women younger than 25 years of age with any cervical finding had infection with Chlamydia, gonorrhea, or both. In this study, a relatively small proportion of women older than 25 years with any cervical finding had *C. trachomatis* or *N. gonorrhoeae* documented (9 to 17%).

Because so many cases of mucopurulent cervicitis are not explained by Chlamydia, GC, or HSV it is now suspected that unrecognized pathogens play a role. Several studies have demonstrated a strong association of BV with cervicitis (152, 155). One study has demonstrated that if mucopurulent cervicitis coexists with BV, combination treatment (e.g., doxycycline and metronidazole) resulted in statistically significant better cure rates of both infections when compared with treating only one of the two conditions (156). The role of *Mycoplasma* and *Ureaplasma* species in cervicitis, including testing or treating for these organisms, remains controversial.

ATROPHIC VAGINITIS

Atrophic vaginitis is a symptomatic vaginal inflammatory condition caused by estrogen-deficient vaginal epithelium. It is important to distinguish it from simple vaginal atrophy. With reduced endogenous estrogen, the epithelium becomes thin and lacking in glycogen, and this contributes to a reduction in lactic acid production and an increase in vaginal pH. This change in the environment encourages the overgrowth of nonacidophilic coliforms and the disappearance of *Lactobacillus* species.

The majority of women are asymptomatic, especially in the absence of coitus. Symptoms include vaginal spotting and soreness, external dysuria, pruritus, and dyspareunia. Burning is a frequent complaint, and intercourse often exacerbates this symptom. On examination, the vaginal surface appears thin, smooth, pale pink, without rugae, and with a predominance of parabasal cells on vaginal smear. The discharge is minimal and may be bloodlike, thick, or watery. The vaginal pH varies from 5.0 to 7.0. Microscopy reveals the absence of organisms, increased leukocytes, and small round parabasal epithelial cells. The normal *Lactobacillus*-dominated flora is replaced by a mixed flora of Gram-negative rods.

Atrophic vaginitis also occurs in women who are postpartum, or who are lactating, and in women with athletic amenorrhea. Medications causing similar symptoms include leuprolide, nafarelin, tamoxifen, danazol, some low-dose oral contraceptives, and contraceptives containing progesterone only such as Depo-Provera and Norplant (157).

Treatment consists primarily of intravaginal estrogen cream inserted into the vagina once daily or every other day for 2 weeks. In patients unwilling or unable to use estrogen, topical vaginal lubricants are an option. A long-lasting lubricant, such as Replens, is preferable to K-Y jelly.

VULVOVAGINOGINGIVAL SYNDROME

Lichen planus is an inflammatory dermatosis that may involve the skin, oral and genital mucous membranes, scalp, and nails. The typical lesions of cutaneous lichen planus are pruritic violaceous papules. The association between lichen planus or lichen sclerosus and vaginitis was first described in the mid-20th century (158, 159). The term *desquamative inflammatory vaginitis* was introduced and eight further cases were added in 1968 (160). A patient with desquamative inflammatory vaginitis and oral lesions was later presented as a case of erosive lichen planus (161). Hence, what has previously been called "desquamative vaginitis" is now known to represent a subtype of erosive lichen planus—the vulvovaginogingival syndrome. The vulvovaginogingival syndrome is a distinct type of erosive lichen planus.

The etiology of lichen planus is unknown, although evidence suggests it is immunologically mediated (162). Although the prevalence of lichen planus is unknown, women comprise 55 to 65% of patients with cutaneous lichen planus, and it generally develops in the sixth decade (163, 164).

The clinical presentation of lichen planus is variable, but typically, patients complain of vulval soreness. They may also describe pruritus, burning, dyspareunia, or ulceration, and often present as persistent vulvovaginitis. Unless the woman has a urogenital complaint, she may not be asked about genital symptoms and a vulvovaginal exam may not be done. This is unfortunate because vulvar involvement was found in 51% of women with cutaneous disease in one study (165). Erosive lichen planus often affects the labia minora and vaginal orifice. In one series, vaginal lesions were seen in 70% of the women examined (166). The vaginal mucosa may be acutely inflamed with a denuded epithelium (167). It may be impossible to place a speculum into the vagina, and contact bleeding from the denuded vaginal walls frequently occurs. A seropurulent exudate and serosanguineous discharge are common. In some women, a vaginal pseudomembrane forms. Cervical involvement may also occur in these patients (168). Although most cases of cutaneous lichen planus spontaneously remit, the erosive form may persist and prove difficult to treat.

The differential diagnosis of erosive lichen planus includes bullous disorders, lichen sclerosus, vulval intraepithelial neoplasia, and lupus erythematosus. Biopsy and immunofluorescent studies are helpful in differentiating between erosive lichen planus and bullous disorders. Plasma cell vulvitis can present with vulval erosions, but oral and vaginal lesions are uncommon in this disorder.

Although there is debate about possible overlap between lichen planus and lichen sclerosis, the latter is not known to affect the vagina—a point that may be useful in distinguishing between the two entities.

Although rare, cases of squamous cell carcinoma and squamous carcinoma in situ arising in vulval lichen planus have been reported (169–172). It is important to follow-up with these patients and to perform an early biopsy of any suspicious lesions.

Management of lichen planus is difficult, and there is no one standard regimen. Ointments may be tolerated better than creams, and clinicians should note that patients using long-term topical treatment may develop a contact sensitivity to these agents. Oral analgesics and low-dose antidepressants may be helpful. Treatment of superimposed infections should be instituted promptly. In one series, the use of 25-mg hydrocortisone suppositories inserted into the vagina twice a day for 2 months resulted in improvement in 16 of 17 women (167). Regular use of vaginal dilators coated with a topical steroid is important to prevent vaginal synechiae (173).

Short courses of oral steroids have also been used in the treatment of vaginal lesions (174). One woman with vulval lichen planus was treated with a solution of oral cyclosporin and olive oil; an improvement was noted in symptoms, clinical signs, and histologic appearances, but her disease relapsed after treatment was stopped (175). Results with either griseofulvin or dapsone in vulval lichen planus have been mixed (166, 174).

ACUTE DERMATITIS

Acute dermatitis is a common affliction with a myriad of sources. In contact dermatitis, the vulva becomes erythematous, pruritic, and often exfoliated from scratching. Common offenders are vaginal hygienic products, laundry detergents, perfumed soaps or toilet paper, tight-fitting and/or synthetic undergarments, and local anesthetic medications. Management includes identifying and eliminating the offending agent and should not rely on topical corticosteroids, which frequently cause local burning. Measures for local relief include sodium bicarbonate sitz baths and topical vegetable oils.

PEDIATRIC VULVOVAGINITIS

The most common causes of vulvovaginitis in the pediatric population include poor hygiene and threadworms (pinworms). Poor hygiene is frequently the cause of vaginal contamination from fecal material; bubble baths, soaps, shampoos, sand, and tight clothing may also cause irritation. Other causes of vulvovaginitis include beta-hemolytic streptococci, shigella, sexually transmitted diseases, foreign bodies, inflammatory dermatoses, and desquamative vulvovaginitis.

Diagnosis, as with an adult, includes a full history and physical examination. Common complaints include pruritus, irritation, pain, dysuria, and discharge. Depending on the severity of the symptoms, examination can be in the frog-leg position, which will often show a scanty discharge traced to poor hygiene. If discharge is persistent, purulent, or recurrent, or if there is a concern about sexual abuse, examination in the knee-chest position is preferable. An otoscope may be helpful in visualizing the vagina and cervix. Often, the child is too uncomfortable for a pelvic examination, and examination under general anesthesia is required.

Treatment of vulvovaginitis in the child and/or adolescent depends on the cause. The use of cotton underpants, avoidance of nylon tights or tight-fitting clothing, frequent handwashing, and "front to back" wiping after urination or defecation may address those cases precipitated by poor hygiene.

Further problems encountered in prepubertal and adolescent girls are discussed in Chapter 2.

Clinical Notes

- The normal vaginal pH is 3.8 to 4.5, there is minimal odor, and the phase of the menstrual cycle influences the quantity of normal discharge.
- All women with complaints of vulvovaginitis should have a directed history, physical examination, and in-office laboratory testing because symptoms alone are an insufficient basis for diagnosis and treatment.
- Office analysis of a woman with symptoms of vulvovaginitis includes a pH of vaginal secretions, an amine or whiff test, and wet mount using both saline and 10% KOH.
- BV accounts for 40 to 50% of all cases of vaginitis among reproductive age women.
- BV can occur in women who have had a hysterectomy.
- Three of four clinical criteria must be met for the diagnosis of BV: milky, homogenous discharge; vaginal pH greater than 4.5, at least 20% of epithelial cells on wet mount are clue; and a positive whiff test.
- Approximately 50% of women with microbiologic evidence of BV are asymptomatic. Treatment of asymptomatic patients is not universally recommended.
- The therapy of choice for BV is metronidazole (Flagyl), 500 mg orally twice a day for 5 to 7 days, or 2 g orally as a single dose. Alternative therapies include clindamycin, 300 mg orally two times a day for 7 days, intravaginal metronidazole gel 0.75% 5 g intravaginally twice a day for 5 days, or clindamycin cream 2% 5 g intravaginally every night for 7 nights.
- It is not currently recommended that sexual partners of women with BV undergo therapy, although some recommend this for women with intractable or recurrent disease.
- Twenty-five to 40% of women with positive vaginal cultures for *Candida* are asymptomatic. About 85 to 90% of yeast isolated from the vagina are *C. albicans* strains.
- Diagnosis of vaginal yeast infection is made by identification of hyphae or budding yeast in vaginal secretions mixed with 10% KOH solution and a normal vaginal pH.

- The presence of Candidal vulvovaginitis in women who are menopausal or breast-feeding, or in prepubertal children, should raise suspicions of underlying diabetes mellitus.
- Up to 33% of patients with recurrent Candidal vulvovaginitis (at least four mycologically proven symptomatic episodes of Candidal vaginitis in a 12-month period with the exclusion of other pathogens) will have a non-*albicans* species present.
- Of topical agents, the imidazole and triazole vaginal preparations are the best broad-spectrum antimycotics.
- Oral agents used for Candidal vulvovaginitis include ketoconazole, 400 mg four times a day for 5 days, itraconazole 200 mg four times a day for 3 days or 400 mg as a single dose, or fluconazole 150 mg as a single dose are all highly effective.
- The incidence of Candidal vulvovaginitis is markedly increased in pregnant women. Vaginal therapy is recommended during pregnancy, not oral therapy.
- Women with recalcitrant Candidal infection require long-term suppressive therapy. Treatment of the sexual partner does not seem to significantly reduce the recurrence rate.
- Trichomoniasis is a source of significant morbidity for women (e.g., atypical PID, cervical neoplasia, enhanced transmission or infection with HIV, preterm labor, postoperative infection).
- Control strategies focusing on reducing *T. vaginalis* may have a significant impact on reducing HIV transmission among both women and men.
- Transmission of trichomonas is higher from men to women and it may be detected in about 5% of newborn girls born to infected mothers.
- Trichomonas is asymptomatic in 50% of women and 90% of men.
- Definitive diagnosis of trichomonas requires demonstration of the organism. The vaginal pH is usually greater than 5, and a gray or yellow-green, malodorous discharge may be present.
- All patients with trichomonas and their recent sexual contacts require therapy, with metronidazole (Flagyl) being the drug of choice. Treatment with vaginal preparations may not result in complete eradication of the organism.
- For (rare) metronidazole resistance, the use of metronidazole, 1 to 2 g four times a day, for 10 to 14 days will usually result in eradication of the organism.
- Atrophic vaginitis is usually asymptomatic but may cause vaginal spotting, dysuria, pruritus, and/or dyspareunia. The vaginal pH is greater than 5. Treatment is with intravaginal estrogen cream or topical lubrication.
- The most common causes of vulvovaginitis in the pediatric population are poor hygiene, threadworms, and foreign body.

REFERENCES

1. Kent HL. Epidemiology of vaginitis. Am J Obstet Gynecol 1991;165(4 pt 2):1168–1176.
2. Larsen B. Vaginal flora in health and disease. Clin Obstet Gynecol 1993;36:107–121.
3. Sobel JD. Vaginal infections in adult women. Med Clin North Am 1990;74:1573–1602.
4. Chaponis RJ, Bresnick PA, Weiss RR, et al. Candid vaginitis: signs and symptoms aid women's self-recognition. J Clin Res Drug Dev 1993;7:17–23.
5. Lipsky MS, Waters T, Sharp LK. Impact of vaginal antifungal products on utilization of health care services: evidence from physician visits. J Am Board Fam Pract 2000;13:178–182.
6. Ferris DG, Hendrich J, Payne PM, et al. Office laboratory diagnosis of vaginitis. J Fam Pract 1995;41: 575–581.
7. Bergman JJ, Berg AO, Schneeweis R, et al. Clinical comparison of microscopic and culture techniques in the diagnosis of Candida vaginitis. J Fam Pract 1984;18:549–552.
8. Krieger JN, Tam MR, Stevens CE, et al. Diagnosis of trichomoniasis: comparison of conventional wet-mount examination with cytologic studies, cultures, and monoclonal antibody staining of direct specimens. JAMA 1988;259:1223–1238.
9. Biswas MK. Bacterial vaginosis. Clin Obstet Gynecol 1993;36:166–176.
10. Eschenbach DA. History and review of bacterial vaginosis. Am J Obstet Gynecol 1993;169:441–445.
11. McCoy MC, Katz VL, Kuller JA, et al. Bacterial vaginosis in pregnancy: an approach for the 1990s. Obstet Gynecol Surv 1995;50:482–488.
12. Mead PB. Epidemiology of bacterial vaginosis. Am J Obstet Gynecol 1993;169:446–449.

13. Amsel R, Totten PA, Spiegal CA, et al. Nonspecific vaginitis: diagnostic criteria and microbial and epidemiologic associations. Am J Med 1983;74:14.
14. Eschenbach DA, Critchlow CW, Watkins H, et al. A dose duration study of metronidazole for the treatment of nonspecific vaginosis. Scand J Infect Dis 1993;40(suppl):73.
15. Joesoef MR, Wiknjosastro M, Norojono W, et al. Coinfection with Chlamydia and gonorrhea among pregnant women with bacterial vaginosis. Int J STD AIDS 1996;7:61–64.
16. Sobel JD. Vulvovaginitis. Dermatol Clin 1992;10:339–358.
17. Spiegal CA, Amsel R, Holmes KK, et al. Diagnosis of *Haemophilus vaginalis* by direct gram stain of vaginal fluid. J Clin Microbiol 1983;18:170.
18. Schwebke JR, Hillier SL, Sobel JD, et al. Validity of the vaginal Gram stain for the diagnosis of bacterial vaginosis. Obstet Gynecol 1996;88(4 pt 1):573–576.
19. Spiegel CA. Bacterial vaginosis. Rev Med Microbiol 2002;13(2):43–51.
20. West B, Morsin L, Van der Loeff MS, et al. Evaluation of a new rapid diagnostic kit (FemExam) for bacterial vaginosis in patients with vaginal discharge syndrome in the gambia. Sex Transm Dis 2003;30(6):483–489.
21. van Belkum A, Koeken A, Vandamme P, et al. Development of a species-specific polymerase chain reaction assay for *Gardnerella vaginalis*. Mol Cell Probes 1995;9:167–174.
22. Hillier S, Holmes KK, Holmes KK, et al., eds. Sexually Transmitted Diseases. 3rd ed. New York: McGraw-Hill, 1999:563–586.
23. Spiegal CA. Bacterial vaginosis. Clin Microbiol Rev 1991;4:485–502.
24. Soper DE. Bacterial vaginosis and postoperative infection. Am J Obstet Gynecol 1993;160:467–469.
25. McDonald HM, O'Loughlin JA, Jolley P, et al. Vaginal infection and preterm labor. Br Obstet Gynecol 1991;98:427–435.
26. Hay PE, Lammont RF, Taylor-Robinson D, et al. Abnormal bacterial colonization of the lower genital tract as a marker for subsequent preterm delivery and late miscarriage. BMJ 1994;308:295–298.
27. Hillier SL, Martius J, Krohn M, et al. A case-control study of chorioamnionitis infection and histologic chorioamnionitis in prematurity. N Engl J Med 1988;319:972–988.
28. Watts DH, Krohn MA, Hillier SL, et al. Bacterial vaginosis as a risk factor for post-cesarean endometriosis. Obstet Gynecol 1990;75:52–58.
29. Briselden AM, Hillier SL. Evaluation of Affirm VP microbial indentification test for *Gardnerella vaginalis* and *Trichomonas vaginalis*. J Clin Microbiol 1994;32:148–152.
30. Bejar R, Curbeol V, Davis C, et al. Pre-mature labor II bacterial sources of phospholipase. Obstet Gynecol 1981;57:479–482.
31. McGregor JA, French JI, Jones W, et al. Bacterial vaginosis is associated with prematurity and vaginal mucinase and sialidase: results of a controlled trial of topical clindamycin cream. Am J Obstet Gynecol 1994;170:1048–1059.
32. Sjöberg I, Häkansson S. Endotoxin in vaginal fluid of women with bacterial vaginosis. Obstet Gynecol 1991;77:265–266.
33. Ralph SG, Rutherford AJ, Watson JD. Influence of bacterial vaginosis on conception and miscarriage in the first trimester: cohort study. BMJ 1999;319:220–223.
34. Brocklehurst P, Hannah M, McDonald H. Interventions for treating bacterial vaginosis in pregnancy. Cochrane Database Syst Rev. 2000;(2):CD000262. Review.
35. Rodrigues AG, Märdh P-A, Pina Vaz C, et al. Is lack of concurrence of bacterial vaginosis and candidosis explained by presence of bacterial amines? Am J Obstet Gynecol 1999;367–370.
36. Schwebke JR. Asymptomatic bacterial vaginosis: response to therapy. Am J Obstet Gynecol 2000;183:1434–1439.
37. Ferris DG, Litaker MS, Woodward L, et al. Treatment of bacterial vaginosis: a comparison of oral metronidazole, metronidazole vaginal get, and clindamycin vaginal cream. J Fam Pract 1995;41:443–449.
38. Joesoef MR, Schmid GP. Bacterial vaginosis: review of treatment options and potential clinical indication for therapy. Clin Infect Dis 1995;20:s72–s79.
39. Greaves WL, Chungafung J, Morris B, et al. Clindamycin versus metronidazole in the treatment of bacterial vaginosis. Obstet Gynecol 1988;72:799–802.
40. Bistoletti P, Fredricsson B, Hagstrom B, et al. Comparison of oral and vaginal Metronidazole therapy for nonspecific bacterial vaginosis. Gynecol Obstet Invest 1986;21:144–149.
41. Hanson JM, McGregor JA, Hillier SL, et al. Metronidazole for bacterial vaginosis. A comparison of vaginal gel vs. oral therapy. J Reprod Med 2000;45:889–896.
42. Hilliers, Lipinski C, Briselden AM, et al. Efficacy of intravaginal 0.75% Metronidazole gel for treatment of bacterial vaginosis. Obstet Gynecol 1993;81:963–967.
43. Covino JM, Black JR, Cummings M, et al. Comparative evaluation of ofloxacin and Metronidazole in the treatment of bacterial vaginosis. Sex Transm Dis 1996;20:262– 264.
44. Durfee MA, Forsyth PS, Hale JA, et al. Ineffectiveness of erythromycin for treatment of *Haemophilus vaginalis*-associated vaginitis: possible relationship to acidity of vaginal secretions. Antimicrob Agents Chemother 1979;16:635–637.
45. Pheifer TA, Forsyth PS, Durfee MA, et al. Nonspecific vaginitis. Role of *Haemophilus vaginalis* and treatment with metronidazole. N Engl J Med 1978;298:1429–1434.
46. Duff P, Lee ML, Hillier SL, et al. Amoxicillin treatment of bacterial vaginosis during pregnancy. Obstet Gynecol 1991;77:431–435.
47. Fuller R. Probiotics in man and animals. J Appl Bacteriol 1989;66:365–378.

48. Elmer GW, Surawicz CM, McFarland LV. Biotherapeutic agents. A neglected modality for the treatment and prevention of selected intestinal and vaginal infections. JAMA 1996;275:870–876.
49. McFarland LV, Surawicz CM, Greenberg RN, et al. A randomized placebo-controlled trial of *Saccharomyces boulardii* in combination with standard antibiotics for *Clostridium difficile* disease. JAMA 1994;271:1913–1919.
50. Antonio MAD, Hillier SL. Repetitive element sequence based PCR DNA fingerprinting of *Lactobacillus crispatus* strain CTV-05 used in a pilot study of vaginal colonization. J Clin Microbiol 2003;41(5):1881–1887.
51. Hillier SL, Wiesenfeld HC, Murray P. A trial of *Lactobacillus crispatus* as an adjunct to metronidazole therapy for treatment of bacterial vaginosis. Poster presented at: annual meeting of the Infectious Disease Society for Obstetrics and Gynecology; August 8–10, 2002; Banff, Alberta, Canada.
52. Bump RC, Zuspan FP, Buerschig WJ, et al. The prevalence, six month persistence, and predictive values of laboratory indicators of bacterial vaginosis (nonspecific vaginitis) in asymptomatic women. M J Obstet Gynecol 1984;150:917–924.
53. Vejtorp M, Bollerup AC, Vejtorp L, et al. Bacterial vaginosis: a double-blind randomized trial of the effect of treatment of the sexual partner. Br J Obstet Gynecol 1988;95:920–926.
54. Moi H, Erkkola R, Jerve F, et al. Should male consorts of women with bacterial vaginosis be treated? Genitourin Med 1988;158:935–939.
55. Joesoef MR, Hillier SL, Wiknjosastro G, et al. Intravaginal clindamycin treatment for bacterial vaginosis: effects on preterm delivery and low birth weight. Am J Obstet Gynecol 1995;173:1527–1531.
56. Vermeulen GM, Bruinse HW. Prophylactic administration of clindamycin 2% vaginal cream to reduce the incidence of spontaneous preterm birth in women with an increased recurrence risk: a randomized placebo-controlled double-blind trial. Br J Obstet Gynecol 1999;106:652–657.
57. Caro-Paton T, Carvajal A, Martin de Diego I, et al. Is metronidazole teratogenic? A meta-analysis. Br J Clin Pharmacol 1997;44:179–182.
58. Burtin P, Taddio A, Ariburnu O, et al. Safety of metronidazole in pregnancy: a meta analysis. Am J Obstet Gynecol 1995;172:525–529.
59. Piper JM, Mitchel EF, Ray WA. Prenatal use of metronidazole and birth defects: no association. Obstet Gynecol 1993;82:348–352.
60. CDC sexually transmitted diseases treatment guidelines 2002. MMWR Recomm Rep 2002;51:RR1–6.
61. Sobel JD. Preliminary analysis of a placebo-controlled trial indicates a substantial protective effect of twice-weekly metronidazole vaginal gel in excess of 70% and associated with significantly enhanced overall cure rate. Paper presented at: Fourth World Conference on Vaginitis; January 10–13, 2004; Playa Herradura, Costa Rica.
62. Sobel JD, Faro S, Force JW, et al. Vulvovaginal candidiasis: epidemiologic, diagnostic and therapeutic considerations. Am J Obstet Gynecol 1998;178:203–211.
63. O'Connor MI, Sobel JD. Epidemiology of recurrent vulvovaginal candidiasis: identification and strain differentiation of *Candida albicans*. J Infect Dis 1986;154:358–363.
64. Centers for Disease Control and Prevention. Sexually transmitted diseases treatment guidelines, 2002. MMWR Morb Mortal Wkly Rep 2002;51(RR6):42–44.
65. Spinillo A, Capuzzo E, Egbe TO, et al. Torulopsis glabrata vaginitis. Obstet Gynecol 1995;85:993–998.
66. Geiger AM, Foxman B. Risk factors for vulvovaginal candidiasis: a case-control study among university students. Epidemiology 1996;7:182–187.
67. de-Oliveira J, Cruz AS, Fonseca AF, et al. Prevalence of *Candida albicans* in the vaginal fluid of Portuguese women. J Reprod Med 1993;38:41–42.
68. Odds FC. Candidosis of the genitalia. In: *Candida* and Candidosis. Baltimore: University Park Press, 1988:124–135.
69. Garsia-Tamayo J, Castillo G, Marinez AJ. Human genital candidosis. Histochemistry, scanning and transmission electron microscopy. Acta Cytol 1982;26:4–14.
70. Sullivan D, Coleman D. *Candida dubliensis*: characteristics and identification. J Clin Microbiol 1998;36:329–334.
71. Nyirjesy P, Vasques JA, Ufberg DD, et al. *Saccharomyces cerevisiae* vaginitis: transmission from yeast used in baking. Obstet Gynecol 1995;86:326–329.
72. Stein GE, Sheridan VL, Magee BB, et al. Use of rDNA restriction fragment length polymorphisms to differentiate strains of *Candida albicans* in women with vulvovaginal candidiasis. Diagn Microbiol Infect Dis 1991;14:459–464.
73. Guaschino S, Michelone G, Stola E, et al. Mycotic vaginitis in pregnancy: a double evaluation of the susceptibility to the main antimycotic drugs of isolated species. Biol Res Pregnancy Perinatol 1986;7:20–22.
74. Spinillo A, Capuzzo E, Nicola S, et al. The impact of oral contraception on vulvovaginal candidiasis. Contraception 1995;51:293–297.
75. Leegaard M. The incidence of *Candida albicans* in the vagina of "healthy young women". How often do they have symptoms? Possible etiological factors. Acta Obstet Gynecol Scand 1984;63:85–89.
76. Sobel JD. Epidemiology and pathogenesis of recurrent vulvovaginal candidiasis. Am J Obstet Gynecol 1985;152:924–935.
77. Schmidt A, Noldechen CF, Mendling W, et al. Oral contraceptive use and vaginal *Candida* colonization. Zentralbl Gynakol 1997;119:545–549.
78. Hooton TM, Roberts PL, Stamm WE. Effects of recent sexual activity and use of a diaphragm on the vaginal microflora. Clin Infect Dis 1994;19:274–278.

79. Jones BM, Eley A, Hicks DA, et al. Comparison of the influence of spermicidal and nonspermicidal contraception on bacterial vaginosis. Candidal infection and inflammation of the vagina—a preliminary study. Int J STD AIDS 1994;5:362–364.
80. Parewijck W, Claeys G, Thiery M, et al. Candidiasis in women fitted with an intrauterine contraceptive device. Br J Obstet Gynecol 1988;95:408–410.
81. Elegbe IA, Elegbe I. Quantitative relationships of *Candida albicans* infections and dressing patterns in Nigerian women. Am J Public Health 1983;73:450–452.
82. Sobel JD. Candidal vulvovaginitis. Clin Obstet Gynecol 1993;36:153–165.
83. Witkin SS, Jeremias J, Ledger WJ. Vaginal eosinophils and IgE antibodies to *Candida albicans* in women with recurrent vaginitis. J Med Vet Mycol 1989;27:57–58.
84. Witkin SS, Jeremias J, Ledger WJ. A localized vaginal allergic response in women with recurrent vaginitis. J Allergy Clin Immunol 1988;81:412–416.
85. Witkin SS, Jeremias J, Ledger WJ. Recurrent vaginitis as a result of sexual transmission of IgE antibodies. Am J Obstet Gynecol 1988;159:32–36.
86. Schaaf VM, Perez-Stable EJ, Borchardt K. The limited value of symptoms and signs in the diagnosis of vaginal infections. Arch Intern Med 1990;150:1929–1933.
87. Mårdh P-A, Novikova N. Who are the women that present with a history suggestive of RVVC and with current symptoms mimicking an attack of the condition, but who remains unproven as genital carriers of *Candida* by culture studies? Int J STD AIDS 2001;12(suppl 2):55.
88. Novikova N, Rodrigues AG, Pina-Vaz C, et al. What are the signs and symptoms in women with RVVC caused by *Candida albicans* and non-albicans strains and do they differ from *Candida* culture-negative cases with a history suggestive of RVVC? Mycoses 2001;44(suppl 1):47–48.
89. Abbott J. Clinical and microscopic diagnosis of vaginal yeast infection: a prospective analysis. Ann Emerg Med 1995;25:587–591.
90. Ledger WJ, Monif GR. A growing concern: inability to diagnose vulvovaginal infections correctly. Obstet Gynecol 2004;103(4):782–784.
91. Nyirjesy P, Seeney SA, Grody MH, et al. Chronic fungal vaginitis: the value of cultures. Am J Obstet Gynecol 1995;173:820–823.
92. Hurley R. Recurrent *Candida* infection. Clin Obstet Gynecol 1981;8:209.
93. Giraldo P, von Nowaskoski A, Gomes FA, et al. Vaginal colonization by *Candida* in symptomatic women with and without a history of recurrent vulvovaginal candidiasis. Obstet Gynecol 2000;95:413–416.
94. Horowitz BJ, Mardh P-A, Nagy E, et al. Vaginal lactobacillosis. Am J Obstet Gynecol 1994;170:857–861.
95. Cibley LJ, Cibley LJ. Cytolytic vaginosis. Am J Obstet Gynecol 1991;165:1245–1249.
96. Sobel JD. Pathogenesis and treatment of recurrent vulvovaginal candidiasis. Clin Infect Dis 1992;14(suppl 1):S80–S90.
97. Donders GGG, Preuen H, Reybrouch R. Impaired tolerance for glucose in women with recurrent vaginal candidiasis. Int J AIDS 2001;12(suppl 2):55.
98. Eckert LO, Hawes SE, Stevens CE, et al. Vulvovaginal candidiasis: clinical manifestions, risk factors, management algorithm. Obstet Gynecol 1998;92:757–765.
99. Lynch ME, Sobel JD, Fidel PL. Role of antifungal drug resistance in the pathogenesis of recurrent vulvovaginal candidiasis. J Med Vet Mycol 1996;34:337–339.
100. Ross RA, Lee ML, Onderdonk AB. Effect of *Candida albicans* infections and clotrimazole treatment on vaginal microflora in vitro. Obstet Gynecol 1995;86:925–930.
101. Ferris DG, Nyirjesy P, Sobel JD, et al. Over-the-counter antifungal drug misuse associated with patient-diagnosed vulvovaginal candidiasis. Obstet Gynecol 2002;99:419–425.
102. Desai PC, Johnson BA. Oral fluconazole for vaginal candidiasis. Am Fam Physician 1996;54:1337–1340.
103. Frega A, Gallog D, Renzi F, et al. Persistent vulvovaginal candidiasis: systematic treatment with oral fluconazole. Clin Exp Obstet Gynecol 1994;21:259–262.
104. Sobel JD. Recurrent vulvovaginal candidiasis. N Engl J Med 1986;315:1455–1458.
105. Odds FC. Resistance of yeasts to azole-derivative antifungals. J Antimicrob Chemother 1993;31:463–471.
106. Ősturland A, Strand A. Resistens mot *Candida*. Redan ett bekymmer. Lakartidningen 1998;95:4476–4477.
107. Wirsching S, Michel S, Morschhauser J. Targeted gene disruption in *Candida albicans* wild-type strains: the role of the MDR1 gene in fluconazole resistance of clinical *Candida* isolates. Mol Microbiol 2000;36:856–865.
108. Maenza JR, Merz WG, Romagnoli MA, et al. Infection due to fluconazole-resistant *Candida* in patients with AIDS: prevalence and microbiology. Clin Infect Dis 1997;24:328–340.
109. Guaschina S, de Seta F, Sartore A, et al. Efficacy of maintenance therapy with topical boric acid in comparison with oral itraconazole treatment of recurrent vulvovaginal candidiasis. Am J Obstet Gynecol 2001;184:598–602.
110. Hammer KA, Carson CF, Riley TV. In vitro activity of essential oils, in particular Melaleuca alternifolia (tea tree) oil and tea tree oil products, against *Candida* spp. J Antimicrob Chemother 1998;42:591–595.
111. Wölner-Hanssen P, Sjöberg I. Warning against a fashionable cure for vulvovaginitis. Tea tree oil may substitute *Candida* itching with allergy itching. Lakartidningen 1998;95:3309–3310.
112. Bisschop MP, Merkus JM, Scheygrond H, et al. Co-treatment of the male partner in vaginal candidosis: a double-blind randomized control study. Br J Obstet Gynecol 1986;93:79–81.
113. Calderon-Marquez JJ. Itraconazole in the treatment of vaginal candidosis and the effect of treatment of the sexual partner. Rev Infect Dis 1987;9:143–145.

114. Cates W. Estimates of the incidence and prevalence of sexually transmitted diseases in the US. Sex Transm Dis 1999;26(suppl):52–57.
115. Martinez-Garcia F, Regardera J, Mayer R, et al. Protozoan infections in the male genital tract [Review]. J Urol 1996;156:340–349.
116. Gopalkrishnan K, Hunduja I, Kumar A. Semen characteristics of asymptomatic males affected by *Trichomonas vaginalis*. J In Vitro Fertil Embryo Transfer 1990;7:165–167.
117. Skerk V, Schonwald S, Krhen J, et al. Aetiology of chronic prostatitis. Int J Antimicrob Agents 2002;19:471–474.
118. Bowden FJ, Garnett G. *Trichomonas vaginalis* epidemiology: parameterising and analyzing a model of treatment interventions. Sex Transm Infect 2000;27:241–242.
119. Hasseltine HC, Wolters SL, Campbell A. Experimental human vaginal trichomoniasis. J Infect Dis 1942; 71:127–130.
120. Weston TET, Nico CS. Natural history of trichomonal infection in males. Br J Vener Dis 1963;39:251–257.
121. Heine P, McGregor JA. *Trichomonas vaginalis*: a reemerging pathogen. Clin Obstet Gynecol 1993;36:137–144.
122. Bramley M. Study of female babies of women entering confinement with vaginal trichomoniasis. Br J Vener Dis 1976;52:58–62.
123. Wölner-Hanssen P, Kreiger JN, Stevens CE, et al. Clinical manifestations of vaginal trichomoniasis. JAMA 1989;261:571–576.
124. Sobel JD. Vaginitis. N Engl J Med 1997;337:1896–1903.
125. Schneider H, Coetzee DJ, Fehler HG, et al. Screening for sexually transmitted diseases in rural South African women. Sex Transm Dis 1998;74(1 suppl):S147–S152.
126. Moodley P, Connolly C, Sturm W. Interrelationships among HIV type 1 infection, bacterial vaginosis, trichomoniasis and the presence of yeasts. J Infect Dis 2002;185:69–73.
127. Kingston MA, Bansal D, Carlin EM. 'Shelf life' of *Trichomonas vaginalis*. Int J STD AIDS 2003;14(1): 28–29.
128. Wendel KA, Erbelding EJ, Gaydos CA, et al. *Trichomonas vaginalis* polymerase chain reaction compared with standard diagnostic and therapeutic protocols for the detection and treatment of vaginal trichomonas. Clin Infect Dis 2002;35:576–580.
129. Petrin D, Delgaty K, Bhatt R, et al. Clinical and microbiological aspects of *Trichomonas vaginalis*. Clin Microbiol Rev 1998;11:300–317.
130. Lossick JC, Kent HL. Trichomoniasis: trends in diagnosis and management. Am J Obstet Gynecol 1991; 135:1217–1222.
131. Lossick JG. Treatment of *Trichomonas vaginalis* infections. Rev Infect Dis 1982;(suppl 4):S801–S818.
132. Schmid G, Narcisi E, Mosure D, et al. Prevalence of metronidazole resistant *Trichomonas vaginalis* in a gynecology clinic. J Reprod Med 2001;46:545–549.
133. Sobel JD, Nagappan V, Nyirgesy P. Metronidazole resistant vag trichomoniasis an emerging problem. N Engl J Med 1999;341:292–293.
134. Pearlman MD, Yashar C, Ernst S, et al. An incremental dosing protocol for women with severe vaginal trichomoniasis and adverse reaction to metronidazole. Am J Obstet Gynecol 1996;174: 934–936.
135. Sobel JD, Nyirfesy P, Brown W. Tinidazole therapy for metronidazole resistant vaginal trichomoniasis. Clin Infect Dis 2001;33:1341–1346.
136. Hamed KA, Studemeister AE. Successful response of metronidazole-resistant trichomonal vaginitis to tinidazole. Sex Transm Dis 1992;19:339–340.
137. Voolmann T, Borcham P. Metronidazole resistant *Trichomonas vaginalis* in Brisbane. Med J Aust 1993; 159:490.
138. Saurina G, DeMeo L, McCormack WM. Cure of metronidazole and tinidazole resistant trichomoniasis with use of high dose oral and intravaginal tinidazole. Clin Infect Dis 1998;26:1238–1239.
139. Lyng J, Christen J. A double-blind study of the value of treatment with a single dose of tinidazole of partners to females with trichomoniasis. Acta Obstet Gynecol Scand 1981;60:199–201.
140. 2002 Sexually transmitted diseases treatment guidelines. MMWR Morb Mortal Wkly Rep 2002;51:44–45.
141. Hook EW. *Trichomonas vaginalis*—no longer a minor STD. Sex Transm Dis 1999;26:388–389.
142. Keith LG, Friberg J, Fullan N, et al. The possible role of *Trichomonas vaginalis* as a "vector" for the spread of other pathogens. Int J Fertil 1986;31:272–277.
143. Grodstein F, Goldman M, Cramer D. Relation of tubal infertility to history of sexually transmitted diseases. Am J Epidemiol 1993;137:577–584.
144. Sorvillo F, Kerndt P. *Trichomonas vaginalis* and amplification of HIV-I transmission. Lancet 1998;351:213–214.
145. Laga M, Monoka Akivuvu M, Tuliza M, et al. Non-ulcerative sexually transmitted diseases as risk factors for HIV-I transmission in women: results from a cohort study. AIDS 1993;7:95–102.
146. Zhang Z, Begg C. Is *Trichomonas vaginalis* a cause of cervical neoplasia? Results from a combined analysis of 24 studies. Int J Epidemiol 1994;23:682–690.
147. Vikki M, Pukkala E, Nieminen P, et al. Gynecological infections as risk determinants of subsequent cervical neoplasia. Acta Oncol 2000;39:71–75.
148. Cotch MF, Pastorek JG II, Nugent RP, et al. *Trichomonas vaginalis* associated with low birth weight and preterm delivery: the Vaginal Infections and Prematurity Study Group. Sex Transm Dis 1997;24:353–360.
149. Klebanoff M, Carey C, Hauth J, et al. Failure of metronidazole to prevent preterm delivery among pregnant women with asymptomatic *Trichomonas vaginalis* infection. N Engl J Med 2001;345:487–493.

150. Brunham RC, Paavonen J, Stevens CE, et al. Mucopurulent cervicitis—the ignored counterpart in women of urethritis in men. N Engl J Med 1984;311:1–6.
151. Nugent RP, Hillier SL. Mucopurulent cervicitis as a predictor of chlamydial infection and adverse pregnancy outcome. The Investigators of the Johns Hopkins Study of Cervicitis and Adverse Pregnancy Outcome. Sex Transm Dis 1992;19:198–202.
152. Paavonen J, Critchlow CW, DeRouen T, et al. Etiology of cervical inflammation. Am J Obstet Gynecol 1986;154:556–564.
153. Paavonen J. Chlamydia trachomatis: a major cause of mucopurulent cervicitis and pelvic inflammatory disease in women. Curr Probl Dermatol 1996;24:110–122.
154. Marrazzo JM, Handsfield HH, Whittington WLH. Predicting chlamydial and gonococcal cervical infection: implications of management of cervicitis. Obstet Gynecol 2002;100(3):579–584.
155. Moi H. Prevalence of bacterial vaginosis and its association with genital infections, inflammation and contraceptive methods in women attending sexually transmitted disease and primary health clinics. Int J STD AIDS 1990;161:129–135.
156. Schwebke JR, Schulien MB, Zajackowski ME. A pilot study to evaluate the appropriate management of patients with coexistent bacterial vaginosis and cervicitis. Infect Dis Obstet Gynecol 1995;3:119–122.
157. Beard MK. Atrophic vaginitis: can it be prevented as well as treated? Postgrad Med 1992;91:257–260.
158. Scheffey LC, Rakoff AE, Lang WR. An unusual case of exudative vaginitis (hydrorrhoea vaginalis) treated with local hydrocortisone. Am J Obstet Gynecol 1956;72:208–211.
159. Gray LA, Barnes ML. Vaginitis in women, diagnosis and treatment. Am J Obstet Gynecol 1965;92:125–134.
160. Gardner HL. Desquamative inflammatory vaginitis: a newly defined entity. Am J Obstet Gynecol 1968; 102:1102–1105.
161. Lynch P. Erosive lichen planus. In: Proceedings of the International Society for the Study of Vulval Disease; September 1975; Mexico.
162. Shiohara T. The lichenoid reaction. An immunological perspective. Am J Dermatopathol 1988;10:252–256.
163. Schmidt H. Frequency, duration and localization of lichen planus. Acta Derm Venereol 1961;41:164–167.
164. Kaplan B, Barnes L. Oral lichen planus and squamous carcinoma. Arch Otolaryngol 1985;111:543–547.
165. Lewis FM, Shah M, Harrington CI. Vulval involvement in lichen planus: a study of 37 women. Br J Dermatol 1996;135:89–91.
166. Ridley CM. Chronic erosive vulval disease. Clin Exp Dermatol 1990;15:245–252.
167. Mann MS, Kaufman RH. Erosive lichen planus of the vulva. Clin Obstet Gynecol 1991;34:605–613.
168. Pelisse M. The vulvo-vagino-gingival syndrome: a new form of erosive lichen planus. Int J Dermatol 1989;28:381–384.
169. Liebowitch M, Neill S, Pelisse M, et al. The epithelial changes associated with squamous cell carcinoma of the vulva: a review of the clinical, histological and viral findings. Br J Obstet Gynecol 1990;97:1135–1139.
170. Lewis FM, Harrington CI. Squamous cell carcinoma arising in vulval lichen planus. Br J Dermatol 1994;131:703–705.
171. Dwyer CM, Kerr RE, Millan DW. Squamous carcinoma following lichen planus of the vulva. Clin Exp Dermatol 1995;20:171–172.
172. Franck JM, Young AW Jr. Squamous cell carcinoma in situ arising within lichen planus of the vulva. Dermatol Surg 1995;21:890–894.
173. Lewis FM. Vulval lichen planus. Br J Dermatol 1998;138(4):569–575.
174. Edwards L. Vulval lichen planus. Arch Dermatol 1989;125:1677–1680.
175. Berrego L, Ruiz-Rodriguez R, Ortiz de Frutos J. Vulvar lichen planus treated with topical cyclosporine. Arch Dermatol 1993;129:794.

CHAPTER 11

Sexually Transmitted Diseases

Lisa M. Hollier

INTRODUCTION

Sexually transmitted diseases (STDs) have plagued man for thousands of years. Disease trends have changed dramatically with the availability of effective screening tests and medical therapy. This chapter details the diagnosis and treatment of the major sexually transmitted infections. Two of the most important components in the management of these patients are evaluation for coexisting infections and patient education. Counseling should emphasize compliance with treatment and prevention of future infections. The prevention messages should take into account specific risk factors for the individual patient and provide specific actions to be taken to reduce disease transmission.

DISEASES CHARACTERIZED BY GENITAL ULCERS

The following sections detail the STDs that are characterized by genital ulcers. Table 11.1 provides a summary of these disorders.

Herpes Simplex

Herpes simplex infection is one of the most prevalent STDs, with serious medical consequences such as neonatal infection and increased risk of acquiring other STDs such as HIV (1, 2). Genital herpes is also associated with considerable psychological and psychosexual morbidity (3).

Approximately 5 million adults in the United States report a history of genital herpes infection. Based on national serologic studies, however, the number of infected Americans is probably much closer to 45 million (4). Genital herpes simplex infection can be caused by either HSV type I (HSV-1), also associated with oral/facial lesions, and HSV type II (HSV-2). Both HSV-1 and 2 can be transmitted to other sites by direct contact with infected secretions or autoinoculation. Asymptomatic shedding is very common, especially in the first year after a primary episode, and probably represents a major source of sexual transmission. Recurrences are more common in men than women, and HSV-2 genital lesions recur more frequently than genital lesions caused by HSV-1 (4, 5).

Clinical Symptoms

Infection with the herpes simplex virus (HSV) may be classified into four groups: primary initial infection, nonprimary initial infection (infection with a new HSV type in a patient who has been previously infected with another type of HSV), recurrent infection, and subclinical infection. Although the primary outbreak of herpes is typically asymptomatic, if symptoms are present, they tend to appear within 2 to 14 days of contact. The lesions may be multiple and bilateral, beginning as papules and progressing to vesicles, then finally shallow, exquisitely painful ulcers.

TABLE 11.1

Characteristics of the Ulcerative Sexually Transmitted Diseases

	Incubation Time (Days)	Adenopathy		Bubo Formation		Ulcer		Ulcer		Bleeds Easily[a]		Scarring	
		Bilateral	Unilateral.	Yes	No	Single	Multiple	Tender	Nontender	Yes	No	Yes	No
Lymphogranuloma venereum	4–21		X (2/3)	X		X			X				X
Chancroid	5–7		X	X		Men	Women	X			X	?	
Herpes	3–7	X			X		X	X			X		X
Primary syphilis	10–90	X			X	X			X		X		X
Granuloma inguinale	8–80	X			X	X			X	X		X	

[a] In the absence of secondary infection.

The lesions may be accompanied by burning pain, inguinal adenopathy, and dysuria. In more than two-thirds of women, a flulike syndrome may be present, with fever and malaise. Acute urinary retention may occur. In 10 to 20% of patients, extragenital lesions are also present (6). The duration of viral shedding averages 7 to 14 days for primary infection. The lesions in primary herpes may require 2 to 6 weeks to resolve completely. After the primary infection, the virus becomes latent in sensory nerve ganglion (7, 8).

When symptomatic, the symptoms of nonprimary initial infections may be less severe than with the primary infection. In addition, systemic symptoms, regional lymphadenopathy, and neuropathy tend to be less common (6).

Initial HSV infections occur at mucoepithelial surfaces, followed by latent infection in sensory ganglia. Recurrent lesions result when the virus becomes reactivated and travels down the sensory nerve to the mucoepithelial surface. Approximately 50% of patients develop recurrent lesions within 6 months of the first episode (9). Trigger factors for recurrent outbreaks vary from person to person but can include fever, menses, emotional stress, or local trauma. Recurrent lesions may be less painful than those of the first episode but can still be quite uncomfortable. Systemic symptoms are uncommon with recurrences. A prodrome, including vulvar burning, tingling, itching, or hypersensitivity, may be present prior to the appearance of lesions. The length of viral shedding is shortened in recurrent infections, usually lasting 3 to 6 days. By the seventh to ninth day, most lesions are healed.

Shedding of the herpes virus can also occur in the absence of symptomatic lesions. In the study by Wald et al. lasting from 1987 to 1992, women with a known history of herpes genital tract infection were asked to submit samples from the genital tract and rectum for at least 60 consecutive days (10). Participants were followed for a median of 105 days. Subclinical shedding of virus occurred in 55% of the women with HSV-2, in 52% of women with both HSV-1 and HSV-2, and in 29% of women with only HSV-1. Among women with genital HSV-2 infection, subclinical shedding occurred on a mean of 2% of the days. In this study, there was a good bit of variability in the rates of subclinical shedding among women with genital herpes. The authors noted that significant correlates of subclinical shedding included (a) short length of time since the acquisition of genital herpes and (b) a high frequency of symptomatic recurrences (10).

Diagnosis

Viral culture is the preferred virologic technique for diagnosis. If possible, the specimen should be obtained from vesicular fluid because cultures obtained from broken or crusted lesions have a higher false-negative rate. Vesicles contain their highest viral concentration in the first 24 to 48 hours of appearance, so cultures are most likely to be positive early in the course of infection (11). The viral medium must be refrigerated for best results, and rapid transport to the laboratory is important. In recurrent infections, up to 50 to 60% of cultures are negative (12). Because viable virus may not be present as lesions begin to heal, a negative culture does NOT rule out the diagnosis of herpes. PCR has been used in research settings but is not widely available (13). Accurate type-specific assays for HSV antibodies are based on the HSV-specific glycoprotein G2 for the diagnosis of infection with HSV-2 and glycoprotein G1 for diagnosis of infection with HSV-1 (14). HerpeSelect-1 ELISA IgG or HerpeSelect-2 ELISA IgG (Focus Technology, Inc.) and HerpeSelect 1 and 2 Immunoblot IgG (Focus Technology, Inc.) are laboratory-based, type-specific assays currently approved by the U.S. Food and Drug Administration (15).

The sensitivities of these serologic tests to detect HSV-2 antibody vary from 80 to 98%. False-negative results may occur, especially during the early stages of infection. The specificities of these assays are 96% or greater.

Typing of the viral isolate can be used in counseling the patient about the anticipated frequency of recurrences because the ability of each virus to cause recurring outbreaks in the anogenital region differs significantly. In the first year after primary infection, the HSV-2 has a median recurrence rate of 5, whereas HSV-1 is associated with a median recurrence rate of 1 (16). The type-specific serologic tests may also be used to confirm a clinical diagnosis of genital herpes, particularly if a false-negative HSV culture is suspected—a common occurrence in patients with recurrent infection or with healing lesions. In addition, these tests can be used to diagnose unrecognized infection and to manage the sex partners of persons with genital herpes.

Serologic surveys in developed countries indicate an ongoing HSV-2 epidemic, with a significant rise in HSV-2 seroprevalence in the last two decades (17, 18). The majority of HSV-2 antibody seropositive individuals either does not manifest symptoms or have unrecognized infection. One study found that only 9.2% of those who were HSV-2 seropositive knew they had been infected with genital herpes (17). This lack of recognition facilitates spread of HSV-2 because the virus is shed intermittently from anogenital sites of most HSV-2-seropositive individuals. Most new infections with HSV-2 are believed to result from exposure during a period of asymptomatic viral shedding (19).

There are increasing reports that the prevalence of HSV-1 genital infection in women is rising (20, 21). Genital infection with HSV-1 is strongly associated with age younger than 25 years and being female. Although most new cases of genital HSV-1 infection are likely to be due to urogenital transmission, there is no evidence suggesting that oral sex practices have changed substantially (22). Recurrence rates associated with genital HSV-1 infections are less frequent and are milder than recurrences associated with HSV-2. Subclinical shedding of HSV-1 is less likely, and this bears directly on the risk of transmission. Prevention strategies for genital herpes may need to be tailored to the patient's etiologic cause of infection and/or recurrences, and for HSV-1, should focus on the risk of unprotected urogenital intercourse, which is frequently perceived as "safe" in the context of sexually transmitted infections.

The use of testing to determine HSV type has been suggested for pregnant women at risk of acquiring herpes in the third trimester, for monogamous couples seeking ways to minimize transmission, for the diagnosis of recurrent genital eruptions, and for identifying HSV as a risk factor for HIV transmission in high-risk patients (23).

Treatment

The first clinical outbreak of herpes may require hospitalization for pain control and possibly bladder catheterization. In addition to topical anesthetics (e.g., viscous lidocaine) applied to the lesions, the use of oral or intravenous narcotics may be necessary. Other symptomatic measures include applying warm compresses and sitting in sitz baths. The current guidelines for antiviral treatment and prophylaxis are listed below (15). Oral treatment can be extended for more than 10 days if lesions are incompletely healed after that time. Intravenous antiviral medication is indicated in severe primary outbreaks or in disseminated herpetic infections.

Following the first outbreak, there are options for further management. Patients may choose to take episodic therapy at the first signs of a recurrent outbreak or they may opt for continuous suppressive therapy. Episodic therapy with acyclovir, famciclovir, or valacyclovir as described in the following sections has been shown to decrease the proportion of patients with outbreaks, reduce the duration of symptoms, and shorten the duration of viral shedding (24). Suppressive therapy reduces the frequency of genital herpes recurrences by 70 to 80% among patients who have frequent recurrences (i.e., at least 6 recurrences per year), and many patients report no symptomatic outbreaks (15, 25). The safety and efficacy of suppressive therapy has been documented among patients receiving daily acyclovir for as long as 6 years and daily valacyclovir or famciclovir for 1 year. In patients with frequent recurrences, suppressive therapy improves quality of life more than episodic treatments (26). Patients on suppressive therapy must be counseled that although recurrences are less frequent, viral shedding still occurs, so they are still capable of transmitting the disease.

First Clinical Episode—Recommended Regimens

Acyclovir 400 mg orally three times a day for 7 to 10 days, *or*
Acyclovir 200 mg orally five times a day for 7 to 10 days, *or*
Famciclovir 250 mg orally three times a day for 7 to 10 days, *or*
Valacyclovir 1 g orally twice a day for 7 to 10 days.

Recurrent Episodes—Recommended Episodic Regimens

Acyclovir 400 mg orally three times a day for 5 days, *or*
Acyclovir 200 mg orally five times a day for 5 days, *or*
Acyclovir 800 mg orally twice a day for 5 days, *or*

Famciclovir 125 mg orally twice a day for 5 days, *or*
Valacyclovir 500 mg orally twice a day for 3 to 5 days, *or*
Valacyclovir 1 g orally once daily for 5 days.

Recurrent Episodes—Recommended Suppressive Regimens

Acyclovir 400 mg orally twice a day, *or*
Famciclovir 250 mg orally twice a day, *or*
Valacyclovir 500 mg orally once daily, *or*
Valacyclovir 1 g orally once daily.
Valacyclovir 500 mg once a day might be less effective than other valacyclovir or acyclovir dosing regimens in patients who have very frequent recurrences (i.e., at least 10 episodes per year).

Severe Primary Infection or Disseminated Infection

Acyclovir, intravenous 5 to 10 mg/kg every 8 hours for 2 to 7 days or until clinical improvement, followed by oral antiviral therapy to complete at least 10 days total therapy.

Special Considerations

Pregnancy

Approximately 2% of susceptible women acquire HSV during pregnancy (27). Among women with a history of recurrent outbreak, 16 to 82% may have a recurrence during pregnancy (28, 29). Because of the potential for neonatal morbidity and mortality with vertically acquired infection, herpes infection in pregnancy is especially important.

A primary outbreak in the first trimester of pregnancy has been associated with chorioretinitis, microcephaly, and skin lesions in rare cases (30). Acyclovir may be administered orally to pregnant women with mild or moderate outbreaks, but for primary infections or severe recurrent outbreaks, intravenous therapy should be administered. The maternal antibody status and the timing of maternal infection influence the risk of neonatal transmission risk. The risk of vertical transmission to the neonate when a primary outbreak occurs at the time of delivery is approximately 30 to 50% (31). Among women with recurrent lesions at the time of delivery, the rate of transmission is only 3%, and for women with recurrent disease and no visible lesions at delivery, the transmission risk has been estimated to be 2/10,000 (31). At the onset of labor, all women should be questioned carefully about symptoms of genital herpes, and all women should be examined carefully for herpetic lesions (15). In the absence of lesions or prodromal symptoms, vaginal delivery is appropriate, excluding other obstetric indications for Cesarean delivery. Patients with typical prodromal symptoms or active lesions in labor should be delivered by Cesarean, regardless of the duration of membrane rupture (32).

Unfortunately, although Cesarean decreases the risk of transmission, it does not negate it altogether. The use of serial viral cultures near term is of no clinical benefit. Other special situations, such as preterm premature rupture of the membranes in patients with genital HSV should be managed in conjunction with a specialist in obstetric infections. Preliminary data suggest that acyclovir prophylaxis late in pregnancy may reduce the frequency of clinical recurrences and possibly also reduce the need for cesarean delivery among women who have genital herpes (33, 34). Tested regimens include acyclovir 400 mg orally three times a day or valacyclovir 500 mg orally twice a day, beginning at 36 weeks and continuing until delivery.

The incidence of neonatal infection is approximately 1 in 3000 to 20,000 live births (32). There are three forms of neonatal infection: disseminated (with the high morbidity and mortality despite appropriate treatment), central nervous system (CNS) only (high morbidity, some mortality despite treatment), and skin/eye/mouth involvement only (low morbidity and almost no mortality with treatment). Preventing neonatal infection is difficult because 70 to 80% of afflicted newborns are born to mothers with no history of prior infection or signs or symptoms at or around the time of delivery (28).

Syphilis

Syphilis is caused by the spirochete, *Treponema pallidum*. After peaking at more than 100,000 cases in 1990, syphilis declined every year thereafter until 2001, when the number of reported cases of primary and secondary (P&S) syphilis increased slightly. In 2001, the rate of P&S syphilis was 2.2 cases per 100,000 population, and a total of 6103 cases were reported (35). Rates are more than 100% higher in men than in women, and non-Hispanic blacks accounted for 70% of the cases in 2001 (35). Syphilis is primarily acquired through sexual contact, although approximately 1000 cases of vertically acquired congenital infections occur each year in the United States. The risk of infection to a partner of an infected person is approximately 30% (36).

Clinical Symptoms

Syphilis has been called "the great imitator." It can present in any stage and with almost any symptoms. Even with its ability to present in myriad ways, the hallmark of primary syphilis remains the chancre, a solitary, indurated, and painless ulceration that occurs at the site of inoculation of the spirochete, typically after an incubation period of 10 to 90 days. It is indurated with a smooth base and raised, firm borders. There is no exudate unless secondary infection occurs. There is little pain or bleeding if the lesion is scraped for a darkfield examination. The chancre may occur in the cervix, vagina, or vulva, or on nongenital sites such as the oropharynx. Multiple chancres can occur, particularly in patients infected with HIV (37). Because the chancre is nontender and can be located on the cervix or in the vagina, it can go unnoticed by the patient. Thus, women may be unaware of the infection until serologic testing is performed. If untreated, the primary chancre resolves spontaneously within 3 to 6 weeks. Patients with a previous history of syphilis and who are re-exposed may not develop a chancre or may only develop a small popular lesion.

In the absence of therapy, the patient develops the secondary stage of syphilis from 6 weeks to 6 months later. Low-grade fever, malaise, lymphadenopathy, and rash characterize secondary syphilis. The primary chancre may still be present in secondary syphilis. Epitrochlear adenopathy, a rare occurrence, should strongly raise suspicions for the diagnosis of syphilis. The nature of the rash in secondary syphilis is variable. It may be macular, maculopapular, papular, pustular, or any variation thereof. With the exception of congenital syphilis, it is never vesicular. It may be quite pronounced or rather unimpressive. It may occur anywhere on the body, including the palms of the hands and soles of the feet. If hair follicles are involved, a temporary, localized alopecia may develop. In warm, moist areas of the body, gray plaques called condyloma lata may develop. They are highly infectious. Lesions of mucus membranes, or mucus patches, may develop as silvery gray, shallow ulcerations with a raised red border. These are also highly infectious. During the secondary stage, there is hematogenous and lymphatic dissemination of the spirochete. If left untreated, the symptoms of secondary syphilis will resolve spontaneously.

An asymptomatic latent phase that is quite variable in duration follows secondary syphilis. The Centers for Disease Control and Prevention (CDC) defines early latent phase as latent infection acquired within 1 year while the World Health Organization (WHO) defines early latent phase as infection of less than 2 years' duration (15, 38). Syphilis is sexually communicable by patients in primary, secondary, or early latent stages. The late latent stage is unlikely to be sexually contagious but can be transmitted to a fetus transplacentally.

If latent syphilis is untreated, about 33% of patients will develop tertiary syphilis with involvement and progressive destruction of the CNS and/or ascending aorta, although almost any organ may be involved. Another expression of tertiary syphilis is gummas, lesions with a coagulated, necrotic center and evidence of small-vessel obliterative endarteritis. These principally appear in the skin, liver, bones, and spleen.

Diagnosis

Diagnostic testing involves a two-step process, beginning with a nonspecific test and concluding with a treponeme-specific test for patients screening positive. The nontreponemal screening tests include the VDRL (Venereal Disease Research Laboratory), RPR (rapid plasma reagin), or ART (automated reagin test). Nontreponemal test antibody titers usually correlate with disease activity, and tests should be reported with a quantitative titer. The RPR has greater than 90%

sensitivity and 98% specificity. In about 2% of patients, a prozone phenomenon occurs, especially in secondary syphilis when the antigenic load is peaking. Therefore, when the index of suspicion is high but the test is reported as negative, it may be useful to contact the lab and request a repeat test with higher than normal dilutions. In addition, the nonspecific tests may be falsely negative early in the course of the infection.

False-positive results may occur with other disease states or physiologic conditions (e.g., pregnancy). Any strong immunologic stimulus (vaccination, acute viral or bacterial infections) may cause a transient false-positive reaction (39). False-positives have also been associated with drug abuse and connective tissue diseases (39). Diseases due to other treponemes (e.g., Lyme disease) may also cause false-positive treponemal test results (40). Because the current incidence of syphilis is so low, the majority of positive screening tests will not be due to treponemal infection.

Treponemal specific tests including FTA-ABS (fluorescent treponemal antibody absorbed) or TP-PA (*Treponema pallidum* particle agglutination test) are necessary to confirm the diagnosis of syphilis after a positive screening result. These tests are specific for *Treponema pallidum* antigens and are reported as positive or negative. The TP-PA is more commonly used than the FTA-ABS because it is less expensive and simpler to perform.

Darkfield examination can be done on specimens obtained directly from syphilitic lesions. This may be the diagnostic method of choice for patients with a chancre because the nonspecific and specific serologic tests may be nonreactive when the chancre first appears.

CNS involvement can occur in any stage of syphilis. If a patient has any neurologic symptoms, regardless of suspected stage of infection, a lumbar puncture is recommended. Lumbar puncture may also be indicated in HIV-positive patients where asymptomatic neurosyphilis may occur or in cases where inadequate treatment (including Benzathine penicillin) was given. More detailed discussion of HIV-infected patients and syphilis is found in Chapter 24.

Treatment

Penicillin G, in benzathine, aqueous procaine, or aqueous crystalline form, is the drug of choice for treatment of all stages of syphilis. Because of the high rate of failure of other treatment modalities, particularly in pregnancy, patients with known penicillin allergy should undergo desensitization with subsequent administration of penicillin. For one oral desensitization protocol, see Table 11.2 (41). The first dose of benzathine penicillin should be given at the completion of the oral protocol.

Recommended (15) Regimen for Adults (Nonpenicillin Allergic or After Desensitization)

PRIMARY, SECONDARY, OR EARLY LATENT STAGE
Benzathine penicillin G, 2.4 million units intramuscularly in a single dose

LATE LATENT STAGE OR SYPHILIS OF UNKNOWN DURATION
Benzathine penicillin G, 2.4 million units intramuscularly once a week for 3 consecutive weeks

NEUROSYPHILIS
Aqueous crystalline penicillin G, 3 to 4 million units intravenously every 4 hours or 18 to 24 million units daily as continuous infusion, for 10 to 14 days

Response to therapy should be monitored with clinical and serologic examination at 6 and 12 months. Titers decrease more quickly in earlier stages of disease, when titers are low, and in patients without a previous history of syphilis. Failure of nontreponemal antibody titers to decrease four-fold at 6 months indicates probable treatment failure in primary or secondary syphilis (15). For patients with latent syphilis, an additional antibody titer should be performed at 24 months post-treatment. Titers should decline at least four-fold by 12 to 24 months after treatment. However, 15% of patients do not meet criterion for serologic cure 12 months after appropriate treatment (42). A four-fold rise in the antibody titer (e.g., 1:4 to 1:16) signifies recurrent infection and retreatment is indicated. With treatment, the nonspecific tests may revert to negative. In the majority of patients, once a specific treponemal test is positive, it stays positive for life. However, after treatment with benzathine penicillin G, up to 24% of those with a positive FTA-ABS test, and up to 13% of those with a positive MHA-TP test, may revert to negative (42).

TABLE 11.2

Oral Penicillin Desensitization Protocol

Dose[a]	Penicillin V Suspension (U/mL)	Amount[b] (mL)	Amount[b] (U)	Cumulative Dose (U)
1	1000	0.1	100	100
2	1000	0.2	200	300
3	1000	0.4	400	700
4	1000	0.8	800	1500
5	1000	1.6	1600	3100
6	1000	3.2	3200	6300
7	1000	6.4	6400	12,700
8	10,000	1.2	12,000	24,700
9	10,000	2.4	24,700	48,700
10	10,000	4.8	48,000	96,700
11	80,000	1.0	80,000	176,000
12	80,000	2.4	164,000	336,700
13	80,000	4.8	320,000	656,700
14	80,000	8.0	640,000	1,296,700

Adapted from Hutto C, Arvin A, Jacobs R, et al. Intrauterine herpes simplex virus infections. J Pediatr 1987;110:97–101, with permission.
[a] Interval between doses: 15 minutes; elapsed time: 3 hours and 45 minutes; cumulative dose: 1.3 million units.
[b] The specific amount of drug is diluted in approximately 30 mL of water and then given orally.
Patients will be desensitized as above. After desensitization, patients will be observed for 30 minutes before parenteral injection of benzathine penicillin.
Patients who have been desensitized previously, who have received their benzathine penicillin intramuscularly, and who are returning for their second shot will not require additional desensitization. Although desensitization is usually lost within 2 days of terminating the penicillin therapy, long-acting benzathine penicillin will sustain the sensitized state for periods up to 3 weeks.

Within hours after antibiotic treatment, patients can develop an acute complication called the Jarisch-Herxheimer reaction. Symptoms include fever, chills, myalgias, headache, tachycardia, hyperventilation, vasodilation, and mild hypotension. Although the reaction occurs in 10 to 25% of patients overall, it is most common in the treatment of secondary syphilis. Symptoms last for 12 to 24 hours and are usually self-limiting. Patients can be treated symptomatically with antipyretics. All patients receiving initial treatment should be counseled regarding this reaction and instructed to report any symptoms they may develop.

Special Considerations

Syphilis in Pregnancy

Testing during pregnancy is recommended at the first prenatal visit, and again in the third trimester, particularly in high-risk populations. Laws also mandate serologic screening at delivery in many states. The only effective treatment for the prevention of congenital syphilis in pregnancy is penicillin G. Treatment of syphilis during pregnancy should consist of the penicillin regimen appropriate for the stage of syphilis. Because the treatment failure rate is increased in patients with secondary syphilis, some experts recommend the use of a second injection of benzathine penicillin G 2.4 million units intramuscularly 1 week after the first to treat early syphilis in pregnancy.

Although titers are generally followed at 6 and 12 months, women with a high risk of reinfection should be followed with monthly titers (15). The decline in titer during pregnancy is similar to nonpregnant patients. The highest congenital infection rate is seen with P&S infections in the mother. Symptomatic fetal infection before 20 weeks of gestation is rare, so treatment of the mother during the first 20 weeks of pregnancy almost ensures the newborn will not be infected. Transmission with fetal neonatal infection occurs in 50 to 67% of cases with maternal primary or secondary syphilis (43). The risk of congenital infection for early latent infection is 40 to 80% and 6 to 14% for late latent infection (43).

When symptoms appear within the first 2 years of life, the disease is termed *early congenital syphilis*. Symptoms occurring after that time constitute *late congenital syphilis*. Early symptoms include hepatosplenomegaly, a maculopapular rash, bone lesions, and nasal discharge or "snuffles." Late manifestations include Hutchinson's triad (Hutchinson's teeth, interstitial keratitis, and eighth-nerve deafness) (44). Penicillin treatment of potentially infected newborns is the main stay of therapy and prevention of adverse sequelae. Quantitative antibody titers should be repeated at 3, 6, and 12 months post-therapy.

Syphilis and Human Immunodeficiency Virus

Given the strong association between HIV and genital ulcer disease, concurrent infection with HIV and syphilis is common. It is believed by some, but not all, that the HIV-infected patient with syphilis may present with greater constitutional symptoms, organ involvement, particularly uveitis, and a significant predisposition to neurosyphilis (45, 46). For most patients with HIV, serologic testing provides accurate information. It has been suggested that patients with HIV and syphilis should be treated more aggressively than patients without HIV. A further discussion of syphilis in HIV-positive patients is found in Chapter 24.

Cerebrospinal Fluid Examination

Patients with neurologic involvement, syphilitic uveitis, and other ocular manifestations should have a CSF evaluation. In addition, most would agree that failure of initial therapy, an antibody titer of greater than or equal to 1:32 in infection known to be more than 1 year in duration, history of nonpenicillin therapy in infection known to be more than 1 year in duration are sufficient grounds for lumbar puncture (15). Discussion regarding the use of lumbar puncture in syphilis for patients who are HIV positive is found in Chapter 24.

There is no single test that can diagnose neurosyphilis. Clinical neurologic findings and combinations of reactive serology, specific abnormalities on examination of the cerebrospinal fluid (e.g., elevated protein and cell count), and/or a reactive VDRL or PCR on cerebrospinal fluid are used. The RPR should not be performed on cerebrospinal fluid for the diagnosis of neurosyphilis. For asymptomatic neurosyphilis, treatment can prevent destruction of the nervous system and the development of symptoms. For symptomatic neurosyphilis, treatment will prevent further destruction but will not reverse the damage that has been done (47).

Lymphogranuloma Venereum

Lymphogranuloma venereum (LGV) is an STD caused by *Chlamydia trachomatous* serotypes L1, L2, and L3 (48). LGV is more common in Central and South America than in North America. In Third World countries it is more common, with some areas reporting an incidence of up to 11% (49).

Clinical Symptoms

The incubation period from exposure to appearance of a painless lesion is about 4 to 21 days. The primary lesion of LGV may be a papule, an ulcer or erosion, a small herpetiform lesion, or nonspecific urethritis (50). In women, the primary lesion occurs most commonly on the posterior aspect of the vagina or cervix, or on the vulva. The lesion usually heals without scarring in several days (50). Approximately 1 to 4 weeks later, the secondary stage begins with tenderness and swelling of the lymph nodes that drain the primary lesion. In women, if the primary lesion is on the vulva, the inguinal and femoral nodes are involved. In 10 to 20% of patients with femoral node involvement, the inguinal ligament may produce a "groove" sign. If the lesion is rectal, the deep iliac nodes are affected; if it is in the upper vagina or cervix, the obturator and iliac nodes become inflamed. The adenopathy, also called buboes, may progress to extensive adenitis; ultimately, about one-third of buboes will rupture, often through multiple draining sinuses. About 20 to

30% of women have the characteristic inguinal involvement (51). Patients may also complain of symptoms consistent with lower abdominal and/or back pain secondary to deep pelvic and lumbar lymph node involvement. Left untreated, the infection continues with tissue destruction and scarring. As a result, sinuses, fistulas, and strictures involving the vulva, perineum, and rectum may develop. At the end stage of the disease, elephantiasis and hypertrophic ulceration occurs.

Diagnosis

A diagnosis of LGV may be difficult, particularly because of the rarity of the condition, but is usually based on positive chlamydial serology for acute infection, isolation of chlamydia from infected tissue, and occasionally on histopathology. Culture of purulent aspirate from buboes may yield the best results, but culture from genital or rectal tissue can be used. Unfortunately, isolation rates are low—only about 30% of cases (52). The complement fixation test for chlamydial antibodies may be used and active LGV infection is generally associated with titers greater than 1:64. There is cross-reactivity between the genotypes of chlamydia. PCR techniques have recently been used to identify the organism (53).

Treatment

Treatment for LGV is doxycycline 100 mg two times a day for 21 days. Alternative regimens include tetracycline, erythromycin, or sulfamethoxazole (15). Aspiration of fluctuant nodes through adjacent healthy skin should be done to prevent sinus tract formation. Surgical excision of affected nodes, however, will only serve to further impair already compromised lymphatic drainage and is not recommended. Antibiotics will help with constitutional symptoms but will only have a limited effect in resolution of buboes.

Recommended Regimen

Doxycycline 100 mg orally 2 times a day for 21 days.

Alternative Regimens

Erythromycin 500 mg orally four times a day for 21 days, *or*
Sulfisoxazole 1000 mg orally two times a day for 21 days, *or*
Tetracycline 500 mg four times a day for 21 days.

Chancroid

Chancroid is a genital ulcer disease caused by *Haemophilus ducreyi*. Although very rare in the United States, major outbreaks have been reported in the last 15 years (54, 55). The disease is highly contagious, and the incubation time varies from 1 day to several weeks, with a median of 5 to 7 days (56).

Clinical Symptoms

Lesions usually begin as small papules and progress over 1 to 3 days to relatively painful ulcers. In women, most of the lesions are located at the entrance to the vagina and may include the fourchette, labia, vestibule, and clitoris (57). Unilateral, tender, inguinal adenopathy is common and present in about 50% of patients (56). Approximately 25% of cases may develop a bubo 7 to 10 days after the appearance of the lesion. Left untreated, the bubo can enlarge and may drain spontaneously or require drainage for resolution of symptoms.

Diagnosis

A definitive diagnosis of chancroid requires the identification of *H. ducreyi* from genital ulcers or infected inguinal nodes. The most reliable material to use for culture is purulent material aspirated from a bubo. Even with special culture media, the sensitivity of culture is less than 80% (15). Although there are no FDA-approved PCR tests, these assays have been developed and used with success (58, 59). Both HSV and syphilis should be ruled out during the diagnostic process.

Treatment

First-line treatment involves azithromycin (Zithromax), ceftriaxone (Rocephin), ciprofloxacin (Cipro), or erythromycin base (Eryc, e-mycin) (15). Patients should be seen for follow-up within 7 days after initiation of treatment—most patients will begin to improve within 3 days. Fluctuant nodes can be aspirated through adjacent healthy skin, if necessary. Partners should also be examined and treated, regardless of symptomatology, and the couple should abstain from any sexual contact until the treatment is completed.

Recommended Regimen

Azithromycin (Zithromax) 1 g orally in a single dose, *or*
Ceftriaxone (Rocephin) 250 mg intramuscularly in a single dose, *or*
Ciprofloxacin (Cipro) 500 mg orally twice a day for 3 days, *or*
Erythromycin base (Eryc, E-mycin) 500 mg orally three times a day for 7 days.

Granuloma Inguinale (Donovanosis)

Granuloma inguinale is a genital ulcer disease caused by *Calymmatobacterium granulomatis*. There are fewer than 100 cases per year in the United States, but it is more frequent worldwide. Granuloma inguinale, or Donovanosis, is endemic in Papua New Guinea, KwaZulu/Natal and Eastern Transvaal, South Africa, parts of India, Brazil, and in the aboriginal community of Australia.

Clinical Symptoms

The incubation time is uncertain, ranging from 1 to 360 days (60). The initial lesion is commonly a small, painless papule or nodule that soon ulcerates and becomes beefy red. The ulcer bleeds easily and, unless secondary infection occurs, is painless. In women, the most common sites involved are the labia and fourchette, although the vaginal walls or cervix may also be involved. It is frequently diagnosed in pregnancy, and it is suspected that pregnancy intensifies the disease (57). Inguinal groin swellings, or pseudobuboes, result from the subcutaneous spread of granulomas into the inguinal region—it is not a true adenitis. Lymphedema and subsequent elephantiasis of the external genitalia may result in severe cases. Healing is often accompanied by scarring. Systemic disease, although rare, does occur and is more common in women, particularly those with primary lesions of the cervix (61). In cases of concurrent infection with another STD, secondary bacterial infection of lesions, or extensive spread of lesions, constitutional symptoms may also be noted.

Although the typical appearance of lesions on the genitalia is well known, Donovanosis is also associated with other lesser well-known appearances and complications. Primary lesions have been reported to occur on the upper arms, chest, legs, bones (especially the tibia), and even the jaw. It may appear as an atypical lesion on the cervix, mimicking cervical cancer, and may extend to the pelvis. Donovanosis has a more aggressive course during pregnancy and should be suspected in women with atypical genital lesions attending antenatal clinics.

Diagnosis

The diagnosis is usually made on clinical grounds but can be confirmed with histologic examination of a biopsy or scrapings taken from the edges of a lesion. It may be readily identified from tissue smears using a rapid Giemsa test. If multiple swabs of the lesion are to be taken to identify the etiology and granuloma inguinale is suspected, the swab for it should be done first to ensure enough cellular material is obtained. The gold standard for diagnosis is demonstration of intracellular Donovan bodies. No serologic tests are currently used for diagnosing this disease.

Treatment

There are few trials to guide the choice of the ideal drug or duration of therapy. The recommended regimens should be continued for at least 3 weeks or until all lesions have completely healed (15). Larger lesions seem to require longer periods of treatment. Patients should be followed until symptoms are resolved. Sexual partners should be evaluated and offered treatment, but the benefit of empiric therapy has not been established (15).

As first-line treatment, the CDC recommends 3 weeks of either trimethoprim-sulfamethoxazole one double-strength tablet orally twice a day or doxycycline 100 mg twice a day, and as second-line treatment, either ciprofloxacin 750 mg twice a day or erythromycin base 500 mg orally four times a day (62). Gentamicin 1 mg/kg IV every 8 hours should be considered if lesions do not respond within the first few days of therapy. The WHO latest draft guidelines recommend azithromycin 1 g orally on the first day, then 500 mg daily or doxycycline 100 mg two times a day as first-line treatment, or alternatively, trimethoprim-sulfamethoxazole one double-strength tablet orally twice a day or erythromycin base 500 mg orally four times a day or tetracycline 500 mg four times a day, with treatment to be continued until all lesions have completely epithelialized (63).

Recommended Regimens

Doxycycline (Vibramycin, Doryx) 100 mg twice a day, *or*
Trimethoprim-sulfamethoxazole (800 mg/160 mg) (Bactrim DS) two tabs twice a day.

Alternative Regimens

Ciprofloxacin (Cipro) 750 mg orally twice a day for at least 3 weeks, *or*
Erythromycin base 500 mg orally four times a day for at least 3 weeks, *or*
Azithromycin 1 g orally once per week for at least 3 weeks.
The erythromycin regimen is recommended for treatment of pregnant patients.

DISEASES CHARACTERIZED BY CERVICITIS

Chlamydia

Chlamydia genital infection is the most common infectious disease reported to state health departments and to the CDC, with adolescent females 15 to 19 years of age having the highest reported rates of chlamydia and gonorrhea (64, 65). The pathogen, *Chlamydia trachomatis*, is an intracellular bacterium that infects women most commonly at the transformation zone of the cervix. The incubation period is 1 to 3 weeks. The majority of female patients with chlamydia are asymptomatic, although some may present with mucopurulent cervical discharge. Chlamydia has been associated with pelvic inflammatory disease (PID), mucopurulent cervicitis, a pneumonialike syndrome in neonates, and a conjunctivitis syndrome in the infant (64).

Diagnosis

The diagnosis is currently made either by culture or rapid diagnostic tests. Although tissue culture is the gold standard in identifying *Chlamydia trachomatis*, rapid diagnostic tests using nucleic acid amplification technology are readily available, accurate, and avoid a number of disadvantages associated with culture (66). Because *C. trachomatis* is an intracellular bacterium, it is essential that cells be included in the sampling, regardless of the diagnostic methodology. Neither cytology nor serology is used for the diagnosis of chlamydial infection. Screening programs using DNA testing on urine samples have proved highly acceptable (67). As a result of the high rate of concurrent infection, any woman being tested for chlamydia should also be screened for gonorrhea (68). Annual screening of all sexually active women ages 20 to 25 is recommended, as is screening of older women with risk factors (15).

Treatment

The recommended regimens for chlamydia cervicitis include azithromycin and doxycycline (15). A study of patients in a health maintenance organization demonstrated that screening and treatment of women with cervical infection with chlamydia may reduce the likelihood of PID (69). Although erythromycin (erythromycin base 500 mg orally four times a day for 7 days) or amoxicillin (500 mg orally three times a day for 7 days) are the recommended treatment regimens for pregnant patients, there is accumulating evidence that azithromycin as a 1-g single dose is a safe and effective therapy in pregnant patients (15, 70). To minimize further transmission and reinfection, patients should be instructed to abstain from sexual intercourse for 7 days after single-dose therapy, or until completion of a 7-day regimen, and should also be instructed to abstain from sexual intercourse until all their sex partners have been treated. Patients should refer their sexual partners for evaluation, testing, and treatment.

Patients do not need to be tested for chlamydia after completing treatment with doxycycline or azithromycin unless they remain symptomatic or reinfection is otherwise suspected. A test of cure can be considered 3 weeks after completion of therapy for patients treated with erythromycin or amoxicillin because treatment failure may be more likely (15).

Recommended Regimens

Azithromycin 1 g orally in a single dose, *or*
Doxycycline 100 mg orally two times a day for 7 days.

Alternative Regimens

Erythromycin base 500 mg orally four times a day for 7 days, *or*
Erythromycin ethylsuccinate (EES) 800 mg orally four times a day for 7 days, *or*
Ofloxacin 300 mg orally two times a day for 7 days, *or*
Levofloxacin 500 mg orally for 7 days.

Neisseria Gonorrhea

Neisseria gonorrhoeae is still a major cause of infectious cervicitis and PID, and in 2001, a total of 361,705 cases of gonorrhea were reported, which reflects a stabilization of rates since 1998 (65). Although men are often symptomatic and usually present early for therapy, significant symptoms in women may not be evident until complications such as PID are present (71, 72). The incubation period after exposure is 3 to 5 days. Risk of transmission from a male to a female after one exposure is high at about 70% (73).

Clinical Symptoms

When women are symptomatic, the most common complaints are a mucopurulent discharge, dysuria, and/or abnormal vaginal bleeding. Mucopurulent discharge is present in about 25% of symptomatic women. In addition to cervicitis, infection may also involve the urethra, Skene's glands, Bartholin's glands, and anus. Approximately 10% of infected women will also have a pharyngeal infection with gonococcus (74). In 15 to 20% of women with pelvic site infection, acute PID will develop. Disseminated gonococcal infection (DGI) occurs in 1 to 2% of patients with gonorrhea and is more common in women than in men (75). Untreated, gonorrhea is associated with severe sequelae, such as infertility, increased incidence of ectopic pregnancy, and chronic pelvic pain. Infertility may occur in as high as 20% of patients without early treatment for pelvic infections caused by *N. gonorrhoeae* (76).

Diagnosis

The diagnosis of gonorrhea is best made either with culture or with nucleic acid amplification tests (NAATs). Rapid diagnostic tests are highly sensitive—detecting up to 98% of infections (77, 78). If culture is done, modified Thayer-Martin media should be used, and the specimen should be placed in an oxygenfree environment. The specimen should not be refrigerated. For either culture or rapid testing, the specimen should be obtained from the discharge in the endocervix. A single endocervical swab will detect up to 90% of infections with gonorrhea, whereas two consecutive endocervical swabs or an endocervical and separate anal swab increase the detection rate to 99%. The use of NAATs for rectal and oropharyngeal specimens has had limited evaluation and is not recommended (79). As antimicrobial resistance increases among gonococcal strains, culture with sensitivity testing provides an advantage over DNA-based technologies.

Treatment

The recommended treatment regimens for uncomplicated gonorrheal infection of the cervix or urethra include cefixime 400 mg orally or ceftriaxone 125 mg intramuscularly in a single dose. Other oral regimens include a single dose of ciprofloxacin 500 mg, ofloxacin 400 mg, and levofloxacin 250 mg.

As a result of increasing resistance, fluoroquinolones are no longer advised for treatment of gonorrhea in Hawaii or California or for infections that may have been acquired in those states (15). The primary recommended treatment option for gonorrhea in Hawaii and California is ceftriaxone (80). Fluoroquinolones are also not recommended for persons younger than 18 years of age because of the theoretical risk of articular joint damage seen in animal models. However, no permanent joint damage attributable to therapy has ever been reported in fluoroquinolone-treated children (81). Therefore, children weighing 45 kg or more can be treated with any adult-recommended regimen.

Approximately 10 to 30% of women with genital gonorrhea are also infected with *C. trachomatis*; therefore, the treatment regimen should also include azithromycin 1 g orally or doxycycline 100 mg orally twice a day for 7 days. Patients do not require a test of cure unless their symptoms are persistent. Resistance testing should be performed at that time. Partners of infected women should be screened and treated to prevent reinfection.

Recommended Regimens

Cefixime (Suprax) 400 mg orally in a single dose, *or*
Ceftriaxone (Rocephin) 125 mg intramuscularly in a single dose, *or*
Ciprofloxacin (Cipro) 500 mg orally in a single dose, *or*
Ofloxacin (Floxin) 400 mg orally in a single dose, *or*
Levofloxacin (Levaquin) 250 mg orally in a single dose.

Treatment should also include antibiotics for chlamydia, as described previously. Because of increasing quinolone resistance among gonococcal strains acquired in the Pacific (including Hawaii and California), quinolones should not be used; rather, ceftriaxone is preferred.

Disseminated gonococcal infections are rare and should be managed in conjunction with an infectious disease specialist.

Pelvic Inflammatory Disease

PID, or acute salpingitis, is the most frequent, acute infection in reproductive age, nonpregnant women. Among sexually active females, the highest rate of infection occurs in those 15 to 19 years of age. It is estimated that 1 million women per year are treated for PID in the United States. Approximately 25% of women who suffer from PID will also experience one or more long-term complications, the most common of which is infertility. Other morbidities include chronic pelvic pain, dyspareunia, increased risk for ectopic pregnancy, and/or tubo-ovarian abscesses. An estimated 150,000 surgical procedures are performed each year specifically for addressing complications of PID. The direct medical costs for PID and its sequelae (e.g., ectopic pregnancy, infertility) were estimated to be $1.88 billion in 1998 (82).

Clinical Symptoms

PID usually occurs as a result of organisms spreading from the vagina and cervix upward to the fallopian tubes and ovaries via the uterine cavity. It is polymicrobial in nature, although the most frequently associated organisms are *C. trachomatis* and *N. gonorrhoea*. Typical features may include fever (temperature higher than 100.4°F), lower abdominal/pelvic pain, and a mucopurulent discharge. On exam, cervical motion tenderness and adnexal tenderness may be present. Leukocytosis (more than 10,000 cells/mm^3) and an elevated erythrocyte sedimentation rate may be present.

Diagnosis

Currently, PID is commonly diagnosed on the basis of clinical history and physical findings. Clinical signs and symptoms are poor predictors of PID, due in part to the wide variety of signs

TABLE 11.3

Diagnostic Considerations for Pelvic Inflammatory Disease

Minimum criteria for initiation of empiric therapy in women at risk
- Uterine/adnexal tenderness *or*
- Cervical motion tenderness
- No other identified cause of illness

One or more of these increases the specificity of the diagnosis
- Fever (oral temperature >101°F [>38.3°F])
- Abnormal cervical or vaginal discharge
- Presence of white blood cells in vaginal discharge
- Elevated erythrocyte sedimentation rate
- Elevated C-reactive protein
- Laboratory proven infection with *Neisseria gonorrhoeae* or *Chlamydia trachomatis*

Adapted from MMWR Morb Mortal Wkly Rep Sexually Transmitted Diseases Treatment Guidelines 2002;51(RR-6):49, with permission.

and symptoms that may be present (83). The most specific criteria for the diagnosis include endometrial biopsy with histopathologic evidence of endometritis and pelvic imaging showing fluid-filled tubes or tubo-ovarian complexes (15).

Laparoscopy is often used as the gold standard for diagnosis in clinical trials; however, it is neither economically feasible nor practical for all patients with suspected PID to undergo this procedure. Diagnostic considerations for PID are presented in Table 11.3. Diagnostic features were recently assessed as part of the PID Evaluation and Clinical Health (PEACH) trial (84). Results from the PEACH study indicate that most women with PID have mucopurulent cervical discharge or evidence of white blood cells on a wet preparation of vaginal fluid (85). Therefore, if the cervical discharge appears normal and no white blood cells are noted on wet preparation, the diagnosis of PID is unlikely and alternative causes of pain should be sought.

The use of traditional imaging studies has been limited primarily to patients with evidence of tubal abscesses. A more recent study of 50 patients evaluated the use of power Doppler ultrasound to detect changes in blood flow associated with tubal inflammation. Power Doppler had a positive predictive value of 91% and a negative predictive value of 100% for PID. Larger studies are needed to assess the usefulness of this technique in clinical practice (86).

The CDC's new PID diagnostic guidelines improve both the sensitivity and specificity of this challenging clinical diagnosis. To enhance sensitivity, the minimum criteria were expanded to "uterine or adnexal tenderness or cervical motion tenderness" (15).

Treatment

The goal of treatment is to prevent infertility, ectopic pregnancy, and other long-term sequelae associated with PID. Although the general population has a 3% rate of infertility, in women who have had at least one episode of treated PID the average infertility rate is 21% (87). The likelihood of infertility is directly related to the number of episodes of PID a woman suffers. With one episode, her risk is 11%; after two, it rises to 34% and with three or more episodes, it rises to 54% (88). The effectiveness of therapy in preventing subsequent infertility is also related to the time between onset of symptoms and treatment of disease. The less time that elapses between the two, the lower the woman's risk of infertility (89).

Of patients treated in the United States, only 20 to 25% are hospitalized. The rest are treated as outpatients. The PEACH study reported outcomes of outpatient treatment of mild to moderate PID with 35 months of follow-up (90). The outcomes of women treated with cefoxitin as a single, intramuscular dose (plus probenecid orally) and oral doxycycline were similar to outcomes among women treated with intravenous cefoxitin and oral doxycycline (90). The CDC has published guidelines for the treatment of PID on an outpatient or hospitalized basis (15). Although

TABLE 11.4

Recommendations for Hospitalization of Patients With Pelvic Inflammatory Disease

- Diagnosis is uncertain, and surgical emergencies such as appendicitis cannot be excluded.
- Patient is pregnant.
- Patient has not responded clinically to oral antimicrobial therapy.
- Patient is unable to follow or tolerate an outpatient oral regimen.
- Patient has severe illness, nausea and vomiting, or high fever.
- Patient has a tubo-ovarian abscess.

Adapted from MMWR Morb Mortal Wkly Rep Sexually Transmitted Diseases Treatment Guidelines 2002;51(RR-6):49, with permission.

the decision about hospitalization is left to the discretion of the health care provider, several criteria for hospital admission based on observational studies are outlined in Table 11.4. If a patient is being treated as an outpatient, a repeat physical examination within 24 to 72 hours is warranted to verify response to therapy. If there has been no improvement in 72 hours, the diagnosis should be confirmed and parenteral treatment begun. An affected woman's sexual partner should also be examined, tested, and treated with a regimen appropriate for both uncomplicated gonorrhea and chlamydia.

Treatment Regimens

The significant changes in recommendations for treatment of PID are outlined as follows:

1. Levofloxacin 500 mg orally once daily for 14 days can be substituted for ofloxacin.
2. Metronidazole 500 mg twice a day for 14 days can also be used to enhance anaerobic coverage.

TABLE 11.5

Outpatient Treatment of Pelvic Inflammatory Disease

Regimen A
Ofloxacin (Floxin) 400 mg orally two times a day for 14 days

or

Levofloxacin 500 mg orally once daily for 14 days

with or without

Metronidazole (Flagyl) 500 mg orally two times a day for 14 days

Regimen B
Ceftriaxone (Rocephin) 250 mg intramuscularly once

or

Cefoxitin (Mefoxin) 2 g intramuscularly plus probenecid 1 g orally in a single dose concurrently once

or

Other parenteral third-generation cephalosporin (e.g., ceftizoxime [Cefizox] or cefotaxime [Claforan])

plus

Doxycycline (Vibramycin, Doryx) 100 mg orally two times a day for 14 days

with or without

Metronidazole (Flagyl) 500 mg orally two times a day for 14 days

Adapted from MMWR Morb Mortal Wkly Rep Sexually Transmitted Diseases Treatment Guidelines 2002;51(RR-6):50, with permission.

TABLE 11.6

Inpatient Treatment of Pelvic Inflammatory Disease

Regimen A
Cefotetan (Cefotan) 2 g intravenously every 12 hours *or* cefoxitin (Mefoxin) 2 g intravenously every 6 hours

plus

Doxycycline (Vibramycin) 100 mg orally or intravenously every 12 hours

Regimen B
Clindamycin (Cleocin) 900 mg intravenously every 8 hours

plus

Gentamicin (Garamycin) loading dose intravenously or intramuscularly (2 mg/kg of body weight), followed by a maintenance dose (1.5 mg/kg) every 8 hours. Single daily dosing may be substituted.

Alternative parenteral regimens
Ofloxacin (Floxin) 400 mg intravenously every 12 hours

or

Levofloxacin 500 mg intravenously once daily

with or without

Metronidazole (Flagyl) 500 mg intravenously every 8 hours

or

Ampicillin/sulbactam (Unasyn) 3 g intravenously every 6 hours **plus** doxycycline (Vibramycin, Doryx) 100 mg intravenously or orally every 12 hours.

These regimens are to be used until at least 24 hours after the patient demonstrates substantial clinical improvement. They may then be changed to doxycycline (Vibramycin) 100 mg orally two times a day for a total of 14 days of treatment. If tubo-ovarian abscess is present, many health care providers use clindamycin (Cleocin) 900 mg orally three times a day or metronidazole 500 mg twice a day for continued therapy with doxycycline.

Adapted from MMWR Morb Mortal Wkly Rep Sexually Transmitted Diseases Treatment Guidelines 2002;51(RR-6):50–51, with permission.

3. The ciprofloxacin plus doxycycline plus metronidazole alternative parenteral treatment regimen is no longer recommended (91).

The outpatient therapy options for treating PID are reviewed in Table 11.5, and the inpatient regimens are reviewed in Table 11.6.

OTHER SEXUALLY TRANSMITTED DISEASES AND INFESTATIONS

Condyloma Acuminata (Genital Warts)

Condyloma acuminata, or genital warts, are caused by human papilloma virus (HPV), and an estimated 500,000 to 1 million new cases occur annually (92). Overall, 1% of sexually active persons in the United States have clinically visible external genital warts (93). The prevalence of subclinical infection with HPV far exceeds the prevalence of visible genital warts, and studies using DNA-based technology (PCR) have found a prevalence of 40% or more (94). At this time, more than 100 types of HPV have been identified, and it is expected that new identification techniques will raise this total to 200 (93). Approximately 40 subtypes are associated with genital infection. Subtypes 6 and 11 are most frequently associated with external genital warts, whereas HPV types 16, 18, 31, 33, 35, and 39 are more frequently associated with genital cancer (95).

Other than HIV infection, HPV infection incurs the highest direct medical costs of all STDs, with an estimated $1.6 billion spent annually in treating external genital warts and cervical atypia due to HPV (96). Close to 250,000 private office visits are made each year by women seeking treatment for conditions related to HPV, and an additional 100,000 to 200,000 visits occur in public health departments and family planning clinics for the same reason (97).

Clinical Symptoms

HPV is seen most frequently in women of reproductive age and is acquired most commonly through sexual contact. The incubation period for external genital warts ranges from 1 month to more than 2 years after HPV exposure. Most warts appear 2 to 4 months after exposure to the virus (98). Up to one in five patients who do develop external genital warts will experience spontaneous regression of the lesions, usually within 1 year of detection (99). Alterations in the patient's immune state predispose to growth of the warts. Condylomata tend to flourish during pregnancy but usually regress postpartum. Patients may complain of pruritus or be asymptomatic. Untreated, the warts may increase in size and proliferate or regress spontaneously. For discussion of the effects of HPV infection on cervical cytology, see Chapter 4.

Diagnosis

Diagnosis is most often made by visualization of the lesions. Although genital warts may appear singly, they typically occur in groups of five to ten lesions. In one long-term study, 66% of women with genital warts had vulvar warts, with some involving the clitoris (100). The second most common sites were the vagina and introitus (37%), followed by the perineum (28%) and the perianal areas (23%). It is less common to see warts in the upper vaginal area and cervix, although it does occur. Although seldom required, if doubt exists about the diagnosis, a biopsy should be performed. Biopsy should also be performed for warts greater than 2 cm in diameter, warts that are pigmented, warts fixed to underlying tissues, or warts that have not responded to two to three consecutive treatments. Although there are genetic probes available to identify HPV subtypes, the clinical utility of these tests in the management of external condyloma has not been determined.

Treatment

The indications for treatment of genital warts include cosmesis, relief of local symptoms, relief of psychological stress caused by the presence of the lesions, and reduction of viral load. Approximately 10 to 20% of patients will have spontaneous resolution of the lesions. Any associated infection(s) should be eradicated prior to treating the warts. It is important to counsel patients that although the warts themselves may be eradicated, the virus, once present, will never be lost from the genital tract. As a result, recurrences of warts are common. Few head-to-head clinical trials are available comparing the various treatment modalities of external genital warts.

Podophyllin (Podocon-25, Podofin) is a cytotoxic agent that is contraindicated during pregnancy. Podophyllin can be used in a 10 to 25% solution once a week. The 2002 Sexually Transmitted Disease Treatment Guidelines (15) eliminate podophyllum resin as a treatment option for vaginal warts due to its transmucosal systemic absorption. It is most effective when used on lesions under 2 cm in size. Podophyllin will cause blanching of the warts shortly after application, and patients will complain of a burning sensation. Chemical burns may be seen in as many as 30 to 50% of patients. They may wash the area within 1 to 4 hours to reduce the severe irritation of the skin that may occur with prolonged exposure. If the warts fail to regress after four applications, an alternative therapy may be needed. Neurologic, hematologic, and febrile complications, including death, have been seen as complications associated with topical podophyllin. Podophyllin should not be used in children. The European Course on HPV Associated Pathology, an expert group of clinicians, pathologists, and virologists, more recently reclassified podophyllin as "not being recommended" because of its lower efficacy and mutagenic properties (101).

Bi- and trichloroacetic acid in up to 85% solution in alcohol is also an effective treatment for small lesions. These solutions are most applicable for acuminate or popular lesions but not large keratinized warts. Solution can be applied with a swab weekly for up to 4 weeks. Repeated therapies are often not tolerated because intense burning may be experienced for up to 10 minutes after therapy. Because of its extremely corrosive nature, ready availability of a neutralizing agent, such as sodium bicarbonate, is recommended in instances of overzealous application or spills. As this is a more liquid solution than podophyllin, some recommend applying petrolatum ointment to the skin around the wart and on the corresponding area contralaterally to avoid extensive irritation. Alternatively, talcum powder or bicarbonate soda may be used to protect the opposing skin or to remove any acid that has not reacted. The patient may wash the solution off after 6 to 8 hours and may find a sitz bath with baking soda effective in relieving any discomfort. There are fewer side effects with this regimen than with podophyllin, and this treatment may be used safely in pregnancy. Neither compound appears to be effective in treating vaginal or cervical warts.

Interferon alpha 2b (Intron A) is an effective therapy given by local injection. It is usually reserved for recurrent and/or resistant genital warts. The maximum dose to be used at any one time is 3 million units. Treatment is usually given three times per week for approximately 3 weeks. When this treatment is offered, patients may have a flu- or virallike syndrome within the first 24 hours (102). With repeated injections, this side effect often subsides. Systemic use of interferon for the treatment of genital warts is not recommended due to the immunosuppression that occurs.

5-Flourouracil (Efudex), 5% cream, may eliminate lesions in 3 to 7 days but is associated with severe side effects, including erythema, edema, and shallow ulcerations of the skin. It should not be used in pregnant women and is not considered a first-line therapy in the treatment of genital warts.

Several regimens are currently available for the patient to apply at home. A purified podophyllin resin, podofilox, is also available as a prescription ointment, Condylox 0.5%, which patients may apply two times a day for 3 consecutive days per week but for no more than 3 weeks. This ointment does not need to be washed off, is less toxic, and is more efficacious than podophyllin 20% (103). It is Category C for pregnancy.

Iquimod (Aldara), 5% cream, can be used topically by the patient three times a week for up to 8 weeks. It should be used at bedtime and washed off in 6 to 10 hours. It is rated Category B in pregnancy. It may elicit a strong local response with erythema, but this usually looks worse than it feels. Complete clearing is found in at least 50% of patients using this therapy.

Cryotherapy is another modality employed in treating genital warts. Lesions are frozen every 1 to 2 weeks, and it is important to freeze just the lesion and not the surrounding skin. Its most common clinical role in HPV is in the treatment of multiple cervical lesions. Burning and ulceration may follow therapy, although it usually resolves in 7 to 10 days with little or no scarring.

Surgical excision via loop electrosurgical excision procedure (LEEP), scalpel excision, scissor excision, punch biopsy, or CO_2 laser are other methods that can be used, particularly when large lesions or perianal lesions are present. If CO_2 laser is used for surgical ablation, the lesions must be destroyed down to the base or the incidence of recurrence will be higher.

Treatment Regimens for HPV

Podophyllin (Podocon-25, Podofin) 10% solution: Apply to warts once or twice weekly.
Condylox 0.5%: Apply twice a day for 3 consecutive days for no more than 3 weeks.
Bi- and trichloroacetic acid, up to 85%: Apply weekly for up to 4 weeks.
Iquimod (Aldara) cream 5%: Apply three times weekly for up to 8 weeks.
Interferon alpha 2b (Intron A): Inject three times weekly for 2 to 3 weeks.
Cryotherapy: Freeze warts every 1 to 2 weeks.
Surgical excision (LEEP, CO_2 laser, or scalpel): Use for large or perianal lesions.

Molluscum Contagiosum

Clinical Symptoms

Molluscum contagiosum is a dome-shaped lesion with central umbilication caused by a member of the Pox virus family. They are found on epithelial surfaces but not on mucosal membranes. Sometimes a curdlike, milky core can be expressed. Lesions are slow growing and usually multiple. Infection is usually self-limiting, lasting 6 to 9 months on average. There are two forms of infection. One is seen in young children resulting from skin-to-skin contact or fomite transmission, whereas the other occurs in adolescents and adults and results from sexual transmission (104).

Diagnosis

Diagnosis of this lesion is primarily made by gross appearance or via skin biopsy. However, skin biopsy is usually only performed when the diagnosis is in question.

Treatment

Effective treatment can be achieved with skin curettage, cryotherapy, expression of the umbilicated core, or excision. Because the latter will cause scarring, it is not routinely recommended. At-home therapeutics are often preferred by parents and children, and include imiquimod, retinoids, and alpha-hydroxy acids. Although a variety of such at-home therapies are available, none are as effective or as rapid acting as in-office therapy (105, 106).

Treatment Regimens

Skin curettage
Cryotherapy
Expression of umbilicated core
Podophyllin
Trichloroacetic acid

Scabies

Scabies is a highly contagious infection caused by *Sarcoptes scabiei*, also known as the itch mite. It is an obligate parasite that burrows into, resides in, and reproduces in human skin. It is worldwide in its distribution and occurs in all races and socioeconomic classes. It is not a vector for other infectious diseases. It is transmitted by intimate contact, often sexual, but casual contact may also incur transmission. Fomites may also be an important means of transmission.

Clinical Symptoms

Most persons with scabies complain of intense pruritus that is worse at night. Areas prone to infection include interdigital spaces, wrists, axillary folds, the periumbilical area, pelvic area, penis, and ankles. In infants or toddlers, the head, neck, palms, and soles may be involved. Infection is usually erythematous, and papules or vesicles may be present with excoriations often seen. Chronic infection may lead to pruritic reddish brown nodules, especially in children. They may not disappear for weeks or months after therapy is completed.

Diagnosis

The classic linear burrows (short, wavy lines that cross skin lines) should be sought to assist in the diagnosis. Formal diagnosis is made by microscopically examining skin scrapings of suspected sites for the organism, eggs, or feces. Skin samples are obtained by either scraping or shaving the superficial layers of skin over a burrow. This is done to a depth sufficient to cause a very small amount of bleeding.

Treatment

The drug of choice for treatment is permethrin (Nix 1% or Elimite 5%) cream, which has a higher cure rate than lindane (107). As a Category B agent, permethrin is safe for use in pregnancy but should not be used in infants younger than 2 months old. Crotamiton (Category C) has less topical absorption than lindane. Lindane should not be used immediately after a bath or shower because this increases the amount of topical absorption, nor should it be used by persons who have extensive dermatitis, pregnant or lactating women, or children younger than 2 years of age. Lindane should be washed off after 6 to 8 hours. Another risk associated with lindane overuse or misuse in children is the risk of seizures.

Despite years of effectiveness, resistant organisms now exist. The CDC more recently added ivermectin, an oral antiparasitic drug used in strongyloidosis, as an acceptable therapeutic option. The most common treatment regimen with ivermectin is with two doses (200 μg/kg per dose) administered 7 to 14 days apart. The optimum dosing regimen remains an issue of controversy (108). Studies have found that two doses of ivermectin have cure rates comparable with those of topical permethrin and lindane (109). This option may be more acceptable and easier to use than creams and lotions that must be applied to almost the entire body overnight.

Household contacts should also be treated, and recently worn clothes and linens should be washed in hot soapy water and placed in a hot dryer. Dry cleaning is also sufficient to kill the mite(s). Fingernails should be trimmed as part of the treatment and patients should be counseled that the itching may persist for up to 2 weeks after therapy.

Treatment Regimens

Permethrin (Nix 1% or Elimite 5% cream): Apply head to toe, avoiding mouth/nose/eyes area, and wash off after 8 to 10 hours.
Crotamiton (Eurax) 10% cream or lotion: Apply from chin to feet for two consecutive nights and wash off 24 hours after second application.
Lindane (Kwell) 1%: Apply from head to toe, avoiding mouth/nose/eyes area, and wash off after 8 to 12 hours.

Pediculosis pubis

Pediculosis pubis is also known as the crab louse. An estimated 3 million cases occur each year in the United States. It may be spread through fomites, although the usual acquisition is through sexual contact. It is one of the most contagious of the sexually transmitted infections—the risk of acquiring pediculosis is 95% with a single sexual encounter (110). The infestation is more common in women than men up to age 19, after which it is more common in men. Incubation time is 30 days.

TABLE 11.7

Sexually Transmitted Diseases: Should the Partner(s) be Treated?

		Treat Partners?		
	Average Incubation	Yes	No	Which Partners?
Herpes	3–7 days		X	
Venereal warts	3–6 months	X	X	Treatment of partners is controversial; unless symptoma, most do not
Molluscum contagiosum	2–7 weeks	X		Partners in last 1–2 months; examine and treat if affected
Lymphogranuloma venereum	4–21 days	X		Last 30 days
Chancroid	5–7 days	X		Immediate
Chlamydia	1 day–several weeks	X		Last 1–2 months
Gonorrhea	3–5 days	X		Immediate
Syphilis	10–90 days (primary)	X		All contacts in primary, secondary, and early latent; late latent and tertiary not sexually communicable
Granuloma inguinale	1–360 days		X	
Pelvic inflammatory disease	Varies by organism	X		Immediate
Pediculosis	30 days	X		Contacts in last month
Scabies	4–6 weeks	X		Contacts in last 4–6 weeks

TABLE 11.8

Treatment Regimens for Sexually Transmitted Diseases

Herpes			
Initial Outbreak	Recurrence	Severe Disease	Prophylaxis
Acyclovir	Acyclovir	Acyclovir, intravenous	Acyclovir
Valacyclovir	Famciclovir		Famciclovir
Famciclovir	Valacyclovir		Valacyclovir

Human Papilloma Virus	
Medical Options	Surgical Options
Podophyllin 10% solution	Cryotherapy
Condylox 0.5%	LEEP excision
Bi- or Trichloroacetic acid, up to 85%	CO_2 laser ablation
5-Fluorouracil, 5% cream	Scalpel excision
Iquimod 5%	
Interferon-alpha 2b	

Molluscum Contagiosum
Options
Skin curettage
Cryotherapy
Expression of umbilicated core
Podophyllin
Trichloroacetic acid

Lymphogranuloma Venereum	
Recommended	Alternative
Doxycycline	Erythromycin
	Sulfisoxazole
	Tetracycline

Chancroid	
Recommended	Comments
Azithromycin	Drain buboes
Ceftriaxone	Do not excise nodes
Ciprofloxacin	
Erythromycin	

Chlamydia	
Recommended	Alternative
Azithromycin	Erythromycin
Doxycycline	Ofloxacin
	Levofloxacin

(continued)

TABLE 11.8 Continued

Treatment Regimens for Sexually Transmitted Diseases

	Gonorrhea			
Recommended	Concurrent			
Cefixime	See regimen for chlamydia			
Ceftriaxone				
Ciprofloxacin				
Ofloxacin				
Levofloxacin				
	Syphilis			
Primary	Secondary	Early Latent	Late Latent	Neurosyphilis
Benzathine penicillin	Benzathine penicillin	Benzathine penicillin	Benzathine penicillin	Procaine penicillin G
	Granuloma Inguinale			
Options	Alternative			
Doxycycline	Ciprofloxacin			
Trimethoprim-sulfamethoxazole	Erythromycin			
	Azithromycin			
	Scabies			
Recommended	Children, Pregnant Women	Infants		
Permethrin	Permethrin	Pyrethrins/piperonyl butoxide		
Crotamiton				
Lindane				
	Pediculosis			
Options				
Permethrin				
Pyrethrin with piperonyl butoxide				
Lindane				

LEEP, loop electrosurgical excision procedure.

Clinical Symptoms

Most patients complain of intense pruritus or irritation in the pubic hair area. Systemic symptoms such as low-grade fever and malaise can occur if there are a significant number of bites from the lice.

Diagnosis

The diagnosis is made by visualizing the lice, larvae, and/or nits with a magnifying glass or fine-tooth comb.

Treatment

All sexual contacts, family members, and close contacts should be treated, even if they are asymptomatic. Recently worn clothing or linens should be washed in hot, soapy water and dried in a hot dryer. Dry cleaning is also acceptable. Petrolatum jelly should be applied to infested eyelashes. After therapy a fine-tooth comb should be used to remove any remaining lice and/or nits. If lice or eggs are found 5 to 7 days after therapy, the treatment should be repeated.

Treatment Regimens

Permethrin (Nix 1% rinse or Elimite 5% cream): Apply to affected areas and wash off after 10 minutes.
Pyrethrin with piperonyl butoxide (Rid): Apply to affected areas and wash off after 10 minutes.
Lindane (Kwell 1% shampoo): Apply for 4 minutes and wash off.

Recommendations for the treatment of the infected patient's partner are summarized in Table 11.7. In addition, a summary of all treatments is provided in Table 11.8.

Clinical Notes

- Primary outbreaks of herpes are often asymptomatic. Eighty percent of patients will suffer a recurrent outbreak the year following the primary outbreak.
- Not all patients are aware of the primary outbreak of herpes or of exposure to the virus.
- Accurate type-specific serologic screening tests for HSV-1 and HSV-2 are now commercially available.
- Acyclovir, famciclovir, and valacyclovir may be used prophylactically to reduce the frequency and severity of recurrences.
- The risk of neonatal infection with herpes is highest in those mothers with an initial outbreak at or around the time of delivery. For recurrent maternal infections, the risk of fetal transmission is much lower.
- Condyloma acuminata is common—up to 20% of patients will have spontaneous resolution of the warts. Both medical and surgical modalities exist to treat it.
- Lymphogranuloma venereum is caused by *Chlamydia* and is a painless ulcer in the early stages. If untreated, it results in fistulas, strictures, and elephantiasis.
- Chancroid, caused by *H. ducreyi*, causes a painful ulcer and subsequent bubo formation.
- *C. trachomatis* infection is often asymptomatic; therefore, adequate detection depends on screening.
- Asymptomatic chlamydia infection is associated with tubal damage, infertility, and chronic pain.
- Gonorrhea is readily transmitted from a male to a female. In 15 to 20% of women, acute PID will result.
- When treating gonorrhea, a regimen effective against *C. trachomatis* should also be given because these two infections are often concurrent.
- Syphilis may present in any fashion and in any organ system. The primary ulcer is painless.
- After treatment for syphilis, titers should be followed for 1 to 2 years to ensure adequate therapy and/or detect reinfection.
- Syphilis is most easily transmitted to the fetus in the primary or secondary stages, although it is also transmissible in the latent phase.
- Granuloma inguinale, or Donovanosis, presents as a nontender ulcer and causes the formation of pseudobuboes.
- PID is a major cause of hospitalization in reproductive age women in the United States. It is also a significant cause of infertility, chronic pelvic pain, and increased risk of ectopic pregnancy.
- Scabies is caused by a mite and is highly contagious. It does not act as a vector for other infectious diseases.
- Pediculosis pubis, or crabs, is a highly contagious STD.

REFERENCES

1. Halioua B, Malkin JE. Epidemiology of genital herpes—recent advances. Eur J Dermatol 1999;9:177–184.
2. Wald A. New therapies and prevention strategies for genital herpes. Clin Infect Dis 1999;28(suppl 1):S4–S13.
3. Mindel A. Psychological and psychosexual implications of herpes simplex virus infections. Scand J Infect Dis 1996;100(suppl):27–32.
4. Fleming DT, McQuillian GM, Johnson RE, et al. Herpes simplex virus type 2 in the United States, 1976 to 1994. N Engl J Med 1997;337:1105–1111.
5. Koelle DM, Benedetti J, Langenberg A, et al. Asymptomatic reactivation of herpes simplex virus in women after the first episode of genital herpes. Ann Intern Med 1992;116:433–437.
6. Corey L, Adams H, Brown Z, et al. Genital herpes simplex viral infection: clinical manifestations, course, and complications. Ann Intern Med 1983;98:958–972.
7. Baringer JR, Swoveland P. Recovery of herpes-simplex virus from human trigeminal ganglions. N Engl J Med 1973;288:648–650.
8. Baringer JR. Recovery of herpes simplex virus from human sacral ganglions. N Engl J Med 1974;291:828–830.
9. Reeves WC, Corey L, Adams HG, et al. Risk of recurrence after first episodes of genital herpes. Relation to HSV type and antibody response. N Engl J Med 1981;305:315–319.
10. Wald A, Zeh J, Selke S, et al. Virologic characteristics of subclinical and symptomatic genital herpes infections. N Engl J Med 1995;333:770–775.
11. Spruance SL, Overall JC Jr, Kern ER, et al. The natural history of recurrent herpes simplex labialis: implications for antiviral therapy. N Engl J Med 1977;297:69–75.
12. Koutsky LA, Stevens CE, Holmes KK, et al. Underdiagnosis of genital herpes by current clinical and viral-isolation procedures. N Engl J Med 1992;326:1533–1539 .
13. Van Doornum GJ, Guldemeester J, Osterhaus AD, et al. Diagnosing herpes virus infections by real-time amplification and rapid culture. J Clin Microbiol 2003;41:576–580.
14. Schmid DS, Brown DR, Nisenbaum R, et al. Limits in reliability of glycoprotein G-based type-specific serologic assays for herpes simplex virus types 1 and 2. J Clin Microbiol 1999;37:376–379.
15. Centers for Disease Control and Prevention. 2002 Sexually Transmitted Disease Treatment Guidelines. MMWR Morbid Mortal Wkly Rep 2002:51(RR–6):1–84.
16. Benedetti JK, Zeh J, Corey L. Clinical reactivation of genital herpes simplex virus infection decreases in frequency over time. Ann Intern Med 1999;131:14–20.
17. Fleming DT, McQuillan GM, Johnson RE, et al. Herpes simplex virus type 2 in the United States, 1976 to 1994. N Engl J Med 1997;337:1105–1111.
18. Kinghorn GR. Epidemiology of genital herpes. J Int Med 1994;2(suppl 1):14A–23A.
19. Mertz GJ, Benedetti J, Ashley R, et al. Risk factors for the sexual transmission of genital herpes. Ann Intern Med 1992;116:197–202.
20. Lamey P-J, Hyland PL. Changing epidemiology of herpes simplex virus type 1 infections. Herpes 1999;6:20–24.
21. Scoular A, Norrie J, Gillespie G, et al. Longitudinal study of genital infection by herpes simplex virus type 1 in western Scotland over 15 years. BMJ 2002;324:1366–1367.
22. Johnson AM, Wadsworth J, Wellings K, et al. Sexual Attitudes and Lifestyles. Oxford: Blackwell Scientific, 1994.
23. Barry G. Herpes serology for dermatologists. Arch Dermatol 2000;136:1158–1161.
24. Spruance SL, Tyring SK, DeGregorio B, et al. A large-scale placebo-controlled, dose-ranging trial of peroral valacyclovir for episodic treatment of recurrent herpes genitalis. Arch Intern Med 1996;156:1729–1735.
25. Reitano M, Tyring S, Lang W, et al. Valacyclovir for the suppression of recurrent genital herpes simplex virus infection: a large-scale dose range-finding study. International Valacyclovir HSV Study Group. J Infect Dis 1998;178:603–610.
26. Patel R, Tyring S, Strand A, et al. Impact of suppressive antiviral therapy on the health related quality of life of patients with recurrent genital herpes infection. Sex Transm Infect 1999;75:398–402.
27. Brown ZA, Selke S, Zeh J, et al. The acquisition of herpes simplex virus during pregnancy. N Engl J Med 1997;337:509–515.
28. Frenkel LM, Garratty EM, Shen JP, et al. Clinical reactivation of herpes simplex virus type 2 infection in seropositive pregnant women with no history of genital herpes. Ann Intern Med 1993;118:414–418.
29. Harger JH, Amortegui AJ, Meyer MP, et al. Characteristics of recurrent genital herpes simplex infections in pregnant women. Obstet Gynecol 1989;73:367–372.
30. Hutto C, Arvin A, Jacobs R, et al. Intrauterine herpes simplex virus infections. J Pediatr 1987;110:97–101.
31. Brown ZA, Benedetti J, Ashley R, et al. Neonatal herpes simplex virus infection in relation to asymptomatic maternal infection at the time of labor. N Engl J Med 1991;324:1247–1252.
32. American College of Obstetricians and Gynecologists (ACOG). Management of Herpes in Pregnancy. ACOG Practice Bulletin. Washington, DC: ACOG, 1999:8.
33. Scott LL, Sanchez PJ, Jackson GL, et al. Acyclovir suppression to prevent cesarean delivery after first-episode genital herpes. Obstet Gynecol 1996;87:69–73.
34. Scott LL, Hollier LM, McIntire D, et al. Acyclovir suppression to prevent recurrent genital herpes at delivery. Infect Dis Obstet Gynecol 2002;10:71–77.

35. CDC. Primary and secondary syphilis—United States, 2000–2001. MMWR Morbid Mortal Wkly Rep 2002;51(43):971–973.
36. Holmes KK, Mardh P-A, Sparling PF, et al. Natural history of syphilis. In: Sexually Transmitted Diseases. New York: McGraw-Hill, 1999:473.
37. Chapel TA. The variability of syphilitic chancres. Sex Transm Dis 1978;5:68–70.
38. World Health Organization (WHO). Guidelines for the Management of Sexually Transmitted Infections. Geneva: WHO, 2003. Available at: www.who.int/hiv/pub/sti/en/STIGuidelines2003.pdf. Accessed July 13, 2005. WHO/HIV_AIDS/2001.01 WHO/RHR/01.10: 38.
39. Hook EW, Marra CM. Acquired syphilis in adults. N Engl J Med 1992;326:1060–1069.
40. Brauner A, Carlsson B, Sundkvist G, et al. False-positive treponemal serology in patients with diabetes mellitus. J Diabetes Complications 1994;8:57–62.
41. Wendel GD Jr, Stark BJ, Jamison RB, et al. Penicillin allergy and desensitization in serious infections during pregnancy. N Engl J Med 1985;312:1229–1232.
42. Romanowski B, Sutherland R, Fick GH, et al. Serologic response to treatment of infectious syphilis. Ann Intern Med 1991;114:1005–1009.
43. Hollier LM, Harstad TW, Sanchez PJ, et al. Clinical characteristics of fetal syphilis. Obstet Gynecol 2001;97:947–953.
44. Hollier LM, Cox SM. Syphilis. Semin Perinatol 1998;22:323–331.
45. Hutchinson CM, Rompalo AM, Reichart CA. Characteristics of patients with syphilis attending Baltimore STD clinics. Multiple high-risk subgroups and interactions with human immunodeficiency virus infection. Arch Intern Med 1991;151:511–516.
46. Musher DM, Hammil RJ, Baughn RE. Effect of human immunodeficiency virus (HIV) infection on the course of syphilis and on the response to treatment. Ann Intern Med 1990;113:872–881.
47. Holmes KK, Mardh P-A, Sparling PF, et al. Late syphilis. In: Sexually Transmitted Diseases. New York: McGraw-Hill, 1999:487.
48. Borchardt KA. Lymphogranuloma venereum. In: Sexually Transmitted Diseases: Epidemiology, Pathology, Diagnosis, and Treatment. 1st ed. Boca Raton: CRC Press, 1997:117.
49. Sischy A, da L'Exposto F, Dangor Y, et al. Syphilis serology in patients with primary syphilis and non-treponemal sexually transmitted diseases in southern Africa. Genitourin Med 1991;67:129–132.
50. Smith EB, Custer RP. The histopathology of lymphogranuloma venereum. J Urol 1950;63:546–548.
51. Torpin et al. Lymphogranuloma venereum in the female: a clinical study of ninety-six consecutive cases. Am J Surg 1939;43:688.
52. Holmes KK, Mardh P-A, Sparling PF, et al. Lymphogranuloma venereum. In: Sexually Transmitted Diseases. 3rd ed. New York: McGraw-Hill, 1999:423.
53. Kellock DJ, Barlow R, Suvarna SK, et al. Lymphogranuloma venereum: biopsy, serology and molecular biology. Genitourin Med 1997;73:399–401.
54. Schmid GP, Sanders LL Jr, Blount JH, et al. Chancroid in the United States: reestablishment of an old disease. JAMA 1987;258:3265–3268.
55. Flood JM, Sarafian SK, Bolan GA, et al. Multi-strain outbreak of chancroid in San Francisco, 1989–1991. J Infect Dis 1993;167:1106–1111.
56. Lewis DA. Chancroid: clinical manifestations, diagnosis, and management. Sex Transm Infect 2003;79:68–71.
57. Plummer FA, D'Costa LJ, Nsanze H, et al. Clinical and microbiologic studies of genital ulcers in Kenyan women. Sex Transm Dis 1985;12:193–197.
58. Tekle-Michael T, Van Dyck E, Abdellati S, et al. Development of a heminested polymerase chain reaction assay for the detection of *Haemophilus ducreyi* in clinical specimens. Int J STD AIDS 2001;12:797–803.
59. Totten PA, Kuypers JM, Chen CY, et al. Etiology of genital ulcer disease in Dakar, Senegal, and comparison of PCR and serologic assays for detection of *Haemophilus ducreyi*. J Clin Microbiol 2000;38:268–273.
60. O'Farrell N. Donovanosis. Sex Transm Infect 2002;78:452–457.
61. O'Farrell N. Donovanosis (granuloma inguinale) in pregnancy. Int J STD AIDS 1991;2:447–448.
62. CDC guidelines on sexually transmitted diseases. MMWR Morbid Mortal Wkly Rep 1998;47:RR02.
63. UNAIDS/WHO Meeting Report (Draft) Advisory Group Meeting on Sexually Transmitted Infections Management; May 11–14, 1999; Geneva.
64. Hollier LM. Chlamydia. In: Gynecology for the Primary Care Physician. Philadelphia: Current Medicine, 1999:57.
65. Centers for Disease Control and Prevention (CDC). Sexually Transmitted Disease Surveillance, 2001. Atlanta: U.S. Department of Health and Human Services, CDC, September 2002:51–57. Available at: http://www.cdc.gov/std/stats01/TOC2001.htm. Accessed July 13, 2005.
66. Black CM. Current methods of laboratory diagnosis of *Chlamydia trachomatis* infections. Clin Microbiol Rev 1997;10:160–184.
67. Pimenta JM, Catchpole M, Rogers PA, et al. Opportunistic screening for genital chlamydial infection. I: acceptability of urine testing in primary and secondary healthcare settings. Sex Transm Infect 2003;79:16–21.
68. Dicker LW, Mosure DJ, Berman SM, et al. Gonorrhea prevalence and coinfection with chlamydia in women in the United States, 2000. Sex Transm Dis 2003;30:472–476.
69. Scholes D, Stergachis A, Heidrich FF, et al. Prevention of pelvic inflammatory disease by screening for cervical Chlamydia infection. N Engl J Med 1996;334:1362–1366.

70. Adair CD, Gunter M, Stovall TG, et al. Chlamydia in pregnancy: a randomized trial of azithromycin and erythromycin. Obstet Gynecol 1998;91:165–168.
71. Mandel GL, Bennett JE, Dolin R. *Neisseria gonorrhea*. In: Principles and Practices of Infectious Diseases. 4th ed. New York: Churchill Livingstone, 1995;1909–1925.
72. Stoval TG, Ling FW. Gonorrhea. In: Gynecology for the Primary Care Physician. Philadelphia: Current Medicine, 1999:47.
73. Lin JS, Donegan SP, Heeren TC, et al. Transmission of *Chlamydia trachomatis* and *Neisseria gonorrhoeae* among men with urethritis and their female sex partners. J Infect Dis 1998;178:1707–1712.
74. Bro-Jornensen A, Jensen T. Gonococcal pharyngeal infections. Report of 110 cases. Br J Vener Dis 1973;49:491–499.
75. Holmes KK, Counts GW, Beaty HN. Disseminated gonococcal infection. Ann Intern Med 1971;74:979–993.
76. Division of STD Prevention. Sexually Transmitted Disease Surveillance, 1994. U.S. Department of Health and Human Services, Public Health Service. Atlanta: Centers for Disease Control and Prevention, September 1995. Available at: http://wonder.cdc.gov/wonder/STD/Title3400.html/. Accessed July 13, 2005.
77. Judson FN. Gonorrhea. Med Clin North Am 1990;74:1353–1366.
78. Ho BS, Feng WG, Wong BK, et al. Polymerase chain reaction for the detection of *Neisseria gonorrhoeae* in clinical samples. J Clin Pathol 1992;45:439–442.
79. Johnson RE, Newhall WJ, Papp JR, et al. Screening tests to detect *Chlamydia trachomatis* and *Neisseria gonorrhoeae* infection—2002. MMWR Recomm Rep 2002;51(RR–15):1.
80. Centers for Disease Control and Prevention. Oral Alternatives to Cefixime for the Treatment of Uncomplicated *Neisseria gonorrhoeae* Urogenital Infections. Available at: http://www.cdc.gov/std/treatment/cefixime.htm. Accessed July 13, 2005.
81. Burstein GR, Berman SM, Blumer JL, et al. Ciprofloxacin for the treatment of uncomplicated gonorrhea infection in adolescents: does benefit outweigh risk? Clin Infect Dis 2002;35:S191–S199.
82. Rein DB, Kassler WJ, Irwin KL, et al. Direct medical cost of pelvic inflammatory disease and its sequelae: decreasing, but still substantial. Obstet Gynecol 2000;95:397–402.
83. Chaparro MV, Ghosh S, Nashed A, et al. Laparoscopy for confirmation and prognostic evaluation of pelvic inflammatory disease. Int J Gynaecol Obstet 1978;15:307–309.
84. Ness RB, Soper DE, Peipert J, et al. Design of the PID Evaluation and Clinical Health (PEACH) Study. Control Clin Trials 1998;19:499–514.
85. Peipert JF, Ness RB, Soper DE, et al. Association of lower genital tract inflammation with objective evidence of endometritis. Infect Dis Obstet Gynecol 2000;8:83–87.
86. Molander P, Sjoberg J, Paavonen J, et al. Transvaginal power Doppler findings in laparoscopically proven acute pelvic inflammatory disease. Ultrasound Obstet Gynecol 2001;17:233–238.
87. Westrom L. Effect of acute pelvic inflammatory disease on fertility. Am J Obstet Gynecol 1975;121:707–713.
88. Westrom L. Incidence, prevalence, and trends of acute pelvic inflammatory disease and its consequences in industrialized countries. Am J Obstet Gynecol 1980;138:880–892.
89. Viberg L. Acute inflammatory conditions of the uterine adnexa. Clinical, radiological, and isotopic investigations of non-gonococcal adnexitis. Acta Obstet Gynecol Scand 1964;43:1–86.
90. Ness RB, Soper DE, Holley RL, et al. Effectiveness of inpatient and outpatient treatment strategies for women with pelvic inflammatory disease: results from the Pelvic Inflammatory Disease Evaluation and Clinical Health (PEACH) Randomized Trial. Am J Obstet Gynecol 2002;186:929–937.
91. Walker CK, Workowski KA, Washington AE, et al. Anaerobes in pelvic inflammatory disease: implications for the Centers for Disease Control and Prevention's guidelines for treatment of sexually transmitted diseases. Clin Infect Dis 1999;28:S29–36
92. Beutner KR, Reitano MV, Richwald GA, et al. External genital warts: report of the American Medical Association consensus conference. Clin Infect Dis 1998;27:796–806.
93. Koutsky LA. Epidemiology of human papillomavirus infection. Am J Med 1997;102:3–8
94. Bauer HM, Ting Y, Greer CE. Genital human papillomavirus infection in female university students as determined by a PCR-based method. JAMA 1991;265:472–477.
95. Chuang TY. Condyloma acuminata (genital warts). An epidemiologic review. J Am Acad Dermatol 1987;16:376–384.
96. American Social Health Association and the Kaiser Family Foundation. Sexually Transmitted Diseases in America: How Many Cases and at What Cost? Menlo Park, CA: Kaiser Family Foundation, 1998.
97. Division of STD Prevention. Sexually Transmitted Disease Surveillance, 1998. Department of Health and Human Services. Atlanta: Centers for Disease Control and Prevention, September 1999. Available at: http://www.cdc.gov/nchstp/dstd/stats_Trends/1998Surveillance/98PDF/Section1.pdf. Accessed July 13, 2005.
98. Ferenczy A. Epidemiology and clinical pathophysiology of condylomata acuminata. Am J Obstet Gynecol 1995;172:1331–1339.
99. Ferenczy A, Mitao M, Nagai N, et al. Latent papillomavirus and recurring genital warts. N Engl J Med 1985;3131:784–788
100. Chuang TY, Perry Ho, Kurland LT, et al. Condyloma acuminatum in Rochester, Minnesota, 1950–1978. Arch Dermatol 1984;120:469–476.
101. Von Krogh G, Lacey CJN, Gross G, et al. European course on HPV associated pathology: guidelines for primary care physicians for the diagnosis and management of anogenital warts. Sex Transm Infect 2000;76:162–168.
102. Clark DP. Condyloma acuminatum. Dermatol Clin 1987;4:779–788.

103. Edwards A, Atma-Ram A. Podophyllotoxin 0.5% vs podophyllin 20% to treat penile warts. Genitourin Med 1988;64:263–265.
104. Felman YM, Nikitas JA. Genital molluscum contagiosum. Cutis 1980;26:28–32.
105. Silverberg N. Pediatric molluscum contagiosum: optimal treatment strategies. Paediatr Drugs 2003;5:505–12.
106. Liota E, Amoth KJ, Buckley R, et al. Imiquimod therapy for molluscum contagiosum. J Cutan Med Surg 2000;4:76–82.
107. Amer M, El-Garib I. Permethrin versus crotamiton and lindane in the treatment of scabies. Int J Dermatol 1992;31:357–358.
108. Vaidhyanathan U. Review of ivermectin in scabies. J Cutan Med Surg 2001;5:496–504.
109. Wendel K, Rompalo A. Scabies and pediculosis pubis: an update of treatment regimens and general review. Clin Infect Dis 2002;35:S146–S151.
110. Letau LA. Nosocomial transmission and infection control aspects of parasitic and ectoparasitic diseases. Part III. Ectoparasites/summary and conclusions. Infect Control Hosp Epidemiol 1991;12:179–185.

CHAPTER 12

Chronic Pelvic Pain

John F. Steege

INTRODUCTION

Chronic pelvic pain is generally defined as pain present in the pelvis more often than not for 6 months or longer. It may be cyclic or continuous in nature. Pain that is present at least 5 days/month occurs in 12% of women of reproductive age and is the reason for hysterectomy in approximately 12% of such procedures (1, 2). Approximately one-half of all operative laparoscopies are performed to investigate problems with pain, many of those chronic in nature (3, 4).

As a multifactorial disease, chronic pelvic pain often challenges the best of clinicians. When organic pathology is detected, its precise relationship to the production of symptoms is often uncertain. The longer the pain has gone on, the more likely treatment will be prolonged and perhaps incompletely successful. For the surgically oriented gynecologist, this problem can be especially frustrating. Surgical solutions are not always apparent, and pain may persist despite a satisfactory anatomic result.

This chapter focuses on new information about pain pathways that may help explain some of these phenomena. It reviews basic elements of history and physical examination pertinent to the various diagnoses and sources of chronic pelvic pain. Current treatments for each disorder are summarized.

PATHWAYS OF PAIN PERCEPTION

Nociceptive pain results from injury to a pain-sensitive structure and is somatic or visceral in origin. Nociceptive signals emerging from pelvic visceral structures travel cephalad through one or more of several routes (5). (Nociceptive signals are peripheral nerve impulses that are destined to produce negatively perceived sensations; "pain" is a brain interpretation of sensations indicative of real or potential tissue damage.) Sympathetic afferent signals arising from the uterus, cervix, and immediately adjacent portions of the uterosacral, broad, and round ligaments travel via the inferior and superior hypogastric plexuses to the sympathetic chain. From there they go to the T10 to T12 levels of the spinal cord. Additional sensation may be provided through the nervi erigentes, or pelvic nerves, which cross the pelvic floor and ultimately join the S2 to S4 segments of the spinal cord. Fibers from both the sympathetic and parasympathetic systems traverse Frankenhauser's plexus and the uterovesical ganglion.

Neuroanatomic work performed in the last century elucidated these pathways, and clinical neurophysiologic work has validated the significance of most of these. What is not always fully appreciated is the degree of biological variability that exists among women. A better understanding of this variability may provide useful clinical information in the future as we attempt to understand unusual pain patterns.

The gate control theory, developed by Melzack and Wall in the 1950s and early 1960s, provides a model to help explain some of the variability in clinical pain patterns (6). It is a useful model of integration of physical and psychological processes into a single scheme. The major contribution of this theory was to suggest that higher centers in the brain have the capacity to *physiologically* down- or upregulate the spinal cord. This regulation may determine the degree to which peripheral nociceptive signals travel cephalad to reach conscious perception.

Building on this theory, further neurophysiologic research has focused on these spinal cord mechanisms (7). It is now known that there are several categories of narcotic receptor sites both in the brain and the spinal cord. In addition, the spinal cord appears to have receptors for local anesthetics and numerous other neurotransmitterlike substances, including cannabinoids.

Many researchers in pain have found the gate theory too limiting. Melzack suggested the term "neuromatrix" to describe a weblike set of communications, ascending and descending, that are involved in nociception, and ultimately, in the perception of pain (8). The newer model allows inclusion of multiple new factors that have been the foci of more recent research on spinal cord and central elements of the pain perception system.

Three clinically important concepts emerge from this evidence: (a) centralization of pain, (b) spinal cord "wind-up," and (c) viscerosomatic convergence (9). Centralization of pain is said to occur when, following extended periods of peripheral nociceptive signal production, changes seem to occur at the spinal cord level that result in ongoing signals sent to the brain despite the dramatic decrease or even absence of peripheral nociception. That is, the brain and spinal cord take over even when the best therapeutic efforts have been made to reduce signals from damaged tissue peripherally. Medical management of the central neurotransmitter processes would seem to be the most appropriate therapeutic intervention for pain that has become centralized.

Spinal cord "wind-up" occurs when repeated, low-level nociceptive stimuli from the periphery elicit progressively more dramatic responses from second-order neurons at the spinal cord level, even though the intensity of the stimuli may remain constant or even be diminished. This phenomenon has been well demonstrated in acute pain models at the animal level (9). There is considerable speculation regarding the impact of this process on chronic pain symptoms. When examining a patient with pain, the tendency for repeated examination to elicit pain from initially nontender areas is a phenomenon consistent with "wind-up."

It has long been observed that visceral organs and portions of the somatic system often share nerve supply from the same level of the spinal cord. (Somatic pain originates from skin, muscles, bones, and joints, and is transmitted along sensory fibers.) Pain from viscera may thus be referred to the appropriate somatic dermatome. With time, however, stimuli applied to somatic structures may sometimes reproduce a nociceptive response perceived as though it emanated from the original offending viscus. For example, pain from a vaginal fornix in a posthysterectomy patient can be referred to a relatively localized area of the abdominal wall. With time, this abdominal wall area may itself become intrinsically tender. Palpation of this spot may reproduce the vaginal apex pain.

There are complex interactions among the reproductive organs, the urinary tract, and the colon. One phenomenon associated with these interactions is viscerovisceral hyperalgesia. In this condition, inflammation or congestion in an organ (e.g., in the reproductive organs), enhances pain in viscera, skin, or muscle that share common spinal cord segments (10–12).

The categorization of pain as *either* mental *or* physical is inaccurate. Pain is an experience wherein psychological factors impact the way pain stimuli reach and are processed by the brain, even when there is an apparent somatic etiology. Pain can produce changes in muscle tone and peripheral hormone concentrations, and invoke autonomic nervous responses.

Although acute pain and chronic pain are quite different physiologic processes, some lessons learned from acute pain management apply well to the management of chronic pain. For example, studies regarding the impact of preemptive analgesia on acute postoperative pain suggest that the ideal postoperative pain regimen is multifaceted. The ideal regimen simultaneously interrupts the nociceptive signals at the peripheral tissue level, blocks receptor sites within the spinal cord, and alters the central perception of pain (13). In many chronic pain conditions, this would also be the ideal regimen. Treatments need to be applied at the peripheral tissue level and include pharmacologic measures directed toward spinal cord and central mechanisms as well.

EVALUATION OF CHRONIC PAIN SYNDROMES

History

Chronic pelvic pain is a symptom, not a specific disease. Its diagnosis is made on the basis of a careful and detailed clinical history. Physical examination supplies additional detail(s) and confirmation of diagnoses, but in the majority of cases, if uncertainty remains, more historical questions need to be asked. A very detailed history enables the physician and patient to formulate a well-designed intervention, especially one that involves surgical treatment.

The history of the present illness should include the character, intensity, and radiation of the pain; the relationship of the pain to the menstrual cycle; and the daily chronologic pattern of the pain. A standard method of quantifying pain severity should be used to measure pain at successive visits. Information regarding previous medical therapies and their associated side effects, and previous procedures and their effect(s) on the pain pattern(s), should be garnered. Some useful generalizations about pain patterns associated with particular kinds of pelvic pathology are listed in Table 12.1.

When pain is prolonged and chronic, it may remain confined to its original site and intensity. All too often, however, the anatomic site of the pain becomes less distinct, and symptoms originating in surrounding organ systems may join the original complaint. For example, a woman who starts with a problem limited to endometriosis may develop functional bowel symptoms, as well as discomforts related to excessive contraction of the pelvic floor musculature. Nociception from a painful posthysterectomy vaginal apex may refer to the lower abdominal wall on the side of the involved fornix. When taking a history of a chronic pain problem, it is useful to pay attention to the precise chronology of the addition of each component of the pain. Asking this type of detailed question will allow the clinician to deduce if the pain intensity is increasing despite relatively stable pathology.

TABLE 12.1

Typical Pain Patterns and Descriptors

Pain Type	History	Physical Examination
Endometriosis	Gradual progression from dysmenorrhea to continuous pain Deep dyspareunia	Tenderness in implant areas
Pelvic congestion	Luteal phase increase Afternoon, evening increase Deep dyspareunia Relieved by lying down "Heavy," "aching"	BLQ and central pelvic pain Tender at ovarian points, broad ligaments
Levator spasm	"Falling out" pressure sensation Afternoon, evening increase Midvaginal dyspareunia Radiates to low back Minimal cyclicity Relieved by lying down	Tender to palpation increased by contraction
Piriformis spasm	Pain on arising, climbing stairs, driving car	Pain on external thigh rotation; palpated externally or transvaginally
Adhesions	Starts 3–6 mo after surgery Localized to adhesions pulling, tugging	Vague thickening Pain on visceral motion

Reprinted from Steege JF. Office assessment of chronic pelvic pain. Clin Obstet Gynecol 1997;40:554–563, with permission.
BLQ, bilateral lower quadrant.

In many instances, taking this type of complete history requires more than one visit. Once the clinician decides that they are dealing with a significant chronic pain problem, the patient should be prepared to attend several visits before the evaluation is complete.

The clinician needs to understand the impact the pain has had on the patient as an individual, on her relationships, and on her work capacities. Psychological and behavioral factors are known contributors to the pain experience. The emotional components may be evaluated by the clinicians' own history and possibly by psychometric evaluation or psychological consultation. The purpose of psychometric instruments is to draw attention to particular problems, such as depression, that might not easily emerge from an interview. However, they are not meant to diagnose psychiatric disorders; that responsibility remains with the clinician. Personality profiles can serve to define an individuals' strengths and weaknesses but do not yield specific diagnoses. Taken as a whole, these instruments will convey to the patient your interest in knowing as much about her as possible before beginning treatment.

The clinician must also ask about past or present experiences with physical and/or sexual abuse. Many studies suggest that histories of abuse are more common in women referred to tertiary care specialty clinics for pelvic pain (14). In the primary care setting, this association is also present, but it is substantially weaker (15). In some cases, a history of abuse serves as a trigger for referral, whereas in others referral is done only if the history is accompanied by complicated psychosocial problems. Women with histories of particularly traumatic or prolonged abuse may develop somatization disorder and/or post-traumatic stress disorder. These women may exhibit dissociative reactions during examination, appearing to have "drifted off," becoming withdrawn, and noncommunicative (16).

Having obtained a history of sexual or physical abuse, the clinician is confronted with a dilemma: is the abuse etiologically related to the person's pain? Or is it an unfortunate, but unrelated, aspect of her life? The full impact of physical and/or sexual abuse in an individual's history requires careful assessment. Great care must be taken that appropriate medical and surgical attention to organic disease is not undermined by overemphasis of a relationship between the patient's pain and her past history of trauma.

Physical Examination

The data provided by the history and observations made during the history-taking process will provide focus for the physical examination. Before and during the history, the clinician may have the opportunity to observe facial expressions, posture, stance, gait, and sitting behavior. For example, a person with levator spasm will often sit forward on the chair and rest more of her weight on one buttock or the other. Sitting perfectly straight often aggravates the pain from this disorder.

The abdominal examination in a woman with chronic pelvic pain may be more informative if done in the following manner. First, inspect the abdominal wall for scars. Then, ask the patient to point to the area of pain with one finger and outline and circle the area involved. Ask her then to press as hard as she feels it is necessary in order to elicit the pain she experiences. Done in this manner, the impact of her anxiety about being examined may be diminished, and a more accurate assessment of tissue sensitivity obtained.

The abdominal wall should then be systematically palpated by the examiner's index finger in an effort to identify local spots of tenderness (pain with pressure), or "trigger points." A trigger point is a hyperirritable spot within a taut band of skeletal muscle fibers that is painful on compression and may give rise to referred pain, tenderness, tightness, and sometimes, local twitch response and autonomic phenomena (17,18). If these areas are found, the patient is asked to contract the abdominal wall by either raising her head or one leg off the table without assistance. If focal pain is exacerbated by this maneuver, there is a reasonable probability that a trigger point or other myofascial abdominal wall component is present. If the pain is reduced, a visceral source is more likely; if the pain is unchanged, then the maneuver is not diagnostic. Mapping these pain locations may be helpful in assessing if the pain corresponds to the distribution of the ilioinguinal or genitofemoral nerves. A diagrammatic record of the examination findings in the chart is also valuable.

TABLE 12.2

Musculoskeletal Screening Examination for Chronic Pelvic Pain

Observation/Maneuver	Typical Abnormal Findings
Gait, stance	Scoliosis
Lateral standing view	One extremity externally rotated; exaggerated kyphosis-lordosis
Sitting	Raised up on one buttock (levator spasm)
With supine flexion of one hip, observe other hip (Thomas test)	Contralateral hip flexes, indicating hip flexor contracture
External rotation of the thigh against resistance (sitting, supine, or during pelvic examination)	Pain on external rotation indicates piriformis syndrome
Psoas flexion and extension	Limited extension and/or pain with flexion indicates psoas shortening ± spasm
Digital vaginal examination	Pain indicates levator spasm

Specific elements of the musculoskeletal examination should be performed to look for piriformis spasm and/or psoas muscle pain. The piriformis originates at the lateral margin of the sacrum, traverses the greater sciatic notch, and inserts on the greater trochanter of the femur. Its function is to externally rotate the thigh. It also forms a muscular bed for the sacral plexus of nerves in the pelvis, and some or all the sciatic nerve goes through the belly of the piriformis in 25% of women. With her hip and her knee partially flexed (i.e., in the stirrups), ask the patient to externally rotate each thigh in turn against resistance. Pain in the posterior hip area with this maneuver suggests piriformis spasm. Irritation of the sciatic nerve by this spasm can cause hyper reflexia and "pseudosciatica," or pain that mimics sciatic nerve compression seen in lumbosacral disc disease.

In the lateral decubitus position, the hip is actively and passively extended and flexed. Pain with these maneuvers suggests a psoas muscle origin. Further elements of the musculoskeletal screening examination are discussed elsewhere (19) (Table 12.2).

The pelvic examination in the patient with chronic pelvic pain is more informative when performed in a careful stepwise fashion. Meticulous attention is paid to each potential contributing organ system. First, place one index finger in the vaginal introitus and ask for voluntary contraction and relaxation. Inability to exert conscious control of the bulbocavernosus muscles suggests vaginismus. This diagnosis should, of course, be corroborated by additional history. The presence of good voluntary control during pelvic examination does not exclude the diagnosis of vaginismus that may occur during sexual situations (20).

Extending the index finger beyond the bulbocavernosus muscle, one can usually palpate the levator muscles on the right and left sides at approximately the 4:30 and 7:30 positions. In the asymptomatic person, a sense of pressure is experienced. When levator spasm is present, gentle palpation on these muscles may reproduce the patient's sense of pelvic pressure (a "falling out" sensation) and/or the pain of dyspareunia. Further verification is obtained when the symptom is exacerbated by voluntary contraction of the levators.

The next step is to press directly on the coccyx, reaching it with the vaginal finger by going around the rectum on either side. External palpation of the coccyx combined with this maneuver will normally allow it to flex and extend through an approximately 30-degree angle. This is normally not a painful maneuver. If pain is present, it may be related to coccydynia or adjacent levator spasm.

The piriformis muscle can be tested by the maneuvers described earlier. When these maneuvers suggest piriformis spasm, this can be further confirmed on pelvic examination. The belly

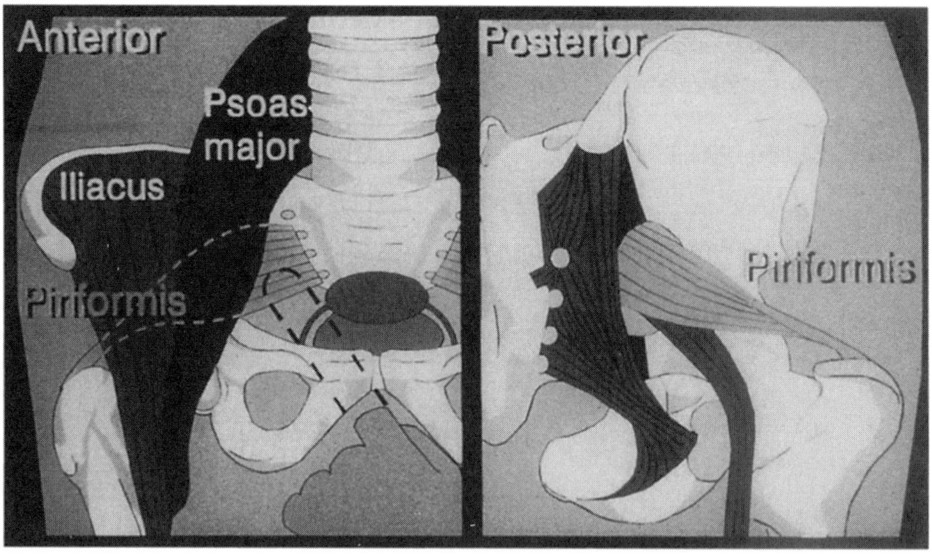

FIGURE 12.1 ● Palpation of the piriformis muscle during vaginal examination. (Reprinted from Barton PM. Piriformis syndrome: a rational approach to management. Pain 1991;47:345–352, with permission.)

of the piriformis can be easily felt transvaginally when the thigh is externally rotated against resistance. When palpation of the piriformis muscle belly reproduces pain, then spasm is likely to be present. A false-positive interpretation of this maneuver can occur if intrinsic cul de sac disease is present because the vaginal examination finger must traverse this area to reach the piriformis muscle (Fig. 12.1).

The anterior vaginal wall, urethra, and bladder trigone should be examined either before or after the muscular examinations just described, depending on the clinical situation. In general, it is best to examine the (likely) nontender areas first. This technique helps minimize the tendency to experience pressure as pain ("wind-up") once pain has been elicited. In many cases, the clinician can make the presumptive diagnosis of chronic urethritis, trigonitis, or interstitial cystitis on the basis of careful history combined with focused digital examination. If complex therapeutic interventions are being contemplated, then cystoscopic confirmation of these presumptive diagnoses should first be obtained. In the asymptomatic patient, pressure on the bladder base creates only urinary urgency without replicating the clinical pain.

Unimanual, single-digit transvaginal examination should continue by testing the intrinsic sensitivity of the cervix to palpation and traction. The adnexal areas are then examined in a similar manner, first unimanually and then adding the abdominal hand. Separating the bimanual exam into three discrete steps (unimanual vaginal exam alone, unimanual external exam of lower abdomen alone, and then examining the pelvis bimanually) helps distinguish internal visceral pain from pain originating from the abdominal wall.

Rather than following a rigid sequence, speculum examination should be done at a time when it makes the most sense, depending on the type of pain under consideration. For example, in the patient with a history suggesting posthysterectomy vaginal apex pain, it is probably wisest to complete the muscular examination and the adnexal palpation *prior* to insertion of the speculum. In this manner, the areas more likely to be nontender are examined prior to the speculum directly touching the potentially sensitive vaginal apex.

In contrast, if the history suggests an adnexal source of pain, then the pelvic examination should begin with the speculum examination (as is traditionally done). The speculum examination is then followed by a pelvic musculoskeletal exam, leaving the adnexal examination for last. To determine if adnexal pathology exists to a sufficient degree to contribute to the pain, the examiner need only palpate with a single vaginal finger. This avoids confusing the diagnostic picture by using the traditional bimanual exam, which may mingle pain signals from the abdominal wall with those from the adnexa. The gynecologist, focusing on the reproductive organs, may interpret all pain as coming from this system, sometimes leading to overtreatment of the adnexa. Having examined the adnexa for pain, the traditional bimanual adnexal exam can then evaluate size, shape, and mobility. Throughout this portion of the examination, the clinician should ask whether any tenderness elicited reproduces the pain of her chief complaint.

Rectovaginal examination remains an essential component of the complete pelvic exam. Insertion of the rectal finger causes the least discomfort if the middle finger is placed gently at the anus and exerts slow, gentle pressure. Some clinicians are taught that having the woman bear down will facilitate insertion of the finger. When most patients "bear down," however, they do a Valsalva maneuver and simultaneously contract the voluntary portion of the anal sphincter. This causes an increase in discomfort and makes digital insertion more difficult. The rectal finger should advance as far as possible, ideally reaching the hollow of the sacrum. In this manner, the entire floor of the posterior cul de sac can be thoroughly evaluated for the presence of irregularities or nodularity that might imply the presence of deep infiltrating endometriosis. To fully evaluate the uterosacral ligaments, a rectovaginal examination is done. The uterosacral ligaments can be more accurately assessed by putting the cervix on traction in an anterior direction with the tip of the vaginal finger, while palpating the stretched uterosacral ligaments with the rectal finger.

After palpation of the uterosacral ligaments, the bimanual portion of the examination is repeated with sequential palpation with the rectovaginal hand, the abdominal hand, and both hands together. When examining areas that are tender, it is useful to pause to inform the patient that examination of the tender area will only last for a count of "one, two, three . . .", and will only begin when she feels ready. By time limiting this portion of the exam and allowing the woman to determine when it will commence, the examination is made more tolerable for the patient. When tenderness is elicited, the clinician should ask whether this reproduces the clinical pain the patient is experiencing.

Office Diagnostic Procedures

Trigger point injections have been well established as a diagnostic and therapeutic technique (21, 22). The trigger point is identified first through palpation and then with the needle before injection. Eliciting the local twitch response, a brisk contraction of the taut band (but not the surrounding normal muscle fibers), is essential for success (23–25). Multiple types of local anesthetics (e.g., 1% lidocaine or 0.25% bupivacaine) have been used with none demonstrably superior to any other. The pain of injection can be substantially reduced by adding sodium bicarbonate (1 mL per 10 mL of 1% lidocaine; 0.2 mL per 30 mL of 0.25% bupivacaine). A 27-gauge tuberculin needle or a 25-gauge, 1.5-in needle is preferable for injection. The use of botulinum toxin A has also been described for abdominal wall trigger point injection with prolonged reductions in pain scores (26, 27). The use of botulinum toxin A is appealing for chronic myofascial pain for its local, temporary muscle paralysis and its reduction of neurogenic inflammatory mediators. If the abdominal wall trigger points can be blocked successfully, then the pelvic examination might be repeated to better understand the contributions of intrapelvic pathology to the patient's pain.

Similarly, local injection can be used to anesthetize the vaginal apex tissue in an effort to determine whether this tissue is intrinsically sensitive, or whether pain elicited from vaginal cuff palpation on bimanual examination emanates from intrapelvic pathology.

Transvaginal ultrasound examination provides very useful information in evaluating acute pelvic pain. Unfortunately, it is less contributory for the evaluation of chronic pelvic pain complaints. The occasional exceptions to this generalization are noted as individual pelvic pain syndromes are discussed in the next section.

SPECIFIC PELVIC PAIN SYNDROMES

Endometriosis

Certain historical stigmata signal the possibility that endometriosis may be present. Severe dysmenorrhea during adolescence with worsening in early adult life should suggest this etiology. With endometriosis, the duration of severe dysmenorrhea may also change. In cases of primary dysmenorrhea not due to endometriosis, the typical pattern is for the first day of menses to be the most painful. This is followed by a roughly 50% reduction in pain on the second menstrual day. If endometriosis develops, the duration of the more severe menstrual cramps may lengthen, and the severe dysmenorrhea may last into the second or third menstrual days. The next change may be the appearance of premenstrual pain, ultimately followed by pain present for almost all the menstrual month, but with continuing premenstrual and menstrual exacerbations. Deep dyspareunia may join the picture at any point along the way, usually appearing perimenstrually at first.

Early in the disease of endometriosis, physical examination may not detect any abnormalities, but when endometriosis is at a stage where deep dyspareunia and severe dysmenorrhea are present, the examination may reveal focal cul de sac tenderness and nodularity of the uterosacral ligaments. Increased attention has been paid more recently to deep infiltrating endometriosis in the cul de sac of Douglas, which may not be readily visualized during laparoscopy (28, 29). The chances of detecting palpable nodularity may be increased by examining the patient during menstruation. At this point, the nodularity may be more palpable and tender.

More recent investigations have suggested that there may be more than one subtype of endometriosis (29). There are two common varieties of endometriosis: one with multiple peritoneal implants, predominantly in the cul de sac or on the ovaries, and a second variety appearing primarily as intraovarian disease, or endometriomas. The intraovarian variety is not frequently associated with dysmenorrhea and pelvic pain, and is often diagnosed by an incidental finding of ovarian enlargement. Pain may appear if the endometrioma(s) become quite large.

A third variety, quite distinct from the other two, consists primarily of deep cul de sac disease. Laparoscopy in such cases may reveal only the mildest signs of peritoneal abnormality, with the bulk of the disease hidden in the retroperitoneal space next to the rectum and at the vaginal apex. This last variety has been called vaginal adenomyosis by some authors (30). It has been described as being potentially due to a Müllerian anomaly rather than resulting from retrograde menstruation (Sampson's theory). Diagnosis of deep, infiltrating cul de sac endometriosis can be quite difficult. Although history and pelvic examination may be suggestive, the use of special magnetic resonance imaging (MRI) techniques may be necessary to accurately detect this disorder. Treatment is believed to be primarily surgical because sex steroid receptor patterns are different in this type of disease when compared with more typical peritoneal disease (31).

Other physical findings of endometriosis may include a fixed, retroverted uterus, as well as generalized pelvic tenderness. Differentiating this diagnosis from chronic pelvic inflammatory disease or other forms of pelvic masses may be difficult.

With the possible exception of new approaches using MRI techniques, imaging studies in general are not very useful in the diagnosis of endometriosis. Transvaginal ultrasound may detect cystic enlargement of the ovaries, but endometriomas may have a variety of different ultrasonic appearances, none of which are unique to this disorder.

Medical management of this disorder most reasonably starts with cyclic oral contraceptives. Continuous oral contraceptives may also be employed, thus avoiding the discomforts of regular menstruation. To go beyond this first order of therapy is to ask the patient to incur significantly greater expense, side effects, and disruption of her normal endocrinologic milieu. For these reasons, most authorities advocate laparoscopic confirmation of the diagnosis prior to embarking on more intrusive medical therapies such as danazol (Danocrine), continuous high-dose progestins, or gonadotropin-releasing hormone (GnRH) agonists (Table 12.3).

More recently, one study has challenged this traditional view. Ling et al. (32) tested the ability of clinicians to diagnose endometriosis on clinical grounds, without laparoscopy. In 95 women, 82% were found to have visual evidence of endometriosis at the time of laparoscopy (biopsy for proof by pathology was not uniformly done). Prior to this surgery, they had been randomly assigned to treatment with leuprolide or placebo. The active drug relieved pelvic pain with equal frequency in women with or without endometriosis. This means that pain relief on leuprolide did not make the diagnosis of endometriosis; that is, laparoscopy was still required. Unfortunately, the study has been widely misinterpreted to mean that when pain goes away on leuprolide, endometriosis is present.

Until more recently, surgical treatment of minimal and mild endometriosis by laparoscopic methods was believed to be equivalent to medical management in improving fertility. However,

TABLE 12.3

Medications Used in Conjunction With GnRH Agonists

Norethindrone	Estrogen + progestin (continuous)
Etidronate	Estrogen + progestin (cyclic)
Norethindrone + etidronate	Calcitonin
Estrogen (oral and transdermal)	Calcium
	Medroxyprogesterone acetate

Reprinted from Metzger DA. An integrated approach to the management of endometriosis. In: Steege JF, Metzger DA, Levy BS, eds. Chronic Pelvic Pain: An Integrated Approach. Philadelphia: WB Saunders, 1998, with permission.

a more recent randomized trial demonstrated a more rapid accomplishment of the desired pregnancy following laparoscopic treatment of the disorder when compared with expectant therapy (33). Similar comparisons of medical and surgical treatments of endometriosis for the purpose of pain relief have not been performed.

Various opinions exist about the appropriate technique for laparoscopic treatment of endometriosis. Electrocoagulation or laser treatment of superficial implants is regarded as sufficient for very small foci of disease. When confluent collections of implants are noted or when active red or purple lesions are found, some surgeons prefer laser vaporization for definitive therapy. Others believe that excision of the entire area of involved peritoneum is the only way to adequately remove the disease to its depths (29). When extensive areas of peritoneum are removed, however, severe peritoneal adhesions may be the sequelae. This may result in trading endometriosis for adhesive disease as the pain etiology.

Women dealing with endometriosis may also develop some of the other chronic pain syndromes described as follows, such as pelvic congestion, musculoskeletal problems, and/or irritable bowel syndrome. Careful attention to the nature and chronology of symptoms will usually allow separate consideration and treatment of these disorders.

Pelvic Adhesions

Intra-abdominal adhesions are found in approximately 30% of autopsied women older than 60 years of age (34). In asymptomatic women undergoing laparoscopic tubal sterilization, adhesions are found in approximately 12% of the women (35). Among women undergoing laparoscopy for chronic pelvic pain, adhesions are found between 45% and 90% of the time (36).

Studies of the impact of adhesiolysis on chronic pelvic pain have been relatively limited. Uncontrolled series suggest that 65 to 85% of treated women obtained significant relief 8 to 12 months after surgery (37, 38). One randomized trial showed adhesiolysis by laparotomy to be superior to diagnostic laparoscopy only in the small percentage of women with dense bowel adhesions (39). This latter study did not evaluate the impact of the laparoscopic approach to adhesiolysis.

These results suggest that certain types of adhesions may play an etiologic role in chronic pelvic pain, but by no means are they always responsible for pain generation. The clinician is left with the challenge of providing a balanced interpretation of the role of adhesions in pain causation and the role of adhesiolysis in the overall pain management plan. Future studies using microlaparoscopic pain mapping under conscious sedation may provide additional information regarding the particular types of adhesions that are most important in pain generation.

The clinical diagnosis of adhesions is quite difficult. It is possible to assess the relative mobility of the pelvic viscera during examination, but adhesions can only be strongly suspected when they are quite extensive. Transvaginal ultrasound is another way to evaluate the mobility of the pelvic organs, but it has low sensitivity and specificity in predicting the presence of adhesions. Sophisticated imaging studies, such as computed tomography scans and MRI, are ineffective in diagnosing adhesions; the gold standard for diagnosing adhesive disease remains diagnostic laparoscopy.

Following laparoscopic adhesiolysis, adhesions will start to reform within 1 to 2 weeks after surgery. Pain may not recur for another several months. The mechanism of this delay is uncertain, but strong possibilities include the time necessary for adhesive tissue to become well collagenized and contract, as well as the time required for neural ingrowth. The overall prevalence of nerve tissue in adhesions is uncertain, as is its role in pain generation.

In summary, treatment of adhesions in some cases may play an important role in the management of chronic pelvic pain. In many situations it is wisest to simultaneously direct treatment efforts to other visceral and somatic sources of the pain, as well as to the affective components, in order to bring about the best resolution.

Adenomyosis

Adenomyosis is a condition in which endometrial glands and stroma grow within the myometrium, usually without direct connection to the endometrium. For true pathologic diagnosis, these glands and stroma must be present three high-powered fields below the basal layer of the endometrium. Adenomyosis is an extremely common condition, generally believed to be present in parous women in their 30s and 40s. Its relationship to symptoms is uncertain because it may be present in as many as 30% of women, most of whom are asymptomatic (40). Its role as a post hoc justification for hysterectomy in a woman with an otherwise anatomically normal pelvis has made it the focus of significant controversy.

Traditionally, the diagnosis has only been possible by histologic examination of the uterine wall. Transvaginal ultrasound, MRI scanning, and myometrial needle biopsy have all been employed in an effort to make a preoperative diagnosis. Although these efforts are encouraging, they lack sufficient resolution and standardized criteria and technique to explain or quantify the pathophysiologic process or relationship between histologic changes and clinical symptoms.

On a clinical basis, it may be useful to use serial pelvic examinations, possibly in combination with transvaginal ultrasound, in evaluating the potential role for adenomyosis as the etiologic source of the woman's pelvic pain. A woman who has a truly substantial amount of this disease will often demonstrate substantial cyclic changes in the size, consistency, and tenderness of the uterine fundus. In the follicular phase, the uterus will be smaller and firmer, whereas immediately premenstrually it will be enlarged as much as 1.5-fold over its baseline, and will be extremely tender and much softer in consistency.

Pharmacologic therapy has been attempted with continuous oral contraceptives, luteal phase progestins, danazol (Danocrine), or GnRH agonists. Although success has not been confirmed by clinical trials, there are patients who report that luteal phase medroxyprogesterone acetate (Provera) provides sufficient reduction of pain and diminution of menometrorrhagia. When any of these therapies are successful, the clinician must decide whether their long-term use makes practical and clinical sense.

Whether hysterectomy is appropriate for this condition is a matter of considerable debate, especially in the current era of managed care. The condition is not life threatening, and when medical therapy works, the discussion of further surgery centers primarily around quality of life issues. In this case, as in many others, the discussion of medical necessity leaves off, and the discussion of personal preferences and cultural expectations begins.

Pelvic Congestion

Since the mid-20th century, this syndrome (and its many different names) has been widely described in the literature. Discomfort has been associated with distention of abnormal pelvic veins. In the early literature, a variety of other pathologic findings were attributed to the process (41, 42). More recent studies indicate the venous distention itself is primarily responsible for the production of symptoms (43, 44).

As much or more than any other gynecologic disorders related to pain, it is in this instance that mind–body interactions have been most intensely debated. Early publications by Taylor described a population of women with enlarged pelvic veins who had otherwise normal pelvic anatomy, but whose psychosocial histories divulged a high prevalence of early deprivation and abuse. He described increases in vascular pelvic congestion (measured by increases in vaginal blood flow detected photometrically) that occurred only during interviews dealing with stressful topics (43, 44). Using similar methodology, however, a later investigator described the same phenomenon in pain-free controls (45).

Documentation of pelvic varices has been primarily demonstrated by transuterine venography (46). In this procedure, radiopaque aqueous contrast material is injected into the uterine fundus transvaginally, and radiographs are taken at closely spaced intervals to document the passage of this contrast through the pelvic veins. Scoring criteria have been developed (47).

The symptom pattern associated with this disorder includes a sensation of pressure low in the pelvis that worsens during the course of the day and premenstrually, deep dyspareunia, and a subset of women who experience menorrhagia. Bladder irritability and altered bowel habits are also found in some series, thus confusing the diagnostic picture (41, 42). Its prevalence is uncertain because reports from experts on pelvic congestion may reflect a higher incidence than what is true for the general population (41, 42). Given the complexity of this disorder, prescription and assessment of therapeutic measures must be done carefully.

Concrete physical examination findings in this disorder are limited. Beard places emphasis on the detection of pain at the "ovarian point" (42). This is located two-thirds of the way from the anterior, superior, iliac spine to the umbilicus. Tenderness in this area may be present in women without other evidence of this disorder and therefore this sign may not be consistently diagnostic. Bimanual examination will reveal a "doughy" consistency to the parametrial areas, and the patient will report these areas as the most sensitive areas in the pelvis. Examination in the premenstrual period may demonstrate substantial change in consistency of this area when compared with a follicular phase examination.

Diagnostic laparoscopy will often miss this diagnosis. Laparoscopy is usually performed early in the day with the patient in the Trendelenburg position. Attempts have been made to examine the pelvis laparoscopically with the patient in the reverse Trendelenburg position using a volume of irrigating fluid to float the bowels out of the way. This approach has not been systematically studied or validated. Diagnostic ultrasound is being evaluated for this disorder, but the technique has been difficult to standardize (48).

Pelvic congestion has been treated by suppressing the menstrual cycle. One study using GnRH agonists with estrogen and progestin add-back therapy did not demonstrate relief (49). Oral contraceptives have been similarly ineffective (50). In contrast, continuous high-dose medroxyprogesterone acetate (Provera) (30 mg four times a day), in combination with a six-session course of psychotherapy has produced a minimum of 50% improvement in three-fourths of the women in one study (51). The psychotherapy focused on stress management and establishment of a better understanding of mind–body interactions. Medroxyprogesterone acetate (Provera) alone showed similar benefits when compared with placebo, but the duration of the effect was much greater when medical therapy was combined with counseling.

Surgical therapy has traditionally involved hysterectomy (52). In the most severe cases, bilateral salpingo-oophorectomy is also recommended. Less radical approaches have included ligation of individual varices, although this has proven relatively unsuccessful. Other techniques are individual ovarian vein ligation or ligation of the entire infundibular pelvic ligament, with the literature describing a modest effect from this latter approach (53).

Although surgical therapy or intense medical therapy remain the mainstays of treatment, pharmacologic therapy with progestins and behavioral methods of stress reduction are central to an effective treatment plan.

Irritable Bowel Syndrome

The symptoms of irritable bowel syndrome (IBS) are frequently misinterpreted as being of gynecologic origin. The International Consensus Criteria require that abdominal pain be relieved by defecation or associated with a change in the frequency or consistency of stools. In addition, two or more of the following symptoms must be present:

TABLE 12.4

Differential Diagnosis of Painful Gastrointestinal Disorders That May Present as Pelvic Pain

Disorder	Symptoms	Diagnostic Test
Lactose intolerance test	Cramping pain, flatulence after milk products	Lactose tolerance
Small bowel bacterial overgrowth and diarrhea growth	Postprandial bloating	Hydrogen breath test
Chronic intestinal pseudo-obstruction	Migratory abdominal pain	Small bowel motility study
Inflammatory bowel disease	Copious diarrhea, sometimes bloody	Endoscopy, x-ray contrast studies
Diverticulosis	Pain, diarrhea	Endoscopy, contrast studies
Bowel endometriosis	Pain with bowel movements, ± alteration of bowel function	Endoscopy, laparoscopy

1. Altered stool frequency
2. Altered stool form
3. Dyschezia or urgency
4. Passage of mucus
5. Bloating (54)

Alternative etiologies can be ruled out with flexible sigmoidoscopy, stool guaiac testing, and hematologic tests that screen for immunologic problems or thyroid dysfunction.

The differential diagnosis includes lactose intolerance, bacterial overgrowth of the small intestine, chronic intestinal pseudo-obstruction, inflammatory bowel disease, diverticular disease, levator ani syndrome (proctalgia fugax), and/or endometriosis affecting the bowel (Table 12.4).

There appears to be a fairly strong association of IBS with dysmenorrhea (55). IBS is more common in women who have undergone hysterectomy in the absence of identifiable gynecologic pathology compared with women who underwent hysterectomy for pathology (56).

In rectal manometric studies, approximately 40 to 60% of IBS patients report pain at levels of distention below the range of normal values (57). Although controversial, this observation may serve as a marker for IBS when combined with other clinical indicators. This lowered pain threshold may reflect a difference in the sensitivity of peripheral stretch receptors or pain afferent pathways. Attempts have been made to correlate these physiologic observations with measures of psychological stress or affective change, with mixed results (57, 58). In addition to the "visceral hyperalgesia" phenomenon suggested by these studies, IBS patients may have increased colonic motility, as well as abnormal small bowel motility (59, 60). None of these physiologic markers is specific enough to be used as a single diagnostic sign of IBS. Fifty to 85% of patients with IBS report that psychological stress exacerbates their bowel symptoms (58). One study found that 53% of women with IBS referred to tertiary care centers had a history of previous sexual abuse compared with 37% of those referred with other organic diagnoses. This same pattern is not seen at a primary care level (61).

The medical management choices for IBS are dictated by the predominant symptom(s) (Table 12.5). If diarrhea is the major symptom, a variety of antispasmodic medications such as diphenoxylate (Lomotil), hyoscyamine (Levsin, Donnatal), and dicyclomine (Bentyl) are used. Desipramine (Norpramin) or other tricyclic antidepressants are also effective and have the added benefit of treating the chronic pain syndrome component of the problem.

TABLE 12.5

Pharmacologic Treatment of Irritable Bowel Syndrome

Symptom	Drug	Daily Dose	Major Side Effects
Diarrhea	Loperamide (Imodium)	Titrate; 4 mg average	Constipation
	Diphenoxylate HCl	20 mg	Euphoria, sedation, dry mouth, constipation
	Hyoscyamine sulfate (Levsin, Donnatal)	<1.5 mg	Dry mouth, blurred vision, dizziness
	Dicyclomine HCl (Bentyl)	80–160 mg	Dry mouth, blurred vision, dizziness
	Desipramine HCl (Norpramin)	150 mg	Dry mouth, sedation, confusional states, hypertension, hypotension, constipation
	Trimipramine maleate (Surmontil)	50 mg	Dry mouth, sedation, confusional states, hypertension, hypotension, constipation
Constipation	Fiber from any source	≥30 g	Bloating, abdominal pain
	Lactuiose (Chronulac, Duphalac)	10–30 g	Bloating
	Sorbitol	10–30 g	Bloating
	Cisapride (Propulsid)	40–80 mg	Dizziness, headaches

Reprinted from Whitehead WE. Gastrointestinal disorders. In: Steege JF, Metzger DA, Levy BS, eds. Chronic Pelvic Pain: An Integrated Approach. Philadelphia: WB Saunders, 1998, with permission.

Constipation is best treated by increased fiber and water intake. Lactose and sorbitol are effective but increase abdominal bloating. A very effective, but more expensive, treatment is cisapride (Propulsid), although it may manifest side effects of dizziness and headaches.

For general pain treatment, the serotonin reuptake inhibitors have not been widely explored, although one study suggests that 5HT3 receptor antagonists (e.g., granisetron HCl [Kytril]) will lower the increased pain sensitivity seen in IBS patients (62).

Psychological treatments for IBS have included relaxation training, cognitive behavioral therapy, hypnosis, and individual psychotherapy. Each modality has research studies that support efficacy, and some studies have used them in one or more combinations (63, 64).

As a matter of practicality, the first-line approach for severe IBS includes dietary change, increased fiber and water intake, an anticholinergic for diarrhea-predominant patients, and tricyclic antidepressants when pain is the major complaint. If these interventions fail, mental health referral should be considered.

Musculoskeletal Problems

There are three basic categories of musculoskeletal pain that may contribute to or create pelvic pain:

1. Dysfunction of the levator ani and/or piriformis muscle(s)
2. Musculoskeletal dysfunction that is secondary to a primary gynecologic source of pain
3. Musculoskeletal dysfunction that is the primary source of pelvic pain but mimics a gynecologic problem

Levator Ani Spasm

Spasm of the levator ani muscle(s) is perhaps one of the most frequently overlooked findings in the patient with pelvic pain. Historically, the person will describe a sensation of her pelvis "falling out," which is worse later in the day. The pain commonly radiates to the lower back or sacral area and may increase premenstrually. This premenstrual increase is less dramatic than that seen with endometriosis or pelvic congestion. The spasm may be relieved by lying down and is aggravated by defecation. Pelvic examination reveals tenderness specific to the levator muscles. This is most readily elicited by vaginal palpation of the pelvic floor in the 4:30 and 7:30 positions with the index finger. To amplify the finding, ask for voluntary contraction of the pelvic floor, such as what might occur during attempts to hold back defecation. The patient should then be asked how closely any discomfort mimics her chief complaint.

In this setting, it may be helpful to teach pelvic floor muscle relaxation exercises. The patient is asked to tighten the pelvic floor for a count of "one" or "two," and relax for a count of "seven" or "eight." In essence, these are "reverse" Kegel exercises. The patient is counseled that when she is standing and notes this sense of pelvic pressure, if she simply lets it "fall out," the pelvic floor will relax.

Piriformis Muscle Spasm

The piriformis muscle originates in the lateral margin of the sacrum and passes through the greater sciatic notch to attach to the greater trochanter of the femur. Its function is to assist in external rotation of the thigh. When this muscle is in spasm, the patient may notice pain on first arising and starting to walk, with climbing stairs, or with driving a car. The pain is present regardless of time of day and phase of the menstrual cycle.

On physical examination, the pain is elicited by (a) externally rotating the entire leg in the supine position or (b) externally rotating the thigh against resistance while transvaginally palpating the piriformis muscle during this maneuver. When cul de sac pathology is present, the transvaginal palpation of the piriformis may yield a false-positive result. In addition to being associated with initial gynecologic problems, piriformis syndrome may develop as a result of athletic injury or other inflammatory conditions such as trochanteric bursitis. As a normal anatomic variant, the sciatic nerve may traverse the belly of the piriformis in up to 20 to 30% of people. With this anatomic variant, when the piriformis goes into spasm, pseudosciatic symptoms may appear.

Treatment for the piriformis syndrome involves range of motion exercises, heat, local massage, deep ultrasound, and other physical therapy techniques. Continuous nonsteroidal anti-inflammatory drugs are also useful and should perhaps be a first-line agent.

The second category of disorders, musculoskeletal dysfunctions that develop as a response to initial gynecologic problems, may include shortening and spasm of the psoas, shortening of the abdominal muscles, and/or a general abnormal posture, including increased lumbar lordosis and an anterior tilt of the pelvis. The original gynecologic problem may promote splinting or cessation of exercise, leading to muscle(s) of abnormal lengths (i.e., longer or shorter). This may induce tissue damage that results in the development of trigger points. Injection therapy for trigger points may not yield long-term results unless they are supplemented by physical therapy techniques aimed at re-establishing normal posture, muscle length, and muscular relaxation.

The musculoskeletal disorders listed previously, as well as others, may develop primarily and not in response to other pain etiologies. When these problems are detected coincidentally with known gynecologic pathology, clinical judgment as to which component is the more likely originator of the pain disorder is difficult.

Urinary Tract Disorders

Problems of the bladder and urethra may be roughly grouped as anatomic, inflammatory, or functional. Although anatomic or structural urologic causes of chronic pelvic pain occur, the majority are either inflammatory or functional in nature.

Problems resulting from pelvic relaxation are the most common structural disorders of the urinary tract. A pronounced cystocele may result in urinary retention and chronic, recurrent urinary tract infection (UTI). Ordinarily, the history and physical examination readily detects this anatomic problem. Postcoital antibiosis, voiding, and occasional daily antibiotic prophylaxis will treat most cases of chronic infection. When possible, surgical repair of the cystocele is most appropriate.

A urethral diverticulum is a relatively infrequent cause of pelvic pain. A bulging mass underneath the urethra may be appreciated, although in many cases urethroscopy and/or a urethrogram with a double balloon Davis catheter is needed. By history, the patient may report dribbling when she stands up after voiding. On examination, even if a bulge cannot be appreciated, an area of focal tenderness along the course of the urethra may be palpable.

Perhaps the largest overall category of bladder problems contributing to chronic pelvic pain is the inflammatory disorders. Chronic, recurrent UTI is perhaps the most common, followed by chronic, bacterial urethritis. In the latter disorder, clean catch urine cultures may yield colony counts significantly less than 100,000 CFU/mL and are erroneously reported as "negative." Diagnosis can be made by historical reports of urethral pain and generalized tenderness to palpation along the entire urethra. A short course of antibiotics may help symptoms subside, but prolonged courses of at least 3 months are often needed to produce long-term relief. Urethral dilation is an outmoded treatment for chronic UTI but may have occasional application in refractory cases of chronic urethritis.

Much attention has been focused on the very difficult problem of interstitial cystitis. This disorder typically presents as frequency, nocturia, urgency, and suprapubic pain, often relieved by voiding. Dyspareunia is present in as many as 60% of female patients. The disorder may present in a mild, intermittent form initially but may gradually progress to a more chronic and disabling pattern over several years.

The diagnosis of interstitial cystitis is made by cystoscopy and hydrodistention under general or regional anesthesia (65). The bladder is distended to 80 cm of water pressure with gravity filling over a period of 1 to 2 minutes, noting final bladder capacity. Typically, total bladder capacity during anesthesia is reduced from a normal value of 800 mL to between 350 and 450 mL. The bladder is then emptied and refilled. At this point, the cystoscope typically reveals glomerulations that look like small petechiae, or submucosal hemorrhages, fissures, and/or ulcers. Quantitatively, the diagnosis is made when these lesions appear in at least three quadrants of the bladder with at least ten glomerulations per quadrant. Bladder biopsy may be performed to rule out other diseases such as eosinophilia, cystitis, endometriosis, chronic cystitis, and carcinoma in situ. The hydrodistention process itself may reduce symptoms in 30 to 60% of patients.

The only U.S. Food and Drug Administration-approved medication for interstitial cystitis is pentosan polysulfate sodium (Elmiran); it purportedly works by repairing the altered permeability of the bladder surface (66). It may take up to 6 months for the maximal effect of pentosan polysulfate sodium to be seen, and only 28 to 32% of patients report improvement with this therapy (67, 68). Other therapies for interstitial cystitis include a host of oral and intravesical agents, as well as general pain management techniques (Table 12.6).

Dietary therapy may contribute to management. This involves adequate food intake, avoidance of soft drinks, caffeine, and citrus juices, as well as a variety of other less well-substantiated recommendations.

Under the heading of functional disorders, chronic intermittent bladder spasm is an uncommon, but not rare, contributor to chronic pelvic pain. Ordinarily, the association with voiding and the suprapubic location of the pain makes the diagnosis. During pelvic examination, the bladder area may be somewhat tender, especially if the patient has just voided prior to the examination. Anticholinergic and antispasmodic agents (e.g., hyoscyamine sulfate [Levsin] or Donnatal) are effective initial therapies, although the sedative side effects of these drugs complicate their use.

Bladder training or the bladder "drill" is often helpful in reducing the inherent irritability of the bladder in both interstitial cystitis and bladder spasm. In this exercise, the patient records the time of each urination over several days and then calculates the average interval. While maintaining a steady fluid intake throughout the day, the patient then voids on a schedule. She gradually increases the voiding interval over weeks or months. This accomplishes a gradual nontraumatic stretching of the bladder wall, and often, a reduction in symptoms.

TABLE 12.6

Treatment Modalities in Interstitial Cystitis

NONSURGICAL	SURGICAL
Pharmacologic	*Endoscopic Procedures*
Antihistamines	Hydrodistention
Anti-inflammatories	Transurethral resection and fulguration
Sodium pentosan polysulfate (Elmiron)	Neodymium:yttrium-aluminum garnet laser
Anticholinergics	*Open Surgical Procedures*
Intravesical	Denervation procedures
Dimethyl sulfoxide (DMSO)	Bladder augmentation procedures
$DMSO_2$ (investigational)	Urinary diversion
DSMO cocktails	
Silver nitrate	
Sodium oxychlorosene (Chlorpactin)	
Cystostat (investigational)	
Cromolyn (a mast cell inhibitor) (investigational)	
OTHER	
Electric stimulation	
Biofeedback	
Transcutaneous electric nerve stimulation	
Epidural block	
Bladder pillar block	

Reprinted from Peters-Gee JM. Bladder and urethral symptoms. In: Steege JF, Metzger DA, Levy BS, eds. Chronic Pelvic Pain: An Integrated Approach. Philadelphia: WB Saunders, 1998, with permission.

Neuropathic Pain

Since the early 1990s, there has been a growing recognition that pain may at times arise from nerves supplying a nociception-producing organ, sometimes even after the organ has been removed. Examples we have seen include intrinsic cervical pain to gentle touch (allodynia) after trauma such as obstetric laceration or loop electrosurgical excision procedure procedures, vulvar vestibulitis, and sensitivity of the vaginal apex (usually one fornix) after hysterectomy. In each case, creatively devising ways to deliver lidocaine 5% ointment to the sensitive area for as many hours of the day as possible has often been helpful. For the cervix, a contraceptive diaphragm can be partly filled with lidocaine and placed in the vagina overnight. For the vaginal apex, commercial lidocaine ointment or a compounded preparation can be delivered to the spot with a vaginal applicator. For the vestibule, ointment can be directly applied with a fingertip or copiously applied to a cotton ball, which is then placed directly on the vestibule, being held in place overnight by the labia (69).

Miscellaneous Causes of Chronic Pelvic Pain

In addition to the previous disorders, a whole host of uncommon and rare conditions may produce pelvic pain. The uncommon categories would include posthysterectomy entrapment of the ovary, ovarian remnant syndrome, and intrinsic vaginal apex pain. The rarer disorders would include true peripheral neuropathies of the pelvis, traumatic neuromas, levator muscle tendinitis, and a variety of other focal pain syndromes of mixed etiology.

Following hysterectomy, reapproximation of the pelvic peritoneum may result in encasement of one or both ovaries in adhesion, sometimes at close proximity to the vaginal apex. During intercourse, percussion of the encased ovary can be quite painful. Incorporating the utero-ovarian ligament in the vaginal apex at the time of vaginal hysterectomy leads to a high frequency of postvaginal hysterectomy deep dyspareunia. For this reason, this surgical technique is no longer recommended. Although suppression of ovarian function may reduce the discomfort, surgical removal is often necessary.

The ovarian remnant syndrome is uncommon but not as rare as previously believed. Clinical series published in the last 15 years have prompted more frequent testing for, and hence diagnosis of, this condition (70–72). In a patient with ostensible bilateral salpingo-oophorectomy, the presence of functioning ovarian tissue is detected by withdrawing replacement hormones for 3 to 4 weeks, and then determining the serum FSH and estradiol levels. If the FSH level is well over 40 and estradiol levels are minimal, then it is highly unlikely that ovarian tissue is present. If premenopausal levels of these hormones are present, then hormonally functional ovarian tissue is present. Complete suppression of the remnant with a GnRH agonist will help determine the degree to which the ovarian remnant contributes to the patient's pain. If the patient is sufficiently close to menopausal age, then suppression with a GnRH agonist (along with add-back estrogen as appropriate) may be continued until menopause is reached. If not, surgical intervention should be contemplated. Let the GnRH agonist wear off, allowing the remnant to grow back to a size that allows easier surgical pursuit. With the best of surgical techniques, there is a 10 to 15% chance of recurrence of the ovarian remnant after careful excision.

After hysterectomy, the vaginal apex may be intrinsically sensitive in the occasional patient. Although granulation tissue can cause this problem in the early postoperative months, localized sensitivity sometimes remains for years thereafter, even after all postoperative inflammation has disappeared. This condition is detected by gently "walking" a cotton-tipped applicator over the vaginal apex during speculum examination. Often, one part of the vaginal apex will be sensitive, whereas other parts will be quite comfortable. A local block with 1% Xylocaine mixed with sodium bicarbonate (1.0 cc of 0.9% sodium bicarbonate with 9 cc of 1% Xylocaine) can accomplish transient and sometimes long-term relief. Blocking the area successfully will confirm the diagnosis. Some patients can adequately cope with this disorder by using 5% Xylocaine ointment delivered by a vaginal applicator. Dose titration is important to accomplish comfortable intercourse without producing genital anesthesia for both partners. If these conservative modalities fail, then surgical revision of the vaginal apex may be helpful.

HYSTERECTOMY FOR PAIN

Referral center clinicians who treat women with chronic pelvic pain often believe hysterectomy for this condition does not work well. Examples of women who are referred for evaluation of pain continuing after surgery, as well as women with chronic pelvic pain of unknown etiology who are referred to a tertiary care center for surgery, cast a negative pall over surgical intervention. However, literature describing outcomes of hysterectomy in women undergoing surgery in primary care settings is encouraging (73, 74). Taken as a whole, positive outcomes are seen in between 80% and 90% of cases in which pelvic pain was a major indication for surgery. This would suggest that, generally speaking, clinicians employ reasonable judgment in selecting patients for surgery. Somewhat more surprising, perhaps, is that even women with chronic pain and depression before surgery and substantially improved in 80% of cases when followed prospectively for 2 years after surgery. Further work needs to be done to determine what measures are needed to improve surgical results in the 20% or so of women who are more compromised at the time they have their surgery. It would seem that recognition of other components of pain would be most helpful, such as musculoskeletal pain, bladder pain, IBS, and so on.

PSYCHIATRIC CONDITIONS ASSOCIATED WITH CHRONIC PELVIC PAIN

Once pain has become chronic, it has a very powerful emotional meaning to the patient and to her family and friends. When concise diagnosis proves elusive, anxiety and fear of the unknown pathologic process can aggravate both the intensity of the pain and the suffering that is its consequence.

When painful events occur to a person who has substantial emotional needs that are unmet, the combination of these circumstances may support the development of one of the following styles of interaction between family members and the patient (71):

1. The pain serves as a proxy for dysfunction in the family that is easier to tolerate than the dysfunctional relationships in the family.
2. The family acts as a re-enforcer of the pain by nurturing and caring for the patient.
3. The patient uses the pain to control the family (with this pattern unwittingly reinforced by the family).
4. The stress of the family life produces psychological effects that predispose the patient to stress and pain (75).

Even when these patterns are present, or when obvious depression is present, this does not necessarily preclude the existence of organic pathology that requires medical and/or surgical therapy.

Much has been said and written about the association of depression with chronic pain of virtually any sort (76, 77). Depression, when associated with pain, may lower the pain threshold, thereby increasing sensitivity to pain, and may be associated with irritability and social withdrawal symptomatology rather than the more dramatic symptoms of overt sadness, sleeplessness, and suicidal ideation. In most instances, the depression can be seen as coevolving with the pain disorder, not as an etiologically important precursor.

Similarly, anxiety disorders may contribute substantially to the intensity of symptoms of pelvic pain but are rarely the sole etiologic agent of the pain. Comanagement with a mental health professional is usually desirable, although the interested and experienced primary care clinician can certainly manage medication approaches for these problems.

Finally, personality disorders, somatization, and hypochondriasis can accompany any of the pelvic pain disorders. A more complete discussion of these psychological aspects of chronic pain is presented elsewhere (78).

GENERAL PRINCIPLES OF PAIN MANAGEMENT

When confronted with chronic pelvic pain, the practitioner is challenged to present all possible modes of therapy in a balanced fashion. In addition, the health care provider must resist the tendency to attribute the entire symptom complex to a single disorder. It is useful to conduct a thorough educational session that creates a list of potentially contributing factors and outlines reasonable therapies. This list can be constructed only at the completion of a thorough history and physical examination, and possibly after some preliminary diagnostic studies.

Even when surgery seems imperative, the clinician should resist the tendency to pursue maximal surgical treatment without consideration of treatment of other components. Pursuit of only one therapeutic modality reinforces the notion that chronic pelvic pain problems can be understood in an either/or fashion (i.e., they are *either* physically caused *or* psychologically based). In the vast majority of situations, both realms are important to explore and treat, and overemphasis of one at the expense of the other is unproductive. For most, if not all, situations, this approach is applicable even when obvious organic pathology exists.

In addition to the specific therapies described for the conditions listed previously, some general principles of medication management deserve review. An individual patient's problem list may require a pharmacologic approach to two or three conditions simultaneously. For example, IBS may require dietary management with fiber and water additions, whereas the pain may require analgesia of either a narcotic or nonnarcotic variety, and a chronic pain syndrome may require antidepressant therapy. It is often useful to begin some or all these medications in close proximity to each other, allowing only enough time between their initiations to evaluate the side effects accurately. Although this may result in polypharmacy initially, it is more likely to produce a greater degree of clinical improvement, thereby accomplishing a better, and perhaps quicker, return to normal function (79).

TABLE 12.7

Narcotics Commonly Used in Chronic Pain Management

Drug Name	Usual Dose Range	Side Effects
Hydrocodone bitartrate with acetaminophen Lortab 2.5/500, 5/500, or 7.5/500 Vicodin 5/750 Lorcet 10/650 Lorcet Plus 7.5/650 (all are scored tablets)	5–10 mg hydrocodone either q6hr or q8hr Can use additional acetaminophen between doses to potentiate effect	Lightheadedness, dizziness, sedation, nausea and vomiting, and constipation (These are common side effects of all narcotics.)
Oxycodone hydrochloride Percocet 5 mg with 325 mg acetaminophen Percodan 4.5 mg with 325 mg aspirin (also contains 0.38 mg oxycodone terephthalate)	1 tablet q6hr or q8hr Additional acetaminophen between doses may serve to potentiate effect	Common effects.
Oxycodone controlled release OxyContin	10–40 mg q12hr	Common effects.
Methadone hydrochloride Dolphine 5- or 10-mg scored tablets	2.5 mg q8hr to10 mg q6hr Commonly 15–20 mg qd	Common effects. Lower extremity edema or joint swelling may occur and require discontinuation. Concurrent use of desipramine may increase methadone blood level. Cautious use in patients on monoamine oxidase inhibitors.
Acetaminophen with codeine Tylenol No. 3, 300 mg acetaminophen with 30 mg codeine	1–2 tablets q6–8hr	Common effects. Constipation very likely. Nausea and vomiting more common than with other narcotics. More common allergy—rash.
Morphine sulfate MS Contin or Oramorph	15–60 mg q12hr; controlled release tablets	Common effects, Higher doses increase risk of respiratory depression.
Fentanyl transdermal system Duragesic	25-μg patch, 1 q72hr Also available in 50 or 75 μg Always start with lowest dose	Common effects. Patch must be kept from heat sources, or dose may be increased. Extreme caution in patients on other central nervous system medications. Respiratory depression can result.

Reproduced from Steege JF. General principles of pain management. In: Steege JF, Metzger DA, Levy BS, eds. Chronic Pelvic Pain: An Integrated Approach. Philadelphia: WB Saunders, 1998, with permission.

Narcotic medications can sometimes be used on a long-term basis in the carefully selected and monitored patient. Table 12.7 describes their general dose levels and common side effects. It is useful to have the patient sign a narcotics "contract," which is basically her promise to obtain controlled substances from only one physician and one pharmacy, and to stick to a rigidly prescribed schedule.

Antidepressant medications have been a mainstay of chronic pain management of all types for many years. The best studied is amitriptyline (Elavil), commonly used in doses of 50 to 75 mg at bedtime. If constipation is a major factor in the patient's pain, a selective serotonin uptake inhibitor (SSRI) such as sertraline (Zoloft) or paroxetine (Paxil) rather than amitriptyline is probably a better initial treatment as SSRIs have fewer anticholinergic side effects.

The clinician dealing with chronic pain syndromes soon recognizes that complete success is often elusive. For the surgically oriented gynecologist who is used to a very high level of positive therapeutic outcome, this realization may prove frustrating. To survive, the successful clinician lowers his or her reward threshold when dealing with chronic pain patients but makes the commitment to continue the positive therapeutic relationship with the patient despite the frustrations involved. Early consultation with a specialist in chronic pain can often be fruitful and should provide the basis for an ongoing collaborative and therapeutic team approach.

Clinical Notes

- Chronic pelvic pain is pain present in the pelvis more often than not for 6 months or longer.
- Centralization of pain occurs when changes take place in the spinal cord that result in ongoing signals being sent to the brain, despite the dramatic decrease or even absence of peripheral nociception.
- Spinal cord "wind-up" occurs when repeated, low-level nociceptive stimuli from the periphery elicit progressively more dramatic responses from second-order neurons at the spinal cord level, even though the intensity of the stimuli may remain constant or even be diminished.
- When pain is prolonged and chronic, the anatomic site of the pain may become less distinct and symptoms originating in surrounding organ systems may join the original complaint.
- Studies suggest an association between a history of abuse and chronic pelvic pain. Care must be taken not to automatically ascribe responsibility to this history for pain that is present.
- Examination of the patient with chronic pelvic pain should include a thorough abdominal examination.
- The sequence of the pelvic examination is determined by the nature, suggested source, and type of pain.
- Trigger points may be treated by injection of local anesthetics; this may also facilitate the pelvic examination.
- Possible pelvic sources for chronic pelvic pain include endometriosis, adhesions, adenomyosis, pelvic congestion, and neuropathic pain.
- Physical examination may not detect any abnormalities early in the disease of endometriosis, although detection of uterosacral nodularity may be enhanced by conduction of the pelvic exam during menstruation.
- Among women undergoing laparoscopy for chronic pelvic pain, adhesions are found between 45 and 90% of the time. Studies on the impact of adhesiolysis suggest laparotomy to be superior to laparoscopy only in cases of dense bowel adhesions.
- The diagnosis of adenomyosis requires histologic examination of the uterine wall. A woman with severe disease may demonstrate substantial cyclic changes in the size, consistency, and tenderness of the uterine fundus.
- The prevalence of pelvic congestion is uncertain and concrete physical findings are limited. Bimanual exam may reveal a "doughy" consistency to the parametrial areas.
- IBS may cause symptoms attributed to a gynecologic origin.

- There appears to be a fairly strong association of IBS with dysmenorrhea.
- The medical management of choice for IBS is determined by the predominant symptoms.
- Levator ani muscle spasm is a frequently overlooked finding in the patient with pelvic pain. If present, it may be helpful to teach pelvic floor relaxation exercises.
- Piriformis muscle spasm causes pain on first arising and starting to walk, climbing stairs, and/or while driving. The pain is not related to time of day or phase of cycle. It may develop as a result of athletic injury or be associated with other inflammatory conditions.
- Musculoskeletal dysfunctions may develop as a response to initial gynecologic problems.
- Urinary tract disorders may also cause pelvic pain; examples would include pelvic relaxation, urethral diverticulum, chronic UTIs, and interstitial cystitis.
- Posthysterectomy pain may occur if the ovaries become encased in adhesions; dyspareunia may be present if the ovaries and/or ovarian adhesions are close to the vaginal apex.
- Other sources of posthysterectomy pain include ovarian remnant syndrome or hypersensitivity of the vaginal apex.
- Depression may be associated with chronic pelvic pain. Similarly, anxiety disorders, personality disorders, somatization, or hypochondriasis may also accompany a pelvic pain disorder.
- Treatment of a patient's pain may require a pharmacologic approach to two or three conditions simultaneously.
- Antidepressants, such as amitriptyline, have been a mainstay of chronic pain management of all types for many years. If the patient suffers constipation, an SSRI may be better initial therapy.

APPENDIX 12.1

International Pelvic Pain Society Pelvic Pain Assessment Form

THE INTERNATIONAL PELVIC PAIN SOCIETY

Professionals engaged in pain management for women

Pelvic Pain Assessment Form

Physician: ____________________

Initial History and Physical Exam *Date:* ____________________

Contact Information

Name: ____________________ Birth Date: __________ Chart Number: __________

Phone: Work: ____________________ Home: ____________________

Is there an alternate contact if we cannot reach you? ____________________

Alternate contact phone number: ____________________

Information About Your Pain

Please describe your pain problem: ____________________

What do you think is causing your pain? ____________________

What does your family think is causing your pain? ____________________

Do you think anyone is to blame for your pain? ❑ Yes ❑ No If so, who? ____________________

Do you think surgery will be necessary? ❑ Yes ❑ No

Is there an event that you associate with the onset of pain? ❑ Yes ❑ No If so, what? ____________________

How long have you had this pain? ❑ < 6 months ❑ 6 months – 1 year ❑ 1 – 2 years ❑ > 2 years

For each of the symptoms listed below, please "bubble in" your level of pain over the last month using a 10-point scale:

0 – no pain 10 – the worst pain imaginable

How would you rate your present pain?	0	1	2	3	4	5	6	7	8	9	10
Pain at ovulation (mid-cycle)	O	O	O	O	O	O	O	O	O	O	O
Pain level just before period	O	O	O	O	O	O	O	O	O	O	O
Pain (not cramps) with period	O	O	O	O	O	O	O	O	O	O	O
Deep pain with intercourse	O	O	O	O	O	O	O	O	O	O	O
Pain in groin when lifting	O	O	O	O	O	O	O	O	O	O	O
Pelvic pain lasting hours or days after intercourse	O	O	O	O	O	O	O	O	O	O	O
Pain when bladder is full	O	O	O	O	O	O	O	O	O	O	O
Muscle/joint pain	O	O	O	O	O	O	O	O	O	O	O
Ovarian pain	O	O	O	O	O	O	O	O	O	O	O
Level of cramps with period	O	O	O	O	O	O	O	O	O	O	O
Pain after period is over	O	O	O	O	O	O	O	O	O	O	O
Burning vaginal pain with sex	O	O	O	O	O	O	O	O	O	O	O
Pain with urination	O	O	O	O	O	O	O	O	O	O	O
Backache	O	O	O	O	O	O	O	O	O	O	O
Migraine headache	O	O	O	O	O	O	O	O	O	O	O
What would be an acceptable level of pain?	O	O	O	O	O	O	O	O	O	O	O

What is the worst type of pain that you have ever experienced?

❑ Kidney stone ❑ Bowel obstruction ❑ Migraine headache
❑ Labor & delivery ❑ Current pelvic pain ❑ Backache
❑ Broken bone ❑ Surgery
❑ Other ____________________

(205) 877-2950 *www.pelvicpain.org* *(800) 624-9676 (if in the U.S.)*

Demographic Information

Are you (check all that apply):

- ❑ Married
- ❑ Widowed
- ❑ Separated
- ❑ Committed Relationship
- ❑ Single
- ❑ Remarried
- ❑ Divorced

Who do you live with? ______________________________

Education: ❑ Less than 12 years ❑ High School graduate ❑ Bachelor's degree ❑ Postgraduate degree

What kind of work are you trained for? ______________________________

What type of work are you doing? ______________________________

Health Habits

Do you get regular exercise? ❑ Yes ❑ No Type: ______________________________

What is your diet like? ______________________________

What is your caffeine intake (number per day, include coffee, tea, soft drinks, etc.)? ❑ 0 ❑ 1–3 ❑ 4–6 ❑ >6

How many cigarettes do you smoke per day? ______________ How many years? ______________

Have you ever felt the need to cut down on your drinking? ❑ Yes ❑ No

Have you ever felt annoyed by criticism of your drinking? ❑ Yes ❑ No

Have you ever felt guilty about your drinking, or about something you said or did while you were drinking? ❑ Yes ❑ No

Have you ever taken a morning "eye-opener" drink? ❑ Yes ❑ No

What is your use of recreational drugs? ❑ Never used ❑ Used in past, but not now ❑ Presently using ❑ Choose not to answer

- ❑ Heroin
- ❑ Amphetamines
- ❑ Marijuana
- ❑ Barbiturates
- ❑ Cocaine
- ❑ Other ______________________

Have you ever received treatment for substance abuse? ❑ Yes ❑ No

Coping Mechanisms

Who are the people you talk to concerning your pain, or during stressful times?

- ❑ Spouse/Partner
- ❑ Relative
- ❑ Support Group
- ❑ Clergy
- ❑ Friend
- ❑ Doctor/Nurse
- ❑ Mental Health Professional
- ❑ I take care of myself

How does your partner deal with your pain?

- ❑ Doesn't notice when I'm in pain
- ❑ Takes care of me
- ❑ Not applicable
- ❑ Withdraws
- ❑ Feels helpless
- ❑ Distracts me with activities
- ❑ Gets angry

What helps your pain?

- ❑ Meditation
- ❑ Relaxation
- ❑ Lying down
- ❑ Music
- ❑ Massage
- ❑ Ice
- ❑ Heating pad
- ❑ Hot bath
- ❑ Pain medication
- ❑ Laxatives/enema
- ❑ Injection
- ❑ TENS unit
- ❑ Bowel movement
- ❑ Emptying bladder
- ❑ Nothing
- ❑ Other ______________________________

What makes your pain worse?

- ❑ Intercourse
- ❑ Orgasm
- ❑ Stress
- ❑ Full meal
- ❑ Bowel movement
- ❑ Full bladder
- ❑ Urination
- ❑ Standing
- ❑ Walking
- ❑ Exercise
- ❑ Time of day
- ❑ Weather
- ❑ Contact with clothing
- ❑ Coughing/sneezing
- ❑ Not related to anything
- ❑ Other ______________________________

Of all of the problems or stresses in your life, how does your pain compare in importance?

❑ The most important problem ❑ Just one of several/many problems

Menses

How old were you when your menses started? ____________________
Are you still having menstrual periods? ❑ Yes ❑ No

Answer the following only if you <u>are</u> still having menstrual periods:

Periods are: ❑ Light ❑ Moderate ❑ Heavy ❑ Bleed through protection

How many days between your periods? ____________________
How many days of menstrual flow? ____________________
Date of last menses? ____________________
Do you have any pain with your periods? ❑ Yes ❑ No
Does pain start the day flow starts? ❑ Yes ❑ No
Starts __________ days before flow starts: ❑ Yes ❑ No
Are periods regular? ❑ Yes ❑ No
Do you pass any clots in menstrual flow? ❑ Yes ❑ No

Bladder

Do you experience any of the following:

Loss of urine when coughing, sneezing, or laughing? ❑ Yes ❑ No
Frequent urination? ❑ Yes ❑ No
Need to urinate with little warning? ❑ Yes ❑ No
Difficulty passing urine? ❑ Yes ❑ No
Frequent bladder infections? ❑ Yes ❑ No
Frequency of nighttime urination: ❑ 0–1 ❑ 2 or more Volume: ❑ Small ❑ Medium ❑ Large
Frequency of daytime urination: ❑ 8 or less ❑ 9–15 ❑ >16 Volume: ❑ Small ❑ Medium ❑ Large
Do you still feel full after urination? ❑ Yes ❑ No

Bowel

Is there discomfort or pain associated with a change in the consistency of the stool (i.e., softer or harder) ? ❑ Yes ❑ No

Would you say that at least one-fourth (_) of the occasions or days in the last 3 months you have had any of the following (Check *all* that apply)

❑ Fewer than three bowel movements *a week* (0–2 bowel movements)
❑ More than three bowel movements *a day* (4 or more bowel movements)
❑ Hard or lumpy stools
❑ Loose or watery stools
❑ Straining during a bowel movement
❑ Urgency – having to rush to the bathroom for a bowel movement
❑ Feeling of incomplete emptying after a bowel movement
❑ Passing mucus (white material) during a bowel movement
❑ Abdominal fullness, bloating, or swelling

[1] <u>The Functional Gastrointestinal Disorders</u>, Drossman, et al. Chapter 4, "Functional Bowel Disorders and Functional Abdominal Pain". 1994.

Gastrointestinal/Eating

Do you have nausea? ❑ No ❑ With pain ❑ Taking medications
❑ With eating ❑ Other ______________________________

Do you have vomiting? ❑ No ❑ With pain ❑ Taking medications
❑ With eating ❑ Other ______________________________

Have you ever had an eating disorder such as anorexia or bulimia? ❑ Yes ❑ No

Short-Form McGill

The words below describe average pain. Place a check mark (✓) in the column which represents the degree to which you feel that type of pain. Please limit yourself to a description of the pain in your pelvic area only.

What does your pain feel like?

Type	***None (0)***	***Mild (1)***	***Moderate (2)***	***Severe (3)***
Throbbing	_____	_____	_____	_____
Shooting	_____	_____	_____	_____
Stabbing	_____	_____	_____	_____
Sharp	_____	_____	_____	_____
Cramping	_____	_____	_____	_____
Gnawing	_____	_____	_____	_____
Hot-Burning	_____	_____	_____	_____
Aching	_____	_____	_____	_____
Heavy	_____	_____	_____	_____
Tender	_____	_____	_____	_____
Splitting	_____	_____	_____	_____
Tiring-Exhausting	_____	_____	_____	_____
Sickening	_____	_____	_____	_____
Fearful	_____	_____	_____	_____
Punishing-Cruel	_____	_____	_____	_____

Melzack, R: The Short-Form McGill Pain Questionnaire, Pain 30:191–197, 1987

Which statement(s) below best describes how you cope with the pain? Check all that apply

- ❑ I count numbers in my head or run a song through my mind
- ❑ I just think of it as some other sensation, such as numbness
- ❑ I pray to God it won't last long
- ❑ I do something active, like household chores or projects
- ❑ I ignore it as best I can
- ❑ I tell myself to be brave and carry on despite the pain
- ❑ I tell myself that it really doesn't hurt
- ❑ I worry all the time about whether it will end
- ❑ I take pain medication
- ❑ Other

SF-36

In general, would you say your health is: O Excellent O Very Good O Good O Fair O Poor

Compared to one year ago, how would you rate your health in general now?

- O Much better now than one year ago
- O Somewhat better now than one year ago
- O About the same as one year ago
- O Somewhat worse now than one year ago
- O Much worse than one year ago

The following items are about activities you might do during a typical day. *Does your health now limit you in these activities? If so, how much?*	Yes, limited a lot	Yes, limited a little	No	Not limited at all
Vigorous activities, such as running, lifting heavy object, participating in strenuous sports				
Moderate activities, such as moving a table, pushing a vacuum cleaner, bowling, or playing golf				
Lifting or carrying groceries				
Climbing several flights of stairs				
Climbing one flight of stairs				
Bending, kneeling, or stooping				
Walking more than a mile				
Walking several blocks				
Walking one block				
Bathing or dressing yourself				

During the *past 4 weeks*, have you had any of the following problems with your work or other regular daily activities *because of your physical health*?

Cut down the amount of time you spent on your work or other activities	O Yes	O No
Accomplish less than you would like	O Yes	O No
Were limited in the kind of work or other activities	O Yes	O No
Had difficulty performing the work or other activities (for example, it took extra effort)	O Yes	O No

During the *past 4 weeks*, have you had any of the following problems with your work or other regular daily activities *because of any emotional problems* (such as feeling depressed or anxious)?

Cut down the amount of time you spent on work or other activities	O Yes	O No
Accomplished less than you would like	O Yes	O No
Didn't do work or other activities as carefully as usual	O Yes	O No

During the *past 4 weeks*, to what extent has your physical health or emotional problems interfered with your normal social activities with family, friend, neighbors, or groups?

O Not at all O Slightly O Moderately O Quite a bit O Extremely

How much bodily pain have you had during the past 4 weeks?

O None O Very mild O Mild O Moderate O Severe O Very severe

During the past 4 weeks, how much did pain interfere with your normal work (including both work outside the home and housework)?

O Not at all O A little bit O Moderately O Quite a bit O Extremely

These questions are about how you feel and how things have been with you *during the past 4 weeks*. For each question, please give the one answer that comes closest to the way you have been feeling. How much of the time during *the past 4 weeks*:	All of the time	Most of the time	A good bit of the time	Some of the time	A little of the time	None of the time
Did you feel full of pep?						
Have you been a very nervous person?						
Have you felt so down in the dumps that nothing could cheer you up?						
Have you felt calm and peaceful?						
Did you have a lot of energy?						
Have you felt downhearted and blue?						
Did you feel worn out?						
Have you been a happy person?						
Did you feel tired?						

During the *past 4 weeks*, how much of the time has your *physical health or emotional problems* interfered with your social activities (like visiting with friends, relatives, etc.?

O All of the time O Most of the time O Some of the time O A little of the time O None of the time

How TRUE or FALSE is each of the following statements for you?	Definitely True	Mostly True	Don't Know	Mostly False	Definitely False
I seem to get sick a little easier than other people					
I am as healthy as anybody I know					
I expect my health to get worse					
My health is excellent					

Personal History

What would you like to tell us about your pain that we have not asked? Comments: ______________________

____

____

____

What types of treatments have you tried in the past for this pain? ❑ Acupuncture ❑ Homeopathic medicine ❑ Physical therapy

❑ Anesthesiologist
❑ Anti-seizure medications
❑ Antidepressants
❑ Biofeedback
❑ Birth control pills
❑ Danazol (Danocrine)
❑ Depo-Provera
❑ Family Practitioner
❑ Herbal medication
❑ Lupron, Zoladex, Synarel
❑ Massage
❑ Meditation
❑ Narcotics
❑ Naturopathic medications
❑ Nerve blocks
❑ Neurosurgeon
❑ Nonprescription medicine
❑ Nutrition/diet
❑ Psychotherapy
❑ Rheumatologist
❑ Skin magnets
❑ Surgery
❑ TENS unit
❑ Trigger point injections
❑ Other __________

What physicians or health care providers have evaluated or treated you for chronic pelvic pain? Include all healthcare professionals, whether they were physicians or not. Do you have any objections to me contacting these healthcare providers? ❑ Yes ❑ No

Physician/Provider	***City, State***

Who is your primary care physician? ______________________

Please list <u>all</u> surgical procedures you've had (***related to this pain***):

Year	***Procedure***	***Surgeon***

Please list all <u>other</u> surgical procedures:

Year	***Procedure***	***Year***	***Procedure***

Please list pain medications you've taken for your pain condition in the past 6 months, and the physicians who prescribed them (use separate page if necessary):

Medication	***Physician***	***Did it help?***
		❑ Yes ❑ No
		❑ Yes ❑ No
		❑ Yes ❑ No
		❑ Yes ❑ No
		❑ Yes ❑ No
		❑ Yes ❑ No
		❑ Yes ❑ No
❑ I have written more medications on a separate page		

Have you ever been hospitalized for anything besides surgery or childbirth? ❑ Yes ❑ No If yes, explain: ________________

Have you had major accidents such as falls or back injury? ❑ Yes ❑ No
Have you ever been treated for depression? ❑ Yes ❑ No Treatments: ❑ Medication ❑ Hospitalization ❑ Psychotherapy

Birth control method: ❑ Nothing ❑ Pill ❑ Vasectomy ❑ Hysterectomy
❑ IUD ❑ Rhythm ❑ Diaphragm ❑ Tubal Ligation
❑ Condom ❑ Other: ____

Is future fertility desired? ❑ Yes ❑ No

How many pregnancies have you had?___________________
Resulting in (#): _______ Full 9 month _______ Premature _______ Abortions (miscarriage) _______ # living children
Any complications during pregnancy, labor, delivery, or post partum period?
❑ 4° Episiotomy ❑ C-section ❑ Post-partum hemorrhaging
❑ Vaginal lacerations ❑ Forceps ❑ Medication for bleeding
❑ Other: ____

Has anyone in your family ever had: ❑ Fibromyalgia ❑ Chronic pelvic pain ❑ Scleroderma
❑ Endometriosis ❑ Lupus ❑ Interstitial cystitis
❑ Cancer ❑ Depression ❑ Irritable Bowel Syndrome
❑ Recurrent Urinary Tract Infections

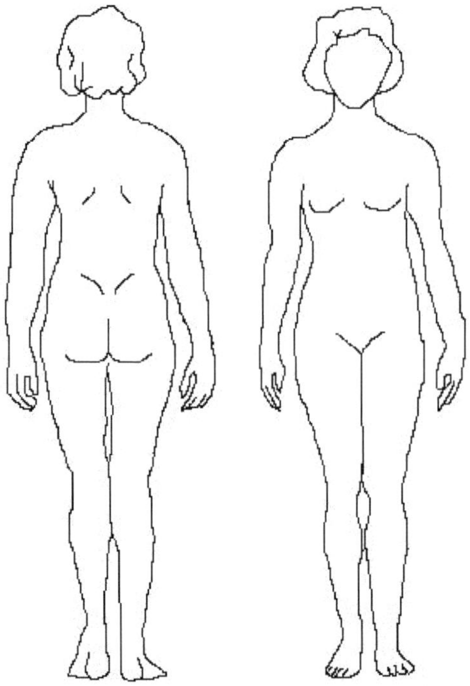

Place an "X" at the point of your most intense pain.
Shade in all other painful areas.

Sexual and Physical Abuse History

Have you ever been the victim of emotional abuse? This can include being humiliated or insulted. ❑ Yes ❑ No ❑ No answer

		As a child (13 and younger)		As an adult (14 and over)	
	Circle an answer for <u>both</u> as a child and as an adult.				
1a.	Has anyone ever exposed the sex organs of their body to you when you did not want it?	Yes	No	Yes	No
1b.	Has anyone ever threatened to have sex with you when you did not want it?	Yes	No	Yes	No
1c.	Has anyone ever touched the sex organs of your body when you did not want this?	Yes	No	Yes	No
1d.	Has anyone ever made you touch the sex organs of their body when you did not want this?	Yes	No	Yes	No
1e.	Has anyone ever forced you to have sex when you did not want this?	Yes	No	Yes	No
1f.	Have you had any other unwanted sexual experiences not mentioned above? If yes, please specify: ______________________	Yes	No	Yes	No

2	When you were a child (13 or younger), did an older person do the following?				
a.	Hit, kick, or beat you?	Never	Seldom	Occasionally	Often
b.	Seriously threaten your life?	Never	Seldom	Occasionally	Often
3	Now that you are an adult (14 or older), has any other adult done the following:				
a.	Hit, kick, or beat you?	Never	Seldom	Occasionally	Often
b.	Seriously threaten your life?	Never	Seldom	Occasionally	Often

Leserman, J., Drossman, D., Li, Z: The Reliability and Validity of a Sexual and Physical Abuse History Questionnaire in Female Patients with Gastrointestinal Disorders. Behavioral Medicine 21:141–148, 1995

Physical Examination – For Physician Use Only

Name: ______________________________ Chart Number: ______________

Height: ________ Weight: _______ BP: __________ LMP: _________ Temp: ________ Resp: _________

ROS, PFSH Reviewed: ❑ Yes ❑ No Physician Signature ______________________________

General: ❑ WNL ❑ Walk ❑ Facial expression
❑ Color ❑ Alterations in posture ❑ Other ______________

NOTE: Mark "Not Examined" as N/E

HEENT ❑ WNL ______ ***Chest*** ❑ WNL ______ ***Heart*** ❑ WNL ______ ***Breasts*** ❑ WNL _________

Abdomen
❑ Non-tender ❑ Incisions ❑ Trigger Points ❑ Ovarian point tenderness
❑ Inguinal tenderness ❑ Inguinal bulge ❑ Suprapubic tenderness ❑ Other ______________

Back
❑ Non-tender ❑ Tenderness ❑ Altered ROM ❑ Alterations in posture

Extremities
❑ WNL ❑ Edema ❑ Varicosities ❑ Neuropathy ❑ Range of motion

Neuropathy
❑ Iliohypogastric ❑ Ilioinguinal ❑ Genitofemoral ❑ Pudendal ❑ Altered sensation

EGBUS/Vagina
❑ WNL ❑ Lesions
❑ Wet prep:
❑ Local tenderness:
❑ Vaginal mucosa:
❑ Posterior fourchette:
❑ Discharge:
Cultures:
❑ GC ❑ Chlamydia ❑ Fungal ❑ Herpes

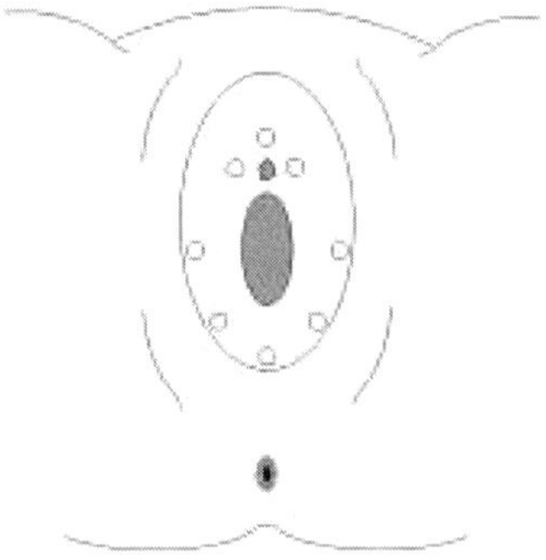

Patient rates allodynia produced by Q-tip for each circle (0-4).
Total Score: ______________

Unimanual pelvic exam
❑ WNL ❑ Cervix
❑ Introitus ❑ Cervical motion
❑ Uterine-cervical junction ❑ Parametrium
❑ Urethra ❑ Vaginal cuff
❑ Bladder ❑ Cul de sac
❑ R ureter ❑ L ureter
❑ R inguinal ❑ L inguinal
❑ Muscle awareness ❑ Clitoral tenderness

Rank muscle tenderness on 0-4 scale
❑ R obturator ______________
❑ L obturator ______________
❑ R piriformis ______________
❑ L piriformis ______________
❑ R pubococcygeus ___________
❑ L pubococcygeus ___________
❑ Total pelvic floor score _______

Bimanual pelvic exam ❑ Absent

Uterus: ❑ Tender ❑ Non-tender

Position ❑ Anterior ❑ Posterior ❑ Midplane

Size ❑ Normal ❑ Other ____________________

Contour ❑ Regular ❑ Irregular ❑ Other ____________________

Consistency ❑ Firm ❑ Soft ❑ Hard

Mobility ❑ Mobile ❑ Hypermobile ❑ Fixed

Support ❑ Well supported ❑ Prolapse

Adnexae

Right	Left
❑ Absent	❑ Absent
❑ WNL	❑ WNL
❑ Tender	❑ Tender
❑ Fixed	❑ Fixed
❑ Enlarged ___________ cm	❑ Enlarged ___________ cm

Rectovaginal

❑ WNL	❑ Nodules	❑ Guaiac positive (negative with quality control)
❑ Tenderness	❑ Mucosal pathology	
❑ Not examined		

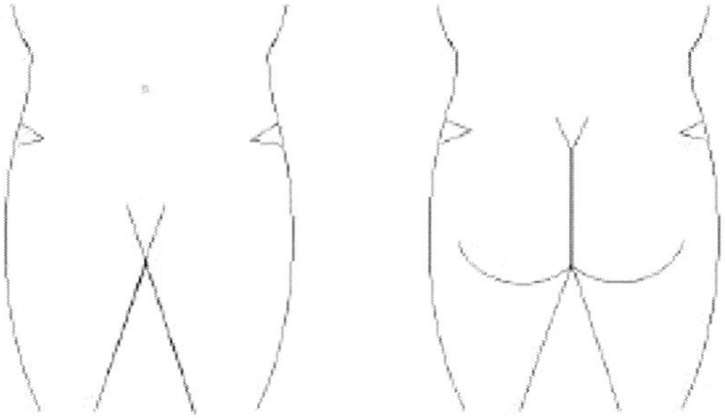

Trigger Points

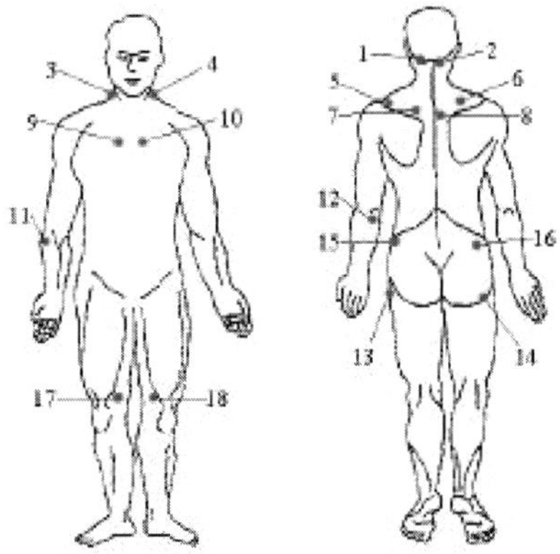

Fibromyalgia

Assessment: ____

____

Diagnostic Plan: ____

____

Therapeutic Plan: ____

____

THE INTERNATIONAL
PELVIC PAIN
SOCIETY
Professionals engaged in pain management for women.

Dear Healthcare Professional:

The Research Committee, headed by Deborah Metzger, M.D., Ph.D., along with the Board of Directors of The International Pelvic Pain Society are proud to present this Pelvic Pain Assessment Form for use in the medical community. This form has been developed by clinicians who treat chronic pelvic pain on a daily basis, and is the culmination of two year's effort. We hope that you find it useful.

The Pelvic Pain Assessment Form is designed to be printed front and back to yield a total of 10 pages on 5 sheets, for your convenience.

It is our desire that this form become a standard in your intake procedures. We solicit your constructive comments. It is only by open communication from the clinician who uses this form consistently that we will improve it. You can phone your comments to the number shown on the form, or e-mail us at pelvicpain@aol.com.

Sincerely,

C. Paul Perry, M.D.,	Deborah Metzger, M.D., Ph.D.
Chairman of the Board of Directors	Chairperson, Research Committee

REFERENCES

1. Jamieson DJ, Steege JF. The prevalence of dysmenorrhea, dyspareunia, pelvic pain, and irritable bowel syndrome in primary care practices. Obstet Gynecol 1996;87:55.
2. Graves EJ. National Hospital Discharge Survey: Annual Summary, 1990. National Center for Health Statistics. Vital Health Stat 1992;13(112).
3. Hulka JF, Peterson HB, Phillips JM, et al. Operative laparoscopy: American Association of Gynecologic Laparoscopists 1991 membership survey. J Reprod Med 1993;38:569.
4. Steege JF, Metzger D, Levy B, eds. Chronic Pelvic Pain: An Integrated Approach. Philadelphia: WB Saunders, 1998.
5. Rogers RM Jr. Basic pelvic neuroanatomy. In: Steege JF, Metzger D, Levy B, eds. Chronic Pelvic Pain: An Integrated Approach. Philadelphia: WB Saunders, 1998.
6. Melzack R. Neurophysiologic foundations of pain. In: Sternback RA, ed. The Psychology of Pain. New York: Raven, 1986:1.
7. Melzack R. Gate control theory: on the evolution of pain concepts. Pain Forum 1996;5:128.
8. Melzack R. From the gate to the neuromatrix. Pain 1999;6(suppl):S121–S126.
9. Cervero F. Visceral pain: mechanisms of peripheral and central sensitization. Ann Med 1995;27:235.
10. Giamberardino MA, Berkley KJ, Affaitati G, et al. Influence of endometriosis on pain behaviors and muscle hyperalgesia induced by a ureteral calculosis in female rats. Pain 2002;95:247–257.
11. Giamberardino MA, Berkley KJ, Iezzi S, et al. Pain threshold variations in somatic wall tissues as a function of menstrual cycle, segmental site and tissue depth in non-dysmenorrheic women, dysmenorrheic women, and men. Pain 1997;71:187–197.
12. Giamberardino MA, DeLaurentis S, Afaitati G, et al. Modulation of pain and hyperalgesia from the urinary tract by allogenic conditions of the reproductive organs in women. Neurosci Lett 2001;304:61–64.
13. Katz J. Pre-emptive analgesia: evidence, current status and future directions. Eur J Anaesthesiol 1995;12(suppl 10):8.
14. Walker EA, Katon W, Harrop-Griffiths J, et al. Relationship of chronic pelvic pain to psychiatric diagnosis and childhood sexual abuse. Am J Psychiatry 1988;145:75.
15. Jamieson D, Steege J. The association of sexual and physical abuse with pelvic pain complaints in a primary care population. Am J Obstet Gynecol 1997;177:1408.
16. Beitchman JH, Zuker KJ, Hood JE, et al. A review of the long-term effects of child sexual abuse. Child Abuse Negl 1992;16:101.
17. Fischer AA. New developments in diagnosis of myofascial pain and fibromyalgia. Phys Med Rehab Clin North Am 1997;8:1–27.
18. Yunus MB, Kalyan-Raman UP, Kalyan-Raman K. Primary fibromyalgia syndrome and myofascial pain syndrome: clinical features and muscle pathology. Arch Phys Med Rehabil 1988;69:451–454.
19. Baker PK. Musculoskeletal problems. In: Steege JF, Metzger D, Levy B, eds. Chronic Pelvic Pain: An Integrated Approach. Philadelphia: WB Saunders, 1998.
20. Lamont JA. Vaginismus. Am J Obstet Gynecol 1978;131:632.
21. Travell JG, Simmons DG. Myofascial Pain and Dysfunction: The Trigger Point Manual. 2nd ed. Baltimore: Williams & Wilkins, 1992.
22. Slocumb JC. Neurological factors in chronic pelvic pain: trigger points and the abdominal pelvic pain syndrome. Am J Obstet Gynecol 1984;149:536.
23. Hong CZ. Consideration and recommendation of myofascial trigger point injection. J Musculoskeletal Pain 1994;2:29–59.
24. Hong CZ. Lidocaine injection versus dry needling to myofascial trigger point: the importance of the local twitch response. Am J Phys Med Rehabil 1997;73:256–263.
25. Gunn CC, Milbrandt WE, Little AS, et al. Dry needling of motor points for chronic low-back pain: a randomized clinical trial with long-term follow-up. Spine 1980;5:279–291.
26. Porta M. A comparative trial of botulinum toxin type A and methylprednisolone for the treatment of myofascial pain syndrome and pain from chronic muscle spasm. Pain 2000;85:101–105.
27. Cheshire WP, Abashian SW, Mann JD. Botulinum toxin in the treatment of myofascial pain syndrome. Pain 1994;59:65–69.
28. Koninckx PR, Martin D. Treatment of deeply infiltrating endometriosis. Curr Opin Obstet Gynecol 1994;6:231.
29. Koninckx PR, Meuleman C, Demeyere S, et al. Suggestive evidence that pelvic endometriosis is a progressive disease, whereas deeply infiltrating endometriosis is associated with pelvic pain. Fertil Steril 1991;55:759.
30. Donnez J, Nissolle M, Casanas-Roux F, et al. Rectovaginal septum endometriosis or adenomyosis: laparoscopic management in a series of 231 patients. Hum Reprod 1995;10:630.
31. Donnez J, Nisolle M, Gillerot S, et al. Rectovaginal septum adenomyotic nodules: a series of 500 cases. Br J Obstet Gynecol 1997;104:1014.
32. Ling FW. Randomized controlled trial of depot leuprolide in patients with chronic pelvic pain and clinically suspected endometriosis. Obstet Gynecol 1999;93:51–58.
33. Marcoux S, Maheux R, Berube S, et al. Laparoscopic surgery in infertile women with minimal or mild endometriosis. N Engl J Med 1997;337:217.
34. Weibel MA, Majno G. Peritoneal adhesions and their relation to abdominal surgery. Am J Surg 1973;126:345.
35. Kresch AJ, Seifer DB, Sachs LB, et al. Laparoscopy in the evaluation of pelvic pain. Obstet Gynecol 1973;64:672.

36. Steege JF. Adhesions and pelvic pain. In: Steege JF, Metzger D, Levy B, eds. Chronic Pelvic Pain: An Integrated Approach. Philadelphia: WB Saunders, 1998.
37. Steege JF, Stout AL. Resolution of chronic pelvic pain after laparoscopic lysis of adhesions. Am J Obstet Gynecol 1991;165:278.
38. Sutton C, MacDonald R. Laser laparoscopic adhesiolysis. J Gynecol Surg 1990;6:155.
39. Peters AAW, Trimbos-Kemper GCM, Admiraal C, et al. A randomized clinical trial on the benefit of adhesiolysis in patients with intraperitoneal adhesions and chronic pelvic pain. Br J Obstet Gynecol 1992;99:59.
40. Vercellini P, Parazzini F, Oldani S, et al. Adenomyosis at hysterectomy: a study on frequency distribution and patient characteristics. Hum Reprod 1995;10:1160.
41. Taylor HC. Vascular congestion and hyperemia, their effect on structure and function in the female reproductive organs. Part II. The clinical aspects of the congestion-fibrosis syndrome. Am J Obstet Gynecol 1949;57:654.
42. Taylor HC. Vascular congestion and hyperemia, their effect on structure in the female reproductive organs. Part III. Etiology and therapy. Am J Obstet Gynecol 1949;57:654.
43. Beard RW, Highman JH, Pearce S, et al. Diagnosis of pelvic varicosities in women with chronic pelvic pain. Lancet 1984;2:946.
44. Beard RW, Reginald PW, Pearce S. Pelvic pain in women. BMJ 1986;293:1160.
45. Osofsky HJ, Fisher S. Pelvic congestion: some further considerations. Obstet Gynecol 1968;31:406.
46. Hughes RR, Curtis DD. Uterine phlebography: correlation of clinical diagnoses with dye retention. Am J Obstet Gynecol 1962;83:156.
47. Kaupilla A. Uterine phlebography with venous compression. A clinical and roentgenological study. Acta Obstet Gynecol Scand 1970;49:33.
48. Giacchetto C, Cotroneo GB, Marincolo F, et al. Ovarian varicocele: ultrasonic and phlebographic evaluation. J Clin Ultrasound 1990;18:551.
49. Gangar KF, Stones RW, Saunder C, et al. An alternative to hysterectomy? GnRH analogue combined with hormone replacement therapy. Br J Obstet Gynaecol 1993;100:360.
50. Allen WM. Chronic pelvic congestion and pelvic pain. Am J Obstet Gynecol 1971;109:198.
51. Farquhar CM, Rogers V, Franks S, et al. A randomized controlled trial of medroxyprogesterone acetate and psychotherapy for the treatment of pelvic congestion. Br J Obstet Gynecol 1989;96:1153.
52. Beard RW, Kennedy RG, Gangar KF, et al. Bilateral oophorectomy and hysterectomy in the treatment of intractable pelvic pain associated with pelvic congestion. Br J Obstet Gynaecol 1991;98:988.
53. Rundqvist E, Sondholm LE, Larsson G. Treatment of pelvic varicosities causing lower abdominal pain with extraperitoneal resection of the left ovarian vein. Lancet 1984;i:339.
54. Thompson WG, Creed F, Drossman DA, et al. Functional bowel disease and functional abdominal pain. Gastroenterol Int 1992;5:75.
55. Crowell MD, Dubin NH, Robinson JC, et al. Functional bowel disorders in women with dysmenorrhea. Am J Gastroenterol 1994;89:1973.
56. Longstreth GF, Preskill DB, Youkeles L. Irritable bowel syndrome in women having diagnostic laparoscopy or hysterectomy. Relation to gynecologic features and outcome. Dig Dis Sci 1990;35:1285.
57. Lembo T, Munakata J, Mertz H, et al. Evidence for the hypersensitivity of lumbar splanchnic afferents in irritable bowel syndrome. Gastroenterology 1994;107:1686.
58. Drossman DA, Sandler RS, McKee DC, et al. Bowel patterns among subjects not seeking health care. Gastroenterology 1982;83:529.
59. Kellow JE, Gill RC, Wingate DL. Prolonged ambulant recordings of bowel motility demonstrate abnormalities in the irritable bowel syndrome. Gastroenterology 1990;98:1208.
60. Kellow JE, Phillips SF. Altered small bowel motility in irritable bowel syndrome is correlated with symptoms. Gastroenterology 1987;92:1885.
61. Drossman DA, Leserman J, Nachman G, et al. Sexual and physical abuse in women with functional or organic gastrointestinal disorders. Ann Intern Med 1990;113:828.
62. Talley NJ. 5-Hydroxytryptamine agonists and antagonists in the modulation of gastrointestinal motility and sensation: clinical implications. Aliment Pharmacol Ther 1992;6:273.
63. Drossman DA, Thompson WG. The irritable bowel syndrome: review and a graduated multi-component treatment approach. Ann Intern Med 1992;116:1009.
64. Guthrie E, Dreed F, Dawson D, et al. A controlled trial of psychological treatment for the irritable bowel syndrome. Gastroenterology 1991;100:450.
65. Peters-Gee JM. Bladder and urethral syndromes. In: Steege JF, Metzger D, Levy B, eds. Chronic Pelvic Pain: An Integrated Approach. Philadelphia: WB Saunders, 1998.
66. Moldwin RM, Sant GR. Interstitial cystitis: a pathophysiology and treatment update. Clin Obstet Gynecol 2002;45:259–272.
67. Mulholland SG, Hanno PM, Parsons CL. Pentosan polysulfate sodium for therapy of interstitial cystitis. Urology 1990;35:522–558.
68. Parsons CL, Benson G, Childs SJ, et al. A quantitatively controlled method to study prospectively interstitial cystitis and demonstrate the efficacy of pentosan polysulfate. J Urol 1993;150:845–848.
69. Zolnoun DA, Hartmann KE, Steege JR. Overnight 5% lidocaine ointment for treatment of vulvar vestibulitis. Obstet Gynecol 2003;102:84–87.
70. Steege JF. Ovarian remnant syndrome. Obstet Gynecol 1987;70:64.
71. Pettit PD, Lee RA. Ovarian remnant syndrome: diagnostic dilemma and surgical challenge. Obstet Gynecol 1988;71:580.

72. Price FV, Edwards R, Buchsbaum HJ. Ovarian remnant syndrome: difficulties in diagnosis and treatment. Obstet Gynecol Surv 1990;45:151.
73. Carlson KJ, Miller BA, Fowler FJ Jr. The Maine Women's Health Study. II. Outcomes of nonsurgical management of leiomyomas, abnormal bleeding, and chronic pelvic pain. Obstet Gynecol 1994;83:566–572.
74. Kjerulff KH, Langenberg PW, Rhodes JC, et al. Effectiveness of hysterectomy. Obstet Gynecol 2000;95:319–326.
75. Payne B, Norfleet M. Chronic pain and the family: a review. Pain 1986;26:1.
76. Aronoff GM. Evaluation and Treatment of Chronic Pain. 2nd ed. Baltimore: Williams & Wilkins, 1992:57.
77. Talbott JA, Hales RE, Yudofsky SC. Textbook of Psychiatry. Washington, DC: American Psychiatric Press, 1988:409.
78. Bashford RA. Psychiatric illness. In: Steege JF, Metzger D, Levy B, eds. Chronic Pelvic Pain: An Integrated Approach. Philadelphia: WB Saunders, 1998.
79. Steege JF. General principles of pain management. In: Steege JF, Metzger D, Levy B, eds. Chronic Pelvic Pain: An Integrated Approach. Philadelphia: WB Saunders, 1998.

CHAPTER 13

Endometriosis

John M. Storment

Since its original description in 1860, endometriosis has been considered a common disorder. It is one of the leading diseases encountered in clinical gynecology and a common cause for hysterectomy. Endometriosis is a condition characterized by ectopic endometrial glands and stroma. Endometriosis commonly presents as a progressive disease whose causes and rational treatment remains enigmatic. The literature on endometriosis is extensive, although often contradictory or inadequate. This chapter reviews the current knowledge on the epidemiology, diagnosis, and treatment of endometriosis. In addition, endometriosis-associated infertility, recurrence, and appropriate hormone replacement after "definitive" surgery are covered.

EPIDEMIOLOGY

Standardized, objective criteria for an accurate diagnosis of endometriosis are difficult to establish because the disease has a variable and nonspecific clinical presentation and natural history. Confirmation of the diagnosis requires laparoscopy or laparotomy. This makes data regarding the prevalence of endometriosis difficult to interpret. Table 13.1 illustrates that the incidence of endometriosis found at surgery varies by the type of surgery performed (1). The variation in published incidence figures also likely reflects diversity in the groups of women entered into the different studies. Best estimates are that endometriosis is present in 5 to 10% of reproductive age women and 25 to 35% of patients with infertility (2). Melis et al. (3) evaluated 305 premenopausal women undergoing surgery for infertility or benign gynecologic disease. Endometriosis was diagnosed in 24.9% of the total study population but was significantly higher in women with infertility, chronic pelvic pain, or benign ovarian cysts. Because endometriosis lesions are not always symptomatic, the mere presence of endometriosis is not diagnostic of disease.

One group assessed the epidemiologic factors linked to endometriosis in infertile women (4). They compared 174 infertile women with 174 fertile women with laparoscopically proven endometriosis. Age at menarche; duration of menstrual flow; age at study; reproductive history, including previous abortion rate and infertility history; family history; and social class were similar in both groups. This report and others discredit prior studies, indicating that endometriosis is seen more frequently in higher socioeconomic groups. Although there is little data of sufficient quality to show socioeconomic or ethnic differences in disease risk, it is known that there is a genetic basis of risk for endometriosis (5).

PATHOGENESIS

There are numerous theories proposed for the origin of endometriosis. No single theory can account for the location of the ectopic endometrium in all cases of endometriosis. For an in-depth discussion of the different theories proposed for the pathogenesis of endometriosis, there

TABLE 13.1

Incidence of Endometriosis by Type of Surgery at Which Diagnosis Was Made

Surgery	Total	No. With Endometriosis	% With Endometriosis
Tubal anastomosis	1860	19	1%
Tubal sterilization	3060	61	2%
Vaginal hysterectomy	858	69	8%
Abdominal hysterectomy	5511	606	11%
Diagnostic laparoscopy for infertility	724	116	16%
Operative laparoscopy	2065	619	31%
Diagnostic laparoscopy for pelvic pain in teenagers	140	74	53%

Adapted from Wheeler JM. Epidemiology and prevalence of endometriosis. Infertil Reprod Med Clin N Am 1992;3:545, with permission.

are several very thorough reviews (6–8). The theories for the histogenesis of endometriosis can be classified into three basic categories: (a) transplantation of endometrial tissue via retrograde menstruation (Sampson's theory), (b) transformation of totipotential cells into endometrial cells, and (c) lymphatic or vascular transport of endometrial fragments. Sampson's theory of retrograde menstruation fails to explain why endometriosis affects such a small percentage of women, given that 75 to 90% of patients with patent tubes display retrograde flow (9). A role for immunologic factors influencing a woman's susceptibility for developing endometriosis has been proposed. One theory proposes that in women with decreased cellular immunity function, the endometriotic cells are "allowed" to implant and grow in ectopic sites (10). This altered cellular immunity may also partially explain the impaired fertility in some patients. Conclusions of studies regarding the role of cellular immunity have been inconsistent (11, 12). Genetic predisposition does appear to influence the development of disease (13). A woman whose sibling has endometriosis has a six-fold increase in risk, and the daughter of a woman with endometriosis has a ten-fold increased risk of endometriosis compared with the general population. In one report, approximately 6 to 7% of first-degree female relatives of women with endometriosis had the disease compared with 1% in a control group (5).

Most endometrial implants are located in the dependent portions of the female pelvis. Two-thirds of patients with endometriosis will have ovarian involvement (14). Other common sites include the pelvic peritoneum, the anterior and posterior cul de sacs, and the uterosacral, round, and broad ligaments. However, endometriosis has been reported in almost every organ in the body, including the brain and lungs. The phenomenon of catamenial pneumothorax has been reported, whereby endometrial implants on the pleura may lead to recurrent pneumothorax at the time of menstruation. In the case of central nervous system implants, catamenial seizures have been reported (15–17). Any symptom with a catamenial pattern of change and/or worsening should raise suspicions of being causally related to endometriosis.

DIAGNOSIS

Classic symptoms of endometriosis include dysmenorrhea, dyspareunia, dyschezia, and/or a history of infertility. Few women present with all these symptoms. Frequently, endometriosis presents as a diagnostic challenge to both the patient and the physician. The diagnosis should be suspected in women who have pelvic pain or are infertile. The pain is believed to arise from enlargement of the implants stretching on the areas of fibrosis often found around the implants. (The implants not only enlarge in response to hormonal stimulation, they bleed into themselves,

TABLE 13.2

Correlation Between Dysmenorrhea Severity and Relative Risk of Endometriosis in One Study

Menstrual Pain	Relative Risk of Endometriosis
None	1.0
Mild	1.7
Moderate	3.4
Severe	6.7

Adapted from Cramer DW, Wilson E, Stillman RJ, et al. The relation of endometriosis to menstrual characteristics, smoking and exercise. JAMA 1985;225:1904, with permission.

causing inflammation and fibrosis in the surrounding tissues.) Pain can be very diffuse or localized and of varying quality. A history of years of painfree menses with a gradual onset and progressive worsening of dysmenorrhea is suggestive of endometriosis. Severe dysmenorrhea is often the only complaint. Symptoms can vary throughout the menstrual cycle or remain constant. Urinary tract complaints may indicate ureteral or bladder involvement and should also be investigated. Low back pain and rectal pain may be due to endometriosis. The degree of pelvic pain is often unrelated to the severity or distribution of endometriosis (15, 18). Perper et al. (19) however, found a very good correlation in the number of endometrial implants and the intensity of dysmenorrhea, and Cramer et al. (20) noted a direct relationship between severity of menstrual pain and relative risk of endometriosis (Table 13.2).

A history of factors that relieve and/or exacerbate the pain must be taken. Many patients derive significant relief from oral contraceptives, indicating that pain could be attributed to pelvic pathology. Although this finding is not uniform, it often helps in the management of this disease. A trial of a gonadotrophin-releasing hormone (GnRH) agonist can also help in the diagnosis. If pain is improved, the pain is likely of reproductive tract origin (21). This approach can therefore allow both diagnosis and treatment to be achieved in one step and possibly avoid surgery.

Physical findings are as variable as subjective complaints. Uterosacral ligament tenderness and nodularity is very specific to endometriosis (22, 23). The finding of tenderness and nodularity of the uterosacral ligaments and/or cul de sac is present in only about one-third of patients. Obliteration of the cul de sac in conjunction with fixed uterine retroversion implies extensive disease. Ovarian involvement may be accompanied with adnexal tenderness and palpable enlargement if endometriomas are present. Endometriomas are cystic structures usually filled with a chocolate-colored fluid. The presence of any adnexal mass should prompt the usual workup, including a pelvic ultrasound. Endometriomas have unique radiologic features that increase the accuracy of diagnosis. The specificity of transvaginal ultrasonography in differentiating endometriomas from other ovarian masses is approximately 90% (24).

Currently, laparoscopy is the standard approach to confirm the presence of endometriosis. Because endometriosis is a specific disease entity, the diagnosis should not be given to a patient unless direct visualization of implants is made at either laparoscopy or laparotomy. It is imperative that the surgeon is skilled in diagnosing the various appearances of implants and in excising or ablating the disease. Although endometriosis is classically described as having either a powder-burn appearance or that of red lesions, implants may be black, blue, white, or even nonpigmented. Implants are usually multiple and, if biopsied, are out of phase with the normal endometrium. Accurate staging of the disease is extremely important to allow comparison of results of various treatments and consistent exchange of information among clinicians.

CA-125 Assay

CA-125 is a glycoprotein expressed on the cell surface of some derivatives of coelomic epithelium (including endometrium) and has been used for monitoring patients with epithelial ovarian cancer. Serum CA-125 levels are often elevated in patients with advanced endometriosis and correlate with patient response to treatment (25, 26). It was believed that CA-125 levels could be used for a marker of recurrence of the disease, but levels that decrease with medical therapy often return to pretherapy levels on cessation of treatment, so the clinical utility of the CA-125 marker is limited (27). It is not sensitive enough to use as a screening test because CA-125 levels can be elevated in other benign conditions, such as early pregnancy, acute pelvic inflammatory disease, leiomyomata, and menstruation.

CLASSIFICATION

Numerous classifications have been proposed for endometriosis. The primary objective of a classification system is to describe certain characteristics of a disease that will respond to treatment in a consistent manner (28). A revised classification system of the American Society for Reproductive Medicine (ASRM) has been proposed based on the surgical findings of 469 patients (Fig. 13.1) (29). Although trends were apparent, this method has not proven to be a sensitive predictor of pregnancy following treatment. There is no method of categorizing endometriosis shown to accurately correlate pain with location and severity of endometriosis. Thus, efforts must continue to develop a useful method of staging this disease (30).

ENDOMETRIOSIS-ASSOCIATED INFERTILITY

Ten to 15% of infertile couples have endometriosis as their only identifiable cause of infertility, and 30 to 40% of women with the disease are infertile (31). Verkauf (32) prospectively described endometriosis in 38.5% of infertile patients compared with 5.2% of controls. Patients with even minimal endometriosis have decreased fecundity compared to normal controls (33, 34). Although these and other similar findings imply an association between endometriosis and infertility, doubts regarding a causal relationship remain. When adnexal adhesions alter tubo-ovarian anatomy, infertility is easily explainable, but in the presence of a few scattered peritoneal implants and no disruption of ovum pickup, an etiologic role is not as clear.

Proposed mechanisms for infertility associated with endometriosis include mechanical, peritoneal, immunologic, and ovulatory factors. Some authors have suggested an association between endometriosis and spontaneous abortion; however, these data are purely observational and likely explained by other factors (35, 36). Alterations in tubal motility due to pelvic adhesions or elevated prostaglandins present in the peritoneal fluid are one possible explanation for the decreased fecundity. Peritubal and peri-ovarian adhesions can alter tubo-ovarian relationships essential for ovum pick-up. Prostaglandins can cause dysmenorrhea, dyspareunia, and pelvic pain. They affect smooth muscle function and may interfere with tubal and uterine motility, resulting in altered transport of gametes or even implantation. Ectopic endometrial implants contain increased levels of prostaglandin F compared with normal endometrium, and some investigators have reported a higher concentration of prostaglandins within the peritoneal fluid of patients with endometriosis (37, 38). Others have found no difference in prostaglandin levels of peritoneal fluid in women with and without endometriosis (39). Because the correlation of impaired fertility with increased levels of prostaglandins remains unproven, this theory remains speculative as an etiology.

Peritoneal fluid of patients with endometriosis contains an increased number of activated macrophages (40). It had been believed that these macrophages might ingest sperm via phagocytosis, but further study failed to demonstrate a difference in the number of motile sperm in peritoneal fluid of patients with endometriosis versus those without (41, 42). Although no in vivo data support an adverse affect on fertility, these macrophages can serve as an additional source of prostaglandins and interleukin-1, possibly altering follicular rupture, tubal motility, and corpus luteum function.

Subtle defects in ovulation have also been attributed to endometriosis. Specifically, impaired folliculogenesis and luteinized unruptured follicle syndrome have been suggested as causes of

AMERICAN SOCIETY FOR REPRODUCTIVE MEDICINE
REVISED CLASSIFICATION OF ENDOMETRIOSIS

Patient's Name ______________________ Date ______________________

Stage I (Minimal) - 1-5
Stage II (Mild) - 6-15
Stage III (Moderate) - 16-40
Stage IV (Severe) - >40
Total ______________

Laparoscopy ________ Laparotomy ________ Photography ________
Recommended Treatment ______________________

Prognosis ______________________

PERITONEUM	ENDOMETRIOSIS	<1cm	1-3cm	>3cm
	Superficial	1	2	4
	Deep	2	4	6
OVARY	R Superficial	1	2	4
	Deep	4	16	20
	L Superficial	1	2	4
	Deep	4	16	20
	POSTERIOR CULDESAC OBLITERATION	Partial		Complete
		4		40
OVARY	ADHESIONS	<1/3 Enclosure	1/3-2/3 Enclosure	>2/3 Enclosure
	R Filmy	1	2	4
	Dense	4	8	16
	L Filmy	1	2	4
	Dense	4	8	16
TUBE	R Filmy	1	2	4
	Dense	4*	8*	16
	L Filmy	1	2	4
	Dense	4*	8*	16

*If the fimbriated end of the fallopian tube is completely enclosed, change the point assignment to 16.

Denote appearance of superficial implant types as red [(R), red, red-pink, flamelike, vesicular blobs, clear vesicles], white [(W), opacifications, peritoneal defects, yellow-brown], or black [(B) black, hemosiderin deposits, blue]. Denote percent of total described as R___%, W___% and B___%. Total should equal 100%.

Additional Endometriosis: ______________________

Associated Pathology: ______________________

To Be Used With Normal Tubes and Ovaries

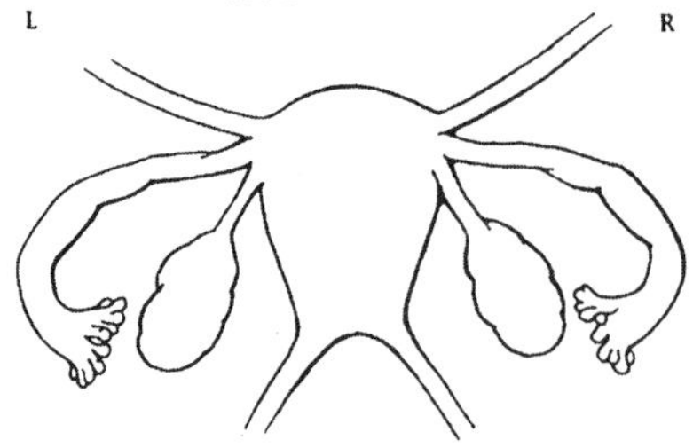

To Be Used With Abnormal Tubes and/or Ovaries

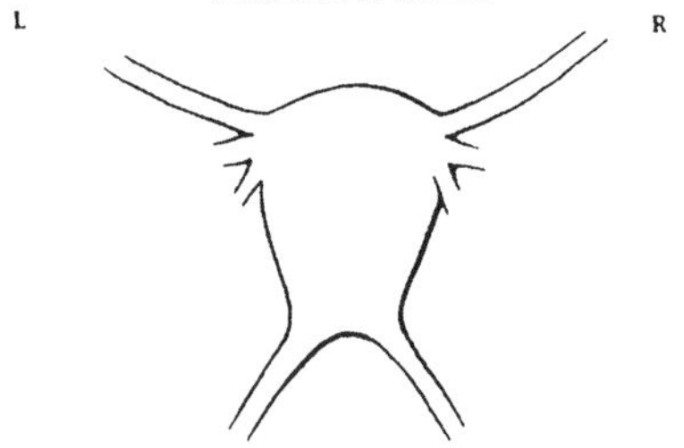

FIGURE 13.1 ● American Society for Reproductive Medicine revised classification of endometriosis. (Property of the American Society for Reproductive Medicine, 1996.)

STAGE I (MINIMAL)

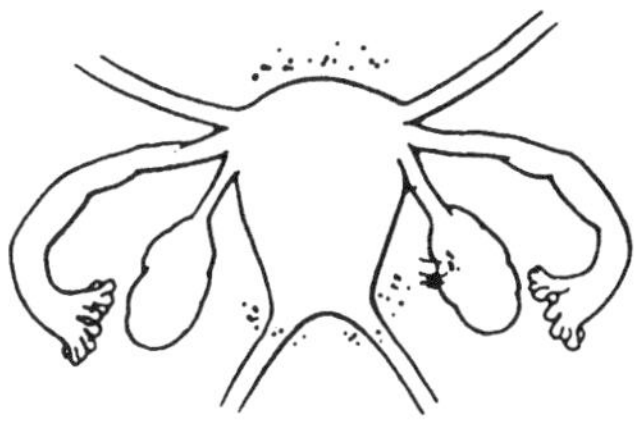

PERITONEUM			
Superficial Endo	–	1-3cm	- 2
R. OVARY			
Superficial Endo	–	<1cm	- 1
Filmy Adhesions	–	<1/3	- 1
TOTAL POINTS			4

STAGE II (MILD)

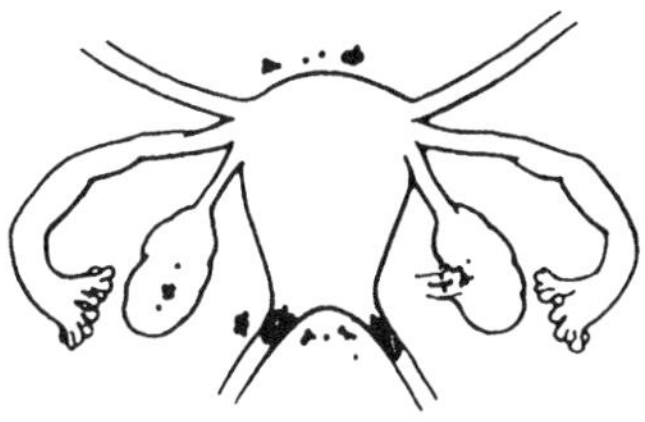

PERITONEUM			
Deep Endo	–	>3cm	- 6
R. OVARY			
Superficial Endo	–	<1cm	- 1
Filmy Adhesions	–	<1/3	- 1
L. OVARY			
Superficial Endo	–	<1cm	- 1
TOTAL POINTS			9

STAGE III (MODERATE)

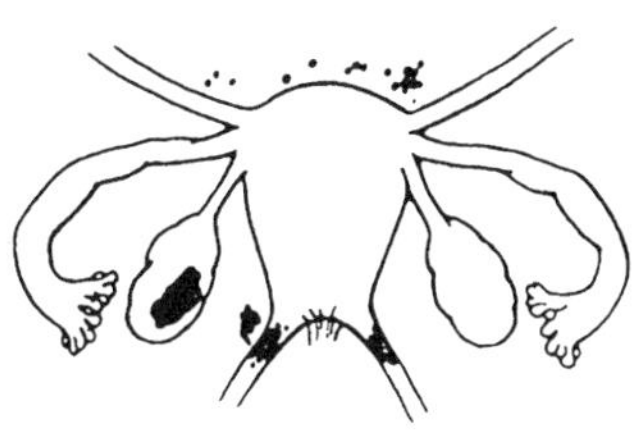

PERITONEUM			
Deep Endo	–	>3cm	- 6
CULDESAC			
Partial Obliteration			- 4
L. OVARY			
Deep Endo	–	1-3cm	- 16
TOTAL POINTS			26

STAGE III (MODERATE)

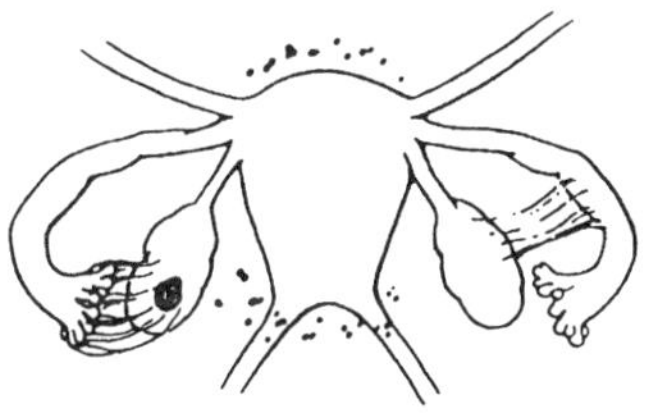

PERITONEUM			
Superficial Endo	–	>3cm	-4
R. TUBE			
Filmy Adhesions	–	<1/3	- 1
R. OVARY			
Filmy Adhesions	–	<1/3	- 1
L. TUBE			
Dense Adhesions	–	<1/3	- 16*
L. OVARY			
Deep Endo	–	<1 cm	-4
Dense Adhesions	–	<1/3	-4
TOTAL POINTS			30

STAGE IV (SEVERE)

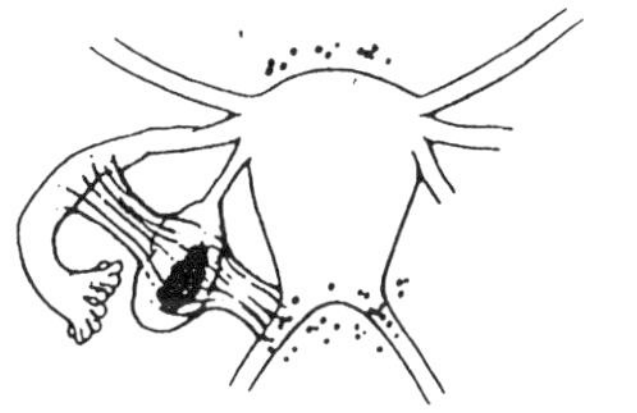

PERITONEUM			
Superficial Endo	–	>3cm	- 4
L. OVARY			
Deep Endo	–	1-3cm	- 32**
Dense Adhesions	–	<1/3	- 8**
L. TUBE			
Dense Adhesions	–	<1/3	-8**
TOTAL POINTS			52

*Point assignment changed to 16
**Point assignment doubled

STAGE IV (SEVERE)

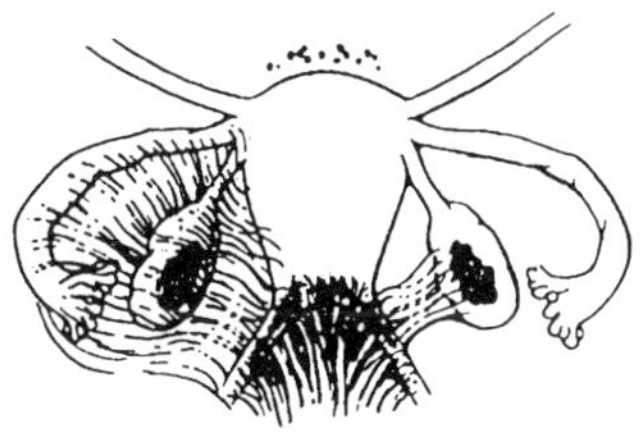

PERITONEUM			
Deep Endo	–	>3cm	- 6
CULDESAC			
Complete Obliteration			- 40
R. OVARY			
Deep Endo	–	1-3cm	- 16
Dense Adhesions	–	<1/3	- 4
L. TUBE			
Dense Adhesions	–	>2/3	- 16
L. OVARY			
Deep Endo	–	1-3cm	- 16
Dense Adhesions	–	>2/3	- 16
TOTAL POINTS			114

Determination of the stage or degree of endometrial involvement is based on a weighted point system. Distribution of points has been arbitrarily determined and may require further revision or refinement as knowledge of the disease increases.

To ensure complete evaluation, inspection of the pelvis in a clockwise or counterclockwise fashion is encouraged. Number, size and location of endometrial implants, plaques, endometriomas and/or adhesions are noted. For example, five separate 0.5cm superficial implants on the peritoneum (2.5 cm total) would be assigned 2 points. (The surface of the uterus should be considered peritoneum.) The severity of the endometriosis or adhesions should be assigned the highest score only for peritoneum, ovary, tube or culdesac. For example, a 4cm superficial and a 2cm deep implant of the peritoneum should be given a score of 6 (not 8). A 4cm deep endometrioma of the ovary associated with more than 3cm of superficial disease should be scored 20 (not 24).

In those patients with only one adnexa, points applied to disease of the remaining tube and ovary should be multipled by two. **Points assigned may be circled and totaled. Aggregation of points indicates stage of disease (minimal, mild, moderate, or severe).

The presence of endometriosis of the bowel, urinary tract, fallopian tube, vagina, cervix, skin etc., should be documented under "additional endometriosis." Other pathology such as tubal occlusion, leiomyomata, uterine anomaly, etc., should be documented under "associated pathology." All pathology should be depicted as specifically as possible on the sketch of pelvic organs, and means of observation (laparoscopy or laparotomy) should be noted.

FIGURE 13.1 ● *(Continued)*

decreased fertility (43, 44). Given that the diagnosis of follicle rupture is so difficult, even in normal ovulatory women, this correlation remains doubtful (45). McBean et al. (46) demonstrated an abnormal transition from follicular to luteal phase in endometriosis patients compared with controls. The resulting abnormalities of oocyte release and progesterone production could be a contributing mechanism of infertility.

Fertilization and implantation rates have been compared between normal women and patients with endometriosis. Although some authors report a decreased fertilization rate in women with endometriosis, others show no correlation (47, 48). An increase in abnormal implantation rates has been reported in patients with endometriosis. This is theorized to be secondary to an embryotoxic environment created by endometriosis (49). Lessey et al. (50) described aberrant integrin expression in the endometrium of patients with endometriosis and proposed this as a possible cause of subfertility.

TREATMENT

There is considerable debate regarding efficacy in treatment of endometriosis. There is no medical therapy to prevent this disease or to selectively destroy the endometrial implants. Medical therapy and conservative surgical therapy (i.e., retention of the uterus and ovaries) must be viewed as palliative, not curative. Much of the controversy involves the appropriate treatments of minimal and mild disease. Severe disease is usually treated surgically, unless the patient desires fertility, in which case in vitro fertilization (IVF) is a common intervention. Numerous trials have been completed that address the question of optimal therapy for endometriosis. Only recently have well-designed, prospective, randomized, controlled studies been introduced to this debate. The presence of a control group that includes patients who do not receive any therapy for endometriosis is essential to demonstrate conclusively that treatment of endometriosis is better than expectant management.

It is imperative that the goal of therapy, either pain relief or improvement of fertility, is outlined before any plan is initiated. Often, this delineation is not clear cut because infertile women may also complain of pelvic pain. It is important to recognize that the diagnosis of endometriosis in an infertile woman does not preclude the presence of other infertility factors for the couple. This is particularly applicable to minimal or mild endometriosis where there is no distortion of pelvic anatomy. For these patients, one reasonable course would be to treat other infertility factors that are present and if no conception occurs, proceed to the use of clomiphene citrate (Clomid) and intrauterine insemination (IUI). (This assumes prior laparoscopic diagnosis with treatment at the same time. If no treatment was provided at the time of laparoscopy, repeat laparoscopy with the use of ablation or resection of implants should be considered.) The ideal treatment would provide pain relief *and* allow pregnancy to occur safely while on treatment. This section reviews treatment options for endometriosis-associated infertility and pelvic pain. Treatment modalities for endometriosis can be classified into four major categories: expectant management, medical therapy, surgical therapy, and assisted reproductive technologies.

Treatment of Endometriosis-Associated Infertility

Expectant Management

Lack of prospective, controlled trials and inconsistency in staging contribute to the uncertainty about endometriosis as a cause of reduced fertility. The cumulative pregnancy rate after 5 years without treatment is 90% in women with minimal disease and is only slightly more in women without endometriosis (51). Based on these findings, many recommend a period of expectant management prior to any therapy (52). This means that additional infertility factors such as ovulatory disorders should be diagnosed and treated. Compared with medical therapy, expectant management is less costly, and avoids treatment-induced anovulation and medication-related side effects. The disadvantages of expectant management are that it does not specifically treat the endometriotic implants, and in the majority of patients who fail to conceive with expectant management, progression of the disease may occur (53). Most studies that address treatment options first categorize patients according to the severity of disease. Classification of endometriosis based on the ASRM revised classification system requires laparoscopic evaluation, which is in itself an intervention. Two randomized controlled trials compared expectant management with surgical correction of endometriosis. Marcoux et al. (54) presented a prospective randomized trial comparing laparoscopic surgery with expectant management after laparoscopic diagnosis of minimal or mild disease. They concluded that monthly fecundity of the surgical treatment group was almost twice that of the expectant management group (30.8% versus 17.7%). In contrast, Parrazzini (55) reported another randomized controlled trial demonstrating a live birth rate of 19.6% in the treatment group and 22.2% in the controls within 1 year of surgery. Combining the results of these two trials statistically still favors surgical treatment over expectant management, with an odds ratio for pregnancy of 1.7 (confidence interval 1.1 to 2.5) (56). It is therefore reasonable to proceed with removal or destruction of endometriosis at the time of surgery to obtain the most immediate improvement in pregnancy rate.

Medical Therapy

The most commonly used medical treatments for endometriosis-associated infertility include danazol (Danocrine), progestins, and GnRH agonists. Although use of ovulation-suppressive agents to treat patients with endometriosis may improve pelvic pain, they will not improve fecundity.

Danazol is a derivative of 17-alpha ethinyl testosterone. It produces a high-androgen, low-estrogen environment that does not support the growth of endometriosis. Benefits of danazol include pain relief and prevention of disease progression (57). Discontinuation of the drug frequently leads to recurrence of symptoms. There is no apparent evidence supporting the use of danazol over expectant management in the treatment of infertility (58, 59).

Progestational agents have not been effective in the treatment of endometriosis-associated infertility (60, 61). Although some reports demonstrate higher pregnancy rates, these were not controlled studies (58). One randomized, double-blind, placebo-controlled study of luteal phase treatment with dydrogesterone (a synthetic progestogen) failed to show any improvement in pregnancy rates over a control group (62).

GnRH agonist is the most recent type of medication introduced for the treatment of endometriosis. These medications are analogs of GnRH that have altered amino acid sequences to prolong their half-life and improve receptor binding (63). The use of GnRH agonist in the treatment of endometriosis relies on its ability to downregulate the gonadotropins and create a hypoestrogenic environment that suppresses endometrial tissue growth. No studies to date have shown an improved pregnancy rate using GnRH agonist versus danazol or expectant management in the treatment of endometriosis-associated infertility (64, 65).

Surgical Treatment

To appropriately assess the effect of surgical treatment of endometriosis on fertility, it is imperative to analyze the data with the proper methodology. Simple pregnancy rates are an inappropriate measure of success because of the variability in the length of patient follow-up. A reported 50% pregnancy rate has a vastly different meaning with 1-month versus 1-year follow-up. A better approach is the use of life table analysis to describe the resulting cumulative pregnancy rate (66). Life table analysis is a statistical method that accounts for variable lengths of follow-up in a study population and for patients lost to follow-up. It is frequently and appropriately applied to the study of infertility and fertility. A life table analysis requires a well-defined starting point. In infertility studies, this is most often the time when the couple registers with an infertility service. In addition, a distinct dichotomous end point must be defined. This is an end point that either occurs or does not and is usually defined as any pregnancy in studies of interest. Last, the life table must have a well-described and limited time interval.

Surgical treatment of severe disease has been shown by appropriate methodologic studies to improve pregnancy rates (67). Success of surgery is directly related to the severity of disease. Treatment of patients with moderate and severe endometriosis results in 60% and 35% pregnancy rates, respectively (66). Pregnancy rates are improved when minimal and mild disease is treated, but likely not as much as with more advanced disease (54, 55). Guzick and Rock (68) demonstrated a rapid rise in the cumulative pregnancy rate with endoscopic laser therapy, but a plateau is reached similar to that seen in other forms of treatment. Their study, however, did not compare surgery with expectant management.

In summary, laparoscopic removal of minimal to mild endometriosis appears to have some benefit. No study to date has addressed whether the same immediate increase in pregnancy rates resulting from surgery could be obtained from a less expensive medical management, such as ovulation induction with IUI. Treatment for severe endometriosis with either laparoscopic surgery or assisted reproductive technologies (ART) significantly improves pregnancy rates (69, 70).

Preoperative or postoperative medical therapy with hormonal suppression is not associated with any improvement in overall pregnancy rates compared with surgical or medical treatment alone (71). Although one study demonstrated a small improvement in pregnancy rate with the use of postoperative danazol, the preponderance of evidence suggests no benefit (72–74).

For women currently seeking pregnancy and diagnosed (incidentally) with mild endometriosis at the time of surgery, it is reasonable to ablate or remove all lesions. For those incidentally diagnosed with more advanced disease, the lesions should definitely be treated at the time of surgery. Postoperative medical therapy (GnRH agonist, Danocrine, medroxyprogesterone acetate) is only effective for pain relief; it is not effective in improving fertility.

Advanced Reproductive Technologies

Because the benefit of conservative surgical treatment of patients with minimal disease still remains controversial, many physicians confronted with such cases have used ART to bypass the unknown mechanisms by which endometriosis may be causing decreased fecundity. For instance, if endometriosis is causing ovulatory dysfunction, treatment with ovulation induction should improve fecundity. If the infertility is secondary to tubal distortion from endometriosis, the use of in vitro fertilization increases the chance of pregnancy.

Superovulation with clomiphene or with human menopausal gonadotropins (hMGs) has been used successfully to treat endometriosis-associated infertility (75–77). Results are not uniform, but it does appear that per-cycle fecundity in women receiving superovulation and IUI is increased over expectant management. In women with documented mild endometriosis, clomiphene–IUI provided improvement in pregnancy rates over expectant management, but not as significant as that seen with hMG–IUI (77). In patients in whom clomiphene–IUI is unsuccessful, hMG–IUI may be considered as the next step in treatment.

IVF should be reserved for patients failing to achieve pregnancy with the aforementioned less invasive methods. As with other indications for IVF, such a decision must take into consideration the age of the couple, their desires, and the duration of infertility. Most studies comparing the use of IVF with expectant management for all stages of endometriosis demonstrate a significant benefit for the treatment group (49, 78).

Treatment of Endometriosis-Associated Pelvic Pain

Optimal treatment of pelvic pain due to endometriosis is challenging. Expectant management, medical treatment with nonsteroidal anti-inflammatory drugs (NSAIDs) and/or hormonal therapies, and surgery (conservative or definitive) have all been used for treatment of pelvic pain secondary to endometriosis.

Prior to initiating any therapy, it is essential to complete a comprehensive history and physical examination. Other, perhaps additional, causes of pelvic pain such as adhesions, leiomyomata, hernias, and gastrointestinal disease should be sought. Routine laboratory tests and physical examination to exclude pelvic inflammatory disease or a sexually transmitted disease is important. Ovarian cancer (which rarely presents as chronic pelvic pain) and abnormalities of the ovary are generally detected by physical examination and/or ultrasonography. Figure 13.2 provides an algorithm for evaluation and management of chronic pain from endometriosis, based on initial history and physical exam findings.

Expectant Management

In a prospective, randomized, double-blind, controlled trial of laser laparoscopy in the treatment of stage I, II, or III disease, Sutton et al. (79) evaluated pelvic pain relief after laparoscopy. This study randomized 63 patients with pelvic pain and endometriosis at the time of laparoscopy

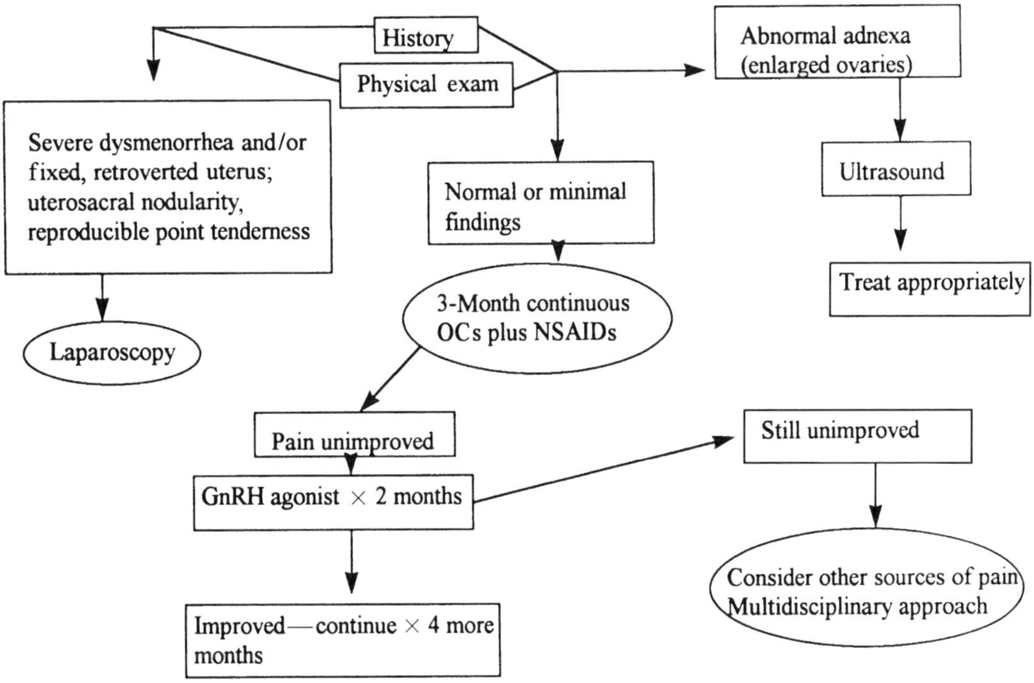

FIGURE 13.2 ● A clinical algorithm for the evaluation and management of chronic pelvic pain suspected to be caused by endometriosis. OCs, oral contraceptives; NSAIDs, nonsteroidal anti-inflammatory drugs; GnRH, gonadotrophin-releasing hormone.

to either laser ablation of endometriotic implants and laparoscopic uterine nerve ablation or expectant management. The patients were unaware of the treatment allocated as was the nurse evaluating them at 3 and 6 months after surgery. Patients with stage II or III disease treated surgically demonstrated significant improvement in pain (74% of laser group versus 20% of expectant management group). There did not appear to be a significant difference between treatment and expectant management in patients with stage I disease (79). Because of the lack of proof of efficacy of treatment and the known risks of surgical complications and adhesion formation, how to address minimal disease encountered in a laparoscopy is a dilemma. Although expectant management of minimal disease is as effective as any other therapy, treating it may also slow or stop progression to a more severe stage.

Medical Treatment

Medical management of pelvic pain secondary to endometriosis includes symptomatic and hormonal therapy. Chronic, cyclic, pelvic pain symptoms of dysmenorrhea, dyschezia, and dyspareunia are characteristic of, although not unique to, endometriosis. Each patient needs to be carefully evaluated to identify the etiology of pelvic pain. The cyclicity of symptoms is not enough to exclude other causes of pain. To help delineate the nature of the pain, a trial of ovarian suppression with a GnRH agonist or danazol may be used. If pain is related to the reproductive tract, patients usually report symptomatic improvement after the first month of amenorrhea. If the frequency and intensity are unchanged, further evaluation of other organ systems is warranted (21).

Symptomatic management of endometriosis requires close interaction between the patient and her physician. Patients who are well informed about their condition and the goals of treatment have a better response to symptomatic management. Various types of prostaglandin synthetase inhibitors can effectively control dysmenorrhea and endometriosis-associated pelvic pain (80). The severity of dysmenorrhea that women with endometriosis suffer does correlate with the amount of prostaglandins produced by the implants (81). To achieve optimal response, the use of mefenamic acid (Ponstel) is recommended (500 mg for the initial dose, then 250 mg every 6 hours as needed). In one study, up to 80% of dysmenorrheic women reported improvement in symptoms using either mefenamic acid or indomethacin (Indocin) (82). Symptomatic therapy should begin 1 to 2 days prior to the onset of menses and continue for the duration of the menstrual process.

Hormonal treatment of endometriosis includes the use of oral contraceptives, danazol, progestins, gestrinone, mifepristone (RU 486), and GnRH agonists. Despite the histologic differences between endometrial implants and the endometrium, estrogen does stimulate the implants to grow; hence, hormonal therapy is employed to interrupt the cycle of stimulation and bleeding. Oral contraceptives have been prescribed in a continuous fashion to promote decidualization of endometriotic implants with resulting pain relief in 75% of patients (21). A monophasic oral contraceptive results in less breakthrough bleeding and active pills should be continued for up to 3 months. If during this 3 months breakthrough bleeding occurs, it is reasonable to discontinue the pill to allow menses to occur and restart active pills 4 to 5 days later.

Danazol has been used successfully in the treatment of endometriosis-associated pelvic pain. Unfortunately, it also displaces testosterone from sex hormone binding globulin, resulting in increased free serum testosterone allowing androgenic side effects to occur. Ultimately, danazol creates a high-androgen, low-estrogen environment that does not allow for growth or cyclical changes in the endometrial implants. Up to 90% of patients with minimal to moderate disease will experience improvement in pain symptoms (83). The recommended effective dose is 800 mg daily (84, 85). Treatment is initiated after menses, and patients should be advised to use barrier contraception for the first few months of therapy. The patient must be told that the chance of spontaneous ovulation is higher in doses less than 600 mg. Therapy is generally continued for 6 months. The induction of amenorrhea appears to correlate with an improved outcome of treatment. Up to 80% of women will experience side effects, including weight gain, fluid retention, acne, decreased breast size, hot flushes, muscle cramps, and emotional liability. In addition, danazol is associated with decreased high-density lipoprotein cholesterol levels. A baseline lipid profile is warranted to ensure the patient does not have pre-existing dyslipidemia. Danazol is contraindicated in women with liver disease. Although symptomatic improvement is common, recurrence rates of up to 30% are reported in the first year after discontinuation of treatment (86). There is no contraindication to repeated courses of danazol. If the side effects are intolerable or if optimal effectiveness was not achieved, another treatment modality should be considered. Women with endometriomas may respond to danazol therapy, but usually require surgical intervention for complete pain relief.

Progestins are also used to suppress ovarian function and are similar to danazol in their effectiveness in treating endometriosis (86, 87). Like danazol, progestins induce decidualization and subsequent atrophy in the implants. The progestins most commonly used to treat endometriosis are medroxyprogesterone acetate (Provera, 10 to 30 mg daily) and norethindrone acetate (Aygestin, 5 to 10 mg daily). Monthly Depo-Provera (150 mg intramuscularly) is also effective and provides reliable contraception to the patient not interested in pregnancy. With oral progestin therapy, ovarian suppression is inconsistent, resulting in variable estrogen levels. Breakthrough bleeding is common and may be treated with ethynyl estradiol (20 mcg/day) or conjugated estrogens (1.25 mg/day) for 1 to 2 weeks. Adverse lipid effects may be seen during progestin therapy. Other side effects include depression, nausea, fluid retention, and breast tenderness. In light of the decreased cost, comparable efficacy, and more tolerable side effects of progestins compared with danazol, many clinicians prescribe this as first-line therapy for endometriosis-associated pelvic pain. A summary of the literature regarding progestin therapy for symptomatic endometriosis suggests that the efficacy for temporary relief is good and is comparable to other treatments with more side effects (88).

The antiprogestational agent mifepristone has been proposed as an alternative agent for treatment of endometriosis (89). Clinical data, however, is lacking and its use in this capacity is discouraged until further studies address its efficacy.

GnRH agonists have been demonstrated to be effective in treating chronic pelvic pain due to endometriosis (90, 91). These agents are effective against endometriosis because of their profound suppression of ovarian function and induction of a hypoestrogenic state. GnRH agonists decrease the secretion of follicle-stimulating hormone and luteinizing hormone. This diminishes production of ovarian steroids to the postmenopausal range within 6 weeks. Trials comparing the efficacy of GnRH agonists with danazol demonstrate equal efficacy in successfully alleviating pelvic pain. Hypoestrogenic side effects occur more frequently with GnRH agonists, and androgenic side effects are more common with danazol.

A long-term consequence of the hypoestrogenic state caused by GnRH agonists is a reduction in trabecular bone density (92). Trabecular bone is found in the distal radius and spine. The addition of progestin alone or in combination with low-dose estrogen (0.625 mg conjugated estrogens or transdermal estradiol 0.025 mg weekly) has been proposed as an effective means of preventing hypoestrogenic symptoms, including loss of bone mineral density. Several studies have evaluated the impact of this "add-back" therapy on the efficacy of pain treatment (93). Those patients with osteoporosis risk factors (strong family history, White or Oriental race, thin, high alcohol intake, or low calcium intake) that cannot be modified should perhaps consider an alternative treatment with a bone-sparing effect. GnRH agonists should not be used in women who already have osteoporosis or who have other medical conditions causing accelerated demineralization of the bone.

During the first 1 to 2 weeks after initial administration of a GnRH agonist, there is a release of gonadotropins that causes an ovarian "flare-up" and resultant increased estradiol production. This flare response, which may exacerbate pain symptoms, can be minimized by initiating therapy on cycle day 1 or just before day 1 of expected menses (94). A pregnancy test should be performed prior to initiating therapy in the luteal phase.

There are no data indicating that extremely low estrogen concentrations have a more pronounced effect on endometriosis than moderately depressed ones. Barbieri (95) proposed a so-called "therapeutic window" for estrogen levels providing end organ response. He determined that an estradiol concentration of 30 to 50 pg/mL is sufficient for reduction in endometriosis without causing deleterious bone loss. This provides a basis for estrogen add-back therapy (96). If no improvement from GnRH agonist is obtained, two possibilities exist. Either severe disease is present or, if treatment was begun empirically, no disease is present.

Surgical Treatment

The most common form of treatment for endometriosis is surgery (96). The goals of conservative surgery are to remove and/or destroy the endometriosis, lyse adhesions if present, and to restore, as much as possible, normal pelvic anatomy. Most forms of endometriosis can be eliminated with laparoscopic intervention, although surgical treatment of endometriosis pain caused by stage I disease may not be superior to expectant management (79). Treatment of minimal or mild disease usually involves laser vaporization or electrocauterization of peritoneal implants. Complete excision of the peritoneum has also been described. Moderate forms of the disease, which include unilateral endometriomas and bilateral small ovarian cysts with limited adhesions, can also be treated successfully at laparoscopy. Standard treatment for severe endometriosis—that is, bilateral large ovarian endometriomas attached by extensive dense adhesions, an obliterated cul de sac, or parametrial infiltration—depends on the laparoscopic expertise of the surgeon (97).

That success of pain control with surgery may or may not be related to the stage of disease reiterates the need for a full diagnostic evaluation of patients suffering from chronic pelvic pain prior to surgery. Because of the expense and the inherent imperfection in visualizing all endometriotic lesions, an empiric trial of GnRH agonist is frequently recommended prior to surgery (Fig. 13.2). Once laparoscopy is chosen as the treatment modality, the patient and surgeon must be prepared for all possible outcomes. It is important to clarify the patient's expectations from surgery, determine her desire for future fertility, and establish a plan of treatment if severe disease is encountered at time of surgery (i.e., patient's preference for conservative surgery versus definitive surgery with hysterectomy and/or oophorectomy).

RECURRENCE OF ENDOMETRIOSIS

Endometriosis may recur after medical therapy, conservative surgical therapy, and even after castration (98). In one long-term follow-up study, rates of recurrence in women treated with GnRH agonists were 37% for minimal disease and 74% for severe disease (99). These rates are similar for patients treated with danazol (100). The recurrence rate 5 years after conservative surgery is close to 40%. Compared with women with oophorectomy for endometriosis, patients undergoing hysterectomy with ovarian conservation have a 6.1 times greater risk of developing recurrent pain and 8.1 times greater risk of reoperation (101, 102).

HORMONE REPLACEMENT THERAPY AFTER "DEFINITIVE" SURGERY

The potential for estrogen replacement therapy to reactivate residual endometriotic implants remains unclear. Some studies indicate that hormone replacement therapy (HRT) does not stimulate recurrence of symptoms related to endometriosis, but others advocate delaying the initiation of HRT for up to 1 year (103, 104). In patients with moderate or severe disease immediately posthysterectomy and bilateral salpingo-oophorectomy, we prescribe combined estrogen/progestin therapy during the first 3 to 6 months postoperatively. Then, if no symptoms have occurred, we initiate estrogen alone. In the rare event of pain recurrence, progestins can be added back to help diminish the pain. The addition of a progestational agent is sometimes recommended even after a hysterectomy because of reported cases of adenocarcinoma arising from endometriotic implants in women treated with unopposed estrogen (105, 106).

Clinical Notes

- Endometriosis affects an estimated 5 to 10% of reproductive age women and 25 to 35% of women with infertility.
- Endometriosis does *not* primarily afflict career-driven women older than 30 years of age, and it *does* occur in women of African American descent.
- Two-thirds of women with endometriosis will have ovarian involvement.
- Classic symptoms of endometriosis include dysmenorrhea, dyspareunia, dyschezia, and/or a history of infertility, but few women will present with all these symptoms.
- The degree of pelvic pain is not related to the severity or distribution of endometriosis, although there may be a correlation in the number of endometrial implants and the intensity of dysmenorrhea.
- Although uterosacral ligament tenderness and nodularity is specific to endometriosis, this finding is present in only about one-third of patients and is usually present late in the course of the disease.
- The diagnosis of endometriosis requires direct visualization of lesions by laparoscopy or laparotomy.
- CA-125 is not a marker that can be reliably used for screening for endometriosis or for following response to therapy.
- The classification system most commonly used is that developed by the ASRM; neither it nor any other method of classification/staging has been proven to accurately correlate pain with location and severity of endometriosis.
- Ten to 15% of infertile couples have endometriosis as the only identifiable cause, and 30 to 40% of women with the disease are infertile.
- The cumulative pregnancy rate after 5 years of expectant management in women with minimal disease is 90%.
- Limited data show an increase in fecundity of women with minimal or mild endometriosis after laparoscopic surgical therapy compared with women undergoing expectant management.
- To date, no studies have shown any difference in improved pregnancy rates in the medical therapy of endometriosis with danazol or GnRH agonists.
- Surgical treatment of moderate or severe disease has been shown to improve pregnancy rates by 60% and 35%, respectively.

- For women receiving superovulation and IUI, per cycle fecundity is increased over expectant management; IVF should be reserved for patients failing to achieve pregnancy after attempts at superovulation and IUI.
- There are data to support the use of surgical therapy in patients with pelvic pain and moderate or severe endometriosis; however, the efficacy of surgical treatment of minimal endometriosis for pelvic pain is more controversial.
- Of the NSAIDs used to treat endometriosis-related pelvic pain, the fenamate class (mefenamic acid) or indomethacin is recommended.
- Oral contraceptives, prescribed in a continuous fashion, have resulted in pain relief in 75% of patients with endometriosis-related pain.
- If danazol is used to treat endometriosis, an initial dose of 800 mg daily, with a decrease to 600 mg daily, is one recommended regimen. With doses of less than 600 mg daily, the chance of spontaneous ovulation is increased.
- Progestins such as medroxyprogesterone acetate 10 to 30 mg daily, norethindrone acetate 5 to 10 mg daily, or Depo-Provera 150 mg intramuscularly monthly may be used to treat endometriosis-related pain.
- Use of GnRH therapy with "add-back" estrogen and progesterone sufficient to maintain an estradiol concentration of 30 to 50 pg/mL may provide pain relief from endometriosis without incurring deleterious bone loss.
- Rates of recurrence for women treated with GnRH agonists or danazol are approximately 35% for minimal disease and 75% for severe disease.
- The recurrence rate 5 years after treatment with conservative surgery is close to 40%.
- For patients with moderate or severe disease who receive hysterectomy with bilateral oophorectomy, one regimen recommends combined estrogen/progestin therapy for 3 to 6 months beginning immediately postoperatively. If no symptoms develop, estrogen alone is initiated thereafter.

REFERENCES

1. Wheeler JM. Epidemiology and prevalence of endometriosis. Infertil Reprod Med Clin N Am 1992;3:545.
2. Cramer DW. Epidemiology of endometriosis. In: Endometriosis. New York: Liss, 1987:5.
3. Melis GB, Ajossa S, Guerriero S, et al. Epidemiology and diagnosis of endometriosis. Ann N Y Acad Sci 1994;74:352–357.
4. Matorras R, Rodriguez F, Pijoan JI, et al. Epidemiology of endometriosis in infertile women. Fertil Steril 1995;63:34–38.
5. Simpson JL, Elias S, Malinack LR, et al. Heritable aspects of endometriosis I. Genetic studies. Am J Obstet Gynecol 1980;137:327.
6. Haney AF. Endometriosis: pathogenesis and pathophysiology. In: Endometriosis. New York: Liss, 1987:23–51.
7. Haney AF. Etiology and histogenesis of endometriosis. In: Endometriosis: Current Concepts in Clinical Management. Philadelphia: Lippincott, 1989:1–49.
8. Brosens I, Vasquez G, Deprest J, et al. Pathogenesis of endometriosis. In: Endometriosis. New York: Springer-Verlag, 1995:9–19.
9. Liu DTY, Hitchcock A. Endometriosis: its association with retrograde menstruation, dysmenorrhea, and tubal pathology. Br J Obstet Gynecol 1986;93:859–862.
10. Steele RW, Dmowski WP, Marmer DJ. Immunologic aspects of human endometriosis. Am J Reprod Immunol 1984;6:33.
11. Dmowski WP. Immunological aspects of endometriosis. Int J Gynecol Obstet 1995;50(suppl 1):3–10.
12. Kennedy S, Mardon H, Barlow D. Familial endometriosis. J Assist Reprod Genet 1995;1:32–34.
13. Damewood MD. Pathophysiology and management of endometriosis. J Fam Pract 1993;37:68–75.
14. Franklin RR, Grunert GM. Extragenital endometriosis. In: Endometriosis. New York: Springer-Verlag, 1995:127–136.
15. Vercellini P, Trespidi L, Giorgi OD, et al. Endometriosis and pelvic pain: relation to disease stage and localization. Fertil Steril 1996;65:299–304.
16. Foster DC, Stern JL, Buscema J, et al. Pleural and parenchymal pulmonary endometriosis. Obstet Gynecol 1991;78:946.
17. Schorlemer GR, Battaglini JW. Pneumothorax in menstruating females. Contemp Surg 1982;20:53.
18. Fedele L, Parazzini F, Bianchi S, et al. Stage and localization of pelvic endometriosis and pain. Fertil Steril 1990;53:155.

19. Perper MM, Nezhat F, Goldstein H, et al. Dysmenorrhea is related to the number of implants in endometriosis patients. Fertil Steril 1995;63:500–503.
20. Cramer DW, Wilson E, Stillman RJ, et al. The relation of endometriosis to menstrual characteristics, smoking and exercise. JAMA 1985;225:1904.
21. Dmowski WP. The role of medical management in the treatment of endometriosis. In: Endometriosis: Advanced Management and Surgical Techniques. New York: Springer-Verlag, 1995:229–240.
22. Matorras R, Rodriguez F, Pijoan JI, et al. Are there any clinical signs and symptoms that are related to endometriosis in infertile women? Am J Obstet Gynecol 1996;174:620–623.
23. Ripps B, Martin DC. Focal pelvic tenderness, pelvic pain and dysmenorrhea in endometriosis. J Reprod Med 1991;7:36.
24. Mais V, Guerriero S, Ajossa S, et al. The efficiency of transvaginal ultrasonography in the diagnosis of endometrioma. Fertil Steril 1993;60:776–780.
25. Ozaksit G, Caglar T, Cicek N, et al. Serum CA125 levels before, during and after treatment for endometriosis. Int J Gynecol Obstet 1995;50:269–273.
26. Barbieri RL, Niloff JM, Bast RC Jr, et al. Elevated serum concentrations of CA-125 in patients with advanced endometriosis. Fertil Steril 1986;45:630.
27. Franssen AMHW, van der Heijden PFM, Thomas CMG, et al. On the origin and significance of serum CA-125 concentrations in 97 patients with endometriosis before, during, and after buserelin acetate, nafarelin, or danazol. Fertil Steril 1992;57:974.
28. Schenken RS, Guzick DS. Revised endometriosis classification: 1996. Fertil Steril 1997;67:815–816.
29. Guzick DS, Silliman NP, Adamson GD, et al. Prediction of pregnancy in infertile women based on the American Society for Reproductive Medicine's revised classification of endometriosis. Fertil Steril 1997;67:822–829.
30. Fedele L, Branchi S, Bocciolone L, et al. Pain symptoms associated with endometriosis. Obstet Gynecol 1992;79:767–769.
31. Burns WN, Schenken RS. Pathophysiology in Endometriosis: Contemporary Concepts in Clinical Management. Philadelphia: Lippincott, 1989:83–126.
32. Verkauf BS. The incidence, symptoms and signs of endometriosis in fertile and infertile women. J Fla Med Assoc 1987;74:671.
33. Toma SK, Stovall DW, Hammond MG. The effect of laparoscopic ablation on Danocrine on pregnancy rates in patients with stage I or II endometriosis undergoing donor insemination. Obstet Gynecol 1992;80: 253.
34. Jansen RPS. Minimal endometriosis and reduced fecundability: prospective evidence from an artificial insemination by donor program. Fertil Steril 1986;46:141.
35. Wheeler JM, Johnston BM, Malinak LR. The relationship of endometriosis to spontaneous abortion. Fertil Steril 1983;39:656–660.
36. Metzger DA, Olive DL, Stohs GF, et al. Association of endometriosis and spontaneous abortion: effect of control group selection. Fertil Steril 1986;45:18–22.
37. Moon YS, Leung PC, Yuen BH, et al. Prostaglandin F in human endometriotic tissue. Am J Obstet Gynecol 1981;141:344–345.
38. Badawy SZ, Cuenca V, Marshall L, et al. Cellular component in peritoneal fluid in infertile patients with and without endometriosis. Fertil Steril 1984;42:704–707.
39. Haney AF, Muscato JJ, Weiberg JB. Peritoneal fluid cell populations in infertility patients. Fertil Steril 1981;35:696.
40. Graf MJ, Dunaif A. Association of reproductive endocrine dysfunction with pelvic endometriosis. Semin Reprod Endocrinol 1985;3:319.
41. Muscato JJ, Hancy AF, Weinberg JB. Sperm phagocytosis by human peritoneal macrophages: a possible cause of infertility and endometriosis. Am J Obstet Gynecol 1982;144:503.
42. Stone SAC, Himsl K. Peritoneal recovery of motile and nonmotile sperm in the presence of endometriosis. Fertil Steril 1986;46:338.
43. Doody MC, Gibbons WE, Buttram VC Jr. Linear regression analysis of ultrasound follicular growth series: evidence for an abnormality of follicular growth in endometriosis patients. Fertil Steril 1988;49:47.
44. Brosens IA, Koninckx PR, Corvelyn PA. A study of plasma progesterone, estradiol, prolactin, and LH levels and the luteal phase appearance of the ovaries in patients with endometriosis and infertility. Br J Obset Gynecol 1978;85:246.
45. Portuondo JA, Pena L, Otaola C. Absence of ovulation stigma in the conception cycle. Int J Fertil 1983;28:52–54.
46. McBean JH, Blackman J, Brumsted JR. Abnormal ovulation in women with endometriosis [Abstract P-168]. American Society of Reproductive Medicine, October 18–22, 1997.
47. Mills MS, Eddowes HA, Cahill DJ, et al. A prospective controlled study on in-vitro fertilization, gamete intrafallopian transfer and intrauterine insemination combined with superovulation. Hum Reprod 1992;7:490–494.
48. Jones HW Jr, Acosta AA, Andrews MC, et al. Three years of in vitro fertilization at Norfolk. Fertil Steril 1984;42:826–834.
49. Arici A, Oral E, Bukulmez O, et al. The effect of endometriosis on implantation: results from the Yale University in vitro fertilization and embryo transfer program. Fertil Steril 1996;65:603–607.
50. Lessey BA, Castelbaum AJ, Sawin SW, et al. Aberrant integrin expression in the endometrium of patients with endometriosis. J Clin Endocrinol Metab 1994;79:643–649.

51. Badawy SZA, El Bakry MM, Samuel F, et al. Cumulative pregnancy rates in infertile women with endometriosis. J Reprod Med 1988;33:757–760.
52. Rodriguez-Escudero FJ, Neyro JL, Corcostegui B, et al. Does minimal endometriosis reduce fecundity? Fertil Steril 1988;50:3.
53. Thomas IJ, Cooke ID. Successful treatment of asymptomatic endometriosis: does it benefit infertile women? Br Med J 1987;294:1117–1119.
54. Marcoux S, Maheux R, Berube S. Canadian Collaborative Group on Endometriosis. Laparoscopic surgery in infertile women with minimal or mild endometriosis. N Engl J Med 1997;337:217–222.
55. Parrazzini F. Ablation of lesions or no treatment in minimal-mild endometriosis in infertile women: a randomized trial—Guppo Italiano per lo Studio dell' Endometriosis 1999. Hum Reprod 14:1332–1334.
56. Schenken RS, Malinak LR. Conservative surgery versus expectant management for the infertile patient with mild endometriosis. Fertil Steril 1982;37:183–186.
57. Dmowski WP, Cohen MR. Antigonadotropin (Danazol) in the treatment of endometriosis: evaluation of post-treatment fertility and three year follow-up data. Am J Obstet Gynecol 1978;130:41.
58. Hull ME, Moghissi KS, Magyar DF, et al. Comparison of different treatment modalities of endometriosis in infertile women. Fertil Steril 1987;47(1):40.
59. Seibel MM, Berger MJ, Weinstein FG, et al. The effectiveness of danazol on subsequent fertility in minimal endometriosis. Fertil Steril 1982;38:534.
60. Tellima S. Danazol and medroxyprogesterone acetate inefficacious in the treatment of infertility in endometriosis. Fertil Steril 1988;50:872.
61. Moghissi KS, Boyce CR. Management of endometriosis with oral medroxyprogesterone acetate. Obstet Gynecol 1976;47:265–267.
62. Overton CE, Lindsay PC, Johal B, et al. A randomized, double blind, placebo-controlled study of luteal phase dydrogesterone (Duphaston) in women with minimal to mild endometriosis. Fertil Steril 1994;62:701–707.
63. Henzl M. Gonadotropin-releasing hormone agonists in the management of endometriosis: a review. Clin Obstet Gynecol 1988;31:4.
64. Fedele L, Bianchi S, Arcaini L, et al. Buserelin versus danazol in the treatment of endometriosis associated infertility. Am J Obstet Gynecol 1989;161:871–876.
65. Marana R., Pailli FV, Muzii L, et al. GnRH analogs versus expectant management in minimal and mild endometriosis-associated infertility. Acta Eur Fertil 1994;25:37–41.
66. Olive DL, Lee KL. Analysis of sequential treatment protocols for endometriosis-associated infertility. Am J Obstet Gynecol 1986;154:613–619.
67. Olive DL, Martin DC. Treatment of endometriosis-associated infertility with CO_2 laser laparoscopy: the use of one- and two-parameter exponential models. Fertil Steril 1987;48:18.
68. Guzick DS, Rock JA. A comparison of danazol and conservative surgery for the treatment of infertility due to mild or moderate endometriosis. Fertil Steril 1983;40:580.
69. Kodama H, Fukuda J, Karube H, et al. Benefit of in vitro fertilization for endometriosis associated infertility. Fertil Steril 1996;66:974–979.
70. Adamson GD, Pasta DJ. Surgical treatment of endometriosis-associated infertility: meta-analysis compared with survival analysis. Am J Obstet Gynecol 1994;171:1488–1505.
71. Donnez J, Nisolle M, Clerckx F, et al. Evaluation of preoperative use of danazol, gestrinone, lynestrenol, buserelin spray, and buserelin implant, in the treatment of endometriosis associated infertility. Prog Clin Biol Res 1990;323:427–442.
72. Wheeler JM, Malinak LR. Postoperative danazol therapy in infertility patients with severe endometriosis. Fertil Steril 1990;53:407–410.
73. Telimaa S, Puolakka J, Ronnberg L, et al. Placebo-controlled comparison of danazol and high-dose medroxyprogesterone acetate in the treatment of endometriosis. Gynecol Endocrinol 1987;1:13–23.
74. Chong AP, Keene ME, Thornton NL. Comparison of three modes of treatment for infertility patients with minimal pelvic endometriosis. Fertil Steril 1990;53:407–410.
75. Fedele L, Bianchi S, Marchini M, et al. Superovulation with human menopausal gonadotropins in the treatment of infertility associated with minimal or mild endometriosis: a controlled randomized study. Fertil Steril 1992;58:28–31.
76. Simpson CW, Taylor PJ, Collins JA. A comparison of ovulation suppression and ovulation stimulation in the treatment of endometriosis-associated infertility. Int J Gynaecol Obstet 1992;57:597–600.
77. Kemmann E, Ghazi D, Corsan G, et al. Does ovulation stimulation improve fertility in women with minimal/mild endometriosis after laser laparoscopy? Int J Fertil Menopausal Stud 1993;38:16–21.
78. Soliman S, Davis S, Collins J, et al. A randomized trial of in vitro fertilization versus conventional treatment for infertility. Fertil Steril 1993;59:1239–1244.
79. Sutton CJG, Ewen SP, Whitelaw N, et al. Prospective, randomized, double-blind, controlled trial of laser laparoscopy in the treatment of pelvic pain associated with minimal, mild, and moderate endometriosis. Fertil Steril 1994;62:696–700.
80. Kauppila A, Ronnberg L. Naproxen sodium in dysmenorrhea secondary to endometriosis. Obstet Gynecol 1985;65:379–383.
81. Owens PR. Prostaglandin synthetase inhibitors in the treatment of primary dysmenorrhea: outcome trials reviewed. Am J Obstet Gynecol 1984;148:96.
82. Olive DL. Medical treatment: alternatives to danazol. In: Endometriosis: Contemporary Concepts in Clinical Management. RS Schenken (ed.). Philadelphia: Lippincott, 1989:189–211.

83. Koike H, Egawa H, Ohtsuka T, et al. Correlation between dysmenorrheic severity and prostaglandin production in women with endometriosis. Prostaglandins Leukot Essent Fatty Acids 1992;46:133.
84. Bayer SR, Siebel MM, Saffan DS, et al. Efficacy of danazol treatment for minimal endometriosis in infertile women: a prospective, randomized study. J Reprod Med 1988;33:179–183.
85. Dmowski WP, Kapetanakis E, Scommegna A. Variable effects of danazol on endometriosis at four low-dose levels. Obstet Gynecol 1982;59:408.
86. Bayer SR, Seibel MM. Medical treatment: Danazol. In: Endometriosis: Contemporary Concepts in Clinical Management. RS Schenken (ed.). Lippincott: Philadelphia, 1989:169–187.
87. Gunning JE, Moyer D. The effect of medroxyprogesterone acetate on endometriosis in the human female. Fertil Steril 1967;18:759–774.
88. Vercellini P, Cortesi I, Crosignani PG. Progestins for symptomatic endometriosis: a critical analysis of the evidence. Fertil Steril 1997;68:393–401.
89. Kettel LM, Murphy AA, Morales AJ, et al. Treatment of endometriosis with the antiprogesterone mifepristone (RU 486). Fertil Steril 1996;65:23–28.
90. Adamson GD, Kwei L, Edgren RA. Pain of endometriosis: effects of nafarelin and danazol therapy. Int J Fertil Menopausal Stud 1994;39(4):215–217.
91. Rock JA, Truglia JA, Caplan RJ. Zoladex endometriosis study group. Zoladex (goserelin acetate implant) in the treatment of endometriosis: a randomized comparison with danazol. Obstet Gynecol 1993;82:198–205.
92. Dawood MY. Considerations in selecting appropriate medical therapy for endometriosis. Int J Gynecol Obstet 1993;40(suppl):S29–S42.
93. Hurst BS, Schlaff WD. Treatment options for endometriosis: medical therapies. Infertil Reprod Clin North Am 1992;3:645–655.
94. Bergqvist IA. Hormonal regulation of endometriosis and the rationales and effects of gonadotrophin-releasing hormone agonist treatment: a review. Human Reprod 1995;10(2):446–452.
95. Barbieri RL. Hormone treatment of endometriosis: the estrogen threshold hypothesis. Am J Obstet Gynecol 1992;166:740–745.
96. Olive DL, Schwartz LB. Endometriosis. N Engl J Med 1993;328(24):1759–1769.
97. Cosignani PG, Vercellini P, Biffignandi F, et al. Laparoscopy versus laparotomy in conservative surgical treatment for severe endometriosis. Fertil Steril 1996;66:70.
98. Koninckx PR, Lesaffre E, Meulaman C, et al. Suggestive evidence that endometriosis is a progressive disease, whereas deeply infiltrating endometriosis is associated with pelvic pain. Fertil Steril 1991;55:759–765.
99. Waller KG, Shaw RW. Gonadotropin-releasing hormone analogues for the treatment of endometriosis: long-term follow-up. Fertil Steril 1993;59:511.
100. The Nafarelin European Endometriosis Trial Group. Nafarelin for endometriosis: a large-scale danazol-controlled trial of efficacy and safety, with 1-year follow-up. Fertil Steril 1992;57:514.
101. Schmidt CL. Endometriosis: a reappraisal of pathogenesis and treatment. Fertil Steril 1985;44:157–173.
102. Wheeler JM, Malinak LR. Recurrent endometriosis: incidence, management, and prognosis. Am J Obstet Gynecol 1983;146:247–253.
103. Thom MH, Studd JW. Procedures in practice. Hormonal implantation. Br Med J 1980;280:848–850.
104. Malinak LR. Proceedings of the ICI conference on endometriosis, Cambridge, 1989. Cranforth, UK: Parthenon, 1990.
105. Reimnitz C, Brand E, Nieberg RK, et al. Malignancy arising in endometriosis associated with unopposed estrogen replacement. Obstet Gynecol 1988;71:444.
106. Heaps JM, Nieberg RK, Berek JS. Malignant neoplasms arising in endometriosis. Obstet Gynecol 1990;75:1023.

CHAPTER 14

Preconception Evaluation and Counseling

Justin P. Lavin, Jr. and John Stewart, Jr.

Preconception counseling began in an attempt to improve the pregnancy outcomes of women with diabetes and has expanded to include patients with myriad other disorders, and ideally, all patients (1–5). Because 50% of pregnancies are unplanned, annual gynecologic or "well-woman" exams offer an optimal opportunity to begin the process of preconception care and education. As the patient begins to contemplate pregnancy more seriously, or if specific problems develop, the counseling can become somewhat more formal and substantially more detailed. This affords the health care provider the opportunity to detect problems that may compromise maternal–fetal well-being in subsequent pregnancies and to initiate appropriate therapeutic interventions. It also provides an opportunity to encourage the adoption of recommended lifestyle changes.

Preconception counseling should encourage a healthy lifestyle, including proper nutrition and at least moderate exercise (2, 6). A detailed reproductive history should be obtained, including menarche, menstrual history, and prior pregnancy outcomes. Particular attention should be paid to modes of delivery, types of anesthesia, and pregnancy-related complications, such as early or repetitive pregnancy loss, ectopic pregnancy, pre-eclampsia, abruption, placenta previa, premature labor, premature rupture of membranes, intrauterine growth restriction (IUGR), isoimmunization, congenital anomalies, or stillbirths. If problems are uncovered, more detailed discussion and planning may be indicated.

The age of both prospective parents should be determined. The association between advanced maternal age and increased risk of fetal aneuploidy should be discussed. Paternal age in the fifth and sixth decades has been associated with the occurrence of new dominant single gene mutations.

The general health history should emphasize diseases and disorders that may lead to adverse maternal or fetal outcomes. The patient should be specifically queried regarding past surgeries, hospitalizations, hypertension, diabetes, cardiac disorders, pulmonary problems such as asthma, and thyroid or other endocrine diseases.

Inadequately controlled pregestational diabetes, phenylketonuria, and congenital adrenal hyperplasia are associated with fetal or newborn malformation and dysfunction (7–9). A complete discussion of the complex therapy of these disorders is beyond the scope of this chapter, but suggestions for corrective action prior to pregnancy are outlined in Table 14.1.

Medications should be reviewed so more appropriate agents may be substituted for known or strongly suspected teratogens (10). Smoking, alcohol abuse, or illegal drug use should be determined and addressed. See Chapter 19 for techniques to assist patients in lifestyle modification. Inquiry should be made regarding prior infectious diseases, including sexually transmitted diseases (STDs), hepatitis, tuberculosis, toxoplasmosis, or cytomegalovirus. HIV screening should be offered to all women contemplating pregnancy (2). The vaccination history should be ascertained. If there is any question, rubella and hepatitis B immunity status can be verified, and if the patient is not immune, vaccination encouraged (2).

TABLE 14.1

Preconception Treatment of Maternal Diseases to Minimize Risk of Associated Fetal or Newborn Malformations and Dysfunction

Pregestational Diabetes
Diet and exercise and insulin therapies to maintain
- Fasting glucose <95 mg/dL
- Postprandial glucose values either
  1 hour <140 mg/dL *or*
  2 hour <120 mg/dL
- Normal glycosylated hemoglobin

Phenylketonuria
Phenylalanine-restricted diet to achieve phenylalanine level <300 μmol/L

Congenital Adrenal Hyperplasia
Steroid replacement therapy, usually with dexamethasone

Next, a genetic history should be obtained. Discussion of family history, ethnic origin, and genetic testing can require extreme patience and tact. Some couples regard prior abnormal outcomes with a sense of guilt or failure. Not infrequently, relevant facts have been hidden from others for years. Discussions should be nonjudgmental, and most authorities recommend nondirectional counseling. The patient and her husband should be questioned to determine if there is any family history of structural anomaly, metabolic disease, chromosomal abnormality, mental retardation, repetitive abortion, stillbirth, or severe neonatal disease. It is often useful to refresh the patient's memory by specifically mentioning some of the more common disorders outlined in Table 14.2.

The majority of U.S. women are employed outside the home, and it is pertinent to ascertain specifics of a woman's profession. Inquiry should include the physical requirements of her job, and if there are any unusual risks or teratogenic exposures, these should be addressed (11). A similar history should be obtained regarding any risky avocations. Chapter 26 reviews occupational and environmental exposures and their effects on gynecologic conditions including fertility, abortion, and pregnancy.

PRECONCEPTION SCREENING FOR RISK OF GENETIC FETAL DISORDERS

During the last decade, advancements in molecular biology have made screening for a myriad of genetic disorders possible. Usually, either direct DNA analysis or linkage analysis by restriction fragment length is employed. At present, testing for most diseases is usually only offered to couples with a positive family history for that specific disease. Some screens are also offered based on ethnicity, as detailed later. Disorders for which screening is currently carried out relatively commonly include cystic fibrosis, Tay-Sachs disease, hemoglobin disorders, Duchenne's dystrophy, most forms of hemophilia, Huntington's chorea, adrenal 21-hydroxylase deficiency, and adult-onset polycystic kidney disease.

The U.S. National Institutes of Health funds a website listing the Genetests database of disorders for which testing is available by DNA analysis. For some conditions, individuals with a large variety of mutations can manifest the same clinical disease, making screening technically difficult and less accurate. Obstetricians will usually want to enlist the aid of a geneticist or genetic counselor to assist with the care of these higher-risk women.

TABLE 14.2

Conditions Associated With Genetic Risk or Teratogenic Potential

Maternal History	
Age ≥35 years	Diabetes
Repetitive abortion	Phenylketonuria
Medications	Congenital adrenal hyperplasia
Substance abuse	
Family History	
Chromosomal Disorders	
Trisomy 21	Trisomy 13
Trisomy 18	Translocations
Metabolic Disorders	
Cystic fibrosis	Tay-Sachs disease
Duchenne muscular dystrophy	Hemoglobinopathies
Thalassemias	
Structural Abnormalities	
Cardiac malformations	Gastroschisis
Neural tube defects	Omphalocele
Hydrocephalus	Skeletal dysplasias
Renal or bladder anomalies	
Miscellaneous	
Family history of mental retardation	

Cystic Fibrosis

In 2001, the American College of Obstetricians and Gynecologists (ACOG) suggested new guidelines for cystic fibrosis carrier screening (12). In contradistinction to other diseases in which testing is usually offered only to couples with a positive family history, ACOG recommended "offering" cystic fibrosis carrier screening not only to individuals with a family history of cystic fibrosis and the reproductive partners of individuals who have cystic fibrosis, but also to couples in whom one or both members are Caucasian and are planning a pregnancy or seeking prenatal care. ACOG also recommended "making available" cystic fibrosis carrier screening to individuals in other racial ethnic groups who are at lower risk and in whom the test may be less sensitive. "Offering" was defined as nonphysician office staff providing information such as a standardized brochure with the recommendation that the information be considered, followed by a discussion with the provider during which the patient is given the opportunity to ask questions and the provider documents the patient's decision. "Make available" was defined as providing the same information but not necessarily following up with a discussion regarding the patient's decision unless the patient has questions. Disease prevalence and carrier risks before and after testing are outlined in Table 14.3.

Cystic fibrosis screening should only be carried out in a laboratory with documented expertise with this test, and the practitioner must provide the laboratory with sufficient demographic data to allow for appropriate interpretation of the results. Because of the complex nature of prenatal diagnosis of cystic fibrosis, if a patient and her partner are identified to be carriers for cystic fibrosis or if there is a family history, most physicians would be well advised to involve a geneticist to assist the couple with decisions regarding prenatal diagnosis.

TABLE 14.3

Cystic Fibrosis Risks for Racial and Ethnic Groups

		Carrier Risk	
Racial/Ethnic Group	Incidence of Cystic Fibrosis	Before Screen	With Negative Screen
Whites	1:3300	1:29	1:140
Ashkenazi Jews	1:3300	1:29	1:930
Hispanics	1:8000–9000	1:44	1:101
African Americans	1:15,300	1:62	1:207
Asian Americans	1:32,100	1:90	Uncertain

Hemoglobinopathies

Persons of Mediterranean, African, Asian, Indian, and Pakistani descent are at increased risk for abnormalities of hemoglobin structure or function, particularly sickle cell disease and alpha and beta thalassemias (13). Initial attempts at screening for hemoglobin disorders in the United States were largely confined to the use of solubility tests such as the Sickledex for the detection of hemoglobin S. The ever-widening ethnic diversity of the American population and the resultant presence of other abnormalities of hemoglobin formation have led to the realization that this limited approach is no longer sufficient. Although a complete discussion of hemoglobin disorders is beyond the scope of this chapter, women at risk should be tested with a complete blood count (CBC). Individuals of Asian or Mediterranean descent who are found to have a hemoglobin less than 11 g/dL, an MCV less than 80 fl, or an MCH less than 27% with normal iron stores should undergo a hemoglobin electrophoresis. All women of African descent should undergo a hemoglobin electrophoresis. If a woman is found to have an abnormal hemoglobin type or hemoglobin A_2 greater than 3.5%, her partner should be tested. Women of Asian descent with the CBC abnormalities listed previously should be offered DNA testing for alpha globulin abnormalities. Of the alpha thalassemia syndromes, the most severe is hydrops fetalis. If a patient is found to have alpha thalassemia, her partner should be tested to determine if he is also positive (13). See Figure 14.1 for a flowchart for testing at-risk populations.

If the couple is found to be at risk for a hemoglobin disorder, or if a woman is at risk and her partner refuses to be tested, prenatal diagnosis by amniocentesis or chorionic villus sampling for DNA analysis should be offered in any ensuing pregnancies.

Tay-Sachs Disease

Individuals of Ashkenazi Jewish, French Canadian, and Cajun descent have a higher risk for Tay-Sachs disease, which is an autosomal recessive disorder caused by a deficiency of the Hex-A form of the enzyme hexosaminidase. This abnormality leads to a lysosomal storage disorder that can result in severe neurologic disease and death in early childhood. Individuals of Eastern European Jewish descent (Ashkenazi Jews) have been reported to have a carrier frequency of 1 in 30. The carrier frequency in the non-Jewish population has been found to be 1 in 300. Gravidas of French-Canadian and Cajun descent have also been reported to have elevated carrier frequencies. Serum screening tests are available for preconception evaluation. Hex-A activity in noncarriers is generally more than 60% and in carriers is usually less than 55%. Carrier screening during pregnancy or while taking oral contraceptives is less accurate, with a higher false-positive rate. Leukocyte testing can be performed in these situations or when serum testing is inconclusive. DNA testing for the α-subunit gene for Tay-Sachs disease is also available but should be reserved for couples who consistently have inconclusive results on serum and leukocyte testing.

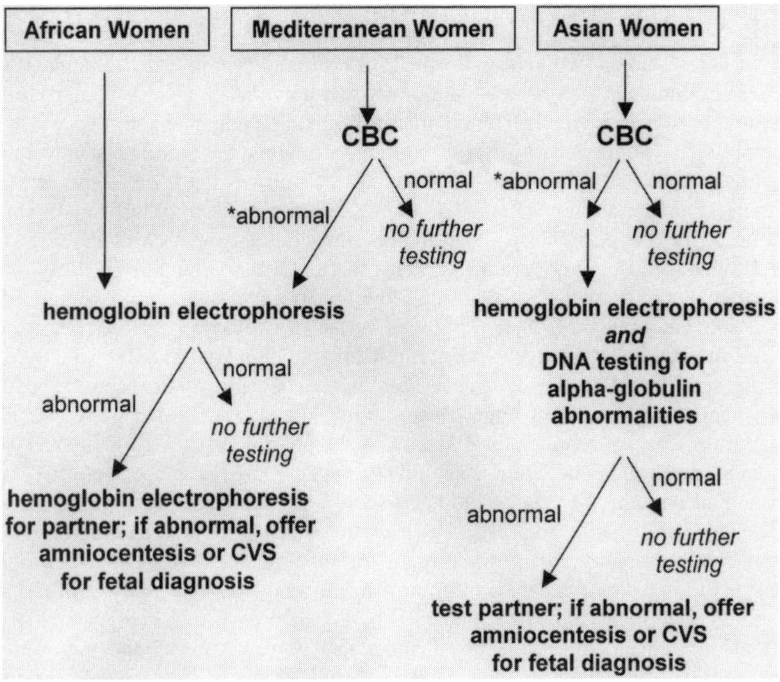

FIGURE 14.1 ● Protocol for prenatal screening for common disorders of hemoglobin formation and function. Women of African, Asian (including the Southeast Asia countries of India and Pakistan), and Mediterranean descent are at higher risk for hemoglobinopathies and their carrier states. CBC, complete blood count, including red blood cell indices. CVS, chorionic villous sampling. *Any of these constitutes an abnormality: hemoglobin <11 g/dL, MCV <80 fl, or MCH <27% with normal iron stores.

ACOG has recommended serum screening of couples from high-risk groups or with a positive family history (14). If only one member of the couple is at high risk, he or she should be screened, and the partner tested only if the screen is positive. Ambiguous results or positive tests in individuals not at high risk should be confirmed by molecular analysis. If both members of a couple test positive, genetic counseling and prenatal diagnosis should be offered.

Neural Tube Defects

Known risk factors for neural tube defects (NTDs) include diabetes mellitus, use of anticonvulsants (whether for seizures or a psychiatric disorder), and family history (first- or second-degree relative diagnosed with a NTD). Only 5% of NTDs occur in families with a positive family history. The daily ingestion of 4 mg of folic acid during the first trimester has been linked to a reduction in the occurrence of NTDs among infants of women at increased risk to conceive a fetus with these malformations. Therefore, 4 mg of folic acid should be prescribed for high-risk women. The use of 0.4 mg of folic acid has been associated with a 50% reduction in NTDs among the infants of families not believed to have an increased risk for NTDs (15). For low-risk women then, folic acid supplementation of 400 μg/day is currently recommended because nutritional sources alone are insufficient. Higher levels of supplementation should not be achieved by taking excess multivitamins because of the risk of vitamin A toxicity. There is limited evidence to indicate that folic acid supplementation may not decrease the risk of NTDs in women with high first-trimester blood glucose levels or high first-trimester maternal temperature, or in women who take valproic acid. NTDs associated with aneuploidy or genetic syndromes are not prevented by folic acid.

PRECONCEPTION PHYSICAL EXAMINATION

A physical examination should be performed with particular attention to findings associated with pre-existing or undiagnosed disease that may suggest potential pregnancy-related problems. Vital signs should be determined. The blood pressure should be obtained with the patient in a seated position after 5–10 minutes of rest. For bedridden patients, the blood pressure can be taken in the left lateral recumbent position, with the patient's arm at the level of the heart. To reduce inaccurate readings, an appropriate size cuff should be used. The cuff length should be 1.5 times the upper arm circumference or should surround at least 80% of the circumference of the arm to avoid falsely high readings; a cuff that is too large may give falsely low readings. The patient should not use tobacco or caffeine for 30 minutes preceding the measurement. A mercury sphygmomanometer is preferable to the use of validated electronic devices. In patients with cardiovascular disease risk factors or in whom the blood pressure is found to be abnormal, blood pressure should be measured at several visits to develop a more accurate baseline.

In patients with diabetes or hypertension, funduscopic examination should be performed to assess the presence of retinopathy. Because of the possible association between gum disease and premature labor, dental hygiene should be evaluated (16). The neck should be checked for goiter and adenopathy. The lungs and heart should be evaluated. In patients with asthma, any baseline wheezing should be noted, and similarly, in patients with cardiac disease, any rales suggestive of pulmonary edema should be carefully evaluated. A systolic murmur grade 3/6 or greater in intensity, a diastolic murmur, cardiomegaly, a persistently split S_2, a persistent arrhythmia, or an increased P_2 accompanied by left parasternal shift (suggestive of pulmonary hypertension) suggests the presence of underlying cardiac disease and the need for further evaluation. Additional signs of cardiac disease include clubbing, cyanosis, and persistent jugular venous distension.

The abdomen should be evaluated and a pelvic examination performed. During a preconception examination, pay particular attention to uterine enlargement and evidence of abnormal cervical architecture or prior damage, and determine the configuration and size of the maternal pelvic bones. Uterine enlargement suggests the need to rule out uterine malformation or myomas. Cervical anomalies may suggest that ultrasonic evaluation of the cervix during pregnancy or cerclage may be appropriate (17). If an adnexal mass is detected, it should be evaluated and, if necessary, treated prior to conception. A Pap smear should be performed. We encourage patients with abnormal Pap smears to delay pregnancy until they can be properly evaluated (18). Testing for gonorrhea and chlamydia infections should be performed in at-risk populations.

The spine and extremities should be evaluated. Particular attention should be paid to any postural abnormalities or deformities that may be aggravated by pregnancy or that may complicate delivery. In some cases, orthopedic or anesthesia consultation may be desired. The deep tendon reflexes should be recorded to provide a baseline in the event that pre-eclampsia develops in subsequent pregnancy.

PRECONCEPTION COUNSELING FOR SPECIFIC CONDITIONS

Recurrent Early Pregnancy Loss

This entity has traditionally been defined as three consecutive pregnancy losses (usually before 12 weeks gestation). It is currently recognized that the 25 to 30% prevalence of recurrence after two consecutive early pregnancy losses is very similar to that encountered after three consecutive losses, and many clinicians may initiate an evaluation for recurrent early pregnant loss (REPL) after two or more consecutive early losses (19). Approximately 2 to 4% of couples with recurrent pregnancy loss have one partner with a genetically balanced structural chromosome rearrangement. Balanced translocations account for the largest percentage of these karyotypic abnormalities. Genetic karyotyping of both partners is recommended in couples suffering from REPL.

The presence of antiphospholipid antibodies in a woman is associated with REPL (20). These autoantibodies may arise de novo or in association with other autoimmune diseases such as systemic lupus erythematosus (SLE). There are two antiphospholipid antibodies for which clinical assays are widely available: lupus anticoagulant and anticardiolipin antibodies. Lupus anticoagulant, despite its name, is associated with clinical thrombosis, not bleeding. It is detected in plasma by using the activated partial thromboplastin time, Russell viper venom time, or kaolin clotting time. The presence of these antibodies causes prolongation of the laboratory test leading to its misnomer as an anticoagulant. Anticardiolipin antibodies are detected by conventional immunoassays. Results are reported as GPL (IgG anticardiolipin), MPL (IgM anticardiolipin), and APL (IgA anticardiolipin) in semiquantitative terms (negative, low positive, medium positive, or high positive). A consensus has been reached that anticardiolipin antibodies are associated with REPL, but there is currently some conflict in the literature as to exactly which subgroup of patients with these antibodies should receive treatment (20).

A variety of treatments for antiphospholipid syndrome, including aspirin alone, aspirin and prednisone, or aspirin and heparin, have been proposed. Because of the increased prevalence of preterm premature rupture of membranes (PPROM) associated with the use of prednisone, its use is not recommended. During pregnancy, women with APL benefit from treatment with low-dose aspirin and heparin, using dosages in the range of 10,000 to 25,000 U/d (19).

Other inherited thrombophilias associated with REPL include factor V Leiden mutation, prothrombin G20210A mutation, homozygosity for the 4G/4G mutation in the plasminogen activator inhibitor, the thermolabile variant of methylenetetrahydrofolate reductase (C677T MTHFR), and autosomal dominant deficiencies of antithrombin, protein C, and protein S (21). At present, there is not a consensus on the prevention of REPL by treatment of these entities. Clinicians may employ supplemental folate in a dose of 4 mg daily to reverse the hyperhomocysteinemia associated with the C677T MTHFR mutation and heparin for the other disorders.

Women with a prior uterine surgery or infection, and women with a suspected uterine malformation may benefit from hysterosalpingogram or hysteroultrasound to evaluate uterine anatomy and rule out Asherman syndrome. Controversy exists over the relationship of Ureaplasma or mycoplasma uterine infection with REPL, and whether testing and treating confers benefit. The diagnosis of luteal phase defect and its association with REPL is also controversial; evaluation for this disorder should be reserved for patients with a suggestive history.

A majority (approximately 50 to 75%) of couples with recurrent pregnancy loss will have no certain diagnosis. Although the number of previous pregnancy losses and maternal age influences the likelihood of successful pregnancy, it is estimated that 60 to 70% of women with unexplained recurrent pregnancy loss will have a successful next pregnancy (19).

Prior Unexplained Stillbirth

Women who have experienced a prior stillbirth are naturally anxious regarding the probability that this tragedy will recur. When a definable underlying cause such as pre-eclampsia, abruption, or chromosomal or structural anomaly has been identified, the patient can be counseled with specific data related to recurrence rate for her disorder as outlined elsewhere in this chapter. Many women present with a history of unexplained stillbirth. Given the absence of an explanation, they are perhaps even more anxious. Weeks and associates (22) evaluated 300 such women using an antepartum testing scheme consisting of either weekly contraction stress tests or semiweekly modified biophysical profile (nonstress test and amniotic fluid index) and reported only one case of recurrent stillbirth. Abnormal and equivocal results led to delivery prior to 36 weeks in four (1.3%) of the women and after 36 weeks in 35 (11.7%) of the women. The authors recommended the initiation of antepartum fetal testing at 32 weeks. Most women find these data extremely reassuring. Some practitioners follow this scheme with the slight modification of initiating antepartum testing 1 week prior to the gestational age at which the patient experienced her prior stillbirth if that has occurred at 28 to 32 weeks' gestation. For a woman with a clear-cut explanation for her prior stillbirth, following a standard disease-specific testing scheme is recommended.

Pre-Eclampsia and Eclampsia

Pre-eclampsia complicates 5 to 8% of pregnancies. Fortunately, eclampsia is much less common. Because of the frightening aspects of this disorder, many women present with questions regarding recurrence risks. Due to the more subjective nature of the diagnosis of mild pre-eclampsia, it is very difficult to find precise data regarding recurrence rates. Chesley (23) followed 225 women with eclampsia and reported that 50% developed recurrent hypertension in subsequent pregnancies. Interestingly, women who experienced eclampsia in their first pregnancy only had a 33% prevalence of hypertension in subsequent pregnancies. Most women had mild disease in subsequent pregnancies, but 5% experienced recurrent eclampsia.

Sibai et al. (24) followed 409 women with severe pre-eclampsia–eclampsia in their first pregnancy and reported that the prevalence of severe pre-eclampsia was 25.9% in second pregnancies and 12.2% in all subsequent pregnancies. These rates were significantly higher than the corresponding 4.6% and 5.0% prevalences of pre-eclampsia experienced by controls (who were normotensive in first pregnancy). A second report from the same institution described 108 women who had severe pre-eclampsia in the second trimester (25). Subsequent pregnancies were complicated by pre-eclampsia in 65% of the patients, and by the second trimester, pre-eclampsia in 21% of these women. These data suggest that earlier onset of disease may confer a higher recurrence risk.

In separate publications, Sullivan et al. (26) and Sibai et al. (27) evaluated recurrence risks among women with HELLP (hemolysis, elevated liver enzymes, and low platelets) syndrome. Sullivan et al. (26) reported some type of hypertensive disorder complicated 48% of 195 subsequent pregnancies, and 27% were affected by recurrent HELLP syndrome. Sibai et al. (27) studied a population of women experiencing HELLP syndrome and subdivided them into two groups, 139 previously normotensive women and 13 chronic hypertensives. The first group experienced 192 subsequent pregnancies with 19% and 3% rates of pre-eclampsia and HELLP, respectively. The second group experienced 20 subsequent pregnancies with corresponding rates of 75% pre-eclampsia and 55% HELLP. This group also experienced quite high rates of other complications, including IUGR (45%), abruption (20%), and perinatal death (40%).

A large number of pharmacologic agents and dietary supplements, including aspirin, calcium, magnesium, zinc, and fish oil have been employed in attempts to lower the occurrence of pre-eclampsia. To date, the consensus of most of the medical community is that these agents are not effective in accomplishing that goal (28). Therefore, frequent prenatal visits may be required to identify early signs and symptoms of developing pre-eclampsia, and to hopefully allow effective intervention.

Women with pre-eclampsia–eclampsia often inquire as to whether they will be more likely to develop hypertension in later life. In his 40-year follow-up of women with eclampsia in their first pregnancy, Chesley et al. (29) observed no increase in chronic hypertension or cardiovascular mortality. In contrast, women who were eclamptic in later pregnancies were at substantially increased risk for these complications. Among the severe pre-eclamptic–eclamptic women followed for a minimum of 2 years in Sibai et al.'s series (24), 14.8% developed chronic hypertension compared with 5.6% of controls. Among the women who developed severe pre-eclampsia in the second trimester, after an average 5.4-year follow-up, 35% had developed chronic hypertension (25). In findings very similar to those of Chesley et al., Sibai et al. (25) observed that if the women developed recurrent severe pre-eclampsia in the second trimester, the prevalence of chronic hypertension was 67% as opposed to 4% among those who remained normotensive.

Abruptio Placenta

Abruption occurs in 0.49 to 1.29% of pregnancies with a mean prevalence of 0.83% (30). This disorder represents a life-threatening condition for both mother and fetus, and therefore, generates significant concern. Unfortunately, the prevalence of abruption is approximately tenfold higher among woman who experienced a prior abruption. Rates of 5.5 to 16.6% have been reported. The corresponding risk after two abruptions increases to 25%. Because of the extremely strong correlation between cigarette smoking and abruption, encouraging smoking cessation among these women is mandatory. Because of the reluctance of many women who abuse illicit drugs to reveal this information to their health care providers, and the association between the use of cocaine and abruptio placenta (31), inquiries about domestic violence and warnings against participation in activities associated with a high probability of physical trauma are also warranted.

Placenta Previa

The prevalence of placenta previa averages 0.5%. Clark summarized the literature regarding risk factors associated with the occurrence of placenta previa and reported that a history of a previous placenta previa is associated with an eight-fold relative risk (30). A previous cesarean is associated with a relative risk of 1.5 to 15, and a prior suction curettage for a voluntary pregnancy termination carries a 1.5-fold increase in risk. Smoking is associated with a 1.4- to 3.0-fold increase in prevalence. Just as with abruption, particular attention should be directed toward encouraging smoking cessation in this population. Because of the strong association between placenta previa in a scarred uterus and placenta accreta or percreta, women with a prior cesarean and a placenta previa should be evaluated with Doppler (and possibly magnetic resonance scanning) to prepare for and minimize complications at repeat cesarean.

PRECONCEPTION COUNSELING FOR SPECIFIC MATERNAL MEDICAL DISORDERS

The following sections detail preconception counseling for women with chronic hypertension, pregestational diabetes, cardiovascular disease, seizure disorders, asthma, renal disease, and SLE. Table 14.4 provides a more general checklist for preconception counseling of women with other medical conditions.

TABLE 14.4

Checklist for Preconception Counseling of Women With Medical Disorders

Effects of pregnancy on the mother's disease and long-term health
Effects of the mother's disease on the pregnancy
Effects of the mother's disease on the fetus
- Possible genetic risk
- Other risks (e.g., early pregnancy loss, intrauterine growth restriction, stillbirth)

Effects of maternal medications on the fetus
Preconception and antepartum care
- Appropriate lifestyle changes
- Possible dietary changes
- Medication changes
- Laboratory or other diagnostic procedures prior to pregnancy
- Frequency of prenatal visits
- Other types of testing required

Management of labor and delivery
Breast-feeding issues
Possible postpartum problems
Contraceptive options
Long-term health implications and planning

Chronic Hypertension

Approximately 1 to 5% of pregnant women are affected by chronic hypertension (32–34). Women with chronic hypertension are at increased risk for cardiovascular complications, pre-eclampsia (particularly if they have underlying renal disease, hypertension for more than 4 years, or pre-eclampsia in a prior pregnancy), abruption, and cesarean delivery. Their offspring exhibit increased rates of growth restriction and perinatal mortality. When proteinuria accompanies hypertension, it suggests underlying renal disease and increased risk for adverse neonatal outcome irrespective of the development of pre-eclampsia (34). A more recent report from the National High Blood Pressure Education Program Working Group on High Blood Pressure in Pregnancy emphasized that most hypertensive pregnant women have essential hypertension, which is usually stage 1 or 2 (systolic pressure 140 to 179 mm Hg or diastolic pressure 90 to 109 mm Hg) (32). If they possess normal renal function, these patients are at low risk to experience the acute cardiovascular consequences of hypertension during pregnancy, and the outcomes for their neonates are usually good.

Woman with chronic hypertension should be evaluated before conception to ascertain potentially reversible causes and possible end organ involvement (e.g., heart or kidney). Particularly, young patients and women with severe hypertension (stage 3, systolic pressure greater than or equal to 180 mm Hg or diastolic pressure greater than 110 mm Hg) are more likely to have secondary hypertension (hypertension due to, e.g., primary renal disease, renovascular hypertension, primary aldosteronism, Cushing syndrome, or pheochromocytoma) and should be evaluated for reversible causes. Women younger than 30 years of age with severe hypertension and no family history of hypertension may warrant Doppler flow studies or magnetic resonance angiography to detect renal artery stenosis. (Negative results from renal ultrasonography do not rule out renal artery stenosis.)

Women with a history of hypertension for several years should be evaluated for target organ damage. Specifically, they should be assessed for left ventricular hypertrophy, ischemic heart disease, retinopathy, and renal disease. Evaluation of such patients may include electrocardiogram, echocardiogram, retinal examination, serum electrolytes, blood urea nitrogen and creatinine, urinalysis, 24-hour urine for protein and creatinine clearance, and renal ultrasound. If abnormalities are detected, referral to an appropriate subspecialist may be warranted.

The risk of fetal loss and accelerated deterioration of maternal renal disease is increased if the patient's serum creatinine is greater than or equal to 1.4 mg/dL. In addition, the risk of fetal loss is elevated ten-fold if maternal hypertension is poorly controlled (32). Therefore, it is important to attempt to adequately control hypertension prior to conception. There is little evidence that patients with stage 1 or 2 hypertension derive maternal or fetal benefit from pharmacologic control of their blood pressure during pregnancy (32, 34). Therefore, many clinicians currently withhold or discontinue pharmacologic antihypertensive therapy, and only start or reinstitute it if the patient blood pressure levels exceed a threshold of 150 to 160 mm Hg systolic or 100 to 110 mm Hg diastolic. Patients with stage 3 disease, with hypertension for several years, with evidence of target organ damage, or who present on a regimen of multiple agents should be started or continued on pharmacologic therapy.

Women with mild hypertension (140 to 179 mm Hg systolic or 90 to 109 mm Hg diastolic pressure) generally do well during pregnancy and do not, as a rule, require antihypertensive medication. When therapy is indicated—when blood pressure exceeds 150 to 160 mm Hg systolic or 100 to 110 mm Hg diastolic or in cases of severe chronic hypertension with systolic pressure greater than or equal to 180 mm Hg or diastolic pressure greater than or equal to 110 mm Hg—most clinicians favor methyldopa (Aldomet) as the first-line agent to treat hypertension during pregnancy because of its lack of significant effect on uteroplacental blood flow and long history of use without adverse effect (32). If methyldopa is insufficient, additional agents such as beta-blockers or calcium channel blockers may be employed. Although there may be increased risk of IUGR associated with the use of beta-blockers, particularly atenolol (Tenormin, a selective beta1-blocker), there has been extensive experience with the use of labetalol (an alpha1-beta1-beta2-blocker) during pregnancy, and most experts suggest that the benefits of this medication outweigh its risks in appropriate patients. The use of calcium channel blockers has not been associated with adverse fetal outcome.

The use of diuretics during pregnancy has been controversial because of the possible reduction in plasma volume and secondary decrease in uterine blood flow, and these medications are usually not employed as first-line antihypertensive agents in patients considering pregnancy. More recently, however, based on a review of data from thousands of patients, the National High Blood Pressure Education Program Working Group on High Blood Pressure in Pregnancy concluded that if diuretics are indicated, they are safe and efficacious agents that can markedly potentiate the response to other hypertensive medications, and therefore, are not contraindicated in pregnancy (32).

Angiotensin-converting enzyme (ACE) inhibitors are contraindicated during the second and third trimesters because they frequently engender fetal renal dysfunction, leading to oligohydramnios and secondary pulmonary hypoplasia. ACE inhibitors should usually be discontinued prior to pregnancy.

Pregestational Diabetes

Since the mid-1980s, women with diabetes mellitus (type 1 or 2) receiving state-of-the-art care have been able to contemplate pregnancy with less than a 4% probability of perinatal mortality and, in the absence of coexistent ischemic heart disease, an exceptionally low probability of maternal death (35, 36). It is important for the patient to understand that this is critically dependent on her level of glycemic control. Poor maternal glycemic control is associated with early pregnancy loss, premature labor, major congenital malformations, macrosomia, and perinatal asphyxia (7, 37–39). Congenital anomalies have come to represent the most important cause of perinatal mortality in pregnancy complicated by diabetes, and early care is important for prevention (40). Women with pregestational diabetes who receive intensive treatment before conception experience a 1% prevalence of congenital malformations versus an 8% prevalence among women who do not receive care until after 8 weeks' gestation. The precise level of glycemic control associated with optimal pregnancy outcome is arguable, but most authorities recommend a fasting serum glucose of less than 95 mg/dL and values 1 or 2 hours postprandial of less than 140 mg/dL or less than 120 mg/dL, respectively, or a mean serum glucose of less than 105 mg/dL (37). Because studies have shown a correlation between glycosylated hemoglobin ($HgbA_{1c}$) levels and the prevalence of both congenital anomalies and spontaneous abortion, patients with diabetes should attempt to achieve the levels of glycemic control outlined previously and to have an $HgbA_{1c}$ level of less than 6.5 for 3 months prior to attempting to conceive. To accomplish these goals, a team approach is often required involving the patient, obstetrician, primary medical physician, maternal–fetal medicine specialist, endocrinologist, diabetic educator, dietician, and/or perinatal nurse clinician (41). A well-developed plan of diet and exercise is required. Most women will need to employ home glucose monitoring at least four times daily; for some women, more extensive glucose monitoring will be required. Because insulin requirements may decrease in the early portion of pregnancy and then increase substantially as pregnancy progresses, insulin doses must be frequently adjusted to avoid both hypoglycemia and hyperglycemia. For a patient with diabetes mellitus for more than a few years prior to conception or with any evidence of vascular disease, a baseline 24-hour urine collection analyzed for protein and creatinine clearance, an ophthalmology consultation, and an electrocardiogram are recommended. Women with pregestational diabetes should be made aware of the extensive patient time (including visits, nonstress tests, and ultrasounds) and commitment required to optimally manage their pregnancies. Their increased risks of pre-eclampsia and cesarean section should be noted. The possibilities of fetal macrosomia or growth restriction, as well as neonatal respiratory distress, hypoglycemia, hypocalcemia, and hyperbilirubinemia should also be reviewed.

Women with diabetes often pose questions regarding the effect of their becoming pregnant on the progression of their underlying disease process. After 20 years, approximately 80% of women with diabetes will exhibit some element of retinopathy (42). The prevalence of retinopathy appears to be influenced by the level of long-term glycemic control, and parity is not a risk factor for the development of retinopathy. It is unusual for women without retinopathy to develop proliferative retinopathy during pregnancy. Approximately one-third of women with background retinopathy and one-half of women with proliferative retinopathy will experience progression of their retinopathy during pregnancy. In many, if not most, patients, regression occurs postpartum. Poor glycemic control at the start of pregnancy, rapid establishment of tight glycemic control, and hypertension increase the risk of progression. Diabetics should be advised that if proliferative retinopathy develops or progresses, photocoagulation will be necessary.

Overt diabetic nephropathy affects approximately 30 to 40% of patients, with a peak incidence occurring 16 years after the onset of diabetes (42). It is often preceded for several years by a stage of microalbuminuria. Many patients with diabetes are prescribed ACE inhibitors to delay the development or progression of diabetic nephropathy. For the reasons outlined previously, ACE inhibitors should usually be discontinued during pregnancy. There is a gathering body of evidence that it is relatively safe to continue these medications up to conception, and in severe cases, perhaps even in the first trimester (37). A woman with diabetic nephropathy may be reassured that although she is at increased risk for developing pre-eclampsia and may experience some deterioration of renal function during pregnancy, renal parameters usually return to prepregnancy levels in the postpartum period, and pregnancy does not appear to adversely affect the long-term progression of diabetic nephropathy (42). Some caution is required in counseling patients with a serum creatinine of greater than or equal to 1.4 mg/dL as outlined in the Renal Disease section.

Women with diabetes are at substantially increased risk for atherosclerosis and coronary artery disease. Diabetic women who have suffered a myocardial infarction during pregnancy or the peripartum period have slightly greater than 50% maternal mortality and perinatal mortality rates (42). In more recent years, a few successful pregnancies have been reported in diabetic women who had experienced a prior myocardial infarction; however, even patients with relatively stable cardiac function after a myocardial infarction appear to be at substantially increased risk for adverse cardiac events, including death in subsequent pregnancies (42, 43). Therefore, such women should be advised to very carefully weigh the risks to their own well-being when contemplating pregnancy.

Cardiovascular Disease

Advances in neonatal intensive care and pediatric cardiovascular surgery have allowed a large number of women with congenital cardiac lesions to reach childbearing age. Currently, maternal cardiac disorders complicate approximately 1 to 3% of pregnancies in industrialized nations (44). In general, the patient's prognosis depends on her specific cardiac lesions, her New York Heart Association (NYHA) classification, the occurrence of various complications during pregnancy, and the skill of her health care providers. Much of the data in the literature predate modern cardiovascular and obstetric management, and therefore, is of questionable value in counseling contemporary patients.

More recently, a prospective trial including 562 patients whose 599 pregnancies did not end in abortion and who received care during pregnancy at 13 Canadian cardiac–obstetric teaching centers has been completed (43). In that report, 46% of the mothers had undergone at least one corrective cardiac surgery, and 4% suffered from pulmonary hypertension. Thirteen percent of the 599 pregnancies were complicated by at least one primary cardiac event defined as pulmonary edema, tachyarrhythmia requiring therapy (two not responding to medicine and requiring electrical cardioversion), bradyarrhythmia requiring therapy, embolic stroke, or cardiac death. Six percent of pregnancies were complicated by a defined secondary cardiac event, either worsening of NYHA class by more than two classes or requiring an urgent cardiac procedure within 6 months of delivery. A total of 99 pregnancies (17%) suffered a primary or secondary cardiac event or both.

The authors were able to construct a scoring system in which 1 point was assigned for each of four cardiac predictors:

- Prior cardiovascular event (heart failure, transient ischemic attack, or stroke before pregnancy) or arrhythmia
- Baseline NYHA class greater than II or cyanosis

- Left heart obstruction (mitral valve area less than 2 cm^2, aortic valve area less than 1.5 cm^2, or left ventricular outflow tract gradient greater than 30 mm Hg by echocardiography)
- Systemic ventricular dysfunction (ejection fraction less than 40%) (43)

No patient had a score greater than 3. The risks of a cardiac event in pregnancy were 5%, 27%, and 75% for women with scores of 0 points, 1 point, and greater than 1 point, respectively. All three cardiac deaths occurred among women with scores greater than or equal to 1.

Twenty percent of the pregnancies experienced at least one adverse neonatal event, defined as premature birth, small-for-gestational-age birthweight, respiratory distress syndrome, intraventricular hemorrhage, or fetal or neonatal death (43). Seven percent of the live births were diagnosed with congenital heart disease (excluding those born to mothers with a recognized genetic syndrome).

Five maternal risk factors predicted an adverse neonatal event:

- NYHA class greater than II or cyanosis at baseline prenatal visit
- Use of anticoagulants during pregnancy
- Smoking during pregnancy
- Multiple gestation
- Left heart obstruction (43)

If none of these was present, the fetal or neonatal death rate was 2%; if one or more was present, the rate was 4%.

A complete discussion of counseling for specific cardiac lesions is beyond the scope of this chapter. Pregnancy is usually relatively uncomplicated in patients with NYHA class I or II, atrial septal defect, ventricular septal defect without pulmonary hypertension, patent ductus arteriosis, pulmonic or tricuspid disease, and Marfan's syndrome with undilated aorta (44). Conversely, most authorities consider pregnancy to be relatively contraindicated in patients with pulmonary hypertension, severe cyanosis, severe congestive failure, advanced ischemic heart disease, Marfan's syndrome with aortic dilation, or severe mitral or aortic stenosis. Other cardiac lesions are intermediate in risk.

Patients with peripartum cardiomyopathy in a prior pregnancy frequently present with questions regarding the advisability of conceiving again. A more recent survey of members of the American College of Cardiology revealed experience with 44 women with a history of this disorder who became pregnant again (45). In 28 patients, ventricular function had returned to normal, and in 16, it was persistently abnormal. In their subsequent pregnancies, clinical symptoms of heart failure occurred in 21% of the former and 44% of the latter women. None of the patients with normal ventricular function died, but 19% of those with abnormal left ventricular function died.

The management of women with mechanical prosthetic valves poses a special concern during pregnancy. These patients require continuous long-term anticoagulation with warfarin. They must be advised that warfarin crosses the placenta, and that congenital anomalies occur in approximately 6% of pregnancies with any exposure and 10 to 12% of those pregnancies in which warfarin therapy is continued beyond 6 weeks' gestation (44, 46). The most common congenital anomaly is warfarin embryopathy, consisting of nasal hypoplasia and stippled epiphyses. In addition, warfarin exposure in the third trimester has been associated with fetal intracranial hemorrhage (47). Overall pregnancy outcomes remain poor among women receiving warfarin during pregnancy (46, 47). A more recent publication described 71 patients treated with warfarin during pregnancy and reported that they experienced 23 pregnancy losses and 5 stillbirths (47).

Because of its large molecular weight, heparin does not cross the placenta. Some investigators have advised the use of heparin or, more recently, fractionated heparin in the first trimester to avoid warfarin embryopathy (48). This practice has been associated with increased risks of maternal valve thrombosis, thromboembolic events, and fatality in comparison to continuous therapy with warfarin (44, 46–48). After appropriate discussion, the patient in consort with her physicians must choose a regimen consisting of subcutaneous heparin (or fractionated heparin) throughout pregnancy, warfarin throughout pregnancy, or heparin (or fractionated heparin) in the first trimester followed by warfarin for the remainder of pregnancy. In the warfarin regimens, heparin is substituted for warfarin at term or shortly before delivery to avoid hemorrhagic complications. This is indeed a difficult choice that pits the welfare of the woman against that of her fetus. Physician support and empathy are required and appreciated.

Seizure Disorders

One in 100 to 200 pregnant women suffer from seizures (49). In a more recent survey, 34% of women with seizures reported never receiving advice regarding the interaction of pregnancy with their seizure disorder (50). This is particularly discouraging because preconception counseling appears to lead to improved neonatal outcomes among the infants of mothers with seizure disorders (51).

There are conflicting data regarding the effect of pregnancy on seizure frequency, but most authors report that a substantial proportion of patients experience an increase in seizure frequency (49). This may be related to physiologic changes of pregnancy, resulting in poorer absorption of oral medications, increased volumes of distribution, altered protein binding of drugs, maternal fatigue, and decreased compliance due to nausea and vomiting. Patients who experience frequent seizures should be informed that they are more likely to experience a pregnancy-related increase in seizure activity. They may also require substantial adjustments in their medication dosage. Patients may be reassured that seizure frequency usually returns to prepregnancy levels after pregnancy.

Many women ask if their child will experience seizures. If a mother has idiopathic epilepsy, the risk that her child will develop seizures is 2 to 4% (52). Offspring of a father with epilepsy do not have any increased seizure risk. Since the initial description of fetal hydantoin syndrome by Hanson and Smith in 1975 (53), hundreds of articles have been published that describe various teratogenic effects of anticonvulsants (49, 51, 52). The prospective mother should be informed that malformations have been reported with all but the newest anticonvulsants (there has not yet been widespread use of these agents among pregnant women). Specific syndromes of dysmorphic features have been described for several drugs, including phenytoin (Dilantin), valproic acid (Depakote), and carbamazepine (Tegretol). Almost all involve facial anomalies, and there is wide overlap among the correlations between specific anomalies and various drugs. Cardiac malformations have been reported to result from exposure to all previous medications. Spina bifida has been reported to occur in 1 to 2% of the infants of women receiving valproate and 1% of the infants of women receiving carbamazepine. Hypoplastic nails have been observed in fetuses exposed to phenytoin and carbamazepine. Neonatal hemorrhage due to decreased vitamin K-dependent clotting factors has been reported in infants of mothers exposed to phenobarbital (Luminal), phenytoin, and primidone (Mysoline). A survey of more recent prospective studies of children exposed to anticonvulsants in utero reported dysmorphic features in 11 to 79% and major malformations in 5 to 11% (52). Most, but not all, studies have suggested that the frequency of malformations is lower with monotherapy compared with multiple drug therapy.

The literature is replete with articles suggesting one antiepileptic or another provides greater fetal safety. When reviewed as a body, given the multiple conflicting claims, it is difficult to substantiate that any specific medication is safer than the others. It may also be appropriate to inform prospective mothers taking antiepileptic drugs that there may be an increased prevalence of learning and developmental abnormalities among their offspring (49, 51, 52), although at present the evidence regarding this issue is conflicting. We currently counsel prospective mothers that this remains an unresolved question.

At least several months before conception (and because of difficulties with contraception among women using antiseizure medications, preferably at the beginning of reproductive capacity), a working relationship needs to be developed between the patient, her neurologist, and her obstetrician. Because nearly all anticonvulsants affect folic acid metabolism, the patient should be started on 4 mg of folate daily at least 3 months prior to attempting conception to reduce the risk of NTDs. If the patient has been seizure free for 2 to 5 years, in consultation with her neurologist, it may be appropriate to attempt to withdraw her seizure medications. It is important for the obstetrician to impress on the woman that it is imperative to control her seizures, that this may require the resumption of anticonvulsants, and that pregnancy should be delayed until reasonable control of seizure activity is achieved. If medication is necessary, most authorities recommend attempting monotherapy with the most appropriate drug at the lowest dosage that will adequately control seizures. The use of serum drug levels to adjust dosage is controversial in well-controlled patients but may prove helpful in women with refractory seizures. Some authorities suggest the substitution of lamotrigine for valproate (51, 52), but this is somewhat controversial (49). Others suggest the administration of vitamin K to the mother for several weeks prior to delivery (52). Again, this is somewhat controversial, and many physicians instead choose to treat the infant immediately after birth.

Asthma

The National Asthma Education Program Working Group on Asthma and Pregnancy has suggested that 1 to 4% of pregnant women suffer from asthma (54), and a 6% prevalence has been reported in a large Canadian population-based study (55). Women with asthma should be informed that asthma will remain stable or even improve for most patients in pregnancy (56, 57). Approximately one-third will experience an exacerbation of asthma symptoms during pregnancy. There are conflicting reports regarding the effect of asthma on maternal complications and neonatal morbidity. Most large population-based studies of women with asthma have reported increased rates of hypertensive disorders, abruption, premature labor, cesarean delivery, prematurity, and IUGR. In contrast, smaller studies of hospitalized patients have revealed less dramatic increases in maternal–fetal problems (58). These discrepancies may be related to both smaller sample size and better disease control in the hospitalized patients.

Most pregnant asthmatic women are initially treated with intermittent use of short-acting inhaled $beta_2$-agonists (i.e., rescue inhalers such as albuterol). The need for rescue inhaler use more than three times per week usually indicates a need for anti-inflammatory treatment with inhaled corticosteroids (54). Inhaled steroids are also usually prescribed if adequate peak flow rates cannot be maintained or if clinical exacerbations continue to occur. The routine use of inhaled steroids has been reported to result in less frequent exacerbations among pregnant women (57). Patients may be reassured that these classes of drugs have been shown to be quite safe from both the maternal and the fetal perspectives. Some patients receive additional pharmacologic therapy with inhaled cromolyn, sympathomimetics, antihistamines or leukotriene inhibitors. None of these are believed to be teratogenic, and thus, may be employed during pregnancy. There is less data regarding the safety of the longer-acting $beta_2$-agonists, and they are probably best avoided unless believed to be necessary by a pulmonary specialist familiar with the care of pregnant women.

Renal Disease

When patients with renal disease seek preconception counseling, it is very important to ascertain the severity of their disease. Women with mild renal disease (usually defined as a serum creatinine less than 1.4 mg/dL) can be reassured that their prognosis for successful pregnancy outcome is very good (59). Pregnancy is becoming more common among women with moderate renal insufficiency (a serum creatinine greater than or equal to 1.4 mg/dL), is now quite common among patients who have undergone renal transplants, and occasionally occurs among patients undergoing dialysis (60). Women with moderate renal disease should be informed that although the precise mechanism is presently uncertain, pregnancy might accelerate the progression of their kidney problem in comparison to the rate of deterioration experienced by women with similar disease who do not become pregnant (59, 60). Prematurity and IUGR remain quite high with reported ranges of 43 to 73% and 22 to 57%, respectively. Maternal pre-eclampsia is also more common. Even so, the probability that their pregnancy will result in a surviving infant is good, reported at 70 to 100%, and to a large extent, appears to depend on the presence or absence of maternal hypertension.

Patients who have undergone a renal transplant and who have been stable for at least 2 years can be reassured that if they become pregnant, they are no more likely to suffer graft rejection (10 to 15% rejection rates) than similar patients who do not conceive (60). Before attempting pregnancy, their renal function should be stable with a serum creatinine less than 2.0 mg/dL, no evidence of ongoing graft rejection, normal or easily controlled blood pressure, 24-hour urine protein less than 500 mg, and immunosuppression drugs at maintenance levels (59). Fetal survival rates have been reported to be substantially improved among renal transplant patients who have a prepregnancy serum creatinine less than 1.4 mg/dL versus those with a creatinine greater than or equal to 1.4 mg/dL (96% versus 75%) (59).

Pre-eclampsia has been reported to occur more frequently in renal transplant patients and is sometimes difficult to differentiate from transplant rejection. IUGR has also been commonly reported. Some clinicians have attributed this to the exposure to azathioprine and cyclosporine used to prevent graft rejection (59, 60). The former drug is also associated with dose-related myelosuppression, but this is usually not a significant problem unless the maternal white blood cell count is less than 7.5 10^9/L. Cyclosporine (Sandimmune, Gengraf) does not appear to be associated with birth defects, but fetuses exposed to this medication have been reported to have higher rates of IUGR than those exposed to other immunosuppressive agents. Prednisone (Deltasone), also used to prevent graft rejection, crosses the placenta and rarely has been reported to result in fetal adrenal insufficiency and thymic hypoplasia. Maternal side effects of corticosteroids have included increased maternal glucose levels resulting in gestational diabetes and, rarely, significant bone demineralization resulting in fracture. Chronic steroid use may also be associated with preterm premature rupture of membranes.

Fertility is low among patients undergoing dialysis, with less than 1% of patients conceiving annually (59). More recent neonatal survival rates among women conceiving while undergoing dialysis have ranged from 50 to 70%. Of children born to women undergoing dialysis, 85% of infants were born premature, 28% had IUGR, and 36% had very low birth weight (60). Maternal hypertensive complications have been very common, occurring in 80% of patients overall and in 40% of patients with stage 3 hypertension or greater. Most disturbingly, occasional maternal deaths have been reported.

Systemic Lupus Erythematosus

SLE occurs in about 1 in 700 of all women but is approximately three times as common among black women. Pregnancy does not appear to alter the long-term course of SLE. The literature examining the relationship between pregnancy and acute exacerbation of SLE has contained conflicting data, with some authors reporting low rates and others quite high rates of SLE flare during pregnancy (61–63). This discrepancy may arise due to the natural flaring and remitting course of the disease, as well as the relatively small sample sizes included in most publications, and there appears to be no clear-cut pattern in the literature. Although this remains an unresolved question, pregnancy among women with well-controlled SLE appears to be associated with a reasonable level of maternal risk.

Thirty percent of women with lupus nephritis will experience a transient deterioration of renal function during pregnancy, and in approximately 7% of women with lupus nephritis, the decrease in renal function is permanent. Pre-eclampsia occurs more frequently among women with SLE and is often difficult to differentiate from deterioration of lupus nephritis. For this reason, as well as the quiescent nature of lupus nephritis before significant deterioration in renal function occurs, all women with SLE should collect a 24-hour urine for protein and creatinine clearance, and their blood should be tested for anti–double-stranded DNA antibodies. These autoantibodies are highly correlated with the occurrence and activity of lupus nephritis.

The woman with lupus can be informed that her ability to conceive should not be inhibited by her disease. She should be cautioned, however, that abortion rates in women with lupus are increased and have been reported to range from 16 to 36% (61). This may be due to the presence of antiphospholipid antibodies and lupus anticoagulant, which should be treated as outlined previously in this chapter. Premature delivery is very frequent among women with SLE, reported in one-fourth to one-half of live births. This may be related to both the increased prevalence of PPROM among women receiving corticosteroids and labor induction for maternal conditions such as pre-eclampsia or flair of underlying SLE (61). IUGR is more common in infants of mothers with SLE than among the general population. Although stillbirths are increased, 96 to 97% of pregnancies that progress beyond 20 weeks result in live births (61, 64).

Neonatal lupus syndrome occurs in a small percentage of the infants of mothers with SLE. It consists of skin lesions, hematologic complications, and cardiac abnormalities. The previously indicated problems are related to the transplacental passage of IgG antibodies. Because maternal antibodies do not persist in the neonate, these conditions, with the exception of the cardiac abnormalities, are usually transient in the newborn period. Sometimes neonatal lupus syndrome presents as fetal heart block in utero manifested by a persistent fetal heart rate of approximately 60 bpm. The occurrence of fetal heart block among women with SLE and Sjögren's syndrome has been highly correlated with the presence of maternal anti-SSA (anti-Rho) and anti-SSB (anti-La) antibodies. The risk of fetal heart block among women with anti-SSA has been reported to be approximately 1 in 20 and increases to 1 in 3 in women with a prior affected infant. Some clinicians recommend testing all mothers with SLE for these antibodies and further suggest weekly fetal heart rates after 20 weeks' gestation in those who test positive for anti-SSA or anti-SSB.

Most women with SLE are treated with oral steroids and nonsteroidal anti-inflammatory drugs (NSAIDs). Potential complications of maternal steroid use are discussed in previous sections of this chapter. NSAIDs have been associated with oligohydramnios and closure of the fetal ductus arteriosus. With normal doses of aspirin, this is very unlikely to occur, but other NSAIDs are probably best avoided if possible. Some women are treated with azathioprine. This medication has also been discussed previously. Antimalarial agents are occasionally employed in SLE; although they have been found to attach to tissue in the fetal eye, there has been no clear-cut evidence to suggest fetal injury.

Clinical Notes

REPRODUCTIVE HISTORY

- Menarche
- Menstrual history
- Deliveries
- Abortions
- Pregnancy complications

GENERAL HEALTH HISTORY

- Medical disorders
- Medications
- Substance abuse
- Infectious disease
- Vaccination history

GENETIC HISTORY

- Family history of anomalies or mental retardation
- Ethnic origin
  - Tay-Sachs disease
  - Hemoglobin disorders
- Maternal and paternal age
- Medical disorders requiring preconception therapy to decrease congenital anomalies
- Family history of metabolic disorders
- Cystic fibrosis screening

OCCUPATION AND AVOCATIONS

PHYSICAL EXAMINATION

- Abnormalities associated with specific diseases
- Uterine or cervical anomalies

LAB

- Pap smear
- STD screening
- Urine protein
- Disease-specific tests

REFERENCES

1. Garcia-Patterson A, Corcoy R, Rigla M, et al. Does preconceptional counseling in diabetic women influence perinatal outcome. Ann Ist Super Sanita 1998;33:333–336.
2. American College of Obstetricians and Gynecologists (ACOG). Primary and Preventive Care: Periodic Assessments. ACOG Committee Opinion 246. Washington, DC: ACOG, 1999.
3. Steel JM, Johnstone FD, Smith AF, et al. Five years experience of a "prepregnancy" clinic for insulin-dependent diabetics. Br Med J 1982;285:353–356.
4. Jack BW, Culpepper L. Preconception care. Risk reduction and health promotion in preparation for pregnancy. JAMA 1990;264:1147–1149.
5. Chamberlain G. The prepregnancy clinic. Br Med J 1980;281:29–30.
6. American College of Obstetricians and Gynecologists (ACOG). Exercise During Pregnancy and the Postpartum Period. ACOG Committee Opinion 267. Washington, DC: ACOG, 2002.
7. Rose BI, Graff S, Spencer R, et al. Major congenital anomalies in infants and glycosylated hemoglobin levels in insulin-requiring diabetic mothers. J Perinatol 1988;8:309–311.
8. Platt LD, Koch R, Hanley WB, et al. The International Study of Pregnancy Outcome in Women with Maternal Phenylketonuria: report of a 12-year study. Am J Obstet Gynecol 2000;182:326–333.
9. Krone N, Wachtert I, Stefanidou M, et al. Mothers with congenital hyperplasia and their children: outcome of pregnancy, birth and childhood. Clin Endocrinol 2001;55:523–529.
10. Koren G, Pastuszak A, Ito S. Drugs in pregnancy. N Engl J Med 1998;338:1128–1137.
11. Mozurkewich EL, Luke B, Avni M, et al. Working conditions and adverse pregnancy outcome: a meta-analysis. Obstet Gynecol 2000;95:623–635.
12. American College of Obstetrician and Gynecologists (ACOG). Preconception and Prenatal Carrier Screening for Cystic Fibrosis. Washington, DC: ACOG, 2001.
13. Stein J, Berg C, Jones J, et al. A screening protocol for a prenatal population at risk for inherited hemoglobin disorders: results of its application to a group of Southeast Asians and blacks. Am J Obstet Gynecol 1984;150:333–341.
14. American College of Obstetricians and Gynecologists (ACOG). Screening for Tay-Sachs Disease. ACOG Committee Opinion 162. Washington, DC: ACOG, 1995.
15. Locksmith G, Duff P. Preventing neural tube defects: the importance of periconceptional folic acid supplements. Obstet Gynecol 1998;91:1027–1034.
16. Jeffcoat MK, Geurs NC, Reddy MS, et al. Periodontal infection and preterm birth: results of a prospective study. J Am Dent Assoc 2001;132:875–880.
17. Althuisius SM, Dekker GA, Hummel P, et al. Final results of the Cervical Incompetence Prevention Randomized Cerclage Trial (CIPRACT): therapeutic cerclage with bed rest versus bed rest alone. Am J Obstet Gynecol 2001;185:1106–1112.
18. Hopkins MP, Lavin JP. Cervical cancer in pregnancy. Gynecol Oncol 1996;63:293.
19. American College of Obstetricians and Gynecologists (ACOG). Management of Recurrent Early Pregnancy Loss. ACOG Practice Bulletin 24. Washington, DC: ACOG, 2001.
20. Lockwood CJ, Rand J. The immunobiology and obstetrical consequences of antiphospholipid antibodies. Obstet Gynecol Surv 1994;49:432–441.
21. Lockwood CJ. Inherited thrombophilias in pregnant patients: detection and treatment paradigm. Obstet Gynecol 2002;99:333–341.
22. Weeks JW, Asrat T, Morgan M, et al. Antepartum surveillance for a history of stillbirth: when to begin. Obstet Gynecol 1995;172:486–492.
23. Chesley LC. Hypertension in pregnancy: definitions, familial factor, and remote prognosis. Kidney Int 1980;18: 234–240.
24. Sibai BM, el-Nazer A, Gonzalez-Ruis A. Severe preeclampsia–eclampsia in young primigravid women: subsequent pregnancy outcome and remote prognosis. Am J Obstet Gynecol 1986;155:1011–1016.

25. Sibai BM, Mercer B, Sarinoglu C. Severe preeclampsia in the second trimester: recurrence risk and long term prognosis. Am J Obstet Gynecol 1991;165:1408–1412.
26. Sullivan CA, Magann EF, Perry KG, et al. The recurrence of the syndrome of hemolysis, elevated liver enzymes, and low platelets (HELLP) in subsequent gestations. Am J Obstet Gynecol 1994;171:940–943.
27. Sibai B, Ramadan MK, Chari RS, et al. Pregnancies complicated by HELLP syndrome (hemolysis, elevated liver enzymes, and low platelets): subsequent pregnancy outcome and long-term prognosis. Am J Obstet Gynecol 1995;172:125–129.
28. American College of Obstetricians and Gynecologists (ACOG). Diagnosis and Management of Preeclampsia and Eclampsia. ACOG Practice Bulletin 33. Washington, DC: ACOG, 2002.
29. Chesley LC, Annitto JF, Cosgrovve BA. The remote prognosis of eclamptic women: sixth periodic report. Am J Obstet Gynecol 1976;124:446–459.
30. Clark SL. Placenta previa and abruptio placentae. In: Creasy RK, Reshik R, eds. Maternal Fetal Medicine: Principles and Practice. 4th ed. Philadelphia: WB Saunders, 1999:616–631.
31. Slutsker L. Risks associated with cocaine during pregnancy. Obstet Gynecol 1992;79:778–789.
32. Report of the National High Blood Pressure Education Program Working Group on High Blood Pressure in Pregnancy. Am J Obstet Gynecol 2000;183:S1–S22.
33. Ferrer RL, Sibai BM, Mulrow CD, et al. Management of mild hypertension during pregnancy: a review. Obstet Gynecol 2000;96:849–860.
34. Sibai BM, Lindheimer M, Hauth J, et al. for The National Institute of Child Health Human Development Network of Maternal-Fetal Medicine Units. Risk factors for preeclampsia, abruptio placentae, adverse neonatal outcomes among women with chronic hypertension. N Engl J Med 1998;339:667–671.
35. Lavin JP, Lovelace D, Miodovnik M, et al. Clinical experience with 107 diabetic pregnancies. Am J Obstet Gynecol 1983;147:742–752.
36. Hanson U, Persson B. Outcome of pregnancies complicated by type 1 insulin-dependent diabetes in Sweden: acute pregnancy complications, neonatal mortality and morbidity. Am J Perinatol 1993;10:330–333.
37. Reece E., Homko C, Miodovnik M, et al. A consensus report of the Diabetes in Pregnancy Study Group of North America Conference, Little Rock, Arkansas, May 2002. J Maternal Fetal Neonatal Med 2002;12:361–364.
38. Miodovnik M, Mimouni F, Dignan PS, et al. Major malformation in infants of IDDM women. Vasculopathy and early first trimester poor glycemic control. Diabetes Care 1988;11:713–718.
39. Miodovnik M, Skillman C, Holyrode JC, et al. Elevated maternal hemoglobin A_{1c} in early pregnancy and spontaneous abortion among insulin-dependent diabetic women. Am J Obstet Gynecol 1985;153:439–442.
40. Centers for Disease Control. Perinatal mortality and congenital malformations in infants born to women with insulin-dependent diabetes—United States, Canada, and Europe, 1940–1988. JAMA 1990;264:437–441.
41. Rosenn B, Miodovnik M, Mimouni F, et al. Patient experience in a diabetic program project improves subsequent pregnancy outcome. Obstet Gynecol 1991;77:87–91.
42. Rosenn BM, Miodovnik M. Medical complications of diabetes mellitus in pregnancy. Clin Obstet Gynecol 2000;43:17–31.
43. Siu SC, Sermer M, Colman JM, et al., on behalf of the Cardiac Disease in Pregnancy (CARPREG) Investigators. Prospective multicenter study of pregnancy outcomes in women with heart disease. Circulation 2001;104:515–521.
44. Gei AF, Hankins GDV. Cardiac disease in pregnancy. Obstet Gynecol Clin North Am 2001;28:465–511.
45. Elkayam U, Tummala PP, Rao K, et al. Maternal and fetal outcomes of subsequent pregnancies in women with peripartum cardiomyopathy. N Engl J Med 2001;344:1567–1571.
46. Ramsey PS, Ramin KD, Ramin SM. Cardiac disease in pregnancy. Am J Perinatol 2001;18:245–265.
47. Cortrufo M, DeFeo M, DeSanto LS, et al. Risk of warfarin during pregnancy with mechanical valve prostheses. Obstet Gynecol 2002;99:35–40.
48. Rowan JA, McCowan LME, Raudkivi PJ, et al. Enoxaparin treatment in women with mechanical heart valves during pregnancy. Am J Obstet Gynecol 2001;185:633–637.
49. Pschirrer ER, Monga M. Seizure disorders in pregnancy. Obstet Clin North Am 2001;28:601–609.
50. Crawford P, Lee P. Gender difference in management of epilepsy—what women are hearing. Seizure 1999;8:135–139.
51. Bets T, Fox C. Proactive pre-conception counseling for women with epilepsy—is it effective? Seizure 1999;8:322–327.
52. Moore SJ, Turnpenny P, Quinn A, et al. A clinical study of 57 children with fetal anticonvulsant syndrome. J Med Genet 2000;37:489–497.
53. Hanson JW, Smith DW. The fetal hydantoin syndrome. J Pediatr 1975;87:285–290.
54. Clark SL and the National Asthma Education Program Working Group on Asthma and Pregnancy. Asthma in pregnancy. Obstet Gynecol 1993;82:1036–1040.
55. Alexander S, Dodds L, Armson BA. Perinatal outcomes in women with asthma during pregnancy. Obstet Gynecol 1998;92:435–440.
56. Tan KS, Thomson NC. Asthma in pregnancy. Am J Med 2001;109:727–733.
57. Wendel PJ, Ramin SM, Barnett-Hamm C, et al. Asthma treatment in pregnancy: a randomized controlled study. Am J Obstet Gynecol 1996;175:150–154.
58. Liu S, Wen SW, Demissie K, et al. Maternal asthma and pregnancy outcomes: a retrospective cohort study. Am J Obstet Gynecol 2001;184:90–96.
59. Jungers P, Choukroun CG, Moynot A, et al. Pregnancy in women with impaired renal function. Clin Nephrol 1997;47:281–288.

60. Hou S. Pregnancy in chronic renal insufficiency and end-stage renal disease. Am J Kidney Dis 1999;33:235–252.
61. Le Huong D, Wechler B, Vauthier-Brouzes D, et al. Outcome of planned pregnancies in systemic lupus erythematosus: a prospective study of 62 pregnancies. Br J Rheumatol 1997;36:772–777.
62. Georgiou PE, Politi EN, Katisimbri P, et al. Outcome of lupus in pregnancy: a controlled study. Rheumatology 2000;39:1014–1019.
63. Lockshin MD. Pregnancy does not cause systemic lupus erythematosus to worsen. Arthritis Rheum 1989;32:665–670.
64. Kleinman D, Katz VL, Kuller JA. Perinatal outcomes in women with systemic lupus erythematosus. J Perinatol 1998;18:178–182.

CHAPTER 15

Contraception

Anthony DelConte

INTRODUCTION

Contraception has been considered since man first recognized the connection between coitus and subsequent pregnancy. Providing control over a woman's reproductive potential can be one of the most important functions of those who regularly provide health care to women. Although there are no perfect contraceptive methods, several types are available: behavioral, mechanical, and hormonal. Each has its own advantages and disadvantages. It is up to the patient to decide which method is best for her, barring any contraindication to her choice. This can be accomplished with the assistance of her health care provider after considering her health history, as well as any psychological and social factors. Not all women are alike in their contraceptive needs, thus the need for different methods for different segments of the population. Prescribing contraceptives to adolescents involves a significant amount of time and resources. Clinicians need to be familiar with how teens think about sex and birth control, what their beliefs are, and how individual teens may make choices based on their lifestyles. At the other end of the reproductive spectrum, choices can be just as complex. The need for safe and effective contraceptive methods remains great in the premenopausal period as evidenced by the high unintended pregnancy rate in this age group.

As we move into the 21st century, several new methods have been introduced. Rather than replacing traditional methods, these new technologies provide more choices and allow women increased opportunity for success and satisfaction with their chosen method. An important benefit of modern contraception is that it promotes the concept of birth control as a fundamental right of women. Control over reproduction has led to further rights for women, in particular, that of a free choice in respect to their sex lives, their method of procreation, and, in more general terms, their way of life. What is taken for granted as an obvious right in the Western world is continually being challenged in cultures where women have not yet achieved their legitimate place in society.

There is no doubt that fertility regulation represents an important contribution to reproductive health. The role of fertility regulation in decreasing maternal mortality has been well documented. This holds true in Western civilization but is even more important in Third World countries, where poverty and malnutrition maintain a dominant place in considerations of health care public policy. Providing access in these areas requires a multidisciplinary effort to overcome the legal, financial, cultural, and societal barriers to providing contraceptive services. Contraceptives are currently being manufactured in at least 27 developing countries. Subsidiaries of multinational companies are often involved in the local production of oral contraceptives (OCs) and condoms, whereas most domestic intrauterine device (IUD) manufacturing ventures have been undertaken by local private companies. External assistance agencies have been active in supporting the local production of contraceptives (1).

NATURAL METHODS

Natural Family Planning (Fertility Awareness-Based Method)

Natural family planning, also known as the rhythm method or periodic abstinence, encompasses three techniques: the calendar rhythm method, the basal body temperature method, and the cervical mucus method. All are based on the fact that pregnancy is possible for only about 7 days of the menstrual cycle (2). The calendar technique requires women to record the length of a menstrual cycle for several months. She then subtracts 19 days from her shortest cycle and 9 days from her longest cycle to determine her fertile period and abstains from intercourse during that time. For example, if a woman's cycle averages 27 to 31 days, her fertile period would start on day 8 ($27 - 19 = 8$) and end on day 22 ($31 - 9 = 22$). This method is not recommended for women whose cycle is less than or equal to 25 days or if it varies by more than 8 days between cycles.

The determination of temperature is a way of estimating the day of ovulation in each cycle. A special thermometer is available, making it easier to determine if there is a rise in basal body temperature. With the rise in progesterone that follows ovulation, there is an increase in the basal body temperature of 0.5 to 1°F. The woman must check the temperature on awakening, but *before* arising, and record the reading on a graph. Abstinence from intercourse starts on the first day of menses and continues until there is at least a 3-day duration, consecutively, of elevated basal body temperature. This technique requires a fairly long period of abstinence. It is worth remembering that weekends, which often involve later hours and arising later, will tend to cause an elevation of the basal body temperature that may approach 0.4 or 0.5°F, so that only persistence of the elevation in following days will be a certain determinant that ovulation has occurred. It is also useful to remember that the progesterone-induced temperature elevation begins only *after* ovulation, which is why its usefulness is mainly retrospective.

In addition to the basal body temperature, the time of ovulation can be identified by the amount and consistency of cervical mucus, and in this case, imminent ovulation can be anticipated before it occurs. Endogenous levels of estrogen and progesterone directly influence the quantity and quality of cervical mucus. Women are taught to recognize these changes. Abstinence is employed during the menses, and then may occur every other day until the first appearance of a larger amount of very thin, slippery mucus. After that, abstinence resumes until 4 days after the last day the almost liquidlike discharge was present. Ovulation can also be determined in advance by urinary measurements of luteinizing hormone and estradiol, but this often requires the expense of three to four determinations per cycle.

The failure rate of natural family planning is usually estimated as 20 to 30% per year, and a principal reason for this is that sperm, after ejaculation, may survive for 6–8 days in the fallopian tube or in the pelvic peritoneal cavity (3). In addition, strict compliance with abstinence may be unreliable and misinterpretations of cervical mucus changes may occur. One study has shown no increase in the spontaneous abortion rate associated with natural family planning (4). Natural family planning methods can be supplemented with the use of over-the-counter ovulation predictor kits to more accurately assess when abstinence is necessary.

Lactational Amenorrhea Method

The contraceptive effect of lactation has been long recognized, but specific knowledge concerning the degree and duration of this effect has been lacking. A quoted consensus statement from 1988 emphasized that women are protected against another pregnancy during the first 6 months postpartum, provided they are breast-feeding and not employing significant nutritional supplement to their infant(s) (5). Lactational amenorrhea method pregnancy rates were 2.9 and 5.9 per 100 women at 6 and 12 months in women supplementing with formula; however, when no supplement was employed, the pregnancy rate was only 0.7 at 6 months (6). One study in Pakistan included 391 women who were breast-feeding and were amenorrheic until 6 months postpartum and had a pregnancy rate of 0.6% and 1.1%, respectively, at 1 year (7). It is obvious that if menstrual periods resume, the risk of conception is increased, but lactation still appears to provide some additional protection against pregnancy, perhaps by imperfect ovulation or endometrial response.

STEROIDAL CONTRACEPTION: ORAL

The development and widespread use of combination oral contraceptives (OCs) was a major breakthrough in the 20th century. Many observers regard this development as second in importance only to the development and use of broad-spectrum antibiotics.

In choosing an OC, the optimal formulation will comprise the lowest effective dose with acceptable bleeding profiles and minimal side effects. OCs impact protein, lipid, and carbohydrate metabolism. In the United States, combination OCs with less than 50 mcg estrogen use ethinyl estradiol (EE) as the estrogenic component. Most women start an OC containing 15 to 35 mcg EE. Among the progestins, there are those related to norethindrone (norethisterone outside the United States), levonorgestrel (LNG), or the more recently introduced drospirenone or dienogest. There is no evidence-based rationale for selecting one formulation over another for any particular patient. The choice depends on the clinician's experience and his or her familiarity with the medical literature. The diverse patient characteristics allow clinicians to offer several options of OCs to patients based on their individual preference and tolerance. However, with most OCs available in the United States, side effects are mild, self-limiting, and tend to resolve over time. Therefore, watchful waiting and reassurance may be a more logical approach to OC prescribing than continued switching from one formulation to another. For a more in-depth comparison of the various OCs, refer to Table 15.1. For information regarding missed pills, see Table 15.2.

For women who are nursing, the combination OC is not recommended because it decreases the quantity of milk, and some amounts of EE may be transferred to the infant. Progestin-only minipills are preferred for lactating women seeking oral hormonal contraception.

Benefits of Oral Contraception

Known benefits of OC use include the prevention of extrauterine pregnancies; reduction in pelvic inflammatory disease, ovarian cysts, and iron-deficiency anemia; and decrease in the rate of ovarian and endometrial cancers. The efficacy of OCs and other methods is depicted in Table 15.3.

Side Effects of Oral Contraceptives

Side effects of OCs are a major source of patient noncompliance and discontinuation. Breast tenderness and nausea, which are estrogen related, are markedly reduced with pills containing less than 50 μg estrogen. When side effects do occur, they will usually decline after the first 3 months of OC use. Patients who persist with nausea may try taking the OC immediately after a meal rather than at night on an empty stomach. In addition, changing to a 20-mcg pill may help.

A more recent Cochrane Review assessed 42 trials, including 3 placebo-controlled randomized clinical trials; none of the randomized trials showed a statistically significant difference in weight gain for OC users compared with the placebo group (8).

Contraception Concerns With Selected Medical Conditions

For many women, the risk–benefit equation is in favor of proper use of combination OCs. For a better understanding of the risks associated with each contraceptive method, as well as the risk of pregnancy, see Table 15.4. For a complete list of absolute contraindications, see Table 15.5. Other disorders that are relative contraindications to the use of OCs are listed in Table 15.6.

Cerebrovascular Disease

OCs are contraindicated in the presence of cerebrovascular disease. OCs increase the risk for stroke in women with other underlying risk factors.

TABLE 15.1

Composition and Activities of Oral Contraceptives

	Progestin and Dose (mg)	Estrogen and Dose (μg)	Activity		
			Endometrial	Progestational	Androgenic
Monophasic					
Brevicon	Norethindrone 0.05	EE 35	I	L	L
Demulen	Ethinyl diacetate 1.0	EE 50	L	H	L
Demulen 1/35	Ethinyl diacetate 1.0	EE 35	L	H	L
Desogen	Desogestrel 0.15	EE 30	I	H	L
Genora 1/35	Norethindrone 1.0	EE 35	I	I	I
Genora 1/50	Norethindrone 1.0	M 50	I	I	I
Levlen	Levonorgestrel 0.15	EE 30	I	I	I
Loestrin 1.5/30	Norethindrone 1.5	EE 30	L	I	I/H
Loestrin 1/20	Norethindrone 1.0	EE 20	L	I	I/H
Lo/Ovral	Norgestrel 0.3	EE 30	I	I	I
Modicon	Norethindrone 0.5	EE 35	I	L	L
Nelova 1/35E	Norethindrone 1.0	EE 35	I	I	I
Nelova 0.5/35E	Norethindrone 0.5	EE 35	I	L	L
Nordette	Levonorgestrel 0.15	EE 30	I	I	I
Norethin 1/35E	Norethindrone 1.0	EE 35	I	I	I
Norethin 1/50M	Norethindrone 1.0	M 50	I	I	I
Norinyl 1/35	Norethindrone 1.0	EE 35	I	I	I
Norinyl 1/50	Norethindrone 1.0	M 50	I	I	I
Norlestrin 1/50	Norethindrone 1.0	EE 50	I	I	I
Norlestrin 2.5	Norethindrone 2.5	EE 50	H	H	H
Ortho-Cept	Desogestrel 0.15	EE 30	I	H	L
Ortho-Cyclen	Norethindrone 0.25	EE 35	L	L	L
Ortho-Novum 1/35	Norethindrone 1.0	EE 35	I	I	I
Ortho-Novum 1/50	Norethindrone 1.0	M 50	I	I	I
Ovcon 35	Norethindrone 0.4	EE 35	I	L	L
Ovcon 50	Norethindrone 1.0	EE 50	H	H	H
Ovral	Norgestrel 0.5	EE 50	H	H	H
Multiphasic					
Jenest 7/14 days	Norethindrone 0.5/1.0	EE 35/35	I	I	I
Ortho-Novum 7/7/7 7/7/7 days	Norethindrone 0.5/0.75/1.0	EE 35/35/35	I	I	I
Ortho-Novum 10/11 10/11 days	Norethindrone 0.5/1.0	EE 35/35	L	L	L
Tri-Cyclen 7/7/7 days	Norgestimate 0.18/0.215/0.25	EE 35/35/35	L	L	L
Tri-Levlen 6/5/10 days	Levonorgestrel 0.05/0.075/0.125	EE 30/40/30	I	L	I

(Continued)

TABLE 15.1 Continued

Composition and Activities of Oral Contraceptives

	Progestin and Dose (mg)	Estrogen and Dose (μg)	Activity		
			Endometrial	Progestational	Androgenic
Tri-Norinyl	Norethindrone	EE	I	I	I
7/9/5 days	0.5/1.0/0.5	35/35/35			
Triphasil	Levonorgestrel	EE	I	L	I
6/5/10 days	0.05/0.075/0.125	30/40/30			
Progestin only					
Micronor	Norethindrone 0.35	None	L	L	L
Nor-QD	Norethindrone 0.35	None	L	L	L
Ovrette	Norgestrel 0.075	None	L	L	L

EE, ethinyl estradiol; H, high; I, intermediate; L, low; M, mestranol.

Migraine and Headache

Patients with a history of migraine headaches should use OCs cautiously. Some patients will note an improvement, whereas some will notice no change; however, approximately 50% of patients will notice a worsening of their condition. One commonly accepted contraindication to the use of OCs is a history of classic migraine (migraine with focal neurologic symptoms or aura lasting more than 1 hour) due to an increased potential for stroke, although the evidence to support this is scant (9). It should be noted that women with a history of migraines have a two- to three-fold increased risk of ischemic stroke, regardless of OC use.

Seizure Disorder

The incidence of epilepsy in the general population is approximately 1%. OCs have no impact on the pattern or frequency of seizures. However, some anticonvulsants can decrease serum concentrations of estrogen and thus may increase the likelihood of intermenstrual bleeding among

TABLE 15.2

Instructions for Patients Who Missed an Oral Contraceptive Pill

Consecutive Pills Omitted	Time in Cycle	Instructions to Patient[a]
1	Any time	Take missed pills immediately and next one at regular time
2	First 2 weeks	Take two pills every day for next 2 days, and then resume taking pills on regular schedule.
2	Third week	Take one pill every day until last day of third week. Dispose of placebos and begin new pack next day.
≥3	Any time	Take one pill every day until last day of that week. Dispose of placebos and begin new pack next day.

[a] Additional contraceptive measures should be used as soon as the omission of oral contraceptive pills is discovered. These additional measures should be used for a least 7 days.

In the event of vomiting, the dose must be repeated.

TABLE 15.3

Percentage of Women With Unintended Pregnancy During First Year of Typical Use and First Year of Perfect Use of Contraception and Percentage Continuing Use at End of First Year, United States

	% of Women Experiencing Unintended Pregnancy Within First Year of Use		% of Women Continuing Use at 1 Year[c]
Method (1)	Typical Use[a] (2)	Perfect Use[b] (3)	(4)
Chance[d]	85	85	
Spermicides[e]	26	6	40
Periodic abstinence	25		63
Calendar		9	
Ovulation method		3	
Symptothermal		2	
Postovulation		1	
Cap[f]			
Parous women	40	26	42
Nulliparous women	20	9	56
Sponge			
Parous women	40	20	42
Nulliparous women	20	9	56
Diaphragm[g]	20	6	56
Withdrawal	19	4	
Condom[h]			
Female (reality)	21	5	56
Male	14	3	61
Pill	5		71
Progestin only		0.5	
Combined		0.1	
IUD			
Progesterone T	2.0	1.5	81
Copper T380A	0.8	0.6	78
LNG 20	0.1	0.1	81
Depo-Provera	0.3	0.3	70
Levonorgestrel implants (Norplant)	0.05	0.05	88
Female sterilization	0.5	0.5	100
Male sterilization	0.15	0.10	100

From Trussell J. Contraceptive efficacy. In: Hatcher RA, Trussell J, Stewart F, et al., eds. Contraceptive Technology. 17th rev ed. New York: Irvington, 1998, with permission.

[a] Among *typical* couples who initiate use of a method (not necessarily for the first time), the percentage who experience an accidental pregnancy during the first year if they do not stop use for any other reason.

[b] Among couples who initiate use of a method (not necessarily for the first time) and who use it *perfectly* (both consistently and correctly), the percentage who experience an accidental pregnancy during the first year if they do not stop use for any other reason.

[c] Among couples attempting to avoid pregnancy, the percentage who continue to use a method for 1 year.

[d] The percentages becoming pregnant in columns (2) and (3) are based on data from populations where contraception is not used and from women who cease using contraception to become pregnant. Among such populations, about 89% become pregnant within 1 year. This estimate was lowered slightly (to 85%) to represent the percent who would become pregnant within 1 year among women now relying on reversible methods of contraception if they abandoned contraception altogether.

[e] Foams, creams, gels, vaginal suppositories, and vaginal film.

[f] Cervical mucus (ovulation) method supplemented by calendar in the preovulatory and basal body temperature in the postovulatory phases.

[g] With spermicidal cream or jelly.

[h] Without spermicides.

TABLE 15.4

Annual Number of Birth-Related or Method-Related Deaths Associated With Control of Fertility Per 100,000 Nonsterile Women, by Fertility Control Method and According to Age

Method of Control and Outcome	15–19	20–24	25–29	30–34	35–39	40–44
No fertility control methods[a]	7.0	7.4	9.1	14.8	25.7	28.2
Oral contraceptives Nonsmoker[b]	0.3	0.5	0.9	1.9	13.8	31.6
Oral contraceptives Smoker[b]	2.2	3.4	6.6	13.5	51.1	117.2
IUD[b]	0.8	0.8	1.0	1.0	1.4	1.4
Condom[a]	1.1	1.6	0.7	0.2	0.3	0.4
Diaphragm/spermicide[a]	1.9	1.2	1.2	1.3	2.2	2.8
Periodic abstinence[a]	2.5	1.6	1.6	1.7	2.9	3.6

[a] Deaths are birth related.
[b] Deaths are method related.
Adapted from Ory HW. Mortality associated with fertility and fertility control. Fam Plann Perspect 1983;15:57–63, with permission.

patients on OCs. For these women, it may be preferable to start them on a 50-mcg EE formulation. If a woman has been started on a 30-mcg EE formulation and develops intermenstrual bleeding, switching to a 50-mcg EE pill may be helpful. Anticonvulsants that do not appear to decrease serum estrogen levels when used concurrently with an OC include valproic acid, gabapentin, lamotrigine, and tiagabine (10).

Cardiovascular Disease

Almost all excess mortality in OC users is due to cardiovascular disease. Most of these deaths are due to myocardial infarction (MI). The morbidity and mortality of cardiovascular diseases

TABLE 15.5

Absolute Contraindications to Oral Contraceptive Use

- Thrombophlebitis/thromboembolic disorders
- History of deep vein thrombophlebitis or thromboembolic disorders
- Cerebral vascular or coronary artery disease
- Known or suspected breast cancer
- Known or suspected endometrial cancer or estrogen-dependent neoplasm
- Abnormal uterine bleeding of unknown etiology
- Cholestatic jaundice of pregnancy or jaundice with prior oral contraceptive use
- Hepatic adenomas, carcinomas, or benign liver tumors
- Known or suspected pregnancy
- Markedly impaired liver function
- Benign or malignant liver tumor that developed during previous use of oral contraceptives or other estrogen-containing products

TABLE 15.6

Relative Contraindications to Oral Contraceptive Use

- Migraine or vascular headache
- Cardiac or renal dysfunction
- Blood pressure ≥90 mm Hg diastolic or ≥160 mm Hg systolic
- Major depressive disorder
- Varicose veins
- Smoker ≥30 years old
- Sickle cell disease or sickle cell–hemoglobin C disease
- History of cholestatic jaundice during pregnancy
- Hepatitis or mononucleosis during past year
- Breastfeeding
- Asthma
- First-degree family history of nonrheumatic cardiovascular disease (fatal or nonfatal) or diabetes at <50 years old
- Use of drugs known to interact with oral contraceptives
- Ulcerative colitis

in OC users is related to the estrogen content and progestin dose and activity of the pill. The cardiovascular disease risk with OC use is most prevalent in women older than 35 years of age who smoke and who have used OCs for long periods of time.

Deep Vein Thrombosis

Although not a major cause of morbidity and mortality in OC users, venous thrombotic disease and pulmonary emboli are known side effects of OC use. Efforts to identify populations at high risk have not yet provided a safe and effective screening method for identification of this group. Currently, a family or personal history of thromboembolic events should raise the clinician's suspicions. In the future, detection of genetic polymorphisms will allow identification of high-risk individuals. Thromboembolic disorders, conditions that predispose to these conditions, and a past history of such problems are contraindications to OC use.

The World Health Organization (WHO) stated that only a small proportion of women with inherited thrombophilias, albeit no personal history of thrombosis, will experience venous thromboembolism (VTE) in association with OC use; however, debate continues to persist about the relative risk these women face (11). Controversy also surrounds the use of combination versus progestin-only OCs or nonhormonal contraception for women known to have deficiencies in protein C, protein S, or antithrombin III. Although the majority of women with the factor V Leiden mutation who use OCs do not experience VTE, there are clinicians who believe a nonestrogen-containing method of contraception is also indicated in this population.

Being severely overweight (body mass index greater than 29 kg/m^2) is an independent risk factor for VTE. In obese women ages 35 years or younger, OC use is appropriate, although there is some evidence that with overweight or obese patients the efficacy of combination OCs with less than 50 mcg EE may be compromised (12).

Hypertension

If a patient has hypertension, it should be controlled (to less than 140/90 mm Hg) prior to beginning OCs because they have the potential to aggravate this condition. That is, increases in blood pressure have been reported in women taking OCs so follow-up evaluation of blood pressure in such a patient is advised. As long as the blood pressure is controlled and no vascular disease is present, OCs are not contraindicated. A history of pregnancy-induced hypertension does not preclude the use of OCs as long as the blood pressure returns to normal postpartum.

Dyslipidemia

Women younger than age 35, in the absence of uncontrolled hypertension, diabetes, or other OC contraindications, may consider OC use, even with low-density lipoprotein cholesterol levels as high as 160 mg/dL (13). An OC with 30 to 35 mcg EE and a low-androgenic activity progestin is preferred for women noted to have dyslipidemia (excluding hypertriglyceridemia) at baseline or who develop it during OC use. If a woman's triglycerides are above 350 mg/dL or in patients with familial hypertriglyceridemia, OCs should be avoided because they may precipitate pancreatitis and/or adversely affect the patient's risk for cardiovascular disease.

Although all oral OCs increase triglyceride levels to some extent, combinations containing EE and norgestimate have been reported to incur less of an increase than most other progestins (14).

Angina and Coronary Atherosclerosis

OCs do not stimulate the atherosclerotic process and may actually inhibit plaque formation. However, OCs are contraindicated in the presence of coronary disease. One study of women younger than 50 years of age who had experienced an MI found that the incidence of angiographically confirmed coronary atherosclerosis in non-OC users was almost twice that of OC users (79% versus 36%, respectively) (15). In addition, there is no increase in the incidence of cardiovascular disease secondary to atherosclerosis in past OC users. Smoking, when combined with OC use, markedly increases the risk of atherogenesis, and this risk increases with age and with the extent of smoking (16). Women with known angina and suspected atherosclerosis, but with no history of prior MI or additional risk factors, may safely use low-dose OCs (17).

Mitral Valve Prolapse

In general, OCs can be safely used by women with mitral valve prolapse (MVP) who are symptom free. OC use should be limited to MVP patients with an echocardiographic-confirmed diagnosis but without mitral regurgitation. A history of thrombotic complications would require another contraceptive method. Long-acting progestins such as injection or implants are safe to use and may provide increased fibrinolytic activity.

Diabetes

Young diabetic women who are free of retinopathy, nephropathy, hypertension, or other complicating vascular disease(s) are appropriate candidates for low-dose contraceptives. It is the progestin component of OCs that is believed to increase insulin resistance. Women with a history of gestational diabetes during their last pregnancy can safely take low-dose OCs. The incidence of frank diabetes developing within 3 years of pregnancy is no higher in women taking these low doses than in those using nonhormonal contraceptive methods (18).

Systemic Lupus Erythematosus

Exacerbations of lupus and increased numbers of flare-ups have been reported with the use of combination OCs. This is believed to be due to the estrogenic component (19).

Sickle Cell Disease

Internationally, recommendations for women with sickle cell disease and OC use vary widely. In the United States, many clinicians think that the risks of pregnancy far outweigh the risks associated with OC use in women with sickle cell disease, and it is often prescribed for this population (20, 21).

Oral Contraceptives and Cancer

Breast Cancer

Fear of developing breast cancer has been a deterrent to the use of both hormonal contraceptives and hormone replacement therapy. The issue has been one of major debate for a number of years. Because the effect of hormone use in case-control studies is relatively small in comparison to other known risks for breast cancer, it is hard to sort out the attributable risk of OCs. A number of case-control and cohort studies have attempted to answer the question with conflicting results. Additional studies will probably add very little to answer this question, even if they are of sufficient power and duration. Although some epidemiologic studies have found a small increase in the diagnosis of breast cancer among current users of OCs (RR = 1.3), once OCs are discontinued this risk declines over 10 years until the risk becomes identical to those who have never used OCs (22). The overwhelming majority of studies do not find an association between OC use and increased relative risk of breast cancer. Overall, the risk of breast cancer in women who take OCs up to the age of 55 appears to be no different from that of nonusers (23). One of the largest controlled studies on a relationship of OCs in breast cancer was conducted by the Centers for Disease Control and Prevention (CDC). The results showed no added risk linked to OC use at a younger age, before a first pregnancy, or in women with benign breast disease or a family of history of breast cancer. In other words, even the addition of OCs to these increased risk groups did not increase the incidence (24). The fact that the CDC analysis confirmed these previously identified risk factors (nulliparity, age at first birth, family history, and history of benign breast disease) reinforces the reliability of the data. OC use by women with a family history of breast cancer in a first-degree relative does not increase their risk of breast cancer (25).

Cervical Cancer

OCs alone do not increase the risk of cervical cancer. However, there may be confounding factors that increase the exposure to human papilloma virus (HPV) and cause an increase in the diagnosis of cervical dysplasias in those using hormonal contraception over those using barrier methods.

Endometrial Cancer

The use of OCs is clearly protective against endometrial cancer. In a WHO study, a review of data from 130 cases and 835 matched controls showed a nearly 50% reduction in the risk of endometrial cancer in women who had ever used OCs (26). This protective effect has been shown to persist for up to 20 years after discontinuation of OCs (27).

Ovarian Cancer

As with endometrial cancer, protection from ovarian cancer may persist for up to 20 years after discontinuation of OCs (28). In addition, the degree of protection is directly related to the duration of OC use. For women who had used OCs for 10 years or more, there is an 80% reduction in their risk for ovarian cancer, but some protection is conferred with as little as 3 to 6 months of use. There does not appear to be any diminution in protection with the use of low-dose (30 to 35 mcg) versus high-dose (50 mcg) OCs (29). There are no current data regarding the risk of ovarian cancer and the use of combination OCs with less than 30 mcg EE.

Clinical Decision Making

Dosing Choices

All oral combination OCs contain formulations using EE in combination with various types of progestins. Clinical choices of a combination OC may be based on either the type of progestin agent in the pill or the dose of EE. Combination OCs containing EE may contain 50 mcg, 34 mcg, 30 mcg, 25 mcg, or 20 mcg. In general, the higher the dose of EE, the better the cycle control, although the type of progestin used in a formulation and the estrogen-progestin ratio may also effect cycle control (30, 31).

In one study of women using a pill with 20 mcg EE and 0.1 mg progestin (Alesse, Levlite) for up to 3 years, the incidence of intermenstrual bleeding, spotting, or both was 23.1% among all cycles, with intermenstrual bleeding occurring only 3.6% of the time. Irregular bleeding was the most common reason patients discontinued with this method of contraception (32). Studies using a different 20-mcg EE pill (Mircette, which contains 20 mcg EE and 150 mcg desogestrel [DSG]) reported a lower intermenstrual bleeding or spotting incidence of only 12% among all cycles, although it was higher in the first cycle (19.1%) and fewer than 3% of the study participants discontinued the contraception due to bleeding complaints (33). In contrast to Alesse, however, it is important to know that Mircette has 21 days of 20 mcg EE, followed by 2 days of placebo tablet, and then 5 days of tablets with 10 mcg of only EE. The use of the additional EE probably contributes to the stabilization of bleeding patterns, even though the overall dose of EE is low.

Although the relationship between EE dose and cycle control is clear, as mentioned previously, the type of progestin and estrogen-progestin ratio are also important in determining the extent of cycle control achieved. In one large open label study, a triphasic OC with 25 mcg EE and DSG (Cyclessa) was compared with a combination triphasic OC containing 35 mcg EE and norethindrone acetate (NETA). The triphasic combination containing 25 mcg EE and DSG had a significantly lower rate of intermenstrual bleeding and spotting (11%) in comparison to the triphasic combination with 35 mcg EE and NETA. These results may be due to the higher progestational activity of DSG compared with NETA, even though the dose of EE was higher in the NETA combination (34).

Overall, OCs with 30 to 35 mcg EE offer very good cycle control with the incidence of intermenstrual bleeding and spotting ranging from approximately 4 to 14% (35, 36). One of the newest agents in the 30- to 35-mcg category, Yasmin, contains 30 mcg EE and 3 mg drospirenone (DRSP), a new progestin with a pharmacologic profile quite similar to that of natural progesterone (37). This newer progestin is reported to have antimineralocorticoid activity similar to a 25-mg dose of spironolactone, and in its preclinical studies, it appears to be antiandrogenic (37, 38).

Use of OCs containing 50 mcg estrogen should be reserved for women requiring additional estrogen to prevent intermenstrual bleeding (e.g., women using drugs that induce hepatic enzymes) or women who have recurring functional ovarian cysts while on OCs containing less than 50 mcg estrogen.

Interactions With Other Drugs

Antimicrobial agents can interact with the pharmacokinetics and efficacy of sex steroid hormones present in OCs (39, 40). Rifampicin (Rifampin) has been shown to decrease circulating levels of EE, resulting in OC failures (41). Certain antibiotics, particularly penicillins and their derivatives and tetracyclines, may diminish the effectiveness of OCs. It is suggested that additional contraceptive measures be used while using these drugs. Other drugs have been implicated in diminishing the efficacy of OCs, but much of this data is anecdotal. A current drug history should be taken when prescribing OCs, and the user should report new medications. For a brief list of various drugs and their interactions with OCs, refer to Table 15.7.

Breast-feeding

Breast-feeding women should avoid the use of combination OCs because small amounts of steroids and/or metabolites have been identified in the milk of nursing mothers. Adverse effects on the child have been reported, including jaundice and breast enlargement. In addition, combination OCs given postpartum may interfere with lactation by decreasing the amount and quality of breast milk. The nursing mother should be counseled to use an alternate method of contraception because breast-feeding provides only partial protection from pregnancy. Combination OCs can be safely started in most women when they have completely weaned their child.

Starting and Stopping the Pill

OCs are available in 21- or 28-day packages. When the patient initiates therapy, she may either start on Sunday (Sunday start) or on the first day of menses (day 1 start), depending on the brand of pill and individual preference. For a Sunday start, the patient is instructed to begin taking her

TABLE 15.7

Interactions of Drugs and Oral Contraceptives

Drug	Mechanism of Action	Management Options
Hydantoins Barbiturates Primidone (Mysoline) Carbamazepine (Tegretol)	Liver enzyme induction	Alternative drug or use a pill regimen with 50 mcg estrogen
Rifampin (Rimactane)	Liver enzyme induction	Use additional contraceptive measures or use a pill regimen with 50 mcg estrogen
Certain antibiotics, particularly: Penicillins and derivatives Tetracyclines Sulfonamides Metronidazole (Flagyl) Nitrofurantoin (Macrodantin)	Possibly diminished enterohepatic circulation of ethinyl estradiol	Use additional contraceptive measures
Griseofulvin (Fulvicin, Grifulvin)	Liver enzyme induction	Use additional contraceptive measures

pills on the first Sunday after the onset of menstruation. If menstruation begins on a Sunday, the first tablet is taken that day. One tablet should be taken daily for 21 consecutive days. During the first cycle, patients are instructed to use backup contraception for the first 7 days. For patients beginning a day 1 start, they are instructed to take their first pill on the first day of menses. Patients are also instructed to take their pills at the same time each day and to use some type of mnemonic or cue to avoid missing pills.

Any time the patient misses two or more tablets, she should also use another method of contraception until she has taken a tablet daily for 7 consecutive days. It is important to continue to take the remaining pills in the package on schedule. If breakthrough bleeding occurs following missed tablets, it will usually be transient. The likelihood of ovulation occurring if only one or two tablets are missed is low. Newer formulations with a decrease in the pillfree interval will decrease the likelihood of ovulation if pills are missed during the early part of the cycle. Further instructions for patients can be found in Table 15.8.

Discontinuation of the Pill

Return to fertility is rapid following discontinuation of today's low-dose OCs. Generally, it is recommended that women wait for the establishment of two to three regular cycles before attempting pregnancy.

Perimenopausal Women and Oral Contraceptives

The transition period of changing hormone patterns, or perimenopausal state, begins about 5 to 10 years before the actual menopause. Characteristics of the perimenopause are irregular cycles, changes in both the volume and the duration of bleeding, and for approximately half the women, the onset of variable vasomotor symptoms. The perimenopausal period is characterized by

TABLE 15.8

Instructions for Patients Who Missed an Oral Contraceptive Pill

Consecutive Pills Omitted	Time in Cycle	Instructions to Patient[a]
1	Any time	Take missed pills immediately and next one at regular time
2	First 2 weeks	Take two pills every day for next 2 days, and then resume taking pills on regular schedule.
2	Third week	Take one pill every day until last day of third week. Dispose of placebos and begin new pack next day.
≥3	Any time	Take one pill every day until last day of that week. Dispose of placebos and begin new pack next day.

[a] Additional contraceptive measures should be used as soon as the omission of oral contraceptive pills is discovered. These additional measures should be used for a least 7 days.
In the event of vomiting, the dose must be repeated.

an increased incidence of anovulatory cycles, resulting in an unopposed estrogen state. This predisposes to dysfunctional uterine bleeding, possible endometrial hyperplasia, and a poorly documented, but frequently observed, accelerated growth of uterine myomata. Although the fertility of women has diminished by age 45, pregnancy is still possible. This is reflected in the fact that the pregnancy termination rate in women 40 to 50 years of age is exceeded only by those women younger than 15 years of age. There continues to be a need for contraception for sexually active women older than age 40 or 45. Aside from permanent sterilization, OCs should be the method of choice for nonsmoking women to regulate menstrual periods and provide contraception. These women often do well on the lowest estrogen dose of 20 μg.

Extended Use of Combined Oral Contraception

In late 2003, the U.S. Food and Drug Administration (FDA) approved Seasonale, a 91-day OC regimen (42). The active tablets contain 0.15 mg LNG and 30 mcg EE. Under this extended-use regimen, the active tablets are taken for 12 weeks, followed by 1 week of placebo tablets. This reduces the number of periods in a given year from 13 with traditional OC to 4. However, women may experience more breakthrough bleeding on the Seasonale regimen, especially in the first few cycles of use. The risks of using Seasonale are similar to the risks of other OC drugs, including risk of pregnancy with missed doses.

STEROIDAL CONTRACEPTION: OTHER

Progestin-Only Contraceptive Pill

The progestin-only pill is an alternative for breast-feeding women and women with conditions that preclude the use of combination OCs, yet they still retain many of the advantages of combined OCs: decreased blood loss, menstrual cramping, and premenstrual syndrome symptoms.

All progestin-only contraceptives cause bleeding pattern changes (43, 44). Three brands of oral progestin-only contraceptive pills are currently available in the United States: two containing 0.35 mg norethindrone (Micronor and Nor-QD), and one containing 0.075 mg norgestrel (Ovrette). These products are particularly useful in women with a contraindication to the use of estrogen. Approximately 40% of patients will ovulate with the progestin levels achieved with a progestin-only regimen. Although the exact mechanism(s) of action are unknown, it is known that the cervical mucus becomes thick and hostile, rendering it relatively impermeable to sperm. In addition, the endometrium is out of phase, making nidation less likely.

Progestin-only contraceptives can be used by almost every woman and have few medical contraindications (active liver disease or liver tumor being one). Early postpartum administration may slow involution of the uterus after delivery and prolong postpartum spotting and bleeding.

Injectables

Depo Medroxyprogesterone Acetate

The principle concern with the use of injectable contraceptives is occasional delayed return of fertility following discontinuation. This is not related to the duration of use. After discontinuing depo medroxyprogesterone acetate (DMPA) (Depo-Provera) to become pregnant, 50% of women conceive promptly (45). In a small proportion of women, fertility is not re-established until as long as 18 months after the last injection. However, the use of DMPA has no permanent impact on the ability to conceive (46). Counseling is required before initiation of this method, which is obviously not ideally suited for simple spacing of pregnancy.

The typical side effects concern menstrual changes, particularly with episodes of unpredictable irregular bleeding during the first months of use. A review of several studies determined that 37.5% of DMPA users experienced irregular bleeding and 27.7% prolonged bleeding in the first 3 to 6 months of use (47). With increasing duration of use, these episodes decrease and amenorrhea becomes common. If breakthrough bleeding persists, the next dose of DMPA can be given early or conjugated estrogens (1.25 mg) may be given daily for 10 to 21 days for several cycles. Approximately 50% of women who use DMPA for 1 year report amenorrhea, and this is an advantage for women troubled with increased or irregular periods. By 3 years, approximately 80% of users are amenorrheic. Women may also complain of breast tenderness, weight gain, and/or depression.

In a placebo-controlled trial, there was no relationship between DMPA and weight change or in the balance of food intake and energy expenditure (48). In another trial comparing weight gain between DMPA users and those using the copper IUD, both groups had significant weight gain, but the DMPA users had greater increases in their weight (49).

Women with sickle cell anemia, congenital heart disease, or those older than 35 who smoke are excellent candidates for DMPA. There is no increase in stroke risk or MI with use of DMPA (46). There is no link with cervical cancer, no increase in breast cancer risk, and a decrease in the incidence of anemia. There does not appear to be any relationship between the use of DMPA and the risk of ovarian cancer. One small study suggested a decreased risk of pelvic inflammatory disease (50). Depo-Provera is an excellent choice for epileptics because the high progestin levels raise the seizure threshold (51).

Women with a history of long-term use of DMPA have lower bone mineral densities than nonusers, although this has not yet been associated with an increase in fracture rate, and two new studies have shown this bone loss to be minimal and reversible (52–54). The effect on lipids has been inconsistent, but the use of DMPA has not been associated with increased risk for MI. DMPA has not been found to increase a woman's risk of thrombotic episodes. DMPA is not teratogenic and is safe for use in lactating women. It may be given immediately postpartum, even in women who are breast-feeding. Women at high risk for developing postpartum depression may not be good candidates for injectable progestin-only methods if there is any concern that progestin might worsen their symptoms.

Lunelle

In comparison to DMPA, the newest injectable contraceptive agent is a combination of an estrogen and progesterone. This new agent, Lunelle, is unique in its use of estradiol cypionate (E_2C) instead of EE in combination with medroxyprogesterone acetate (MPA). E_2C results in no increases in hepatic clotting factor synthesis and fewer adverse lipoprotein fraction alterations than with EE-based formulations (55). Each injection contains 5 mg E_2C and 25 mg MPA in 0.5 mL of an aqueous suspension. The regimen approved is for monthly (every 27 to 33 days) deep intramuscular injection into the gluteus or deltoid.

The contraceptive efficacy of Lunelle is comparable to that of oral combination, although more women using Lunelle may experience amenorrhea than those using combination OCs (1 to 4% versus less than 1%) (56). If the injection is received within 5 days of the onset of menses and subsequent injections occur within 33 days after the previous injection, a backup method of contraception is not warranted.

Body weight does not appear to affect the efficacy of MPA/E_2C, nor is there any difference if the injection site is deep into the deltoid, gluteus, or quadriceps muscles (57). No data regarding the effects of MPA/E_2C on bone mineral density are yet available.

During the first several months, users typically experience four bleeding episodes, each of 4 to 5 days' duration, but with continued use of Lunelle, the bleeding pattern more closely mimics that of normal menses and monthly bleed occurs approximately 20 days after each injection (58).

In contrast to DMPA, Lunelle is associated with regular menses in more than two-thirds of long-term users (58). The rate of discontinuation due to bleeding irregularities with Lunelle is less than 50% of that seen with DMPA (59). Another advantage of Lunelle is the rapid return to fertility on discontinuation; MPA levels are undetectable 60 days after discontinuation. In one study, 53% of women had conceived within 6 months of discontinuation and 83% by 12 months (60). This is in marked contrast to the average 9 to 10 months seen after discontinuation of Depo-Provera.

Use of the MPA/E_2C injection has been associated with weight gain. In a trial comparing MPA/E_2C with oral combination OCs, weight gain with use of the injection ranged from 2 to 8 lb (61).

In late 2002, the pharmaceutical manufacturer of Lunelle had initiated a voluntary recall of Lunelle Monthly Contraceptive Injection (MPA and E_2C injectable suspension) in prefilled syringes due to a lack of assurance of full potency and possible risk of contraceptive failure. Lunelle packaged in vials is not affected by this recall.

Implants

The six-rod LNG implant system (Norplant) was developed by the Population Council in the 1960s and was available in the United States from 1991 to 2000. Norplant consists of six soft plastic implants, 34 × 2 × 2.4 mm each, filled with 36 mg LNG. The original, overall daily rate of release is 85 mcg, which gradually declines to approximately 30 mcg by the fifth year of use (62). Insertion and removal of the implants is usually a minor office procedure performed under local anesthesia. The implants should be inserted within 5 to 7 days after the onset of the menstrual period and immediately inhibit ovulation. Circulating progestin levels are sufficient to prevent ovulation in most women using implants. However, there is a degree of luteal activity manifested by low progesterone levels. In addition to impaired oocyte maturation, progestin-induced unfavorable cervical mucus is sufficient to prevent conception even when ovulation occurs (63, 64). Annual pregnancy rates among implant users average 0.8/100 during the entire 5 years of use, less than what is seen in some OCs. After removal of the implants, serum progestin levels fall to undetectable amounts within 1 week (65).

Menstrual changes are the most common side effect of implants, and many women will experience an irregular bleeding pattern during the first year following insertion; however, this declines to about one-third by the fifth year. During the entire 5 years, 5 to 10% of women will experience amenorrhea. Norplant has no major impact on the lipid profile, carbohydrate metabolism, coagulation factors, or liver function. Women using medications that induce microsomal liver enzymes (e.g., phenytoin, phenobarbital, rifampin, carbamazepine) have an increased risk of pregnancy secondary to lower blood levels of norgestrel. Although the Norplant system was removed from the U.S. market in August 2000, a more recent study confirmed its safety and efficacy (66). Withdrawal from the U.S. market occurred when lower than expected release rates of LNG in specific lots were demonstrated; there are no current plans to begin redistribution of Norplant.

The promising future of implant contraceptive may lie with the single 3-keto-desogestrel implant (Implanon) or the two-rod LNG implant system (Jadelle). The single-rod system releases etonogestrel at decreasing rates for a period of 3 years, and insertion is done with a disposable trocar, obviating the need for an incision. The efficacy of Implanon has been quite high, and side effects include irregular bleeding, headaches, and weight gain (67). The two-rod system, Jadelle, contains a total of 150 mg LNG (75 mg/rod) and may be effective for 5 years of use (68).

Vaginal Contraceptive Ring

A novel vaginal delivery system for administering combination estrogen/progestin has been developed and has received marketing approval in the United States. The NuvaRing system consists of a flexible nonbiodegradeable vaginal ring containing etonogestrel and EE. Etonogestrel (or 3-keto-desogestrel) is the active metabolite of the gonane progestin desogestrel. In OCs, desogestrel is a prodrug that must be converted to 3-keto-desogestrel for biological activity.

The vaginal ring should be kept refrigerated before dispensing, and clinicians should be aware that it has a shelf-life of only 4 months. The vaginal ring (outside diameter is 54 mm) is inserted by the woman and worn continuously for 3 weeks, after which it is removed for 1 week to allow for a withdrawal bleed. After this 1 week, a new devise is inserted. The device can be inserted on days 1 to 5 of the menstrual cycle. In clinical trials, about 18% of the women and 30% of the men reported feeling the ring occasionally during intercourse. If this is a problem, the ring can be removed for intercourse but must be replaced within 3 hours. If the ring remains outside the vagina for longer than 3 hours, its efficacy may be compromised. If it is removed or expelled from the vagina for longer than 3 hours, a backup method of contraception for 1 week is recommended (69). If the ring is left in the vagina for more than 3 weeks, ovulation may continue to be inhibited for up to 2 weeks after the recommended-use period (70).

The ring releases minimal amounts of EE into the circulation, yet maintains efficacy and cycle control comparable to the OC. Clinically, there is less breakthrough bleeding with the ring than with any other hormonal contraceptive method, and although there appears to be no diminished efficacy with increasing body weight, it has not been studied in women weighing more than 200 lb (71).

For current noncontraceptive users starting use of the ring, an additional nonhormonal method of contraception is recommended for the first week following the first insertion. If switching directly from OCs, the ring can be inserted any time after the last active tablet is taken. When switching from another method of birth control, the ring can be inserted when the previous method is discontinued.

In two clinical trials evaluating the safety and efficacy of the vaginal ring, pregnancy rates were between 1 and 2 per 100 woman-years of use (72). If displacement of the ring occurs, the patient may rinse it off and reinsert it within 3 hours of expulsion.

On removal of the ring, follicle-stimulating hormone levels began to rise almost immediately, and return to ovulation can be expected in several weeks (73).

The most frequently reported side effects with the ring were vaginitis (13.7%), headache (11.8%), and leukorrhea (5.9%) (71). It is currently not known if the ring has a different thromboembolic risk than oral combination OCs.

Oil-based local antifungal vaginal therapy has been shown to increase blood levels of the ring's active ingredients but should not have any effect on contraceptive efficacy. Tampons and water-based spermicides such as nonoxynol-9 (N-9) do not alter serum levels of the active hormones. There is no risk of toxic shock syndrome from the ring because the ethyl-vinyl-acetate ring is nonabsorbent. In one study of the ring, the incidence of vaginitis was 13.7%, which is approximately 5% higher than would be expected in the general population (73).

If backup nonhormonal contraception is used, diaphragms should be avoided because the contraceptive ring can preclude proper placement of the barrier contraceptive.

This novel method, although not for every woman, will be a useful choice for some.

Combination Hormonal Contraceptive Patch (Transdermal System)

A combination contraceptive patch (Ortho Evra) has more recently been introduced into the U.S. market. This transdermal system consists of a 20-cm^2 matrix-type patch containing norelgestromin (the primary active metabolite of norgestimate) and EE. Norelgestromin, like LNG, is an active metabolite of orally administered norgestimate. Direct comparisons with OC delivery doses should not be made because of the differences in pharmacokinetic activity between parenteral and oral delivery. Due to its continuous delivery system, the patch is not associated with any peaks or valleys of serum hormonal concentrations.

The Evra system uses a 28-day (4-week) cycle in which a new patch is applied each week for 3 weeks. There is a 7-day period in which no patch is worn (corresponding to the 7-day pillfree interval with OCs). Patients may use a first-day or Sunday start. If a first-day start is used, no backup method of contraception is needed. If a Sunday start is used, a backup method of contraception for the next 7 days is advised. In three large clinical trials with more than 22,000 cycles of use, the pregnancy rate (Pearl index) was approximately 1 per 100 woman-years of use.

The start day is also referred to as the patch change day. A woman may change this day during the fourth week by applying a new patch early on the desired day. If a woman is in the first week of her cycle and has forgotten to apply a new patch, she should apply one as soon as she remembers but also use a backup method of contraception for the next 7 days. She should also note that her patch change day for successive weeks has also been changed. If she is in week 2 or 3 of her cycle, has forgotten to change the patch, and less than 48 hours have elapsed between her patch change day and recognition of the error, she simply needs to place a new patch. A backup method of contraception is not necessary, and her original patch change day remains the same. If more than 48 hours has passed, she should replace the patch, use a backup method of contraception, and note that her patch change date has changed.

If a woman is interested in changing from OCs to the patch, she should apply the patch on the first day of her menses. No backup method of contraception is needed. If she is past the first day of withdrawal bleeding, she may apply the patch and use a backup method of contraception for the next week.

If the patch detaches (occurrence rate, 1.1%), it should be replaced immediately. Hormonal release from the patch is not significantly affected by treadmill exercise or exposure to cold water, whirlpool, or sauna. Efficacy and side effect profiles are not affected by the anatomic site of application (abdomen, buttocks, torso, or upper outer arm), although it should not be placed on the breasts (74). Placement of the patch in an area where the skin stays taught (i.e., is not prone to wrinkle with movement or positions) is highly recommended. Makeup, lotions, or body oils should not be applied to where the patch will be placed, and on placement, the patch should be pressed firmly for 10 seconds to ensure complete adherence by all edges.

Efficacy of the contraceptive patch is lower in women weighing more than 198 lb or 90 kg, although this may not be completely related to the delivery system because a similar decrease in efficacy has been noted in women weighing more than 198 lb or 90 kg who are using combination OCs (12, 75). Clinical studies with the patch have shown a minimal effect on body weight with patch use (76). Contraindications, warnings, and precautions are similar to combination OCs.

In the first two cycles of use, the patch was associated with a significantly higher incidence of breast discomfort (which was primarily mild to moderate in nature) in comparison to the OC. By the end of the second cycle, there was no significant difference in breast discomfort between the two modalities (77). The patch should not be applied to any skin disruptions (e.g., eczema or seborrheic lesions).

NONSTEROIDAL CONTRACEPTION

Intrauterine Contraception

Millions of users worldwide suggest that insertion of an IUD by an appropriately experienced practitioner in a properly selected parous patient constitutes the closest thing to an ideal contraceptive currently available. Yet, only 1% of U.S. women use IUDs (78). Jack Lippes of Buffalo developed the first truly modern IUD in 1962. This was a polyethylene device with a single filament thread as a tail. This quickly became the most widely used IUD by the late 1960s. Introduction and use of the Dalkon Shield and inappropriate selection of patients led to a high incidence of pelvic infections and large class-action lawsuits. The Dalkon Shield no longer marketed in the US after 1974, but lawsuits related to IUD use were ultimately extended to the copper-based IUD devices. Most of these lawsuits were successfully defended, but the cost of defense and threats of continued legal actions led to the withdrawal of copper IUDs from the market in 1986.

The availability of the progesterone-containing IUD (Progestasert) continued. The T- shaped Progestasert releases 65 μg progesterone per day for more than 1 year. Although the manufacturer recommends replacement in 1 year, significant empirical experience has shown that its effectiveness is probably closer to 18 months.

In 1988, a new copper-containing IUD with an increased amount of copper added to the arms began to be marketed as ParaGard (Fig. 15.1). Shortly thereafter, a LNG-containing IUD (Mirena) became available first in Europe and was later marketed in the United States.

The mechanism of action of IUDs is not as an abortifacient, a common misperception. A sterile inflammatory response to the foreign body in the uterus produces tissue injury of a minor degree, but sufficient enough to be spermicidal. In a more recent study, interleukin and tumor necrosis factor cytokines in the endometrial cavity were obtained at curettage or at hysterectomy. These cytokines are increased in all IUD users. The copper IUD, in particular, was associated

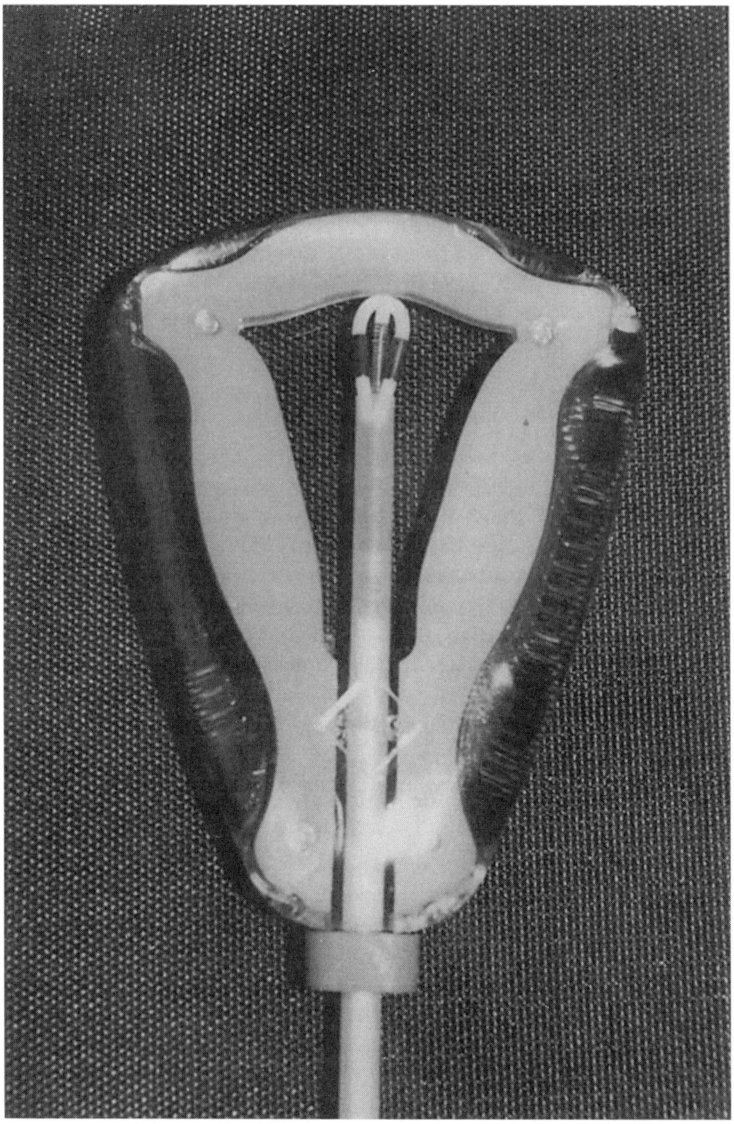

FIGURE 15.1 ● Copper IUD (ParaGard) readied for placement.

with an increased concentration of endometrial cytokines, and this may well be its significant mechanism of action (79). These changes are believed to be primarily spermicidal in nature, although the inflammatory response also prevents implantation.

In addition to increasing local cytokines, the progestin IUD thickens the cervical mucus, creating a barrier to sperm penetration through the cervix. Its proposed major mechanism of action is inhibition of implantation and inhibition of sperm capacitation and survival. Removal of the IUD, particularly if it is done premenstrually to allow "cleansing" of the endometrium, is followed by normal conception rates for the next cycle and thereafter.

A 1987 review of a first year trial of experience in parous women showed that in the first year of use, the copper T (Tcu-380A) experienced an expulsion rate of 5% and a removal rate, usually for pain or bleeding, of 14%, whereas the progesterone IUD (ParaGard) experienced an expulsion rate of 2.7% and a removal rate of 9.3% (80). Half of all expulsions occur during the first year of use. The progesterone IUD may decrease blood flow by 40 to 50% and improve dysmenorrhea so its use may be preferable in women experiencing heavy or painful periods. Over time, copper IUDs are associated with stable ovulatory bleeding patterns, but prolonged bleeding is common in the first few months (81).

The ectopic pregnancy rate for noncontraceptive users is 3 to 4.5 per 1000 woman-years; for progesterone IUD users, 6.8 per 1000 woman-years; and for the copper-containing IUD, 0.2 per 1000 woman-years (82, 83).

The Progestasert IUD has an annual pregnancy failure rate of 2% for total pregnancies compared with 0.8% for the ParaGard (82). The copper IUD is effective for 10 years, and expulsion rates decrease to 0.4 to 3.7% per year by the tenth year; the cumulative net pregnancy rate for the copper IUD after 7 years of use is 1.5 per 100 women-years (84). The copper T is a more effective and semipermanent device; the progesterone T is better tolerated in the first year of use and is perhaps more suitable for child spacing.

The Mirena IUD releases 20 mcg LNG daily and has been approved for up to 5 years of use. Although irregular spotting or bleeding may occur in the first few months, this usually diminishes over time. The number of bleeding and spotting days is also decreased, and about 30% of LNG IUD users become amenorrheic by 2 years of use (81, 85–87). Two large clinical trials in Finland and Sweden with more than 1600 women and 45,000 cycles of use have demonstrated cumulative 5-year pregnancy rates of less than 0.7 per 100 women.

The majority of women who continue to have cyclical menses with the LNG IUD have ovulatory progesterone levels, but only 58% of these women have normal growth and rupture of ovarian follicles on ultrasound exam. Of the women who do not have cyclical menses, 29% have growth and rupture of follicles (88). It is not surprising then that women using the LNG IUD more commonly develop large (greater than 3 cm) ovarian cysts. In one study, all these cysts spontaneously resolved over a 4-month period, and it is believed the formation of these cysts is of limited significance (89). These findings are similar to what has been seen with the subdermal LNG implants (90).

There is some evidence for the use of Mirena as a substitute for oral progestin in hormone therapy, and it may be an excellent transition from contraception to hormone therapy (91). Use of the LNG IUD has been shown to induce epithelial atrophy and stromal decidualization when used in postmenopausal women in conjunction with estrogen for up to 5 years (92).

The IUD is recommended for the parous woman in a mutually monogamous relationship with no history of pelvic inflammatory disease and a desire for long-term contraception. IUDs may be used safely in a nulliparous and/or nulligravida woman if both she and her partner are monogamous. The incidence of pain, bleeding, and/or syncope may be higher at the time of insertion in nulliparous women. For a list of contraindications to placement and use of the IUD, refer to Table 15.9. The patient should be cautioned at the time of insertion that if there is a change in that relationship, strong consideration should be given to IUD removal and use of another contraceptive method.

When pregnancy is diagnosed in the presence of an IUD, the location of the pregnancy (intra- or extrauterine) should be determined and the device removed as soon as possible, regardless of whether pregnancy continuation is planned. The earlier the pregnancy is diagnosed, the better, because there is a greater likelihood of successful removal when the strings are still accessible in the enlarging uterus. If there is no evidence of infection and the strings are easily seen, this

TABLE 15.9

Contraindications to Use of Copper T-380A or Progesterone-Releasing IUD

Contraindications To Use Of Both

Known or suspected pregnancy

Abnormalities of uterus that distort uterine cavity, including uterus with cavity <6 cm or >10 cm on sounding

Presence or history of pelvic inflammatory disease or sexually transmitted diseases

Patient or partner has multiple sexual partners

Known or suspected uterus or cervical malignancy, including unresolved abnormal Pap smear

Conditions or treatments that increase susceptibility to infection

Genital bleeding of unknown etiology

Genital actinomycoses

Untreated acute cervicitis or vaginitis, including bacterial vaginosis

Postpartum endometritis or septic abortion in past 3 months

Valvular heart disease (may use in mitral valve prolapse, but if mitral regurgitation is present, give prophylactic antibiotics at time of insertion)

Anticoagulant therapy

Severe anemia

Severe dysmenorrhea and/or menstruation (more significant contraindication for copper IUD than for progesterone IUD)

Contraindications Specific To Copper T-380A IUD

Wilson's disease

Known allergy to copper

can be done in the office or clinic setting. Women who become pregnant with an IUD in place have an increased rate, approximately 50%, of spontaneous abortion. After removal of the IUD, the spontaneous abortion rate decreases to about 30%.

If the IUD cannot be easily removed, a therapeutic abortion should be offered to the patient. The risk of life-threatening septic abortion in the second trimester is increased 20-fold if the IUD is left in utero. Removal of an IUD in an infected, pregnant uterus should be accomplished only after intravenous antibiotic blood levels have been achieved. It should be done in an area where emergency measures are available, in case septic shock ensues. Studies have not shown any increase in congenital anomalies associated with the presence of an IUD in utero during pregnancy.

The IUD can be inserted safely at any time after delivery, abortion, or during menses. There is a higher rate of expulsion immediately postpartum, although this can be decreased with high fundal placement. Insertion of the IUD during the period of lactational amenorrhea has the advantage of not being associated with a spotting problem often encountered during the first cycle after insertion. The usually atrophic endometrium tolerates the IUD very well. While menstruating, the ideal time for insertion is at the end of a menstrual period or within 2 to 3 days thereafter. For women at low risk of occult sexually transmitted diseases (STDs), there is probably no benefit of prophylactic antibiotics prior to insertion of the IUD. Most think that administration of doxycycline (Doryx, Vibramycin, 200 mg) 1 hour prior to insertion may give some protection against insertion-associated pelvic infection. Directions for placement of the copper and progesterone IUDs are found in Appendices 15.1 and 15.2.

The patient is to check for the IUD string monthly, and the practitioner checks for it at the time of gynecologic examination. If it is not present, an ultrasound should be done to confirm intrauterine location. If the ultrasound does not show it, a flat plate abdominal radiograph is taken.

If the IUD is intra-abdominal/extrauterine, it must be physically retrieved. An intra-abdominal IUD can cause serious problems, including bowel obstruction or perforation. Removal should be done as soon as possible after the diagnosis is made. Copper IUDs, in particular, elicit a strong inflammatory response that may make laparoscopic removal quite difficult. Perforation of the uterus usually occurs at the time of insertion, so it is important to identify the strings a few weeks afterward.

To remove an IUD, the strings are grasped with either a ring forceps or uterine dressing forceps and firm traction is exerted. If the string(s) cannot be seen, a cytobrush in the endocervical canal may help in extracting them. If further maneuvers are necessary, a paracervical block should be given. Visualization of the IUD with sonography or hysteroscopy may be necessary to facilitate removal.

BARRIER METHODS OF CONTRACEPTION

Diaphragm

The diaphragm can be an effective method of contraception. Diaphragm failure rates for the first year are estimated at 13 to 23% (93).When used faithfully, the failure rate is probably closer to 6%. The diaphragm is fitted by the practitioner in the office, preferably using actual diaphragms rather than rings. There are three types of diaphragms: the flat metal spring, all-flex arcing type, or hinged arcing type. Sizes range from 50 to 105 mm in diameter, with most women using a size between 65 and 80 mm.

To fit the diaphragm, place the middle finger against the vaginal wall and posterior cul de sac. Lift the hand anteriorly until the index finger is against the back of the symphysis pubis. Mark this point with the thumb to approximate the necessary diameter of the diaphragm. Insert the corresponding ring or diaphragm. Both the practitioner and patient are to assess the fit. If it is too tight, a smaller size is chosen. If it is expelled with increased intra-abdominal pressure, a larger size is needed. The practitioner should instruct and observe the patient in the insertion process, and check for proper placement.

The diaphragm should be placed no more than 6 hours before intercourse. It should be left in the vagina for about 6 hours, but no more than 24 hours, after coitus. Additional spermicide should be placed intravaginally without removing the diaphragm for each additional episode of intercourse. Oil-based lubricants should not be used with the diaphragm. After it is removed, it should be washed with soap and water, rinsed, and dried. Powders should never be used on the diaphragm. Periodic checks for leaks should be done. The diaphragm should not be exposed to light or extreme temperatures during storage.

The incidence of urinary tract infections (UTIs) among diaphragm users is about twice that of women using OCs. This may be due to pressure on the urethra with the diaphragm in place or increased colonization of the vagina with *Escherichia coli* (94, 95). Voiding after intercourse is helpful in avoiding UTI. A single postcoital dose of prophylactic antibiotics may also be used. There are some parous women with relaxation of the anterior vaginal wall in whom proper fitting is difficult, although the flat metal spring diaphragm may be tried in such instances. Well-motivated, properly fitted and instructed women find the diaphragm a very acceptable method of contraception. The diaphragm reduces the incidence of STDs, as well as cervical neoplasia, presumably by reducing acquisition of HPV and other pathogens (96). With a change in weight greater than 10 lb or after each pregnancy, the woman may need to be refitted with a diaphragm of another size.

Cervical Cap

Currently, the cervical cap devices approved for use in the United States include the cavity rim cervical cap, the Prentif, FemCap, and the Lea's Shield. Prentif comes in four sizes based on internal diameter size: 22, 25, 28, and 31 mm. FemCap is available in three sizes based on internal diameter size: 22, 26, and 30 mm. The Lea's Shield comes in only one size and does not require fitting by a clinician. Although Prentif is a latex cervical cap, FemCap and Lea's Shield are both made of medical-grade silicone. The silicone caps are advantageous for women with latex allergies, and silicone is believed to resist odor formation.

A practitioner experienced in the use of this device must fit the Prentif and FemCap to the size of the cervix. The dome of the cervical cap covers the cervix and the rim fits snugly into the vaginal fornices. The brim adheres and conforms to the vaginal walls. Approximately 50% of women can be properly fitted. Women with a long cervix, short cervix, small cervix, or one that is too anterior may not be suitable candidates for the cap. Unlike the diaphragm, the cervical cap may be used in women with relaxation of the anterior vaginal wall.

Women should be advised to check placement of the device prior to and after intercourse to confirm correct positioning; the possibility of emergency contraception in the event of dislodgment during intercourse should also be discussed. A follow-up exam after prescribing is recommended, and the patient should wear the device into the office so the clinician can confirm proper placement. If a speculum is used to determine proper placement, it should be inserted only halfway into the vagina to avoid inadvertent dislodgment of the cervical cap.

Prior to use, the cervical cap should be filled one-third with spermicidal jelly or cream, applied to the inside of the cap, which is then positioned over the cervix by hand or with a special applicator. The cap should be inserted no less than 20 minutes and no more than 4 hours prior to intercourse. It is advised that women insert the cervical cap prior to sexual arousal because lengthening of the vagina on arousal may make insertion and proper placement more difficult. After insertion and after each act of coitus, the cervix should be checked to ensure it is covered. The FemCap and Prentif should not be removed any less than 6 hours after intercourse (the Lea's Shield must be left in place for a minimum of 8 hours), and all cervical caps may be left in place for up to 48 hours. The Lea's Shield has an anterior loop to facilitate removal and the FemCap has an anterior strap for this purpose as well; however, removal of the Prentif or FemCap is done by exerting pressure on the rim to break the seal and easily removing it. Squatting seems to be the best position for removal of these devices. Cleaning of the device is best done with a mild antibacterial soap. Heat, synthetic detergents, organic solvents, or sharp objects should not be used for cleaning purposes. The device should be inspected regularly for signs of puncture, perforation, or wear.

With FemCap, the past obstetric history can predict the necessary size about 85% of the time with nulliparous women most often using the small size, with parous women with abdominal modes of delivery requiring the medium, and with parous women with a history of vaginal delivery requiring the large size. In clinical trials with the FemCap, it was noted that the risk of pregnancy was twice as high for parous women using the large device in comparison to nulliparous women using the small device or parous women using the medium-size device. For this reason, parous women requiring the larger size should be strongly counseled about an increased risk for pregnancy when relying on the FemCap as the sole means of contraception (97–99).

When used with a spermicide, Prentif first-year failure rates with perfect use are approximately 9%, but with typical use failure rates are estimated at 20% for nulliparous women and 26 to 40% for parous women (100). The failure rate for the Lea's Shield and typical use is estimated to range between 9% and 15% (101). Like other vaginal barrier methods, the cap is associated with increased incidence of UTIs, bacterial vaginosis, and vaginal candidiasis when used with a spermicide (102). Cervical caps do not decrease the risk of transmission of STDs. They have been associated with disruption of the cervicovaginal epithelium, although the actual clinical ramifications of this are unclear.

The cervical cap should not be used in women with active vaginal, cervical, or pelvic infections or vaginal or cervical lesions. Use of the cap during menstruation is discouraged because of the possibility of an increased risk of toxic shock syndrome and endometriosis; this possibility is theoretical, and no clinical evidence exists to disprove or support this to date.

Male Condom

Male condoms are the third most popular contraceptive method employed by married couples in the United States, following sterilization and oral contraceptives. First-year failure rates with condom use are reported to be 8 to 15%, although use of the condom by highly motivated couples has a failure rate of 2 to 4% (84, 103). Contraceptive failure rates are lower in women older than the age of 30 years, those who seek to prevent pregnancy rather than delay it, and women of higher socioeconomic-economic status and level of education.

Most current condoms are made of latex, although the "natural skin" male condoms are made of lamb's intestine, and newer materials such as polyurethane are also used. Allergic reactions to latex or chemicals in the latex can occur, either immediately or as delayed reactions.

Clinicians should never assume pre-existing knowledge on proper condom use on the part of their patients. It is important to place the condom on the penis before any genital contact occurs. Uncircumcised men must pull the foreskin back prior to placement. Before unrolling and applying the condom, air should be squeezed out of the reservoir and the tip of the condom should extend beyond the end of the penis. The condom must be withdrawn prior to loss of the erection. Condoms may break during vaginal intercourse or withdrawal; slipping and tearing are more common with polyurethane condoms than with latex ones, but polyurethane condoms are suitable for latex-sensitive users, and because they are thinner may offer enhanced sensitivity (104). The principle disadvantage to the use of the condom relates to an interruption of sexual foreplay, which can be minimized by incorporating its application during foreplay.

Although water-based lubricants can be used with any type of condom, petroleum-based lubricants should not be used with natural skin or latex condoms because they markedly decrease the strength of condoms, even with only brief exposure times. Polyurethane condoms may be used with any type of lubricant.

Male condom use has risen since the mid-1980s in the United States primarily as an HIV protection method. A meta-analysis of 25 studies found that male condoms offered a protective efficacy of 84 to 87% (102, 105). The latex condom is the only male condom shown to effectively prevent HIV transmission; condoms made from lamb intestines are permeable to virus particles, such as HIV and herpes (102). Theoretically, polyurethane condoms may offer similar HIV protection as the latex condoms, but this has not been clinically confirmed yet. Users must realize that to reduce the risk of HIV transmission, latex male condoms must be used with each and every act of sex.

In addition to the decreased transmission of HIV, latex condoms also offer good protection against other viral and bacterial STDS such as *Neisseria gonorrhea*, *Chlamydia trachomatis*, and trichomonas infections (106). Debate exists as to the extent of protection they may offer in preventing transmission of the herpes and HPVs if virus particles are located on the groin or vulvar areas (107, 108).

Female Condom

The FDA approved the female condom in 1994 (Fig. 15.2). There are several studies that evaluated its utilization and effectiveness. One study included female employees of two hospitals in Cape Town, South Africa. Twenty-three of 52 participants used all ten of the devices issued to them, 21 stated that they or their partner(s) did not enjoy using the method, and an additional 9 had other problems with it. One problem that has been reported is that the device is noisy. Sexual responsivity, however, was the same or better in 52%, and overall acceptability was 52%. Compared with the male condom, 50% of the women and 44% of their partners considered the device as good, or better than, the male condom (109). In the initial U.S. trial, there was a pregnancy rate of 15% in 6 months, although with perfect use the pregnancy rate is probably 3% (110). The female condom should not be used with a male condom because this may increase slippage and/or breakage (102).

Current experience shows that the female condom is an acceptable method for some couples. Although intended for single use only, some women reuse them for financial reasons. The female condom may be used for up to eight cycles of vaginal intercourse (and subsequent washing, drying, and relubrication with use) without any significant compromise to its structural integrity (111). A clear advantage is that it is a female-controlled contraceptive that provides protection against STDs, including HIV. Directions regarding placement of the female condom can be found in Appendix 15.3.

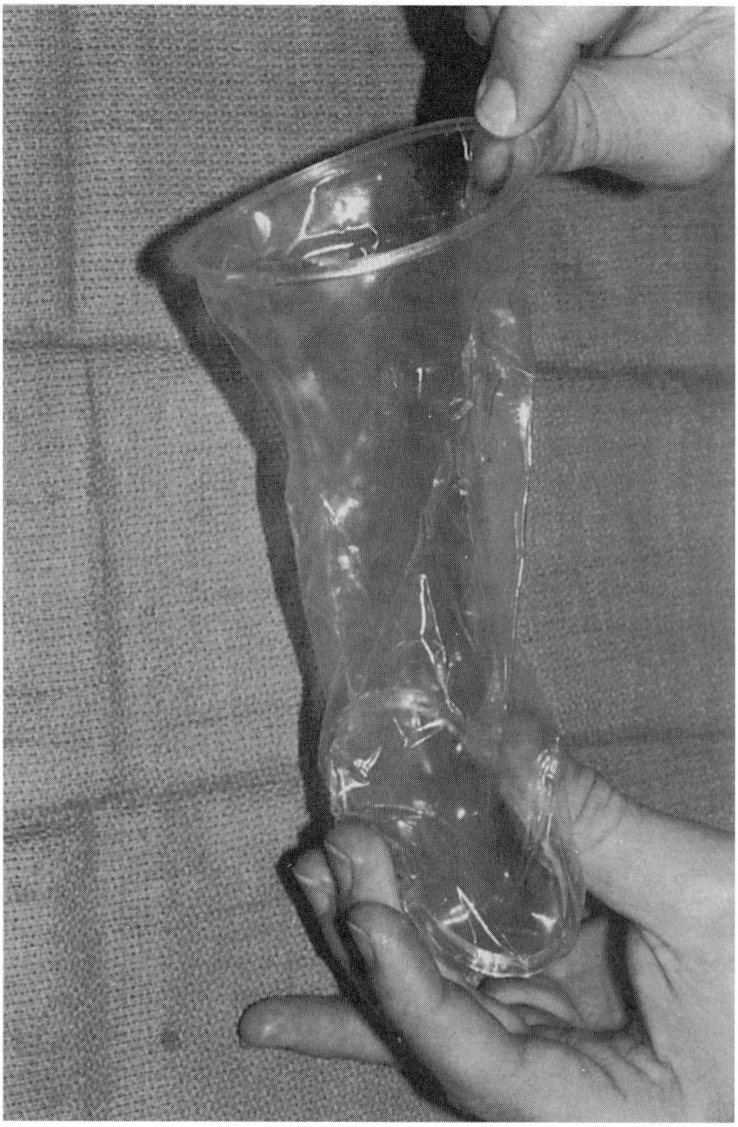

FIGURE 15.2 ● Female condom.

Sponge

The over-the-counter Today contraceptive sponge was withdrawn from the U.S. market in 1995 due to manufacturing issues. Although it will be re-released to the general market, it is currently available via the Internet. The Today sponge is a physical and a chemical barrier that fits closely over the cervix, absorbs semen, and releases spermicide. Another similar sponge that can be ordered via the Internet is the Protectaid sponge, which contains three spermicides, including a lower dose of N-9 that may reduce mucosal irritation. Whereas the Today sponge can be inserted immediately before coitus or up to 24 hours in advance, the Protectaid sponge should be inserted no more than 12 hours in advance. Both sponges should be left in the vagina for 6 hours after intercourse.

Failure rates for the sponge are similar to use of spermicide alone and are higher than diaphragm use (100). As with the cervical cap, parous women experience failure rates approximately double those of nonparous women (100, 112).

SPERMICIDES

Spermicides are supplied as jellies, creams, foams, melting suppositories, foaming tablets, and soluble films. Nonoxynol-9 (N-9) is the active ingredient in almost all spermicides available in the United States, and it works by disrupting the integrity of the sperm cell membrane (102). Most spermicides employ N-9 in concentrations ranging from 3 to 20%. N-9 is not absorbed from the vagina. Other spermicides such as octoxynol-9 or menfegol, are offered in some over-the-counter vaginal contraceptives, usually with 60 to 100 mg per vaginal application, but the FDA has stated that their efficacy and safety remain unproven.

Timing of the application of the spermicide is an important determinant of efficacy and although some must be inserted no more than 1 hour before coitus, others simply require enough time to melt or dissolve intravaginally prior to coitus. All must be reapplied for each act of intercourse. Aerosol foams offer the best protection as the jellies, and melting suppositories provide poor intravaginal distribution (113). The jelly, cream, and foam preparations are good for use up to 80 minutes prior to intercourse. The tablets and suppositories are good for 1 hour or less.

Efficacy of spermicides is highly product and user dependent. Failure rates with perfect use are approximately 6%, whereas overall failure rates are approximately 26%. Unfortunately, the correct use of spermicides does not correlate with years of experience of use (100).

Occasionally, spermicides may cause allergic reactions or yeast infections and may promote UTIs through alterations of the normal bacterial flora of the vagina (102).

Since the mid-1980s, spermicides, including N-9, have been recommended for the prevention of STDs, including HIV. However, more recent studies indicate that N-9 causes an increase in genital ulcers and vaginal inflammation (114, 115). This raised concerns regarding the possibility of increasing the risk of HIV transmission. Several randomized trials have been performed more recently to evaluate the effectiveness of N-9 in prevention of STDs. Three different preparations of N-9 have been examined, including film, gel, and vaginal sponge. These investigators concluded that N-9 is not effective in preventing gonorrhea, chlamydia, trichomoniasis, syphilis, or HIV infection (114, 116, 117). In addition, in one study using vaginal sponges with N-9, there was nearly a 50% increase in the transmission of HIV compared with the placebo group (116). As a result of these findings, the CDC no longer recommends the use of spermicides containing N-9 for vaginal or anal intercourse (118).

The use of spermicides does not increase the risk for spontaneous abortion, birth defects, or low birth weight (119).

EMERGENCY CONTRACEPTION

Emergency contraception, also known as postcoital contraception or the "morning after" pill, has been available for more than 30 years. Two products, Preven and Plan B, are currently approved by the FDA for the use of emergency contraceptive. Preven is simply the Yuzpe regimen (two OC tables, each with a combination of EE and LNG), which includes a pregnancy test and patient instructions. Plan B, a newer product, is a progestin-only formulation (LNG).

A more recent WHO-sponsored study demonstrated that the LNG regimen is more effective than the Yuzpe method. The proportion of pregnancies prevented in the LNG group was 85% (compared with the predicted rate that would have occurred with no emergency contraception), whereas the Yuzpe method prevented only 57% of pregnancies (120).

Treatment efficacy of emergency contraception is related in part to the timing of the first dose and the sexual exposure. The sooner after exposure the first dose of emergency contraception is administered, the greater the efficacy. For both regimens, the greatest protection against pregnancy is offered within the first 24 hours after unprotected sex.

Side effects are also less with the LNG-only regimen. About 50% of users of the Yuzpe regimen experience nausea and 20% report vomiting in comparison to 23% and 6%, respectively, for the LNG-only regimen (121).

As a practical matter, it is recommended that an antiemetic be taken 1 hour prior to the first postcoital OC dose (122). Such a proactive approach is more effective than simply taking the

TABLE 15.10

Emergency Contraceptive Regimens

Conjugated estrogens (Premarin) 30 mg twice a day × 5 days *or* 10 mg four times a day × 5 days *or* 25 mg IV immediately and again 24 h later
Ethinyl estradiol (Estinyl) 2.5 mg twice a day × 5 days *or* 5 mg four times a day × 5 days
Oral contraceptive regimens[a]
Ovral two tablets immediately and again 12 h later
Levlen, Levora, Lo/Ovral, Nordette, Tri-Levlen, or Triphasil four tablets immediately and again 12 h later

[a] In the event of vomiting, the dose must be repeated.

antiemetic if needed to relieve the nausea after taking the regimen and is often necessary with use of Preven.

Both WHO and the International Planned Parenthood Federation find no absolute evidence-based contraindications to the use of emergency contraception, except for a known established pregnancy (e.g., a positive pregnancy test). The FDA-approved labeling in the United States does list clotting problems, ischemic heart disease, stroke, migraine, liver tumors, breast cancer, and breast biopsies as contraindications. Because the duration of therapy is short, the usual medical contraindications to long-term use of steroidal contraceptives are probably not applicable to emergency contraception (123).

Other formulations marketed for use as combination OCs have been studied for the use as emergency contraceptives. For additional information on other regimens that may be useful for emergency contraception, see Table 15.10.

Insertion of copper IUDs within 5 days of unprotected sex is another method of providing emergency contraception. An emergency IUD insertion reduces the risk of pregnancy by about 99%. It is not a method recommended for nulliparous women or women at risk of having an STD.

STERILIZATION

Female Sterilization

Sterilization is one of the most common methods of contraception in the United States. Most procedures are done in an outpatient surgical setting, although some are done in private offices. The mortality rate for sterilization is 1.5 per 100,000 procedures. This is lower than the mortality associated with childbirth (10 per 100,000) (124). The average failure rate in the first year is 0.5% for female sterilization and 0.1 to 0.15% for male sterilization, with the actual rate being operator, patient, and technique dependent (125). Techniques that rely on more equipment have a higher failure rate secondary to technical problems (126, 127). Female patients younger than 35 years have a higher failure rate, as do women who are not lactating at the time of the procedure.

With sterilization currently being readily available, careful consideration and counseling is in order. This is particularly true of women younger than 30 years, and the procedure should generally be limited to the patient who is presumably in a long-term relationship. These criteria are obviously not the case when a disease is present that could be worsened by the complication of subsequent pregnancy. The median age at sterilization is 30, and there is a higher incidence of regret in women sterilized before age 30 and among those who divorce and remarry. In certain ethnic cultures, a woman incapable of bearing children may be considered "damaged" to some degree. The question needs to be asked, "What if something happened to your partner, or to one of your children—would this change your mind?" The decision should be regarded as irrevocable and unseemly optimism for the possibility of uncomplicated reversal should be faced with facts of insurance payments, the increase in risk of ectopic pregnancy, and the greatly diminished chance of success in the event of any type of cauterization procedure. An informed consent should state the risk of failure and the increased rate of ectopic pregnancy in that event.

Currently, the four most commonly used methods of sterilization in the United States include sterilization in conjunction with cesarean section or other abdominal surgery, immediate postpartum partial salpingectomy, minilaparotomy, or laparoscopy. An interval minilaparotomy approach would certainly be appropriate if the patient's history or pelvic findings suggested the possibility of significant pelvic adhesions and perhaps distortion of anatomy.

A more recently published, multicentered, prospective, cohort study involving 10,685 women was reported from the U.S. Collaborative Review of Sterilization (CREST). The CREST data show that failures continue beyond the first year: by 5 years, more than 1% of women had a sterilization failure, and by 10 years, 1.8% failed (128). It is well known that the risk of ectopic pregnancy after tubal sterilization is greatly increased. Failures of sterilization are associated with a higher rate of ectopic pregnancies, with the incidence depending on the surgical procedure originally performed. Bipolar cauterization has a higher incidence of ectopic pregnancy associated with tubal failures than mechanical occlusion (129). Another study found 7.3 tubal pregnancies per 1000 procedures, and found that bipolar tubal coagulation before the age of 30 had a probability of ectopic pregnancy 27 times greater than women of similar age who underwent postpartum partial salpingectomy (130). The same study also showed that a history of tubal sterilization does not rule out the possibility of ectopic pregnancy, even 10 years after the procedure (130). The overall risk for ectopic pregnancy in sterilized women, however, is still lower than if they were not sterilized.

The first suggestion of a "post-tubal syndrome" was in 1951 (131). The CREST multicenter prospective study on this subject showed that of patients interviewed immediately prior and again poststerilization for up to 5 years, 35% report higher levels of menstrual pain, 49% reported very heavy increase in menstrual flow, and 10% reported increased spotting between periods. This was at the fifth year; the first year showed a lesser degree of pain and hypermenorrhea (132). It is obvious that aging of the cohort may be a factor, as well as the fact that it takes such changes a significant time to develop. In similar, paired studies of poststerilization on women conducted several years apart, both Rulin and DeStephano showed an increased prevalence of pain in the latter studies (133–136).

There have been anecdotal reports about the prevalence of hysterectomy after sterilization. Hilliset al. reported that the cumulative probability of undergoing hysterectomy within 14 years after sterilization was 17% (137). The highest likelihood occurred among women who reported a history of endometriosis or noted prolonged bleeding prior to sterilization. Not surprisingly, women with gynecologic disorders were at greater risk of hysterectomy than were women without these disorders (137). Women may be reassured that there is no detrimental effect on sexual response associated with tubal sterilization (138).

In 2002, the FDA approved a nonsurgical method of permanent female sterilization. In this procedure a special catheter is inserted into the fallopian tubes via the vagina, cervix, and uterus, and a small metal implant (Essure) is deposited. The implants induce scar tissue formation, blocking the fallopian tubes, and preventing fertilization of the egg. Women must use alternate forms of contraception at least for 3 months after the procedure and until proper implant placement is confirmed by hysterosalpingography.

Male Sterilization

Permanent surgical sterilization of men is done in the office and is safer, easier, and less expensive then surgical sterilization of women. In the "no scalpel" technique, a sharpened dissection forceps is used to pierce the skin and dissect the vas deferens. Complications are uncommon but may include some bleeding, hematoma formation, infection, or local reactions to anesthetics or sutures. A patent reanastomosis is achieved in approximately 86 to 97% of men seeking reversal of the vasectomy, although their fertility rates are considerable less due to a variety of issues.

Clinical Notes

- Natural family planning, also known as the rhythm method or periodic abstinence, encompasses three techniques: the calendar rhythm method, the basal body temperature method, and the cervical mucus method.
- Oral contraceptives impact protein, lipid, and carbohydrate metabolism.
- In lactating women, the combination OC is not recommended because it decreases the quantity of milk and some amounts of EE may be transferred to the infant.
- Progestin-only minipills are preferred for lactating women seeking oral hormonal contraception.
- One commonly accepted contraindication to the use of OCs is a history of classic migraine (migraine with focal neurologic symptoms or aura lasting more than 1 hour) due to an increased potential for stroke, although the evidence to support this is scant.
- There is no impact of OCs on the pattern or frequency of seizures in women with epilepsy.
- Some anticonvulsants can decrease serum concentrations of estrogen and thus may increase the likelihood of intermenstrual bleeding among patients on OCs.
- The cardiovascular disease risk with OC use is most prevalent in women older than 35 years who smoke and who have used OCs for long periods of time.
- For women with hypertension, if their blood pressure is controlled and no vascular disease is present, OCs are not contraindicated.
- If a woman's triglycerides are above 350 mg/dL or in patients with familial hypertriglyceridemia, OCs should be avoided because they may precipitate pancreatitis and/or adversely affect the patient's risk for cardiovascular disease.
- In general, OCs can be safely used by women with MVP who are symptom free.
- Young diabetic women who are free of retinopathy, nephropathy, hypertension, or other complicating vascular disease(s) are appropriate candidates for low-dose contraceptives.
- Overall, the risk of breast cancer in women who take OCs until they are 55 years of age appears to be no different from that of nonusers.
- Antimicrobial agents can interact with the pharmacokinetics and efficacy of sex steroid hormones present in OCs.
- The risks of using Seasonale are similar to the risks of other OC drugs, including risk of pregnancy with missed doses.
- Progestin-only contraceptives can be used by almost every woman and have few medical contraindications (active liver disease or liver tumor being one).
- Women with sickle cell anemia, congenital heart disease, or those older than 35 who smoke are excellent candidates for DMPA.
- There is no increase in stroke risk or MI with use of DMPA.
- The contraceptive efficacy of Lunelle is comparable to that of oral combination, although more women using Lunelle may experience amenorrhea than those using combination OCs.
- The NuvaRing system consists of a flexible nonbiodegradeable vaginal ring containing etonogestrel and EE. The vaginal ring should be kept refrigerated before dispensing, and clinicians should be aware that it has a shelf-life of only 4 months.
- There is less breakthrough bleeding with the vaginal contraceptive ring than with any other hormonal contraceptive method.
- The efficacy of the vaginal contraceptive ring has not been studied in women weighing more than 200 lb.
- There is no increase in risk of toxic shock syndrome with the vaginal contraceptive ring because it is not absorbent.

- The contraceptive patch system uses a 28-day (4-week) cycle in which a new patch is applied each week for 3 weeks. There is a 7-day period in which no patch is worn (corresponding to the 7-day pillfree interval with OCs).
- Hormonal release from the contraceptive patch is not significantly affected by treadmill exercise, or exposure to cold water, whirlpool, or sauna. Nor is it affected by the anatomic site of application (abdomen, buttocks, torso, or upper outer arm), although it should not be placed on the breasts.
- The Mirena IUD releases 20 mcg LNG daily and has been approved for up to 5 years of use.
- The progesterone IUD may decrease blood flow by 40 to 50% and improve dysmenorrhea so its use may be preferable in women experiencing heavy or painful periods.
- The copper IUD is effective for 10 years.
- If a pregnancy occurs with an IUD in place, the device should be removed as soon as possible, regardless of whether termination or pregnancy continuation is planned.
- Women who become pregnant with an IUD in place have an increased rate, approximately 50%, of spontaneous abortion. After removal of the IUD, the spontaneous abortion rate decreases to about 30%.
- Male condoms are the third most popular contraceptive method employed by married couples in the United States, following sterilization and OCs.
- Because there is evidence that N-9 may actually increase the risk of HIV transmission, the CDC no longer recommends the use of spermicides containing N-9 for vaginal or anal intercourse.
- The average failure rate in the first year is 0.5% for female sterilization and 0.1 to 0.15% for male sterilization, with the actual rate being operator, patient, and technique dependent.

APPENDIX 15.1

Placement of the Copper IUD

1. Can be inserted whenever pregnancy has been reliably excluded, including immediately postpartum or after abortion.
2. Confirm uterine size and position on examination.
3. Clean cervix and upper vagina with antiseptic.
4. Apply topical anesthesia or paracervical block to cervix; place tenaculum on anterior lip of cervix for traction (if uterus is extremely retroverted, placing tenaculum on posterior lip of cervix may be more helpful).
5. Sound the uterus; do not place IUD if uterus sounds to less than 6 cm or greater than 9 cm.
6. Document IUD lot number in chart and open IUD package, keeping contents sterile.
7. Wear sterile gloves; load the IUD into the insertion tube with the arms of the "T" folded *downward* into tube; do not leave the IUD in the insertion tube with the arms folded for more than 5 minutes.
8. Insert solid tube into bottom of insertion tube until it touches the bottom of the IUD.
9. Adjust the flange of the insertion tube to depth of uterus and to the plane in which the arms will open. Make sure the horizontal arms and long axis of the flange lie in the same horizontal plane.
10. Place insertion tube into cervix/uterus until it touches fundus of uterus. The flange should be at the cervix. Hold solid rod stationary and retract the insertion tube no greater than 0.5 inch to release the arms.
11. Hold insertion tube still and remove solid rod only. After the solid rod is out, remove the insertion tube. Cut threads 2.5 to 4 cm beyond os. Measure and record the length of the strings.

APPENDIX 15.2

Placement of Progesterone IUD

1. Able to insert in latter part of menstrual period or for 1 to 2 days after menses has finished. If being used postpartum, uterine involution must be complete. It is not to be placed immediately postabortion or postpartum.
2. Confirm uterine size and position on examination.
3. Clean cervix and upper vagina with antiseptic.
4. Apply topical anesthesia or paracervical block to cervix; place tenaculum on anterior lip of cervix for traction (if uterus is extremely retroverted, placing tenaculum on posterior lip of cervix may be more helpful).
5. Sound the uterus; do not place IUD if uterus sounds to less than 6 cm or greater than 9 cm.
6. Document IUD lot number in chart and open IUD package, keeping contents sterile.
7. Use the cocking device to fold the arms against the stem by pressing insert straight down on a solid surface. Do not leave cocked for more than 5 minutes.
8. Adjust the inserting tube for the curvature of the uterus; if anteverted, the numbers face up, if retroverted, the numbers face down.
9. Check that the thread-retaining plug at the end of the tube is secure.
10. Wear sterile gloves; place into cervix/uterus until it reaches fundus. The number at the cervix on the inserter should equal the depth noted on the sounding of the uterus.
11. Hold the arm of the inserter still and squeeze the wings of the thread-retaining plug to remove it.
12. Withdraw inserter. Measure shorter of the two threads. The IUD is at the fundus if the length of the shorter thread is equal to the difference between 9 cm and the uterine depth in centimeters noted on sounding. Cut other thread usual length and record.

APPENDIX 15.3

Placement of the Female Condom

1. After removing the condom from the package, check to ensure the lubrication is spread evenly inside the pouch from the bottom to the top. If more lubricant is necessary, add two drops from the additional lubricant that is supplied. (Some women may need more than two drops.)
2. Check that the inner ring is at the bottom, closed end of the pouch.
3. Hold the condom with the open end hanging down toward the ground. Squeeze the inner ring with your thumb and middle finger. It should look like a long, narrow "O".
4. With the other hand, separate the labia so the vagina is accessible. The hand holding the condom pushes the inner ring and pouch up into the vagina until the entire inner ring is just behind the pubic bone. (This is the same placement one uses for a diaphragm.) The condom should be inserted straight into the vagina; in other words, it should not be twisted. About 1 inch of the open end should remain in place outside the vagina.
5. During sex, the outer ring may move from side to side, which is normal. However, if it begins to slide or slip or is noisy during sex, add more lubricant.
6. If the outer ring begins to be pushed into the vagina, the female condom should be replaced, with extra lubricant around the opening of the new pouch or on the penis.
7. To remove the condom, squeeze and twist the outer ring, keeping the sperm and semen inside the pouch. The condom is not designed to be flushed down a toilet—it must be placed in the trash. It should *not* be reused.
8. A new condom must be used with every act of sex. The female condom must be replaced with a new one with a subsequent episode of sex.
9. The female condom should not be used at the same time as a male condom. If used simultaneously, neither product will stay in place.

REFERENCES

1. Garza-Flores J. Reversible contraception: issues faced by emerging countries. Int J Gynaecol Obstet 1998;62(suppl 1):S37–S40.
2. Brown JB, Blackwell LF, Billings JJ, et al. Natural family planning. Am J Obstet Gynecol 1987;157:1082–1089.
3. Brown JB, Holmes J, Barker G. Use of the home ovarian monitor in pregnancy avoidance. Am J Obstet Gynecol 1991;165:2008–2011.
4. Roetzer J. Natural family planning and pregnancy outcome. Int J Fertil 1988;33(suppl):40–42.
5. Bohler E. Breast feeding as family planning in a global perspective. Tidsskr Nor Laegeforen 1997;117:701–704.
6. Kennedy KI, Visness CM. Contraceptive efficacy of lactational amenorrhea. Lancet 1992;330:227–230.
7. Kazi A, Kennedy KI, Visness CM, et al. Effectiveness of the lactational amenorrhea method in Pakistan. Fertil Steril 1995;64:717–723.
8. Gallo MF, Grimes DA, Schulz KF, et al. Combination contraceptives: effects on weight [Cochrane Review]. In: The Cochrane Library. Issue 2. Oxford: Update Software, 2003.
9. Mattson RH, Rebar RW. Contraceptive methods for women with neurologic disorders. Am J Obstet Gynecol 1993;169:2027–2032.
10. American College of Obstetricians and Gynecologists (ACOG). The use of hormonal contraception in women with coexisting medical conditions. ACOG practice bulletin, no. 18, July 2000. Int J Gynaecol Obstet 2001;75:93–106.
11. Winkler UH. Role of screening in vascular disease in pill users: the hemostatic system. In: Evidence-guided Prescribing of the Pill. Cranforth, UK: Parthenon, 1996:109–120.
12. Holt VL, Cushing-Haugen KL, Daling JR. Body weight and risk of oral contraceptive failure. Obstet Gynecol 2002;99:820–827.
13. Knopp RH, LaRosa JC, Burman RT Jr. Contraception and dyslipidemia. Am J Obstet Gynecol 1993;168:1994–2005.
14. Speroff L, DeCherney A, and the Advisory Board for the New Progestins. Evaluation of a new generation of oral contraceptives. Obstet Gynecol 1993;81:1034–1047.
15. Engel HJ, Engel E, Lichtlen PR. Coronary atherosclerosis and myocardial infarction in young women—role of oral contraceptives. Eur Heart J 1983;4:1–6.
16. Mileikowsky GN, Nadler JL, Huey F, et al. Evidence that smoking alters prostacyclin formation and platelet aggregation in women who use oral contraceptives. Am J Obstet Gynecol 1988;159:1547–1552.
17. Sullivan JM, Lobo RA. Considerations for contraception in women with cardiovascular disorders. Am J Obstet Gynecol 1993;168:2006–2011.
18. Kjos SL, Shoupe D, Douyan S, et al. Effect of low-dose oral contraceptives on carbohydrate and lipid metabolism in women with recent gestational diabetes: results of a controlled, randomized, prospective study. Am J Obstet Gynecol 1991;163:1822–1827.
19. Jungers P, Dougados M, Pelissier C, et al. Influence or oral contraceptive therapy on the activity of systemic lupus erythematosus. Arthritis Rheum 1982;25:618–623.
20. Goldzieher JW, Zamah NM. Oral contraceptive side effects: where's the beef? Contraception 1995;52:327–335.
21. Freie HMP. Sickle cell diseases and hormonal contraception. Acta Obstet Gynecol Scand 1983;62:211–217.
22. Collaborative Group on Hormonal Factors in Breast Cancer. Breast cancer and hormonal contraceptives: further results. Contraception 1996;54(suppl 3):1–106.
23. Thomas DB. Oral contraceptives and breast cancer: review of the epidemiologic literature. Contraception 1991;43:597–642.
24. The Cancer and Steroid Hormone Study of the Centers for Disease Control and the National Institute of Child Health and Human Development. Oral contraceptive use and risk of breast cancer. N Engl J Med 1986;315:405–411.
25. Murray PM, Stadel BV, Schlesselman JJ. Oral contraceptive use in women with a family history of breast cancer. Obstet Gynecol 1989;73:977–983.
26. Thomas DB. The WHO Collaborative Study of Neoplasia and Steroid Contraceptives: the influence of combined oral contraceptives on risk of neoplasms in developing and developed countries. Contraception 1991;43:695–710.
27. Jick SS, Walker AM, Jick H. Oral contraceptives and endometrial cancer. Obstet Gynecol 1993;82:931–935.
28. Rosenberg L, Palmer JR, Zauber AG, et al. A case-control study of oral contraceptive use and invasive epithelial ovarian cancer. Am J Epidemiol 1994;139:654–661.
29. CDC/National Institute of Child Health and Development. The cancer and steroid hormone study: the reduction of ovarian cancer associated with oral contraceptive use. N Engl J Med 1987;316:650–655.
30. Rosenberg MJ, Waugh MS, Stevens CM. Smoking and cycle control among contraceptive users. Am J Obstet Gynecol 1996;174:628–632.
31. Cedars MI. Triphasic oral contraceptives: review and comparison of various regimens. Fertil Steril 2002;77:1–14.
32. Archer DF, Maheux R, DelConte A, et al. Efficacy and safety of a low-dose monophasic combination of oral contraceptive containing 100 mcg levonorgestrel and 20 mcg ethinyl estradiol (Alesse). Am J Obstet Gynecol 1999;181:39–44.

33. Mircette Study Group. An open-label, multicenter, noncomparative safety and efficacy study of Mircette, a low-dose estrogen-progestin oral contraceptive. Am J Obstet Gynecol 1998;179:2–8.
34. Kaunitz AM. Efficacy, cycle control and safety of two triphasic oral contraceptives: Cyclessa (desogestrel/ethinyl estradiol) and Ortho-Novum 7/7/7 (norethindrone/ethinyl estradiol): a randomized clinical trial. Contraception 2000;61:295–302.
35. Parsey KS, Pong A. An open-label multicenter study to evaluate Yasmin, a low-dose combination oral contraceptive containing drospirenone, a new progestogen. Contraception 2000;61:105–111
36. Sulak P, Lippman J, Siu C, et al. Clinical comparison of triphasic norgestimate/35 mcg ethinyl estradiol and monophasic norethindrone acetate/20 mcg ethinyl estradiol: cycle control, lipid effects, and user satisfaction. Contraception 1999;59:161–166.
37. Fuhrmann U, Krattenmacher R, Slater EP, et al. The novel progestin drospirenone and its natural counterpart progesterone: biochemical profile and antiandrogenic potential. Contraception 1996;54:243–251.
38. Muhn P, Krattenmacher R, Beier S, et al. Drospirenone: a novel progestogen with antimineralocorticoid and antiandrogenic activity. Pharmacological characterization in animal models. Contraception 1995;51:99–110.
39. Shenfield GM, Griffin JM. Clinical pharmacokinetics of contraceptive steroids: an update. Clin Pharmacokinet 1991;20:15–37.
40. Orme ML. The clinical pharmacology of oral contraceptive steroids. The Third SK&F Prize Lecture, University of London, December 1981. Br J Clin Pharm 1982;14:31–42.
41. Back DJ, Breckenridge AM, Crawford FE, et al. The effect of rifampicin on the pharmacokinetics of ethinylestradiol in women. Contraception 1980;21:135–143.
42. U.S. Food and Drug Administration. FDA Approves Seasonale Oral Contraceptive. FDA Talk Paper, September 5, 2003. Available at: http://www.fda.gov/bbs/topics/ANSWERS/2003/ANS01251.html. Retrieved July 22, 2005.
43. d'Arcangues C. Management of vaginal bleeding irregularities induced by progestin-only contraceptives. Hum Reprod 2000;15(suppl):24–29.
44. Meckstroth KR, Darney PD. Implantable contraception. Obstet Gynecol Clin North Am 2000;27:781–815.
45. Schwallie PC, Assenze JR. The effect of depo-medroxyprogesterone acetate on pituitary and ovarian function, and the return of fertility following its discontinuation: a review. Contraception 1974;10:181–202.
46. Kaunitz AM. Injectable contraception: new and existing options. Obstet Gynecol Clin North Am 2000;27: 741–780.
47. Fraser IS. Vaginal bleeding patterns in women using once-a-month injectable contraceptives. Contraception 1994;49:399–420.
48. Pelkman CL, Chow M, Heinback RA, et al. Short-term effects of progestational contraceptive drug on food intake resting energy expenditure, and body weight in young women. Am J Clin Nutr 2001;73:19–26.
49. Bahamondes L, Castillo SD, Tabares G, et al. Comparison of weight increase in users of depot medroxyprogesterone acetate and copper IUD up to 5 years. Contraception 2001;64:224–225.
50. Gray RH. Reduced risk of pelvic inflammatory disease with injectable contraceptives. Lancet 1985;1:1046.
51. Mattson RH, Cramer JA, Caldwell BV, et al. Treatment of seizures with medroxyprogesterone acetate. Neurology 1984;34:1255–1258.
52. Cundy T, Reid OR, Roberts H. Bone density in women receiving depot medroxyprogesterone for contraception. Br Med J 1991;303:13–16.
53. Tang OS, Tang G, Yup PSF, Li B. Further evaluation of long-term depot-medroxyprogesterone acetate use and bone mineral density: a longitudinal cohort study. Contraception 2000;62:161–164.
54. Petitti DB, Piaggio G, Mehta S, et al. Steroid hormone contraception and bone mineral density: a cross-sectional study in an international population. Obstet Gynecol 2000;95:736–744.
55. United Nations Development Programme/United Nations Population Fund/World Health Organization/World Bank, Special Programme of Research, Development and Research Training in Human Reproduction Task Force on Long-Acting Systemic Agents for Fertility Regulation. Comparative study of the effects of two once-a-month injectable steroidal contraceptives (Mesigyna and Cyclofem) on lipid and lipoprotein metabolism. Contraception 1997;56:193–207.
56. Garceau RJ, Wajszczuk CJ, Kaunitz AM, for the Lunelle Study Group. Bleeding patterns of women using Lunelle monthly contraceptive injections (medroxyprogesterone acetate and E_2C injectable suspension) and Ortho-Novum 7/7/7 oral contraceptive (norethindrone/ethinyl estradiol triphasic). Contraception 1999;60:179–187.
57. Rahimy MH, Cromie MA, Hopkins NK, et al. Lunelle monthly contraceptive injection (medroxyprogesterone acetate and E_2C injectable suspension): effects of body weight and injection sites on pharmacokinetics. Contraception 1999;60:201–208.
58. World Health Organization Task Force on Long-Acting Systemic Agents for Fertility Regulation. A multicentered phase III comparative study of two hormonal contraceptive preparations given once-a-month by intramuscular injection: II. The comparison of bleeding patterns. Contraception 1989;40:531–551.
59. World Health Organization. Facts about once-a-month injectable contraceptives: memorandum from a WHO meeting. Bull World Health Organ 1993;71:677–689.
60. Bahamondes L, Lavin P, Ojeda G, et al. Return of fertility after discontinuation of the once-a-month injectable contraceptive Cyclofem. Contraception 1997;55:307–310.
61. Kaunitz AM, Garceau RJ, Cromie MA. Comparative safety, efficacy, and cycle control of Lunelle monthly injection (medroxyprogesterone acetate and E_2C injectable suspension) and Ortho-Novum 7/7/7 oral contraceptive (norethindrone/ethinyl estradiol triphasic) Lunelle group. Contraception 1999;60:179–187.

62. Robertson DN, Sivin I, Nash HA, et al. Release rates of levonorgestrel from Silastic capsules, homogeneous rods and covered rods in humans. Contraception 1983;27:483–495.
63. Shoupe D, Horenstein J, Mishell D, et al. Characteristics of ovarian follicular development in Norplant users. Fertil Steril 1991;55:766–770.
64. Croxatto HB, Diaz S, Salvatierra AM, et al. Treatment with Norplant subdermal implants inhibits sperm penetration through cervical mucus in vitro. Contraception 1987;36:193–201.
65. Croxatto HB, Diaz S, Pavez M, et al. Clearance of levonorgestrel form the circulation following removal of Norplant subdermal implants. Contraception 1988;38:509–523.
66. Meirik O, Farley TMM, Sivin I. Safety and efficacy of levonorgestrel implant, intrauterine device, and sterilization. Obstet Gynecol 2001;97:539–547.
67. Darney PD, Speroff L. New methods. Dialog Contracept 2001;7:1–4.
68. Sivin I, Alvaraz F, Mishell Dr, et al. Contraception with two levonorgestrel rod implants. Contraception 1998;8:275–282.
69. NuvaRing package insert. Oss, The Netherlands: N.V. Organon, 2001.
70. Mulders TMT, Dieben TOM. Use of the novel combined contraceptive vaginal ring NuvaRing for ovulation inhibition. Fertil Steril 2001;75:865–870.
71. Roumen FJ, Apter D, Mulders TM, et al. Efficacy, tolerability and acceptability of a novel contraceptive vaginal ring releasing etonogestrel and ethinyl oestradiol. Hum Reprod 2001;16:469–475.
72. Roumen F. Contraceptive efficacy and tolerability with a novel combined contraceptive vaginal ring, NuvaRing. Eur J Contracept Reprod Health Care 2002;7(suppl 2):19–24.
73. Mulders TM, Dieben TO, Bennink HJ. Ovarian function with a novel combined contraceptive vaginal ring. Human Reprod 2002;17:2594–2599.
74. Zacur HA, Hedon B, Mansour D, et al. Integrated summary of Ortho Evra/Evra contraceptive patch adhesion in varied climates and conditions. Fertil Steril 2002;77:S32–S35.
75. Zieman M, Guilegaud J, Weisberg E, et al. Contraceptive efficacy and cycle control with the Ortho Evra/Evra transdermal system: the analysis of pooled data. Fertil Steril 2002;77:S13–S18.
76. Sibai BM, Odlind V, Meador M, et al. A comparative and pooled analysis of the safety and tolerability of the contraceptive patch (Ortho Evra/Evra). Fertil Steril 2002;7(2 suppl 2):S19–S26.
77. Audet M-C, Moreayu M, Koltun WE, et al, for the ORTHO EVRA/EVRA 004 Study Group. Evaluation of contraceptive efficacy and cycle control of a transdermal contraceptive patch vs. an oral contraceptive: a randomized controlled trial. JAMA 2001;285:2347–2354.
78. Mosher W, Martinez GM, Chandra A, Abma JC, Willson JJ. Use of contraception and use of family planning services in the United States, 1982–2002. Advance data from vital and health statistics; no 350, National Center for Health Statistics, Hyattsville, MD, 2004.
79. Ammala M, Nyman T, Strengell L. Effect of intrauterine contraceptive devices on cytokine messenger ribonucleic acid expression in the human endometrium. Fertil Steril 1995;63:773–778.
80. Sivin I, Schmidt F. Effectiveness of IUDs: a review. Contraception 1987;36:55–84.
81. Suvisaari J, Lahteenmaki P. Detailed analysis of menstrual bleeding patterns after postmenstrual and postabortal insertion of a copper IUD or a levonorgestrel-releasing intrauterine system. Contraception 1996;54:201–208.
82. Franks AL, Beral V, Cates W Jr. Contraception and ectopic pregnancy risks. Am J Obstet Gynecol 1990;63:1120–1123.
83. Sivin I. Dose and age-dependent ectopic pregnancy risk with intrauterine contraception. Obstet Gynecol 1991;78:291–298.
84. World Health Organization. Task force on the safety and efficacy of fertility regulating methods. The Tcu 380, Tcu 220 Multiload 250 and Nova T IUD at 3, 5 and 7 years of use: results from 3 randomized multicenter trials. Contraception 1990;42:141–159.
85. Anderson K, Odlind V, Rybo G. Levonorgestrel-releasing and copper-releasing (Nova T) IUDs during five years of use: a randomized comparative trial. Contraception 1994;49:56–72.
86. Luukkainen T, Toivonen J. Levonorgestrel-releasing IUD as a method of contraception with therapeutic properties. Contraception 1995;52:269–276.
87. Sivin I, Stern J. Health during prolonged use of levonorgestrel 20 mcg/d and the copper TCu 380Ag intrauterine contraceptive device a multicenter study. International Committee of Contraception Research (ICCR). Fertil Steril 2004;61:70–77.
88. Barbosa I, Olsson SE, Odlind V, et al. Ovarian function after seven years' use of a levonorgestrel IUD. Adv Contracept 1995;11:85–95.
89. Jarvela I, Tekay A, Jouppila P. The effect of a levonorgestrel-releasing intrauterine system on uterine artery blood flow, hormone concentrations and ovarian cyst formation in fertile women. Hum Reprod 1998;13:3379–3383.
90. Shaaban MM, Segal S, Salem HT, et al. Sonographic assessment of ovarian and endometrial changes during long-term Norplant use and their correlation with hormonal levels. Fertil Steril 1993;59:998–1002.
91. Ronnerdag M, Odlind V. Health effects of long-term use of the intrauterine levonorgestrel-releasing system. Acta Obstet Gynecol Scand 1999;78:716–721.
92. Suvanto-Luukkonen E, Kauppila A. The levonorgestrel intrauterine system in menopausal hormone replacement therapy: five year experience. Fertil Steril 1999;72:161–163.
93. Grady WR, Haywood MD, Yagi J. Contraceptive failure in the United States: estimates from the 1982 National Survey of Family Growth. Fam Plann Perspect 1986;18:200–209.

94. Fihn SD, Lathan RH, Roberts P, et al. Association between diaphragm use and urinary tract infections. JAMA 1986;254:240–245.
95. Hooton TM, Hillier S, Johnson C, et al. *Escherichia coli* bacteriuria and contraceptive method. JAMA 1991;265:64–69.
96. Wright WH, Vessey MP, Kenward B, et al. Neoplasia and dysplasia of the cervix uteri and contraception: a possible protective effect of the diaphragm. Br J Cancer 1978;38:273–279.
97. Mauck CK, Baker JM, Barr SP, et al. A phase I study of FemCap used with and without spermicide. Postcoital testing. Contraception 1997;56:111–115.
98. Mauck C, Callahan M, Weiner DH, Dominik R. A comparative study of the safety and efficacy of FemCap, a new vaginal barrier contraceptive, and the Ortho All-Flex diaphragm. The FemCap Investigators' Group. Contraception 1999;60:71–80.
99. U.S. Food and Drug Administration, Center for Devices and Radiological Health. FemCap summary of safety and effectiveness data [P020041]. March 28, 2003. Available at: http://www.fda.gov/cdrh/pdf2/P020041b.pdf. Retrieved July 22, 2005.
100. Trussell J, Vaughan B. Contraceptive failure, method-related discontinuation and resumption of use: results from the 1995 National Survey of Family Growth. Fam Plann Perspect 1999;31:64–72.
101. Mauck C, Glover LH, Miller E, et al. Lea's Shield: a study of the safety and efficacy of a new vaginal barrier contraceptive used with and without spermicide. Contraception 1996;53:329–335.
102. Gilliam MLL, Derman RJ. Barrier methods of contraception. Obstet Gynecol Clin North Am 2000;27:841–858.
103. Trussell J, Hatcher RA, Kates W Jr, et al. Contraception failure in the United States: an update. Stud Fam Plann 1990;21:51–54.
104. Cook L, Nanda K, Taylor D. Randomized crossover trial comparing the eZ-on plastic condom and a latex condom. Contraception 2001;63:25–31.
105. Davis KR, Weller SC. The effectiveness of condoms in reducing heterosexual transmission of HIV. Fam Plann Perspect 1999;31:272–279.
106. Centers for Disease Control and Prevention. Nonoxynol-9 spermicide contraception use—United States, 1999. MMWR Morb Mortal Wkly Rep 2002;51:389–392.
107. Fleming DT, McQuillan GM, Johnson RE, et al. Herpes simplex virus type 2 in the United States, 1976–1994. N Engl J Med 1997;337:1105–1111.
108. Armstrong Gl, Schillinger J, Markowitz L, et al. Incidence of herpes simplex virus type 2 infection in the United States. Am J Epidemiol 2001;153:912–920.
109. Sapire KE. The female condom (Femidon)—A study of user acceptability. S Afr Med J 1995;85:1081–1084.
110. Trussell J, Sturgen K, Strickler J, et al. Comparative efficacy of female condom and other barrier methods. Fam Plan Perspect 1994;26:66–72.
111. Beksinska ME, Rees HV, Dickson-Tetteh KE, et al. Structural integrity of the female condom after multiple uses, washing, during and relubrication. Contraception 2001;63:33–36.
112. Trussell J, Strickler J, Vaughan B. Contraceptive efficacy of the diaphragm, the sponge and the cervical cap. Fam Plann Perspect 1993;25:100–105.
113. Johnson V, Masters WH. Intravaginal contraceptive study. Phase II. Physiology. West J Surg Obstet Gynecol 1963;71:144–153.
114. Roddy RE, Zekeng L, Ryan K, et al. A controlled trial of nonoxynol-9 film to reduce male-to-female transmission of sexually transmitted diseases. N Engl J Med 1998;339:504–510.
115. Stafford MK, Ward H, Flanagan A, et al. Safety study of nonoxynol-9 as a vaginal microbicide: evidence of adverse effects. J Acquir Immune Defic Syndr Hum Retrovirol 1998;17:327–331.
116. Kreiss J, Ngugi E, Holmes, et al. Efficacy of nonoxynol-9 contraceptive sponge use in preventing heterosexual acquisition of HIV in Nairobi prostitutes. JAMA 1992;268:447–482.
117. Richardson BA, Lavreys, Martin HL, et al. Evaluation of a low-dose nonoxynol-9 gel for the prevention of sexually transmitted diseases. Sex Transm Dis 2001;28:394–400.
118. Centers for Disease Control and Prevention. Sexually transmitted diseases treatment guidelines 2002. MMWR Morbid Mortal Wkly Rep 2002;51:1–78.
119. Linn S, Schoenbaum SC, Monson RR. Lack of association between contraceptive usage and congenital malformation in offspring. Am J Obstet Gynecol 1983;147:923–928.
120. Task Force on Postovulatory Methods of Fertility Regulation. Randomized controlled trial of levonorgestrel versus the Yuzpe regimen of combined oral contraceptives for emergency contraception. Lancet 1998;352:428–433.
121. Trussell J, Elerston C, Stewart F. The effectiveness of the Yuzpe regimen of emergency contraception. Fam Plann Perspect 1996;28:58–64, 87.
122. Raymond EG, Creinin MD, Barnhart KT, et al. Meclizine for prevention of nausea associated with use of emergency contraceptive pills: a randomized trial. Obstet Gynecol 2000;95:271–277.
123. Webb A. How safe is the Yuzpe method of emergency contraception? Fertil Control Rev 1995;4:16–18.
124. Escobedo LF, Peterson HB, Grubbs GS, et al. Case fatality rate for sterilization in United States hospitals. Am J Obstet Gynecol 1989;160:147–150.
125. Trussell J, Kowal. The essentials of contraception. In: Contraceptive Technology. 17th ed. New York: Ardent Media, 1998:211–247.
126. Mosher WE, Pratt WF. Contraceptive use in the United States, 1973–1988. Advance data from vital and health statistics. No 182. Hyattsville, MD: National Center for Health Statistics, 1990.

127. Cheng M, Wong YM, Rochat R, et al. Sterilization failure in Singapore: an examination of ligation techniques and failure rates. Stud Fam Plann 1977;8:109–115.
128. Peterson HB, Jhisen X, Hughes JM, et al. A risk of pregnancy after tubal sterilization: findings from the U.S. Collaborative Review of Sterilization (CREST). Am J Obstet Gynecol 1996;174:1161–1168.
129. McCausland A. High rate of ectopic pregnancy following laparoscopic tubal coagulation failure. Am J Obstet Gynecol 1980;136:97–101.
130. Peterson HB, Jhisen X, Hughes JM, et al. The risk of ectopic pregnancy after tubal sterilization. N Engl J Med 1997;336:762–767.
131. Williams EL, Jones HE, Merrel RE. The subsequent course of patients sterilized by tubal ligation. Am J Obstet Gynecol 1951;61:423–426.
132. Wilcox LS, Martinez-Schnell B, Peterson, HB, et al. Menstrual function after tubal sterilization. Am J Epidemiol 1992;135:1368–1381.
133. Rulin MC, Turner JH, Dunworth R, et al. Post-tubal sterilization syndrome—a misnomer. Am J Obstet Gynecol 1985;151:13–19.
134. Rulin MC, Davidson AR, Philliber, SG, et al. Changes in menstrual symptoms among sterilized in comparison women: a prospective study. Obstet Gynecol 1989;74:149–154.
135. DeStefano F, Huezo CM, Peterson HB, et al. Menstrual changes after tubal sterilization. Obstet Gynecol 1983;62:673–681.
136. DeStefano F, Pearlman JA, Peterson HB, et al. Long-term risk of menstrual disturbances after tubal-sterilization. Obstet Gynecol 1985;152:835–841.
137. Hillis HD, March-Banks, PA, Taylor GP. Tubal sterilization and long-term risk of hysterectomy findings from the U.S. Collaborative Review of Sterilization. The U.S. Collaborative Review of Sterilization Working Group (CREST). Obstet Gynecol 1997;89:609–614.
138. Kjer J. Sexual adjustment to tubal sterilization. Eur J Obstet Gynecol 1990;35:211–214.

CHAPTER 16

Infertility and Recurrent Pregnancy Loss

John M. Storment

INFERTILITY

Infertility is a condition affecting more than 5 million couples annually with important medical, economic, and psychological implications (1). The care of the infertile couple must be based on an accurate assessment of factors affecting the fertility of both partners. The postponement of marriage and delay of pregnancy in marriage in the post–World War II generation are largely responsible for the increase in consultations for the evaluation of infertility (1). With the increased availability of services and improved diagnostic and therapeutic management, more couples are now able to access infertility services.

EPIDEMIOLOGY

A couple is said to be infertile if they have been trying to achieve a pregnancy for more than 1 year without success. This definition is arbitrary, and many couples achieve pregnancy after 12 months with no abnormalities and no outside intervention. Infertility is classified by the woman's history. Primary infertility implies no antecedent pregnancy, and secondary infertility is defined by a history of any pregnancy, including abortions and ectopic pregnancies. Fecundity (f) is the most useful statistic pertaining to reproduction. It represents the probability of conception per month of effort and is calculated by dividing the number of conceptions (C) by the person-months of exposure (T).

$$f = C/T \tag{16.1}$$

It must be remembered that even in infertile populations, fecundity is almost never zero, and for fertile couples, it is only approximately 0.20. Thus, it is useful to consider infertility as simply a reduction in fecundity to less than the general population. The evaluation of infertile couples should be designed to identify factors that are responsible for diminished fecundity, and treatment should be limited to therapy proven to restore fecundity toward normal. Counseling patients is made easier when tests and treatments are discussed using these terms.

Estimating the prevalence of infertility is not straightforward because inconsistencies in epidemiologic reports make it difficult to assess any trends in fecundity. Between 1965 and 1988, the prevalence appeared to remain stable at approximately 13% of U.S. women who are 15 to 44 years of age (excluding surgically sterilized individuals). Approximately half of these couples will never succeed in having as many children as they want (2). Although the prevalence of infertility has remained at approximately 13 to 15% of the U.S. population since the mid-1980s, more couples are seeking medical and surgical services for impaired fecundity. The number of childless women who are 35 to 44 years old increased by more than 1 million from 1982 to 1988 (3). Women were 2 to 3 years older in 1990 than in 1979 when they delivered their first child, and significantly more women never had a child (3).

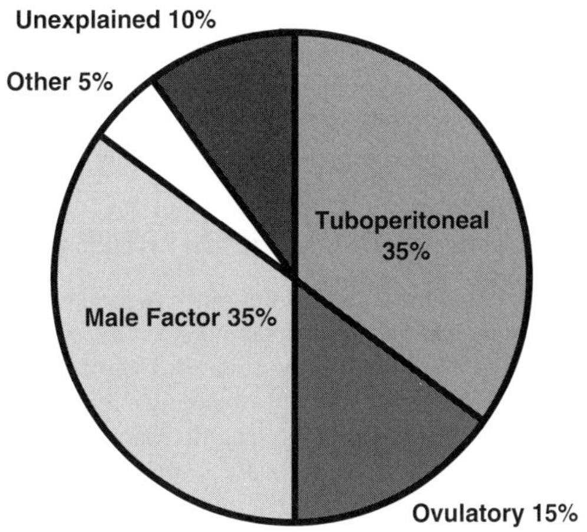

FIGURE 16.1 • Causes of infertility among U.S. couples.

Differences in the distribution of primary and secondary infertility have a direct impact on the use of fertility services because women with primary infertility are more likely to use medical services than women with secondary infertility. Overall, about half of all infertile couples will seek treatment, although only 25% will obtain assistance from an infertility specialist (4). Approximately half of couples with infertility eventually conceive. Likelihood of conception is influenced by several factors, including the duration of infertility, the causes of infertility, and the age of the woman at the time of treatment.

The distribution of causes of infertility among U.S. couples is shown in Figure 16.1.

Age and Infertility

A woman's fertility is known to decline after the age of 35. It is estimated that between 1980 and 2010, the number of U.S. women who are 35 to 45 years old will increase from 13 to 19 million. This alone will contribute to the increase in number of women older than age 35 seeking treatment for infertility. The gynecologist must be aware of age-related fecundity to properly counsel patients and must know when referral to a specialist should not be delayed.

The classic study of the Hutterites who live in Montana, the North and South Dakotas, and parts of Canada provides demographic information regarding natural fertility rates and aging (5). This sect is unique because contraception is denounced and, because of the arrangement of their community, there is no incentive to limit the size of families. Tietze (5) examined the demographics of this population to derive conclusions about natural fertility rates. The infertility rate was only 2.4%. A decline in fertility with age was demonstrated with 11% of the women infertile by age 34, 33% infertile by age 40, and 87% infertile by age 45. The mean age at the last pregnancy was 41 years.

The decline in fertility as women age can be attributed to several factors. With aging, there is an increase in the frequency of gynecologic and systemic disease, such as endometriosis, pelvic infection, leiomyomata, smoking, diabetes, and obesity. The potential for oocytes to be fertilized and develop normally is compromised with increasing age. Swartz and Mayaux (6) reported on 2193 women with azoospermic husbands treated by donor insemination. The cumulative pregnancy rates were 73%, 74%, 62%, and 54% for age groups younger than 25 years ($n = 371$), 26 to 30 years ($n = 1079$), 31 to 35 years ($n = 599$), and older than 35 years ($n = 144$), respectively. The decline between age groups becomes significant at about age 35, and pregnancies are rarely reported after age 45.

Significant changes in ovarian and uterine physiology begin to occur at age 35. The reasons include loss of oocyte integrity and decreased uterine receptivity after age 30 (7). Before embarking on infertility workup of women 35 years of age and older, proper counseling involving the risks of pregnancy loss with advancing maternal age is essential. The known spontaneous abortion rate increases to approximately 30% at age 35. Among successful pregnancies, trisomies and other chromosomal disorders are significantly increased.

A prompt and full investigation of fertility status should be offered immediately to women older than age 35 who are complaining of difficulty conceiving so any correctable conditions can be treated as soon as possible. Although it is difficult to select an arbitrary time at which no treatment should be offered, appropriate counseling should involve realistic expectations of conception based on the patient's age.

INVESTIGATION OF THE INFERTILE COUPLE

A standardized approach to the investigation of the infertile couple allows for a complete evaluation of each potential cause of infertility. Consistent application of a standard algorithm (Fig. 16.2) provides useful information that can help eliminate unnecessary and costly diagnostic tests. Initially, obtaining a thorough history is essential to guide the remainder of the workup. There are many specific examples of when historical information is useful. Identification of an ovulatory patient can be made by eliciting a history of regular menstrual cycles and premenstrual molimina (8). Diethylstilbestrol (DES)-exposed women have a significantly higher incidence of primary infertility, even with a structurally normal reproductive tract. Smoking, marijuana, and cocaine can reduce fecundity in men and women (9). Chapter 26 reviews occupational and environmental exposures associated with decreased fecundity. Some centers find it helpful to distribute a detailed questionnaire to patients before their first visit to obtain information that is sometimes difficult to express in an office interview. Such a questionnaire is available from the American College of Obstetricians and Gynecologists or the American Society for Reproductive Medicine.

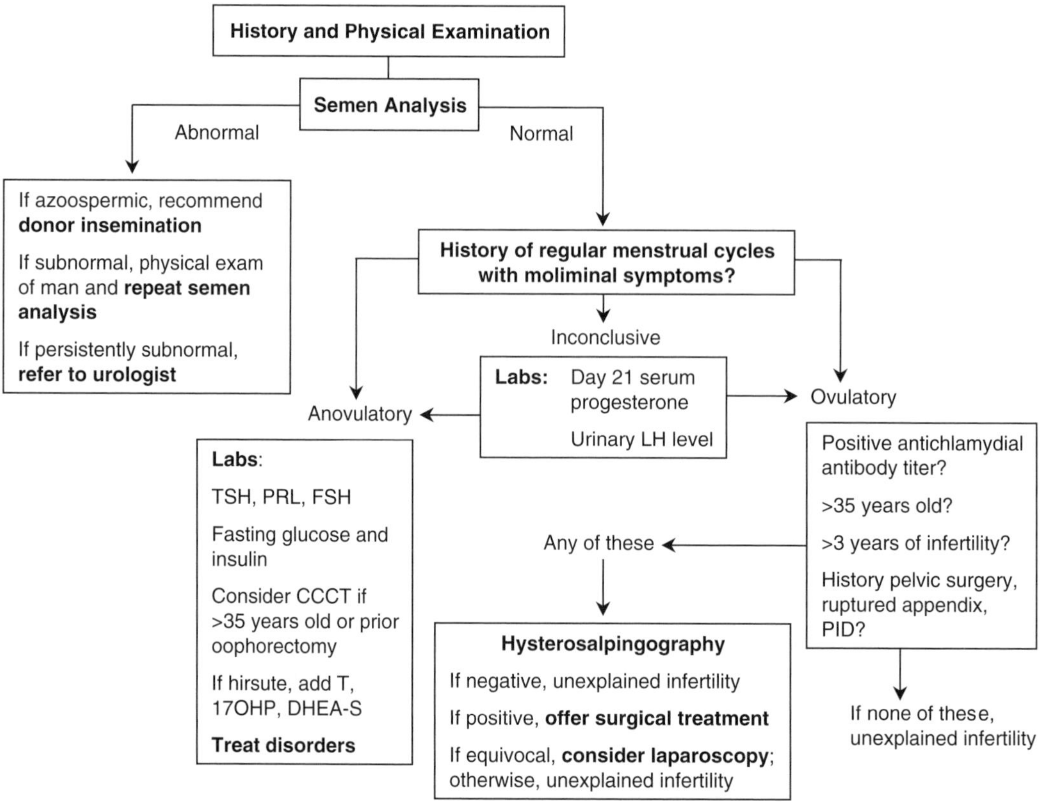

FIGURE 16.2 ● An algorithmic approach to the investigation of an infertile couple. CCCT, clomiphene citrate challenge test; DHEA-S, dehydroepiandrosterone sulfate; FSH, follicle-stimulating hormone; 17OHP, 17-hydroxyprogesterone; LH, luteinizing hormone; PID, pelvic inflammatory disease; PRL, prolactin; T, total testosterone; TSH, thyroid-stimulating hormone.

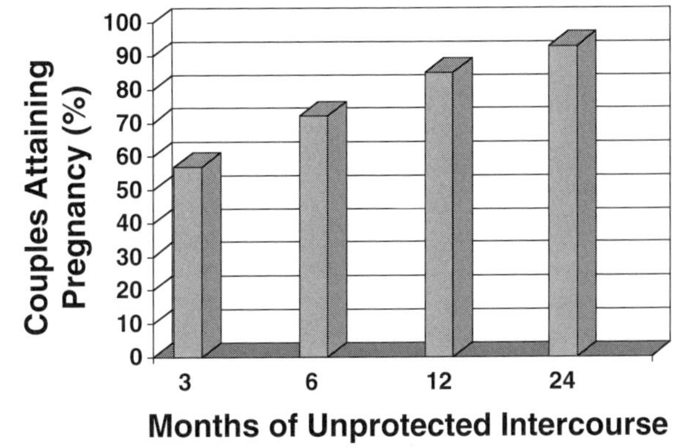

FIGURE 16.3 • Natural history of conception. Within 2 years of unprotected intercourse, approximately 90% of average couples will attain pregnancy. The remaining 10% are clinically defined as infertile. (Reprinted from MRC Vitamin Study Research Group. Lancet 1991;338:131–137, with permission.)

The first office visit should include counseling regarding the couple's identifiable problems and provide a realistic estimate of likelihood for conception (Fig. 16.1). A discussion of the statistics associated with human reproduction is useful, pointing out that the probability of conception in an ovulatory cycle is only 25% under ideal circumstances (10). The time required for conception to occur in couples who will attain pregnancy without medical intervention is shown in Figure 16.3.

After the initial discussion, a plan outlining appropriate laboratory testing should be reviewed. In addition, women with a negative rubella titer should be immunized, and HIV testing should be offered to all couples. Folic acid can also be prescribed at this time to decrease the risk of fetal neural tube defects (11). Some recommend screening for thyroid disease with a serum thyroid-stimulating hormone (TSH) because undiagnosed maternal hypothyroidism is associated with adverse fetal neuropsychological development (12). A more complete discussion of preconception counseling is covered in Chapter 14.

The evaluation should be individualized for each couple based on the initial history; a common approach may include laboratory assessment of ovulation, evaluation of reproductive tract anatomy, and semen analysis. Diagnosis of sterility is simple, but diagnosis of subfertility can be quite arduous. The difficulty is compounded by a lack of consensus regarding which diagnostic tests should be performed. The outcome of primary interest to the infertile couple is pregnancy, and the merit of diagnostic tests lies in their ability to predict this outcome (8). The European Society for Human Reproduction and Embryology provides recommendations for establishing a manner with which to evaluate infertility (13). In this practical way, we can divide the most commonly used diagnostic tests into three categories based on the correlation of an abnormal test result with impaired fecundability: valid correlation, inconsistent correlation, and not apparently correlated (Table 16.1). Treatment effectiveness can best be assessed in randomized clinical trials because conception without therapy can occur in most subfertile couples over time.

FEMALE FACTOR INFERTILITY

Anovulatory Infertility

Ovulatory dysfunction and anovulation affect 15 to 25% of all infertile couples seeking therapy. Unfortunately, the only absolute proof of normal ovulation is a subsequent pregnancy. The process leading to ovulation is comprised of several components; disruption of any of these can impede ovulation or the capacity of a mature oocyte to fertilize. Treatment of ovulation disorders remains one of the most successful of all infertility treatments (Table 16.2).

Evaluation

The woman who reports infrequent, irregular menses and no moliminal symptoms (or who gives an unclear history of her menstrual cycles) should be evaluated for anovulation (Fig. 16.4). An understanding of normal hormonal events that regulate the ovulatory process is essential

TABLE 16.1

Diagnostic Tests Commonly Used to Assess Impairment of Fecundability

Abnormal Test Results That have a Validated Correlation with Impaired Fecundability [a]
Semen analysis
Assessment of tubal patency by hysterosalpingogram or laparoscopy
Laboratory assessment of ovulation

Abnormal Test Results That are Not Consistently Correlated with Impaired Fecundability [b]
Postcoital test
Laparoscopic finding of minimal or mild endometriosis
Cervical mucus penetration test
Antisperm antibody assays
Zonafree hamster egg penetration test

Abnormal Test Results That Do Not Appear to be Correlated with Impaired Fecundability [c]
Endometrial biopsy for dating
Asymptomatic varicocele repair (infertility alone is not considered a symptom)
Falloposcopy

[a] In these diagnostic tests, when the test is unequivocally abnormal (azoospermia, bilateral tubal occlusion, or anovulation), fertility is definitely impaired without therapy.
[b] For these diagnostic tests, abnormal results are frequently associated with subsequent fertility without therapy.
[c] For these diagnostic tests, either there are data that confirm the lack of a correlation with pregnancy or such follow-up studies do not exist.

to determine which of the many tests devised for ovulation detection should be used. The trophic effects of both follicle-stimulating hormone (FSH) and luteinizing hormone (LH) result in maturation of ovarian follicles. Release of both FSH and LH from the anterior pituitary is controlled by gonadotropin-releasing hormone (GnRH), which is produced in the hypothalamus in a pulsatile fashion. The ovulatory process is characterized by a rapid midcycle rise in LH that culminates in the LH peak. A consensus from previous reports places the onset of the serum LH surge approximately 36 to 38 hours before ovulation (14). FSH also increases midcycle but to a

TABLE 16.2

Major Causes of Infertility and Treatment Outcomes

Cause of Infertility	Frequency (%)	Posttreatment Conception at 2 Years (%)
Anovulation	21	
Amenorrhea	7	96
Oligomenorrhea	14	78
Anatomic Cause		19
Male Factor		
Oligospermia	15	11
Azoospermia	6	0
Unexplained Causes	28	72

Adapted from Hull MG, Glazener CM, Kelly NJ, et al. Population study of causes, treatment, and outcome of infertility. BMJ 1985;291:1693–1697.

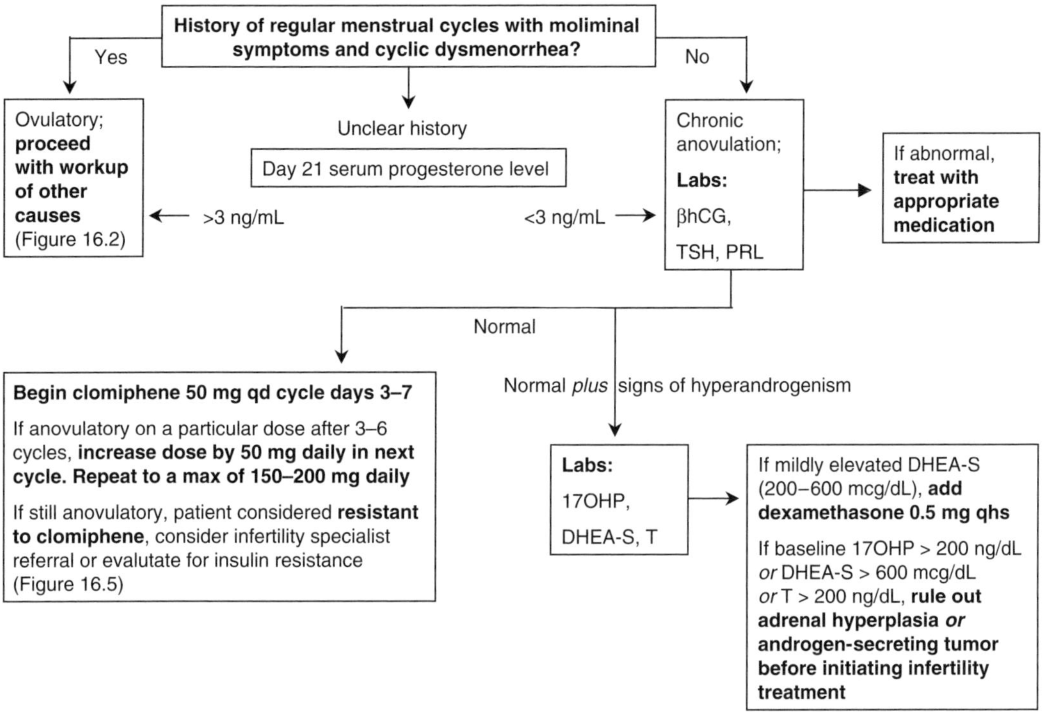

FIGURE 16.4 ● Workup for anovulatory infertility. *β*hCG, beta human chorionic gonadotropin; DHEA-S, dehydroepiandrosterone sulfate; 17OHP, 17-hydroxyprogesterone; PRL, prolactin; T, total testosterone; TSH, thyroid-stimulating hormone.

lesser degree than does LH. The luteal phase is characterized by a rise in the concentration of progesterone, with maximal concentration reached about 8 days after the LH peak. The menstrual cycle length is variable, with the variation residing in the follicular phase. The luteal phase is consistently 12 to 14 days.

Detection of serum progesterone greater than 3 ng/mL on day 21 suggests a secretory endometrium and is presumed to indicate ovulation (15). One report indicated that midluteal progesterone levels greater than 8.8 ng/mL were present in more than 95% of spontaneous conception cycles (16). Because of the extreme variability in progesterone secretion throughout the luteal phase in normal patients, it is not practical to make assumptions that a higher level of progesterone indicates a "better" ovulation than a lower level.

Detection of an LH surge seems to offer a greater degree of reliability and allows the patient to appropriately time intercourse (17). There is a lag of approximately 4 to 6 hours between serum and urinary LH surges, and most surges begin between 5:00 AM and 9:00 AM. More than 90% of ovulation episodes can be detected by a single urinary test performed that midafternoon or early evening (18). Several studies have confirmed the sensitivity, specificity, and utility of home ovulation monitoring kits (19, 20). The one-step urinary LH kits are easier for patients to use than a multistep urinary LH kit and correlate quite well with the multistep kit in determining the onset of ovulation (21). The amenorrheic or oligomenorrheic woman should be worked up and treated for the cause of her anovulation or infrequent ovulation, as discussed later in this section. These same home tests may be used to predict ovulation when necessary as part of assisted reproductive therapies.

Basal body temperature charting has long been used because of its simplicity, but its variability and inconvenience restrict its efficacy as a diagnostic test. The World Health Organization (WHO) defines a shift in basal body temperature as three consecutive daily temperatures 0.4°F higher than the previous six daily temperatures. This is considered confirmation that ovulation has occurred (22). Physical release of the ovum probably occurs on the day before the first day of temperature elevation; hence, this test provides only retrospective evidence of ovulation.

Histologic evidence of secretory endometrium detected by endometrial biopsy is indicative of ovulation and corpus luteum formation. The endometrial biopsy is performed 2 to 3 days prior to the expected period. A good correlation has been noted between biopsy results, the time of the basal body temperature nadir, and midcycle LH surge, indicating this test is reliable for determining presence of ovulation (23). However, it is not effective for diagnosing luteal phase deficiency. Because of a lack of intra- and interobserver consistency, the endometrial biopsy fails to provide useful information other than the presence of ovulation (24). Disadvantages of endometrial sampling include expense and patient discomfort.

The use of transvaginal sonography is recognized as a reliable technique for monitoring follicular development. Ovulation is deemed to have occurred if the follicle reached a mean diameter of 18 to 25 mm and subsequently changed in sonographic density or demonstrated sonographic evidence of follicular collapse (25). However, its use as an initial diagnostic test for all infertile women is not cost effective.

Specific tests ordered to determine the cause of anovulation should depend partly on the physical examination of each patient. Serum prolactin and TSH levels are routine tests for all patients in whom the cause of anovulation is uncertain. In addition, determination of the serum FSH concentration will identify cases where amenorrhea is secondary to ovarian failure. It is reasonable to assess the gonadotropin levels on any patient in whom the cause of anovulation is not apparent, but especially in women older than age 30. In patients demonstrating significant signs of androgen excess, total testosterone, dehydroepiandrosterone sulfate (DHEA-S), and 17-hydroxyprogesterone levels are necessary to rule out androgen-secreting tumors of either the ovary or adrenal, or the possibility of late-onset congenital adrenal hyperplasia. A total testosterone level greater than 200 ng/dL or a DHEA-S level greater than 700 mcg/dL requires further medical evaluation to rule out tumor before proceeding with infertility treatments. A 17-hydroxyprogesterone level of greater than 800 ng/dL is virtually diagnostic of 21-hydroxylase deficiency as a cause of adrenal hyperplasia and should be referred to an endocrinologist; a level of 200 to 800 ng/dL requires adrenocorticotropic testing for confirmation of the diagnosis.

In cases of amenorrhea, a progestin challenge test (medroxyprogesterone acetate [Provera] 10 mg daily for 10 days) can help determine the etiology. When withdrawal bleeding occurs, the outflow tract is patent, and sufficient estrogen production has stimulated endometrial growth. This is most indicative of polycystic ovary syndrome (PCOS). When no withdrawal bleeding occurs and a normal outflow tract has been identified, the most likely etiology is hypothalamic dysfunction.

Women with PCOS are insulin resistant, and the resultant hyperinsulinemia exacerbates the reproductive abnormalities of this condition. Because some of these patients may benefit from agents that reduce circulating insulin levels, some experts recommend that women with PCOS signs and symptoms be screened with fasting glucose and insulin levels. A fasting glucose-to-insulin ratio of less than 4.5 is considered abnormal (26).

Classification and Treatment of Anovulatory Disorders

Classification of ovulatory disorders can be made based on the level of FSH and prolactin. The appropriate treatment is determined by the outcome of these tests.

Hypogonadotropic Anovulation

These patients demonstrate low FSH levels, normal prolactin concentrations, and no withdrawal bleeding after a progesterone challenge test. The most common type of hypogonadotropic hypogonadism is idiopathic. If causes such as anorexia, excessive exercise, or stress are elucidated, treatment with appropriate counseling should be initiated. If instead the cause is primary pituitary failure, ovulation induction with gonadotropins is indicated. Patients demonstrating panhypopituitarism will also demonstrate other symptoms in addition to anovulation.

Patients with hypothalamic ovulatory failure can be treated with pulsatile GnRH or human menopausal gonadotropins and referred to a reproductive endocrinologist. Pure FSH is not indicated for patients with hypogonadotropic hypogonadism because some LH is required for ovulation (27). Clomiphene (Clomid, Serophene) is not an effective treatment for anovulation in these cases.

Normogonadotropic Anovulation

These patients have a normal FSH concentration (with either normal or high LH levels) and demonstrate withdrawal bleeding in response to the progesterone challenge test. The majority of these patients have PCOS. PCOS is characterized by chronic anovulation, hyperandrogenism, and insulin resistance (28). Interventions that reduce circulating insulin levels in women with PCOS may restore normal reproductive endocrine function. In patients with body mass index (BMI) greater than 30, weight loss and exercise is the initial recommended treatment for this etiology of anovulation. To calculate BMI, use the following equation (see Figure 19.1 for a BMI chart using pounds and inches):

$$\text{BMI} = \text{weight (kg)} \div \text{height}^2\ (\text{m}^2) \tag{16.2}$$

Patients who lower their BMI show marked improvement in pregnancy rates with weight reduction alone and frequently need no further therapy (29).

The traditional and standard therapy for anovulatory infertility is clomiphene. Clomiphene is believed to interfere with the normal negative feedback of estradiol on the hypothalamic-pituitary axis (30). When this inhibitory effect is impeded, pituitary FSH and LH is increased. The increased FSH stimulates folliculogenesis by promoting proliferation of granulosa cells and increased intrafollicular estrogen production. Insulin-sensitizing agents such as metformin (Glucophage) have been shown to increase the frequency of spontaneous ovulation, menstrual cyclicity, and the ovulatory response to clomiphene (31, 32).

The recommended starting dose of clomiphene is 50 mg/day beginning on cycle day 3, 4, or 5 and continuing for a total of 5 days. In patients with irregular menses, micronized progesterone (200 mg daily for 10 days) or medroxyprogesterone acetate (10 mg daily for 10 days) can be given and clomiphene started on cycle day 3 after initiation of the withdrawal bleed. Documentation of ovulation is usually made with either urinary LH monitoring or a luteal progesterone level. If clomiphene is taken on cycle days 3 through 7, ovulation usually occurs between days 12 and 15 (33). Therefore, the LH surge would begin about day 11 or 12. If there is no ovulation, the dose should be increased by 50-mg increments (to a maximum of 200 mg) until ovulation is achieved (Table 16.3). If ovulation occurs, the same clomiphene dose should be continued until pregnancy occurs or for a maximum of three to six cycles. Pregnancy is less likely to occur with doses greater than 150 mg; therefore, it is prudent to consider alternative treatments for ovulation induction when 150 mg does not result in ovulation (34). Ninety-five percent of conceptions with clomiphene will occur within six ovulatory cycles (35).

Approximately 70% of women treated with clomiphene for anovulatory infertility will ovulate, and 30 to 40% will become pregnant (36). (The pregnancy rate depends on additional infertility factors.) The twin gestation rate is approximately 10% (37). There does not appear to

TABLE 16.3

Clomiphene Use for Anovulatory Infertility

- Clomiphene 50 mg orally every day, cycle days 3 to 7.
- If ovulatory (detected either by urinary luteinizing hormone, serum luteal progesterone, or spontaneous menses), continue with same dose for three to six cycles.
- If no ovulation, increase dose by 50 mg daily in next cycle, reassess as previously, and increase another 50 mg or continue dose as indicated in subsequent cycles.
- If no ovulation on 150 mg, check fasting glucose and insulin, and prescribe metformin if indicated. Also, consider referral to reproductive endocrinologist for gonadotropin therapy. May also choose to increase to 200 mg daily, days 3 to 7, and assess ovulation.

be an increase in congenital malformations with clomiphene use (38). Dickey et al. (39) observed a small increase in spontaneous abortions in patients using clomiphene compared with spontaneous pregnancies (24% versus 20%). Dickey and Holtkamp (37) provided a more thorough review of clinical observations and pregnancy outcomes with clomiphene use.

The side effects of clomiphene include hot flushes, abdominal bloating, breast discomfort, nausea and vomiting, visual changes, headache, and alopecia. These require discontinuation of treatment for only a small percentage of patients.

Insulin Resistance Treatment for Clomiphene-Resistant Anovulation

Not all women will ovulate in response to clomiphene; thus, they will require some adjuvant therapy. A large proportion of women with PCOS demonstrate peripheral resistance to insulin independent of their weight. The degree of insulin resistance is generally more profound in obese patients. Insulin resistance usually results in a compensatory hyperinsulinemia, which contributes to the ovarian hyperandrogenism commonly seen in women with PCOS and may directly interfere with ovulation. Correction of the hyperinsulinemia in PCOS patients increases the rate of spontaneous ovulation and can also decrease ovarian androgen production. Although it is generally recommended that patients not responding to clomiphene be referred to a reproductive specialist, the evaluation for and treatment of insulin resistance is often initiated in the gynecologist's or primary care physician's office.

Treatment with metformin, the insulin-sensitizing agent studied in most detail, lowers serum insulin levels and increases menstrual cyclicity and fertility rates. Studies supporting this finding have prompted future therapy to focus on correcting or minimizing the insulin resistance (31, 32). In one study, 89% of women who were previously unresponsive to clomiphene alone ovulated when given metformin alone or in combination with clomiphene (40).

Although metformin may result in increased ovulation rates in any clomiphene-resistant patient, it is prudent to screen for insulin resistance prior to beginning therapy. Some authors propose evaluating patients for hyperinsulinemia with a fasting glucose to fasting insulin ratio; a ratio of less than 4.5 is consistent with insulin resistance (26). A fasting insulin of greater than 20 is also consistent with insulin resistance. Figure 16.5 provides an algorithm for the evaluation and initial treatment of insulin resistance in the clomiphene-resistant patient. Insulin resistance is closely linked to hyperandrogenism, glucose intolerance, diabetes, and cardiovascular disease, so it is important for general health maintenance, not just for treatment of infertility, to screen for it in this population (41).

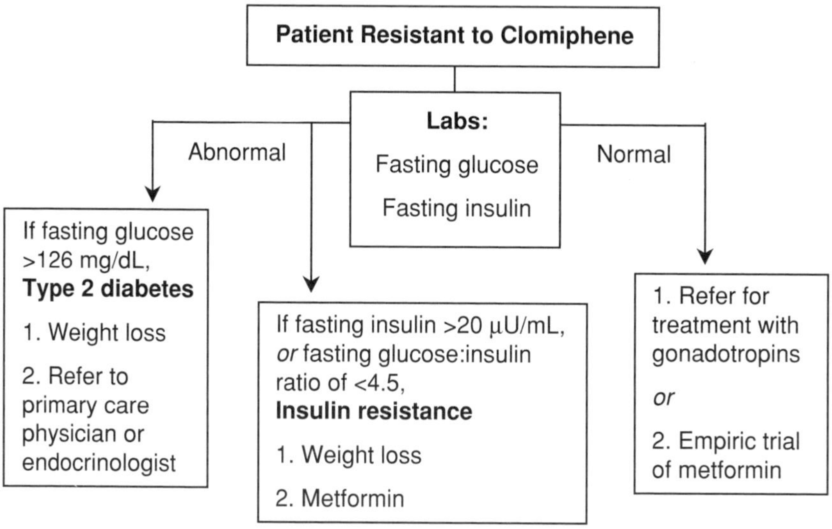

FIGURE 16.5 ● Initial approach to the anovulatory patient resistant to clomiphene.

Metformin is contraindicated in patients with a known hypersensitivity to the drug or any of its components and in patients with renal disease or acute or chronic metabolic lactic acidosis. It should also not be given with other medications that affect renal function because they may affect metformin pharmacology. The drug should be discontinued prior to major surgical procedures (i.e., when food and water are restricted). It should also be temporarily withheld in patients undergoing radiologic procedures involving parenteral administration of iodinated contrast materials. In addition, because alcohol can potentiate the risk of lactic acidosis in patients on metformin therapy, they should be counseled to avoid excessive alcohol intake.

The most common side effects of metformin include nausea, vomiting, diarrhea, and heartburn. These can be minimized by starting with a low dose (500 mg) and increasing the dose by 500 mg weekly in a stepwise fashion to a maximum of 500 mg three times daily with meals. The wholesale cost for 30 days of treatment with metformin (Glucophage) 500 mg three times daily is about $50 (42). An extended-release preparation (Glucophage XR) is titrated from 750 to 1500 mg with the evening meal. The extended-release preparation has fewer gastrointestinal side effects and the convenience of once-daily dosing. Although it is generally recommended to be discontinued as soon as pregnancy is diagnosed, metformin is a pregnancy Category B medication.

The high pregnancy loss rates associated with PCOS are believed to be, at least in part, related to insulin resistance. Jakubowicz et al. (43) found that treatment with metformin compared with a control group decreased the incidence of miscarriage from 42 to 9%. Metformin taken throughout pregnancy has also been shown to decrease the incidence of gestational diabetes (44). Because this is a relatively new use of this medication, it is prudent to consult with a maternal–fetal medicine specialist prior to continuing its use beyond conception.

Other antihyperglycemic agents such as rosiglitazone (Avandia) and pioglitazone (Actos) have been proposed for use for the clomiphene-resistant patient, but these have not been studied as well and are pregnancy Category C. In one double-blind, placebo-controlled, randomized pilot trial with rosiglitazone, 14 of 25 (56%) women on rosiglitazone and placebo successfully ovulated, whereas 10 of 13 (77%) women on rosiglitazone and clomiphene citrate successfully ovulated. All women in this small trial demonstrated resistance to ovulation induction using clomiphene citrate. The authors of the trial believed rosiglitazone increased sex hormone binding globulin levels, and these increased levels improved insulin sensitivity and decreased hyperandrogenemia, both conditions that are associated with anovulation (45). Some drugs in this class have been associated with severe adverse side effects when taken alone or in combination with other medications in small numbers of patients. Only clinicians familiar with the use and contraindications to these drugs should prescribe them for use in infertility patients.

Other Adjuvant Therapies for Clomiphene-Resistant Anovulation

Other medications have also been proposed for the clomiphene-resistant patient. Options include adrenal steroid therapy and gonadotropins with or without a GnRH agonist or GnRH antagonist. There is even the option of a surgical approach to treatment of PCOS with laparoscopic ovarian diathermy or "ovarian drilling" (46). It is generally recommended that patients not responding to clomiphene be referred to a reproductive specialist.

In patients with a DHEA-S value of 200 to 600 mcg/mL, Daly et al. (47) reported improved pregnancy rates with the concurrent administration of dexamethasone (Decadron) 0.5 mg every morning. (DHEA-S levels greater than 600 require further medical evaluation to rule out tumor.) It is believed suppression of the androgenic milieu may improve the response to clomiphene therapy. A more recent reference found benefit for those with normal DHEA-S levels (48).

In patients who ovulate in response to clomiphene therapy but still do not conceive, there is a high incidence of other associated infertility factors (35). Prior to further therapy, it is essential that at least a semen analysis and a hysterosalpingogram are completed to rule out other causes of infertility. Failure to ovulate with 100 to 150 mg of clomiphene may result from an abnormal LH surge, in which case the addition of 10,000 units of intramuscular human chorionic gonadotropin (hCG) timed with follicular ultrasounds may facilitate ovulation. Dominant follicles should approach a mean diameter of 18 to 20 mm prior to hCG administration during clomiphene-induced cycles (49, 50).

The standard treatment for patients not responding to clomiphene and/or metformin is gonadotropin therapy. Gonadotropin therapy provides good per-cycle and cumulative pregnancy rates in hypogonadotropic anovulation (25% and 91.2%, respectively) but carries a higher risk of multiple pregnancies and ovarian hyperstimulation. In normogonadotropic patients who failed to ovulate on clomiphene, the per-cycle and cumulative pregnancy rates are 12% and 30%, respectively (51, 52). The human menopausal gonadotropin medications are available as purified FSH alone (Follistim, Gonal F, Bravelle) or a combination of FSH and LH (Repronex, Pergonal).

Intramuscular or subcutaneous injections of gonadotropin(s) are usually initiated on cycle day 2 and continued for several days. Follicular growth is monitored by ultrasound, and estradiol levels are followed daily until optimal stimulation has occurred (usually 6 to 10 days), with subsequent injection of hCG to stimulate ovulation.

The incidence of multiple pregnancies with the use of human menopausal gonadotropins can be as low as 10% with careful monitoring, but rates as high as 40% are reported (52). Ovarian hyperstimulation syndrome is characterized by excessive weight gain, ascites, and intravascular depletion. Most patients with ovarian hyperstimulation syndrome have mild symptoms and can be managed as outpatients. There is no risk of teratogenic effects on the fetus.

Hypergonadotropic Hypogonadism

This group includes all variants of ovarian failure, including premature menopause and ovarian resistance. FSH concentrations are usually greater than 20 mIU/mL in repeated measurements (51). The patient usually displays hypoestrogenic signs and symptoms, and does not respond to the progesterone challenge. If she is younger than 40 years of age, this indicates premature ovarian failure. In women younger than 30 years of age, a karyotype should be obtained to rule out the presence of a Y chromosome and to evaluate for the presence of Turner's syndrome (45 XO). If a Y chromosome is detected, extirpation of the gonads is warranted to prevent possible malignant transformation (52). If Turner's syndrome is detected, she is at risk for other abnormalities and should be referred to a reproductive specialist. Treatment of infertility in these patients requires assisted reproductive technologies (donor oocyte with in vitro fertilization [IVF]).

Hyperprolactinemia

The incidence of hyperprolactinemia in patients with secondary amenorrhea is 23% and in subjects with oligomenorrhea is 8%. The mechanism of anovulation is believed to be an impaired gonadotropin pulsatility and derangement of the estrogen-positive feedback effect on LH secretion in hyperprolactinemic patients (53). When prolactin levels exceed 20 to 25 ng/mL, the measurement should be repeated under basal conditions (i.e., early morning sampling). If it is still elevated, hypothyroidism should also be ruled out with a TSH level. If prolactin is elevated in the absence of a thyroid disorder, imaging of the pituitary with computed tomography or magnetic resonance imaging should be performed to diagnose empty sella, microadenoma, or macroadenoma. Prolactin concentration can be increased by stress, or by a normal breast or pelvic examination. These events may lead to false positives if the test is inappropriately timed.

The standard medication for the treatment of hyperprolactinemia in the United States is bromocriptine (Parlodel). Bromocriptine is an ergot alkaloid derivative with dopamine receptor agonist activity that directly inhibits prolactin secretion. If there is no anatomic abnormality of the pituitary and the goal of treatment is ovulation, bromocriptine is usually started at 1.25 mg orally at bedtime for 1 week and then increased to 2.5 mg twice daily. After 1 week on this dose (2.5 mg), ovulatory status should be evaluated. In the absence of ovulation, the dose can be increased in 1.25-mg increments (54). After ovulation is established, the medication is maintained until the patient becomes pregnant. Bromocriptine is usually discontinued after a positive pregnancy test but can be used safely during pregnancy. Most patients who conceive do so within six ovulatory cycles with the average being two cycles (55). If there is a pituitary adenoma, this should be treated prior to attempts at pregnancy.

Bromocriptine has been advocated in the anovulatory patient with normoprolactinemic galactorrhea (56). In the absence of galactorrhea or an abnormal prolactin level, however, there remains inadequate data to support the addition of bromocriptine to an ovulation induction regimen.

Side effects of bromocriptine include nausea, headache, and faintness due to orthostatic hypotension. These effects are minimized by gradually increasing the dose. Taking it with food is recommended to avoid gastrointestinal side effects. Vaginal administration of bromocriptine has been associated with fewer side effects but with similar effectiveness (57).

A newer dopamine agonist, cabergoline (Dostinex), can be given just once or twice a week and is more effective in normalizing prolactin and restoring menses than bromocriptine, and is significantly better tolerated. However, it is not yet recommended as first-line therapy for patients seeking fertility because adequate safety data in pregnancy are not available (58).

Tuboperitoneal Infertility

Approximately 40% of all infertile women will demonstrate an abnormality of the uterus, cervix, and/or fallopian tubes. To date, the best assessment of pelvic anatomic causes of infertility is with a thorough history and physical exam, as well as a hysterosalpingogram (59). The hysterosalpingogram is the test of choice to assess uterine and fallopian tube contour and tubal patency, and should be part of the standard evaluation of the infertile couple. The antichlamydial antibody titer has also been proposed as an integral part of the initial evaluation and workup, and is discussed more extensively as follows (60). If an anatomic abnormality is detected, the decision to proceed with reparative surgery or IVF should be based on the specific defect, the clinical and financial resources available, and the desires of the patient.

Evaluation

A history of pelvic inflammatory disease (PID), ectopic pregnancy, septic abortion, ruptured appendix, or tubal and/or other pelvic surgery should prompt suspicion for a possible anatomic cause for infertility. Clearly, PID has had the greatest impact on the increasing incidence of tubal infertility. The classic studies of Westrom (61) correlated the number of episodes of PID with the subsequent infertility rate. An 11% incidence of involuntary infertility was associated with one episode of salpingitis; 23% after two episodes; and 54% after three or more episodes. Physical exam should be directed at detecting decreased mobility of adnexa and uterosacral nodularity to help predict the presence of extensive adhesive disease or endometriosis.

Antichlamydial Antibody Titer

Genital infection with *Chlamydia trachomatis* remains the single most important cause of tubal pathology. Damage to the ciliated epithelium from *Chlamydia* results in impaired tubal transport. Many cases go undetected and untreated because 50 to 80% of women with these infections are asymptomatic (62). Thus, even without a history of recognized salpingitis, subclinical disease is a common cause of decreased fertility. Because of this, serologic *C. trachomatis* antibody testing has been introduced as a means of detecting tuboperitoneal pathology. In a meta-analysis evaluating all studies comparing *Chlamydia* antibody titers and laparoscopy for tubal disease, Mol et al. (63) confirmed that the discriminative capacity of antibody testing is at least as good, if not better, than the hysterosalpingogram. Using newer techniques to detect antibodies specific to *C. trachomatis* (enzyme-linked immunoabsorbent assay or microimmunofluorescence), Debekausen et al. (64) found that 75% of patients with antibody levels of greater than 1:8 had tubal abnormalities at laparoscopy. Although tuboperitoneal pathology can result from other causes (previous surgery, endometriosis, or PID from nonchlamydial micro-organisms), *C. trachomatis* antibody testing is an important component of the standard infertility evaluation.

Hysterosalpingography

Hysterosalpingography is important in the diagnostic evaluation of the infertile woman. It is the first-line radiologic examination and provides immediate information about the appearance of the endocervical canal, the uterine cavity, and the fallopian tube lumina. Ideally, the gynecologist should perform the exam, but it is often the radiologist who completes the hysterosalpingogram.

The procedure involves placing a single-tooth tenaculum on the anterior lip of the cervix followed by insertion of the infusion device attached to a syringe filled with 10 to 20 mL of contrast material. Usually, only 5 to 10 mL of dye is needed to adequately evaluate the uterine cavity and tubal lumen. To allow full visualization of the uterine cavity, the metal speculum should be removed prior to injection of contrast. After attachment of the cannula, the contrast should be slowly injected under fluoroscopic observation. Traction should be applied to the cervix to bring the uterus parallel to the x-ray film. In the absence of proximal tubal obstruction, one should carefully observe filling of both fallopian tubes. If one or both tubes fail to be visualized, prone positioning has been useful in allowing the contrast to fill the tubal lumens (65). Spill of contrast into the peritoneal cavity should be documented. Collection of dye around the distal tube that does not spill into the cavity with changing patient position may suggest peritubal adhesions. Rarely are more than three films needed. A preliminary scout film adds little to the interpretation of the study. A delayed film may be taken to demonstrate late spillage.

Various instruments have been designed for and other methods adapted to the performance of the hysterosalpingogram. A lidocaine paracervical block can sometimes decrease patient discomfort but is not routinely recommended. In parous women, a hysterosalpingogram balloon catheter (Ackrad Laboratories, Inc., Cranford, NJ) may be required to prevent leakage of dye back through the cervix. Nonsteroidal anti-inflammatories are frequently prescribed 30 minutes prior to the procedure to decrease uterine cramping during injection of the contrast. Prophylactic antibiotics (doxycycline 100 mg twice a day for 3 days prior to the hysterosalpingogram) are warranted in women with a prior history of pelvic infection, specifically *Chlamydia* (66, 67).

The specific dye used has been the subject of many reports, most of which compared the therapeutic effects of water-based versus oil-soluble contrast media (68–71). Most, but not all, concluded that the ethiodized oil-soluble contrast media (Ethiodol) provides a slight advantage in improving the pregnancy rate for patients with unexplained infertility in the months following the procedure. Because of the rare possibility of granuloma formation with the oil-based dye, therapeutic Ethiodol is generally used only after bilateral patency has been demonstrated with the water-soluble contrast.

Hysterosalpingography provides extremely useful information in the early evaluation of the infertile female. If bilateral proximal occlusion is shown with a history of chlamydia, one could reasonably avoid laparoscopy and proceed with IVF. If it shows bilateral distal occlusion with no hydrosalpinx, one might attempt tuboplasty. There is a good correlation between hysterosalpingogram findings and tubal patency at laparoscopy, with sensitivity greater than 90% and specificity of 84% reported (72). Hysterosalpingography can demonstrate congenital and acquired lesions of the uterus but is associated with false-positive and false-negative results, precluding its use as the sole method of diagnosing uterine anomalies (73). For assessment of the uterine cavity, clinicians may also use sonohysterography in lieu of hysterosalpingogram, but the sonohysterography cannot help determine fallopian tube patency. When used in conjunction with a thorough history, physical examination, and antichlamydial antibody titers, the hysterosalpingogram is an important adjunct in the assessment of most anatomic causes of infertility.

Based on current evidence, a hysterosalpingogram should be obtained in the workup for infertility in the following cases:

- Positive antichlamydial antibody titer
- History of PID, pelvic surgery, or ruptured appendix
- Greater than 3-year history of infertility
- Patient older than 33 years
- Greater than four cycles of treatment for anovulation without success

Postcoital Test

The postcoital test (also known as the Sims-Hühner test) provides information about the interaction between the sperm and cervical mucus. Despite its frequent use over the past century as a tool to evaluate cervical factor infertility, its validity as a predictor of future pregnancy has been debated. Some authors assert a strong association between the results of the postcoital test and pregnancy rates, whereas others claim it merely confirms the occurrence of intercourse (74–76). A review of the literature by Griffith and Grimes concluded that this test suffers from lack of standard methodology, a lack of a uniform definition of normal, and unknown reproducibility (77).

Cervical factors as a cause of infertility may exist, but a valid test to correctly diagnose them has yet to be discovered. The postcoital test should never be a substitute for a semen analysis because morphology cannot be adequately evaluated in the postcoital test, and the correlation between postcoital sperm motility and total motile sperm count (from semen analysis) departs from linearity in the lower range of sperm count values (77). The postcoital test may be used if there is clinical suspicion of a hostile cervical factor (most likely immunologic in nature).

Office (Diagnostic) Hysteroscopy

Evaluating the uterine cavity for abnormalities responsible for infertility has traditionally been done with hysterosalpingography. However, because of the high false-positive rate of hysterosalpingogram findings for intrauterine abnormalities (i.e., radiographic findings not confirmed at endoscopy), other modes for detecting intrauterine lesions have been proposed. Hysteroscopy performed in the operating room is the gold standard for identifying such lesions but carries the burden of added expense. Office hysteroscopy with carbon dioxide or saline as the distention medium has been proposed as a method to detect endometrial abnormalities (78). This technique can complement the hysterosalpingogram in differentiating endometrial polyps from submucous myomas, or by validating the presence of intrauterine adhesions or congenital anomalies.

Sonohysterography

Fluid contrast ultrasound or sonohysterography has been proposed as a tool in the diagnosis of intrauterine lesions. In light of high false-positive rates with hysterosalpingography and office hysteroscopy, this technique has been proposed as an inexpensive alternative for detecting intrauterine abnormalities (79, 80). It involves the insertion of either a pediatric Foley or hysterosalpingogram catheter into the uterine cavity with subsequent introduction of sterile saline while visualizing with the transvaginal ultrasound. Findings at sonohysterography correlate well with confirmatory diagnosis at hysteroscopy (in the operating room) or after hysterectomy. Sonohysterography offers greater than 85% sensitivity and specificity in diagnosing intracavitary lesions (81). Rubin et al. (80) reported a 64% incidence of intrauterine abnormalities in patients with primary infertility. Although it is still controversial whether these abnormalities are causal for infertility, all patients should be screened for such lesions. Sonohysterography appears to be an effective modality to use for this screening.

Laparoscopy

Laparoscopy was once included in the initial workup of the standard infertility evaluation. Because of expense and risk–benefit analyses, there appears little role for a diagnostic laparoscopy in the early evaluation of the infertile couple. Based on current evidence, only patients with a history and physical exam compatible with endometriosis, positive antichlamydial antibody titer, or abnormalities displayed on the hysterosalpingogram or other studies should undergo laparoscopy for infertility. Even then, the decision to proceed with either laparoscopy or IVF should be made on an individual basis. In older women, because of the rapid decline of fertility potential with advancing age, efforts should be directed toward the treatment method that provides the highest likelihood of success within the shortest time interval (82).

Treatment of Tubal Disease

When the clinician has completed the diagnostic evaluation of infertility, the next step is to estimate the baseline prognosis without therapy and then determine whether treatment can increase the likelihood of pregnancy. There is a wide range of tubal pathology in patients with documented sequelae of PID. Proximal tubal disease, diagnosed most commonly by hysterosalpingogram, has historically been treated with laparotomy. Excision of the uterine cornua with reimplantation of the tube or reimplantation of the nondiseased proximal portion of the tube into the back of the uterus are two methods that have been described (83). More recently, hysteroscopic cannulation of the proximal tube has been reported and appears to be a promising technique. Early studies report a 30% pregnancy rate after cannulation (84–86).

The appropriate therapy for distal disease depends on a number of factors. Patient age, severity of distal disease, and availability of assisted reproductive technologies are all significant in determining prognosis of subsequent fertility. Several studies assessed pregnancy rates based on degree of tubal damage seen at laparoscopy or indicated on the basis of hysterosalpingography (87, 88). The best prognostic factor was fallopian tube thickness. Tubal diameters greater than 2.5 cm measured by hysterosalpingogram are associated with a lower pregnancy rate (22%) than normal-diameter tubes (less than 1.5 cm) (48%) (88). For women whose distal tubes have a diameter greater than 3 cm measured at laparoscopy, the prognosis for a term pregnancy following tubal reconstruction is extremely poor (16%) compared with patients with mild disease (80%) (87).

Dlugi et al. (89) reported on success of laparoscopic procedures for distal disease. Patients with repair of bilateral disease with neosalpingostomy had significantly lower 2-year pregnancy rates compared with patients with unilateral disease (9% versus 32.8%). They also concluded that with severe adhesive disease (American Fertility Society score greater than 23), pregnancy rates were significantly reduced (89). Eight of their 113 patients underwent a second surgical procedure with an intrauterine pregnancy rate of 25%. Most reports agree that patients with severe tubal disease, as defined by the American Fertility Society (90) or the criteria of Rock et al. (91), have poor pregnancy rates after repair and recommendations for IVF should be made. Although IVF and tuboplasty have not been compared in a formal prospective study, IVF appears to be superior to surgical intervention for women with severe tubal disease (92). IVF offers delivery rates of 15 to 20% per cycle and an overall delivery rate of greater than 70% of women with tubal factor infertility with four cycles of treatment. This is superior to surgery for severe disease (93).

Treatment of endometriosis-associated infertility has been the subject of many trials of therapy with ovulation suppression and laparoscopic ablation of endometriosis implants (94). The data suggest that surgical correction of moderate to severe disease is effective in improving pregnancy rates. One prospective randomized trial assessed whether laparoscopic treatment of minimal or mild endometriosis improved cumulative pregnancy rates over expectant management of similar disease and concluded that an improvement in pregnancy rate was evident 36 weeks after laparoscopy (95). However, longer follow-up of these patients may demonstrate that the difference is no longer seen and that the benefit of surgery is only transient. Regardless, if stage I or II endometriosis is encountered in the infertile patient, it is recommended that it be resected or thoroughly ablated. (See Chapter 13 for more information on the staging and treatment of endometriosis.)

Treatment of Intrauterine Disease

Infertility due to leiomyomata is a diagnosis of exclusion primarily because their relationship to one another is so poorly understood. Prior to treating an asymptomatic fibroid in an infertile patient, all other causes of infertility should be addressed. The location of the myoma should be determined because it appears that subserosal fibroids have minimal impact on fertility but can cause other gynecologic symptoms (96, 97). Submucosal fibroids greater than 2 cm should be removed because the size of the fibroid has been implicated as prognostic of conception rate (98). Some studies indicate that in the absence of an intrauterine filling defect and no history of pregnancy losses, fibroids less than 10 cm in the widest dimension should not be removed prior to documented reproductive failure. However, a more recent evaluation of 67 patients with fibroids and no other infertility factors determined that regardless of location, removal of fibroids greater than 4 to 5 cm resulted in improved pregnancy and full-term delivery rates (99). In patients with large fibroids (greater than 10 to 12 cm) and no pregnancy losses, appropriate counseling is essential, and myomectomy is indicated if all diagnostic tests reveal no other cause of infertility.

Asherman's syndrome (the presence of intrauterine adhesions usually resulting from a postpartum dilation and curettage) can result in infertility. Treatment with hysteroscopic resection has been reported to result in an 80% term pregnancy rate (100). For a more detailed discussion of Asherman's syndrome, refer to the Recurrent Pregnancy Loss section.

Endometrial polyps, although frequently diagnosed by various imaging studies, have no clear association with infertility but should be removed if other gynecologic symptoms are present. If they are discovered incidentally at hysteroscopy, polypectomy is warranted for histologic analysis.

Special Topics in Female Infertility

Luteal Phase Deficiency

The luteal phase of the menstrual cycle is the period of time between ovulation and the onset of menses. The luteal phase is characterized by progesterone secretion by the corpus luteum. Most cases of luteal phase deficiency are attributed to inadequate secretion of progesterone; however, decreased endometrial response to progesterone can also result in a luteal phase deficiency (101).

Although a number of clinical tests have been proposed to diagnose luteal phase deficiency, they all suffer from lack of validation and standardization. Despite strict criteria for making a histologic diagnosis of luteal phase defect, there remains significant disparity in pathologists' interpretations of the endometrial biopsy. Even the same pathologists re-reading endometrial biopsy slides a second time disagreed with 75% of their own original diagnoses (102).

It is likely that a luteal phase defect simply reflects the release of an abnormal oocyte. The resulting low progesterone and retarded endometrial maturation occur as a result of abnormal ovulation. Measuring luteal progesterone approximately 7 days after ovulation can give useful information about the preceding ovulation, but supplementation with exogenous progesterone support will not likely improve pregnancy outcome (103). A luteal progesterone level of greater than 3 ng/mL is evidence that ovulation occurred (15). First-trimester progesterone values above 25 ng/mL suggest a normal intrauterine pregnancy 98% of the time, whereas pregnancies with values below 5 ng/mL are almost always nonviable.

Despite improved diagnostic testing for luteal phase deficiency, it remains unproven that luteal phase support with progesterone or hCG supplementation offers any improvement in pregnancy rates (104). Numerous trials comparing progesterone, clomiphene, and gonadotropin therapy for luteal phase deficiency have been described. A disordered luteal phase is likely a reflection of abnormal follicular development, and treatment should be directed at correction of folliculogenesis with either clomiphene or gonadotropins.

Ovulation Induction and Ovarian Cancer Risk

Case reports of ovarian carcinoma in infertile women have raised interest about a potential causative relationship between ovulation induction and cancer. Because ovarian cancer is a relatively rare disease and ovarian cancer associated with fertility drug use even more rare, examination of this connection is limited to case reports and retrospective case–control studies. Current available data fail to reveal a causal effect, although nulliparous women with refractory infertility may harbor a high risk of ovarian cancer irrespective of their use of fertility medication(s) (105). Close clinical surveillance of patients before, during, and after treatment of infertility is recommended. Some recommend a baseline ultrasound before any clomiphene use, repeating an ultrasound with the onset of new and unexplained symptoms, and encouraging yearly exams with the patient advising their physician(s) that they have taken clomiphene in the past.

Treating Infertility in Women of Advanced Reproductive Age

Female fertility begins to decline many years prior to the onset of menopause, despite continued regular ovulatory cycles. In addition, the risk of spontaneous abortion increases with a woman's age. Although age-related changes in fecundity have been documented in several populations, there is significant variability in the timing of onset of diminished reproductive potential for individual women. Since 1990, there has been a greater than ten-fold rise in the number of cases of IVF performed for women older than 40 years (93). Elevated day 3 (basal) FSH and estradiol concentrations are independent predictors in determining prognosis for conception. Although it may vary slightly between different laboratories, follicular phase FSH greater than 10 mIU/mL or serum estradiol greater than 80 pg/mL indicates poor prognosis for conception (106). The clomiphene citrate challenge test (CCCT) is another test of ovarian reserve and has been validated in assisted reproduction and the general infertility population (107). It involves measuring day 3 FSH, administration of clomiphene 100 mg daily from days 5 to 9, followed by repeat FSH on day 10. The test result is considered abnormal if either the basal or day 10 FSH level is above 12 IU/L. The rationale behind this test is that women with adequate ovarian reserve should develop a cohort of follicles producing adequate estradiol and inhibin to suppress the FSH. It is logical to first obtain a basal FSH in the infertile patient older than age 30. If the result is less than 12 IU/L, a CCCT is warranted. If either the day 3 or the day 10 level is elevated (greater than 12 IU/L), appropriate counseling of a poor prognosis for conception is warranted (less than 5% chance of conception). FSH results can vary between laboratories, and clinicians should know the critical values for their respective labs. A single elevated day 3 FSH value implies poor prognosis for pregnancy, even when values in subsequent cycles are normal (108, 109).

MALE FACTOR INFERTILITY

At least 30 to 40% of all infertility is attributable to abnormalities of male reproductive function. For this reason, it is important to evaluate the male partner as an integral part of the infertility workup. The semen analysis should always be included as an initial screening test. A history of fathering a prior pregnancy is inadequate to rule out abnormalities of the semen. The quality limits designed to discriminate infertile from fertile men are constantly being re-examined and redefined. The WHO normal values are seen in Table 16.4 (110). These values help identify patients who should not experience decreased fecundity. However, the predictive value of sub-normal semen analysis parameters is limited except in the case of azoospermia. No diagnostic test of sperm function can unequivocally predict the potential for fertilization to occur.

Although many techniques have been proposed to evaluate different etiologies of male factor infertility, only the semen analysis has proven to be a reproducible predictor of impaired fertility.

History and Physical Exam

During the initial history, the sexual habits of the couple should be ascertained. KY-Jelly and other lubricants can be spermatotoxic and result in impaired motility or count (111). Timing and frequency of intercourse should also be addressed. Some authors recommend intercourse every 48 hours during midcycle (112). A history of childhood illnesses, abnormal testicular development (specifically undescended testicles), or trauma to the genitourinary organs should also be obtained. Impaired testicular function may result from any generalized insult (viremia, fever). It takes approximately 72 days for the sperm to reach the caudal epididymis after the initiation of spermatogenesis, and the effects of any adverse events may not be demonstrated in the ejaculate for 1 to 3 months. A history of a delay in pubertal development and maturation can suggest an endocrinopathy such as hypogonadotropic hypogonadism or adrenal dysfunction. Other factors contributing to impaired spermatogenesis include a history of chemotherapy or

TABLE 16.4

World Health Organization Normal Values for Semen Analysis

Volume	$\geq$2.0 mL
Sperm concentration	$\geq$20 million/mL
Motility	$\geq$50% with forward progression *or*
	$\geq$20% with rapid progression within 60 min of ejaculation
Morphology	$\geq$30% normal focus
White blood cells	<1 million/mL
Immunobead	<20% spermatozoa with adherent particles
Mixed agglutination reaction test	<10% spermatozoa with adherent particles

Data from Laboratory Manual for the Examination of Human Semen and Sperm—Cervical Mucus Interaction. 3rd ed. Cambridge: Cambridge University Press, 1992:44–45, with Permission.

radiation, tuberculosis, exposure to environmental toxins, or drugs (specifically sulfasalazine [Azulfidine], calcium channel blockers, cimetidine [Tagamet], alcohol, marijuana, and/or exogenous androgenic steroids). Elevated temperatures also impair spermatogenesis, and routine use of hot tubs should be discouraged.

A detailed clinical assessment should be performed with particular regard to the evaluation of the genitalia. The presence of hypospadias, abnormally small testes, or the presence of a varicocele should be noted. Testicular volumes in normal men are usually in excess of 15 mL and are frequently in excess of 30 mL. Assessment for varicocele should be performed with the patient in the supine and standing positions using the Valsalva maneuver. An enlarged prostate can suggest prostatitis, which could affect semen quality. Androgen deficiency may be evidenced by decreased body hair, gynecomastia, or eunuchoid proportions, and if any of these findings are present, an exploration of an endocrine abnormality is indicated.

Laboratory Evaluation

Semen Analysis

The most important laboratory investigation in male infertility is the semen analysis. Some authors recommend a period of abstinence for several days before collection to maximize the quality of the specimen (113). However, not abstaining from the normal frequency of ejaculation may be a more accurate reflection of semen quality during intercourse. A period of abstinence is generally recommended only with a prior result of oligospermia. Collection by masturbation into a sterile container is the most commonly recommended method, although coitus interruptus or a spermicidal-free condom can be used if the man cannot or will not masturbate. The specimen should be protected from temperature extremes and delivered to the laboratory within an hour of collection.

Interpretation of the semen analysis results is important to the prognosis of future conception. These values (Table 16.4) help identify patients who should not have decreased ability to induce pregnancy. However, unless there is azoospermia, the predictive value of subnormal semen parameters is limited (12). Morphology consistently seems to be a good predictor of fertilization. One report demonstrated marked decrease in fertilization when the normal morphology was less than 40%, although the current WHO cut-off point is 30% (114). No single category in the semen analysis can be used as a sole predictor of fertility (115). Some reports combine the motility and count for a total motile count:

$$\text{Total motile count} = (\text{sperm/mL}) \times (\%\ \text{motile}) \times (\text{volume in mL}) \qquad (16.3)$$

This measurement is often used to evaluate a washed specimen for intrauterine insemination. Pregnancy rates are improved in specimens with a total motile sperm count that exceeds 5×10^6 (116).

Abnormalities of any parameter in the semen analysis warrant attention. However, treatment of such abnormalities remains unproved in enhancing the pregnancy rate of the involved couple. Therefore, prior to initiating any therapy, it is prudent to completely assess both partners involved.

Tests of Sperm Function

No functional test has yet been validated that can unequivocally predict the fertilization capacity of spermatozoa. (In other words, nothing is more predictive than a normal or abnormal semen analysis based on WHO criteria.) Despite this, many tests have been proposed for the assessment of sperm functionality. The sperm penetration assay, the hemizona assay, in vitro tests of penetration into mucus, sperm mannose-ligand receptor levels, and measurement of the acrosome reaction have all been used. However, because they do not provide any valid information to predict fecundity, they should not be included in the routine assessment of the infertile couple.

Sperm Antibodies

Sperm are very immunogenic. Because sperm antibodies develop only after specific instances, testing should be limited to a distinct population. Men with a history of testicular trauma, vasectomy reversal, or who have evidence of clumping on the semen analysis are candidates for evaluation. An immunologic reaction directed against the sperm has been implicated as a cause of decreased motility (117). Diagnosis is usually made with the immunobead test to identify the presence of antibodies on the sperm. Various forms of treatment have been used, including antibiotics, immunosuppression, testosterone therapy, sperm washing and intrauterine insemination, IVF, and donor insemination. One effective method involves sperm washing and intrauterine insemination of washed sperm with or without concomitant ovulation induction. When compared with corticosteroid immunosuppression, intrauterine insemination is associated with a higher pregnancy rate with fewer side effects (118). If this is unsuccessful, IVF, with or without micromanipulation, should be considered.

Treatment Options for Male Factor Infertility

Approximately 6% of infertile men have conditions for which specific therapy of confirmed benefit is available (e.g., the treatment of hypogonadotropic hypogonadism) (119, 120). Treatment of most infertile men usually involves methods to use the amount of sperm available rather than futile efforts at improving sperm concentration or motility.

Varicocele Repair

Although varicoceles are associated with infertility, many men with varicoceles father children. The literature is replete with studies both supporting and opposing the view that the repair of varicoceles results in increased pregnancy rates. Because the repair is a surgical procedure, it is not possible to perform a double-blind controlled study. Most urologic studies on the evaluation of varicocelectomy are flawed because they fail to outline the evaluation of the female partners of the men in the studies.

Varicocelectomy does appear to have a beneficial effect on sperm density (121, 122). Some studies also report a favorable effect on fertility, although this is an inconsistent finding in the literature (123, 124). The American Society of Reproductive Medicine proposes that surgical intervention should be recommended if the patient is symptomatic with pain or for couples with reduced sperm count and otherwise unexplained infertility (125, 126). An individualized approach is warranted with referral to a urologist when necessary.

Intrauterine Insemination

Treatment of male factor infertility with intrauterine insemination of prepared spermatozoa has been evaluated by a meta-analysis of eight reported trials in which pregnancy was an outcome measure (120). The odds ratio suggests no increase in fertility is obtained with the use of intrauterine insemination alone for therapy. However, when combined with gonadotropin-stimulated cycles, the addition of intrauterine insemination increased the monthly pregnancy rates as much as 8% (127, 128).

Intrauterine insemination is performed after separation of motile from nonmotile spermatozoa and other material in the seminal plasma that might have detrimental effects on fertilization. One procedure is described in Table 16.5. Although a variety of techniques have been used for sperm preparation for intrauterine inseminations, the appropriate choice should be the one most familiar

TABLE 16.5

One Method for Preparation of Spermatozoa for Intrauterine Insemination

The semen is collected by masturbation into a sterile container. After liquefaction, the ejaculate is placed into 10 mL of warmed Ham's 10 (GIBCO, Grand Island, NY) and centrifuged at 300 *g* for 10 min. If a pellet is not obtained, it is resuspended and spun for an additional 10 min. The supernatant is discarded, and the pellet is resuspended in roughly 0.3 mL of Ham's 10 solution. The sperm suspension is introduced into the uterine cavity with a pediatric feeding tube (C.R. Bard, Inc., Cranston, RI) after first confirming adequete count and motility.

to and least time consuming for the physician. Despite the diversity of sperm preparations, no single method has proven superior in improving fecundity.

Other Therapies

Assisted reproductive technology provides additional therapies for couples with male factor infertility. Most recently, the advent of intracytoplasmic sperm injection (ICSI) provides a unique treatment opportunity for couples whose infertility is secondary to severe oligospermia. The live birth rate per embryo transfer is reported to be between 30% and 40%, depending on the age of the woman and if other infertility factors are present (129).

Another technique, therapeutic donor insemination, involves many emotional, ethical, and legal issues. The success rate varies between fresh and frozen samples, but in women younger than 30 years old, the 6-month cumulative pregnancy rates are approximately 40 to 50% for frozen specimens (130). The use of fresh specimen for therapeutic donor insemination is discouraged because of the need for a quarantine period to ensure absence of any transmittable disease(s). Prior to insemination, the involved couple should be appropriately counseled regarding all pertinent legal and social issues involved with this procedure.

UNEXPLAINED INFERTILITY

Unexplained infertility is a diagnosis of exclusion. It is a term applied to an infertile couple for whom standard investigations (semen analysis, tubal patency assessment, and laboratory assessment of ovulation) yield normal results. It is estimated that 10 to 15% of infertile couples will ultimately reach this clinical diagnosis.

Without treatment, up to 60% of couples with unexplained infertility will conceive within 3 years (131). After 3 years of infertility, the pregnancy rate without treatment decreases by 2% for every month (24% for each additional year) of infertility (132). Patient age is a critical factor in determining fecundity. Tietze (5) reported 11% of women at the age of 34 were infertile compared with 33% at age 40 and 87% by age 44. Thus, in women older than 30 with greater than 3 years of unexplained infertility, spontaneous conception is unlikely. Up to 40% of patients with the diagnosis of unexplained infertility display abnormal CCCTs, indicating diminished ovarian reserve. This simple tool can therefore aid the clinician in determining which protocol, if any, to initiate and the length of treatment (133).

Treatment Options for Unexplained Infertility

In couples with unexplained infertility, no biological abnormality is evident, and thus only empirical treatments are relevant. Bromocriptine and danazol (Danocrine) as empiric therapy have no effect on fecundity (8). Although psychological factors have been suggested as causative agents of unexplained infertility, there are no controlled trials showing counseling to be effective. Four trials, to date, have examined the use of clomiphene as empiric treatment and the combined data suggest an improvement in fecundity (8). One of these trials revealed that the greatest relative increase resulted when clomiphene was given to women who had been infertile for more than 3 years (134).

Intrauterine insemination when used in unstimulated, natural cycles has been proposed as a means to increase fecundity in couples with unexplained infertility. Unfortunately, few studies demonstrate a clear benefit of intrauterine insemination alone. When used with clomiphene, Deaton et al. (135) described significantly improved per-cycle fecundity (9.7%) compared with controls (3.3%). Clomiphene 50 mg was administered during cycle days 5 to 9, and 10,000 units hCG intramuscularly were added when an estimated follicular diameter of greater than 18 mm on ultrasound was reached. An intrauterine insemination using washed sperm was performed 36 hours after the hCG injection. Although this regimen may augment fertility, treatment should be limited to three cycles. No pregnancies occurred during the fourth cycle in this study, and no other study has demonstrated benefit of treatment beyond this interval.

Superovulation and intrauterine insemination has also been demonstrated to be of benefit in the treatment of unexplained infertility (136). Immunotherapy with corticosteroids has demonstrated additional benefit to couples treated with this combination therapy, but risks of serious complications, such as aseptic necrosis of the femoral neck, osteoporosis, and increased susceptibility to infection preclude it from routine use (137). A detailed description of different gonadotropin regimens and various assisted reproductive technologies for the treatment of unexplained infertility is beyond the scope of this chapter. Based on available data, a rational treatment plan for affected couples includes up to three cycles of clomiphene in combination with hCG and intrauterine insemination. If unsuccessful, the next steps would include superovulation with intrauterine insemination followed by IVF. A cumulative pregnancy rate of 40% can be achieved using this regimen.

RECURRENT PREGNANCY LOSS

Traditionally, recurrent pregnancy loss has been defined as three consecutive spontaneous abortions. However, it is usually appropriate to initiate an evaluation of the couple after two such losses (138). Recognizing that the spontaneous cure rate is high and the probability of a subsequent successful pregnancy outcome is usually greater than 50%, the focus of the physician should be directed toward obtaining a thorough history and providing adequate counseling to the couple prior to initiating diagnostic tests or suggesting therapy.

EPIDEMIOLOGY

Of all recognized human pregnancies, 15 to 20% will end in spontaneous abortion. The actual incidence of spontaneous pregnancy loss is greater when early, unconfirmed pregnancies are included. One group tested daily urine specimens from 221 healthy women attempting to conceive with ultrasensitive hCG assays and determined that the total rate of pregnancy loss after implantation was 31% (139). These estimates do not include instances where fertilized oocytes fail to implant.

Statistics regarding pregnancy outcome are beneficial when counseling patients during early gestation. Regan et al. (140) studied the course of pregnancy in women with ultrasonographically confirmed intrauterine gestations. The overall incidence of spontaneous abortion was 12%, and half occurred before 8 weeks' gestation. The miscarriage rate was only 5% in primigravidas and 14 % in multigravidas (141). Prior successful pregnancy was associated with a 5% loss, whereas women whose last pregnancy aborted had a subsequent loss 20% of the time. This increased to 24% in the women in whom all previous pregnancies ended in spontaneous abortions. Thus, the most relevant predictive factor for pregnancy outcome in a subsequent pregnancy is past reproductive history.

Poland et al. (142) also reported a 20% spontaneous abortion rate in women with one prior spontaneous abortion, but in women reporting three or more consecutive abortions, the chance of a subsequent loss increased to 50%. These figures are similar to those reported by James (143), who added that women with at least one live birth followed by three or more losses had only a 30% chance of subsequent pregnancy loss.

ETIOLOGY

The mere presence of an etiologic factor does not signify that it is the definitive cause of recurrent miscarriage. Determination and initiation of appropriate therapy should be based only on the expectation that eradication of identified risk factors will enhance the likelihood of a subsequent live birth.

Genetic Factors

Several large studies indicate the incidence of a fetal chromosomal anomaly in first trimester spontaneous abortions exceeds 50% (144, 145). In addition, 30% of second-trimester abortions and 3% of stillbirths demonstrate abnormal karyotypes. The vast majority of these are due to errors in gametogenesis (chromosomal nondisjunction during meiosis), fertilization (triploidy), or the first division of the fertilized ovum (tetraploidy or mosaicism). Only about 5% are due to structural abnormalities such as translocation (141). Aneuploid conceptions are reported to occur more frequently in pregnancies subsequent to recurrent pregnancy loss compared with a control group (1.6% versus 0.3%) (136).

Autosomal trisomy (of chromosomes 13, 16, 18, 21, and 22) is the most common abnormal karyotype (50%), followed by monosomy X (20%), triploidy (15%), tetraploidy (10%), and structural abnormalities (5%). Recall that trisomy is the addition of an extra chromosome to a haploid set of chromosomes, or $2n + 1$, whereas triploidy is when three full haploid sets of chromosomes—or $3n$—are present in all cells. The most common monosomy is 45 XO (Turner's syndrome) (144).

Parental chromosomal abnormalities are an infrequent cause of recurrent pregnancy loss. The reported incidence of major chromosomal abnormalities in either parent varies from 3 to 5%. Half of these anomalies are due to balanced translocation, and one-fourth are due to Robertsonian translocation. Translocation and inversion are associated with a higher risk of pregnancy wastage and are indications for prenatal diagnosis in subsequent pregnancy (146). However, these couples should not be dissuaded from attempting further pregnancies.

Effect of Maternal Age

Advanced maternal age has been associated with an increased frequency of spontaneous abortion and with an increase in chromosomal defects (147). Studies in pregnancies derived from oocyte donation indicate that the age of the donor, and thus the age of the oocyte, is the most important factor in determining the risk of miscarriage (148). Decreased endometrial receptivity is relatively less important (149).

Müllerian Anomalies

Patients with recurrent miscarriage exhibit a higher than average incidence of uterine anomalies. The least frequent uterine anomaly, the unicornuate uterus, is associated with the greatest incidence of miscarriage (about 50%) (150). The most common uterine anomaly is the arcuate uterus, followed by the septate uterus, and then the bicornuate uterus. The septate or bicornuate uterus is associated with a 30% rate of pregnancy loss (151). It has been suggested that hysteroscopic resection of a septum thicker than 1 cm results in a subsequent successful delivery in more than 80% of subsequent pregnancies (152). However, there have been no prospective randomized trials to confirm this finding.

Diethylstilbestrol Exposure In Utero

Women exposed to DES during fetal life have impaired reproductive function compared with control subjects. The exact mechanism, although not fully understood, is believed to be a decreased surface area or altered shape of the endometrial cavity. No intervention, including prophylactic cervical cerclage, has been shown to decrease the overall rate of recurrent loss in these women.

Leiomyoma

Buttram and Reitter (153) established that a myomectomy performed for recurrent abortion decreased the loss rate from 40 to 20%. They recommended a myomectomy in women with recurrent pregnancy loss if no other causes could be found. They reiterated the notion that any fibroid greater than 2 cm is a potential cause of abortion. In the investigation of recurrent pregnancy loss, a transvaginal ultrasound is usually performed. If submucous or large intramural fibroids are present, a hysteroscopic resection or abdominal myomectomy is usually offered (154).

The nulliparous female with asymptomatic fibroids offers a clinical dilemma. It seems reasonable that if the fibroids involve a significant portion of the endometrium or compromise the tubal ostia, removal is warranted. Although not based on prospective data, Buttram and Reitter advocated myomectomy for asymptomatic patients with uteri measuring greater than 12 weeks in size (152).

Incompetent Cervix

The classic description of the incompetent cervix is painless dilation of the internal os leading to pregnancy loss, usually in the second trimester. A history of excessive mechanical cervical dilation at the time of a prior dilation and curettage has been previously described as a cause of cervical incompetence. Now, however, for the majority of cases, incompetent cervix is believed to result from a congenital defect in the cervical tissue. The diagnosis of incompetent cervix is best made by a history of second-trimester loss(es) accompanied by spontaneous rupture of membranes but without antecedent uterine contractions.

Asherman's Syndrome

Asherman's syndrome is usually suspected by history and/or characteristic filling defects on hysterosalpingography. The diagnosis is confirmed with hysteroscopy. Intrauterine adhesions are almost always related to a prior dilation and curettage after a pregnancy-related event. Symptoms include menstrual irregularities, infertility, and recurrent abortion. This syndrome is also associated with premature labor, abnormal placentation, and abnormal fetal lie. Many patients may be asymptomatic. The recommended treatment is lysis of the adhesions during hysteroscopy. The abortion rate has been reported to decrease as much as 80% after appropriate treatment (154). Some authors recommend placement of a pediatric Foley catheter in the uterine cavity that is then removed 3 to 5 days after surgery. They also recommend conjugated estrogen (Premarin) 2.5 mg orally twice daily for 30 to 60 days after hysteroscopic resection and 1 week of prophylactic antibiotics, usually doxycycline (Vibramycin). During the last week of estrogen therapy, medroxyprogesterone acetate 10 mg daily for 10 days is added (155).

Endocrine Causes

Progesterone Deficiency

There is no established consensus on the pathophysiology of luteal phase defects, the method of diagnosis, or its proper treatment. Low hCG and progesterone levels after implantation appear to be the result, not the cause, of pregnancy loss in the majority of cases. Although no randomized controlled trials have had sufficient statistical power to detect a benefit with the use of progesterone vaginal suppositories or intramuscular progesterone in preventing pregnancy loss, a meta-analysis of these studies indicates there is evidence to support progesterone therapy to decrease pregnancy loss (156). The discrepancy among various trials probably arises from the heterogeneity of causes of luteal inadequacy.

Treatment should be directed at restoring normal folliculogenesis and luteal support. Because of the emotional impact of pregnancy loss, and despite a lack of supporting evidence, many clinicians offer empiric treatment with clomiphene (50-mg tablets daily on cycle days 3 to 7), followed by progesterone suppositories (50 mg per vagina daily beginning after ovulation and continuing through 10 weeks' gestation). Giving micronized progesterone pills intravaginally (200-mg tablets placed intravaginally each night before bed) is more cost effective than the prepackaged progesterone gels (157).

Abnormal Thyroid Hormone

Although the traditional workup of recurrent pregnancy loss includes evaluation of thyroid status, several large trials fail to demonstrate clear-cut data on the effects of hypothyroidism and spontaneous abortion. However, the high frequency of hypothyroidism justifies screening with a serum TSH level (158).

Polycystic Ovarian Syndrome

Women with PCOS have increased difficulty achieving pregnancy compared with the general population, but the exact nature of the relationship between PCOS and recurrent pregnancy loss is unclear. Some have demonstrated that women with a history of recurrent miscarriage have higher levels of androgens, both with and without evidence of PCOS (159). The hyperinsulinemic state of PCOS is hypothesized to contribute to early loss during pregnancy, and in one trial, the administration of metformin during pregnancy to women with a history of miscarriage was shown to reduce the first-trimester loss rate in women with PCOS (43). In a large trial of more than 2000 women with a history of recurrent miscarriage, the prevalence of PCOS was 40.7%, although the live birth rate was similar among women with PCOS compared with women with normal ovarian morphology, and neither elevated serum LH nor testosterone levels were associated with an increased miscarriage rate. The criteria sufficient to determine which women with PCOS have a good or poor prognosis of future successful pregnancies remain unknown (160).

Diabetes Mellitus

Diabetes mellitus is traditionally mentioned in association with an increased abortion rate, but it has been determined in a controlled trial that diabetes with good glucose control (with diet or insulin) does not increase the risk of spontaneous abortion (150). Patients in good control with oral agents prior to conception will probably also have improved outcomes. Diabetes with poor glycemic control is associated with an increased risk of early pregnancy loss, and there is a direct correlation between hemoglobin A_{1C} levels and the rate of abortion.

Immunologic Factors

The successful outcome of pregnancy depends on the development of adequate placental circulation. Patients with antiphospholipid antibodies (lupus anticoagulants and anticardiolipin antibodies) are at increased risk for venous and arterial thrombosis, resulting in an increased rate of spontaneous abortion and/or intrauterine fetal death. Antiphospholipid antibody syndrome is diagnosed with the following criteria (161):

Persistent positivity in tests for lupus anticoagulant and/or anticardiolipin antibody, *plus* one of the following:

- Three or more consecutive spontaneous losses before week 10 of gestation
- One or more premature births (before 34 weeks) due to severe pre-eclampsia or impaired fetal growth
- One or more unexplained intrauterine deaths beyond 10 weeks' gestation

Overall, antiphospholipid antibodies are present in 10 to 15% of patients with recurrent pregnancy loss; anticardiolipin antibodies are more common than lupus anticoagulants. In patients with antiphospholipid antibodies, the fetal loss rate approaches 70% (162).

Other causes of inherited thrombophilias include activated protein C resistance, antithrombin III deficiency, hyperhomocysteinemia, and factor V Leiden mutation. These thrombophilias are a group of genetic disorders of blood coagulation that can result in an increased risk of thrombosis. Although most investigators agree that there is an association between the presence of these antibodies and markers of thrombophilias with pregnancy loss, optimal treatment regimens have not been well defined.

The goal of each treatment for antiphospholipid syndrome is to decrease the placental infarction, thrombosis, and fibrin deposition believed to be responsible for pregnancy loss. A commonly used regimen of prednisone 20 to 60 mg daily with 80 mg aspirin appears to improve pregnancy outcome significantly but carries with it the morbidity of prolonged corticosteroid use (163). Some studies have shown that heparin (5000 units subcutaneously, twice daily) combined with aspirin (80 mg) results in better outcome than therapy with low-dose aspirin alone (164). This combination therapy may reduce pregnancy loss in women with antiphospholipid antibodies by 54%. Whether this treatment is beneficial to those patients with recurrent pregnancy loss with one of the other thrombophilic disorders, but with negative antiphospholipid antibodies, is not known and should be administered on an individualized basis. Another trial demonstrated that aspirin (80 mg) is as effective as heparin plus aspirin (165). Because low-dose aspirin has few side effects, it remains a reasonable empiric treatment with potentially significant benefit for patients with recurrent pregnancy losses.

Infectious Factors

Various infectious agents have been postulated to be etiologic factors for abortion. However, they likely play only a coincidental role in spontaneous abortion because there have been no placebo-controlled trials proving benefit with antibiotic therapy.

Environmental Factors

Women who smoke more than 14 cigarettes per day have a 1.7 relative risk for spontaneous abortion (166). The influence of alcohol on abortion rate is very small, with only the heavy users demonstrating a slightly increased risk. However, both smoking and alcohol have other adverse effects on organogenesis and should be avoided during attempts to achieve pregnancy and once pregnancy has occurred.

DIAGNOSIS, TREATMENT, AND COUNSELING

The expected probability of a woman having three consecutive miscarriages is 0.3 to 0.4%, but the actual incidence range is 0.4 to 0.7%, indicating a distinct cause of recurrent pregnancy loss in some patients. The abortuses of women with greater than three losses are more likely to be chromosomally normal. Regardless of the cause, women with greater than three losses and no liveborn children still have a greater than 50% chance of a successful pregnancy. These facts are essential in counseling couples suffering from recurrent pregnancy loss.

A diagnostic regimen (Table 16.6) should begin with a thorough history and physical examination, with specific questions regarding exact gestational age at loss and any possible symptoms of cervical incompetence. Pertinent blood tests include TSH level, tests to detect lupus anticoagulant activity, and antiphospholipid antibodies. If the patient is diabetic, a hemoglobin A_{1C} is useful in reflecting the level of glucose control. A hysterosalpingogram or sonohysterogram should be performed to diagnose uterine anomalies. If these tests reveal no abnormalities, parental karyotypes can be performed. These tests are very expensive, however, and offer little on which to base a change in management, other than heightened genetic counseling and any appropriate studies during the subsequent pregnancy.

TABLE 16.6

Workup for Recurrent Pregnancy Loss

History
Past reproductive history (including history of early pregnancy losses)
Previous uterine surgery (including dilation and curettage)
History of thyroid disease or uncontrolled diabetes
History of diethylstilbestrol exposure
Exposure to cigarette smoke or environmental toxins
Alcohol intake
Laboratory Tests
Thyroid-stimulating hormone
Lupus anticoagulant or activated partial thromboplastin time and anticardiolipin antibody titers
Hemoglobin A_{1C} (if patient is diabetic)
Patient and partner karyotypes (optional)
Hysterosalpingogram or sonohysterogram
Factor V Leiden mutation (if indicated by history)

Sympathetic and frequent counseling has improved pregnancy outcome as much or more than any therapeutic intervention, especially in those patients in which an abnormality can not be identified (167). Unexplained recurrent pregnancy loss is a very frustrating condition, both for the couple and for the practitioner. Many new, as of yet unproved, therapeutic modalities will arise as possible therapies. Therefore, it is imperative that an evidence-based approach as described here serve as a guideline for diagnosis and treatment.

Clinical Notes

INFERTILITY

EPIDEMIOLOGY

- Approximately 13% of U.S. women who are 15 to 44 years old (excluding sterilized women) are infertile.
- Approximately half of all infertile couples will eventually conceive. Evaluation of an infertile couple should be individualized, but both the man and the woman should be evaluated.
- The probability of conception in an ovulatory cycle is about 25% under ideal circumstances.

ANOVULATORY INFERTILITY

- Ovulatory dysfunction and anovulation affect 15 to 20% of all infertile couples seeking therapy.
- Women with infrequent, irregular menses should be evaluated for anovulation. If ovulation is uncertain from the history, tests are performed to determine if ovulation occurs.
- Tests for ovulation include plasma progesterone levels, urinary LH tests, use of basal body temperature charts, endometrial biopsy, and/or transvaginal sonography.
- Labs ordered to determine the etiology of anovulation include a TSH and prolactin. When indicated, androgen levels and/or 17-hydroxy progesterone levels are obtained.
- In infertility due to hypogonadotropic anovulation, the FSH levels are low, the prolactin is normal, and there is no withdrawal bleed after a progesterone challenge test. Treatment may involve a GnRH pump or use of human menopausal gonadotropins.
- In infertility due to normogonadotropic anovulation, the FSH level is normal, and there is a withdrawal bleed in response to a progesterone challenge. Most of these patients have PCOS. Initial treatment is with clomiphene, 50 mg daily starting on cycle day 3, 4, or 5 and continuing for a total of 5 days. About 70% of women treated will ovulate with 15 to 40% becoming pregnant. Clomiphene-resistant patients may require adjuvant therapy; options include insulin-sensitizing agents, adrenal steroid therapy, gonadotropins, and/or referral to a reproductive specialist.
- In infertility due to hypergonadotropic hypogonadism, FSH levels are usually greater than 20 mIU/mL, and there is no response to a progesterone challenge. In women younger than 40, this indicates premature ovarian failure. In a woman younger than 30, a karyotype must be done. Treatment involves assisted reproductive technologies.
- In infertility due to hyperprolactinemia, the basal morning prolactin levels exceed 20 to 25 ng/mL. If no concurrent thyroid disorder is present, imaging studies to rule out a prolactinoma must be done. Treatment is with bromocriptine, starting at 1.25 mg orally nightly for 1 week and increasing thereafter to 2.5 mg twice daily. If ovulation still does not occur, the dose is increased in 1.25 increments.

TUBOPERITONEAL INFERTILITY

- Forty percent of all infertile women will demonstrate an abnormality of the uterus, cervix, and/or fallopian tubes. Assessment for these potential causes includes an extensive history and physical exam, as well as hysterosalpingography, and some investigators also advocate an antichlamydial antibody titer.

- Most studies show an improvement in pregnancy rate for patients with unexplained infertility with use of the oil-based dye in hysterosalpingography, although the possibility of granuloma formation exists. Some use the oil-based dye therapeutically, but only after bilateral patency has been demonstrated with the water-soluble contrast.
- The postcoital test may be used if there is suspicion of a hostile cervical factor contributing to the infertility.
- The office hysteroscopy may be used to detect intrauterine lesions, although some prefer sonohysterography for this. Sonohysterography does not, however, provide any information about tubal patency.
- Laparoscopy should be reserved for patients with a history and physical compatible with endometriosis, a positive antichlamydial antibody titer, or abnormalities of the uterus and/or tubes noted on imaging studies.
- Proximal tubal disease was previously treated with laparotomy, although hysteroscopic cannulation shows great promise as an effective therapy.
- With distal tubal disease, the best prognostic factor for pregnancy is the thickness of the tubal wall. For diameters greater than 3 cm, the likelihood of term pregnancy after tubal reconstruction is very poor—only 16%. Most patients with severe tubal disease have poor pregnancy rates after repair, and IVF should be recommended.
- The relationship between fibroids and infertility is poorly understood. Most agree that if the fibroid does not impinge on the uterine cavity (i.e., there is no filling defect on hysterosalpingography), there are no previous pregnancy losses, and the fibroids are less than 10 to 12 cm wide, no intervention is necessary. Myomectomy could be justifiable if all diagnostic tests show no other cause of infertility.
- Treatment of Asherman's syndrome (intrauterine adhesions) results in an 80% term pregnancy rate. Therapy is done via hysteroscopic lysis of adhesions.

SPECIAL TOPICS IN FEMALE INFERTILITY

- Controversy regarding the existence and/or clinical significance of luteal phase deficiency continues. If luteal phase support with progesterone or hCG supplementation improves, pregnancy rates remain unproven.
- Current data fail to reveal a cause-and-effect relationship between ovulation induction and ovarian cancer risk, but until the issue is more fully researched, close clinical surveillance of patients before, during, and after treatment of infertility with these agents is recommended. In the infertile patient older than 30, a basal FSH should be obtained. If it is less than 12 IU/L, a clomiphene citrate challenge test is performed. If day 3 or 10 FSH levels are greater than 12 IU/L, the prognosis for conception is very poor.

MALE FACTOR INFERTILITY

- A semen analysis should always be included as an initial screening test for male factor infertility. A careful history and physical exam are also done. No other tests of sperm function have provided clinicians with a valid method to predict fecundity and so should be discouraged from clinical use.
- For men with a history of testicular trauma, vasectomy reversal, or with clumping on the semen analysis, a test for sperm antibodies may be indicated. If antibodies are found, one effective method of therapy involves sperm washing and intrauterine insemination of the washed sperm, either with or without ovulation induction. If this fails, IVF should be considered.
- Although varicoceles are associated with infertility, many men with varicoceles father children. Some propose that surgical intervention be limited to men reporting pain with the varicocele or for couples with reduced sperm counts and otherwise unexplained infertility.
- The data indicate that treatment for male factor infertility via intrauterine insemination with washed sperm increases fertility only when combined with gonadotropin-stimulated cycles.

- For men with severe oligospermia, intracytoplasmic sperm injection may result in clinical pregnancy rates per cycle of up to 30%.

UNEXPLAINED INFERTILITY

- Ten to 15% of infertile couples will ultimately be diagnosed with unexplained infertility. Without treatment, up to 60% of couples with unexplained infertility will conceive within 3 years.
- One treatment regimen includes clomiphene for days 5 to 9, followed by an injection of hCG to induce ovulation and performance of intrauterine insemination with washed sperm 36 hours later. This regimen should not be used beyond three cycles because there is no benefit.
- Superovulation and intrauterine insemination has been demonstrated to be of benefit in the treatment of unexplained infertility. If this fails, IVF should follow.

RECURRENT PREGNANCY LOSS

- Defined as three pregnancy losses, all at less than 20 weeks gestation, but it is appropriate to initiate evaluation after two such losses.
- Abortions may be attributable to genetic factors, maternal age, müllerian anomalies, uterine anomalies, endocrine causes, or immunologic or environmental factors, or a cause may never be identified.
- Patients and physicians should be encouraged and patients should be counseled that women with three recurrent pregnancy losses still have a greater than 50% chance of successful pregnancy.

REFERENCES

1. Mosher WD, Pratt EF. The demography of infertility in the United States. In: Asch RH, Studd JW, eds. Annual Progress in Reproductive Medicine. Pearl River, NY: Parthenon, 1993:37–43.
2. Mosher WD, Pratt WF. Fecundity and infertility in the U.S. 1965–82. National Center for Health Statistics Advance Data. Vital and Health Statistics. Washington, DC: Public Health Service, 1985:104.
3. Healy DL, Trounson AO, Andersen AN. Female infertility: causes and treatment. Lancet 1994;343:1539–1544.
4. Hirsch MB, Mosher WD. Characteristics of infertile women in the United States and their use of infertility services. Fertil Steril 1987;47:618–625.
5. Tietze C. Reproductive span and rate of reproduction among Hutterite women. Fertil Steril 1957;8:89–95.
6. Federation COS, Swartz D, Mayaux MJ. Female fecundity as a function of age: results of artificial insemination in 2193 nulliparous women with azoospermic husbands. N Engl J Med 1982;306:404–406.
7. Collins JA, Crosignani PG. Unexplained infertility: a review of diagnosis, prognosis, treatment efficacy and management. Int J Gynecol Obstet 1992;39:267–275.
8. Magyar DM, Boyers SP, Marchall JR, et al. Regular menstrual cycles and premenstrual molimina as indicators of ovulation. Obstet Gynecol 1979;53:411–414.
9. Hull MGR, Glazener CMA, Kelly NJ, et al. Population study of causes, treatment and outcome of infertility. BMJ 1985;291:1693–1697.
10. Guttmacher AF. Factors affecting normal expectancy of conception. JAMA 1956;161:855–860.
11. MRC Vitamin Study Research Group. Prevention of neural tube defects: results of the Medical Research Council vitamin study. Lancet 1991;338:131–137.
12. Haddow JE, Palomaki GE, Allan WC, et al. Maternal thyroid deficiency during pregnancy and subsequent neuropsychological development of the child. N Engl J Med 1999;341:549–555.
13. The European Society for Human Reproduction and Embryology (ESHRE) Workshops. Guidelines to the prevalence, diagnosis, treatment and management of infertility, 1996. Hum Reprod 1996;11:1779–1802.
14. Fritz MA, McLachlan RI, Cohen NL, et al. Onset and characteristics of the midcycle surge in bioactive and immunoactive luteinizing periovulatory ovarian steroid hormone secretion. J Clin Endocrinol Metab 1992;75:489–493.
15. Israel R, Mishell DR Jr, Stone SC, et al. Single luteal serum progesterone assay as an indicator of ovulation. Am J Obstet Gynecol 1972;112:1043–1106.
16. Hull MGR, Savage PE, Bromham DR, et al. The value of a single serum progesterone measurement in the midluteal phase as a criterion of a potentially fertile cycle ("ovulation") derived from treated and untreated conception cycles. Fertil Steril 1982;37:355–360.
17. Miller PB, Soules MR. The usefulness of a urinary LH kit for ovulation prediction during menstrual cycles of normal women. Obstet Gynecol 1996;87:13–17.

18. Batzer FR, Corson SL. Indications, techniques, success rates, and pregnancy outcome: new directions with donor insemination. Semin Reprod Endocrinol 1987;5:45–52.
19. Behre HM, Kuhlage J, Gassner C, et al. Prediction of ovulation by urinary hormone measurements with the home use ClearPlan Fertility Monitor: comparison with transvaginal ultrasound scans and serum hormone measurements. Hum Reprod 2000;15:2478–2482.
20. Guermandi E, Vegetti W, Bianchi MM, et al. Reliability of ovulation tests in infertile women. Obstet Gynecol 2001;97:92–96.
21. Nielsen MS, Barton SD, Hatasaka HH, et al. Comparison of several one-step home urinary luteinizing hormone detection test kits to OvuQuick. Fertil Steril 2001;76:384–387.
22. World Health Organization. Temporal relationships between ovulation and defined changes in the concentration of plasma estradiol-17B luteinizing hormone, follicle stimulating hormone and progesterone. I. Probit analysis. Am J Obstet Gynecol 1980;138:383–390.
23. Lundy LE, Lee SG, Levy W, et al. The ovulatory cycle: a histologic, thermal, steroid and gonadotropin correlation. Obstet Gynecol 1974;44(1):14–25.
24. Scott R, Snyder RR, Strickland DM, et al. The effect of interobserver variation in dating endometrial histology on the diagnosis of luteal phase defects. Fertil Steril 1988;50;888–892.
25. Batzer FR. Ultrasonographic indices of ovulation. J Reprod Med 1986;31:764–769.
26. Legro RS, Finegood D, Dunaif A. A fasting glucose to insulin ratio is a useful measure of insulin sensitivity in women with polycystic ovary syndrome. J Clin Endocrinol Metab 1998;83:2694–2698.
27. Balasch J, Miro F, Burzaco J. The role of luteinizing hormone in human follicle development and oocyte fertility: evidence from in-vitro fertilization in a woman with long-standing hypogonadotropic hypogonadism and using recombinant human follicle stimulating hormone. Hum Reprod 1995;10:1678–1683.
28. Rosenfielf RL. Current concepts of polycystic ovary syndrome. Bailleres Clin Obstet Gynaecol 1997;11:335–347.
29. Clark AM, Ledger W, Galletly C, et al. Weight loss results in significant improvement in pregnancy and ovulation rates in anovulatory obese women. Hum Reprod 1995;10:2705–2712.
30. Kerin JF, Lieu JH, Phillipou G, et al. Evidence for a hypothalamic site of action of clomiphene citrate in women. J Clin Endocrinol Metab 1985;61:265–268.
31. Diamanti-Kandarakis E, Kouli C, Tsikanateli T, et al. Therapeutic effects of metformin on insulin resistance and hyperandrogenism in polycystic ovary syndrome. Eur J Endocrinol 1998;138:269–274.
32. Valazquez E, Acosta A, Mendoza SG. Menstrual cyclicity after metformin in polycystic ovary syndrome. Obstet Gynecol 1997;90:392–395.
33. March CM. Ovulation induction. J Reprod Med 1993;38:335–346.
34. O'Herlihy C, Pepperell RJ, Brown JB, et al. Incremental clomiphene therapy: a new method for treating persistent anovulation. Obstet Gynecol 1981;58:535–539.
35. Gysler M, March CM, Mishell DR, et al. A decade's experience with an individualized clomiphene treatment regimen including its effect on the postcoital test. Fertil Steril 1982;37:164–167.
36. Lobo RA, Granger LR, Davajan V, et al. An extended regimen of clomiphene citrate in women unresponsive to standard therapy. Fertil Steril 1982;37:762–766.
37. Dickey RP, Holtkamp DE. Development, pharmacology and clinical experience with clomiphene citrate. Hum Reprod Update 1996;2:483–506.
38. Shoham Z, Zosmer A, Insler V. Early miscarriage and fetal malformations after induction of ovulation (by clomiphene citrate and/or human menopausal gonadotropins), in vitro fertilization, and gamete intrafallopian tube transfer. Fertil Steril 1991;55:1–11.
39. Dickey RP, Taylor SN, Curole DN, et al. Incidence of spontaneous abortion in clomiphene pregnancies. Hum Reprod 1996;11:2623–2628.
40. Nestler JE, Jakubowics DJ, Evans WS, et al. Effects of metformin on spontaneous and clomiphene-induced ovulation in polycystic ovary syndrome. N Engl J Med 1998;338:1876–1880.
41. Tsilchorozidou T, Overton C, Conway G. The pathophysiology of polycystic ovary syndrome. Clin Endocrinol 2004;60:1–17.
42. Kutteh WH. Treating PCOS related infertility with insulin sensitizing agents. OBG Manage 2000;12:106–116.
43. Jakubowicz DJ, Iuorno MJ, Jakubowicz S, et al. Effects of metformin on early pregnancy loss in the polycystic ovary syndrome. J Clin Endocrinol Metab 2002;87:524–529.
44. Glueck CJ, Goldenberg N, Wang P, et al. Metformin during pregnancy reduces insulin, insulin resistance, insulin secretion, weight, testosterone and development of gestational diabetes: prospective longitudinal assessment of women with polycystic ovary syndrome from preconception throughout pregnancy. Hum Reprod 2004;19:510–521.
45. Ghazeeri G, Kutteh WH, Bruer-Ash M, et al. Effect of rosiglitazone on spontaneous and clomiphene citrate-induced ovulation in women with polycystic ovary syndrome. Fertil Steril 2003;79:562–566.
46. Takeuchi S, Futamura N, Takubo S, et al. Polycystic ovary syndrome treated with laparoscopic ovarian drilling with a harmonic scalpel: a prospective, randomized study. J Reprod Med 2002;47:816–820.
47. Daly DC, Walters CA, Soto-Albors CE, et al. A randomized study of dexamethasone in ovulation induction with clomiphene citrate. Fertil Steril 1984;41:844–848.
48. Parsanezhad ME, Alborzi S, Motazedian S, et al. Use of dexamethasone and clomiphene citrate in the treatment of clomiphene citrate-resistant patients with polycystic ovary syndrome and normal dehydroepiandrosterone sulfate levels: a prospective, double-blind, placebo-controlled trial. Fertil Steril 2002;78:1001–1004.

49. Blacker CM. Ovulation stimulation and induction. Endocrinol Metab Clin North Am 1992;21:57–84.
50. Pepperell BJ. A rational approach to ovulation induction. In: Wallach EE, Kempers RD, eds. Modern Trends in Infertility and Conception Control. Vol. 3. Chicago: Year Book Medical, 1985:250–285.
51. Baird DT. Amenorrhoea, anovulation and dysfunctional uterine bleeding. In: Degroot LJ, ed. Endocrinology. London: WB Saunders, 1995:2059–2079.
52. Layman LC, Reindollar RH. The genetics of hypogonadism. Infertil Reprod Med Clin North Am 1994;1:53–68.
53. Matsuzaki T, Azuma K, Irahara M, et al. Mechanism of anovulation in hyperprolactinemic amenorrhea determined by pulsatile gonadotropin-releasing hormone injection combined with human chorionic gonadotropin. Fertil Steril 1994;62:1143–1149.
54. Collins JA, Hughes EG. Pharmacologic interventions for the induction of ovulation. Drugs 1995;50:480–494.
55. Al-Suleiman SA, Najashi S, Rahman J, et al. Outcome of treatment with bromocriptine in patients with hyperprolactinemia. Aust N Z J Obstet Gynecol 1989;29:176–179.
56. Padilla SL, Person GK, McDonough PG, et al. The efficacy of bromocriptine in patients with ovulatory dysfunction and normoprolactinemic galactorrhea. Fertil Steril 1985;44:695–698.
57. Vermesh M, Fossum GT, Lketzky OA. Vaginal bromocriptine: pharmacology and effect on serum prolactin in normal women. Obstet Gynecol 1988;72:693–698.
58. Biller BM. Hyperprolactinemia. Int J Fertil Womens Med 1999;44:74–77.
59. Bahamondes L, Bueno JGR, Hardy E, et al. Identification of main risk factors for tubal infertility. Fertil Steril 1994;61:478–482.
60. Dabekausen YAJM, Evers JLH, Land JA, et al. *Chlamydia trachomatis* antibody testing is more accurate than hysterosalpingography in predicting tubal factor infertility. Fertil Steril 1994;61:833–837.
61. Westrom L. Incidence, prevalence, and trends of acute pelvic inflammatory disease and its consequences in industrialized countries. Am J Obstet Gynecol 1980;138:880–892.
62. Cetin MT, Vardar MA, Aridogan N, et al. Role of *Chlamydia trachomatis* infections in infertility due to tubal factor. Indian J Med Res 1992;95:139–143.
63. Mol BW, Dijkman B, Wertheim P, et al. The accuracy of serum chlamydial antibodies in the diagnosis of tubal pathology: a meta-analysis. Fertil Steril 1997;67:1031–1037.
64. Debekausen Y, Evers J, Land J, et al. *Chlamydia trachomatis* antibody testing is more accurate than hysterosalpingography in predicting tubal factor infertility. Fertil Steril 1994;61:833–837.
65. Spring DB, Boll DA. Prone hysterosalpingography. Radiology 1980;136:235–236.
66. Stumpf PG, March CM. Febrile morbidity following hysterosalpingography: identification of risk factors and recommendations for prophylaxis. Fertil Steril 1980;33:487–492.
67. Pittaway DE, Winfield AC, Maxson W, et al. Prevention of acute pelvic inflammatory disease after hysterosalpingography: efficacy of doxycycline prophylaxis. Am J Obstet Gynecol 1983;147:623–626.
68. Rasmussen F, Lindequist S, Larsen C, et al. Therapeutic effect of hysterosalpingography: oil- versus water-soluble contrast media. A randomized prospective study. Radiology 1991;179:75–78.
69. Schwabe MG, Shapire SS, Haning RV Jr. Hysterosalpingography with oil contrast medium enhances fertility in patients with infertility of unknown etiology. Fertil Steril 1983;40:604–606.
70. Alper MM, Garner PR, Spence EH, et al. Pregnancy rates after hysterosalpingography with oil and water soluble contrast media. Obstet Gynecol 1986;68:6–9.
71. Mackey RA, Glass RH, Olson LE, et al. Pregnancy following hysterosalpingography with oil and water soluble dye. Fertil Steril 1971;22:504–507.
72. Krynicki E, Kaminski P, Szymanski R, et al. Comparison of hysterosalpingography with laparoscopy and chromopertubation J Am Assoc Gynecol Laparosc 1996;3(suppl):S22–S23.
73. Raziel A, Arieli S, Bukovsky I, et al. Investigation of the uterine cavity in recurrent aborters. Fertil Steril 1994;62:1080–1083.
74. Hull MGR, Savage PE, Bromham DR. Prognostic value of the postcoital test: prospective study based on time-specific conception rates. Br J Obstet Gynaecol 1982;89:299–305.
75. Eimers JM, te Velde ER, Gerritse R, et al. The validity of the postcoital test for estimating the probability of conceiving. Am J Obstet Gynecol 1994;171:65–70.
76. Griffith CS, Grimes DA. The validity of the postcoital test. Am J Obstet Gynecol 1990;62:615–620.
77. Collins JA, So Y, Wilson EH, et al. The postcoital test as a predictor of pregnancy among 355 infertile couples. Fertil Steril 1984;41:703–708.
78. Nagele F, O'Connor H, Daview A, et al. 2500 outpatient diagnostic hysteroscopies. Obstet Gynecol 1996,88:87–92.
79. Hutchins CJ. Laparoscopy and hysterosalpingography in the assessment of tubal patency. Obstet Gynecol 1977;49:325–327.
80. Rubin RD, Hurst BS, Schlaff WE. Predictive value of fluid contrast ultrasound (sonohysterography) in diagnosis of intrauterine lesions. Poster, American Society for Reproductive Medicine, University of Colorado Health Sciences Center, Denver, Co, 1996, P–121.
81. Ayida G, Chamberlain P, Barlow D, et al. Uterine cavity assessment prior to in vitro fertilization: comparison of transvaginal scanning, saline contrast, hysterosonography and hysteroscopy. Ultrasound Obstet Gynecol 1997;10:59–62.
82. Benadiva CA, Kligman I, David O, et al. In vitro fertilization versus tubal surgery: is pelvic reconstructive surgery obsolete? Fertil Steril 1995;64:1051–1061.

83. Musich JR, Behrman SJ. Surgical management of tubal obstruction of the uterotubal junction. Fertil Steril 1983;40:423–441.
84. Risquez F, Confino E. Transcervical tubal cannulation, past, present, and future. Fertil Steril 1993;60:211–226.
85. Das K, Nagel TC, Malo JW. Hysteroscopic cannulation for proximal tubal obstruction: a change for the better. Fertil Steril 1995;63:1009–1015.
86. Honore GM, Holden AE, Schenken RS. Pathophysiology and management of proximal tubal blockage. Fertil Steril 1999;71:785–795.
87. Schlaff WD, Hassiakos DK, Damewood MD, et al. Neosalpingostomy for distal tubal obstruction: prognostic factor and impact of surgical technique. Fertil Steril 1990;54:984–990.
88. Donnez J, Casanas-Roux F. Prognostic factors of fimbrial microsurgery. Fertil Steril 1986;46:1089–1092.
89. Dlugi AM, Reddy S, Saleh WA, et al. Pregnancy rates after operative endoscopic treatment of total (neosalpingostomy) or near total (salpingostomy) distal tubal occlusion. Fertil Steril 1994;62:913–920.
90. The American Fertility Society. The American Fertility Society classification of adnexal adhesions, distal tubal occlusion, tubal occlusion secondary to tubal ligation, tubal pregnancies, Müllerian anomalies and intrauterine adhesions. Fertil Steril 1988;49:944–955.
91. Rock JA, Katayama P, Martin EJ, et al. Factors influencing the success of salpingostomy techniques for distal fimbrial obstruction. Obstet Gynecol 1978;52:591–596.
92. Holst N, Maltau JM, Forsdahl F, et al. Handling of tubal infertility after introduction of in vitro fertilization: changes and consequences. Fertil Steril 1991;55:140–143.
93. Society for Assisted Reproductive Technology, American Society for Reproductive Medicine. Assisted reproductive technology in the United States and Canada: 1993 results generated from the ASRM/ART Registry. Fertil Steril 1995;64:13–21.
94. Hughes EG, Fedorkow DM, Collins JA. A quantitative overview of controlled trials in endometriosis-associated infertility. Fertil Steril 1993;59:963–970.
95. Marcoux S, Maheux R, Berube S, et al. Laparoscopic surgery in infertile women with minimal or mild endometriosis. N Engl J Med 1997;337:217–222.
96. Farrer-Brown G, Beilby JOW, Tarbit MH. Venous changes in the endometrium of myomatous uteri. Obstet Gynecol 1971;38:743–751.
97. Deligdish L, Lowenthal M. Endometrial changes associated with myomata of the uterus. J Clin Pathol 1970;23:676–680.
98. Buttram VC Jr. Uterine leiomyomata-aetiology, symptomatology and management. Prog Clin Biol Res 1986;225:275–296.
99. Sudik R, Husch K, Steller J, et al. Fertility and pregnancy outcome after myomectomy in sterility patients. Eur J Obstet Gynecol Reprod Biol 1996;65:209–214.
100. Valle RF, Sciarra JJ. Intrauterine adhesions: hysteroscopic diagnosis, classification, treatment, and reproductive outcome. Am J Obstet Gynecol 1988;158:1459–1470.
101. Spirtos NJ, Yruewicz EC, Moghisi KS, et al. Pseudocorpus luteum insufficiency: a study of cytosol progesterone receptors in human endometrium. Obstet Gynecol 1985;65:535–540.
102. Li TC, Dockery P, Rogers AW, et al. How precise is histologic dating of endometrium using the standard dating criteria? Fertil Steril 1989;51:759–763.
103. Goldstein P, Berrier J, Rosen S, et al. A meta-analysis of randomized controlled trials of progestational agents in pregnancy. Br J Obstet Gynaecol 1989;96:265–274.
104. Soliman S, Daya S, Collins J, et al. The role of luteal phase support in infertility treatment: a meta-analysis of randomized trials. Fertil Steril 1994;61:1068–1076.
105. Bristow RE, Karlan BY. Ovulation induction, infertility and ovarian cancer risk. Fertil Steril 1996;66:499–507.
106. Pearlstone AC, Fournet N, Gambone JG, et al. Ovulation induction in women age 40 and older: the importance of basal follicle stimulating hormone level and chronological age. Fertil Steril 1992;58:674–679.
107. Scott RT, Leonardi MR, Hofmann GE, et al. A prospective evaluation of clomiphene citrate challenge test screening of the general infertility population. Obstet Gynecol 1993;82:539–544.
108. Scott RT Jr, Hofmann GE, Oehninger S, et al. Intercycle variability of day 3 follicle stimulating hormone level and its effect on stimulation quality in in vitro fertilization. Fertil Steril 1990;54:297–302.
109. Martin JS, Nisker JA, Tummon IS, et al. Future in vitro fertilization pregnancy potential of women with variably elevated-day 3 follicle stimulating hormone levels. Fertil Steril 1996;65:1238–1240.
110. World Health Organization. Laboratory Manual for the Examination of Human Semen and Sperm-Cervical Mucus Interaction. 3rd ed. Cambridge: Cambridge University Press, 1992:44–45.
111. Goldenberg RL, White R. The effect of vaginal lubricants on sperm motility in vitro. Fertil Steril 1975;26: 872–873.
112. Fisch H, Lipshultz LI. Diagnosing male factors of infertility. Arch Pathol Lab Med 1992;116:398–405.
113. Matilsky M, Battino S, Ben-Ami M, et al. The effect of ejaculatory frequency on semen characteristics of normospermic and oligospermic men from an infertile population. Hum Reprod 1993;8:71–73.
114. Mahadevan MM, Trounson AOL. The influence of seminal characteristics on the success rate of human in vitro fertilization. Fertil Steril 1984;42:400–405.
115. Bartoov B, Eltes F, Pansky M, et al. Estimating fertility potential via semen analysis data. Hum Reprod 1993;8:65–70.
116. Huang HY, Lee C, Lai Y, et al. The impact of the total motile sperm count on the success of intrauterine insemination with husbands spermatozoa. J Assist Reprod Genet 1996;13:56–63.

117. Adeghe JA. Male subfertility due to sperm antibodies: a clinical overview. Obstet Gynecol Surv 1992;48:481–488.
118. Lahteenmaki A, Veilahti J, Hovatta O. Intrauterine insemination versus cyclic low dose prednisolone in couples with male antisperm antibodies. Hum Reprod 1995;10:142–147.
119. Nachtigall LB, Boepple PA, Pralong FP, et al. Adult onset idiopathic hypogonadotropic—a treatable form of male infertility. N Engl J Med 1997;336:410–405.
120. O'Donovan PA, Vandkerckhove P, Lilford RJ, et al. Treatment of male infertility: is it effective? Review and meta-analysis of published randomized controlled trials. Hum Reprod 1993;8:1209–1222.
121. Gorelick JI, Goldstein M. Loss of fertility in men with varicocele. Fertil Steril 1993;59:613–616.
122. Laven JSE, Haans LCF, Mali W, et al. Effects of varicocele treatment in adolescents: a randomized study. Fertil Steril 1992;58:756–762.
123. Marks JL, McMahon R, Lipshultz LI. Predictive parameters of successful varicocele repair. J Urol 1986;136:609–612.
124. Madgar I, Weissenberg R, Lunenfeld B, et al. Controlled trial of high spermatic vein ligation for varicocele in infertile men. Fertil Steril 1995;63:120–124.
125. Schlesinger MH, Wilets IF, Nager HM. Treatment outcome after varicocelectomy: a critical analysis. Urol Clin North Am 1994;21:517–529.
126. Hargreave TB. Debate on the pros and cons of varicocele treatment: in favor of varicocele treatment. Hum Reprod 1995;10(suppl):151–157.
127. Gregoriou O, Vitoratos N, Papadias C, et al. Pregnancy rates in gonadotrophin stimulated cycles with timed intercourse or intrauterine insemination for the treatment of male subfertility. Eur J Obstet Gynecol Reprod Biol 1996;64:213–216.
128. Melis GB, Pauletti AM, Ajossa S, et al. Ovulation induction with gonadotropins as sole treatment in infertile couples with open tubes: a randomized prospective comparison between intrauterine insemination and timed vaginal intercourse. Fertil Steril 1995;64:1088–1093.
129. U.S. Department of Health and Human Services, Center for Disease Control and Prevention (CDC). 2001 Assisted Reproductive Technology Success Rates. National Summary and Fertility Clinic Reports. Atlanta, Ga: CDC, December 2003. Available at: www.cdc.gov/reproductivehealth/. Accessed July 26, 2005.
130. Shenfiel F, Doyle P, Valentine A, et al. Effects of age, gravidity and male infertility status on cumulative conception rates following artificial insemination with cryopreserved donor sperm: analysis of 2998 cycles of treatment in one center over 10 years. Hum Reprod 1993;8:60–64.
131. Lobo RA. Unexplained infertility. J Reprod Med 1993;38:241–249.
132. Crosignani PG, Collins J, Cooke ID, et al. Unexplained infertility. Hum Reprod 1993;8:977–980.
133. Scott RT, Leonardi MR, Hofmann GE, et al. A prospective evaluation of clomiphene citrate challenge test screening of the general infertility population. Obstet Gynecol 1993;82:539–544.
134. Glazener CMA, Coulson C, Lambert PA, et al. Clomiphene treatment for women with unexplained infertility: placebo-controlled study of hormonal responses and conception rates. Gynecol Endocrinol 1990;4: 75–83.
135. Deaton JL, Gibson M, Blackmer KM, et al. A randomized, controlled trial of clomiphene citrate and intrauterine insemination in couples with unexplained infertility or surgically corrected endometriosis. Fertil Steril 1990;54:1083–1088.
136. Dodson WC, Whitesides DB, Huges CL Jr, et al. Superovulation with intrauterine insemination in the treatment of infertility: a possible alternative to gamete intrafallopian transfer and in vitro fertilization. Fertil Steril 1987;48:441–445.
137. Kim CH, Cho YK, Mok JE. The efficacy of immunotherapy in patients who underwent superovulation with intrauterine insemination. Fertil Steril 1996;65:133–138.
138. Berry CW, Brambati B, Eskes TKAB, et al. The Euro-Team Pregnancy Protocol (ETPP) for recurrent miscarriage. Hum Reprod 1995;10:1516–1520.
139. Wilcox AJ, Weinberg CR, O'Connor JF, et al. Incidence of early loss of pregnancy. N Engl J Med 1988;319:189–194.
140. Regan L, Braude PR, Trembath PL. Influence of past reproductive performance on risk of spontaneous abortion. Br Med J 1989;299:541–545.
141. Mishell DR. Recurrent abortion. J Reprod Med 1993;38:250–259.
142. Poland BJ, Miller JR, Jones DC, et al. Reproductive counseling in patients who have had a spontaneous abortion. Am J Obstet Gynecol 1977;127:685–691.
143. James WH. On the possibility of segregation in the propensity to spontaneous abortion in the human female. Ann Hum Genet 1961;25:207–210.
144. McDonough PG. Repeated first-trimester loss: evaluation and management. Am J Obstet Gynecol 1985;153:1–6.
145. Boue J, Boue A, Lazar P. Retrospective and prospective epidemiological studies of 1500 karyotyped spontaneous human abortions. Teratology 1975;12:11–26.
146. De Braekeleer M, Dao TN. Cytogenetic studies in couples experiencing repeated pregnancy losses. Hum Reprod 1990;5:519–528.
147. Guerro R, Rojas OI. Spontaneous abortion and aging of human ova and spermatozoa. N Engl J Med 1975;293:573–575.
148. Levran D, Ben-Schlomo I, Dor J, et al. Aging of endometrium and oocytes: observations on conception and abortion in an egg donation model. Fertil Steril 1991;56:1092–1094.

149. Check JH, Askari HA, Fisher C, et al. The use of a shared donor oocyte program to evaluate the effect of uterine senescence. Fertil Steril 1994;61:252–256.
150. Heinonen PK, Saarikoski S, Pystynen P. Reproductive performance of women with uterine anomalies. Acta Obstet Gynecol Scand 1982;61:157–162.
151. Buttram VC, Gibbons WE. Müllerian anomalies: a proposed classification (an analysis of 144 cases). Fertil Steril 1979;32:40–46.
152. Fedele L, Arcaini L, Parazzini F, et al. Reproductive prognosis after hysteroscopic metroplasty in 102 women: life table analysis. Fertil Steril 1993;59:768–772.
153. Buttram VC, Reiter RC. Uterine leiomyomata: etiology, symptomatology, and management. Fertil Steril 1981;36:433–435.
154. Valle RF, Sciarra JJ. Intrauterine adhesions: hysteroscopic diagnosis, classification, treatment and reproductive outcome. Am J Obstet Gynecol 1988;158:1459–1470.
155. March CM, Israel R. Intrauterine adhesions secondary to elective abortion: hysteroscopic diagnosis and management. Obstet Gynecol 1976;48:422–424.
156. Goldstein P, Berrier J, Rosen S, et al. A meta-analysis of randomized control trials of progestational agents in pregnancy. Br J Obstet Gynecol 1989;96:265–274.
157. Friedler S, Raziel A, Schachter M, et al. Luteal support with micronized progesterone following in-vitro fertilization using a down-regulation protocol with gonadotrophin-releasing hormone agonist: a comparative study between vaginal and oral administration. Hum Reprod 1999;14:1944–1948.
158. Montoro M, Collea JV, Frasier SD, et al. Successful outcome of pregnancy in women with hypothyroidism. Ann Intern Med 1981;94:31–34.
159. Okon MA, Laird SM, Tuckerman EM, et al. Serum androgen levels in women who have recurrent miscarriages and their correlation with markers of endometrial function. Fertil Steril 1998;69:682–690.
160. Rai R, Backos M, Rushworth F, et al. Polycystic ovaries and recurrent miscarriage—a reappraisal. Human Reprod 2000;15:612–615.
161. Wilson WA, Gharavi AE, Kolke T. International consensus statement on preliminary classification criteria for definite antiphospholipid syndrome: report of an internal workshop. Arthritis Rheum 1999;42:1309–1311.
162. Regan L, Rai R. Thrombophilia and pregnancy loss. J Reprod Immunol 2002;55:163–180.
163. Blumenfeld Z, Brenner B. Thrombophilia-associated pregnancy wastage. Fertil Steril 1999;72:765–774.
164. Empson M, Lassere M, Craig JC, et al. Recurrent pregnancy loss with antiphospholipid antibody: a systematic review of therapeutic trials. Obstet Gynecol 2002;99:135–144.
165. Furquharson RG, Quenby S, Greaves M. Antiphospholipid syndrome in pregnancy: a randomized, controlled trial of treatment. Obstet Gynecol 2002;100:408–413.
166. Kline J, Stein ZA, Susser M, et al. Smoking: a risk factor for spontaneous abortion. N Engl J Med 1977;297:793–796.
167. Stray-Pedersen B, Stray-Pedersen S. Etiologic factors and subsequent reproductive performance in 195 couples with a prior history of habitual abortion. Am J Obstet Gynecol 1984;148:140–146.

CHAPTER 17

Surgical and Medical Abortion

Mitchell D. Creinin

INTRODUCTION

Abortion can be accomplished by surgical or medical techniques in an office setting (Table 17.1). The phrase *medical abortion* refers to early abortion (usually before 9 weeks' gestation) (1), not for medically induced second-trimester terminations, which are referred to as *labor induction abortion*. Medical abortion allows a woman to have a safe, effective abortion without an invasive surgical procedure. Whereas medical abortion is obviously an outpatient process, the location at which various providers perform surgical abortion services varies by geographic location and gestational age. Most surgical abortions (95% in 2000) are provided in an office or clinic setting (2). Approximately 20% of abortion providers perform surgical abortions in their private office (2). Most women receive services during a single visit. Physicians who provide abortion as part of their routine practice, including those who provide services in a clinic setting, generally have very low complication rates. Such providers tend to be very experienced, were trained in residency, and perform procedures in this setting on patients who are generally healthy (3). Paradoxically, abortions performed in hospitals have higher complication rates than do clinic abortions, in part because of higher-risk patients, residents in training, and less experienced surgeons (4).

In 2000, more than half of abortions (58%) were obtained at 8 weeks' gestation or less, and 88% were performed before 13 weeks (5). Suction curettage (also called vacuum aspiration) accounted for nearly all abortions. Medical abortions, according to the Centers for Disease Control and Prevention (CDC), accounted for approximately 1% of all abortions. Access to abortion services remains a problem in the United States. Abortion providers cluster in metropolitan areas. About one-third of women of reproductive age live in the 87% of U.S. counties without an abortion provider (2). Among the nation's 276 metropolitan areas, 86 have no providers (2). About one-fourth of women have to travel 50 miles or more to reach a clinic (6); this geographic barrier hinders both service provision (7) and follow-up in the event of complications.

UNDERSTANDING ABORTION PROVISION

Preabortion counseling is an important part of both medical and surgical abortion care. Patient counseling must first stress early pregnancy options to ensure a woman is certain about her decision to have an abortion. Preprocedural counseling, including appropriate screening, counseling, and support, may assume a larger role for medical abortion because the patient is a more active participant in the abortion process. If the woman is less than 9 weeks' gestation, a medical abortion is an option. However, medical abortion is not a means to make abortion an easier decision for a woman uncertain about whether to continue the pregnancy. If she is uncertain, then the decision about abortion technique must be delayed until she has reached a firm decision, even if the delay means that she will be unable to choose a medical option.

TABLE 17.1

Comparative Features of Medical and Surgical Abortion

Medical Abortion
- Usually avoids invasive procedure
- Requires two or more visits
- Days to weeks to complete
- Available during early pregnancy
- High success rate (95%)
- Requires follow-up to ensure completion of abortion
- Patient participation throughout a multiple-step process
- Usually avoids anesthesia

Surgical abortion
- Involves invasive procedure
- Usually requires one visit
- Complete in a predictable period of time
- Available during early pregnancy
- High success rate (99%)
- Does not require follow-up in all cases
- Patient participation in a single-step procedure
- Allows use of sedation if desired

Adapted from Breitbart V. Counseling for medical abortion. Am J Obstet Gynecol 2000;183:S26–S33.

Once a woman is sure she wants an abortion, counseling can then focus on the methodologic options; this discussion needs to include the risks, benefits, and side effects of the options available to her. Providing this information is necessary for the woman to give informed consent for the procedure. It is important to emphasize the necessity of follow-up and number of visits for a medical abortion. When discussing medical abortion, it is important to discuss issues of bleeding, cramping, and length of time to complete the abortion. Bleeding will be much heavier than with menses (and potentially with severe cramping) and is best described to patients as comparable to a miscarriage. Even more important, it must be emphasized that medical abortion, regardless of the regimen, does not work as well as early surgical abortion, which has a failure rate (reaspiration) ranging from less than 1% (8) to around 2% (9). Regardless of the abortion method chosen, the counselor and physician must comply with all local and federal regulations.

Provision of abortion, regardless of method, requires accurate assessment of gestational age. In a 1997 survey of provider members of the National Abortion Federation, 66% of clinics routinely use ultrasound to confirm gestational age prior to surgical abortion (10). The remaining providers perform a pelvic examination and use ultrasound examination only when clinically indicated. For medical abortion, pretreatment vaginal ultrasonography is the standard of care in the United States, which is quite different than the practice in France, where only about 30% of patients have ultrasound scanning for any reason (11). The French use ultrasound examination only during preabortion screening when pelvic examination reveals a discrepancy between uterine size and dating by last menstrual period, or when a patient presents with bleeding or symptoms suggestive of ectopic pregnancy.

In contrast to surgical abortion, medical abortion is typically considered a "failure" when a surgical evacuation is performed to complete the abortion for any reason, including incomplete abortion, continuing (viable) pregnancy, hemorrhage, or patient request (12). However, surgical abortion is only a "failure" if a continuing pregnancy occurs; if a repeat aspiration is required for an incomplete abortion or hematometra, these are considered complications, not method failure. Given these definitions of "failure," depending on the gestational age and treatment regimen, medical abortion has lower overall efficacy than surgical abortion. Still, the ability to terminate a pregnancy without surgery is an important alternative early in pregnancy when the patient wants to avoid a surgical procedure, does not have access to a provider for a surgical abortion, or has limited access to a clinician trained in early surgical abortion.

Women who have decided to terminate their pregnancy tend to be happy with their choice of method, either medical or surgical, when they are given the opportunity to make their own choice (13). The most common reason a woman wants to have a medical abortion is because of a desire to avoid some aspect of a surgical procedure (13–16). Thus, one would expect acceptability studies to have positive results—that is, because the study participants were actively seeking an alternative to surgical abortion, they were likely to be happy with their choice. Accordingly, mifepristone regimens would be preferred for a next abortion by 80 to 96% of women overall (16, 17).

Randomized trials of acceptability are only helpful for counseling women who are truly unsure whether they prefer to have a medical or surgical abortion. Henshaw et al. (13) randomized women at or less than 63 days' gestation who had no preference as to the method of their abortion to aspiration under general anesthesia ($n = 96$) versus mifepristone 600 mg followed 48 hours later by misoprostol 400 mcg orally ($n = 99$). Almost all (98%) women who had a surgical abortion would opt for the same procedure in the future as compared with 78% of those having a medical abortion. However, the issue of acceptability of the medical abortion procedure appeared to have been limited to those women at more than 49 days' gestation; 20 of the 21 women who would choose surgical abortion were at more than 49 days' gestation. Because the medical abortion regimen used in this study is one that is not clinically used beyond 49 days' gestation (18), these findings only confirm that women with no preference tend to be happy with either method early in pregnancy. Interestingly, Creinin (19) randomized 50 women at or less than 49 days' gestation to medical or surgical abortion. The surgical abortion method was manual vacuum aspiration with local anesthesia in the office. The medical abortion regimen was methotrexate 50 mg/m^2 intramuscular followed 5 to 6 days later with misoprostol 800 mcg vaginally. The misoprostol was self-administered at home and was repeated 1 to 2 days later, if needed. Of the women randomized to a surgical abortion, 92% (95% CI 81%, 100%) stated they would choose a surgical for a next abortion, whereas only 63% (95% CI 43%, 82%) of women randomized to a medical abortion would choose that option in the future ($p < 0.001$).

SURGICAL ABORTION

Background

Most abortions performed today use suction aspiration, a technique introduced into the United States during the late 1960s. When abortion was legalized in the United States, a significant proportion of procedures were still performed with sharp curettage. By 1976, the proportion of procedures performed by sharp curettage had dropped to 10% and has remained in the 2 to 3% range since 1989 (5). Suction aspiration procedures can safely be performed until around 14 to 15 weeks' gestation. Procedures after 15 weeks are generally performed by dilation and evacuation procedure. The discussion that follows focuses solely on the use of surgical abortion techniques using suction aspiration.

Instruments Necessary for Provision of Surgical Abortion

Suction curettage, the predominant procedure performed for early surgical abortion, does not require a special room other than what clinicians already have available in their general gynecologic office practice. As with any gynecologic examination, an examination table with stirrups and good lighting is necessary. Surgical equipment includes a speculum, swabs for cleansing the vagina and cervix, needle and syringe for application of cervical anesthesia, cervical tenaculum, rigid dilators, uterine curette, and a suction source. Although most of these instruments are readily available in any gynecologist's office, slight modifications can help make the procedure easier for the surgeon and the patient.

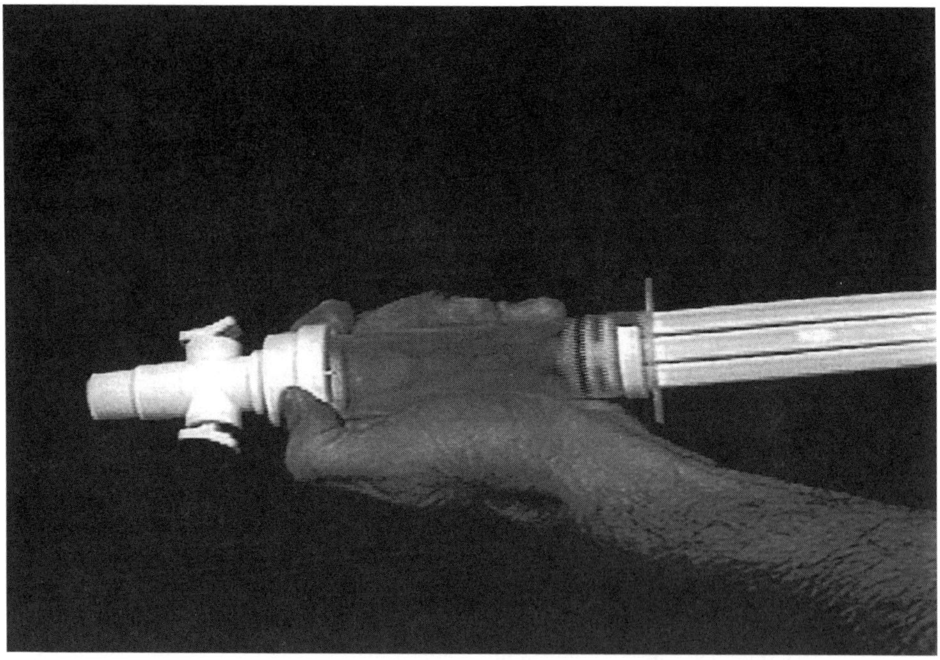

FIGURE 17.1 ● Manual vacuum aspiration syringe (IPAS, Carrboro, NC).

- Speculum: Many experienced providers find that a snub-nose or Moore-Graves style speculum makes the procedure easier. This speculum is shorter and allows the cervix to be pulled down without meeting resistance from the speculum blades high in the vagina. The angle between the cervix and uterine body can be straightened more, easing the ability to dilate the cervix. Theoretically, this could also reduce the risk of perforation.
- Tenaculum: Although most clinicians are accustomed to a toothed tenaculum, tenacula with blunt teeth, called atraumatic or Bierer tenacula, are less likely to tear through the cervix when excessive traction is applied. Rather, these tenacula will slip off without lacerating the cervix. As one would expect, with experience, a surgeon will find that slippage of the atraumatic tenaculum is relatively rare.
- Suction source: Electrical vacuum has been the mainstay of uterine aspiration for decades. Although initially popular, manual vacuum aspiration became rarely used as the 1970s advanced. With advances in design and renewed interest in early surgical abortion, the manual vacuum aspiration procedure has garnered renewed interest (20). Although multiple studies have shown no benefit to patient satisfaction or procedure outcome (21, 22), manual vacuum aspiration is inexpensive and allows the general gynecologist to have an inexpensive, easy-to-use source of suction. Both vacuum methods provide 55 to 60 mmHg negative pressure. The 60-cc manual vacuum syringe (Fig. 17.1) will begin to lose this pressure when it is about 80% filled. For procedures beyond 7 weeks, more than one pass with the manual vacuum syringe is commonly required. In such circumstances, either multiple syringes can be used, one after the other, or a single syringe that is emptied and reloaded for each pass can be used.

An hour or two prior to the procedure, most patients are given preoperative prostaglandin synthetase inhibitors to decrease uterine cramping and augment pain relief (23, 24). Administration of prophylactic antibiotics is widely used by providers (10), although the general benefit of such a practice is still in question. Although a single meta-analysis (25) has implied that generalized prophylaxis is cost beneficial, the evaluation included studies using multiple, different antibiotic regimens and many protocols that actually involved treatment and not simply prophylaxis.

Overview of Surgical Abortion Technique Using Suction Aspiration

The technique of surgical abortion involves insertion of the speculum followed by antiseptic preparation of the operative field. The operative field is the entire area inside the speculum. Cleansing with iodine or a comparable antiseptic solution only needs to be performed of the vagina and cervix (i.e., the area inside the speculum). Microbiological studies demonstrate that 99% of bacteria are killed within 5 minutes after vaginal application of iodine or chlorhexidine (26). Interestingly, a small but underpowered study by Lundh et al. (27) found that cleansing with chlorhexidine digluconate prior to cervical dilation did not decrease the incidence of a diagnosis of postabortal infection.

Nuances of surgical technique will vary from provider to provider. However, the overall concepts of what procedures need to be performed to complete the surgical abortion are the same. After the speculum is placed and the operative field cleansed, local anesthetic is commonly applied, either in a paracervical or intracervical fashion. Local anesthesia is the most common approach to pain control. In a more recent survey of providers, 58% used paracervical block with or without oral premedication, 32% combined paracervical block with intravenous sedation, and 10% used general anesthesia (10). Local anesthesia is both safer and less expensive than general anesthesia, although pain relief is not complete. Data as to the actual benefit of local anesthesia for women receiving procedures without intravenous sedation or general anesthesia are conflicting (28–30). Most women have discomfort similar to bad menstrual cramps during the operation with local anesthesia alone. The cramping typically resolves soon after the operation is finished, and most women feel cramping similar to that of a menstrual period by the time of discharge.

Cervical dilation is most commonly performed using graduated metal or plastic dilators. In more recent years, use of misoprostol, a prostaglandin E_1 derivative, to soften and open the cervix prior to the abortion has grown in popularity. Administration of misoprostol may be done orally, vaginally, or sublingually (31–35). However, use of misoprostol may result in side effects for the patient. No large trials have been performed to demonstrate whether provision of misoprostol prior to a suction aspiration abortion, as compared with rigid dilation, results in lower rates of complication or improves patient acceptability of the procedure.

After cervical dilation is accomplished, a plastic cannula is introduced into the uterine cavity and connected to the suction source to perform the abortion. Cannulas range in size from 4 to 16 mm in diameter and come in rigid and flexible forms. Preferences for cannula type and size for an individual procedure will vary based on the surgeon's preferences, level of experience, and patient characteristics. Typically, a cannula size in millimeters equal to the gestational age in weeks can safely and quickly evacuate the uterine contents using suction aspiration. However, an experienced provider can, when necessary, easily empty the uterus with a cannula that is 1 or 2 mm smaller in diameter if dilation be less than ideally desired.

The source of vacuum is commonly an electrical pump or a handheld syringe. Typical overall procedure time is usually less than 5 minutes. Standard practice is for the physician to inspect the aspirated tissue for the presence of chorionic villi and a gestational sac. A gestational sac at 4 weeks approximates the size of a large pea, at 6 weeks it is similar in size to a dime, and at 8 weeks it is about the size of a quarter. Use of a magnifying glass, microscope, or even a colposcope may facilitate identification of the gestational sac and villi. Identifying the gestational sac is important to ensure an inadvertent chorionic villus sampling did not occur in lieu of an abortion. If the gestational age is 9 weeks or greater, fetal tissue should be easily identifiable. Formal pathology examination of the products of conception is medically unnecessary (36). Typically, the woman is monitored after the abortion in a recovery area for about 30 minutes. Before discharge, a woman who is Rh negative should receive Rh immunoglobulin. All women should receive information about warning signs of possible postabortion complications and emergency contact numbers should these occur, as well as contraceptive information and/or a contraceptive method in hand. Many women resume their usual activities the same day as the abortion, although some prefer to wait another day before returning to work or school.

Common practice has included a follow-up visit that is usually scheduled in 2 or 3 weeks following the procedure. Typically, contraceptive issues are further discussed, and the patient is examined to ensure no complications have occurred. However, evidence supporting the benefit of this visit is lacking, and only about half of the women opt to return (37). A pelvic examination is unnecessary for an asymptomatic woman. Likewise, no laboratory tests are indicated. Most important, full contraceptive counseling should have been accomplished at the time of the procedure. Hence, a "routine follow-up examination" after a surgical abortion is not warranted for all women.

Complications of Suction Abortion

In countries where abortion is legal, accessible, and performed in correct medical settings, complication rates are extremely low. One of the largest evaluations of complications in early surgical abortion was reported from three clinics specializing in abortion services in New York City. Minor complications were experienced by 0.846% of patients, and 0.071% required hospitalization (3). Suction abortion-related complications are increased in women with a history of a prior abortion (RR = 1.6) or multiparity (RR = 1.3); however, the attributable risk for such women is still relatively small (38).

Large series of outpatient procedures by experienced clinicians document that mild infection and reaspiration are the most common complications (Table 17.2) (3, 39). Treatment of infection can typically be performed on an outpatient basis unless evidence of sepsis is present. Significant bleeding from a suction abortion is rare and is most commonly the result of uterine atony. Oxytocics such as methylergonivine or prostaglandin analogs (15-methyl $F_{2\alpha}$ or misoprostol) are effective treatments; oxytocin receptors are not present in the uterus in sufficient quantity for oxytocin to be effective during early gestation. If bleeding persists, incomplete evacuation, cervical injury, or uterine perforation should be suspected.

Uterine perforation, though, is more commonly a complication that is recognized by the surgeon during the procedure when the instruments in the uterus do not meet the resistance of the uterine wall. Typically, experienced surgeons can still complete a suction abortion when a perforation occurs. Often, ultrasound guidance can assist with the completion of the procedure. Women often quickly recover because most perforations are midline and rarely cause significant bleeding. As long as the patient remains clinically stable, hospitalization or other surgical procedures (e.g., laparoscopy) are not indicated. If a significant perforation occurs requiring surgical intervention, hysterectomy is rarely necessary.

TABLE 17.2

Rate of Complications of Early Surgical Abortion

Minor Complications	
Mild infection	1:216 (0.005%)
Reaspiration	1:575 (0.002%)
Amenorrhea from cervical stenosis	1:6071 (0.0002%)
Cervical laceration requiring repair	1:9444 (0.0001%)
Seizure	1:25,086 (0.00004%)
Major Complications [a]	
Incomplete abortion	1:3617 (0.0003%)
Sepsis	1:4722 (0.0002%)
Uterine perforation	1:10,625 (0.00009%)
Uterine bleeding	1:14,166 (0.00007%)
Incomplete evacuation	1:28,333 (0.00003%)
Heterotopic pregnancy	1:42,500 (0.00002%)

[a] Implies hospitalization required due to complication.

Adapted from Hakim-Elahi E, Tovell HM, Burnhill MS. Complications of first-trimester abortion: a report of 170,000 cases. Obstet Gynecol 1990;76:129–135, with permission.

A complication unique to suction abortion is hematometra, or "clots in the uterus." This infrequent problem is a result of small tears in the cervical canal that result during the dilation process. A clot forms over the tear that is adherent to the cervical canal and blocks the normal egress of blood from the uterine cavity after the procedure. With acute hematometra, patients will most commonly complain of no bleeding and severe lower abdominal or rectal pressure. On examination, the uterus is enlarged, boggy and tender, and often bigger in size than before the procedure. Simple dilation to allow blood to flow or aspiration to remove the clots will resolve the problem. Routine use of methylergonivine to reduce this complication (or prevent atony) is of no benefit (40). Many providers add a small amount of vasopressin (1 or 2 U) with the cervical anesthetic based on anecdotal reports of decreased problems with hematometra; however, no studies have been published to prove the benefit of this treatment with suction aspiration procedures.

MEDICAL ABORTION

Background

Medical abortion is a relatively new technology. In Europe and China, a clinically useful medical alternative to surgical abortion has been present since 1988. Mifepristone in combination with a prostaglandin analog has been used in France, Sweden, the United Kingdom, and China by more than 3 million women for abortion up to 63 days' gestation. Beginning in late 1998, many other European countries approved mifepristone for sale and use, followed in September 2001 by the United States. In the remainder of the world, the combination of mifepristone and a prostaglandin analog are not available because of political and economic restrictions on access to mifepristone. As such, alternative regimens such as methotrexate and misoprostol or misoprostol alone have been developed, which have similar, although slightly lower, efficacy (41, 42).

Although the idea of using medications to induce menses or cause abortion dates back centuries, medically proven regimens have only been found in the last 50 years. In 1950, the folic acid antagonist 4-aminopteroylglutamic acid (Aminopterin) was shown to induce embryonic demise and resorption in mice and rats during the first week of gestation (43). In the 1970s, natural prostaglandins such as PGE_2 and $PGF_{2\alpha}$ were found to be very effective at inducing abortion early in pregnancy when administered vaginally (44). However, use of these medications in regimens that resulted in high efficacy caused intolerable nausea, vomiting, diarrhea, fever, and pain, necessitating premedication with analgesic, sedative, antiemetic, and antidiarrheal medications (45). Prostaglandin analogs were developed in the mid-1970s and 1980s with more selective action on the myometrium so lower doses could be used to effect abortion; gastrointestinal side effects were not as severe but still occurred with high frequency, limiting the clinical utility of these agents (46, 47).

Mifepristone, a progesterone receptor modulator, was developed by accident by investigators working on compounds to block glucocorticoid receptors. Mifepristone is a derivative of norethindrone that binds to the progesterone receptor with an affinity greater than progesterone itself (48, 49), without activating the receptor. During early pregnancy, mifepristone induces decidual necrosis that decreases hCG secretion; these events lead to subsequent detachment of the products of conception from the uterus and bleeding. Mifepristone effects endometrial blood vessels, increases prostaglandin release, and sensitizes the uterus and cervix to the effects of prostaglandins (e.g., induction of uterine contractions, cervical softening, and dilation) (50–52).

Clinical testing of mifepristone as a medical abortion agent began in 1982, and by 1988, mifepristone was licensed in France for use in combination with a prostaglandin analog for early abortion. In the United States, laboratory and clinical researchers studied mifepristone up until 1989, when its import into the United States was banned. Once mifepristone was no longer available in the United States, even under research protocols, investigators searched for alternative medications to provide a medical abortion, such as methotrexate (53). Whereas previously prostaglandin analogs used alone were believed to cause intolerable side effects thus precluding their use as medical abortion agents, the unavailability of mifepristone in some countries and the growing use of medical abortion in other areas led researchers to reconsider their view of prostaglandin analogs as medical abortifacients. Consequently, renewed interest

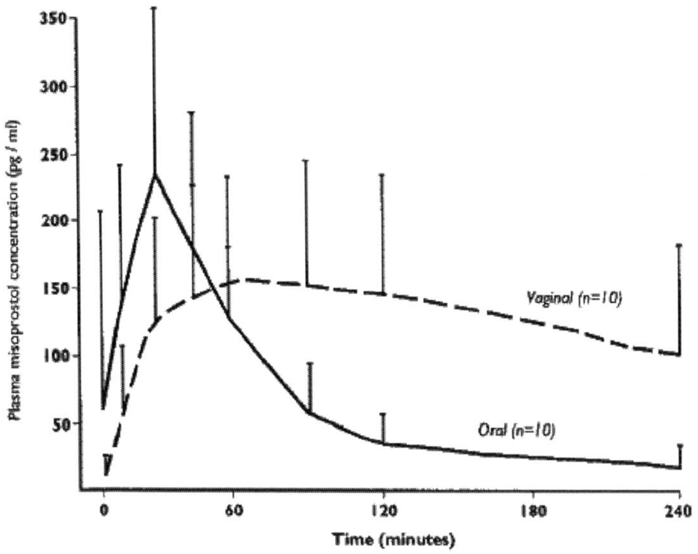

FIGURE 17.2 ● Mean plasma concentrations of misoprostol acid over time with oral *(solid line)* and vaginal *(dotted line)* administration. Error bars represent one standard deviation. (Reprinted from Zieman M, Fong SK, Benowitz NL, et al. Absorption kinetics of misoprostol with oral or vaginal administration. Obstet Gynecol 1997;90:88–92, with permission.)

in prostaglandin analogs, specifically misoprostol, generated further studies of these agents as alternative medical abortion regimens.

The most commonly used medical abortion regimen throughout the world today is mifepristone, followed by a prostaglandin analog. Misoprostol is the prostaglandin analog most commonly used with mifepristone because of its safety, low cost, and stability at room temperatures. Although misoprostol is an oral tablet, it can also be placed in the vagina, which leads to slower absorption, a lower peak serum level, and a greater area under the curve (total amount of drug in the serum over time) as compared with oral misoprostol (Fig. 17.2) (54). In addition, vaginal administration may have direct cervical and uterine effects. Clinically, vaginal administration of misoprostol results in greater efficacy (primarily for gestations more than 49 days) and lower rates of continuing pregnancy than oral administration (55, 56).

In areas without access to mifepristone, methotrexate and misoprostol or misoprostol alone are acceptable alternatives (Table 17.3). Mifepristone regimens result in higher rates of complete abortion and cause expulsion more rapidly than those using methotrexate and misoprostol or misoprostol alone (41, 42). In addition, mifepristone and misoprostol, especially in developing countries, are actually cheaper than misoprostol alone (57). Given the secondary importance of these other regimens as compared with the mifepristone-misoprostol regimen, they are not discussed.

Mifepristone-Misoprostol for Medical Abortion

Standard Regimen

Mifepristone is standardly used in clinical practice as a single 600-mg oral dose followed by a prostaglandin analog. Although initially used with the prostaglandin analog gemeprost throughout Europe, randomized trials have demonstrated the superiority of regimens using misoprostol (58). The regimen approved by the U.S. Food and Drug Administration includes mifepristone 600 mg, followed approximately 48 hours later by misoprostol 400 mcg orally in women up to 49 days' gestation. The patient is supposed to return 2 days after mifepristone administration to receive mifepristone if, in the opinion of the provider, the pregnancy has not already expelled. She can remain in the office for observation or return home after misoprostol ingestion. The patient then returns for a follow-up evaluation and, if the pregnancy is not completely expelled, a suction aspiration should be performed. The vagueness of the protocol in the package labeling leaves a lot of room for interpretation by the provider, including how long to observe a patient

TABLE 17.3

Comparison of Medical Abortion Regimens

Regimen	Mechanism of Action	Doses	Routes of Administration	Comments
Mifepristone plus misoprostol	Mifepristone: decidual necrosis, cervical softening, increase in uterine contractility, increase in prostaglandin sensitivity Misoprostol: cervical dilation and uterine contractility	Mifepristone: 200–600 mg Misoprostol: 400–800 mcg at varying intervals	Mifepristone: oral Misoprostol: vaginal or oral (sublingual and buccal less well studied)	Most effective and best studied medical regimens; cost of mifepristone is a disadvantage
Methotrexate plus misoprostol	Methotrexate: toxic to trophoblast Misoprostol: same as previously	Methotrexate: 50 mg/m^2 of body surface area or 50 mg orally, single dose Misoprostol: 800 mcg at varying intervals	Methotrexate: intramuscular or oral Misoprostol: vaginal	Widely available and inexpensive; immediate expulsion in only 70%; limited availability of parenteral methotrexate due to OSHA regulations regarding handling
Misoprostol alone	Same as previously	Previous doses may be repeated over several days as needed	Same as previously	Widely available and inexpensive; requires multiple visits in short period of time; nausea, vomiting, and fever can occur with repeated doses

OSHA, Occupational Safety & Health Administration.

if she stays in the office, how to perform the evaluation for expulsion, and what is the definition of "complete."

Three large-scale studies examined the mifepristone-misoprostol combination for medical abortion. A French study first evaluated 873 women up to 49 days' gestation in two consecutive studies during which all women received mifepristone 600 mg orally followed approximately 48 hours later by misoprostol 400 mcg orally (59). Women in the second study were also eligible to receive an additional 200 mcg of misoprostol orally if abortion had not occurred within 4 hours. Overall, 4% of women aborted solely from the mifepristone. Complete abortion rates were 97 to 99% and did not differ statistically between the studies. Uterine bleeding averaged 9 to 10 days, and one woman required a transfusion. Approximately 80% of women reported cramping for which about 15% received a nonopiate analgesic. After taking the misoprostol, 40% of the women experienced nausea, 15% vomiting, and 10% diarrhea. Another French trial using the same basic regimen in 1108 women up to 63 days' gestation had similar results (60). Complete abortion rates were highest at lower gestational age: 98% up to 42 days' gestation, 95% from 42 to 49 days' gestation, 93% from 50 to 56 days' gestation, and 87% from 57 to 63 days' gestation. Similarly, continuing pregnancy rates increased with advancing gestational age with a rate of 5% in the highest gestational age range.

TABLE 17.4

Outcome of Treatment with Mifepristone 600 mg Followed by Misoprostol 400 mcg Orally for Abortion in the US Population Council Clinical Trial

Outcome	Pregnant ≤ 49 Days (N=827)	Pregnant 50–56 Days (N=678)	Pregnant 57–63 Days (N=510)	All Pregnancies (<63 Days) N=2015
Percent Success				
Completed pregnancy termination with mifepristone alone	5%	2%	0.8%	3%
Completed pregnancy termination with both agents	87%	81%	76%	82%
Overall pregnancy termination	92%	83%	77%	85%
Percent Failure (surgical intervention needed)				
Ongoing pregnancy	1%	4%	9%	4%
Incomplete abortion	5%	8%	7%	6%
Medical indication (e.g., hemorrhage)	2%	4%	4%	3%
Patient request	1%	2%	2%	2%
Overall Failure	8%	17%	22%	15%

Adapted from Spitz IM, Bardin CW, Benton L, et al. Early pregnancy termination with mifepristone and misoprostol in the United States. N Engl J Med 1998;338:1241–1247, with permission.

The largest clinical trial combining mifepristone 600 mg and misoprostol 400 mcg orally was the U.S. Population Council study (61). All participants had a vaginal ultrasound examination to confirm gestational dating; otherwise, the protocol was similar to that used in common practice in France. The overall effectiveness in the 2015 women evaluated was significantly worse using this treatment regimen for women with gestations more than 49 days (Table 17.4). The time of expulsion was known for 1468 subjects; 50% aborted within 4 hours and 84% within 24 hours after misoprostol administration. Vaginal bleeding averaged 17 days; 9% of women had bleeding lasting more than 30 days. Four women received blood transfusions; one subject each through 49 days and at 57 to 63 days' gestation, and two subjects at 50 to 56 days' gestation.

"Alternative" Regimens

Despite the early acceptance in France and most other countries of the standard regimen of mifepristone 600 mg followed 48 hours later by a prostaglandin analog in the clinic or office in women up to 49 days' gestation (62), investigators questioned whether alternative regimens using these agents would cause fewer side effects, be less expensive, or be more acceptable to providers and patients. The innovations studied have involved lower doses of mifepristone, the use of misoprostol vaginally, home administration of the misoprostol, and altering the timing of the misoprostol dose.

Lower Doses of Mifepristone

Two randomized trials have demonstrated the clinical equivalence of 200-mg and 600-mg doses of mifepristone in combination with misoprostol (63, 64). The larger and more recent trial included women up to 63 days' gestation who received either mifepristone 200 mg ($n = 792$) or 600 mg ($n = 797$), followed 48 hours later by misoprostol 400 mcg orally (64). Complete abortion rates were similar for both groups (89% and 88%, respectively) and, as in the U.S. Population Council study (61), were gestational age dependent: up to 42 days, 92%; 43 to 49 days, 89%;

50 to 56 days, 87%; and more than 56 days, 80%. Side effects were not different between the groups. In addition to these randomized trials, three large studies using mifepristone 200 mg combined with misoprostol 800 mcg vaginally in more than 4000 women have also confirmed the efficacy of the lower dose of mifepristone (65–67). As clinical trials demonstrate no difference in efficacy between the two dosages, the lower dose should be used because it is less expensive. All Rh-negative patients should receive Rh-immune globulin when the mifepristone is ingested.

Vaginal Misoprostol

El-Rafaey (68) first reported the use of vaginal misoprostol in combination with mifepristone in 1994, followed by a randomized trial in 263 women up to 63 days' gestation comparing mifepristone 600 mg followed 800 mcg orally or vaginally 48 hours later (55). Slightly less than 3% of patients aborted from just the mifepristone, 95% aborted with the vaginal misoprostol and 87% with oral misoprostol. Moreover, 93% of the vaginal misoprostol group aborted within 4 hours as compared with 78% of the oral misoprostol group.

Ashok et al. (65) reported a retrospective evaluation of 2000 women who received mifepristone 200 mg, followed 36 to 48 hours later by misoprostol 800 mcg vaginally. In 928 women up to 49 days' gestation and 1072 women from 50 to 63 days' gestation, complete abortion occurred in 98.5% (95% CI 97.7, 99.3%) and 96.7% (95% CI 95.7, 97.8%), respectively. Continuing pregnancy occurred in only 0.2% (95% CI 0, 0.5%) and 0.8% (95% CI 0.2, 1.3%), respectively. Schaff et al. (66, 67) published two reports evaluating a 200-mg dose of mifepristone followed 48 hours later by 800 mcg vaginal misoprostol. In the first trial, which included 933 women with pregnancies up to 56 days' gestation, complete abortion occurred in 97% and 96% of women up to 49 days ($n = 660$) and 50 to 56 days' gestation ($n = 273$), respectively (66). The rates of continuing pregnancy were only 0.3% and 1.1%, respectively. In the second trial, which included 1237 women with pregnancies up to 63 days' gestation, complete abortion occurred in 98%, 97%, and 96% of women up to 49 days ($n = 578$), 50 to 56 days' gestation ($n = 251$), and 57 to 63 days' gestation ($n = 308$), respectively (67). As in the first trial, the rates of continuing pregnancy were similar and extremely low (0.2%, 0.4%, and 1.0%, respectively).

Home Administration of Misoprostol

Multiple investigators have published reports of successful use of self-administered misoprostol in medical abortion regimens using mifepristone (17, 56, 66, 67, 69–71). In three large trials using mifepristone 200 mg and misoprostol 800 mcg vaginally (66, 67, 70), 90% of subjects in all studies found home use of misoprostol acceptable, regardless of prior abortion experience (67), gestational age (67), or time between mifepristone and misoprostol use (70). A total of 4 (0.1%) participants in two studies (66, 67) experienced adverse events in the hours after misoprostol administration. Two of these women presented for an emergent aspiration for heavy bleeding, but neither required a blood transfusion. One woman had a syncopal episode while bleeding and fell and broke her nose. One patient had a vasovagal reaction to cramping and was treated with intravenous fluids. Only the latter occurrence (1 out of approximately 4500 women) would have necessarily been avoided with in-office observation.

Time Interval Between Mifepristone and Misoprostol

Based on the initial clinical trials using mifepristone and a prostaglandin analog, the standard time to administer the prostaglandin analog after mifepristone is 36 to 48 hours. However, regimens with a shorter interval between mifepristone and misoprostol administration, if effective, would lessen the amount of time necessary for a medical abortion to occur and, potentially, increase acceptability. In addition, because approximately half of women bleed during the 48 hours after mifepristone administration (61, 66), administering the drugs on the same day would decrease such an undesirable side effect. There are no studies that identify the time interval at which the increased reactivity to prostaglandin analogs occurs in a pregnant uterus.

Creinin et al. (71) investigated earlier administration of the misoprostol using the standard doses of mifepristone and misoprostol in a randomized trial. Eighty-six women up to 49 days' gestation received mifepristone 600 mg, followed on the same day (group 1) or 2 days later (group 2) by misoprostol 400 mcg orally. Women who received misoprostol on the same day as the mifepristone received a second misoprostol dose at the standard 48-hour interval if expulsion had not occurred. Complete abortion at 24 hours after the misoprostol occurred in 21 of 42 (50%, 95% CI 35, 65%) women in group 1 and 40 of 44 (91%, 95% CI 82, 99%) women in group 2 ($p < 0.0001$).

Schaff et al. (70) performed a multicenter randomized trial in 2295 women up to 56 days' gestation who self-administered misoprostol 800 mcg vaginally 24, 48, or 72 hours after taking mifepristone 200 mg orally. Follow-up occurred within 8 days after the mifepristone. The misoprostol dose was repeated if vaginal ultrasound examination did not confirm expulsion. Complete medical abortion occurred in 98% (95% CI 97, 99%), 98% (95% CI 97, 99%), and 96% (95% CI 95, 97%), respectively. In addition, the time waiting for expulsion was acceptable in 86%, 79%, and 76%, respectively ($p = 0.001$).

The investigators followed this study with a randomized trial to compare oral and vaginal dosing of misoprostol 24 hours after administration of mifepristone 200 mg (56). Women up to 63 days' gestation were randomized to use either two doses of oral misoprostol 400 mcg taken 2 hours apart or misoprostol 800 mcg vaginally. Women returned for follow-up within 5 days and received vaginal misoprostol if a continuing pregnancy was present. Of the 1144 women who complied with their random assignment, complete abortion by the first follow-up visit occurred in 90% and 97%, respectively ($p = 0.001$). By the second follow-up visit, the complete abortion rates were 95% and 99%, respectively ($p = 0.001$). There were minimal differences in side effects. Despite the lower efficacy, women preferred the oral route.

More recently, Pymar et al. (72) and Fox et al. (73) reported that using mifepristone 200 mg and misoprostol 800 mcg vaginally 6 to 8 hours apart caused expulsion within 24 hours in approximately 90% of women through 63 days' gestation. These studies led to a multicenter, randomized trial of 1180 who received the misoprostol either 6 to 8 hours or 23 to 25 hours following the mifepristone (17). Complete abortion rates were statistically equivalent (96% and 98%, respectively). Surprisingly, side effects were significantly more common after mifepristone administration in the women who received misoprostol 23 to 25 hours later. In addition, nausea, vomiting, and heavy bleeding were significantly greater after misoprostol treatment in the women who received misoprostol 23 to 25 hours after the mifepristone. Pain and subject acceptability were similar between groups.

Providing Medical Abortion

General Information

Current published research supports the use of mifepristone orally in a dose of 200 or 600 mg. Clinical trials demonstrate no difference in efficacy between the two dosages; thus, the lower dose should be used because it is less expensive. All Rh-negative patients should receive Rh-immune globulin when the mifepristone is ingested. The upper limit of gestational age acceptable for using a mifepristone regimen for abortion depends on the type and route of administration of the prostaglandin analog. Regimens using misoprostol 400 mcg orally are effective through 49 days' gestation. When misoprostol 800 mcg is administered vaginally following mifepristone, the regimen is clinically effective through 63 days' gestation. The patient can safely and effectively administer misoprostol herself, either orally or vaginally. The misoprostol, when administered vaginally, can be used between 6 and 72 hours after the mifepristone with equal efficacy; however, patients tend to prefer earlier administration. In addition, administration at 6 to 8 hours results in significantly fewer side effects from the abortion process.

Medical contraindications to abortion with mifepristone include confirmed or suspected ectopic pregnancy, intrauterine device (IUD) in situ, chronic systemic corticosteroid administration, adrenal failure, known coagulopathy, allergy to mifepristone, and inherited porphyria. Mifepristone has not been demonstrated clinically to affect asthma, but severe asthmatic patients may require chronic corticosteroid use, which contraindicates mifepristone use.

Misoprostol should be avoided in women with an allergy to misoprostol, uncontrolled seizure disorder, and acute inflammatory bowel disease. In addition, because of a lack of data regarding the safety of these agents in women with significant medical conditions, special considerations should be used before providing medical abortion to women with severe anemia; severe liver, renal, or respiratory disease; uncontrolled hypertension; and cardiovascular disease (angina, valvular disease, arrhythmia, or cardiac failure). Asthma is not a contraindication because misoprostol is a weak bronchodilator. The use of misoprostol during the first trimester for medical abortion has been sparsely evaluated in women with a prior cesarean section (74). Large trials would be needed to better assess this potential risk.

Although medical contraindications are infrequent, social or psychological contraindications to medical abortion are more common. Women are not good candidates for medical abortion if they do not want to participate in their abortion or take responsibility for their care, are anxious to have the abortion over quickly, cannot return for follow-up visits, or cannot understand the instructions because of language or comprehension barriers. Other nonmedical criteria to be considered are access to a phone in case of an emergency and distance from emergency medical treatment (i.e., suction curettage for hemorrhage).

A follow-up evaluation is typically performed 10 to 15 days after misoprostol administration to ensure there are no complications. Expulsion can be confirmed by clinical history or ultrasonography. Interestingly, earlier follow-up can be performed if vaginal ultrasonography is used to confirm expulsion. More recently, Rossi et al. (75) reported that no physical or ultrasound examination may be necessary. When both the clinician and patient believed the gestational sac had passed for 880 women treated with mifepristone and vaginal misoprostol, expulsion was confirmed by sonography in 99% of cases. Typically, European, Chinese, and U.S. clinical trial protocols have included a surgical aspiration if the abortion is not complete by this follow-up visit. However, this intervention is not necessary, and additional doses of misoprostol or simply waiting (if the pregnancy is not viable) is an acceptable alternative (17, 69).

Vaginal bleeding after a medical abortion using mifepristone varies among studies. Davis et al. (76) specifically followed 138 women with bleeding diaries with the intent of ascertaining accurate bleeding patterns. Mifepristone 200 mg and misoprostol 800 mcg vaginally were administered as part of a larger trial comparing misoprostol administration 1, 2, or 3 days after the mifepristone (67, 70). Patients reported bleeding for a mean of 14 days and spotting for a mean of 10 days. Overall, women had bleeding or spotting for an average of 24 days, much longer than what is typically reported in efficacy studies. Twenty percent of women had bleeding or spotting that lasted more than 35 days. Gestational age was directly related to the length of bleeding, with a mean total number of days of bleeding or spotting at 19 days in gestations less than 6 weeks and 25 days for equal to or greater than 6 weeks. In addition, there was no significant difference in bleeding duration based on contraceptive method started after expulsion. Two interesting studies from China have also demonstrated that it is safe to offer women combined hormonal contraception 1 day after misoprostol administration (77, 78). Use of oral contraceptives did not effect abortion outcome, duration of vaginal bleeding, or blood loss as collected on sanitary pads.

Even though heavy bleeding is expected, it is helpful to identify for the patient how much bleeding is considered too much. An easy reference for the patient to use is soaking of two pads per hour for 2 hours in a row. This is not a point at which intervention is necessary, but a time when it is good to check in with the care provider. Whether it is imperative for the patient to seek emergency care depends at that point on how the patient is feeling, her baseline hemoglobin, if the bleeding seems to be slowing, and how far she is from emergency treatment. It may be helpful for the clinician to talk to the patient at 20- to 30-minute intervals until the bleeding slows as long as she is feeling all right; of course, this depends on the factors stated previously.

Excessive bleeding is rare when medical abortion is restricted to pregnancies less than 49 menstrual days. The mean duration of bleeding is less than 2 weeks, but some women bleed until their next menstrual period. Because medical abortion is not 100% effective, 24-hour availability of surgical abortion services for cases of hemorrhage due to retained products of conception is a necessity. This is no different than what is required when patients are primarily treated by surgical abortion. Clinicians other than obstetrician-gynecologists who want to provide medical abortion services must work in conjunction with an obstetrician-gynecologist or be trained in surgical abortion in order to offer medical abortion treatment.

Patients are supplied with appropriate instructions and oral narcotic analgesics. Patients should use ibuprofen or acetaminophen initially and only use oral narcotics, if necessary. The use of a nonsteroidal anti-inflammatory drug such as ibuprofen is not contraindicated and does not decrease the likelihood of abortion after prostaglandin analog administration (79).

Teratogenicity

Congenital anomalies in continuing pregnancies that do not have a surgical abortion is a concern. There has been no evidence of a teratogenic effect of mifepristone. However, misoprostol use in the first trimester has been associated with two specific types of anomalies. Five cases of a frontal and/or temporal defect in the skull without other anomalies were described in women who had taken misoprostol 400 to 600 mcg orally and/or vaginally (80). Gonzalez et al. (81) reported on seven cases of limb abnormalities, four of whom also had a diagnosis of Möbius sequence (masklike faces with bilateral sixth and seventh nerve palsy and frequently coincident micrognathia). The mothers all had taken misoprostol 200 to 1800 mcg orally or vaginally between 4 to 12 weeks amenorrhea to attempt abortion. The authors suggested that these anomalies may represent a vascular disruption defect. There were three other children born with similar anomalies after maternal misoprostol ingestion. Two children had limb deficiencies (one with Möbius sequence), and one child had Möbius sequence; the gestational ages at the time of ingestion were not reported. Because misoprostol is the common agent used with mifepristone or alone, the potential for teratogenicity is an important issue for both types of medical abortion regimens. Wiebe (82) reported six cases of limb reduction abnormalities in fetuses examined after failed abortion with methotrexate and misoprostol. These findings are consistent with the teratogenicity of misoprostol in medical abortion regimens. Schuler et al. (83) published a prospective analysis of 86 misoprostol-exposed and 86 unexposed infants and found no significant difference in the rates of major or minor anomalies. However, they reported a significantly increased risk of spontaneous abortion after misoprostol exposure (17% versus 6%, respectively [RR 3.0, 95% CI 1.1, 7.9]). This study is severely limited by small sample size.

As such, it must be emphasized to the patient before she begins a medical abortion that the agents being used to effect the abortion can cause anomalies in the ongoing pregnancy. Thus, she must be certain of her decision to have an abortion and be willing to have a surgical abortion if the medications do not cause expulsion and the pregnancy is still viable.

CONCLUSION

Surgical and medical abortion procedures are easily provided in an office setting. Surgical abortion offers a fast and safe option for ending an unwanted pregnancy. Some women, though, are very willing to accept a slightly lower efficacy rate in exchange for avoiding a surgical procedure. Mifepristone followed 6 to 72 hours later by vaginal misoprostol is currently the most effective medical abortion regimen available to women. These agents can safely effect abortion through 63 days' gestation. The major side effects with any of these regimens are gastrointestinal. Bleeding lasts a variable duration but has been most accurately described as averaging 2 to 3 weeks in total. Suction curettage is very rarely necessary as an emergency procedure following medical abortion using these agents.

Provision of abortion services requires training to understand how to properly counsel and inform patients of what to expect during their procedure, how to handle questions, how to manage pain, and when to intervene in cases of heavy or prolonged bleeding. The latter point is of primary concern for women having a medical abortion, especially because they are most commonly doing so because of a strong desire to avoid a surgical procedure.

Clinical Notes

- Most surgical abortions (95% in 2000) are provided in an office or clinic setting.
- Abortions performed in hospitals have higher complication rates than do clinic abortions, in part because of higher-risk patients, residents in training, and less experienced surgeons.
- In 2000, more than half of abortions (58%) were obtained at 8 weeks' gestation or less, and 88% were performed before 13 weeks.

- Medical abortion is considered a "failure" when a surgical evacuation is performed to complete the abortion for any reason, including incomplete abortion, continuing (viable) pregnancy, hemorrhage, or patient request.
- Surgical abortion is considered a "failure" if a continuing pregnancy occurs; if a repeat aspiration is required for an incomplete abortion or hematometra, this is considered a complication, not method failure.
- The most common reason a woman wants to have a medical abortion is because of a desire to avoid some aspect of a surgical procedure.
- Suction aspiration procedures can safely be performed until around 14 to 15 weeks' gestation. Procedures after 15 weeks are generally performed by dilation and evacuation procedure.
- Administration of prophylactic antibiotics in an elective abortion is widely used by providers, although the general benefit of such a practice is still in question.
- For practitioners experienced with using suction D&C for abortion, mild infection and reaspiration are the most common complications.
- The most commonly used medical abortion regimen throughout the world today is mifepristone (a single 200- or 600-mg oral dose) followed by a prostaglandin analog.
- Misoprostol (800 mcg vaginally up to 63 days' gestation) is the prostaglandin analog most commonly used with mifepristone because of its safety, low cost, and stability at room temperatures. It is given within 6 to 72 hours of mifepristone ingestion.
- Medical contraindications to abortion with mifepristone include confirmed or suspected ectopic pregnancy, IUD in situ, chronic systemic corticosteroid administration, adrenal failure, known coagulopathy, allergy to mifepristone, and inherited porphyria.
- Severe asthmatic patients may require chronic corticosteroid use, which contraindicates mifepristone use.
- Misoprostol should be avoided in women with an allergy to misoprostol, uncontrolled seizure disorder, and acute inflammatory bowel disease. Asthma is not a contraindication.
- Because medical abortion is not 100% effective, 24-hour availability of surgical abortion services for cases of hemorrhage due to retained products of conception is a necessity.
- Special considerations should be given to women with severe anemia; severe liver, renal, or respiratory disease; uncontrolled hypertension; and cardiovascular disease (angina, valvular disease, arrhythmia, or cardiac failure) before providing medical abortion.
- There has been no evidence of a teratogenic effect of mifepristone.
- Misoprostol use in the first trimester has been associated with two specific types of anomalies: frontal and/or temporal defect in the skull without other anomalies and limb abnormalities.
- All Rh-negative patients undergoing either a surgical or a medical abortion should receive Rh-immune globulin.

REFERENCES

1. Creinin MD. Medical abortion regimens: historical context and overview. Am J Obstet Gynecol 2000;183: S3–S9.
2. Finer LB, Henshaw SK. Abortion incidence and services in the United States in 2000. Perspect Sex Reprod Health 2003;35:6–15.
3. Hakim-Elahi E, Tovell HM, Burnhill MS. Complications of first-trimester abortion: a report of 170,000 cases. Obstet Gynecol 1990;76:129–135.
4. Grimes DA, Cates W Jr, Selik RM. Abortion facilities and the risk of death. Fam Plann Perspect 1981;13:30–32.
5. Elam-Evans LD, Strauss LT, Herndon J, et al. Abortion surveillance—United States, 2000. In: *Surveillance Summaries*, November 28, 2003. MMWR Morbid Mortal Wkly Rep 2003;52:1–32.
6. Henshaw SK, Finer LB. The accessibility of abortion services in the United States, 2001. Perspect Sex Reprod Health 2003;35:16–24.
7. Shelton JD, Brann EA, Schulz KF. Abortion utilization: does travel distance matter? Fam Plann Perspect 1976;8;260–262.
8. Creinin MD, Edwards J. Early abortion: surgical and medical options. Curr Prob Obstet Gynecol Fertil 1997;20:6–32.
9. Paul ME, Mitchell CM, Rogers AJ, et al. Early surgical abortion: efficacy and safety. Am J Obstet Gynecol 2002;187:407–411.

10. Lichtenberg ES, Paul M, Jones H. First trimester surgical abortion practices: a survey of National Abortion Federation members. Contraception 2001;64:345–352.
11. Paul M, Schaff E, Nichols M. The roles of clinical assessment, human chorionic gonadotropin assays, and ultrasonography in medical abortion practice. Am J Obstet Gynecol 2000;183:S34–S43.
12. Winikoff B, Ellertson C, Clark S. Analysis of failure in medical abortion. Contraception 1996;54:323–327.
13. Henshaw RC, Naji SA, Russell IT, et al. Comparison of medical abortion with surgical vacuum aspiration: women's preferences and acceptability of treatment. BMJ 1993;307:714–717.
14. Creinin MD, Burke AE. Methotrexate and misoprostol for early abortion: a multicenter trial. Acceptability. Contraception 1996;54(1):19–22.
15. Cameron ST, Glasier AF, Logan J, et al. Impact of the introduction of new medical methods on therapeutic abortions at the Royal Infirmary of Edinburgh. Br J Obstet Gynaecol 1996;103:1222–1229.
16. Winikoff B, Ellertson C, Elul B, et al. Acceptability and feasibility of early pregnancy termination by mifepristone-misoprostol. Results of a large multicenter trial in the United States. Arch Fam Med 1998;7:360–366.
17. Creinin MD, Fox MC, Teal S, et al. A multicenter, randomized comparison of misoprostol 6 to 8 hours versus 24 hours following mifepristone for abortion through 63 days gestation. Obstet Gynecol 2004;103:851–859.
18. Newhall EP, Winikoff B. Abortion with mifepristone and misoprostol: regimens, efficacy, acceptability and future directions. Am J Obstet Gynecol 2000;183:S44–S53.
19. Creinin MD. Randomized comparison of efficacy, acceptability and cost of medical versus surgical abortion. Contraception 2000;62:117–124.
20. Goldberg AB, Dean G, Kang MS, et al. Manual versus electric vacuum aspiration for early first-trimester abortion: a controlled study of complication rates. Obstet Gynecol 2004;103:10–17.
21. Dean G, Cardenas L, Darney P, et al. Acceptability of manual versus electric aspiration for first trimester abortion: a randomized trial. Contraception 2003;67:201–206.
22. Bird ST, Harvey SM, Beckman LJ, et al. Similarities in women's perceptions and acceptability of manual vacuum aspiration and electric vacuum aspiration for first trimester abortion. Contraception 2003;67:207–212.
23. Suprapto K, Reed S. Naproxen sodium for pain relief in first-trimester abortion. Am J Obstet Gynecol 1984;150:1000–1001.
24. Wiebe ER, Rawling M. Pain control in abortion. Int J Gynaecol Obstet 1995;50:41–46.
25. Sawaya, GF, Grady D, Kerlikowske K, et al. Antibiotics at the time of induced abortion: the case for universal prophylaxis based on a meta-analysis. Obstet Gynecol 1996;87:884–890.
26. Vorherr H, Vorherr UF, Mehta P, et al. Antimicrobial effect of chlorhexidine and povidone-iodine on vaginal bacteria. J Infect 1984;8:195–199.
27. Lundh C, Meirik O, Nygren KG. Vaginal cleansing at vacuum aspiration abortion does not reduce the risk of postoperative infection. Acta Obstet Gynecol Scand 1983;62:275–277.
28. Miller L, Jensen MP, Stenchever MA. A double-blind randomized comparison of lidocaine and saline for cervical anesthesia. Obstet Gynecol 1996;87:600–604.
29. Egziabher TG, Ruminjo JK, Sekadde-Kigondu C. Pain relief using paracervical block in patients undergoing manual vacuum aspiration of uterus. East Afr Med J 2002;79:530–534.
30. Gomez PI, Gaitan H, Nova C, et al. Paracervical block in incomplete abortion using manual vacuum aspiration: randomized clinical trial. Obstet Gynecol 2004;103:943–951.
31. Singh K, Fong YF, Prasad RN, et al. Randomized trial to determine optimal dose of vaginal misoprostol for preabortion cervical priming. Obstet Gynecol 1998;92:795–798.
32. Saxena P, Salhan S, Sarda N. Comparison between the sublingual and oral route of misoprostol for pre-abortion cervical priming in first trimester abortions. Hum Reprod 2004;19:77–80.
33. Inal MM, Ertopcu K, Arici A, et al. The effect of oral versus vaginal misoprostol on cervical dilatation in first-trimester abortion: a double-blind, randomized study. Eur J Contracept Reprod Health Care 2003;8:197–202.
34. Hamoda H, Ashok PW, Flett GM, et al. A randomized controlled comparison of sublingual and vaginal administration of misoprostol for cervical priming before first-trimester surgical abortion. Am J Obstet Gynecol 2004;190:55–59.
35. Tang OS, Mok KH, Ho PC. A randomized study comparing the use of sublingual to vaginal misoprostol for pre-operative cervical priming prior to surgical termination of pregnancy in the first trimester. Hum Reprod 2004;19:1101–1104.
36. Paul M, Lackie E, Mitchell C, et al. Is pathology examination useful after early surgical abortion? Obstet Gynecol 2002;99:567–571.
37. Grossman D, Ellertson C, Grimes DA, et al. Routine follow-up visits after first-trimester induced abortion. Obstet Gynecol 2004;103:738–745.
38. Beuhler JW, Schulz KF, Grimes DA, et al. The risk of serious complications from induced abortion: do personal characteristics make a difference? Am J Obstet Gynecol 1985;153:14–20.
39. Hodgson JE, Portmann KC. Complications of 10,453 consecutive first-trimester abortions: a prospective study. Am J Obstet Gynecol 1974;120:802–807.
40. de Groot AN, van Dongen PW, Vree TB, et al. Ergot alkaloids: current status and review of clinical pharmacology and therapeutic use compared with other oxytocics in obstetrics and gynecology. Drugs 1998;56:523–535.
41. Jain JK, Dutton C, Harwood B, et al. A prospective randomized, double-blinded, placebo-controlled trial comparing mifepristone and vaginal misoprostol to vaginal misoprostol alone for elective termination of early pregnancy. Hum Reprod 2002;17:1477–1482.
42. Wiebe E, Dunn S, Guilbert E, et al. Comparison of abortions induced by methotrexate or mifepristone followed by misoprostol. Obstet Gynecol 2002;99:813–819.

43. Thiersch JB. Therapeutic abortions with a folic acid antagonist, 4-aminopteroyglutamic acid (4-amino P.G.A.) administered by the oral route. Am J Obstet Gynecol 1952;63:1298–1304.
44. Karim SMM. Once a month vaginal administration of prostaglandin E_2 and $F_{2\alpha}$ for fertility control. Contraception 1971;3:173–183.
45. Mocsary P, Csapo AJ. Menstrual induction with $PGF_{2\alpha}$ and PGE_2. Prostaglandins 1975;10:545–547.
46. Bygdeman M, Bremme K, Christensen N, et al. A comparison of two stable prostaglandin E analogues for termination of early pregnancy and for cervical dilatation. Contraception 1980;22:471–482.
47. Smith SK, Baird DT. The use of 16,16-dimethyl-*trans*-Δ^2-PGE_1 methyl ester (ONO 802) vaginal suppositories for the termination of early pregnancy. A comparative study. Br J Obstet Gynaecol 1980;87:712–717.
48. Lahteemnaki P, Heikinheimo O, Croxatto H, et al. Pharmacokinetics and metabolism of RU 486. J Steroid Biochem 1987;27:859–863.
49. Skafar DF. Differences in the binding mechanism of RU 486 and progesterone to the progesterone receptors. Biochemistry 1991;30:10829–10831.
50. Kelly RW, Healy DL, Cameron MJ, et al. RU 486 stimulation of PGF_{2a} production in isolated endometrial cells in short term culture. In: Beaulieu EE, Siegel S, eds. The Antiprogestin Steroid RU 486 and Human Fertility Control. New York: Plenum, 1985:259–262.
51. Herrmann WL, Schindler AM, Wyss R, et al. Effects of the antiprogesterone RU 486 in early pregnancy and during the menstrual cycle. In: Beaulieu EE, Siegel S, eds. The Antiprogestin Steroid RU 486 and Human Fertility Control. New York: Plenum, 1985:259–262.
52. Spitz IM, Bardin CW. Clinical pharmacology of RU-486—an antiprogestin and antiglucocorticoid. Contraception 1993;48:403–444.
53. Creinin MD, Darney PD. Methotrexate and misoprostol for early abortion. Contraception 1993;48:339–348.
54. Zieman M, Fong SK, Benowitz NL, et al. Absorption kinetics of misoprostol with oral or vaginal administration. Obstet Gynecol 1997;90:88–92.
55. El-Rafaey H, Rajasekar D, Abdalla M, et al. Induction of abortion with mifepristone (RU 486) and oral or vaginal misoprostol. N Engl J Med 1995;332:983–987.
56. Schaff EA, Fielding SL, Westhoff C. Randomized trial of oral versus vaginal misoprostol at one day after mifepristone for early medical abortion. Contraception 2001;64:81–85.
57. Creinin MD, Shore E, Balasubramanian B, et al. The true cost differential between mifepristone and misoprostol compared to misoprostol alone for medical abortion. Contraception 2005;71:26–30.
58. Bartley J, Brown A, Elton R, et al. Double-blind randomized trial of mifepristone in combination with vaginal gemeprost of misoprostol for induction of abortion up to 63 days gestation. Hum Reprod 2001;16:2098–2102.
59. Peyron R, Aubény E, Targosz V, et al. Early termination of pregnancy with mifepristone (RU 486) and the orally active prostaglandin misoprostol. N Engl J Med 1993;328:1509–1513.
60. Aubény E, Peyron R, Turpin CL, et al. Termination of early pregnancy (up to 63 days of amenorrhea) with mifepristone (RU486) and increasing doses of misoprostol. Int J Fertil Menopausal Stud 1995;40(suppl 2): 85–91.
61. Spitz IM, Bardin CW, Benton L, et al. Early pregnancy termination with mifepristone and misoprostol in the United States. N Engl J Med 1998;338:1241–1247.
62. Jones RK, Henshaw SK. Mifepristone for early medical abortion: experiences in France, Great Britain and Sweden. Perspect Sex Reprod Health 2002;34:154–161.
63. McKinley C, Thong KJ, Baird DT. The effect of dose of mifepristone and gestation on the efficacy of medical abortion with mifepristone and misoprostol. Hum Reprod 1993;8:1502–1505.
64. World Health Organization Task Force on Post-ovulatory Methods of Fertility Regulation. Comparison of two doses of mifepristone in combination with misoprostol for early medical abortion: a randomised trial. Br J Obstet Gynaecol 2000;107:524–530.
65. Ashok P, Penney G, Flett G, et al. An effective regimen for early medical abortion: a report of 2000 consecutive cases. Hum Reprod 1998;13:2962–2965.
66. Schaff EA, Eisinger SH, Stadalius LS, et al. Low-dose mifepristone 200 mg and vaginal misoprostol for abortion. Contraception 1999;59:1–6.
67. Schaff EA, Fielding SL, Eisinger SH, et al. Low-dose mifepristone followed by vaginal misoprostol at 48 hours for abortion up to 63 days. Contraception 2000;61:41–46.
68. El-Rafaey H. Early induction of abortion by a combination of oral mifepristone and misoprostol administered by the vaginal route. Contraception 1994;49:111–114.
69. Schaff EA, Stadalius LS, Eisinger SH, et al. Vaginal misoprostol administered at home after mifepristone (RU486) for abortion. J Fam Pract 1997;44:353–360.
70. Schaff EA, Fielding SL, Westhoff C, et al. Randomized trial of vaginal misoprostol administered 1, 2, or 3 days after mifepristone for early medical abortion (<56 days gestation). JAMA 2000;284:1948–1953.
71. Creinin MD, Schwartz JL, Pymar HC, et al. Efficacy of mifepristone followed on the same day by misoprostol for early termination of pregnancy: report of a randomised trial. Br J Obstet Gynaecol 2001;108:469–473.
72. Pymar HC, Creinin MD, Schwartz JL. Mifepristone followed on the same day by vaginal misoprostol for early abortion. Contraception 2001;64:87–92.
73. Fox MC, Creinin MD, Harwood B. Mifepristone and vaginal misoprostol on the same day for abortion from 50 to 63 days' gestation. Contraception 2002;66:225–229.
74. Xu J, Chen H, Ma T, et al. Termination of early pregnancy in the scarred uterus with mifepristone and misoprostol. Int J Gynaecol Obstet 2001;72:245–251.

75. Rossi B, Creinin MD, Meyn LA. The ability of the clinician and patient to predict the outcome of mifepristone and misoprostol medical abortion. Contraception 2004;70:313–317.
76. Davis A, Westhoff C, De Nonno L. Bleeding patterns after early abortion with mifepristone and misoprostol or manual vacuum aspiration. J Am Med Womens Assoc 2000;55:141–144.
77. Tang OS, Gao PP, Cheng L, et al. A randomized double-blind placebo-controlled study to assess the effect of OC pills on the outcome of medical abortion with mifepristone and misoprostol. Hum Reprod 1999;14:722–725.
78. Tang OS, Xu J, Cheng L, et al. The effect of contraceptive pills on the measured blood loss in medical termination of pregnancy by mifepristone and misoprostol a randomized placebo controlled trial. Hum Reprod 2002;17:99–102.
79. Creinin MD, Shulman T. Effect of non-steroidal anti-inflammatory drugs on the action of misoprostol in a regimen for early abortion. Contraception 1997;56:165–168.
80. Fonseca W, Alencar AJC, Mota FSB, et al. Misoprostol and congenital malformations. Lancet 1991;338:56.
81. Gonzalez CH, Vargas R, Perez AB, et al. Limb deficiency with or without Möbius sequence in seven Brazilian children associated with misoprostol use in the first trimester of pregnancy. Am J Med Genet 1993;47:59–64.
82. Wiebe ER. Abortion induced with methotrexate and misoprostol: a comparison of various protocols. Contraception 1997;55:159–163.
83. Schuler L, Pastuszak A, Sanseverino TV, et al. Pregnancy outcome after exposure to misoprostol in Brazil: a prospective, controlled study. Reprod Toxicol 1999;13:147–151.

CHAPTER 18

Urogynecology and Pelvic Floor Dysfunction

Alfred E. Bent

INTRODUCTION

Lower urinary tract problems can create significant changes in a woman's psychological and physical well-being, and can also incur significant financial costs. As the population ages in America, the number of women suffering from lower urinary tract problems will increase. Women may experience embarrassment, depression, and loss of self-esteem and productivity as a result of lower urinary tract disorders. At times, the symptoms associated with these disorders may lead to social isolation. It is extremely important that all providers of health care to women inquire about the existence of any urinary symptoms during visits because many women are embarrassed to mention these issues directly to their health care provider.

Although all gynecologists receive training in the evaluation and treatment of urologic conditions that affect the lower genitourinary tract in women, it is only in the last decade that the specific specialty of urogynecology has emerged as an accredited area of training and study within the field of obstetrics and gynecology. These specialists are of great service to women who suffer from complex or recurrent urogynecologic problems, but for a large number of women, the evaluation and treatment of many common urogynecologic problems can be done in the outpatient stetting by gynecologists and other primary care providers. This chapter offers a review of the common causes and types of urogynecologic disorders, their evaluation, and office-based treatment approaches.

URINARY TRACT INFECTION

Acute Urinary Tract Infection

Urinary tract infection (UTI) is the most common bacteria infection. The highest incidence of acute, uncomplicated UTI is in sexually active women from 20 to 40 years of age and in postmenopausal populations. It is estimated that 27 to 48% of women with one UTI will experience recurrent infection (1).

Ideally, the patient is seen in the office. There are occasions when phone consultation and treatment may have to be arranged, and this has been shown to be economically effective and therapeutically adequate in many cases (2, 3). The presence or absence of elevated temperature, history of chills, flank tenderness, and suprapubic tenderness is determined. Vaginal infection is excluded based on vaginal or external itching or irritation, followed by local evaluation for signs of vulvovaginal inflammation. If appropriate, potassium hydroxide and saline wet preparations are obtained to rule out yeast, trichomoniasis, and bacterial vaginosis. Specimens may be obtained for chlamydia and gonorrhea testing.

Symptoms and Evaluation

Symptomatic UTI is diagnosed when there are clinical symptoms caused by the bacteria in the urinary tract, such as urinary frequency, urgency, painful voiding, and hematuria. These symptoms vary, depending on the site of infection. Asymptomatic UTI exists when organisms can be isolated in sufficient numbers from the urine, but the patient manifests no symptoms of infection. The term bacteriuria may be used interchangeably with the phrase "asymptomatic UTI."

The urine is evaluated in the office setting by dipstick or microscopic assessment (4). The simplest test is one of the dipstick methods. The nitrite test detects greater than 10^5 colony-forming units (CFU)/mL in 60% of cases (5). Combined bacteria and leukocyte strips detect greater than 10^5 CFU/mL in 79 to 85% of cases (5–8). Microscopy of unspun urine for white blood cells, red blood cells, and bacteria can be commenced at 100× power and refined at 400× power. Although effective diagnosis can be made without a counting chamber, one study using a mirrored counting chamber correctly identified 23 of 24 UTIs confirmed by culture, and 286 of 318 sterile urine samples (9). The diagnosis of a symptomatic UTI should be confirmed in the office without further laboratory evaluation, and treatment commenced without delay (10).

The indications for urine culture and sensitivity testing are as follows:

- Failure of therapy
- Recurrent infections
- Suspected pyelonephritis
- Diagnosis when the presence of UTI is not certain after office evaluation
- Pregnancy
- Medically high-risk patients such as the elderly and those with immune compromise

A single midstream clean catch urine culture with a growth of 10^5 CFU/mL is considered 85% accurate for the presence of significant bacterial growth, but in the presence of symptoms, is considered confirmatory (11, 12). Counts as low as 10^2/mL in symptomatic women are relevant when *Enterobacteriaceae* are grown, but this is not necessarily the case with other microorganisms (13). Subsequent studies have shown that lower bacterial counts can be important; this applies even to symptomatic women in whom 30 to 50% have fewer than 10^5 organisms/mL (13). A catheterized urine specimen is considered positive with a growth of 100 CFU/mL (14).

Pathology

The normal genitourinary tract, excluding the distal urethra, is sterile. Most infections (80 to 85%) are caused by strains of *Escherichia coli* (4). *Staphylococcus saprophyticus* is a common cause of infection in young sexually active women. Other organisms include *Aerobacter aeruginosa*, *Klebsiella*, and *Pseudomonas*. A growth of *Proteus* suggests calculus disease.

The organisms isolated in patients with asymptomatic infections vary slightly from those isolated from patients with symptomatic UTIs. Evidence suggests a higher frequency of infection with coagulase-negative staphylococci and *Enterococcus* species in asymptomatic UTI. Despite the absence of symptoms in these patients, there is a host immune or inflammatory response in most individuals with asymptomatic bacteriuria (15, 16). Asymptomatic bacteriuria appears to be benign and is not associated with the development of hypertension or renal failure, nor is it associated with increased mortality. It is, however, associated with an increased risk for invasive infection, such as bacteremia and septic shock, when there is trauma to the infected genitourinary tract.

Treatment

Ancillary measures in treating UTI include increased fluid intake, use of urinary analgesics (Table 18.1), and occasionally a mild anti-inflammatory or analgesic. The treatment for initial or interval UTI in the nonpregnant patient is a 3- to 5-day course of one of several medications (Table 18.2), such as nitrofurantoin (Macrodantin, Macrobid) or trimethoprim/sulfamethoxazole (Bactrim, Bactrim DS). A one-dose treatment has previously been shown to be somewhat effective, but a 3-day course is much more likely to provide effective therapy and is as effective as

TABLE 18.1

Urinary Analgesics

Phenazopyridine (Pyridium, many other trade names)
- 100 to 200 mg orally as needed up to three times per day
- May turn urine, contact lenses orange
- May invalidate urinary dipstick analysis

Urised (combination of methenamine, phenyl salicylate, methylene blue, benzoic acid, atropine, and hyoscyamine)
- Two tabs orally as needed up to twice a day
- Do not use in combination with sulfa antibiotics
- May turn urine, contact lenses blue

Hyoscyamine (Levsin, Cystospaz, many other trade names)
- 0.125 to 0.25 mg orally as needed up to four times daily
- Extended-release formulations: 0.375 to 0.75 mg orally every 12 hours
- Maximum dose is 1.5 mg/day

Flavoxate (Urispas)
- 100 to 200 mg orally as needed up to four times daily

longer sources extending 5 to 10 days (17). The only exception might be nitrofurantoin where a 5- to 7-day course is usually recommended (18). The use of fluoroquinolones should be reserved for resistant or recurrent infections, although resistant organisms have led to widespread use of these preparations (19). Short courses of fluoroquinolones, including single-dose therapy, have proved effective in uncomplicated infections (20).

TABLE 18.2

First-Line Antibiotics for Urinary Tract Infections

Nitrofurantoin
- Furadantin 50 mg—four times a day
- Macrobid 100 mg—twice a day

Trimethoprim/sulfamethoxazole (TMP/SMX, Bactrim, Septra)
- Regular strength tablets (80/400)—two tablets twice a day
- Double strength tablets (160/800)—one tablet twice a day

Cephalosporins
- First generation: cephalexin (Keflex) 250–500 mg four times a day
- First generation: cephadroxil (Duricef) 500 mg twice a day
- Second generation: cefuroxime (Ceftin) 250 mg twice a day

Fluoroquinolones
- Ciprofloxacin (Cipro) 250 mg twice a day
- Levofloxacin (Levaquin) 500 mg daily
- Norfloxacin (Noroxin) 400 mg twice a day

Ampicillin with clavulanate
- Augmentin 250 to 500 mg two to three times a day

A test of cure is not required after treatment of simple UTI and is not cost effective. Patients with recurring infections or symptoms require cultures, and perhaps other diagnostic approaches, for correct diagnosis and treatment.

Recurrent Urinary Tract Infection

The major behavioral factors associated with recurrent UTI are sexual activity and contraceptive use. Increased frequency of sexual intercourse is associated with increased frequency of acute cystitis. The use of spermicides and the diaphragm (even without the concurrent use of spermicides) are risk factors for infection. Oral contraceptives and condoms without spermicides do not appear to increase the risk of infection (1, 21).

If a patient has had three or more infections in a 12-month period, prophylaxis is recommended. An anatomic defect leading to recurrent infections is usually determined in childhood after repeat infections. It is rare for local cystitis to lead to structural kidney damage, but if there is pre-existing structural damage, this will predispose to recurrent infections. Invasive testing (cystoscopy, intravenous pyelography, and renal ultrasound) is not usually required prior to commencing prophylaxis. Testing is recommended for the elderly and for those who fail prophylaxis, as well as in children.

Nitrofurantoin 50 or 100 mg once daily offers excellent prophylaxis against *Escherichia coli* without risk of overgrowth of yeast organisms in the vagina. The risk of resistance of *E. coli* to nitrofurantoin is only 2%, compared with 9% for trimethoprim/sulfamethoxazole. If preferred, it may be given after intercourse, rather than daily. Alternative once-a-day medications include one regular strength tablet of trimethoprim/sulfamethoxazole, norfloxacin (Noroxin) 400 mg, and cephalexin (Keflex) 250 mg. Tetracycline, penicillin, regular ampicillin, and erythromycin are not good drugs for treating or preventing UTI.

Acute Nonobstructive Pyelonephritis

Acute uncomplicated pyelonephritis involves the same bacterial organisms as those seen in acute UTI, with *E. coli* being the predominant infectious organism (22). The major determinant of the occurrence of acute pyelonephritis appears to be organism-specific virulence factors; the production of specific adhesions by infecting *E. coli* (P fimbriae) is highly correlated with uncomplicated pyelonephritis relative to other clinical presentations of UTI (23).

One of the most common causes of sudden illness and shocklike status in the elderly is pyelonephritis. It may present with chills, high fever, and gastrointestinal (GI) upset. The patient can present in shock with altered sensorium. After admission and the initiation of fluid therapy, systemic treatment is commenced with intravenous cephalosporins, gentamicin, ciprofloxacin, or Levaquin. Ampicillin is not an appropriate choice of therapy. Recovery is usually rapid, and once stable, the patient can be discharged and continued on a 10- to 14-day course of appropriate oral therapy.

Special Populations

Patients With Diabetes

Although diabetic women have an increased prevalence of asymptomatic bacteriuria, diabetic men do not (24). The presence of asymptomatic bacteriuria correlates strongly with other variable indicatives of the *duration* of the diabetes but not the *control* of the diabetes. Hence, there is an increased prevalence in women with retinopathy or neuropathy but not with elevated hemoglobin A1C levels (24). When symptomatic UTIs appear in people with diabetes, the presentation may be more severe compared with nondiabetic patients. Clinical presentations such as emphysematous cystitis or pyelonephritis, papillary necrosis, and perinephric abscess are seen almost only in diabetic patients.

Patients With Indwelling Urethral Catheters

An indwelling urethral catheter increases a patient's risk for a complicated UTI, with the incidence of infection close to 5% per day. Infection rates are higher in individuals who do not receive antimicrobials in the first 4 days of catheterization. Although most infections are asymptomatic, severe complications can, and do, occur (25). Patients with long-term indwelling catheters (i.e., in place for more than 1 month) will always have bacteriuria, with usually two to five organisms present. The types of organisms present constantly change, so the duration of infection for any specific isolate is variable (25, 26).

Patients in Long-Term Care Facilities

There is a high prevalence of asymptomatic bacteriuria in women who live in long-term care facilities, even in the absence of an indwelling catheter. Although *Escherichia coli* remains the most common infecting organism, other *Enterobacteriaceae, Pseudomonas aeruginosa, Enterococcus* species, and group B streptococci comprise the other common isolates. There is no evidence that asymptomatic bacteriuria is detrimental to patients in long-term care facilities. Evidence of UTI is still, however, one of the most common reasons for antibiotic administration in nursing homes, and UTIs are the most common source of bacteremia in this population (15).

INCONTINENCE

Urinary incontinence (UI), as defined by the International Incontinence Society, is involuntary loss of urine that is objectively demonstrable and that is severe enough to constitute a social or hygienic problem (27). UI affects women of all ages, its prevalence increases as women age, and current estimates put the prevalence at close to 55% (28).

Women suffering from incontinence may experience embarrassment, depression, loss of self-esteem, loss of productivity, and at times, social isolation due to their disease. Unfortunately, many women are reluctant to discuss their symptoms with a physician or have found their physician ill equipped to address these problems. One study showed that only 37% of patients with incontinence reported their symptoms to their doctor, and it is believed this under-reporting may be due to embarrassment, acceptance of the disorder as a natural part of aging, or being unaware that treatment exists (29, 30).

The onset and progression of UI, and its attendant psychological stress, is associated with an increased risk in comorbid psychiatric disorders (31). Compared with the general population, the incontinent population has a higher prevalence of panic disorder (2% versus 7%) and depression (6% versus 16%) (32, 33). Study shows that the onset of panic disorders is directly proportional to the extent that incontinence alters a patient's lifestyle, and the incidence of depression is also related to the degree of incontinence. Although major depression is significantly more common in patients with urge incontinence compared with those with stress incontinence, the highest rate is among patients with mixed incontinence (32, 34, 35).

The annual cost of UI for women in the United States is triple the amount for men and is estimated at $12.4 billion. The majority of these funds are used by noninstitutionalized women older than 65 years of age (36). Most of these resources are used for maintaining patients with chronic incontinence, rather than for diagnosis and treatment of the condition.

UI can be divided into three broad areas: (a) bladder storage failure also known as overactive bladder (OAB) or detrusor overactivity, (b) failure of the urinary sphincter mechanism, and (c) failure of neural control mechanisms that result in disruption of the normal urethral and bladder voiding or storage function. UI results when either the sphincter muscle does not close properly or when the bladder contracts inappropriately. Effective treatment for UI requires distinguishing between a variety of etiologies to diagnose and appropriately treat the incontinence (Table 18.3).

The cause of UI is multifactorial with recognized risk factors, including age, parity, vaginal delivery, advancing age, history of diabetes or frequent UTIs, and obesity (37–40). More recent investigations have focused on the possible link between incontinence, pelvic floor disorders, and predisposing genetic factors. In a study by Elia et al., women with UI were more likely to have at least one family member who also had incontinence in comparison to women who were continent (41). These findings were consistent with those observed in other studies (42). Guong et al. found that although African American women had lower rates of genuine stress incontinence (GSI) in comparison to Hispanic, white, or Asian women (three groups that had

TABLE 18.3

Differential Diagnosis of Urinary Incontinence

Genuine stress incontinence
Hypermobility (anatomic)
Intrinsic sphincter deficiency
Overactive bladder
Motor urge incontinence
Sensory urge incontinence
Detrusor dyssynergia
Detrusor hyper-reflexia
Detrusor hyperactivity with incomplete contractility
Mixed incontinence
Bypass of the continence mechanism
Fistula
Diverticulum
Ectopic ureter
Overflow incontinence
Functional

similar rates), the rate of detrusor instability in African American women was higher than in the other three groups (43).

Although UI is commonly associated with some degree of pelvic floor prolapse, the prolapse is not the causal agent of the incontinence. Patients with severe pelvic organ prolapse may have no complaints of UI, but on correction of the defect on examination, with use of a pessary, or after surgical correction, symptoms of UI may become manifest.

Evaluation

Most patients presenting with UI require only a basic evaluation for making a presumptive diagnosis (44). This consists of history, physical examination, a 3-day urolog (24-hour voiding diary) (Fig. 18.1), residual urine determination, and urinalysis. The history should include a detailed urologic history, with questions related to subjective assessment of urine volume, frequency of fluid intake and voiding, UI episodes, and precipitating factors. In addition, a detailed gynecologic, obstetric, medical, neurologic, and surgical history is obtained. Clinicians should review the patient's medications, including over-the-counter medications, because many agents can compromise urinary tract function and may predispose to UI (Table 18.4).

History and Physical Examination

History alone is not sufficient to diagnose the etiology of the patient's UI. In one study, reliance on history alone to identify GSI resulted in misdiagnosis in 25% of patients (45). The history is a "screening device" to assist in identification of patients who need further evaluation.

The physical exam is done to exclude any related pathology, assess the pelvic support, and reproduce the incontinence. Clinicians should note the patient's body habitus, mental status, and gait and balance. A neurologic assessment is important in the physical examination; up to 33% of patients with demyelinating diseases (e.g., Parkinson's disease, multiple sclerosis) present with loss of bladder control.

VOIDING DIARY

Time	Amount Voided	Activity	Leak Volume	Urge Present	Amount/Type of Intake

FIGURE 18.1 ● Example of a voiding diary or urolog. Patients are instructed to complete the diary for 24 to 72 hours. (Reprinted from Ostergard DR, Bent AK. Urogynecology and Urodynamics: Theory and Practice. 4th ed. Baltimore: Williams & Wilkins, 1996:682, with permission.)

The neurologic screening should include a simple but comprehensive assessment of the lumbosacral spinal segments. The T10 to S4 nerve roots are primarily responsible for control of micturition. An examination of the lower extremity functions dependent on these nerve roots provides indirect evidence regarding bladder function (Fig. 18.2). Motor function can be assessed by flexion and extension maneuvers against resistance at the ankle, knee, and hip. Pelvic floor muscle tone can be determined by voluntary contraction of the rectal sphincter and vagina. Normal sensation in the upper leg and perineal dermatomes confirms intact sensory innervation of the lower urinary tract.

Finally, reflex contraction of the pelvic floor in response to light stroking of the anus or clitoris (also known as the "anal wink" reflex or bulbocavernosus reflex) provides evidence of the integrity of the sacral reflex center. It should be noted, however, that this reflex is not detectable in up to 30% of otherwise normal women (46). A rectal exam should also be done to assess sphincter tone and to rule out fecal impaction, which is associated with UI in the elderly. Findings suggestive of neurologic deficits should be referred for formal neurologic evaluation.

Inspection of the anterior and posterior vaginal walls using the lower blade of a bivalve vaginal speculum will facilitate identification of any cystocele, rectocele, or enterocele. A defect in the anterior vaginal wall support does not confirm the diagnosis of genuine stress incontinence. Fischer-Rasmussen reported no correlation between the presence of genital prolapse and the diagnosis of GSI (sensitivity 72%, specificity 46%) (18). The possibility of a urethral diverticulum

TABLE 18.4

Common Medications Associated with Urinary Incontinence

Medications That May Cause Stress Incontinence by Decreasing Urethral Smooth or Skeletal Muscle Tone
α-Methyldopa (Aldomet)
Prazosin (Minipress)
Phenothiazines
Diazepam (Valium)
Sympathomimetics (decongestants)
Calcium channel blockers
Medications That May Cause Overflow Incontinence with Urinary Retention by Relaxation of the Detrusor Muscle
Antihistamines
Anticholinergic therapies
Antidepressants
Antispasmodics
Medications That May Worsen Urge Incontinence by Exacerbating Detrusor Instability
Alcohol
Caffeine
Medications That May Worsen Urge and Stress Incontinence
Diuretics

or urinary fistula must also be considered during the examination. Palpation of the urethra and bladder trigone may reveal tenderness consistent with acute or chronic inflammation of either structure. Bimanual examination should be performed to detect coexistent adnexal or uterine pathology.

During the pelvic exam, the urethra should be evaluated for hypermobility; this is done via the "Q-tip test." The Q-tip test is performed by cleansing the urethral meatus with a Betadine swab followed by placement of a sterile cotton swab coated in 2% lidocaine gel. The Q-tip is passed through the bladder neck and then pulled gently back to rest at the urethrovesical junction (UVJ). The straining or coughing angle of the arm of the Q-tip compared with the horizontal axis is the measurement of urethral or bladder neck mobility. A straining angle greater than 30 degrees is indicative of poor anatomic support of the UVJ and urethral hypermobility but does not necessarily confirm the diagnosis of genuine stress incontinence.

Because the purpose of anti-incontinence procedures is to elevate the UVJ back to its normal intra-abdominal position, it is essential that a defect in support of the junction is demonstrated before surgical intervention is contemplated. In patients with a negative Q-tip test, the diagnosis of GSI should be seriously questioned. More sophisticated radiographic or urodynamic studies are indicated prior to undertaking surgery in this group of patients.

While in the lithotomy position, the patient should be asked to cough or strain, and the loss of any urine associated with these efforts should be noted. The patient should then be asked to stand and cough or strain, while the clinician observes for any loss of urine.

Urolog

A voiding diary, or urolog, is one of the most important aspects of the urogynecologic investigation (Fig. 18.1). Patients are sent home with a voiding chart and instructions, as well as a measuring container that can fit on her toilet seat. She is asked to record the time and volume of her spontaneous voids over a 24- to 72-hour time period. Additional information regarding urgency prior to voids, frequency of incontinent episodes, activity precipitating incontinence,

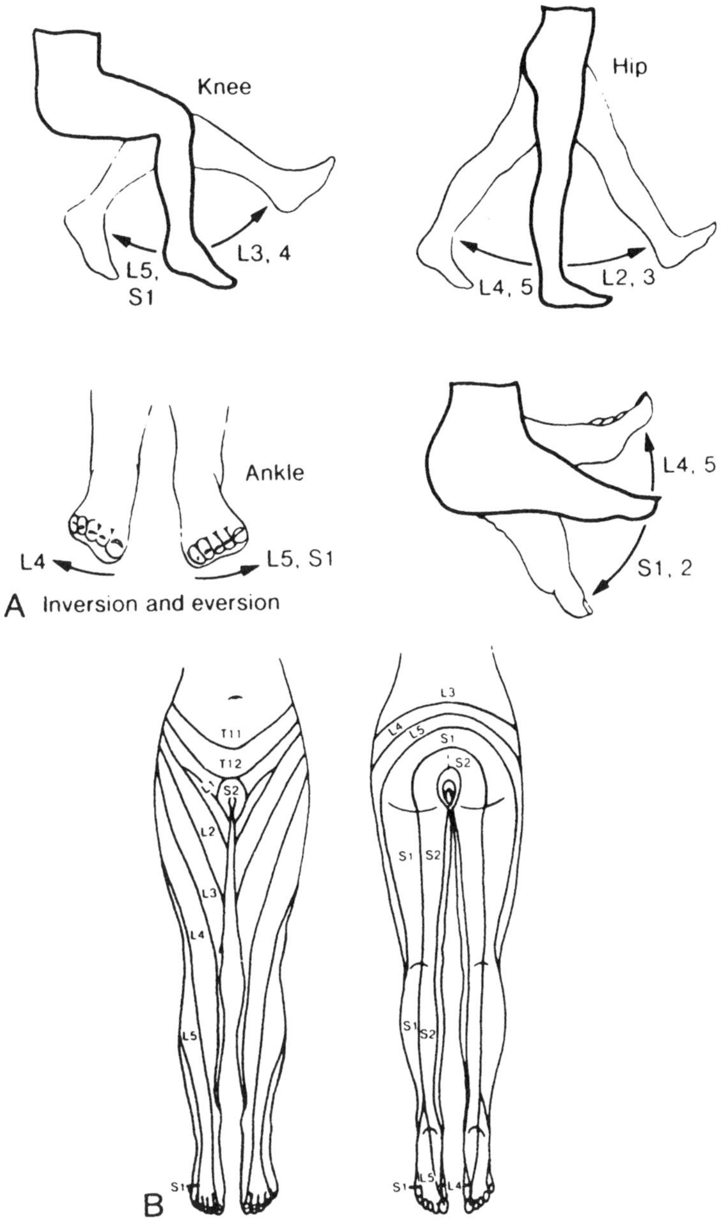

FIGURE 18.2 ● **A:** Patient maneuvers that assess the integrity of motor innervation of the lower extremities from T10 to S4. **B:** Sensory innervation of the lower extremities. (Reprinted from Ostergard DR, Bent AK. Urogynecology and Urodynamics: Theory and Practice. 4th ed. Baltimore: Williams & Wilkins, 1996:101–102, with permission.)

and the type and volume of fluid intake are also recorded. From this journal, vital information regarding the patient's normal voiding pattern, functional bladder capacity, and the severity of her incontinence episodes or irritative symptoms can be obtained. The findings from the urolog can be used to adjust fluid intake in older patients with nocturnal frequency or to begin a timed voiding schedule in a woman with detrusor instability. Occasionally, the voiding pattern may alert the clinician to the possibility of diabetes insipidus or anxiety-related diurnal frequency

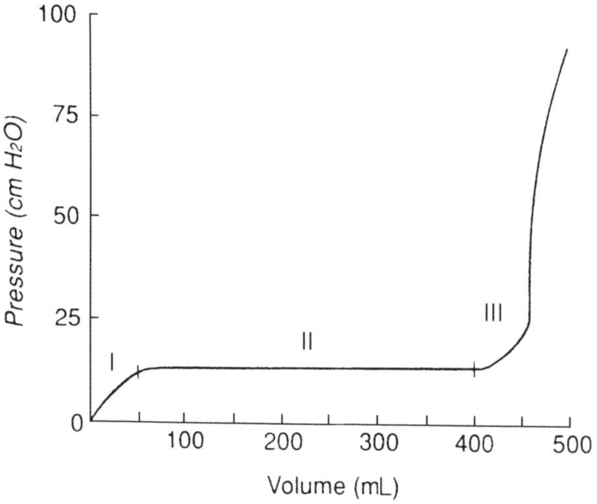

FIGURE 18.3 ● The three phases of a single-channel cystometrogram. Phase I is the small rise in intravesical pressure during the initial phase of filling. Phase II is the plateau phase characterized by an increase in bladder volume without a rise in bladder pressure. Phase III is the increase in intravesical pressure due to a detrusor contraction for voluntary voiding at the end of the study. (Reprinted from Ostergard DR, Bent AK. Urogynecology and Urodynamics: Theory and Practice. 4th ed. Baltimore: Williams & Wilkins, 1996:116, with permission.)

in a patient who sleeps through the night without problems. Thus, a urolog is an inexpensive, noninvasive evaluation of lower urinary tract function that should be obtained early in the course of all urologic evaluations.

Urologic Testing

Patients with complaints of UI need to undergo urologic testing. These tests range from simple "eyeball" urodynamics to sophisticated multichannel synchronous video/pressure/flow/electromyelography studies. The basic office evaluation includes an assessment of voiding, detrusor function during bladder filling, and determination of the adequacy of the proximal urethral sphincter. The patient should come to the visit with a comfortably full bladder. The order of tests is to have the patient empty her bladder in private with the voided volume recorded, and then to catheterize the bladder for residual urine determination and microscopic urinalysis. Postvoid residual volumes of 50 mL or less are considered normal with those greater than 200 mL suggestive of urinary retention. The clinical significance of volumes between 50 and 200 mL is unclear.

The catheter used to check for postvoid residual may be left in place to allow for performance of a simple office cystometrogram (CMG). Cystometry is a pressure–volume relationship recorded during bladder filling. The three main phases of single-channel cystometry are shown in Figure 18.3. Office cystometry (Fig. 18.4) is performed by attaching a 50-mL syringe (without the piston) to the catheter and holding the syringe at bladder height. The patient sits or stands while saline is poured into the syringe and allowed to run into the bladder by gravity. The volume at which the patient first senses bladder filling, as well as maximum bladder capacity, are recorded. Ideally, the patient will fill to a minimum of 350 mL. During the filling process, any fluctuations in the syringe water column should be noted. This simple office test is essentially a single-channel CMG and is easily performed.

The purpose of single-channel cystometry, or even simple office cystometry, is to detect the presence of detrusor instability, which occurs in 8 to 63% of incontinent women (47). Women with OAB symptoms can show variable findings on filling cystometry. The bladder may show unstable phasic contractions (of any amplitude) that cannot be suppressed (detrusor instability), a tonic rise in bladder pressure (reduced bladder compliance), or a stable but low capacity as a result of pain or urgency; or it may have normal function (stable, normal compliance, good capacity) (48). The incidence of unstable contractions is increased by making filling cystometry more provocative (e.g., faster filling speed, change in posture from supine to standing, ice-water filling, and hand washing).

Supine, single-channel cystometry will detect approximately 50 to 60% of patients with an unstable bladder (49–51). The accuracy of this test may be improved an additional 20 to 40% by performing the cystometrics:

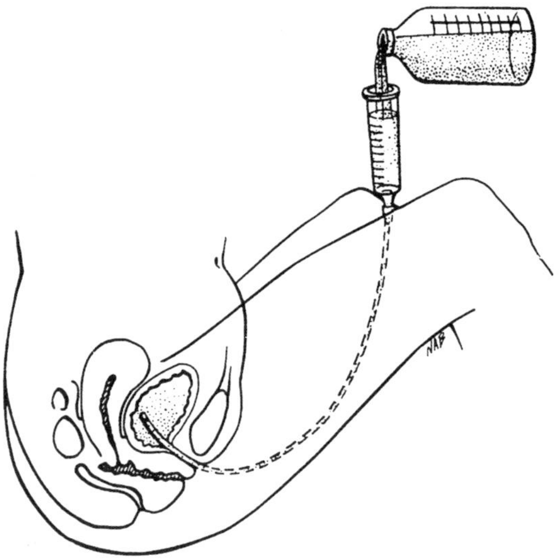

FIGURE 18.4 ● "Poor man's" cystometrogram for office evaluation of bladder filling function. With the patient in sitting or standing position with a catheter in the bladder, the bladder is filled by gravity by pouring sterile water into the syringe (no more than 100 mL/min). A rise in the fluid level associated with urgency or leakage is suggestive of detrusor instability. (Reprinted from Walters MD, Karram MM. Clinical Urogynecology. St. Louis: Mosby, 1993:55, with permission.)

- To maximum bladder capacity
- In the standing position
- With the detrusor provoking maneuvers of repetitive coughing and heel bounce

Multichannel urodynamics are a group of sophisticated urologic tests using microtransducer catheters to simultaneously record urethral, vesical, and intra-abdominal (via a vaginal catheter) pressures, and electromyographic activity of the pelvic floor. Information can be obtained by subtracted urethrocystometry, urethral pressure profilometry, instrumented voiding studies, and electromyographic recordings of the urethral sphincter. Approximately 10% of patients with lower urinary tract dysfunction will require multichannel urodynamic testing to elucidate their diagnosis. Referral for multichannel urodynamic testing should be made for patients with the conditions listed in Table 18.5. Women older than age 65 are candidates for urodynamic testing due to the higher prevalence of detrusor instability and urethral incompetence in this group of patients.

The stress test may be easily performed after the CMG. A stress test is performed in the lithotomy or standing position, and enough fluid (300 mL) needs to be placed into the bladder before declaring a negative test result. Loss of urine during the stress test is strongly suggestive

TABLE 18.5

Indications for Multichannel Urodynamic Testing

History	*Examination*
Incontinent women older than age 65	Neurologic abnormality
Prior anti-incontinence surgery	Postvoid residual >100 mL
History of neurologic disease	Incontinent women with negative stress test, negative Q-tip test, and/or normal cystometrogram
Continuous urinary leakage	Maximum bladder capacity < 350 mL or > 800 mL
Mixed stress and urge incontinence	
Suspected urethral diverticulum	
Suspected urethral spasm	
Suspected low-pressure urethra	

of genuine stress incontinence. If a slight amount of urine is lost a few seconds after the stress effort, this may indicate the presence of detrusor instability.

If the history and physical exam, in conjunction with office testing, fail to identify a diagnosis of UI, the patient should be referred to a urologic center. Multichannel studies should be considered in patients for whom the results of simpler diagnostic tests are inconclusive, when empirical treatments are unsuccessful, or in patients who have had previous corrective surgery for UI, who have known or suspected neurologic disorders, or who have a history of radical pelvic surgery.

Genuine Stress Incontinence

Genuine stress incontinence (GSI), also referred to as stress urinary incontinence (SUI), is an involuntary loss of urine that occurs with physical exertion. Patients with GSI often complain of urine loss with cough, sneeze, lifting, and physically strenuous activity. It is common in women of all ages, and the volume of urine loss may increase with age. In one study, one-third of the 450 female Army service members surveyed indicated that they experienced GSI during exercise and in field training exercises (52).

Sphincter incompetence and dysfunction of the bladder outlet are the underlying causes of GSI. GSI is a result of three inter-related factors: muscle weakness, a decrease in collagen composition, and neuromuscular damage that is probably due to weakened pelvic support. The levator ani muscles provide posterior support to the urethra as the intra-abdominal pressure increases. If this muscle is weak, the increasing intra-abdominal pressure forces the urethra to descend and open, resulting in a loss of urine. The other factor involved in the development of GSI is the collagen composition of the pelvic structures, which is believed to be genetic in origin, although it is known that estrogen deficiency can result in weakened collagen. The neuromuscular damage associated with GSI often occurs during vaginal delivery but is also associated with the aging process. Women who have had one vaginal birth are 2.5 times more likely to report GSI than nulliparous women, and the rate of GSI increases with parity (53).

Patients who have had prior surgery or who have a positive stress test with an empty bladder may have intrinsic sphincter deficiency (ISD), a condition in which the urethral sphincter cannot retain urine in the bladder. This results in loss of urine even during minimal physical exertion. This may be a congenital condition or acquired after trauma, radiation, or development of a sacral cord lesion. These patients should be evaluated further and will most likely need to be referred for management. If a patient does not have urethral hypermobility, but has GSI, then she needs evaluation for ISD and possible periurethral bulking therapy.

Treatment of Genuine Stress Incontinence

Conservative therapy should be offered to all patients with stress incontinence, although it is expected that only one-fourth to one-third of patients will accept the challenge (54, 55).

Pelvic Floor Exercise (Unassisted)

One modality of treatment consists of pelvic floor muscle training (PFMT) by repeated contraction of the muscles of the pelvic floor, primarily the pubococcygeus (56). Strengthening pelvic floor muscles has proved effective in 50 to 90% of women with GSI (57–59). Unfortunately, many women have difficulty identifying and isolating the pelvic floor muscles and find the need for daily practice too burdensome. As a result, the compliance rate with this therapy ranges from 60 to 90% (60). It is important to note that for pelvic muscle exercises to be effective, they must be performed without any Valsalva movement or accessory muscle involvement. Pelvic floor muscle exercises are of little utility for the patient with denervation injury or anatomic muscle detachments.

There are several schedules of exercise programs: (a) squeeze and hold the pelvic floor muscles up to 10 seconds; (b) relax 15 seconds; (c) repeat ten squeezes in each of the lying, sitting, and standing positions; (d) perform ten quick flicks (rapid contraction and release of the muscle) in each position; and (e) repeat the program three times daily. Patients are often unable to simply translate verbal or written instructions regarding PFMT. In one study, verbal instruction alone on Kegel exercises (with the instruction to "contract the muscles you would use if you were trying to stop your stream") resulted in appropriate contraction of the pelvic floor in only 60% of patients; 25% of the women substituted a counterproductive Valsalva maneuver (61). The physician cannot assume patients can identify the appropriate muscles unless they are directly tested during a digital vaginal examination or through the use of different vaginal or rectal sensing devices. For many private practices, patients are asked to perform PFMT with weekly instruction from a personal trainer or coach, such as a physiotherapist or nurse continence specialist. The physiotherapy sessions should consist of four to eight visits with the therapist followed by continued home therapy for a total of 12 weeks. A once-daily maintenance program is essential to preserve the effect of therapy. Reported cure rates through the use of PFMT in women with stress, urge, or mixed incontinence range from 31 to 97% (62–64).

A PFMT program may be assisted by biofeedback, such as with a vaginal probe or a set of vaginal cones (65). Starting with the lowest weight cone (20 g), patients insert the cones and maintain them intravaginally for 15 minutes, twice daily, by contracting their pelvic floor muscles. When they can retain a weight without difficulty, they progress to the next higher group (up to 100 g). One study found that vaginal weights and pelvic floor exercises were similarly effective and resulted in reducing GSI by 40 to 60% (66). Other behavioral tools, such as bladder retraining programs (discussed later in the chapter), can also be added to the program.

Pelvic Floor Exercise (Assisted)

If patients fail the previous PFMT program or are unable to perform the necessary regimen as outlined, portable biofeedback monitors may be prescribed to assist with pelvic muscle exercises done at home. One such biofeedback program is functional electrical stimulation (FES). This therapy uses a vaginal probe, connected to a 9-volt battery source and energy modulator. A setting of 20 to 50 Hz is used, with a cycle of 5 seconds on and 5 to 10 seconds off. It is somewhat less effective than PFMT, but it can be very useful in identifying the appropriate pelvic muscles for contraction. It will not work if there is no innervation to the muscles (67).

One available form of in-office therapy is the use of magnetic neuromodulation. The patient sits in a chair that contains a device that produces pulsing magnetic fields. These pulses depolarize the motor neuron membranes and induce nerve impulses that cause the muscles of the pelvic floor to contract. With this modality, all nerves in the path of the field are activated. This is in contrast to pelvic floor electrical stimulation, which requires direct transcutaneous injection for the current to penetrate and stimulate muscles. Treatment sessions with magnetic neuromodulation consist of two phases, 10 minutes at 5 Hz and 10 minutes at 50 Hz, with a rest period in between. The total treatment time is about 30 minutes, and most patients receive treatments twice weekly for 8 weeks.

Intravaginal Support Devices

There are pessary devices that can be inserted into the vagina to support the bladder neck and hence control GSI. The incontinence ring and incontinence dish pessaries are most commonly used in patients with SUI. Examples of incontinence pessary rings include the Milex incontinence rings (Milex Products, Inc., Chicago, IL) and the Cook balloon-inflated continence rings (Cook Ob/Gyn, Spencer, IN). A Hodge pessary with or without support, depending on the presence of a cystocele, may also be used. Pessaries are particularly helpful for the athlete who needs temporary protection while playing tennis or golf, jogging, or doing aerobics.

The optimum method of care for the vagina and the frequency of pessary removal needs to be tailored for each patient. Lubrication of either the pessary or vagina is usually needed prior to insertion. The pessary should be removed and cleaned every 4 to 6 weeks, depending on the pressure and amount of discharge, type of pessary, and patient comfort level. For periodic disinfection, the pessary may be either autoclaved with 5 lb of pressure at 250°F for 10 minutes, boiled for 15 minutes, or cold sterilized with Cidex.

Patients must be counseled that an incontinence pessary may cause discomfort, tissue erosion, and urinary obstruction. They may also be difficult for the elderly patient to manage because of the dexterity required to manipulate the device.

Introl (UroMed, Needham, MA) is a silicone vaginal prosthesis with two prongs that support the bladder neck on either side of the urethra. It is used for stress and mixed incontinence. It mimics the effects of urethropexy and is available in 16 sizes. The device must be fitted by a physician. The patient needs to remove and clean the device once every 24 hours, and it must be removed for intercourse. In one clinical trial, 80% of women were reportedly dry (68).

An alternative to pessaries is to use one or two tampons inside a condom. This exerts pressure against the bladder neck and can be effective in maintaining continence (69). Although specially designed tampons (e.g., Contrelle Continence Tampon, Coloplast A/S, Humlebaek, Denmark) are available, simple menstrual tampons may work as well for some women.

Newer agents include the disposable vaginal devices or "continence guards," which are made of polyurethane foam with high tissue compatibility. Examples include the Contrelle Activguard (Coloplast, Humlebaek, Denmark) (previously known as the Conveen Contiguard) and the Contiform (Free Spirit Unlimited Pty Ltd., Contiform Trading, Australia). The Contrelle Activguard is an arch-shaped polyurethane foam device that is inserted into the vagina; it has two wings to support the bladder neck. Each Activguard can only be used once. It is inserted with an applicator. The Contiform has a slightly different shape. The Contiform device comes in four different sizes, is placed into the vagina, and molds to the vaginal walls, thus providing expansive support in the vagina for the urethra and other pelvic structures. Contiform may be used for up to 30 days before it needs to be replaced. These devices can be left in for up to 16 hours and do not need to be removed to urinate.

Urinary Control Pads

Urinary control pads such as the Miniguard Patch (UroMed Corp., Needham, MA) prevent, rather than absorb, urine loss in women with mild to moderate GSI. They are small triangular foam pads with hydrophilic adhesive on one side and are not much larger than a postage stamp. The adhesive side is applied against the intralabial epithelium (over the urethral meatus), anterior to the vaginal introitus. In its final placement, it fits between the labial folds and provides pressure around the urethral opening to prevent leakage. It should not cause irritation or discomfort during use or removal. It is a single-use product and falls off when the woman voids. The patch may be worn for up to 5 hours at a time and through the night. It should not be used in women with known UTI, vaginal infections, urge, or other forms of incontinence. Clinical trials demonstrated that 52% of women reported complete dryness, and 82% improved as defined by the decrease in the number of incontinence episodes per week and pad test leakage (70).

Urinary Control Devices

The FemAssist (Insight Medical Corp., Boston, MA) and the Bard Cap Sure Continence Shields (Bard Urological Division, Covington GA) are soft suction silicone caps that are placed externally over the external urethral meatus. An ointment is applied to the inner surface to create a vacuum seal that holds the cap in place. Suction from the device creates negative pressure, inducing coaptation of the urethral walls, and increasing urethral pressure. It does not act as a reservoir to collect urine when leakage occurs. The placement does not have to be exact, and after the device is in place, the labia fold over it and the device cannot be seen or felt. When the patient needs to urinate, the suction cap is easily pulled off, and the cap may then be washed with soap and water and reapplied.

The FemAssist device can, according to the manufacturer, be reused for up to 1 week. Although the expense of FemAssist is offset somewhat by its reusability, its efficacy is limited, and many patients discontinue use of the device because of discomfort. Moore et al. enrolled 97 patients in a study of the FemAssist, of whom only 57 (57%) completed the 1-month trial. Of the 57 women who completed 1 month of use, 27 (47%) were continent on pad testing. It had equal benefits for women with stress, urge, or mixed incontinence (71).

In one study of patients with stress incontinence, CapSure reduced urine loss by 96% within 1 week, and 82% of patients were completely dry. Side effects include irritation and UTIs, although they are not severe (72).

Urethral Occlusion Insert

The Reliance Urinary Control Insert (UroMed Corp., Norwood, MA) is a soft, balloon-tipped, small, catheterlike insert that is fitted inside the urethra. It has a balloon at its proximal end that is inflated with a small amount of air to aid retention. The balloon rests above the bladder neck, obstructing the flow of urine. The balloon can be deflated by an attached string, allowing removal of the device and voiding. The device is disposable and is approved by the U.S. Food and Drug Administration (FDA).

Objective measurement of urine loss in a multicenter clinical study revealed that 92% of patients achieved an 80% decrease in urine loss, and 80% were completely dry (73). In a separate study by Sand et al., urine loss was reduced or eliminated in 91% of 63 women who answered a validated questionnaire (74). Complications associated with the Reliance device include bacteriuria in 30% of users, gross hematuria in 24%, and mucosal irritation in 9%. Other problems reported with this method include migration of the device into the bladder and risk of UTI (75).

The FemSoft Insert (Rochester Medical Products, Stewartville, MN) is a sterile disposable, single-use intraurethral device that consists of a narrow silicone tube enclosed in a soft mineral oil-filled silicone sleeve. The sleeve forms a balloon on the tip of the insert. As it is placed into the urethra, the fluid in the balloon is transferred toward the external retainer to facilitate introduction into the length of the urethra. Once the tip enters the bladder, the fluid returns to fill the balloon at the tip, thus forming a mechanical barrier to retain urine within the bladder. The device comes with a disposable applicator and lubricating gel, is easily removed for normal voiding and should be removed at least once every 6 hours. It is available in different diameter sizes and lengths.

In a study of the FemSoft Insert, results for 1 to 2 years of follow-up for all study participants (mean 15 months) showed a statistically significant reduction in both incontinence episodes and amount of urine loss. In the study, 81% of women reported they never or rarely experience incontinence while the FemSoft Insert was in place, and the authors concluded its efficacy was exceeded only by surgical intervention. The long-term results showed women in the study were highly satisfied with the product's ease of use, comfort, and dryness. Significant improvements in quality of life were also observed (76).

Bioinjectables

Injections of bulking materials that help support the urethra are used for patients with GSI caused by intrinsic sphincter deficiency alone or with urethral hypermobility but who still have good pelvic muscle support and functional bladders. It is particularly useful for elderly women, who have stress incontinence without excessive vaginal prolapse. Any coexisting bladder instability or hyperactivity should be medically treated and managed prior to having the procedure; otherwise, it is likely to fail. A variety of agents have been used to produce a bulking effect in the proximal urethra, including collagen, autologous fat, and polytetrafluoroethylene.

The most common bulking agent currently used is a glutaraldehyde cross-linked bovine collagen (Contigen, Bard Urological Division). A skin test should be performed on the patient at least 4 weeks prior to the injection. The collagen is injected either transurethrally through a cystoscope or periurethrally into the submucosa of the proximal urethra. The procedure is done in the office and takes about 20 to 40 minutes. Patients, or their caregivers, must be taught to self-catheterize because this may be necessary for a few days after the procedure.

Patients whose incontinence does not improve with five injection procedures (five separate treatment sessions) are considered treatment failures, and no further treatment by collagen implant is covered. Collagen implants should not be used in patients with bladder neck or urethral strictures until such strictures have been corrected. Physicians using this technique must be comfortable and skilled with the use of a cystoscope and have completed a collagen implant training program.

Various local complications have been described following transurethral or periurethral collagen injection therapy, including sterile and nonsterile abscess formation and periurethral pseudocyst development (77–79). Postprocedural abscesses are typically characterized by early onset of pain and irritative voiding symptoms following injection. Periurethral pseudocysts usually follow distal migration of the collagen, resulting in a small nontender collagen-filled mass at the meatus. A single case report of the formation of a urethral diverticulum after collagen injection therapy has been reported (80). An increase in autoimmune disease has been reported in a small number of cases, and the procedure may not be appropriate for patients with certain cardiac conditions. Patients may experience immediate improvement followed by a temporary relapse after a week or so. Generally, it takes about 1 month for the full benefits to be apparent. The collagen is absorbed over time, so injections usually need to be repeated every 6 to 18 months. Collagen injections are not very beneficial after radiation therapy.

In a study by Steele et al, periurethral collagen injections were used in a series of 40 women with urinary incontinence due to ISD with or without accompanying urethral hypermobility. Both groups required similar numbers of procedures and amounts of collagen to achieve dryness. Urethral hypermobility does not preclude the use of collagen injections in women with SUI (81).

Autologous fat has also been used as a bulking agent, is readily available and is biocompatible. It is inexpensive when compared with collagen and has no problem with migration. The main disadvantage is its variability of absorption. Excellent short-term results have been reported (82).

Another technique being explored uses saline-filled microballoons as the periurethral bulking agent (UroVive, UroSurge, Inc., Coralville, IA). In a study by Marberger et al., 19 women with both hypermobility and ISD were treated and followed for 1 year; 79% reported significant improvement. In this approach, anywhere between one and five balloons (an average of three) are injected at the 3-, 9-, and 12-o'clock positions. The balloons appear to have excellent biocompatibility, incur no tissue reaction, and provide long-lasting coaptation (83).

Absorbency Products

Absorbance products are designed to absorb and contain urine. The urine-holding capacity of absorbency products varies; it is not standardized. The most common types of products used include pads, guards, undergarments and protective underwear, and briefs. The pad is attached to the woman's underwear or panties. The undergarments have elasticized legs with a belt attached with buttons or Velcro. Diaperlike products have elasticized legs and self-adhesive tabs. Pantlike products, or briefs, are also available, and they contain built-in absorbent materials.

Medical Therapies

Alpha Adrenergic Stimulators

Definitive medical therapy is currently lacking for GSI. Most current medical agents (alpha-adrenergic stimulators) are ineffectual, although in off-label usage some patients have reported improvement with phenylpropanolamine, Ornade, and pseudoephedrine (84). It has also been found that a local estrogen effect combined with an alpha-adrenergic agonist may increase this response (85).

Estrogen

Estrogen has been shown to improve vascular flow to the bladder neck, enhance perineal neurologic function, and correct atrophy of the vaginal mucosa (86, 87). Although multiple observational studies using oral and vaginal routes of hormone administration have reported improvement in incontinence symptoms, more recent prospective randomized studies have less convincing conclusions (88, 89). It may be that early estrogen use will help prevent incontinence and later use may be useful as an adjunct to other therapies.

Tricyclic Antidepressants

Because they have anticholinergic and alpha-adrenergic properties, tricyclic antidepressants may also be used for the treatment of GSI or urge incontinence. Typically, imipramine (Tofranil) is given at a dose of 10 to 25 mg, twice or three times daily. In elderly patients, doses should be kept as low as possible because of the risk of orthostatic hypotension.

Duloxetine

Duloxetine is a new agent, a balanced serotonin and norepinephrine reuptake inhibitor that increases the local concentration of these neurotransmitters equally at their receptor site. This results in a prolonged contraction of the striated rhabdosphincter muscle surrounding the urethra. Contraction of the rhabdosphincter is weak under normal conditions, but when duloxetine is used in the presence of bladder irritation, there is an eightfold increase in periurethral striated muscle electromyographic activity (85). In phase II testing of 553 women, there was significant improvement in the median incontinence episode frequency with duloxetine versus placebo. There were no clinically severe side effects in the duloxetine group; however, nausea was reported as the most common adverse effect resulting in discontinuation of therapy (90).

Overactive Bladder (Urge Incontinence)

Previously referred to as detrusor instability or urge incontinence, OAB is a common condition that affects women of all ages. The precise prevalence of this specific disorder is not known; however, the prevalence of incontinence due to OAB as a result of both urge and mixed incontinence in the United States is estimated to be approximately 17% (91). Part of the difficulty in determining the prevalence of OAB is whether the definition is based on urodynamics, the International Continence Society classification system, or on symptoms of frequency, urgency, and incontinence. Studies do suggest that the prevalence of OAB increases linearly with age (92, 93).

OAB is characterized by involuntary contractions of the detrusor muscle that occur during the filling phase and in the absence of local pathologic factors. These contractions result in urinary frequency, urgency, or urge incontinence (either alone or in combination). Until more recently, OAB was diagnosed only in patients with incontinence. As a result of this, a large subset of patients was not diagnosed despite having symptoms of frequency or urgency.

Symptoms

The three typical symptoms of OAB include urinary frequency, urinary urgency, and urge incontinence. Urgency is the sudden compelling desire to void. Urge incontinence is the involuntary leakage of urine accompanied by or immediately preceded by urgency. The most common symptom reported by patients with OAB is frequency of urination, with nighttime episodes (nocturia) being the most disruptive to their lives. The aforementioned symptoms may occur alone or in combination. Patients with symptoms of OAB may limit fluid intake and may void at frequent intervals to avoid accidents.

The symptoms of OAB may be caused by a number of conditions affecting the lower urinary tract, including

- Lower UTI—The most common cause of urinary symptoms is lower UTI.
- Neurogenic—Conditions that cause inappropriate activation of the sacral reflex arc may cause bladder overactivity; examples include stroke, Parkinson's disease, multiple sclerosis, tumors, and spinal cord lesions.
- Stress incontinence
- Fluid intake—Patients may limit fluid intake, but prolonged fluid depletion can lead to bladder irritability.
- Diet—It has been suggested that artificial sweeteners and certain acidic foods may cause sensory urgency in some patients.
- Bowel function—There may be a link between irritable bowel syndrome and OAB. Constipation in particular is believed to irritate the bladder.
- Atrophic vaginitis—There is much debate about the role of menopause and estrogen loss as significant contributors (94).
- Smoking—In in vitro studies, nicotine produces a phasic contraction of isolated bladder muscle probes (95, 96).
- Age—Bladder capacity, urethral compliance, and flow rates decrease with age. No gender bias has been found (97).
- Drugs—Medications that may be associated with OAB include diuretics, phenothiazines, opioids, and alcohol.

OAB is an associated risk factor for accidents and depression. Hurrying to get to the toilet increases the risk of falls by 30% and the risk of fractures by 3% (98, 99). Nocturia is a significant risk in unsteady patients, who may fall on their way to the toilet or may be only half awake and have difficulty mobilizing in the dark. Depression is also said to occur in 60% of people with OAB (100). Studies suggest a link between the serotonergic neuronal systems in anxiety and depression because descending serotonin pathways from the brain inhibit bladder contractions. This suggests a biochemical link between depression and OAB.

OAB affects almost every facet of a patient's life: social, physical, occupational, sexual, and psychological. Most studies looking at the impact on quality of life by type of incontinence have found urge incontinence to have a greater impact than stress incontinence on psychological, social, and physical functioning (101, 102). This is most likely due to the unpredictable nature of OAB and, when it is accompanied by urge incontinence, usually larger volumes of urine are lost than what occurs with GSI.

One survey found that most people with chronic symptoms of OAB complained only of frequency and urgency; and only one-third of those surveyed discussed urge incontinence with their physicians (103). In one study, among patients seeking medical care for OAB, 44% had experienced symptoms for 5 years or more before presenting and 88% for at least 1 year before presenting. Common coping strategies employed by these patients included avoiding social interaction, toilet mapping, carrying spare clothing, and avoiding long journeys, all of which can lead to social exclusion (104).

A baseline evaluation for patients with symptoms of OAB includes a thorough history to characterize the nature of the voiding dysfunction. The physical exam should focus on GI, gynecologic, neurologic, and urologic evaluations. A urinalysis should be performed. In most patients with OAB, an analysis of symptoms is sufficient for establishing a working diagnosis and initiating treatment. For more complicated disease, the assessment may include the use of a voiding diary, anatomic evaluation of the urinary tract and nervous system, residual urine measurement, and sophisticated urodynamics studies.

Treatment

In contrast to treatments available for stress incontinence, of which several have a long-term cure rate of higher than 80%, medical and surgical treatments for urge incontinence currently achieve long-term cures in a far smaller proportion of patients (105–107).

Bladder Retraining

Initial conservative therapy is offered in the form of bladder retraining; this treatment restores a normal bladder pattern (44, 58, 108). The overall aim of bladder retraining is to increase the time interval between voids. Before any bladder re-education process can start, however, a baseline bladder diary is essential. The voiding diary, or urolog, is used to assess current voiding patterns, frequency, and voided volumes. (A sample diary is shown in Figure 18.1.) The bladder diary can also be used to determine longest time between voids. The largest volume of urine voided can be noted, as an indirect measure of how much the bladder can hold.

Bladder retraining is best performed in conjunction with a therapist. In one approach to bladder retraining, the patient is asked to void every 1 to 1.5 hours by the clock, depending on the normal voiding interval as determined by a 24-hour diary. It is important that most voids occur prior to a strong urge to urinate, and the program ends for the day at bedtime. After 1 week, the voiding interval is increased by 15 minutes. The process continues for 4 to 8 weeks, and the patient records voiding times each day. Eventually, the voiding interval is 2.5 to 3 hours. PFMT (Kegel exercises) are also taught to control sudden voiding urges. In clinical studies, 75 to 80% of bladder retraining participants reported improvement in bladder control (109, 110). The term "bladder retraining" has been applied to a variety of scheduled voiding regimens, including timed voiding, prompted voiding, habit training, and patterned urge responses toileting (Table 18.6).

Pelvic Floor Exercises (Assisted and Unassisted)

Refer to the previous section on GSI for a complete discussion of these techniques. There is evidence for a positive correlation between the number of daily pelvic floor contractions and improvement rates for OAB (62, 111).

Functional Electrical Stimulation

If patients have not obtained control with bladder retraining or medication, then it is feasible to use a trial of FES (112). The settings in this case are 5 to 20 Hz, with a cycle of 5 seconds on and 5 to 10 seconds off. There is an expected response of 50% (113). If these therapies have been unsuccessful, then one may have to consider sacral neuromodulation. This form of nerve stimulation requires an implanted electrode at sacral nerve root three, and a pacing device inserted under the skin of the buttock (114).

TABLE 18.6

Types of Bladder Retraining Schedules

- *Timed voiding*—This approach uses a fixed schedule of toileting. It is particularly useful for clients who are unable to toilet independently. For example, it is used for debilitated older people, usually with a two-hourly interval, and can be used in conjunction with triggers such as running water or tapping the thigh.
- *Prompted voiding*—This approach involves prompts at regular intervals. It is particularly useful for patients who have some awareness but do not ask to go to the toilet. It is used most often in institutionalized settings; patients are asked whether they need to go to the toilet at regular intervals, but are only taken if they want to go (110, 197, 198).
- *Habit training*—This approach encourages a pattern of toileting depending on habit. The pattern should be based on the individual habit; a bladder diary will help establish a pattern (199).

Medications

Medication is often combined with bladder drills to obtain quicker and more effective results. Most drugs used to treat OAB either directly or indirectly decrease the uninhibited detrusor contractions that are characteristic of OAB. Common types of drug therapies and their potential actions are listed in Table 18.7.

Although a wide variety of agents have been used to treat OAB, antimuscarinics are most commonly prescribed for this condition. The antimuscarinic drugs commonly used for OAB are hyoscyamine (Urimax, Prosed DS, NuLev, Arco-Lase Plus), oxybutynin (Ditropan, Ditropan XL), propantheline (Pro-Banthine), and tolterodine (Detrol) (Table 18.8).

Oxybutynin

Oxybutynin (Ditropan) is considered the "gold standard" pharmacologic agent for the treatment of OAB. It effectively reduces intravesical pressure and the frequency of bladder contractions while increasing bladder capacity (115). Due to poor uroselectivity, systemic anticholinergic effects with oxybutynin immediate-release formulation result in up to an 80% discontinuation rate (116). The most common complaint responsible for discontinuance is dry mouth, whereas constipation, dizziness, and central nervous system (CNS) effects are less frequently reported (117).

The extended-release formulation of oxybutynin, Oxybutynin XL, has the benefit over immediate-release formulation of decreasing the incidence and severity of dry mouth, but there is no significant reduction in the incidence of other anticholinergic side effects, such as somnolence, dizziness, and constipation (117). The usual dose of Oxybutynin XL is 5 to 10 mg.

TABLE 18.7

Types of Drug Therapies Commonly Used in the Treatment of Urge Incontinence

Type of Drug	Potential Action
Diuretics	Cause brisk filling of bladder
Anticholinergics	Impair detrusor contraction
Sedatives or hypnotics	Cause confusion
Narcotics	Impair detrusor contraction
α-Adrenergic agonists	Increase tone of internal sphincter
α-Adrenergic antagonists	Decrease tone of internal sphincter
Calcium channel blockers	Decrease detrusor contraction

TABLE 18.8

Medications for Overactive Bladder

Medication	Strength (mg)	Dose/Frequency
Ditropan XL	5, 10, 15	5–30 daily
Detrol LA[a]	2, 4	2–6 daily
Hyoscyamine	0.125	0.125 twice to four times a day
Dicyclomine	10, 20	10–20 twice to four times a day
Oxybutynin[b]	5	5–10 twice to four times a day
Propantheline[b,c]	15, 30, 60	15–60 twice to four times a day

[a] Uroselective.
[b] Lacks uroselectivity.
[c] Excess adverse effects.
Has uroselectivity:

A newer transdermal patch formulation, Oxybutynin TDS (Oxytrol), was more recently approved by the FDA. Avoidance of hepatic and GI drug metabolism minimizes serum levels of the active metabolite, N-desethyloxybutynin, which is responsible for severe anticholinergic side effects. In a phase III clinical trial of patients with OAB, there was no significant difference in the incidence of dry mouth, constipation, CNS disturbances, or visual changes in the oxybutynin-TDS group compared with placebo. The most common side effect of oxybutynin-TDS was pruritus and erythema at the cutaneous application site. A discontinuation rate of 10.2% was associated with this reaction (118).

Intravesicular oxybutynin has been found to be effective in patients with urge incontinence who have spinal cord disease, have detrusor hyperactivity secondary to indwelling catheters, and who failed conventional therapy. Hence, most studies of this delivery method are small. Self-catheterization to instill the medication is required three to four times a day. This method is cumbersome for the general population of people with OAB (119, 120).

Tolterodine

Tolterodine (Detrol) is the first agent designed specifically for OAB. It exhibits selectivity for the muscarinic receptors in the urinary tract system in contrast to those in the salivary glands. This selective affinity results in fewer and less intense episodes of dry mouth than what occurs with Oxybutynin. In addition, tolterodine has a lower incidence of other adverse events including: headache, fatigue, GI symptoms, and CNS symptoms (121, 122).

Clinical trials in patients using tolterodine for OAB demonstrate a reduction in incontinence episodes and increase in bladder capacity (122). In 12-month studies, tolterodine decreased voiding frequency by 20% and the number of incontinence episodes by 74% (123). Use of tolterodine is contraindicated in patients with severe urinary retention, gastric retention, and uncorrected narrow-angle glaucoma. Patients taking drugs that inhibit CYP3A4, such as nefazodone (Serzone) and fluvoxamine (Luvox), should not take dosages of tolterodine in excess of 1 mg twice a day (124).

With the use of either Oxybutynin or tolterodine, studies show that most patients have a 60 to 70% response rate, but medications must be continued long after the therapeutic response (125–127).

Trospium

Trospium (Indevus Pharmaceuticals, Lexington, MA), a new antimuscarinic, was submitted for FDA approval for the indication of OAB in April 2003. It is highly selective for the muscarinic receptors in the bladder, and because this drug does not undergo hepatic metabolism by the cytochrome P-450 system at therapeutic levels, 80% of the drug is excreted unchanged in the bladder (128, 129). As a result, a large percentage of the drug acts directly on the bladder (129).

Theoretically, its hydrophilic design will minimize passage of the drug across the blood-brain barrier, thus reducing CNS effects (130).

Tricyclic antidepressants

As mentioned in the preceding section, because of effectiveness in decreasing bladder contractility and increasing outlet resistance, tricyclic antidepressants have been used in the treatment of OAB and stress incontinence. In patients with mixed incontinence, imipramine 150 mg daily has been recommended (131). With its sedating effect, use of imipramine often improves nocturnal incontinence as well. The disadvantage of tricyclic antidepressants is their narrow safety profile; in elderly patients, doses should be kept as low as possible because of the risk of orthostatic hypotension.

Antispasmodics

Although it has been used for OAB, the mechanism of flavoxate hydrochloride (Urispas) is not well defined (132). It is not currently recommended for OAB, and randomized, placebo-controlled studies showed no benefit over placebo in the treatment of OAB (133).

Alpha-adrenergic Antagonists

Past off-label therapy with alpha-adrenergic antagonists has had limited success in the treatment of OAB (134).

Calcium Channel Blockers

Calcium channel blockers depress bladder contractility. It is believed these drugs possess potential for therapy as intravesical agents or in combination with other anticholinergic agents (135).

Detrusor Sphincter Dyssynergia

Detrusor sphincter dyssynergia is a condition characterized by simultaneous contraction of both the bladder and urethral sphincter muscle (internal or external), so voiding cannot occur (136). The urethral sphincter muscle may suddenly relax, and then incontinence occurs. Consequently, clinical effects range from retention to complete incontinence. Detrusor-sphincter dyssynergia usually presents with incomplete emptying, and patients may describe the passage of urine as being drop by drop, painful, and an accompanying sense of bladder spasm (stranguria).

This condition is common in patients with multiple sclerosis (MS). In fact, more than 80% of MS patients have symptoms of lower genitourinary tract dysfunction, and among patients who have had the disease for longer than 10 years, more than 96% have urologic findings (137–140). Among patients with MS, detrusor sphincter dyssynergia highly correlates with cervical plaque formation and increased cerebrospinal fluid myelin basic protein ($p < 0.05$) (137, 140, 141). In sharp contrast to the associated upper tract dysfunction with dyssynergia in spinal cord injury patients, detrusor sphincter dyssynergia in the MS population is more commonly associated with local symptoms of incomplete emptying, elevated postvoid residuals, bladder calculi, and infection (136, 140, 142–145). The hyper-reflexia and degree of external sphincter spasm in MS may also be less severe than that seen in spinal cord injury patients (144, 145).

The proper method for diagnosing detrusor sphincter dyssynergia is unclear, and there is debate about the roles of urethral versus anal electromyography, wire or patch electrodes, urethral pressure gradients, and video urodynamic urethral assessments. Of these options, electromyography is commonly used (136, 146, 147). Urethral pressure profilometry has a limited role in the assessment of detrusor sphincter dyssynergia. Studies using profilometry have demonstrated urethral pressures that have failed to correlate reliably with neurologic dysfunction in MS (144, 148). Urodynamic evaluation may facilitate the decision for clean intermittent catheterization by defining bladder storage capabilities and selecting the optimum catheterization interval.

Treating patients with detrusor sphincter dyssynergia conservatively with alpha-1 blocking agents (prazosin) and muscle relaxants (diazepam, baclofen, dantrolene) has had mixed results (149, 150). Patients may do well with an antispasmodic medication such as Ditropan XL or Detrol LA, and anecdotal success has been reported with tizanidine, a new spasmolytic with centrally acting alpha-2 adrenergic properties. Clean intermittent catheterization has been the primary treatment for patients with emptying difficulties and may aid in bladder rehabilitation (151).

Mixed Incontinence

Mixed incontinence involves a combination of symptoms of urge and stress incontinence. Approximately one-third of elderly women with urge incontinence have symptoms or signs of stress incontinence (152). The diagnosis is generally based on symptoms rather than pure urodynamic findings.

Conservative intervention with combined pelvic floor muscle training and bladder retraining is an ideal first line approach. FES may also help both conditions. With its anticholinergic and alpha-adrenergic effects, imipramine may be used for the treatment of mixed incontinence. If symptoms of urge incontinence are predominant, consideration should be given to the use of oxybutynin as first-line therapy.

Although there is no foolproof way to determine relative severity of either GSI or OAB, a decision is made as to which is the predominant problem, and further therapy is usually directed in this manner. If the clinical history and urodynamic findings suggest that GSI is the predominant problem, surgery may be beneficial. For symptoms of urge incontinence that remain postoperatively, treatment for OAB may be indicated.

Detrusor Hyperactivity With Incomplete Contractility

Detrusor hyperactivity with incomplete contractility (DHIC) is common in the elderly. In this condition, the bladder will contract uncontrollably, but the emptying is incomplete. The patient's bladder fills more quickly because it is never completely empty. Medical therapy aggravates the retention; therapies to try include double voiding, Credé maneuver, and intermittent self-catheterization in conjunction with an antispasmodic such as flavoxate (Rispas) (153).

Overflow Incontinence

Overflow incontinence occurs when bladder pressure remains low or the outlet pressure remains high, causing the bladder to distend and spill small (or large) amounts of urine. Overflow incontinence does not occur until the residual amount of urine is somewhere in excess of 350 mL, and the urine at that point creates enough pressure in the bladder to overcome the urethral resistance and leakage occurs. Low bladder pressures are often caused by lower motor neuron disease, and high outlet pressures occur most often with an obstructive cause. Causes of overflow incontinence secondary to low bladder pressure include diabetes mellitus, stroke, MS, pelvic trauma or extensive pelvic surgery, and spinal trauma or lesions. High outlet pressures may occur with urethral stricture or detrusor dyssynergia. Patients may note frequent or continuous dribbling, the bladder may be palpable on exam and urodynamic studies will reflect decreased flow rates.

Treatment may employ intermittent or continuous catheterization, double voiding, or relaxation exercises.

Bypass of the Continence Mechanism

Fistula Formation

Vesicovaginal fistulas usually result from local trauma and necrosis, following prolonged labor or an iatrogenic event during gynecologic surgery. In the latter case, fistulas are typically supratrigonal and occur mainly when the procedure is technically difficult, or the ability of local tissue healing is altered by fibrosis, infection, or previous radiotherapy (154). Leakage of urine may start immediately after surgery, or even up to 30 days after. The leakage is constant: day and night. Fistulas require advanced evaluation and management. Vesicovaginal fistulas always represent a distressing medical condition for the patient and demand much attention. Several surgical techniques have been used in these cases with failure rates ranging from 4 to 35%

(155–157). Full discussion of fistula formation and surgical repair is beyond the scope of this text.

Urethral Diverticulum

Urethral diverticulum in women is uncommon and usually presents between the third and fifth decades, although it has been reported in neonates and young women (158). Although it is reported to occur in 1 to 6% of all women, the true incidence is likely much higher because the diagnosis of urethral diverticulum is not always straightforward, and many urethral diverticula are believed to be asymptomatic (159, 160). Urethral diverticulum may be congenital or acquired. Most cases in women are acquired, resulting from infection of the paraurethral glands with subsequent rupture into the urethral lumen. Other etiologies include urethral injury during childbirth or surgery and repetitive trauma secondary to catheterization.

The pathognomonic presentation of postvoid dribbling, urethral pain, tender periurethral mass and/or expression of pus from the urethra on physical examination is actually uncommon (161). Most patients present with nonspecific, refractory, lower urinary tract symptoms that are unrelated to the diverticulum size or number. Urethral diverticulum can cause various symptoms and be misdiagnosed as more common conditions, including cystitis, stress incontinence, and infected periurethral glands (162). Ganabathi et al. reported SUI as an initial symptom in 62% of women with urethral diverticula (158).

Many women undergo extensive evaluation and empirical treatments before correct diagnosis is established (158). Clinical awareness and a high index of clinical suspicion are essential for ordering proper diagnostic tests to make the definitive diagnosis and formulate a treatment plan.

Historically, voiding cystourethrogram and double balloon pressure urethrography were the initial imaging tests of choice. Although these techniques are valuable for diagnosing urethral diverticulum, they have limitations. Urethrography may be time consuming and difficult to perform. Also, it is only adequate when the neck of the diverticulum is sufficiently patent to enable diverticulum filling with contrast material. If a diverticulum is filled with pus or debris, this may prevent adequate filling with contrast medium and an appropriate diagnosis (163). Furthermore, both of these techniques use ionizing radiation and require urethral catheterization.

Cystourethroscopy is the only diagnostic tool that allows direct inspection of the urethra and bladder. It may be used to locate the diverticulum communication site and assess any associated neoplasm(s) or bladder stones. Although it is commonly used, its usefulness for diagnosing this entity has been questioned. For example, if the diverticulum neck is hidden between collapsed urethral folds or does not fully communicate with the urethral lumen, its usefulness as a diagnostic tool is significantly decreased (162). Furthermore, it is not helpful for evaluating diverticulum size or shape, or the appearance of the diverticulum wall (162). Like voiding cystourethrogram and double balloon urethrography, cystourethroscopy is also invasive and increases the risk of UTI.

Magnetic resonance imaging (MRI) and endoluminal MRI have a high degree of accuracy for evaluating urethral diverticulum. Although they have high sensitivity, as well as excellent positive and negative predictive value, their primary disadvantage is relatively high cost. For this reason, these tests are usually reserved for cases with equivocal findings in which clinical findings are strongly suggestive of urethral diverticulum (164–167).

Currently, transvaginal ultrasound is the preferred initial method of evaluation. Compared with other diagnostic tools, including voiding cystourethrogram, MRI, and cystoscopy, transvaginal ultrasound is less expensive (160). Furthermore, the ability to image in different orientations helps clarify the spatial relationship of the diverticulum to the urethra.

The approach to patients with a urethral diverticulum varies depending on the presenting symptoms. Some diverticula are asymptomatic and require no treatment. Acute inflammation of the diverticular sac often presents as a tender suburethral swelling, and purulent material can be expressed from the urethral meatus on massage of the anterior vaginal wall. An inflamed diverticulum may be managed initially by either transvaginal aspiration of the purulent material, followed by a 7- to 10-day course of antibiotics designed to cover uropathogens, or by urethral dilation with transvaginal massage to express the purulent contents of the diverticular sac. Surgical procedures to repair a diverticulum are best postponed until any acute inflammation has subsided.

The operative approach depends on the location of the sac in relationship to the maximum urethral pressure point, which is determined by urethral pressure profilometry. Thus, preoperative urodynamics with urethral pressure profiles are essential.

Functional Incontinence

Functional incontinence occurs when a patient would otherwise be continent but, because of physical or cognitive problems or use of various medications, is unable to reach the toilet facilities in time. This may occur secondary to decreased mobility due to severe arthritis, weakness (from strokes or deconditioning), contractures, or the use of physical restraints. Functional incontinence may also be caused by medications, impaired cognition (e.g., from delirium or dementia), or excessive distance of the patient from the toilet facilities. Patients with peripheral edema from any cause often have fluid shifts at night from recumbency, resulting in nocturia. Generally, patients with functional incontinence have normally functioning urinary systems, and the incontinence is a result of some external factor. Therefore, it is important to distinguish this type of incontinence from other types to appropriately manage it and to address any other coexisting forms of incontinence that may be present. It is, then, a diagnosis of exclusion, and as such, requires complete assessment and treatment of all other potential causes of incontinence.

IRRITATIVE BLADDER PROBLEMS

Although UI primarily affects women older than age 35, women of all ages may suffer from conditions that produce irritative bladder complaints. Patients typically report significant urinary urgency and frequency, which may be associated with dysuria, suprapubic pressure, pain on distention of the bladder, nocturia, postvoid fullness, or dyspareunia. These symptoms may be difficult to distinguish from those associated with an OAB. These symptoms may be episodic in nature, or they may be chronic with acute exacerbations. The conditions most commonly associated with irritative bladder symptoms are acute UTI, acute urethritis, chronic urethritis (urethral syndrome), interstitial cystitis, or detrusor instability. Nonurologic etiologies should also be considered, including vaginal infection (e.g., chlamydia), acute or chronic vulvitis, or atrophic vaginitis.

Urethral Syndrome

Urethral syndrome, or frequency dysuria syndrome, is characterized by frequency dysuria and suprapubic discomfort without any objective finding of urologic abnormalities (168). The etiology is uncertain, although there are numerous theories. Urinary frequency in this syndrome occurs during the day more than during the night. Dysuria or constant suprapubic discomfort is partially relieved by voiding. Patients may also report of difficulty in starting urination, slow stream, and a feeling of incomplete emptying of the bladder. Evaluation includes negative urinalysis/urine culture and normal residual urine determination. The 24-hour voiding diary usually shows frequent daytime voiding of small amounts, but minimal nighttime activity. Cystourethroscopy is normal.

Acute dysuria of less than 2 weeks' duration and associated with urine culture of less than 10^5 bacteria/mL is referred to as "the acute urethral syndrome." The recognition of the specific etiologic diagnosis of this syndrome has led to the more rational evaluation and management of these women. The usual differential diagnosis includes unsuspected pyelonephritis, cystitis, gonococcal infection, chlamydia infection, and vaginitis. These conditions are usually collectively referred to as "dysuria-pyuria syndrome" because all are associated with pyuria, which is considered to be a more reliable index of infectious etiology than is quantitative urine culture.

Chronic urethral syndrome is defined as recurrent irritative urinary symptoms without pyuria, or less than 10^2 bacteria/mL in urine culture. Currently theorized etiologies include hormonal imbalances, a reaction to certain foods, environmental chemicals (e.g., douches, bubble bath, soaps, contraceptive gels, condoms), hypersensitivity following UTI, and traumatic sexual intercourse. Regardless of the initial pain-causing event, the patient has both involuntary spasms and voluntary tightening of the pelvic musculature during the painful episode, which, in addition to any residual irritant or reinjury, starts a vicious cycle of worsening dysfunction of the pelvic floor musculature. Often, the original cause of the pain has healed, but the pelvic floor dysfunction persists and is worsened by patient anxiety and frustration with the condition.

If an infective etiology is suspected, then a course of doxycycline 100 mg twice daily for 10 days, or azithromycin daily for 5 days (Z-Pak), is recommended. The patient is commenced on daily urinary tract prophylaxis with nitrofurantoin 50 to 100 mg daily. If this treatment regimen is not effective, then the next course is amitriptyline (Elavil) 10 to 12.5 mg given as a single dose at 6 PM. The dose is increased every 2 to 3 weeks until the dose is 25 to 50 mg. Six weeks may be needed for therapeutic effect, and the drug, if effective, is continued for 1 to 2 years. The time of administration cannot be stressed enough because there is severe tiredness with onset after 4 or 5 hours (not until patient goes to bed) that lasts 8 to 10 hours (usually over by the next morning when she gets up).

During symptom flare-up, interval treatment may be provided using Cystospaz, Urised, or Pyridium plus for 1 to several days as shown in Table 18.1. Some patients may respond to a combination of diazepam 2 mg two to three times a day and doxazosin (Cardura) 1 to 4 mg per day or prazosin (Minipress). Urethral dilatation and massage is an old therapy with few current indications, other than those patients who have responded to this therapy in the past and who return intermittently requesting retreatment.

Many patients are treated repetitively with only temporary relief of symptoms. The nonspecific nature of these complaints may result in misdiagnosis when recurrent symptoms are attributed to the same condition. It is essential that the physician take a careful, detailed history and re-evaluate each episode to explore the possibility of other causes for the patient's irritative bladder complaints.

Interstitial Cystitis

Interstitial cystitis (IC) is a predominantly female condition (9:1) that has an estimated prevalence ranging from 30 to 500 cases per 100,000 (169, 170). The diagnostic criteria for IC are controversial and often ill defined, the treatment is frequently unsuccessful, and there is a lack of objective and subjective tests to predict or monitor response to treatment (170). Generally agreed criteria for the diagnosis of IC are symptoms of frequency (more than eight voids per day) and urgency, usually with pain; awake bladder capacity less than 350 mL; and the cystoscopic findings of mucosal fissuring or tearing (Hunner's ulcer) seen during, or glomerulations (petechial hemorrhages) seen after, bladder distention.

The initial insult or insults that lead to interstitial cystitis remain unknown. The pathophysiology of interstitial cystitis is incompletely understood, although altered epithelial permeability, mast cell activation, and sensory afferent nerve upregulation play critical roles. However, an altered bladder epithelial permeability results in a complex cascade of changes and interactions involving urinary cations (e.g., potassium), sensory nerves, activated mast cells, detrusor muscle overactivity, and spinal cord sensitization. The resultant vicious circle of inflammation and nerve sensitization leads to the chronicity that is the hallmark of interstitial cystitis. Many patients with interstitial cystitis also have associated diseases such as allergies, autoimmune diseases, fibromyalgia, other rheumatic diseases, and irritable bowel syndrome. Urinary frequency and urgency, as well as urodynamically confirmed detrusor instability, have been shown to be significantly more common among women with irritable bowel syndrome than controls (171). The overlap between these various conditions suggests a common pathophysiology mediated by immune, endocrine, and neurologic (sensory afferent and autonomic) dysfunction.

There is a continuing debate over the role of infectious organisms in interstitial cystitis. The bacterial flora of the lower urinary tract in interstitial cystitis and the urethral syndrome was found to be considerably different from those of healthy women (172). The significance of these findings is uncertain because it is possible that the inflamed, damaged bladder and urethral mucosa in these conditions can cause increased bacterial adherence and colonization.

Interstitial cystitis is suspected when a patient has a voiding diary with 15 to 25 voids per day, with amounts less than 200 mL and often as low as 30 to 45 mL, nocturia three to six times, and pain on bladder filling. Diagnosis may be confirmed by CMG and cystoscopy with bladder distention under anesthesia. The treatment protocol is complex for these patients, and frequently includes a combination of pentosan (Elmiron), amitriptyline, hydroxyzine (Atarax, Vistaril), and bladder instillation of heparin. Approximately 40% of patients with interstitial cystitis treated with hydroxyzine self-report an improvement in symptoms, and this rate rises to 55% in patients with bladder mastocytosis on biopsy or a history of allergies. The ability of hydroxyzine to inhibit the neurogenic activation of bladder mast cells explains its clinical efficacy in treating interstitial cystitis (173). These patients require subspecialty management.

Atrophic Urethritis

Atrophic changes subsequent to estrogen deficiency after menopause may cause genital tract atrophy, especially the mucosal lining of the vagina and urethra. Symptoms include irritative voiding symptoms such as urgency, frequency, and pressure sensation. Loss of mucosal coaptation and pelvic support may cause stress incontinence. Likewise, vaginal atrophy causes vaginal dryness and dyspareunia, and can lead to local infection. Estrogen administration causes engorgement within the submucosal vascular plexus, and may enhance the efficiency of periurethral smooth and striated muscle.

Topical treatment is commenced with a vaginal estrogen tablet twice weekly, or estrogen cream one-fourth to one-third applicator at bedtime two to three times per week, and maintained once or twice weekly indefinitely.

VOIDING DYSFUNCTION

Symptoms of voiding dysfunction include obstructive voiding (inability to void, voiding with high residual, altering stature or voiding position, recurrent infection), irritative symptoms (frequency, urgency, urge incontinence, infection), and nocturnal symptoms.

Obstructive Voiding

Obstructive voiding is seldom spontaneous, except as related to pelvic organ prolapse or impacted retroverted uterus of pregnancy. Most causes are iatrogenic and occur in direct relation to recent surgery (174). The patient evaluation in the postoperative case need not be complex. A normal evaluation preoperatively followed by surgery and development of obstructive symptoms in association with a high postvoid residual urine determination makes the diagnosis. An acceptable postvoid residual urine determination is 100 mL, although larger volumes can be normal in the patient with a large bladder capacity and no adverse sequelae.

Symptomatic patients are managed by intermittent self-catheterization four to six times per day, depending on residual urine volumes and patient comfort. Antibiotic prophylaxis is usually not given because of the risk of culturing resistant organisms. Medications to improve postoperative voiding obstruction are seldom helpful, although some patients have improved with a trial of medication using either urecholine, diazepam, an alpha blocker, or a combination of two medications (Table 18.9).

The failure of medical therapy necessitates a surgical takedown of the prior repair. If synthetic material is used for bladder neck suspension, release may be most satisfactory in the first few weeks after surgery.

Nocturnal Polyuria Syndrome

Nocturnal polyuria syndrome refers to a change in urine volume ratios when comparing daytime to nighttime voiding (175). Normally two-thirds of urine is excreted from 8 AM to 12 PM. Once the volume ratios change to one-half of the urine volume excreted from 12 AM to 8 AM, the diagnosis of nocturnal polyuria syndrome is made (176). The normal presence of the antidiuretic hormone, vasopressin, allows one to rest comfortably overnight as concentrated urine is formed. The body fluid excess is excreted in daytime. With aging, the ability to concentrate urine declines, and daytime fluid retention and borderline cardiac function may aggravate the situation.

The urolog diary is the diagnostic method of choice, and both large amounts voided overnight and total nighttime volume are assessed. Treatment consists of fluid restriction after 6 PM,

TABLE 18.9

Medications for Voiding Dysfunction With Incomplete Bladder Emptying

Drug	Dose (mg)	Schedule	Effect
Bethanechol (Urecholine)	25–50	Three to four times a day	Stimulates bladder to contract Stimulates urethral closure
Doxazosin (Cardura)	1–8	Once daily	Relaxes urethral smooth muscle
Prazosin (Minipress)	2	Three times a day	Relaxes urethral smooth muscle
Diazepam (Valium)	2	Daily to three times a day	Relaxes pelvic and striated sphincter muscle

daytime rest period especially after diuretic administration, and consideration of desmopressin (DDAVP) 100 to 200 mcg 1 hour prior to bedtime (177). Serum sodium may drop in some patients on DDAVP, so medical status must be evaluated. If patients have nocturnal enuresis, imipramine 12.5 to 50 mg 1 hour prior to bedtime may be beneficial. Side effects must be observed carefully.

URETHRAL ABNORMALITIES

Urethral Caruncle

Urethral caruncle is an inflammatory process that develops on the posterior aspect of the urethral meatus. It is red, may be as large as 1 to 2 cm, and can be symptomatic with bleeding and/or pain. Treatment for symptomatic caruncle is direct application of estrogen cream daily for 2 to 4 weeks. Failure to ameliorate symptoms may require local excision, laser vaporization, or cryotherapy.

Urethral Prolapse

Urethral prolapse is a protrusion of urethral mucosa circumferentially around the urethral meatus. It appears as a red ring around the urethral opening. Treatment (also for children) is daily, local application of estrogen cream for 3 to 6 weeks. Excision is rarely required.

PELVIC ORGAN PROLAPSE

Pelvic organ prolapse with SUI is a major health care problem. An American woman's lifetime risk for having a surgical procedure for pelvic prolapse or UI is estimated to be 11.1% (178). It has been estimated that one-half of parous women lose pelvic floor support, resulting in some degree of prolapse, and that of these women, 10 to 20% seek medical care (179). The chance of a woman having a prolapse increases with age (178). Women with SUI frequently have coexistent findings of pelvic floor prolapse, such as cystocele, rectocele, uterine, or vaginal vault prolapse. As a result, at least 40 to 60% of patients undergoing surgery for SUI will also require an additional procedure at the time for pelvic prolapse (180).

The coexistence of SUI and/or pelvic organ prolapse occurs as a result of pelvic floor weakening. It is generally believed that pelvic organ prolapse is multifactorial in etiology. Pelvic floor defects may result from the stretching and tearing of the endopelvic fascia and the levator muscles and perineal body that occur as a result of childbirth. In addition, partial pudendal and perineal neuropathies are also associated with labor. These neuropathies may lead to impaired nerve transmission to the muscles of the pelvic floor, which may predispose them to decreased tone, leading to further sagging and stretching (181). Other medical conditions that may result in prolapse are those associated with increases in intra-abdominal pressure (e.g., obesity, chronic pulmonary disease, smoking, constipation). Certain rare abnormalities in connective tissue (collagen), such as Marfan disease, have also been linked to genitourinary prolapse (182). Risk factors for pelvic organ prolapse include multiparity, obesity, chronic cough, and alterations in collagen metabolism (181, 183). Women with urogenital prolapse may present with a variety of lower urinary tract symptoms, including irritative or obstructive symptoms and UI. Urogenital prolapse may affect the urethra by pulling open the posterior urethral wall and causing sphincteric incontinence by mechanically obstructing the urethra or by dissipating the effects of abdominal pressure on the urethra (184–186). Furthermore, by an unknown mechanism prolapse may be associated with detrusor instability.

Continent women with severe urogenital prolapse may become incontinent after prolapse is reduced (185–189). Bai et al. demonstrated the inverse relationship between the degree of pelvic organ prolapse and the risk of symptomatic SUI, recognizing the potential effects of the former on the latter (190). Using a Smith-Hodge pessary and pressure transmission measurements Bergman et al. noted a 36% rate of occult stress incontinence in 67 women with severe cystocele (189). Similarly, using a ring pessary to reduce prolapse, Rosenzweig et al. unmasked occult stress incontinence in 59% of 22 women with severe cystocele (187). Ghoneim et al. used a vaginal pack to unmask stress incontinence associated with urogenital prolapse. In their series, 11 of 16 women (68%) had stress incontinence after prolapse reduction (191). Therefore, it is widely recognized that to accurately diagnose SUI in a patient with pelvic organ prolapse, one must perform a careful gynecologic examination and similarly consider the performance of urodynamic studies after reduction of any pelvic prolapse (192).

A site-specific physical evaluation is essential. Methods for noting pelvic floor relaxation include (a) the Baden halfway system; (b) the International Continence Society classification, using the Pelvic Organ Prolapse Quantification (POPQ) system; and (c) the revised New York Classification system (193–195). Research purposes are best served by performing a POPQ assessment (194). In clinical practice, it has been considered more expedient to use the Baden-Walker system, which also relates the severity of the defects in relation to the hymenal ring, as shown in Table 18.10 (196).

Pelvic organ prolapse may be managed conservatively or surgically. Pelvic exercises and pessaries are the current mainstays of nonsurgical management of pelvic organ prolapse. The pessary should be fitted to the patient, and different devices are often used to treat the same process in different patients. Although routine Kegel exercises can improve pelvic floor muscle tone and GSI, no evidence in any prospective, blinded, randomized trials indicates that improvement of pelvic floor muscle tone leads to regression of prolapse. A discussion of surgical repair for pelvic organ prolapse is beyond the scope of this text.

TABLE 18.10

Baden-Walker Pelvic Prolapse Severity Guide

Grade 0—Support greater than 2 cm above the hymenal ring
Grade 1—Defect descends to within 1 cm of hymenal ring
Grade 2—Defect descends to hymenal ring
Grade 3—Defect descends 1 cm beyond hymenal ring
Grade 4—Defect extends 2 cm or more beyond hymenal ring; the uterus may be completely outside the vagina

Adapted from Scotti RJ, Flora R, Greston WM, et al. Characterizing and reporting pelvic floor defects: the revised New York classification system. Int Urogynecol J Pelvic Floor Dysfunct 2000;11:48–60, with permission.

Clinical Notes

- Almost any disorder of the urogenital system may be assessed by a basic evaluation consisting of history, physical examination, voiding diary, residual urine determination, and urinalysis. A presumptive diagnosis is made, and therapy commenced.
- UTIs are managed by a 3- to 5-day course of Macrobid, cephalosporin, or trimethoprim/sulfamethoxazole. Recurrent infections may require prophylaxis with a daily dose or postintercourse dose of nitrofurantoin, trimethoprim/sulfamethoxazole, cephalosporin, or fluoroquinolone.
- UI usually comes down to distinguishing between stress incontinence and OAB. Conservative therapy is offered initially, and medications such as Detrol LA and Ditropan XL can be very helpful for OAB. Surgery may be considered for stress incontinence if conservative therapy fails.
- Prolapse should be considered with respect to symptoms it causes and to alterations it makes in voiding or continence.
- Sensory disorders of urethral etiology may be managed with estrogen supplement in the appropriate patient. A course of antibiotic therapy and sometimes ongoing antibiotic suppression is then tried. Once infective causes have been eliminated or treated, the approach is modification of the sensory neurologic input by using Elavil in the early evening (e.g., 6 PM). A course of diazepam combined with an alpha-blocker such as Cardura or Minipress may bring relief. Treatment then becomes more divergent and generally requires specialist care.
- Interstitial cystitis, a painful bladder disorder, requires specialist care for optimal outcome.
- Voiding dysfunction immediately after surgery or obstetric delivery is managed with catheter care. After 1 week, the patient should be instructed in self-catheterization. Obstruction after antecedent incontinence surgery may require surgical takedown (i.e., urethrolysis). Medication is occasionally helpful, as long as obstruction from surgery is not the prime cause.
- Nocturia may be managed with fluid restriction, diuretic therapy, daytime rest period, and bedtime DDAVP.
- Conditions such as urethral caruncle and urethral prolapse generally respond to topical estrogen therapy.

REFERENCES

1. Hooton TM, Scholes D, Hughes JP, et al. A prospective study of risk factors for asymptomatic urinary tract infection in young women. N Engl J Med 1996;335:468–474.
2. Barry HC, Hickner J, Ebell MH, et al. A randomized controlled trial of telephone management of suspected urinary tract infections in women. J Fam Pract 2001;50:589–594.
3. Saint S, Scholes D, Fihn SD, et al. The effectiveness of a clinical practice guideline for the management of presumed uncomplicated urinary tract infection in women. Am J Med 1999;106:634–641.
4. Karram MM. Lower urinary tract infection. In: Urogynecology and Urodynamics: Theory and Practice. 4th ed. Baltimore: Williams & Wilkins, 1996;387–408.
5. Wu TC, Williams EC, Koo SY, et al. Evaluation of three bacteriuria screening methods in a clinical research hospital. J Clin Microbiol 1985;21:796–814.
6. Bixler-Forrell E, Bertram MA, Bruckner DA. Clinical evaluation of three rapid methods for the detection of significant bacteriuria. J Clin Microbiol 1985;22:62–68.
7. Needham CA. Rapid detection methods in microbiology: are they right for your office? Med Clin North Am 1987;71:591–605.
8. Dalton MT, Comeau S, Rainnie B, et al. A comparison of the API Uriscreen with the Vitek Urine identification-3 and the leukocyte esterase or nitrite strip as a screening test for bacteriuria. Diagn Microbiol Infect Dis 1993;16:93–97.
9. Vickers D, Ahmad T, Coulthard MG. Diagnosis of urinary tract infection in children: fresh urine microscopy or culture? Lancet 1991;338:767–770.
10. Young JL, Soper DE. Urinalysis and urinary tract infection: update for clinicians. Infect Dis Obstet Gynecol 2001;9:249–255.
11. Kass EH. Bacteriuria and diagnosis of infections of the urinary tract. Arch Intern Med 1967;100:709–714.
12. Stamm WE. Measurement of pyuria and its relation to bacteriuria. Am J Med 1983;75:53–58.
13. Kunin CM, Hua TH, White L, et al. A reassessment of the importance of "low-count" bacteriuria in young women with acute urinary symptoms. Ann Intern Med 1993;119:454–460.

14. Stamm WE, Counts GW, Running KR, et al. Diagnosis of coliform infection in acutely dysuric women. N Engl J Med 1982;307:463–467.
15. Nicolle LE. Asymptomatic bacteriuria in the elderly. Infect Dis Clin North Am 1997;11:647–662.
16. Zhanel GG, Nicolle LE, Hardking GKM, for the Manitoba Diabetic Urinary Infection Study Group. Prevalence of asymptomatic bacteriuria in women with diabetes mellitus. Clin Infect Dis 1995;21:316–322.
17. Hooton TM, Winter C, Tiu F, et al. Randomized comparative trial and cost analysis of 3-day antimicrobial regimens for treatment of acute cystitis in women. JAMA 1995;273:41–45.
18. Gupta K, Scholes D, Stamm WE. Increasing prevalence of antimicrobial resistance among uropathogens causing acute uncomplicated cystitis in women. JAMA 1999;281:736–738.
19. Garrison J, Hooton TM. Fluoroquinolones in the treatment of acute uncomplicated urinary tract infections in adult women. Expert Opin Pharmacother 2001;2:1227–1237.
20. Richard GA, Mathew CP, Kirstein JM, et al. Single-dose fluoroquinolone therapy of acute uncomplicated urinary tract infection in women: results from a randomized, double-blind, multicenter trial comparing single-dose to 3-day fluoroquinolone regimens. Urology 2002;59:334–339.
21. Foxman B. Recurring urinary tract infection: incidence and risk factors. Am J Pub Health 1990;80:331–333.
22. Talan DA, Stamm WE, Hooton TM, et al. Comparison of ciprofloxacin (7 days) and trimethoprim/sulfamethoxazole (14 days) for acute uncomplicated pyelonephritis: a randomized, double-blind trail. JAMA 2000;2843:1583–1590.
23. Svanborg C, Godaly G. Bacterial virulence in urinary tract infection. Infect Dis Clin North Am 1997;11:513–530.
24. Zhanel GG, Harding GKM, Nicolle LE. Asymptomatic bacteriuria in patients with diabetes mellitus. Clin Infect Dis 1991;13:150–154.
25. Warren JW. Catheter-associated urinary tract infections. Infect Dis Clin North Am 1997;11:609–622.
26. Warren JW, Tenney JH, Hoopes JM, et al. A prospective microbiologic study of bacteriuria in patients with chronic indwelling urethral catheters. J Infect Dis 1982;146:719–723.
27. Abrams P, Blaives JG, Stanton SL, et al. The standardization of terminology of lower urinary tract function. Scand J Urol Nephrol 1998;114(suppl):5–19.
28. Thom D. Variation in estimates of urinary incontinence prevalence in the community: effects of differences in definition, population characteristics, and study type. J Am Geriatr Soc 1998;46:473–480.
29. Burgio K, Ives D, Locher J, et al. Treatment seeking for urinary incontinence in older adults. J Am Geriatr Soc 1994;42:208–212.
30. Hiral K, Sumi T, Kanaoka Y, et al. Female urinary incontinence: diagnosis, treatment and patients' concerns. Drugs Today 2002;38:487–493.
31. Bogner H, Gallo J, Sammel M, et al. Urinary incontinence and psychological distress in community-dwelling older adults. J Am Geriatr Soc 2002;50:489–495.
32. Melville J, Walker E, Katon W, et al. Prevalence of comorbid psychiatric illness and its impact on symptom perception, quality of life, and functional status of women with urinary incontinence. Am J Obstet Gynecol 2002;187:80–87.
33. Kessler R, Berglund P, Demler O. The epidemiology of major depressive disorder results from the national comorbidity survey replication. JAMA 2003;289:3095–3105.
34. Bogner H, Gallo J, Swartz K, et al. Anxiety disorders and disability secondary to urinary incontinence among adults over age 50. Int J Psychiatry Med 2002;32:141–154.
35. Nygaard I, Turvey C, Burns T, et al. Urinary incontinence and depression in middle-aged United States women. Obstet Gynecol 2003;101:149–156.
36. Wilson L, Brown J, Shin G, et al. Annual direct cost of urinary incontinence. Obstet Gynecol 2001;98:398–406.
37. Milson I, Ekelund P, Molander U, et al. The influence of age, parity, oral contraception, hysterectomy and menopause on the prevalence of urinary incontinence in women. J Urol 1993;149:1459–1462.
38. Persson J, Hanssen PM, Rydhstroem H. Obstetric risk factors for stress urinary incontinence: a population-based study. Obstet Gynecol 2000;96:440–445.
39. Brown JS, Grady D, Ouslander JG, et al. Prevalence of urinary incontinence associated risk factors in postmenopausal women. Obstet Gynecol 1999;94:66–70.
40. Bump RC, Sugerman HJ, Fantl JA, et al. Obesity and lower urinary tract function in women: effect of surgically induced weight loss. Am J Obstet Gynecol 1992;167:392–399.
41. Elia G, Bergman J, Dye TD. Familial incidence of urinary incontinence. Am J Obstet Gynecol 2002;187:53–55.
42. Mushkat Y, Bukowsky I, Langer R. Female urinary stress incontinence: does it have a family prevalence? Am J Obstet Gynecol 1996;174:617–619.
43. Guong TH, Korn AP. A comparison of urinary incontinence among African American, Asian, Hispanic, and white women. Am J Obstet Gynecol 2001;184:1083–1086.
44. Urinary Incontinence Guideline Panel. Urinary Incontinence in Adults: Clinical Practice Guideline Update. AHCPR Pub. No. 96–0686. Rockville, MD: Agency for Health Care Policy and Research, Public Health Service, U.S. Department of Health and Human Services, March 1996.
45. Jensen JK, Nielson FR Jr, Ostergard DR. The role of patient history in the diagnosis of urinary incontinence. Obstet Gynecol 1994;83:904–910.
46. Blaivas JG. The bulbocavernosus reflex in urology: a prospective study of 299 patients. J Urol 1981;126:197–199.

47. Sutherst JR, Brown MC. Comparison of single and multichannel cystometry in diagnosing bladder instability. BMJ 1984;288:1720–1722.
48. Abrams P, Blaivas JG, Stanton SL, et al. The standardisation of terminology of lower urinary tract function. Br J Obstet Gynaecol 1990;97(suppl 6):1–16.
49. Arnold EP. Cystometry-postural effects in incontinent women. Urol Int 1974;29:185–186.
50. Sand PK, Hill RC, Ostergard DR. Supine urethroscopic and standing cystometry as screening methods for the detection of detrusor instability. Obstet Gynecol 1987;70:57–60.
51. Frigerio L, Ferrari A, Candiani GB. The significance of the stop test in female urinary incontinence. Diagn Gynecol Obstet 1981;3:301–304.
52. Sherman RA, Davis GD, Wong MF. Behavioral treatment of exercise-induced urinary incontinence among female soldiers. Mil Med 1997;162:690–694.
53. Jolleys JV. Reported prevalence of urinary incontinence in women in a general practice. BMJ 1988;296:1300–1302.
54. Sommer P, Bauer T, Nielsen KK, et al. Voiding patterns and prevalence of incontinence in women. Br J Urol 1990;6:12–15.
55. Wilson P, Bø K, Bourcier A, et al. Conservative management in women. In: 1st International Consultation on Incontinence. Plymouth, UK: Health Publication Ltd., 1999:227–294.
56. Bø K. Pelvic floor muscle exercise for the treatment of stress urinary incontinence: an exercise physiology perspective. Int J Urogyn Pelv Floor Dysfunc 1995;6:282–291.
57. Fantl JA, Newman DK, Colling J, et al. Urinary incontinence in adults: acute and chronic management. Clin Pract Guidel 1996;2:1–154.
58. Fantl JA, Wyman JF, McClish DK, et al. Efficacy of bladder training in older women with urinary incontinence. JAMA 1991;265(suppl 5):609–613.
59. Burgio KL, Locher JL, Goode PS, et al. Behavioral vs drug treatment for urge urinary incontinence in older women. JAMA 1998;280:1995–2000.
60. Holmes DM, Stone AR, Barry PR, et al. Bladder training 3 years on. Br J Urol 1983;55:660–664.
61. Bump RC, Hurt WG, Fantl JA, et al. Assessment of Kegel pelvic muscle exercise performance after brief verbal instruction. Am J Obstet Gynecol 1991;165:322–327.
62. Nygaard IE, Kreder KJ, Lepic MM, et al. Efficacy of pelvic floor muscle exercises in women with stress, urge, and mixed urinary incontinence. Am J Obstet Gynecol 1996;174:120–125.
63. Bø K, Talseth T, Holme I. Single-blinded, randomized, controlled trial of pelvic floor exercises, electrical stimulation, vaginal cones, and no treatment in management of genuine stress incontinence in women. BMJ 1999;318:487–493.
64. Weatherall M. Biofeedback of pelvic floor muscle exercises for female genuine stress incontinence: a meta-analysis of trials identified in a systematic review. BJU Int 1999;83:1015–1016.
65. Laycock J, Brown J, Cusack C, et al. Pelvic floor re-education for stress incontinence: comparing three methods. Br J Community Nurs 2001;6:230–237.
66. Cammu H, Van Nylen M. Pelvic floor exercises versus vaginal weight cones in genuine stress incontinence. Eur J Obstet Gynecol Reprod Biol 1998;77:89–93.
67. Kralj B. Conservative treatment of stress urinary incontinence with functional electrical stimulation. Eur J Obstet Gynecol Reprod Biol 1999;85:53–56.
68. Davila GW, Ostermann KV. The bladder neck support prosthesis: a nonsurgical approach to stress incontinence in adult women. Am J Obstet Gynecol 1994;171:206–211.
69. Nygaard I. Prevention of exercise incontinence with mechanical devices. J Reprod Med 1995;40:89–94.
70. Eckford SD, Jackson SR, Lewis PA, et al. The continence pad—a new external urethral occlusion device in the management of stress incontinence. Br J Urol 1996;77:538–540.
71. Moore KH, Simons A, Dowell C, et al. Efficacy and user acceptability of the urethral occlusive device in women with urinary incontinence. J Urol 1999;162:464–468.
72. Bellin P, Smith J, Poll W, et al. Results of a multicenter trial of the CapSure (Re/Stor) continence shield on women with stress urinary incontinence. Urology 1998;51:697–706.
73. Staskin D, Bavendam T, Miller J, et al. Effectiveness of a urinary control insert in the management of stress urinary incontinence: early results of a multicenter study. Urology 1996;47:629–636.
74. Sand PK, Staskin D, Miller J, et al. Effect of a urinary control insert on quality of life in incontinent women. Int Urogynecol J Pelvic Floor Dysfunct 1999;10:100–105.
75. Choe JM, Staskin DR. Clinical usefulness of urinary control urethral insert devices. J Urol 1999;161:1043–1044.
76. Sirls LT, Foote JE, Kaufman JM, et al. Long-term results of the FemSoft Urethral Insert for the management of female stress urinary incontinence. Int Urogynecol J 2002;13(suppl 2):88–95.
77. Sweat SD, Lightner DJ. Complications of sterile abscess formation and pulmonary embolism following periurethral bulking agents. J Urol 1999;161:93–96.
78. McLennan MT, Bent AE. Suburethral abscess: a complication of periurethral collagen injection therapy. Obstet Gynecol 1998;92:650–652.
79. Wainstein MA, Klutke CG. Periurethral pseudocyst following cystoscopic collagen injection. Urology 1998;51:835–836.
80. Clemens JQ, Bushman W. Urethral diverticulum following transurethral collagen injection. J Urol 2001;166:626.
81. Steele AC, Kohli NJ, Karam MM. Periurethral collagen injection for stress urinary incontinence with & without urethral hypermobility. Obstet Gynecol 2000;95:327–331.

82. Santarosa RP, Blaivas JG. Periurethral injection of autologous fat for the treatment of sphincteric incontinence. J Urol 1994;151:607–611.
83. Pycha A, Klinger CH, Haitel A, et al. Implantable microballoons: an attractive alternative in the management of intrinsic sphincter deficiency. Eur Urol 1998;33(suppl 5):469–475.
84. Collste C, Lindskog M. Phenylpropanolamine in the treatment of female stress urinary incontinence: double-blind, placebo-controlled study in 24 patients. Urology 1987;30:398–403.
85. Thor K, Katofiasc M. Effects of duloxetine, a combined serotonin and norepinephrine reuptake inhibitor, on central neural control of the lower urinary tract function in the chloralose-anesthetized female cat. J Pharmacol Exp Ther 1995;274:1014–1024.
86. Tsai E, Yang C, Chen H, et al. Bladder neck circulation by Doppler ultrasonography in postmenopausal women with urinary stress incontinence. Obstetr Gynecol 2001;98:52–56.
87. Foster D, Palmer M, Marks J. Effect of vulvovaginal estrogen on sensorimotor response of the lower genital tract: a randomized controlled trial. Obstet Gynecol 1999;94:232–237.
88. Grady D, Brown J, Vittinghoff E, et al. Postmenopausal hormones and incontinence: the heart and estrogen/progestin replacement study. Obstet Gynecol 2001;97:116–120.
89. Jackson S, Shepherd A, Brooks S, et al. The effect of oestrogen supplementation on post-menopausal urinary stress incontinence. Br J Obstet Gynecol 1999;106:711–718.
90. Norton P, Zinner N, Yalcin I, et al. Duloxetine versus placebo in the treatment of stress urinary incontinence. Am J Obstet Gynecol 2002;187:40–47.
91. Stewart W, Herzog AR, Wein A, et al. Prevalence and impact of overactive bladder in the US: results from the NOBLE program. Neurourol Urodyn 2001;20:406–408.
92. Milsom I, Abrams P, Cardozo L, et al. How widespread are the symptoms of an overactive bladder and how are they managed? A population-based prevalence study. BJU Int 2001;87:760–766.
93. Hampel C, Wienhold D, Benken N, et al. Definition of overactive bladder and epidemiology of urinary incontinence. Urology 1997;50(suppl 6A):4–14.
94. Rekers H, Drogendijk AC, Valkenburg H, et al. Urinary incontinence in women from 35–79. Eur J Obstet Gynecol Reprod Biol 1992;43:229–234.
95. Hisayama T, Shinkai M, Takayanagi I, et al. Mechanism of action of nicotine in isolated urinary bladder of guinea pig. Br J Pharmacol 1988;95:465–472.
96. Koley B, Koley J, Saha JK. The effects of nicotine on spontaneous contraction of cat urinary bladder in situ. Br J Pharmacol 1984;83:347–355.
97. Wyman J, Fantl JA, McClish DK, et al. Quality of life following bladder training in older women with urinary incontinence. Int Urogynecol J Pelvic Floor Dysfunct 1997;8:223–229.
98. Brown J. Urinary incontinence: does it increase risk for falls and fracture? J Am Geriatric Soc 2000;48:721–724.
99. Stevenson B, Mills EM, Welin L, et al. Falls risk factors in acute care settings: a retrospective study. Can J Nurs Res 1998;30:97–111.
100. Zorn BH, Montgomery H, Pieper K, et al. Urinary incontinence and depression. J Urol 1999;162:82–84.
101. Lenderking WR, Nackley JF, Anderson RB, et al. A review of the quality-of-life aspects of urinary urge incontinence. Pharmacoeconomics 1996;9:11–23.
102. Simeonova Z, Milsom I, Kullendorff AM, et al. The prevalence of urinary incontinence and its influence on the quality of life in women from an urban Swedish population. Acta Obstet Gynecol Scand 1999;78:546–551.
103. Abrams P, Wein AJ. The overactive bladder: a widespread and treatable condition. Stockholm: Erik Sparre Medical AB, 1998:1–60.
104. Brocklehurst J. Urinary incontinence in the community: analysis of a Mori poll. BMJ 1993;306:832–834.
105. Chaikin DC, Rosenthal J, Blaivas JG. Pubovaginal fascial sling for all types of stress urinary incontinence: long-term analysis. J Urol 1998;150:1312–1316.
106. Anderson RU, Mobley D, Blank B, et al. Once daily controlled versus immediate release oxybutynin chloride for urge urinary incontinence. J Urol 1999;161:1809–1812.
107. Appell RA, Sand P, Dmochowski R, et al. Prospective randomized controlled trial of extended-release oxybutynin chloride and tolterodine tartrate in the treatment of overactive bladder: results of the OBJECT study. Mayo Clin Proc 2001;76:358–363.
108. Butler RN, Maby JI, Montella JM, et al. Urinary incontinence: primary care therapies for the older woman. Geriatrics 1999;54:31–34, 39–40, 43–44.
109. Wyman JF, Harkins SW, Fantl JA. Psychosocial impact of urinary incontinence in the community-dwelling population. J Am Geriatr Soc 1990;38:282–288.
110. Burgio K, Matthews KA, Engel BT. Prevalence, incidence and correlates of urinary incontinence in healthy, middle-aged women. J Urol 1991;146:1255–1259.
111. Lagro-Janssen TL, Debruyne FM, Smits AJ, et al. Controlled trial of pelvic floor exercises in the treatment of urinary stress incontinence in general practice. Br J Gen Pract 1991;41:445–449.
112. Yamanishi T, Yasuda K, Sakakibara R, et al. Randomized, double–blind study of electrical stimulation for urinary incontinence due to detrusor overactivity. Urology 2000;55:353–357.
113. Brubaker L. Electrical stimulation in overactive bladder. Urology 2000;55(suppl 5A):17–32.
114. Bosch JL, Groen J. Sacral nerve neuromodulation in the treatments of patients with refractory motor urge incontinence: long-term results of a prospective longitudinal study. J Urol 2000;163:1234–1235.
115. Yarker YE, Goa KL, Fitton A. Oxybutynin. A review of its pharmacodynamic and pharmacokinetic properties, and its therapeutic use in detrusor instability. Drugs Aging 1995;6:243–262.

116. Kelleher C, Cardozo L, Khullar V, et al. A medium-term analysis of the subjective efficacy and treatment for women with detrusor instability and low bladder compliance. Br J Obstet Gynaecol 1997;104:988–993.
117. Anderson R, Mobley D, Blank B, et al. Once daily controlled versus immediate release oxybutynin chloride for urge urinary incontinence. J Urol 1999;161:1809–1812.
118. Dmochowski R, Davilla G, Zinner N, et al. Efficacy and safety of transdermal oxybutynin in patients with urge and mixed urinary incontinence. J Urol 2002;168:580–586.
119. Fowler C. Intravesical treatment of overactive bladder. Urology 2000;55(suppl 5A):60–64.
120. Frohlich G, Burmeister S, Wiedermann A. Intravesicular instillation of trospium chloride, oxybutynin and verapamil for relaxation of the bladder detrusor muscle. Arzneimittelforschung 1998;48:486–491.
121. Abrams P, Freeman R, Anderstrom C, et al. Tolterodine, a new antimuscarinic agent: as effective but better tolerated than oxybutynin in patients with overactive bladder. Br J Urol 1998;81:801–810.
122. Appell RA. Clinical efficacy and safety of tolterodine in the treatment of overactive bladder: a pooled analysis. Urology 1997;50(suppl 6A):90–96.
123. Messelink EJ. Treatment of the overactive bladder with tolterodine, a new muscarinic receptor antagonist. BJU Int 1999;83(suppl 2):48–52.
124. Ruscin JM, Morgenstern NE. Tolterodine use for symptoms of overactive bladder. Ann Pharmacother 1999;33:1073–1082.
125. Rovner ES, Wein AJ. Modern pharmacotherapy of urge urinary incontinence in the USA: tolterodine and oxybutynin. BJU Int 2000;86(suppl 2):44–53.
126. Hartnett NM, Saver BG. Is extended-release oxybutynin (Ditropan XL) or tolterodine (Detrol) more effective in the treatment of an overactive bladder? J Fam Pract 2001;50:571.
127. Dmochowski RR, Appell RA. Advancements in pharmacologic management of the overactive bladder. Urology 2000;56(suppl):41–49.
128. Gulliford G, Bidmead J. Management of incontinence. Pharm J 2001;267:230–232.
129. Fusgen I, Hauri D. Trospium chloride: an effective option for medical treatment of bladder overactivity. Int J Clin Pharmacol Ther 2000;38:223–234.
130. Booth C, Pascoe D. A comparison of newer drug treatments for urinary incontinence. Hosp Pharm 2002;9: 69–75.
131. Klutke J, Bergman A. Nonsurgical treatment of stress urinary incontinence. In: Ostergard's urogynecology and pelvic floor dysfunction. 5th ed. Baltimore: Lippincott Williams & Wilkins, 2003:450–452.
132. Guarneri L, Robinson E, Testa R. A review of flavoxate: pharmacology and mechanism of action. Drugs Today 1994;30:91–98.
133. Chapple C, Parkhouse H, Gardener C, et al. Double-blind, placebo-controlled, cross-over study of flavoxate in the treatment of idiopathic detrusor instability. Urology 1990;66(suppl 5A):491–494.
134. Andersson K, Appell R, Awad S, et al. Pharmacological treatment of urinary incontinence. In: Incontinence, 2nd International Consultation on Incontinence. Plymouth, UK: Plymbridge Distributors Ltd., 2002:479–511.
135. Wein A, Rovner E. Pharmacologic management of urinary incontinence in women. Urol Clin North Am 2002;29:537–550.
136. Blaivas JG, Bhimani G, Labib KB. Vesicourethral dysfunction in multiple sclerosis. J Urol 1979;122:342–347.
137. Goldstein I, Siroky MB, Sax S, et al. Neurourologic abnormalities in multiple sclerosis. J Urol 1982;128:541–545.
138. Andersen JT, Bradley WE. Abnormalities of detrusor and sphincter function in multiple sclerosis. Br J Urol 1976;48:193–198.
139. Bradley WE. Urinary bladder dysfunction in multiple sclerosis. Neurology 1978;9:52–58.
140. Koldewijn EL, Hommes OR, Lemmens WAJG, et al. Relationship between lower urinary tract abnormalities and disease related parameters in multiple sclerosis. J Urol 1995;154:169–173.
141. Blaivas JG. The neurophysiology of micturition: a clinical study of 550 patients. J Urol 1982;127:958–963.
142. Beck RP, Warren KG, Whitman P. Urodynamic studies in female patients with multiple sclerosis. Am J Obstet Gynecol 1981;139:273–276.
143. Franz DA, Towler MA, Edlich RF, et al. Functional urinary outlet obstruction causing urosepsis in a male multiple sclerosis patient. J Emerg Med 1992;10:281–284.
144. Gonor SE, Carroll DJ, Metcalfe JB. Vesical dysfunction in multiple sclerosis. Urology 1985;25:429–431.
145. Blaivas JG, Sinha HP, Zayed AA, et al. Detrusor external sphincter dyssynergia: a detailed electromyographic study. J Urol 1981;125:542–548.
146. Siroky MB, Krane RJ. Neurologic aspects of detrusor-sphincter dyssynergia, with reference to the guarding reflex. J Urol 1982;127:953–957.
147. Dibenedetto M, Yalla SV. Electrodiagnosis of striated urethral sphincter dysfunction. J Urol 1979;122:361–365.
148. Bakke A, Myhr KM, Gronning M, et al. Bladder, bowel and sexual dysfunction in patients with multiple sclerosis—a cohort study. Scand J Urol Nephrol 1996;179(suppl):61–66.
149. Nordling J. Alpha-blockers and urethral pressure in neurological patients. Urol Int 1978;33:304–309.
150. O'Roirdan JI, Doherty C, Javed M, et al. Do alpha-blockers have a role in lower urinary tract dysfunction in multiple sclerosis? J Urol 1995;153:1114–1116.
151. Kornhuber HH, Schutz A. Efficient treatment of neurogenic bladder disorders in multiple sclerosis with initial intermittent catheterization and ultrasound-controlled training. Eur Neurol 1990;30:260–267.
152. Ouslander JG, Leach G, Staskin D, et al. Prospective evaluation of an assessment strategy for geriatric urinary incontinence. J Am Geriatr Soc 1989;37:715–724.

153. Resnick NM, Yalla SV. Detrusor hyperactivity with impaired contractile function. An unrecognized but common cause of incontinence in elderly patients. JAMA 1987;257:3076–3081.
154. Turner-Warwick R. Urinary fistulas in the female. In: Campbell's Urology. 5th ed. Philadelphia: WB Saunders, 1986:2718.
155. Demirel A, Polat O, Bayraktar Y, et al. Transvesical and transvaginal reparation in urinary vaginal fistulas. Int Urol Nephrol 1993;25:439–444.
156. Blaivas JG, Heritz DM, Romanzi LJ. Early versus late repair of vesicovaginal fistulas: vaginal and abdominal approaches. J Urol 1995;153:1110–1113.
157. Ayhan A, Tuncer ZS, Dogan L, et al. Results of treatment in 182 consecutive patients with genital fistulas. Int J Gynaecol Obstet 1995;48:43–47.
158. Ganabathi K, Leach GE, Zimmern PE, et al. Experience with the management of urethral diverticulum in 63 women. J Urol 1994;152:1445–1452.
159. Leach GE, Trockman BA. Surgery for vesicovaginal and urethrovaginal fistula and urethral diverticulum. In: Campbell's Urology. 7th ed. Philadelphia: WB Saunders, 1998:1135–1153.
160. Wang AC, Wang CR. Radiologic diagnosis and surgical treatment of urethral diverticulum in women. A reappraisal of voiding cystourethrography and positive pressure urethrography. J Reprod Med 2000;45:377–382.
161. Kerr LA. Management of female urethral diverticula. AUA News 2002;2:1.
162. Siegel CL, Middleton WD, Teefey SA, et al. Sonography of the female urethra. AJR Am J Roentgenol 1998;170:1269–1274.
163. Martensson O, Duchek M. Translabial ultrasonography with pulsed colour-Doppler in the diagnosis of female urethral diverticula. Scand J Urol Nephrol 1994;28:101–104.
164. Kim B, Hricak H, Tanagho EA. Diagnosis of urethral diverticulum: value of MR imaging. AJR Am J Roentgenol 1993;161:809–815.
165. Blander DS, Rovner ES, Schnall MD, et al. Endoluminal magnetic resonance imaging in the evaluation of urethral diverticula in women. Urology 2001;57:660–665.
166. Mouritsen L, Bernstein I. Vaginal ultrasonography: a diagnostic tool for urethral diverticulum. Acta Obstet Gynecol Scand 1996;75:188–190.
167. Fontana D, Porpiglia F, Morra I, et al. Transvaginal ultrasonography in the assessment of organic diseases of female urethra. J Ultrasound Med 1999;18:237–241.
168. Abrams P, Cardozo L, Fall M, et al. The standardisation of terminology of lower urinary tract function: report from the standardisation sub-committee of the International Continence Society. Neurourol Urodyn 2002;21:167–178.
169. Held PJ, Hanno PM, Wein AJ, et al. Epidemiology of interstitial cystitis. In: Interstitial Cystitis. New York: Springer-Verlag, 1990:29–48.
170. Curhan GC, Speizer FE, Hunter DJ, et al. Epidemiology of interstitial cystitis: a population based study. J Urol 1999;161:549–552.
171. Monga AK, Marrero JM, Stanton SL, et al. Is there an irritable bladder in the irritable bowel syndrome? Br J Obstet Gynaecol 1997;104:1409–1412.
172. Haarala M, Kiilholma P, Lehtonen OP. Urinary bacterial flora of women with urethral syndrome and interstitial cystitis. Gynecol Obstet Invest 1999;47:42–44.
173. Minogiannis P, El-Mansoury M, Betances JA, et al. Hydroxyzine inhibits neurogenic bladder mast cell activation. Int J Immunopharmacol 1998;20:553–563.
174. Germain MM, Ostergard DR. Overflow incontinence. In: Urogynecology and Urodynamics: Theory and Practice. 4th ed. Baltimore: Williams & Wilkins, 1996:427–432.
175. Asplund R. The nocturnal polyuria syndrome (NPS). Gen Pharmacol 1995;26:1203–1209.
176. van Kerrebroeck P, Abrams P, Chaikin D, et al. The standardization of terminology in nocturia: report from the Standardisation Subcommittee of the International Continence Society. Neurourol Urodyn 2002;21:179–183.
177. Kallas HE, Chintanadilok J, Maruenda J, et al. Treatment of nocturia in the elderly. Drugs Aging 1999;15:429–437.
178. Olsen AL, Smith VJ, Bergstrom JO, et al. Epidemiology of surgically managed pelvic organ prolapse and urinary incontinence. Obstet Gynecol 1997;89:501–506.
179. Beck RP. Pelvic relaxation prolapse. In: Principles and Practice of Clinical Gynecology. New York: Wiley, 1983:677–685.
180. Raz S, Erickson DB. SEAPI QMM incontinence classification system. Neurourol Urodynam 1992;11:187–200.
181. Smith AR, Hosker GL, Warrell DW. The role of partial denervation of the pelvic floor in the aetiology of genitourinary prolapse and stress incontinence of urine. A neurophysiological study. Br J Obstet Gynaecol 1989;96:24–28.
182. Norton P, Baker J, Sharp H, et al. Genito-urinary prolapse: relationship with joint mobility. Neuro Urodyn 1990;9:321–322.
183. Rechberger T, Donica H, Baranowski W, et al. Female urinary stress incontinence in terms of connective tissue biochemistry. Eur J Obstet Gynecol Reprod Biol 1993;49:187–191.
184. Arnold EP, Webster JR, Loose H, et al. Urodynamics of female incontinence: factors influencing the results of surgery. Am J Obstet Gynecol 1973;117:805–813.
185. Richardson DA, Bent AE, Ostergard DR. The effect of uterovaginal prolapse on urethrovesical pressure dynamics. Am J Obstet Gynecol 1983;146:901–905.

186. Bump RC, Fantl JA, Hurt WG. The mechanism of urinary continence in women with severe uterovaginal prolapse: results of barrier studies. Obstet Gynecol 1988;72:291–295.
187. Rosenzweig BA, Pushkin S, Blumenfeld D, et al. Prevalence of abnormal urodynamic test results in continent women with severe genitourinary prolapse. Obstet Gynecol 1992;79:539–542.
188. Fianu S, Kjaeldgaard A, Larson B. Preoperative screening for latent stress incontinence in women with cystocele. Neurourol Urodyn 1985;4:3–8.
189. Bergman A, Kooning PP, Ballard CA. Predicting postoperative urinary incontinence development in women undergoing operation for genitourinary prolapse. Am J Obstet Gynecol 1988;158:1171–1175.
190. Bai SW, Jeon MJ, Kim JY, et al. Relationship between stress urinary incontinence and pelvic organ prolapse. Int Urogynecol J Pelvic Floor Dysfunct 2002;13:256–260.
191. Ghoneim GM, Walters F, Lewis V. The value of the vaginal pack test in large cystoceles. J Urol 1994;152:931–934.
192. Chaikin DC, Groutz A, Blaivas JG. Predicting the need for anti-incontinence surgery in continent women undergoing repair of severe urogenital prolapse. J Urol 2000;163:531–534.
193. Baden WF, Walker TA. Genesis of the vaginal profile: a correlated classification of vaginal relaxation. Clin Obstet Gynecol 1972;15:1048–1054.
194. Bump RC, Mattiasson A, Bo K, et al. The standardization of terminology of female pelvic organ prolapse and pelvic floor dysfunction. Am J Obstet Gynecol 1996;175:10–17.
195. Scotti RJ, Flora R, Greston WM, et al. Characterizing and reporting pelvic floor defects: the revised New York classification system. Int Urogynecol J Pelvic Floor Dysfunct 2000;11:48–60.
196. Baden W, Walker T. Surgical repair of vaginal defects. Philadelphia: JB Lippincott, 1992.
197. Colling J, Ouslander J, Hadley BJ, et al. The effects of patterned urge-response toileting on urinary incontinence among nursing home residents. J Am Geriatr Soc 1992;40:135–141.
198. Schnelle JF, Newman DR, Fogarty T. Management of patient continence in long-term care nursing facilities. Gerontologist 1990;30:373–376.
199. Smith P, Smith L. Continence training in intellectually disabled. In: Promoting Continence: A Clinical and Research Resource. 2nd ed. London: Baillière Tindall, 2003.

CHAPTER 19

Lifestyle Modification

Jimmy D. Acklin

Many medical problems are the result of human behaviors and lifestyles, and many problems could be lessened in severity or avoided altogether if healthier lifestyles were chosen or made easier to choose. Although this seems obvious and easy on the surface, there is probably nothing more difficult for humans to do than to change long ingrained behaviors and addictions. Physicians in practice are faced with a frustrating array of unhealthy behaviors and very few tools with which to affect change.

These behaviors include the obvious, such as smoking, overeating, not exercising, and substance abuse, but noncompliance with treatments and failure to keep follow-up appointments are also modifiable patient behaviors. Some behaviors, such as failure to wear seat belts or sexual risk taking, may not be apparent in the medical setting until the patient presents with obvious medical consequences. Screening patients for detrimental behaviors is the practicing physician's responsibility. Knowledge of the basic principles of behavior change and of resources available to help patients achieve change are important tools for assisting patients.

Historically, detrimental health behaviors and their treatment were assumed to be the same for both men and women, and medical knowledge generally was based on studies that were done on male populations. However, evidence has steadily accumulated that the incidence, causes, and consequences of negative behaviors and even treatment for these behaviors in women bear important differences compared with men.

In this chapter, general behavior change is explored, followed by specific behavior-related illnesses and modifications that may be beneficial. Making psychotherapists of primary care physicians is not the goal of this chapter. Instead, the goal is to provide physicians with the tools to recognize behaviors that are contributing to ill health, help the patient to recognize these problem behaviors, and assist the patient in following through with plans for behavior change, which may well include counseling or therapy by a professional in this field.

IDENTIFYING BEHAVIORS WITH NEGATIVE HEALTH CONSEQUENCES

Before a physician can help a patient change an unhealthy behavior, the behavior must be identified. Some problem behaviors are obvious and need only be clarified or quantified by the physician. Other behaviors are much less obvious or are completely hidden, and the physician must rely on patient self-reporting to identify the problem. Patients may present to the physician asking for help with smoking cessation or weight loss, but few patients will visit the physician's office stating that they need help with a drug or alcohol habit. Women rarely ask directly for help dealing with an abusive partner or how to avoid sexually transmitted diseases (STDs), although subtle signs may point to these issues. The physician must be alert for early signs of unhealthy behaviors and include screening questions for them at routine office visits. Familiarity with techniques for eliciting information from patients, while making them feel safe in yielding the information, is a necessary first step in positive behavioral change or lifestyle modification.

The annual gynecologic or "well-woman" exam is an ideal setting for screening for behaviors with negative health consequences because the focus of the visit is already on prevention. The annual interval lends itself to at least a cursory review of medical, family, and social history changes in the past year. Changes that occur may be conversation openers for exploring behavioral effects.

Questioning the patient while she is comfortably seated in a chair (not on the exam table), fully clothed, and with the physician seated (not standing or appearing hurried) will demonstrate that the physician is truly interested and is taking time to understand and help. The presence of others in the room during the interview is not conducive to completely honest answers. The physician must ask questions in a nonjudgmental fashion and listen attentively to the patient's reply. Questions about the severity or quantity of a problem are important, but it is often more telling to ask the patient her perspective and assessment of the problem, how she feels about the problem, and if she believes it is causing or contributing to other problems in her life.

Generally, identifying the problem and addressing the patient's feelings are all that can be accomplished at a health maintenance visit, and follow-up visits should be scheduled to further address the problem and explore possible solutions, unless acute intervention is needed for the patient's immediate safety. Asking the patient to return for a visit that will focus solely on the unhealthy behavior and the most effective ways to address changing that behavior underscores the significance of the need to consider, and hopefully implement, lifestyle change.

Some patients may be willing to identify problems more readily on a written questionnaire of past medical history, family history, and review of systems. Others may be more forthcoming with personal information only verbally. Written and verbal assurances of the confidentiality of the patient's information, the safety of the physician–patient relationship, and that the physician will not inform others (family, police, employers) of problems identified may help put the patient at ease and ensure honesty in her responses.

AFFECTING BEHAVIOR CHANGE: THE TRANSTHEORETICAL MODEL

There are many theories or models regarding human health behavior, but most of these models are attempts at explaining behaviors, with little or no emphasis on changing behaviors. The transtheoretical model (1) proposes that changing health-related behaviors involves progression through five distinct stages. This model was initially developed to address smoking cessation but can be applied to most problem behaviors in primary care practices. These five stages are *precontemplation, contemplation*, *preparation, action,* and *maintenance*. Obviously, the maintenance stage has no end; it continues indefinitely, although it may be marked by periodic relapses.

Each stage is characterized by a well-defined set of beliefs or actions that can be identified in the patient, as well as needs that must be met before a patient can proceed to the next stage (Table 19.1). Using this model, the health care provider identifies a patient's current stage and barriers to be overcome in moving to the next stage. Identifying any form of barriers and overcoming them is important in decreasing the time a patient spends in any one stage, and this prevents stagnation. It is vitally important to note that this model is applied to behaviors, not persons. The health care provider's role is only to be a catalyst for change. It is the patient who must go through the process of advancing from one stage to another. Health care providers, as well as patients, must be diligent in interpreting successes and setbacks as reflections of a behavior pattern, and not imbue them with personalized meanings or values.

The *precontemplation* stage is characterized by minimization or denial of the problem behavior and a reluctance to discuss risky behaviors. The patient has no plans for changing her behavior in the foreseeable future, and from her perspective, her behavior is not fundamentally detrimental or deterministic to her health. Precontemplators may acknowledge the dangers of their behavior in general, but minimize the consequences to themselves. The patient in the precontemplation stage will frequently view the behavior as not personally dangerous because of "off-setting" good behaviors. When pressured, the precontemplator may become angry,

TABLE 19.1

Stages of Change Related to Behavioral Modification Attempts

Stage of Change	Patient Characteristics	Provider Interventions to Promote Change
Precontemplation	Exhibits denial, reluctance, argumentativeness	Ask about patient's thoughts, express concern, ask patient to think about situation between visits
Contemplation	Open to talk about problem, weighs pros and cons, thinks about change, experiments with brief change, no firm plans	Reinforce benefits of change, assist in listing pros, ask about barriers to commitment to change
Preparation	Understands need for change, sees pros as greater than cons, sees obstacles and possible solutions, may delay time commitment	Reinforce pros, help with overcoming barriers, assist with timetable for change and public commitment
Action	Follows plan for change and commits to overcoming barriers, resisting slips and relapses	Help with slips, point out past mistakes to avoid in future, provide close follow-up, help with commitment in weak moments
Maintenance	Change is accomplished, focus changes to preventing relapse, begin to experience positive aspects of change	Provide positive reinforcement with every encounter, ask about benefits of change frequently, help avoid slips or relapse, reinforce long-term benefits and permanence of change
Relapse	Returns to problem behavior after some resolution, may give up if frustrated, may identify self as failure	Reinforce the learning that occurs with relapse, find methods to avoid the specific cause of relapse, reinforce return to plan of action

argumentative, or defensive. This stage may also be marked by a lack of patient confidence in her ability to change.

The physician must cautiously explore the precontemplator's assessment of the relationship of the behavior to the problem. For example, asking "How do you think your weight affects your blood pressure?" is less threatening than stating "You really need to lose some weight." The patient asked the first question is put in the position of contemplating the relationship between behavior and health, helping to move her toward the next stage. A strict demand to change behavior often angers the patient, skips two important stages of change, and is doomed to failure.

For some patients, asking permission to discuss the behavior may be very beneficial because this allows the patient to choose the topic of discussion and also reinforces the necessity of her willingness to discuss change in order to effect change. Most patients will give the permission, but the clinician must be prepared to move on to another topic easily if the patient refuses.

The goal with precontemplators is to begin the process of thinking about the behavior in the context of their medical conditions, not to affect a complete change right away. The physician might also ask a patient to continue to think or read about her problems as "homework" for their next outpatient visit. This may facilitate the patient's movement toward the next stage of change, which is contemplation.

Once the patient begins to consider the relationship between her behavior and her physical health, she has entered the *contemplation* stage. There is still no commitment to change, but the patient begins to see the need for change. This stage is one of ambivalence and wavering. A patient may be frustrated by the conflict between her desire to change and her lack of knowledge of how to effect the desired change. Confidence may be easily eroded in this stage, and slipping back to the precontemplation stage is common.

The clinician's goal in the contemplation stage is to continue to keep the patient focused on the behavior and associated health consequences, and to explore with the patient the obstacles that prevent moving toward preparation. Patients gain insight into necessary actions to overcome barriers if they are first asked to consider what is holding them back from making the desired change. Making some small sacrifices at this point may empower patients in this ambivalent stage and encourage progress to the next stage. For example, counting calories for just the noon meal for a few days, or not smoking for at least 30 minutes after awakening for 1 week, may be a small increment that the patient can achieve easily, boosting morale, confidence, and self-esteem during a stage in which wavering is very common. These small experiments at changing behaviors for limited times and in limited ways slowly help move the patient toward the preparation stage.

The *preparation* stage is marked by a commitment to changing behavior. A date for affecting change will be set for the not too distant future, and preparations are made for the ultimate action stage. Detailed plans for change are formulated. The patient in the preparation stage may make small changes in behavior to "test the water," such as reducing or limiting but not eliminating the undesired behavior. This stage is also characterized by an increase in confidence in one's ability to achieve the goal, although confidence may vary significantly from time to time. In this stage, the patient attempts to foresee those problems that might cause a relapse back to the previous behavior and makes plans to avoid or confront those problems to prevent relapse.

It is important to remind the patient that prior experience with relapse gives the patient a distinct advantage, and also to remind her that for most individuals, several attempts are made before the behavior is modified or eliminated. Each effort helps her gain experience toward the final goal of changing or eliminating the behavior on a permanent basis.

During the preparation stage, a timeline for change is set and a plan is constructed with the patient to determine what will be needed for success. The physician can assist the patient in prospectively identifying or recognizing pitfalls that might result in a less than fully successful effort, and in proactively planning a route to avoid or overcome these anticipated challenges. For example, the clinician will assist the patient in finding a low stress time frame for smoking cessation, prescribe any medications planned for use in the cessation attempt, and provide instructions in their usage. Cold feet are common as the "quit date" approaches, and the patient should be reassured that her decision to try to effect the change is the right thing to do and that feelings of anxiety or nervousness before attempting any change are normal.

Behavioral change attempt is not a reflection of a patient's value or self-worth, it is the action of replacing an unhealthy behavior with a better one. For patients who remain focused on the possibility of failure, reiterate that a relapse is an opportunity to learn how to strengthen the overall plan for changing the behavior. Efforts to affect change should be focused on strengthening the patient's image of herself, her perceptions and feelings of control in her life, and should not be framed in terms of pleasing or disappointing the health care provider or anyone else. A follow-up clinic visit or phone call should be arranged shortly after the agreed-on "quit date." Encourage the patient to share her commitment to change with those who can provide her with positive support and encouragement.

The *action* stage begins when the patient makes the desired change. This stage may vary in length for different problem behaviors and individuals. The clinician should positively reinforce any successful behavioral change efforts and should be very supportive during the entire action phase. Chart notes should be made to remind the clinician to ask about the patient's progress at follow-up visits. "Slips" are to be proactively discussed: the one cigarette, a rich dessert, or a missed day of exercise. Prepare the patient to recover rapidly from a "slip," forgive herself, and learn from the "slip" to prevent a full relapse.

Unfortunately, the most common end to the action stage is *relapse*. Supportive counseling for the patient at the moment of relapse may be helpful in progressing rapidly back to the action stage, with a short preparation stage for laying better plans for the next attempt. Although not common, some patients will transition from the action stage to the maintenance stage, with no bouts of relapse.

The action stage melds into the *maintenance* stage as the patient's focus changes from avoiding the undesired behavior to avoiding relapse and maintaining the gains made through the action stage. There is no end point for the maintenance stage, although the amount of focus the patient must give to avoiding relapse may decrease over time. It is important to continue to ask about successes, ask about any "slips" that occurred and how they were handled, and make plans for future slips. Watch for signs of decreasing enthusiasm for her healthier behaviors, especially if the desired health effects are not forthcoming, such as the patient who experiences weight loss, but whose blood pressure remains high. Focus on the other positive effects the patient is experiencing and encourage continued efforts.

Relapses can lead to discouragement and feelings of failure. The vast majority of those who relapse will find themselves in the contemplation or preparation stage, but some will revert to the precontemplation stage. Those who revert to the contemplation or preparation stages are well poised for another attempt at behavior change, given the right encouragement and counseling (2). The physician should attempt to refocus the patient's attention, not on the unsuccessful effort, but on the learning made available by the failed attempt and the success that it could bring on the next attempt. Focus on the details of the event or emotions that led to the relapse and assist the patient in finding new ways to overcome the obstacle with the next attempt. Remind the patient that successful behavior change generally occurs after multiple efforts, and that with knowledge gained from a relapse, she is smarter about herself and closer to her goal of behavioral change.

SMOKING CESSATION

Tobacco use, especially cigarette smoking, is the leading cause of preventable death in the United States. Women now account for 39% of all smoking-related deaths each year in the United States (3). Lung cancer is the leading cause of cancer-related death among women, having surpassed breast cancer in 1987. In women, smoking is also associated with increased risk for breast, cervical, and vulvar cancer, as well as cancer of the mouth, esophagus, pancreas, bladder, and kidney. As of 2004, lung cancer incidence rates continue to increase among women, while they are declining in men. Lung cancer accounts for 12% of new cancer diagnoses in women, but 25% of cancer related deaths (4). Adult men and women smokers are estimated to lose an average of 13.2 and 14.5 years of life, respectively, because of smoking (5).

Despite laws prohibiting sales of cigarettes and tobacco products to people younger than 18 years old, more than one-third of all adult smokers start smoking by age 14 and nearly all before age 18 (6). Girls tend to start smoking earlier than boys, and women have lower quitting rates than men (6, 7). The prevalence of smoking has an inverse relationship to education level in women (8).

Although female smokers face the same general health risks as male smokers, there are some unique sex-related hazards. Smoking has been associated with a number of reproductive abnormalities, including increased menstrual irregularities, reduced fertility, diminished lactation, earlier menopause, and higher rates of osteoporosis (9). Smoking increases the risk of age-related macular degeneration in women (10).

The most recent U.S. guidelines for treating tobacco use and dependence delineate several recommendations for clinicians and are the result of the review of more than 6000 individual articles on cessation therapy (11, 12). The U.S. Public Health Service statement includes the following points:

- Tobacco use is a chronic, long-term condition that often requires repeated and long-term, intervention efforts. Effective treatments exist that can produce long-term or even permanent abstinence. All health care providers should address tobacco addiction at every clinic visit, even if only briefly.
- Every patient should be offered brief interventions to increase their motivation to quit. If they are currently willing to quit, pharmacotherapy should be offered to assist with their efforts. Patients who have recently quit should receive supportive therapy to prevent relapse.
- Tobacco users should be identified and documented at each health care encounter, and appropriate intervention offered.

- Brief tobacco-dependence interventions are effective at promoting eventual behavioral change. As little as 3 minutes spent discussing smoking can substantially impact the patient's willingness to quit smoking.
- There is a dose-response relationship between the intensity of tobacco dependence counseling and its effectiveness. That is not to say treatment efforts should be harsh, but they should be intense, sustained, and followed up with brief interventions aimed at encouraging cessation, supporting efforts, or applauding successes.
- Three types of counseling were found to be especially effective and should be used for all smokers. These are problem solving and skills training, provision of social support as part of the treatment, and securing social support outside the treatment setting.
- Many effective pharmacotherapeutic options are available (Table 19.2), and in the absence of contraindications, at least one should be offered in all cessation efforts. These treatments include bupropion (Wellbutrin) and nicotine replacement systems such as patches, gum, nasal spray, and inhalers. All have been shown to dramatically increase success rates in smoking cessation, especially when used in a setting of ongoing supportive therapy.

TABLE 19.2

Medications Used for Smoking Cessation

Medication	Dose	Benefits	Possible Adverse Effects	Pregnancy Class
Bupropion SR	150 mg every day for 3 days, then twice a day Start 1–2 wk before quit date Use 12–26 wk or more	Reduces nicotine cravings Convenient dosing	Dry mouth, Sleep disturbances Decreased seizure threshold	B
Nicotine gum	2–4 mg/pc, chew q1–2h Use 10–15 pc/day initially, then taper	Peaks and troughs simulate nicotine levels of smoking Helps with oral habit Variety of flavors	Sore mouth and throat from vigorous chewing; "chew and park" recommended Dental work harm	D
Nicotine patch	1 patch/day Tapering or constant dose Use 8–12 wk	Easy to use Concealable	Skin rashes Note: Steady dose does not mimic nicotine levels of smoking	D
Nicotine inhaler	6–16 cartridges/day (80 inhalations per cartridge) Taper over 3–6 mo	Predictable control Peaks and troughs simulate smoking Keeps hands and mouth busy	Mouth and throat irritation Note: Cartridges are temperature sensitive	D
Nicotine nasal spray	1 spray/nare 8–40 times/day	Fastest acting Peaks and troughs simulate smoking	Nose irritation Allergy aggravation Note: Do not swallow or inhale Avoid with asthma	D

OTC, over the counter; Rx, prescription.

- Tobacco dependence treatments are both clinically effective and cost effective compared with other medical and disease prevention interventions; as such, insurers and purchasers should provide reimbursement for effective counseling and pharmacologic treatments for smoking cessation.

The clinical practice guidelines (12) for treating tobacco use and dependence are divided into two categories, based on patient's interest in treatment. For those patients willing to quit smoking, there are the "5 As":

- Ask—identify all tobacco users at each office visit
- Advise—in a clear and personal way, advise all tobacco users to quit
- Address—the patient's willingness to consider an attempt at cessation and the level of commitment
- Assist—the patient with training, counseling, and support for an effort at cessation
- Arrange—schedule follow-up contact with the patient to continue to support efforts for cessation.

For those unwilling to consider smoking cessation, there are the "5 Rs":

- Relevance—in a personal way, identify for the patient the reasons they need to stop; relate these to their illness, health, or life values
- Risks—identify the risks associated with continued tobacco use
- Rewards—help the patient develop a list of positive benefits to be gained from smoking cessation
- Roadblocks—help the patient identify barriers to their cessation attempt and possible mechanisms for overcoming those barriers
- Repetition—repeat the "5Rs" at each patient visit, if only briefly, to emphasize and motivate the patient for an attempt at cessation.

Following these guidelines, along with the strategies for change mentioned earlier, should give the clinician tools to assist the patient in their smoking cessation thoughts or endeavors.

ALCOHOL AND DRUG ABUSE

Abuse of alcohol and drugs, both prescription and illegal, is widespread in American culture. An estimated 22.0 million Americans ages 12 or older (9.4% of the total population) in 2002 depended on or abused alcohol, drugs, or both. Of these, 3.2 million were classified with dependence on or abuse of both alcohol and illicit drugs, 3.9 million were dependent on or abused illicit drugs but not alcohol, and 14.9 million were dependent on or abused alcohol but not illicit drugs (13). Table 19.3 clarifies some of the terms used in the literature: addiction, abuse, and dependence.

Unfortunately, the abuse of these substances often remains hidden until a cataclysmic event uncovers the problem. Abuse of substances and dependency on them cause significant medical,

TABLE 19.3

Definitions of Commonly Used Alcohol and Substance Abuse Terms

Abuse	Departure from the societal norms of use without the presence of physiologic tolerance
Dependence	The substance plays a central role in the patient's life
Addiction	Use of the substance has created physiologic tolerance Nonuse results in withdrawal symptoms Desire for use results in compulsive substance-seeking behavior

social, and legal problems. Health care providers must be aware of the earliest signs of substance dependency and abuse problems, and attempt to intervene at the earliest opportunity. The pressure to hide habits of substance abuse is particularly heightened for women because they bear an undue social stigma if they are abusers (14). Female substance abusers are frequently victims of past sexual or physical abuses. Up to 70% of women in substance or alcohol abuse treatment report that they were repeatedly sexually abused as children (15, 16). Other studies indicate that women with alcohol abuse problems are frequently victims of physical abuse, either as a cause or consequence of their alcohol abuse (17).

The direct and indirect costs of substance abuse are estimated at $58 billion annually. The specific individual health outcomes either related or secondary to alcohol abuse are well known: hypertension, cardiomyopathy, cirrhosis and hepatic failure, renal disease, and many cancers, including breast cancer (18). Other substances of abuse have identifiable consequences for the abuser as well: methamphetamine is linked to hypertension and stroke, cocaine may induce acute myocardial infarction, and opioid abuse is linked to renal and hepatic disease.

Viewed from an individual patient standpoint, the evidence to support the need to avoid or cease the abuse of alcohol and other substances is compelling. It is only further bolstered by evidence linking substance abuse to the overall health of the population: more than four times as many American women die of substance abuse-related disease than of breast cancer (19, 20). Alcohol intoxication is associated with approximately 50% of the nation's traffic fatalities and homicides every year. For these and many other reasons, clinicians must be prepared to intervene in the arena of substance abuse.

Alcohol Dependence and Abuse

An estimated 6 million American women meet the diagnostic criteria for alcohol dependency or abuse (21). Although men are more likely to enter alcohol treatment through social programs or peer-oriented settings, women are more likely to seek help from a physician or mental health care provider prior to treatment entry than men (22–24). Rates of lifetime alcohol dependence or abuse among women in primary care settings are approximately 23%; in outpatient gynecology practices, prevalence rates of current abuse or dependence range from 12 to 20% (24, 25).

Many women with an alcohol problem will present to their primary care provider with nonspecific health complaints, nervousness, or insomnia (26). Physicians prescribe psychoactive substances more readily for women than for men with the same complaints; for women with alcohol use disorders, a sedative drug prescription represents an increased risk for a secondary addiction to be incurred (27).

Alcoholism is a common but complex disease with a high rate of heritability. Although studies have consistently supported the existence of a moderate genetic influence in men, evidence for the role of genetic factors in alcoholism in women has varied across studies (28). A genetic influence on alcohol use disorders is probable in some but not all women with alcohol use disorders, and the patterns of heritability in women may differ significantly compared with men (29, 30).

In the Stockholm adoption study, there appeared to be two patterns of heredity relevant to alcohol use disorders in women. The more common type of inheritance, type 1, was seen in both men and women, and was characterized by adult onset and less severe alcohol abuse. Alcohol abuse in either the biological mother or father increased the risk for alcohol problems three-fold in the adoptees. The less common type 2 pattern of heredity was only seen in men and was characterized by severe, early-onset alcohol abuse, was associated with criminality in both the biological father and son, and seemed to impart a stronger hereditary influence than the type 1 pattern (31, 32).

Alcohol dependence and abuse is further complicated by the frequency of other comorbid disorders, including anxiety, depression, and personality disorders. Comorbid disorders are estimated to occur in up to 80% of clinical research populations and 50% of community samples (33–35).

The comorbidities present in women dependent on or abusive of alcohol differ from those found in men with the same disease: women have higher rates of comorbid anxiety and affective disorders, and men have higher rates of comorbid abuse of other drugs, conduct disorder, and antisocial personality disorder (35). The onset of psychiatric disorders precedes the onset of

TABLE 19.4

Gender-Specific Definitions for Both Moderate and At-Risk Drinking

	Men	Women
Moderate drinking for age younger than 65 years	≤2 drinks/day	≤1 drink/day
Moderate drinking for age older than 65 years	≤1 drink/day	≤1 drink/day
At-risk drinking	≥14 drinks/wk or ≥4 drinks/occasion	≥7 drinks/wk or ≥3 drinks/occasion

From the National Institute on Alcohol Abuse and Alcoholism (NIAAA), 1995.
2005 Dietary Guidelines for Americans. US Dept Health & Human Services & US Dept Agriculture at: http://www.health.gov/dietary guidelines.

substance abuse, including alcohol, more often in women than in men (36, 37). It is unclear if the presence of one disorder (e.g., alcoholism) increases the risk for another disorder (e.g., depression) or if the risk factors for both disorders are the same.

Table 19.4 defines moderate and at-risk drinking levels based on age and gender. Age is an important predictor of substance abuse, with per capita consumption peaking under the age of 50 and declining with increasing age. Younger women report higher rates of substance abuse, and older women lower rates (35). Elderly alcoholics are more likely to have recently seen a physician than their younger cohorts but are less likely to have been diagnosed or be receiving treatment. An important clue that alcohol dependency or abuse may be a problem for the elderly patient is a change in functional status. The CAGE questionnaire (discussed later in this section) has been validated for use among the elderly (38).

It is estimated that 12% of older American women regularly drink in excess of recommended guidelines and are considered at-risk drinkers; older women are also the largest users of sedatives and narcotic agents (39). The elderly are more sensitive to the acute effects of alcohol, and dysphoria, rather than euphoria, is the predominant mood associated with alcohol dependency or abuse for them. Because the elderly are often taking prescribed substances and are more likely to have chronic medical conditions, they are more likely to have alcohol interactions with prescribed drugs.

Although women are less likely than men to abuse alcohol, women are more susceptible to alcohol-induced diseases (liver disease, cardiovascular disease, and brain damage) and are more likely to suffer alcohol-associated trauma due to accidents or violence (40). Women may be more susceptible to the effects of alcohol than men at the same level of drinking and exhibit the complications of alcohol abuse earlier in their abuse than men (41, 42). In a more recent prospective study of a large population followed for 12 years, daily ingestion of 7 to 13 beverages (84 to 156 g alcohol) in women raised the risk of alcohol-induced liver disease and cirrhosis, whereas a similar increase in risk in men was only seen with daily ingestion of 14 to 27 beverages (168 to 324 g) (43). This susceptibility may lead to a phenomenon known as "telescoping"; telescoping is defined as "an accelerated medical, physiologic, and psychologic progression of alcoholism in women compared to men given the same duration and intensity of drinking careers" (20).

Several explanations have been offered for the increased susceptibility of women to alcohol-related organ injury. There is a gender difference in ethanol pharmacokinetics that is manifested as higher blood ethanol levels in women after drinking. A gender difference in alcohol elimination rates may increase the level of acetaldehyde in the liver and in the blood in women compared with men. Differences in portal and peripheral blood endotoxin levels that produce proinflammatory cytokines may exist between men and women, and there may be a gender-based difference of alcohol metabolism in the liver. Differences of brain neurosteroid levels may also play a role in the differences in cognitive deficits seen after alcohol abuse in women compared with men (44).

Like men, women experience a decreased risk of both fatal and nonfatal coronary artery disease events with light-to-moderate drinking (less than two drinks per day), with this decreased risk being most apparent in women at highest risk for coronary artery disease (45, 46). However, for women younger than 55 years of age, heavy alcohol ingestion (more than two drinks per day) increases the risk of death from cardiovascular disease. The risk for nondrinkers (less than one drink per week) in women younger than 55 years of age is 3.5%, compared with 11.2% for heavy female drinkers younger than age 55 (47). Given the known potential harmful effects of alcohol and the lack of any randomized, controlled trials on the subject, the endorsement of alcohol drinking at any level for protection from coronary heart disease cannot be recommended.

Alcoholic women are more susceptible to developing myopathy and cardiomyopathy than alcoholic men. Myopathy has been found in one-half of alcoholic women, and among asymptomatic alcoholic women, a lower mean ejection fraction and larger ventricular mass in comparison to control women has been noted (48).

Alcohol abuse among women is also associated with an increased risk of breast cancer, dysmenorrhea, infertility, irregular menses, and spontaneous abortions (18, 49–53).

Because they more commonly seek help from a health care provider, a visit with a primary care provider represents an important opportunity for screening and possible entry into treatment for women with alcohol use problems. Screening and brief interventions for alcohol use disorders by primary care providers are effective in reducing future alcohol consumption (54, 55). The U.S. Preventive Services Task Force endorses the use of a self-report screening test for alcohol disorders in the primary care setting (56). Commonly used tools include the CAGE questionnaire, the Alcohol Use Disorders Identification Test (AUDIT), and the TWEAK questionnaire (57–59). These are outlined in Appendix 19.1. A literature review supports use of the AUDIT for screening for at-risk, hazardous, and harmful drinking, and use of the CAGE for screening for lifetime and current abuse or dependence disorders (54). (This same study however, noted that in many of the reviewed articles, there was a lack of inclusion of women or a failure to breakdown results by gender in the studies.) Bradley et al. (60) performed the first systematic review and performance description of alcohol screening questionnaires in women and found that while the CAGE is relatively insensitive in predominantly white female populations, the TWEAK and AUDIT performed adequately in African American or white women when lower than usual cut points were used. Although this review did not clearly define which screening test is optimal for women, it did recommend lowering the cut points for a positive response in women to the following: TWEAK greater than or equal to 2 points; AUDIT greater than or equal to 4 points; and CAGE greater than or equal to 1 point (60). In using any of these tools or others, further questioning about quantity and frequency of drinking should follow a positive screen.

Drug and Illicit Substance Abuse

Issues related to drug and substance abuse are very similar to that of alcohol abuse; in fact, they are often grouped together under the heading of "alcohol and substance abuse" because they share so many similarities in etiologic theory, diagnosis, life-altering or life-threatening complications, and treatment approaches. Although men are more likely to report current illicit drug use than women (10.3% versus 6.4%), women who depend on or abuse drugs or illicit substances are more likely to have a history of parental alcohol or drug abuse then men (13). Childhood sexual abuse is a strong marker for adult drug abuse in women, and it is estimated that 30 to 75% of women in substance abuse treatment have a history of sexual trauma, leading many to believe that sexual trauma is a key contributor to women's drug abuse (61–63). Substance abuse problems in adulthood in women are associated with rape, intimate partner violence, and greater physical aggression in dating (17). Women who abuse drugs often have low levels of self-esteem and an enhanced feeling of powerlessness. Minority women, in particular, may face additional cultural or language barriers that preclude or impede their diagnosis and treatment.

Adults who use illicit drugs are more than twice as likely to have significant mental illness as adults who do not use illicit drugs. In 2002, among adults using illicit drugs in the past year, 17.1% had a significant mental illness in that year, compared with a rate of 6.9% among nonusing adults (13).

Treatment of substance abuse problems must not focus solely on the substance being abused and its potential health complications, but must also incorporate therapy for the myriad of other health risks associated with substance abuse.

Treatment of Alcohol and Other Substance Dependency or Abuse

Treatment of Alcohol Dependency or Abuse

There is evidence that a brief, office-based intervention in the primary care setting is associated with sustained reductions in alcohol consumption in women of childbearing age. Fleming et al. (55) studied intervention with two 15-minute physician-delivered counseling visits that included advice, education, and contracting with use of a scripted workbook. This reduced both 7-day alcohol use and binge drinking episodes during the 4-year follow-up period. In a separate meta-analysis of 12 randomized controlled trials, women who received a brief intervention were more likely to moderate alcohol use than men (64). Women have higher rates of abstinence when treated in a medical setting compared with a peer-oriented setting (e.g., Alcoholics Anonymous) (65).

Treatment of Other Substance Dependency or Abuse

Successful treatments for substance dependency or abuse, either alone or in combination with alcohol dependency or abuse, often use a combination of the biomedical and psychosocial approaches. The social models of substance abuse assert that environment and the relationships a patient has within that environment are key factors in determining if a person engages in substance use. In fact, the initiation of substance use usually results from interactions with family, peers, and neighborhood, whereas substance abuse occurs within the context of friends and lovers, and often results in social isolation. Regardless of the drug, female substance abusers are more likely to have been initiated into use of the drug by a male user, and this drug use is often associated with an intimate relationship (66, 67).

Among persons ages 12 or older in 2002, males were more likely than females to receive treatment for an alcohol or illicit drug problem in the past year (2.1% versus 0.9%, respectively) (13). Women are more reluctant to seek help and may need special considerations, such as child care facilities (14). Female drug users report feeling pressured by a spouse or lover to use drugs and encounter more opposition to seeking treatment than their male counterparts (68). In addition, the male partners of women who depend on or abuse substances are less likely to give support when the woman is in treatment (69).

It has only been more recently that substance abuse treatment programs have attempted to develop models for treatment that are not male oriented, focus less on re-entry into the workplace, and focus more on strengthening or renewing emotional relationships and improving self-esteem. These are factors of significant importance to women in recovery (70).

Although some studies have shown benefit for women treated in a gender-specific setting, whether specialized female-only treatment programs have better outcomes compared with traditional programs is still unresolved (71–73). Finding a treatment program specifically designed for women is challenging. Currently, the Substance Abuse & Mental Health Services Administration (SAMHSA) of the U.S. Department of Health and Human Services does have a substance abuse treatment facility locator on its website.

Pharmacotherapy should almost never be the sole treatment modality for any substance abuse problem. Many medications have been used in the treatment of detoxification and withdrawal (benzodiazepines, antidepressants, clonidine) as replacements for the medication to which the patient is addicted (methadone, nicotine replacement systems), as modifiers of altered neurochemistry in the addiction-prone patient (antidepressants, acamprosate, amantadine, Parlodel), or as antagonists to the addictive substance (buprenorphine, naloxone, naltrexone). Although these may be used in conjunction with other therapies in a carefully structured treatment program, they should never be simply prescribed to the patient to self-treat her addiction.

Perhaps the most important tool for the primary care provider is the knowledge of treatment programs and support systems geared toward women with abuse problems, and to work with the patient to recognize the problem and the importance of treatment. The key to successful treatment of the substance abuser is to find the right combination of many modalities, and to support the patient through the cessation attempt, initial period of sobriety, and thereafter.

OBESITY

Obesity has become pandemic in the United States. Currently, two out of every three American adults are either overweight or obese, compared with one in every four in the 1960s (74). The problem of obesity is more prevalent in women than in men and in African American or Mexican American women than in women of Caucasian descent (75). Women in the lowest socioeconomic strata are 50% more likely to be obese than those of higher status.

Obesity is a significant contributor to a myriad of medical conditions, including premature mortality, coronary artery disease, hypertension, dyslipidemia, sleep apnea, type 2 diabetes, and many cancers (gallbladder, uterine, cervical, ovarian, and breast) (76). More than 280,000 deaths related to obesity occur annually in the United States, and if current trends continue, obesity will overtake smoking as the leading cause of preventable deaths (77). Obesity is associated with greater morbidity and poorer quality of life measures than smoking, alcohol use disorders, and poverty (78). The social consequences of obesity are likewise significant; in one study, obese women were less likely to marry, more likely to live in poverty, and had lower incomes than comparable groups with normal weights (79). Obese persons frequently suffer from discrimination (80).

Changes in both diet and lifestyle have contributed significantly to the increased incidence of obesity. The size of food portions sold or served has increased over time, and lifestyles have become increasingly sedentary (81).

Most of the studies indicate that weight gradually increases over the lifespan for women. Although only 20% of women in their 20s are overweight, 50% of women between the ages of 50 and 59 are overweight (75). The incidence of obesity in women increases during the childbearing years, and weight gain during pregnancy is the primary predictor of weight retention after pregnancy (82, 83).

There is a propensity toward weight gain during menopause, and there is a tendency to gain it in an abdominal distribution in lieu of a gynecoid distribution. The use of hormone therapy in menopause has been shown to positively influence fat distribution and does not adversely affect body composition or energy balance (84–86). Decreased energy expenditure (associated with decreasing muscle mass) and less physical activity in later years is consistently related to weight gain (87).

Obesity is a complex disease, representing an interaction between the environment, genetics, and metabolism. These interactions interface in the biology of body energy balance (88). An energy balance over the years yields a constant body weight, but even a 1% error in kcal intake per year ($\sim$ 10,000 kcal) in a nonobese person results in a gain of 2.5 lb per year and, over a lifetime, leads to overweight or obesity (89).

One of the common theories regarding obesity is the "set point" theory, which postulates that a decrease in energy consumption may be met with opposing changes in body metabolism as a means of resistance. The obesity literature has shown that metabolism may decline by as much as 15% more than the percentage of body weight loss (90). As a result, overweight and obesity may be maintained despite the best efforts of the patient to lose weight.

Genetics of obesity influence the regulatory mechanisms of body weight in both humans and animals. Human studies indicate that 80% of body mass index (BMI) variance is genetic (90). Twin studies have demonstrated that even when raised in different environments, twins have similar body weights. Adoption studies have likewise demonstrated that an individual's weight more closely reflects the weight of the biological parent than the adoptive parent (91).

An increase in adipose tissue mass is associated with insulin resistance, a phenomenon that primarily involves the uptake and metabolism of glucose by skeletal muscle (92). Research into insulin resistance has led to the identification and naming of many adipocyte secretory products (e.g., leptin, resistin, adiponectin); these secretory products are categorized as adipokines (93–95). Evidence is increasing that these adipokines are important determinants of insulin resistance, either through endocrine or autocrine effects.

Human obesity is clearly related to leptin, a circulating anorexic polypeptide, and leptin production. Most of the obesity seen in humans is probably not due to a deficiency of leptin but is more likely associated with receptor disorders (88). Studies of the effect of peripheral administration of leptin, signaling pathways of leptin, and even brain uptake and transport of leptin are ongoing (96–98).

Environment plays an important role in the pathogenesis of overweight and obesity. The data on socioeconomic status and weight reflect many environmental influences such as poor nutritional knowledge, a diet high in high-fat foods, and limited access to exercise programs or facilities, coupled with an unsafe environment for outdoor physical activity (99). Because behavior determines dietary composition and exercise habits, it therefore also influences weight. Numerous studies have demonstrated that obese individuals are less physically active than their thinner counterparts, and that this is a contributor to, not a consequence of, obesity (100).

It is important for clinicians to recognize the genetic, behavioral, and environmental factors influencing a patient's obesity, and to assist her toward a personalized and reasonable goal. Even modest weight losses can lead to tremendous benefits in health and well-being. Diabetes and hypertension both show significant beneficial responses to small changes in weight. All patients should be encouraged to recognize the importance of dietary choices and exercise in helping them attain a healthy weight.

The diagnosis of obesity is most commonly defined by BMI:

$$\text{BMI} = \text{weight (kg)} \div (\text{height [m]})^2 \tag{19.1}$$

or

$$\text{BMI} = (\text{weight [lb]} \times 703) \div (\text{height [in]})^2$$

Figure 19.1 provides a BMI chart using U.S. pounds and inches. A BMI less than 18 kg/m^2 is considered underweight, 19 to 25 is ideal, greater than 25 is overweight, and greater than 30 is obese.

Although this measure is clinically useful, it tends to overdiagnose obesity in young athletic persons (with higher bone density and muscle mass quantities) and underdiagnose obesity in the elderly. BMI also fails to take into account the percentage of body fat, which is the ultimate determination of obesity. Use of skin calipers to measure the skinfold thickness is the most convenient way to estimate body fat percentage—although underwater weighing is the most accurate—and many health and exercise clubs offer this service. The average young adult man and woman with regular activity levels have 15% and 25% body fat, respectively. Elite women athletes may have as low as 12% body fat. Generally, men and women with body fat percentages greater than 20% and 30%, respectively, are considered obese.

Body fat distribution is important in predicting poor health consequences. Android obesity, in which the body fat is distributed more about the waist, rather than the hips, is strongly associated with increased risk for diabetes, hypertension, and coronary artery disease, as well as all-cause mortality (101). The National Institutes of Health has suggested using the waist circumference instead of the waist–hip ratio. A waist circumference greater than 88 cm (35 inches) in women is associated with more visceral fat, a more atherogenic type of fat, and with increased insulin resistance (102). In women with a BMI greater than 35 kg/m^2, the waist circumference loses its predictive power. In a patient with a BMI less than or equal to 35 kg/m^2, changes in the waist circumference over time are useful predictors of changes in risk for cardiovascular disease (103).

Gynecoid obesity, in which the weight is more heavily distributed on the hips and legs, is less strongly associated with disease states. Although distribution of body fat is largely genetic, modifiable behavioral determinants of android obesity have been demonstrated. Smoking, high-fat diets, lack of exercise, and stress tend to result in android obesity, and modification of these factors can greatly decrease morbidity associated with this pattern (104).

The evaluation for obesity begins with a through history of weight trends and dietary habits, determination of the BMI and waist circumference, a careful medical history and physical examination, and a lab evaluation geared toward the causes and complications of obesity. A review of current medications should be included because some categories of drugs are known to contribute to weight gain. Examples of such agents include antidepressants, antiepileptics, antipsychotics, glucocorticoids, and some progestins.

Body Weight (lb)

Height (in)																	
58	91	96	100	105	110	115	119	124	129	134	138	143	148	153	158	162	167
59	94	99	104	109	114	119	124	128	133	138	143	148	153	158	163	168	173
60	97	102	107	112	118	123	128	133	138	143	148	153	158	163	168	174	179
61	100	106	111	116	122	127	132	137	143	148	153	158	164	169	174	180	185
62	104	109	115	120	126	131	136	142	147	153	158	164	169	175	180	186	191
63	107	113	118	124	130	135	141	146	152	158	163	169	175	180	186	191	197
64	110	116	122	128	134	140	145	151	157	163	169	174	180	186	192	197	204
65	114	120	126	132	138	144	150	156	162	168	174	180	186	192	198	204	210
66	118	124	130	136	142	148	155	161	167	173	179	186	192	198	204	210	216
67	121	127	134	140	146	153	159	166	172	178	185	191	198	204	211	217	223
68	125	131	138	144	151	158	164	171	177	184	190	197	203	210	216	223	230
69	128	135	142	149	155	162	169	176	182	189	196	203	209	216	223	230	236
70	132	139	146	153	160	167	174	181	188	195	202	209	216	222	229	236	243
71	136	143	150	157	165	172	179	186	193	200	208	215	222	229	236	243	250
72	140	147	154	162	169	177	184	191	199	206	213	221	228	235	242	250	258
BMI	**19**	**20**	**21**	**22**	**23**	**24**	**25**	**26**	**27**	**28**	**29**	**30**	**31**	**32**	**33**	**34**	**35**

FIGURE 19.1 ● Body mass index (BMI) chart. A person with a BMI less than 18 kg/m^2 is considered to be underweight, 19 to 25 is ideal, more than 25 is overweight, and more than 30 is obese. Note that the BMI fails to correlate well with the gold standard measurement—body fat percentage. Using body fat percentages, the definition of obesity is different for men and women (more than 20% and more than 30%, respectively).

The key to all weight loss programs is the patient's motivation and desire to lose weight. Using the transtheoretical model for change described earlier, frequent but brief discussions about a patient's current weight status and its effects on her health may help move the patient toward contemplation of change (2). Using the stages-of-change model, clinicians should positively support any motivation the patient may have for change, help her make progress in her efforts, and offer specific guidance. Goals for weight loss should be attainable, such as loss of 5 to 10% of current body weight, or 2 BMI units, over a period of 6 months, although in women with a BMI greater than or equal to 35, greater weight loss is desirable. Attainment of these weight loss goals, in combination with lifestyle changes (increased exercise, improved diet composition) that can be sustained for the long term is far preferable to the seemingly impossible goal of attaining "ideal" body weight. Modest weight losses are sufficient to significantly reduce blood pressure, improve glycemic control, improve the lipid profile, and decrease morbidity and mortality (105–107). Setting appropriate goals for weight loss may diminish the rate of relapse.

Obesity requires long-term management. Losing weight may be achieved through dietary and physical activity changes and behavior modification; maintaining weight loss is achieved through increased physical activity. Other therapies, such as pharmacotherapy or surgical therapies, may be beneficial for the morbidly obese population but are not indicated for overweight to moderately obese patients. Behavior change to maintain the weight loss long term is most critical, and without this intervention, any plan is apt to fail.

Dietary Modification for Obesity

Dietary modification to reduce caloric intake and modify the form of calories consumed is absolutely necessary for success in treating obesity. There is considerable controversy regarding type of diet a patient should undertake.

Currently, the most commonly recommended diet is a low-fat, low-calorie diet based on the U.S. Department of Agriculture's food guide pyramid. A diet based on this pyramid limits fat to 30% of daily caloric intake and protein to 15%, leaving carbohydrates (mostly complex carbohydrates and fiber) at greater than 55%. Total caloric intake to affect weight loss is generally recommended at 1200 to 1500 calories per day for women and 1500 to 1800 calories per day for men.

For morbidly obese patients, some obesity experts advocate a very low-calorie diet initially. These plans generally use a liquid diet, restricted to 400 to 800 calories per day, with an emphasis on higher protein and very low fat percentages. Use of these diets requires careful monitoring by the physician and should probably be restricted to patients with BMI greater than 30 mg/kg^2 or patients requiring rapid preoperative weight loss. Although these diets resulted in a very rapid loss of weight initially, there was no significant difference in the weight loss maintained at 1 year compared with more conventional plans (104).

There is an increased risk of gallstone formation in patients on very low-calorie liquid diets, low-calorie diets, or after gastric bypass surgery, and Caucasian women may be at increased risk for this adverse effect (108). Approximately 50% of patients undergoing rapid weight loss will develop gallstones or biliary sludge (108, 109). Ursodiol (Actigall), a natural bile salt that decreases the amount of cholesterol secreted by the liver into bile, is the only U.S. Food and Drug Administration-approved therapy for prevention of gallstones in obese patients experiencing rapid weight loss with a very low-calorie diet.

Over the last few years, interest has been increasing in low-carbohydrate diet plans. These sharply curtail carbohydrate intake, while liberalizing the intake of protein, and in some cases, fats. Although conclusive research has not yet been completed, preliminary results from two studies have been published and indicate that a low-carbohydrate diet may result in more weight loss, decreased triglycerides, and improved insulin sensitivity compared with a low-fat diet. Both studies emphasized that the results were based on relatively short-term follow-up and small groups, and that larger-scale clinical studies were needed to determine the long-term safety and efficacy of low-carbohydrate, high-protein, high-fat diets (110, 111).

Before recommending a specific diet plan, the physician may want to refer the patient for consultation with a registered dietician for a thorough evaluation of the patient's diet, education about basic dietary principles, and recommendations regarding specific diet plans for the patient.

Some very successful programs combine moral support, behavioral and dietary modifications, and teaching. For many patients, this represents the most convenient mechanism for healthy, maintainable weight loss. Commercial programs such as Weight-Watchers, Jenny Craig, and Taking Off Pounds Sensibly (TOPS) have been very successful at helping large numbers of patients to lose weight and maintain this loss for long periods, with sustained support, counseling, diet and exercise instruction, and peer interaction. Costs for these programs may vary considerably, and the physician who refers such programs should be aware of the local group's success, leadership, diet plans, and educational and support programs. A similar (but lower-cost) behavioral support for a patient attempting weight loss would be to offer her weigh-in appointments with nursing staff every 1 to 2 weeks.

Physical Activity

Exercise must be included in any weight loss plan to increase the basal metabolic rate, burn extra calories, and improve cardiovascular health. Aerobic exercise is recommended for its cardiovascular benefits. Anaerobic (e.g., weight-lifting) exercise builds muscle mass that increases the basal metabolic rate. Although there is little evidence to support the theory that exercise promotes short-term weight loss, there is abundant evidence that exercise is critical in maintaining weight loss (112–114). Exercise in general preserves lean body mass, lowers body fat percentage, and improves lipid profiles (115). Aerobic exercise decreases blood pressure, improves endogenous insulin production, and is associated with decreased mortality, even when not associated with weight loss (116).

Behavior Modification for Obesity

The best weight loss programs help the patient identify the causes of weight gain and assist them in achieving better control over situations that cause overeating. These programs may include one-on-one sessions, group therapy, or physician counseling. The goals of behavior modification for obesity include identifying situations that trigger eating, improving exercise habits, conscientious food shopping, and differentiating between hunger and cravings. Key techniques of behavioral modification include self-monitoring with use of a food diary, stimulus control or "mindful eating," reinforcement, and relapse prevention (117).

Pharmacotherapy for Obesity

Pharmacotherapy should be undertaken cautiously, if at all, bearing in mind that although these agents may help produce an initial loss of weight, the ultimate goal is permanent weight loss, not simply to attain a short-lived goal. Medication for obesity should generally not be started until after a lifestyle modification program has been initiated. In general, pharmacologic modalities have limited use in weight loss and should never be used as the sole therapeutic modality for obesity.

Phentermine (Adipex-P, Ionamin, Phentride, Phentercot, Teramine, Pro-Fast, OBY-Trim), fenfluramine (not available in the United States), dexfenfluramine (not available in the United States), orlistat (Xenical), sibutramine (Meridia), diethylpropion (Tenuate), and dextroamphetamine (Dexedrine, Dextrostat) have all been studied and found to be effective in short-term weight loss. Although their short-term use may help a patient see immediate weight loss benefits and be motivational to the patient, discontinuation of the medication often leads to weight gain and loss of motivation.

Some of these agents have been found to be safe for longer-term use but, with the exception of orlistat, all have been demonstrated to raise blood pressure in some patients or may cause nervousness, insomnia, irritability, and palpitations. Some, such as diethylpropion, may contribute to the development of primary pulmonary hypertension. Many have the potential for abuse or dependency.

Orlistat is a pancreatic lipase inhibitor and is taken with meals. It works in the gut to reduce the absorption of dietary fat by approximately 30%. Orlistat also decreases the absorption of fat-soluble vitamins such as vitamins A, D, E, and even beta-carotene, so it is recommended that patients using orlistat take a daily multivitamin containing these fat-soluble vitamins 1 to 2 hours before or after ingestion of the drug. In a 2-year trial, an average of 7.8% weight loss was observed in the orlistat group compared with a 4.6% weight loss in the placebo-treated group (118). Side effects of orlistat include flatus, abdominal pain, and fecal urgency or incontinence. Side effects are related to dietary fat intake, so a higher-fat diet is associated with more side effects, although side effects often diminish over time. Supplementation with nightly psyllium (a fiber bulking agent) may minimize side effects of orlistat (117). Orlistat is contraindicated in patients with chronic malabsorption syndrome or cholestasis and in patients taking cyclosporine.

Sibutramine (Meridia) acts in the central nervous system to suppress the reuptake of norepinephrine and serotonin at the nerve endings. Although originally developed as an antidepressant, it increases satiety during meals. In one trial, 43% of patients on a program of diet, exercise, and sibutramine (10 mg) maintained more than 80% of their weight loss over 2 years, compared with 16% of those using diet and exercise alone (119). Patients who do not lose at least 4 lb within 4 weeks of starting sibutramine will probably not respond well in the long run and should discontinue its use. Side effects of sibutramine are generally mild and usually resolve within a few weeks. They include dry mouth, insomnia, headache, constipation, and restlessness.

Some patients using sibutramine have a clinically insignificant elevation in blood pressure and heart rate, although for a smaller number of patients this elevation may be excessive. This is often seen in the first 4 weeks of treatment and requires cessation of the therapy. Sibutramine should be used cautiously in patients with a history of hypertension and should not be given to patients with uncontrolled or poorly controlled hypertension.

More recently, attention has turned to other medications as options for the long-term treatment of weight problems, particularly in patients with other medical conditions requiring pharmacologic treatment. In obese patients with type 2 diabetes mellitus, many medications (e.g., insulin) contribute to weight gain, but metformin (Glucophage) facilitates weight loss by enhancing satiety in a dose-dependent fashion, and in combination with orlistat, has been shown to significantly reduce weight and improve lipid profiles in obese patients (117).

Topiramate, a medication used for seizures and mood stabilization (e.g., in bipolar disorder), has the side effect of weight loss for many patients (120). Bupropion (Wellbutrin), unlike many antidepressants, does not cause weight gain. In one study, overweight and obese women treated with bupropion demonstrated a 12% weight loss after 24 weeks of treatment (200 mg twice a day) (121).

Surgical Therapy for Obesity

Surgical interventions may be considered for patients with a BMI greater than 40 kg/m^2 who fail other methods of treatment, particularly if serious obesity-related complications are present (102). For patients with a BMI of 35 to 40 kg/m^2 with severe, life-threatening complications (sleep apnea or cardiomyopathy), surgery may also be considered.

SEXUAL RISK REDUCTION

Humans have been plagued by STDs for millennia. Open discussion of sexual behavior and STDs, however, is considered taboo in many cultures and societies. In the United States, this began to change with the recognition of HIV/AIDS as an STD, with high mortality in the early years of the epidemic. Subsequent to this, public discussions about sexual behaviors, frank talk about exactly what represented sexual risk taking, and public debates about "safer sex" became more mainstream topics of conversation.

The link between a history of STD and subsequent sexual behavior is poorly understood. A self-reported history is clearly a marker of past sexual behavior at high risk for HIV infection in the general population; whether it is also a marker for current high-risk behavior is yet to be determined. Surveys assessing the link between a self-reported history of STD and subsequent sexual behavior are contradictory, with one demonstrating an increase in condom use and the other not (122, 123). Other studies have used repeated STDs as an indicator of persistent at-risk sexual behavior in STD patients, but this assumption is not upheld in all studies (124–126).

Discussing a patient's sexual history at the time of any gynecologic exam is an opportunity for assessing past and present levels of sexual risk taking for that woman. This information provides an opportunity for counseling and opens the door for any future sexual concerns the patient might have. Most patients are willing to discuss their sexuality when asked in a private, nonthreatening, and nonjudgmental fashion.

Although it is important to keep in mind that counseling on a health risk does not have a mechanistic effect on subsequent risk reduction, there are numerous methods for decreasing risk. For high-risk sexual behavior, abstinence is quite effective, but it is not a choice many adult women may make. Although encouraging abstinence is important for adolescent populations, a more practical method is needed once a (young) woman becomes sexually active. For example, limiting the number of sexual partners is one means of curtailing sexual risk-taking behavior, but it is important for health care providers to be aware of the roles that recreational substances, mental health states, and environmental pressures play in determining a woman's number of sexual partners (127, 128). Alcohol and drug use among adolescents, in particular, diminish decision-making skills and put adolescent girls at risk for irresponsible sexual behaviors (129–131).

For all patients, discussions of their sexual behaviors must be confidential, with the exception of mandatory reporting of specific STDs to public health authorities. Information and discussion about sexual behaviors should be presented in a fashion individualized for a patient's age and relationship status. Information should also be culturally appropriate, sensitive to a patient's sexual orientation, and presented in words and phrases that are nonjudgmental and clearly understood.

Clinical Notes

- Identification of lifestyle problems
  - Routinely ask questions about health behaviors
  - Remain vigilant for subtle signs of unhealthy behaviors
  - Provide patient education materials that prompt questions
  - Reassure the patient that her information is confidential
- Behavior change: the transtheoretical model
  - Assess stage of change for individual patient behaviors: precontemplation, contemplation, preparation, action, maintenance (and relapse)
  - Assist patient in moving progressively through changes
  - Regular follow-up visits
  - Anticipate and make plans for "slips"
  - Aggressively intervene with relapses, use relapses as learning opportunities for future attempts
- Smoking cessation
  - Often requires repeated and long-term intervention
  - Address smoking status and motivation to quit at each visit
  - Regular, brief interventions eventually lead to cessation efforts
  - Offer pharmacologic support for the "action" stage
  - Combined psychosocial, behavioral, and pharmacologic support offers best results for long-term cessation
- "5As" for those motivated to make a cessation attempt
  - Ask—about tobacco use
  - Advise—all smokers to quit
  - Address—the patient's willingness to quit
  - Assist—with education, support, medications, and therapy
  - Arrange—for close frequent follow-up
- "5Rs" for those not yet motivated to quit
  - Relevance—give personalized reasons to quit
  - Risks—give information about patient's personal risks
  - Rewards—explain the benefits they could expect with cessation
  - Roadblocks—anticipate problems preventing attempt at cessation
  - Repetition—discuss the 5Rs repeatedly
- Alcohol and drug abuse
  - Alcohol problems are increasing in adolescent girls and older women
  - Women are more likely to seek help in health care settings
  - Women have higher all-cause mortality at lower levels of alcohol consumption than men
  - Psychiatric comorbidities (especially depression) are more common in women with alcohol problems than in men
  - Past or current history of sexual or physical abuse places women at increased risk for alcohol problems and/or relapse

- Women with alcohol problems are more likely to be left by their partners than men with alcohol problems
- Mothers who suffer alcohol problems perceive losing custody of their children as a major barrier to treatment
- Treatment
  - Gender-specific or gender-sensitive treatment programs
  - Special needs of women in treatment
  - Medications
  - Match treatment program to patient needs

- Obesity
  - Rapidly increasing incidence in the United States
  - Use BMI and waist circumference as diagnostic tools, body fat percentage if available
  - Fat distribution is important predictor
    - Android (apple) shape—high risk for diabetes, cardiovascular disease
    - Gynecoid (pear) shape—less risky pound for pound
  - Treatment
    - Reasonable, attainable, modest goals of 5 to 10% body weight
    - Dietary modification, healthy, 1200 to 1500 calories per day
    - Moderate exercise plan to burn 1000 to 1500 calories per week and to sustain losses achieved via diet
    - Behavior modification therapy to sustain new eating habits
    - Long-term support
    - Pharmacotherapy and surgical interventions used sparingly for very select patients
- Physical activity
  - Benefits physical, psychological, and social health
  - Benefits not limited to the overweight population
- Sexual risk reduction
  - Gynecologic exams are good settings for assessing risk
  - Question patients nonjudgmentally, tailor questions to patient needs
  - Educate about relative risks of sexual behaviors
  - Prevention and risk reduction

APPENDIX 19.1

Alcohol Screening Questionnaires

CAGE

C Have you ever felt you ought to cut down on your drinking?

A Have people ever annoyed you by criticizing you about your drinking?

G Have you ever felt bad or guilty about your drinking?

E Have you ever had a drink in the morning (eye opener) to steady your nerves or get rid of a hangover?

Scoring: 1 point for each yes response.

Audit

The following questions pertain to your use of alcoholic beverages during the past year. A drink refers to a can or bottle of beer, a glass of wine, a wine cooler, or one cocktail or shot of hard liquor.

1. How often do you have a drink containing alcohol? (Never, 0 points; ≤ monthly, 1 point; 2–4 times/month, 2 points; 2–3 times/week, 3 points; 4 or more times/week, 4 points)
2. How many drinks containing alcohol do you have on a typical day when you are drinking? (1–2 drinks, 0 points; 3–4 drinks, 1 point; 5–6 drinks, 2 points; 7–9 drinks, 3 points; ≥10 drinks, 4 points)
3. How often do you have more than six or more drinks on one occasion? (Never, 0 points; <monthly, 1 point; monthly, 2 points; weekly, 3 points; daily or almost daily, 4 points)
4. How often during the last year have you found that you were not able to stop drinking once you had started? (Points given as in question 3)
5. How often during the last year have you failed to do what was normally expected from you because of drinking? (Points given as in question 3)
6. How often during the last year have you needed a first drink in the morning to get yourself going after a heavy drinking session? (Points given as in question 3)
7. How often during the last year have you had a feeling of guilt or remorse after drinking? (Points given as in question 3)
8. How often during the last year have you been unable to remember what happened the night before because you were drinking? (Points given as in question 3)
9. Have you or someone else been injured as a result of your drinking? (No, 0 points; yes, but not in the past year, 2 points; yes, during the past year, 4 points)
10. Has a relative, friend, doctor, or other health care worker been concerned about your drinking or suggested you cut down? (Points given as in question 9)
11. Scoring: Sum all points.

TWEAK

T Tolerance: How many drinks can you hold ("hold" version; ≥6 drinks indicates tolerance), or how many drinks does it take before you begin to feel the first effects of alcohol ("high" version; ≥3 equals tolerance)

W Worried: Have close friends or relatives worried or complained about your drinking in the past year?

E Eye openers: Do you sometimes take a drink in the morning when you first get up?

A Amnesia: Has a friend or family member ever told you about things you said or did while you were drinking that you could not remember?

K Kut down: Do you sometimes felt the need to cut down on your drinking?

Scoring: 2 points each for tolerance or worried; 1 point each for eye opener, amnesia, or kut down; sum all points.

REFERENCES

1. Prochaska JO, DiClemente CC. Stages and processes of self-change of smoking: toward an integrative model of change. J Consult Clin Psychol 1983;51:390–395.
2. Prochaska JO, DiClemente CC, Norcross JC. In search of how people change: applications to addictive behaviors. Am Psychol 1992;47:1102–1114.
3. Centers for Disease Control and Prevention. Women and smoking: a report of the surgeon general. MMWR Recomm Rep 2002;51(RR12):1–30. Available at: www.cdc.gov/mmwr. Accessed July 27, 2005.
4. Jemal A, Tiwari RC, Murray T, et al. CA Cancer J Clin 2004;54:8–29. Also avail at http://caonline.amcancersoc.org/cgi/content/full/ 54/1/8.
5. Centers for Disease Control and Prevention. Annual smoking-attributable mortality, years of potential life lost and economic costs—United States, 1995–1999. MMWR Morb Mortal Wkly Rep 2002;51:300–303.
6. New York State Women and Tobacco Task Force. Women talk to women about tobacco: a report of the Women and Tobacco Task Force. Commission for a Healthy New York, 1995.
7. Department of Cancer Control and Epidemiology, Roswell Park Cancer Institute. Survey of Alcohol, Tobacco and Drug Use in Ninth Grade Students in Erie County, 1992. Buffalo, NY: Roswell Park Cancer Institute, 1992.
8. Pierce JP, Fiore MC, Novotny TE, et al. Trends in cigarette smoking in the United States: educational differences are increasing. JAMA 1989;261:56–60.
9. U.S. Department of Health and Human Services. The Health Benefits of Smoking Cessation: A Report of the Surgeon General. DHHS Publication No. (CDC) 90-8416G. Rockville, MD: U.S. Department of Health and Human Services, 1990.
10. Seddon JM, Willett WC, Speizer SE, et al. A prospective study of cigarette smoking and age related macular degeneration in women. JAMA 1996;276:1141–1146.
11. Fiore MC, Bailey WC, Cohen SJ, et al. Treating Tobacco Use and Dependence: Clinical Practice Guideline. Rockville, MD: U.S. Department of Health and Human Services, Public Health Service, 2000.
12. Anderson JE, Jorenby DE, Scott WJ, et al. Treating tobacco use and dependence: an evidence-based clinical practice guideline for tobacco cessation. Chest 2002;121:932–941.
13. Chen P, Dai L, Gordek H, et al., for the Substance Abuse and Mental Health Services Administration (SAMHSA). 2002 National Survey on Drug Use and Health: Questionnaire Dwelling Unit-Level and Person Pair-Level Sampling Weight Calibration. Available at: www.drugabusestatistics.samhsa.gov/nhsda. Accessed July 28, 2005.
14. Gomberg ES. Alcoholic women in treatment: the questions of stigma and age. Alcohol Alcohol 1988;23:507–514.
15. National Institutes of Health, National Institute on Drug Abuse (NIDA). Drug Abuse and Addiction Research: 25 Years of Discovery to Advance the Health of the Public. The Sixth Triennial Report to Congress from the Secretary of Health and Human Services. September 1999.
16. Wilsnack SC, Bogeltanz ND, Klassen AD, et al. Childhood sexual abuse and women's substance abuse: national survey findings. J Stud Alcohol 1997;58:264–271.
17. Miller BA, Downs WR, Testa M. Interrelationships between victimization experiences and women's alcohol use. J Stud Alcohol 1993;11:109–117.
18. Smith-Warner SA, Spiegelman D, Yaun SS, et al. Alcohol and breast cancer in women: a pooled analysis of cohort studies. JAMA 1998;279:535–540.
19. Blumenthal SJ. Women and substance abuse: a new national focus. National Institute on Drug Abuse. Bethesda, MD. Available at: http://www.nida.nih.gov/. Accessed July 28, 2005.
20. Brienza RS, Stein MD. Alcohol use disorders in primary care: do gender-specific differences exist? J Gen Intern Med 2002;17:387–397.
21. National Institute on Alcohol Abuse and Alcoholism. Eighth Special Report to the U.S. Congress on Alcohol and Health. Washington, DC: Department of Health and Human Services, 1993.
22. Weisner C, Schmidt L. Gender disparities in treatment for alcohol problems. JAMA 1992;268:1872–1876.
23. Amodei N, Willilams JF, Seale JP, et al. Gender differences in medical presentation and detection of patients with a history of alcohol abuse or dependence. J Addict Dis 1996;15:19–31.
24. Buschsbaum DG, Buchanan RG, Poses RM, et al. Physician detection of drinking problems in patients attending a general medicine practice. J Gen Intern Med 1992;7:517–521.
25. Halliday A, Bush B, Cleary P, et al. Alcohol abuse in women seeking gynecologic care. Obstet Gynecol 1986;68:322–326.
26. Thom B. Sex differences in help-seeking for alcohol problems: barriers to help-seeking. Br J Addict 1986;81:777–788.
27. Parran T Jr. Prescription drug abuse: a question of balance. Med Clin North Am 1997;81:967–978.
28. Prescott CA. Sex differences in the genetic risk for alcoholism. Alcohol Res Health 2002;26:264–273.
29. Kendler KS, Heath AC, Neale MC, et al. A population-based twin study of alcoholism in women. JAMA 1992;268:1877–1882.
30. Hill SY, Smith TR. Evidence for genetic mediation of alcoholism in women. J Subst Abuse Treat 1991;3:159–174.
31. Bohman M, Sigvardsson S, Cloninger CR. Maternal inheritance of alcohol abuse: cross-fostering analysis of adopted women. Arch Gen Psychiatry 1981;38:965–969.
32. Sigvardsson S, Bohman M, Cloninger CR. Replication of the Stockholm Adoption Study of Alcoholism. Confirmatory cross-fostering analysis. Arch Gen Psychiatry 1996;53:681–687.

33. Mustanski BS, Viken RJ, Kaprio J, et al. Genetic influences on the association between personality risk factors and alcohol use and abuse. J Abnorm Psychol 2003;112:282–289.
34. Ueno S. Genetic polymorphisms of serotonin and dopamine transporters in mental disorders. J Med Invest 2003;50:25–31.
35. Kessler RC, Crum RM, Warner LA, et al. Lifetime co-occurrence of DSM-III-R alcohol abuse and dependence with other psychiatric disorders in the National Comorbidity Survey. Arch Gen Psych 1997;54:313–320.
36. Schuckit MA, Tipp JE, Bergman M, et al. Comparison of induced and independent major depressive disorders in 2,945 alcoholics. Am J Psychiatry 1997;154:948–956.
37. Dunne FJ, Galatapoulus C, Schipperheijn JM. Gender differences in psychiatric morbidity among alcohol misusers. Compr Psychiatry 1993;34:95–101.
38. Buchsbaum DG, Buchanan RG, Welsh J, et al. Screening for drinking disorders in the elderly using the CAGE questionnaire. J Am Geriatr Soc 1992;40:662–665.
39. Wysowski DK, Baum C. Outpatient use of prescription sedative-hypnotic drugs in the United States, 1970 through 1989. Arch Intern Med 1991;151:1779–1783.
40. National Institute on Alcohol Abuse and Alcoholism (NIAAA). Are women more vulnerable to alcohol's effects? Alcohol Alert 1999;46:1–4.
41. Frezza M, Di Padova C, Pozzato G. High blood alcohol levels in women: the role of decreased gastric alcohol dehydrogenase activity and first-pass metabolism. N Engl J Med 1990;322:95–99.
42. Saunders JB, Davis M, Williams R. Do women develop alcoholic liver disease more readily than men? BMJ 1981;282:1140–1143.
43. Becker U, Deis A, Sorensen TIA, et al. Prediction of risk of liver disease by alcohol intake, sex and age: a prospective population study. Hepatology 1996;23:1025–1029.
44. Sato N, Lindros KO, Baraona E, et al. Sex difference in alcohol-related organ injury. Alcohol Clin Exp Res 2001;25(suppl):40–45.
45. Garg R, Wagener DK, Madans JH. Alcohol consumption and risk of ischemic heart disease in women. Arch Intern Med 1993;153:1211–1216.
46. Stampfer MJ, Colditz GA, Willett WC, et al. A prospective study of moderate alcohol consumption and the risk of coronary disease and stroke in women. N Engl J Med 1988;319:267–273.
47. Hanna E, DuFour MC, Elliot S, et al. Dying to be equal: women, alcohol and cardiovascular disease. Br J Addict 1992;87:1593–1597.
48. Urbano-Marquez A, Estruch R, Fernandez-Sola J, et al. The greater risk of alcoholic cardiomyopathy and myopathy in women as compared to men. JAMA 1995;274:149–154.
49. Acker C. Neuropsychological deficits in alcoholics. The relative contribution of gender and drinking history. Br J Addict 1986;81:393–403.
50. Kuper H, Ye W, Weiderpass E, et al. Alcohol and breast cancer risk: the alcoholism paradox. Br J Cancer 2000;83:949–951.
51. Wilsnack SC, Klassen AD, Wilsnack RW. Drinking and reproductive dysfunction among women in a 1981 national survey. Alcohol Clin Exp Res 1984;8:451–458.
52. Bahamondes L, Bueno JG, Hardy E, et al. Identification of main risk factors for tubal infertility. Fertil Steril 1994;61:478–482.
53. Harlap S, Shiono PH. Alcohol, smoking, and incidence of spontaneous abortions in the first and second trimester. Lancet 1980;2:173–176.
54. Fiellin D, Reid MC, O'Connor P. Screening for alcohol problems in primary care: a systematic review. Arch Intern Med 2000;160:1977–1989.
55. Fleming MF, Barry KL, Manwell LB, et al. Brief physician advice for problem alcohol drinkers: a randomized controlled trial in community-based primary care practices. JAMA 1997;277:1039–1045.
56. U.S. Preventive Services Task Force. Guide to Clinical Preventive Services: Report of the U.S. Preventive Services Task Force. 2nd ed. Baltimore: Williams & Wilkins, 1996:567–582.
57. Baber TF, Kranzler HR, Lauerman RJ. Early detection of harmful alcohol consumption: comparison of clinical, laboratory, and self-report screening procedures. Addict Behav 1989;14:139–157.
58. Ewing JA. Detecting alcoholism: the CAGE questionnaire. JAMA 1984;252:1905–1907.
59. Chan AW, Pristach EA, Welte JW, et al. Use of the TWEAK test in screening for alcoholism/heavy drinking in three populations. Alcohol Clin Exp Res 1993;17:1188–1192.
60. Bradley KA, Boyd-Wickizer J, Powell SH, et al. Alcohol screening questionnaires in women: a critical review. JAMA 1998;280:166–171.
61. Boyd C. The antecedents of women's crack cocaine abuse: family substance abuse, sexual abuse, depression and illicit drug use. J Subst Abuse Treat 1993;10:433–438.
62. Paone D, Chavkin W. The impact of sexual abuse: implications for drug treatment. J Women Health 1992;1:149–153.
63. Ladwig G, Anderson M. Substance abuse in women: relationship between chemical dependency of women and past reports of physical and/or sexual abuse. J Addict 1989;24:739–754.
64. Wilk AI, Jensen NM, Havighurst TC. Meta-analysis of randomized controlled trials addressing brief interventions in heavy alcohol drinkers. J Gen Intern Med 1997;12:274–283.
65. Piazza NJ, Vrbka JL, Yeager RD. Telescoping of alcoholism in women alcoholics. Int J Addict 1989;24:19–28.
66. Henderson D, Boyd C. Women and illicit drugs: sexuality and crack-cocaine. Health Care Women Int 1995;16:113–124.

67. Henderson D, Boyd C, Mieczkowski T. Gender, relationships, and crack-cocaine: a content analysis. Res Nurs Health 1994;7:265–272.
68. Beckman L, Amaro H. Personal and social difficulties faced by women and men entering alcoholism treatment. J Stud Alcohol 1986;47:135–145.
69. Higgins S, Budney A, Bickel W. Participation of significant others in outpatient behavioral treatment predicts greater cocaine abstinence. Am J Drug Alcohol Abuse 1994;20:47–56.
70. The National Center on Addiction and Substance Abuse at Columbia University. Under the Rug: Substance Abuse and the Mature Woman. June 1998. Available at: http://www.casacolumbia.org/absolutenm/templates/PressReleases.asp?articleid=165&zoneid=49. Accessed July 28, 2005.
71. Dahlgren L, Willander A. Are special treatment facilities for female alcoholics needed? A controlled 2-year follow-up study from a specialized female unit (EWA) versus a mixed male/female treatment facility. Alcohol Clin Exp Res 1989;13:499–504.
72. Copeland J, Hall W, Didcott P, et al. A comparison of a specialist women's alcohol and other drug treatment service with two traditional mixed sex services: client characteristics and treatment outcome. Drug Alcohol Depend 1993;32:81–92.
73. Ashley OS, Marsden ME, Brady TM. Effectiveness of substance abuse treatment programming for women: a review. Am J Drug Alcohol Abuse 2003;29:19–53.
74. Flegal KM, Carroll MD, Ogden CL, et al. Prevalence and trends in obesity among US adults, 1999–2000. JAMA 2002;288:1723–1727.
75. Kuczmarski RJ, Fiegal KM, Campbell SM, et al. Increasing prevalence of overweight among US adults: the National Health and Nutrition Examination Surveys, 1960–1991. JAMA 1994;272:205–211.
76. Manson JE, Colditz GA, Stampfer MJ, et al. A prospective study of obesity and risk of coronary heart disease in women. N Engl J Med 1990;322:882–889.
77. Allison DB, Fontaine KR, Manson JE, et al. Annual deaths attributable to obesity in the United States. JAMA 1999;282:1530–1538.
78. Sturm R, Wells KB. Does obesity contribute as much to morbidity as poverty or smoking? Public Health 2001;115:229–235.
79. Gortmaker SL, Must A, Perrin JM, et al. Social and economic consequences of overweight in adolescence and young adulthood. N Engl J Med 1993;329:1008–1012.
80. Fontaine, KR, Cheskin LJ, Baroski I. Health-related quality of life in obese persons seeking treatment. J Fam Pract 1996;43:265–270.
81. Nestle M. Increasing portion sizes in American diets: more calories, more obesity. J Am Diet Assoc 2003;103:39–40.
82. Williamson DF, Madans J, Pamuk S, et al. A prospective study of childbearing and 10-year weight gain in U.S. white women 25 to 45 years of age. Int J Obesity 1994;18:561–569.
83. Smith DE, Lewis CE, Caveny JL, et al. Longitudinal changes in adiposity associated with pregnancy: The CARDIA Study. JAMA 1994;271(22):1747–1751.
84. Anderson EJ, Lavoie HB, Strauss CC, et al. Body composition and energy balance: lack of effect of short-term hormone replacement in postmenopausal women. Metabolism 2001;50:265–269.
85. Price TM, O'Brien SN, Welter BH, et al. Estrogen regulation of adipose tissue lipoprotein lipase—possible mechanism of body fat distribution. Am J Obstet Gynecol 1998;178:101–117.
86. Hassager C, Christiansen C. Estrogen/gestagen therapy changes soft tissue body composition in postmenopausal women. Metabolism 1989;38:662–665.
87. Simkin-Silverman LR, Wing RR. Weight gain during menopause. Is it inevitable or can it be prevented? Postgrad Med 2000;108:47–50, 53–56.
88. Campfield LA, Smith FJ. The pathogenesis of obesity. Baillieres Clin Endocrinol Metab 1999;13:13–30.
89. Rosenbaum M, Leibel RL, Hirsch J. Obesity. N Engl J Med 1997;337:396–406.
90. Leibel RL, Rosenbaum M, Hirsch J. Changes in energy expenditure resulting from altered body weight. N Engl J Med 1995;332:621–628.
91. Stunkard AJ, Sorensen TIA, Hanis C, et al. An adoption study of human obesity. N Engl J Med 1986;314:193–198.
92. DeFronzo RA, Jacot E, Jequier E, et al. The effect of insulin on the disposal of intravenous glucose: results from indirect calorimetry and hepatic and femoral venous catheterization. Diabetes 1981;30:1000–1007.
93. Flier JS. The adipocyte. Storage depot or node on the energy information superhighway? Cell 1995;80:15–18.
94. Kern PA. Potential role of TNF[alpha] and lipoprotein lipase as candidate genes for obesity. J Nutr 1997;127(suppl):1917–1922.
95. Hotamisligil GS, Spiegelman BM. Tumor necrosis factor [alpha]: a key component of the obesity-diabetes link. Diabetes 1994;43:1271–1278.
96. Heymsfield SB, Greenberg AS, Fujioka K, et al. Recombinant leptin for weight loss in obese and lean adults: a randomized, controlled, dose-escalation trial. JAMA 1999;282:1568–1575.
97. Campfield LA, Smith FJ. Overview. Neurobiology of OB protein (leptin). Proc Nutr Soc 1998;57:429–440.
98. Caro JF, Kolaczynski JW, Nyce MR, et al. Decreased cerebrospinal-fluid/serum leptin ratio in obesity: a possible mechanism for leptin resistance. Lancet 1996;348:159–161.
99. Vivian M. Focus on primary care evaluation, management, and treatment of obesity in women. Obstet Gyn Surv 2001;56:650–663.
100. Shah M, Jeffery RW. Is obesity due to overeating and inactivity, or to a different metabolic rate? Ann Behav Med 1991;13:73–81.

101. Lapidus L, Bengtsson C, Larsson B, et al. Distribution of adipose tissue and risk of cardiovascular disease and death: a 12-year follow-up of participants in the population study of women in Gothenburg, Sweden. BMJ 1984;289:1261–1263.
102. U.S. Department of Health and Human Services, Public Health Service, National Institutes of Health, National Heart, Lung, and Blood Institute. The Practical Guide: Identification, Evaluation, and Treatment of Overweight and Obesity in Adults. NIH Publication No. 00-4084, October 2000.
103. Lemieux S, Prud'homme D, Bouchard C, et al. A single threshold value of waist girth identifies normal-weight and overweight subjects with excess visceral adipose tissue. Am J Clin Nutr 1996;64:685–693.
104. Wing RR, Marcus MD, Salata R, et al. Effects of a very-low-calorie diet on long-term glycemic control in obese type 2 diabetic subjects. Arch Intern Med 1991;151:1334–1340.
105. Wing RR, Koeske R, Epstein LH, et al. Long-term effects of modest weight loss in type II diabetic patients. Arch Intern Med 1987;147:1749–1753.
106. Blackburn GL, Read JL. Benefits of reducing revisited. Postgrad Med J 1984;60:13–18.
107. Williamson DF, Pamuk E, Thun M, et al. Prospective study of intentional weight loss and mortality in never-smoking overweight US white women aged 40–64 years. Am J Epidemiol 1995;141:1128–1141.
108. Shiffman ML, Sugerman HJ, Kellum JM, et al. Gallstone formation after rapid weight loss: a prospective study in patients undergoing gastric bypass surgery for treatment of morbid obesity. Am J Gastroenterol 1991;86:1000–1005.
109. Liddle RA, Goldstein RB, Saxton J. Gallstone formation during weight-reduction dieting. Arch Intern Med 1989;149:1750–1753.
110. Foster GD, Wyatt HR, Hill JO, et al. A randomized trial of a low-carbohydrate diet for obesity. N Engl J Med 2003;348:2082–2090.
111. Samaha FF, Iqbal N, Seshadri P, et al. A low-carbohydrate as compared with a low-fat diet in severe obesity. N Engl J Med 2003;348:2074–2081.
112. Jeffery RW, Wing RR. The effects of an enhanced exercise program on long-term weight loss. Obes Res 2001;9(suppl 3):O193.
113. Kayman S, Bruvold W, Stern JS. Maintenance and relapse after weight loss in women: behavioral aspects. Am J Clin Nutr 1990;52:800–807.
114. Lee IM, Rexrode KM, Cook NR, et al. Physical activity and coronary heart disease in women. JAMA 2001;285:1447–1454.
115. Leon AS, Sanchez OA. Response of blood lipids to exercise training alone or combined with dietary intervention. Med Sci Sports Exerc 2001;33:S502–S515.
116. Mensink GBM, Ziese T, Kok FJ, et al. Benefits of leisure-time physical activity on the cardiovascular risk profile at older age. Int J Epidemiol 1999;28:659–666.
117. Klauer J, Aronne L. Managing overweight and obesity in women. Clin Obstet Gynecol 2002;45:1080–1088.
118. Sjostrom L, Rissanen A, Andersen J. Randomized placebo-controlled trial of orlistat for weight loss and prevention of weight regain in obese patients. Lancet 1998;352:167–172.
119. James WP, Astrup A, Finer N. Effect of sibutramine on weight maintenance after weight loss a randomised Trial STORM Study Group. Sibutramine Trial of Obesity Reduction & Maintenance. Lancet 2000;356:2119–2125.
120. Roy Chengappa KN, Levine JD, Rathore D. Long-term effects of topiramate on bipolar mood instability, weight change and glycemic control. Eur Psychiatry 2001;16:186–190.
121. Gadde KM, Parker CB, Maner LG, et al. Bupropion for weight loss. Obesity Res 2001; 9:544–551.
122. Fleisher JM, Senie RT, Minkoff H, et al. Condom use relative to knowledge of sexually transmitted disease prevention, method of birth control, and past or present infection. J Community Health 1994;19:395–407.
123. O'Campo P, Deboer M, Faden RR, et al. Prior episode of sexually transmitted disease and subsequent sexual risk-reduction practices. A need for improved risk-reduction interventions. Sex Transm Dis 1992;19:326–330.
124. Prins M, Hooykaas C, Coutinho RA, et al. Incidence and risk factors for acquisition of sexually transmitted diseases in heterosexuals with multiple partners. Sex Transm Dis 1994;21:258–267.
125. Richert CA, Peterman TA, Zaidi AA, et al. A method for identifying persons at high risk for sexually transmitted infections: opportunity for targeting intervention. Am J Public Health 1993;83:520–524.
126. The Italian MEGIC Group. Determinants of cervical *Chlamydia trachomatis* infection in Italy. Genitourin Med 1993;69:123–125.
127. Freeman RC, Parillo KM, Collier K, et al. Child and adolescent sexual abuse history in a sample of 1,490 women sexual partners of injection drug-using men. Women Health 2001;34:31–49.
128. Toltzis P, Stephens RC, Adkins I, et al. Human immunodeficiency virus (HIV)-related risk-taking behaviors in women attending inner-city prenatal clinics in the mid-west. J Perinatol 1999;19:483–487.
129. Carr-Gregg MR, Enderby KC, Grover SR. Risk-taking behaviour of young women in Australia: screening for health-risk behaviours. Med J Aust 2003;178:601–604.
130. Scivoletto S, Tsuji RK, Abdo C, et al. Use of psychoactive substances and sexual risk behavior in adolescents. Subst Use Misuse 2002;37:381–398.
131. Flisher AJ, Kramer RA, Hoven CW, et al. Risk behavior in a community sample of children and adolescents. J Am Acad Child Adolesc Psychiatry 2000; 39:881–887.

CHAPTER 20

Integration of Complementary and Alternative Medicine in the Gynecology Office

Michèle G. Curtis

INTRODUCTION

Modern medicine prides itself on being scientific. Increasingly, clinicians are admonished to practice evidence-based medicine, which is purported to be a more scientific medicine than that previously relied on. Evidence-based medicine demands that the clinical practice of medicine be based on scientific knowledge that has been ascertained through the use of certain scientific and methodologic rules.

One of the basic foundations of Western medicine's perspective is that the cause of illness is primarily physical and it is the mission of Western medicine to cure disease. Western or contemporary biomedicine is based on four principal tenets:

1. *Objectivism*: The observer is separated from the observed.
2. *Reductionism*: Complex phenomena are explainable by reducing or deconstructing them to their smaller component parts.
3. *Positivism*: All information can be derived from physically measurable data.
4. *Determinism*: Knowledge of scientific law and conditions allows us to make accurate predictions regarding the ensuing phenomena.

Science, however, is constantly changing as scientists discover discrepancies between metaphysical reality and the scientific models devised through intellectual activity. Ultimately, the four tenets of knowing inherent to the Western medical system are not always applicable. According to the Heisenberg uncertainty principles, objectivism is ultimately not possible, because the act of observing a phenomena necessarily influences the behavior of the phenomena that is being observed. Interactions between humans and their environments are multidirectional, transactional, synergistic, oppositional, and not amenable to simple reductionistic explanations. The tenets of positivism and determinism work only if we have the requisite tools—both intellectually and materialistically—to ask the appropriate questions. In its attempts to be more scientific, Western medicine "underestimates the individuality of patients and pigeon-hole[s] (sic) them within a clinical pseudo-democracy" (1). This approach values typology, not variation and individuality.

In contrast, most other medical traditions are based on the basic tenet that what differentiates each of us as individuals is central to our health and to healing. Healing is the work of the body, and the fundamental role of medicine is to help the body do this. Health or healing practices derived from non-Western medical systems or health philosophies are referred to as complementary and alternative medicine (CAM) modalities. Most forms of CAM embrace two primary principles: the body and emotions are maintained by a life force, and the body is essentially self-healing. Hence, the theories of disease in non-Western medical traditions are usually all encompassing (i.e., they do not distinguish the mind as being separate from the body). Symptoms are seen as a reflection of an imbalance that is affecting the whole system. CAM seeks to prevent disease, as well as to maintain health through balancing internal resources with external natural and social environmental forces. The basic tenets of CAM are as follows:

- The body heals itself.
- The body is an energetic system, and disruptions in this system lead to illness.
- Nutrients and natural products provide sustenance for the body and are also incorporated into the body.
- Plants are an important part of nature relative to human health.
- The body is uniquely individual.

Origins of some medical systems are ancient (traditional Chinese medicine, Ayurvedic medicine), whereas others had their beginnings in the mid-19th century (homeopathy, osteopathy).

Health care systems are based on theories and facts that differ significantly across cultures. Hence, signs and symptoms are interpreted differently in different health care systems. All health care systems, however, are subject to change and modification; as new knowledge is gained and new theories formed, alternative systems of reality are proposed. The concept of numerous models of reality is not a trivial one. Careers and reputations have been fought for, won, and lost in defending the prevailing reality. As an example, it took Simmelweiss 37 years to convince Austrian physicians to wash their hands when they went from the autopsy room to the delivery room (and he nearly lost his license to practice medicine three times). The model of reality currently in use by a system colors the assumptions and application of logic brought to the problems that are viewed through the lens of the prevailing model. Yet, even the facts that constitute the prevailing model of reality are constantly changing over time. Clearly then, there is room for multiple realities in the arena of health and health care.

It would be a mistake to conclude that Western medicine is only reductionistic and CAM is singularly holistic. In fact, to varying degrees, each contains elements of both approaches. The key to using any health care approach or system effectively is to understand its limitations. Perhaps the biggest stumbling block to integrating Western medicine and CAM is the issue of mechanism of action. The demand on the part of allopathic purists to be able to quantitatively measure objective improvements in disease activity as the only form of validating a therapeutic benefit peremptorily precludes the possibility of ever integrating CAM and allopathy. New approaches to measurement, including subjective measurements, and new perspectives of viewing how success is measured will be needed if an integrative approach to health, health care, and medicine is to truly be created and practiced.

It is clearly beyond the scope of this chapter to discuss every modality of CAM or to cover in great detail even one modality. Instead, it is the intent of this chapter to provide a brief overview of several other systems of health care and various CAM modalities. In addition, there is a brief review of some of the CAM modalities used for common office gynecology concerns. For the reader interested in a listing of websites, databases, and journals where he or she can obtain more information on CAM, see Appendix 20.1.

USE OF COMPLEMENTARY AND ALTERNATIVE MEDICINE MODALITIES IN THE UNITED STATES

In 1993, Eisenberg et al. published their findings in a landmark study on the use of CAM in the United States. They found that 34% of Americans had used at least one unconventional therapy or remedy in the past year, and one-third of these people visited unconventional therapists (2). The use of CAM has continued to grow in America, and it is currently estimated that Americans spend at least $10 billion annually on CAM, most of it coming out of their own pockets (3).

As part of the larger 2002 National Health Interview Survey, the National Center for Complementary and Alternative Medicine (NCCAM) and the Center for Disease Control and Prevention's National Center for Health Statistics developed a survey with questions regarding the 27 types of CAM therapy commonly used in the United States. The survey was designed to look at usage rather than safety or effectiveness. The survey was administered to more than 31,000 representative U.S. adults older than 18 years of age and found that 36% of them used some form of CAM in 2002. Similar to other reports, the survey results showed CAM use was greater among women, individuals with higher education, people who had been hospitalized within the last year, and former smokers (4).

CAM therapies were most often used for back pain, colds, neck pain, joint pain or stiffness, and anxiety or depression. Only 12% of respondents sought CAM therapies from a licensed CAM practitioner.

The ten most commonly used CAM therapies and approximate percent of U.S. adults using each therapy are listed:

- Prayer for own health, 43%
- Prayer by others for the respondent's health, 24%
- Natural products (e.g., herbs, other botanicals), 19% (an increase from earlier studies in the 1990s)
- Deep breathing exercises, 12%
- Participation in prayer group for own health, 10%
- Meditation, 8%
- Chiropractic care, 8%
- Yoga, 5%
- Massage, 5%
- Diet-based therapies, 4%

The most commonly used natural products were echinacea, ginseng, gingko biloba, and garlic supplements (5). Reasons that respondents used CAM were several:

- 55% of adults who used CAM believed it would help them when used in conjunction with conventional medical therapy.
- 50% believed it would be interesting to try.
- 28% believed conventional medicine would not help them.
- 26% used CAM because a conventional medical practitioner had recommended it.
- 13% used CAM because conventional medicine was too expensive (5).

Methodologic Issues in Controlled Trials of Complementary and Alternative Medicine

One of the criticisms of CAM is that it lacks clinical trials and is not "evidence based"; however, this is not true. There are many peer-reviewed journals reporting on clinical trials, as well as many basic research endeavors into understanding and evaluating the mechanisms of action, safety, and efficacy of various CAM approaches. The number of randomized controlled trials (RCTs) of CAM treatments has nearly doubled every 5 years (6). The Cochrane Library now includes more than 60 systematic reviews of CAM interventions, including 11 that specifically address issues in obstetrics and gynecology (7).

Although the randomized, double-blind trial is considered by many to be the gold standard in medical research, there have been suggestions that a different methodology is needed for the evaluation of CAM therapies (8). Difficulties in constructing trials for CAM modalities are reflective of several issues: (a) the use of alternative theoretic frameworks, (b) use of unconventional diagnostic systems, (c) difficulties in blinding the trials, (d) difficulties in defining an appropriate placebo control, (e) use of individually tailored treatment and individual measures of response, and (f) difficulty in finding outcome measures that reflect the particular perspective of complementary practitioners.

Although CAM is often derided for not being evidence based, deficiencies abound in orthodox medical research as well (9–11). There are known difficulties in the interpretation, feasibility, and ethics of controlled trials. These difficulties include (a) the blinding of subjects and/or clinicians is not always feasible, (b) participation in the study itself may affect behavior and outcome,(c) trial participants may not truly represent the general population, (d) treatments are artificially standardized, (e) there is inadequate attention to individual responses, (f) outcome measures often do not reflect patient's concerns, and (g) various ethical issues in the design and methodology of the trial may exist (12–15). Other problems encountered include type I and type II errors, unblinded observations of subjective outcomes, and inappropriate group comparisons (e.g., multiple, subgroup, and/or post-hoc analyses). Bloom and his coworkers used traditional literature search techniques to identify as many RCTs of CAM as they could. Using a 100-point scale, they assessed the methodologic quality of these trials. They identified a total of 258 RCTs, with an average score of 44.7. When the authors applied this same process to RCTs from the standard medical literature, the average score was 45 (16).

The Growing Recognition of CAM and Its Significance

In 1992, the U.S. National Institutes of Health (NIH) Office of Alternative Medicine was established. In 1998, Congress gave this office full NIH center status (NCCAM) with an annual budget of more than $70 million. For FY2005, its budget is expected to exceed $121 million. NCCAM is "dedicated to exploring complementary and alternative healing practices in the context of rigorous science, training complementary and alternative medicine (CAM) researchers, and disseminating authoritative information to the public and professionals" (17). An increasing number of U.S. medical schools are offering coursework in CAM: 64% offered classes in CAM in 1998, but only one-third of the classes were part of the required curriculum (18). Currently, the only published set of guidelines for curriculum in CAM for physicians is for family practice residency-level education, endorsed in 2000 by the Society of Teachers in Family Medicine (19).

NONALLOPATHIC HEALTH CARE SYSTEMS

Medical systems are embedded in their cultures. As a result, certain aspects of a medical system believed to be meaningful to one group may be meaningless to another group in another cultural setting. When confronted with a new idea, a common reaction is to "translate" the idea into familiar terms or concepts.

When allopathic practitioners attempt to extract therapeutic options from other traditional systems, such as Ayurvedic, Tibetan, or Traditional Chinese Medicine, a common mistake is to assume identical terms in different systems have identical meanings. The problem is that substituted English language terms differ significantly from the original foreign language terms. For example, the English translated terms of the "organs" such as "kidney" or "liver" do not necessarily correspond in Chinese medicine to the same medical anatomic sites or substrates in allopathic medicine. In Chinese medicine, these terms refer to collections of processes with physiologic, psychological, and emotional manifestations. Hence, it would be a mistake to assume that a Chinese medicine diagnosis of "deficient kidney yen" implies renal failure in allopathic medicine. "Identical" or "translatable" terms often have different meanings in the context of different medical systems.

Ayurveda

As a medical practice, Ayurveda is more than 5000 years old. "Ayur" means longevity and "veda" means knowledge. In the Ayurvedic tradition, spiritual and physical health are inextricably intertwined. Indian medicine is based in part on the principle of a fundamental relationship between the microcosm and the macrocosm. Comprehending and understanding the world is essential to comprehending and understanding humans, and vice versa. In Ayurveda, the cosmos is comprised of five basic elements: earth, air, fire, water, and space. In humans, these five elements occur as the three doshas or forces. The human body is made up of the three doshas (vata, pitta, and kapha), the seven dhatus (tissues), and three malas (waste products).

Health is achieved by maintaining equilibrium among the three doshas. Each person has some of each dosha and a doshic proclivity. A person's doshic tendency determines what illnesses they are prone to, and knowing this, a person can seek to avoid them.

Vata, also referred to as vayu or wind, is derived from air and space. It is associated with metabolic energy, and is responsible for all bodily movement and nervous functions. Its principal location in the body is in the colon, and when disrupted, complaints of gas and muscular or nervous energy leading to pain may be voiced.

Pitta, or bile, is derived from fire and water, and is associated with catabolic fire energy. Pitta is responsible for many things, including digestion, temperature, hunger, thirst, mental activity, courage, and the activity of enzymes and hormones. It resides principally in the stomach, and disruption may lead to inflammation.

Kapha or shleshman, or phlegm, is derived from water and earth, and is associated with anabolic nutritive activity. It regulates Pitta and Vata and is responsible for keeping and maintaining the body's strength, solidity, and sexual power, among other things. Kapha controls patients. Its principal seat is in the lungs, and when disrupted, there may be swelling with or without discharge.

In Ayurveda, the malas are the waste products of food and drink the body has digested and processed. There are three principle malas: urine, feces, and sweat. In this medical system, to avoid an accumulation of malas, a person should have a daily bowel movement and urinate six times per day.

In Ayurveda, digestion is the most important function that occurs in the body. Problems in diet and digestion are among the central causes of all disease. When there is a decrease in enzyme activity, Ama is formed. All diseases inevitably come from Ama. Ama is produced when food or drink is improperly digested; it lodges in different parts of the body, blocking the channels (srotas) that all substances, including the life force (prana), circulate through. Ama mixes with the doshas that circulate through the pathways it may be blocking, and it may gravitate to a weak or stressed organ or to the site of the disease manifestation. Internal diseases begin with Ama, and external diseases produce Ama. The primary course of therapy in Ayurveda is to eliminate Ama and restore balance to the doshas.

Ayurvedic diagnosis involves a preliminary examination using visual observation, touch, interrogation, and assessment of the patient's type of physical constitution and mental status. The physical examination may involve a detailed examination of the pulse; because it is a highly specialized art, not every Ayurvedic physician uses pulse examination. Examination of the urine is also undertaken in a fairly formalized manner.

In addition to examination of the patient, the disease is examined using a five-step process. The etiology of the disease is assessed, as well as its early signs and symptoms. The manifest signs and symptoms are reviewed and exploratory therapy to determine the precise nature of the malady and suitable treatment is undertaken.

Therapies are individualized and based on detailed histories and examinations. In Ayurveda, there are two courses of therapy: prophylactic and therapeutic. The cornerstone of Ayurvedic medicine is not the eradication of disease per se, it is the prevention of illness through diet, herbs, and meditation. If there is a doshic imbalance, purification therapy, alleviation therapy, or a combination of these is prescribed.

Although there are no states that provide licensing specifically for Ayurvedic practitioners in the United States, several states have passed laws that liberalize and decriminalize CAM. In India, government boards regulate the certification and licensing of Ayurvedic practitioners.

Traditional Chinese Medicine

Chinese medicine may be referred to as "traditional," but it would be wrong to assume this means little has changed in this medical system over time. In fact, Chinese medicine has undergone significant changes and developments over the centuries. New ideas have been embraced and old ones discarded as new technologies, information, and even exposure to other medical systems have been introduced. Although many aspects of Chinese medicine are consistent with the system overall, others are rather contradictory. As a result, conflicting concepts of disease etiology, methods and systems of diagnosis, and treatment are juxtaposed in Chinese medicine, and the clinician relies on the perspective he or she believes to be the most applicable.

Fundamental concepts of Chinese medicine include yin and yang, the five phases, qi, and the essential substances of the body, essence and spirit, and zang and fu, or viscera and bowels. Yin and yang express the idea of opposing but complementary phenomena that exist in a state of dynamic equilibrium.

The concept of qi (also spelled ch'i) is crucial to Chinese medicine. Qi exists in all living things, and Chinese medicine sees life as a network of interconnected and intersecting qi. Qi pervades all things, acting as both a material substance and a force. Qi is mobile, and obstruction or blockage of qi's movement through channels in the body contributes to the formation of illness. There are different types of qi in the body, and although debate centers around their number and categories, the basic functions include activation, warming, defense, transformation, and containment.

There are four traditional categories of diagnostics in Chinese medicine: inspection, listening and smelling, inquiry, and palpation. The process of diagnosis includes a detailed assessment of the overall presentation of the individual, pulse reading, and consideration of the tongue's appearance. The tongue is inspected for its color, shape, markings, and coating. When listening and smelling the practitioner notes the quality of speech, breath and other sounds, and the odors of the body, breath, and excreta. Inquiry involves taking a comprehensive history from the patient.

Palpation includes examining the pulse, the body, and the acupuncture points. Pulse diagnosis is done on the radial arteries of the left and right wrists. The pulse is divided into three parts, and each pulse position helps shed light on the status of the organs and the channels. By analyzing the pulse, the practitioner can assess the quality of qi and blood at different locations in the body.

Based on an analytic integration of the information gathered, the clinician then constructs a configuration of the disease based on pattern identification that will enable him or her to prescribe the appropriate therapies. A single biomedical disease diagnosis may be associated with a large number of Chinese diagnostic patterns. Each pattern would be treated in a different way; hence, there may be one disease but different treatments. The reverse may also be true; many different diseases may be covered under one pattern. In this case, therefore, there may be many diseases but one treatment.

Once a diagnosis has been determined and, if necessary, a pattern has been identified, therapy is begun. Chinese medicine treats the condition with opposing measures. Hence, cold is treated with heat and vice versa. Therapeutic measures in Chinese medicine may include acupuncture and moxibustion, cupping and bleeding, Chinese massage (Tui Na), qi cultivation (Qigong), Chinese herbal medicine (Zhong Yao), and dietetics. Herbs are used according to their effects on specific parts of the body.

The physical exercises used in TCM combine movement and meditation. Qigong combines both, but the use of breath is its major focus. Qigong is used to cleanse and strengthen the body, as well as promote qi circulation. T'ai chi chu'an promotes the flow of qi through a meditative type of slow and graceful movement.

Homeopathy

The practice of homeopathy was introduced by Dr. Samuel Hahnemann (1755–1843). In a series of "provings," Hahnemann gave substances to groups of healthy people in doses sufficient to invoke symptoms without causing irreparable harm. A symptom picture of each substance was then assembled that differentiated it from other substances. On the basis of these experiments, Hahnemann concluded that (a) medicinal substances invoke a standard array of signs and symptoms in healthy people, and (b) the medicine whose symptom picture most closely resembled the illness being treated was the one most likely to elicit a curative or therapeutic response in the patient. This second conclusion became known as the Hahnemannian law of similars or "Let likes be cured by likes."

In homeopathy, illness is perceived to be the organism's attempt to heal itself. Homeopathic remedies therefore are chosen to fit the illness as closely as possible and are used in the smallest possible dose. Remedies are established through provings, whereby a volunteer ingests a substance and then records its effects.

Homeopathic remedies are designed to stimulate a self-healing mechanism, not to correct a specific abnormality. As such, if a substance causes symptoms at high concentrations, the same substance in minute doses can help heal a person suffering from an illness characterized by those symptoms. This is one of the more controversial tenets held by homeopathy: the smaller the dose of the treatment substance, the more potent its effect. Preparation of a homeopathic remedy involves the process of dilution, also known as potentization, in which the solution is repeatedly diluted and shaken. This series of dilutions and shakings are called succession of the solution. Succession is believed to make the therapeutic effect of the solution more powerful. Homeopathic remedies commonly come in × (10) or c (100) potencies. A 5× potency would mean that the original matter had been diluted one part in ten, five successive times. Remedies are often so diluted that the final solution may contain no molecules of the original substance. Commercially available remedies are most commonly 6, 12, and 30 × or c potencies. Remedies are usually not taken for more than 2 to 3 days.

Because homeopathy is based on tenets that do not fit within conventional science, it is highly criticized. There is no proven scientific explanation for the mechanism of action of homeopathic medicine, but there are theories. Based on findings in quantum mechanics, some have suggested that the electromagnetic energy in the homeopathic remedies interacts with the body on some level (20). Physical chemists have hypothesized the memory of water theory, which suggests that the structure of the water/alcohol solution is altered by the medicinal substance during the process of dilution and retains this altered structure even after the medicine dissolves. This theory has some support from chaos theory because one basic tenet of this is that very small changes can affect very large systems.

Severely ill patients should not stop taking conventional medicines during homeopathic treatment, although if possible this is optimal. During homeopathic therapy, the use of medicinal herbs, exposure to mothballs and other aromatic substances, initiation of acupuncture, and chiropractics should be avoided.

For both acute and chronic conditions, the remedy is stopped once the reaction is apparent; it should be repeated only when the reaction has subsided. Because homeopathy treats the person rather than the illness, two individuals presenting with the same diagnosis may receive different homeopathic remedies. Patients should be aware that their symptoms may initially worsen on initiation of therapy before they improve.

There is good evidence for the use of homeopathic measures in the treatment of postoperative ileus and allergic rhinitis (21, 22). For the treatment of influenza, two separate randomized, double-blind, placebo-controlled trials showed use of the homeopathic treatment Oscillococcinum (Anas Barbariae, Hepatis and Cordis Extractum HPUS 200c) was shown to be significantly better than placebo in the alleviation of symptoms in mild to moderate cases (23, 24).

Naturopathy

Naturopathy is a medical system based on the principle *Vis Medcatrix Naturae*, or the healing power of nature. This system is not associated with any particular therapy per se, but with a philosophy of life, health, and disease. In this system, symptoms accompanying a disease are not due to the causative agents, but result from the organism's reaction(s) to the agent(s) and reflect its attempt to heal itself. Symptoms are therefore viewed as a constructive response. The role of the physician is to facilitate the body's ability to heal itself, not to assume control over the body's functions.

Naturopaths practice as primary care providers and use natural medicines and interventionist therapies as needed. Clinical nutrition serves as the foundation for naturopathic medicine. Naturopaths may also use acupuncture, hydrotherapy, physical medicine, and counseling and lifestyle modification techniques to achieve the desired results. Depending on state law, they may perform outpatient surgery, give vaccines, and prescribe a limited number of drugs.

Because naturopathy is based on multiple philosophies, naturopathic doctors or NDs study the pathologic origins of illness, as well as the clinical, physical, and laboratory sciences taught in conventional medical education. The naturopathic curriculum requires 4 additional years of schooling after receipt of a baccalaureate degree. Like most allopathic schools, the first 2 years are spent on the basic sciences, whereas the last 2 involve introduction and practice of the clinical sciences of diagnosis and treatments. Their training also includes clinical nutrition, botanical medicine, Oriental medicine, homeopathy, and other medical approaches and modalities.

Naturopathic providers can be licensed or registered in more than ten states in the United States. There are currently four accredited naturopathic schools in the United States, in Washington, Oregon, Arizona, and Connecticut (25).

Chiropractic

Chiropractic is a health care system based on the idea that illness results from vertebral subluxation (a spinal misalignment that causes abnormal nerve transmission), and the best treatment approach is manual manipulation of the subluxated vertebrae. The theory of subluxations maintains that health problems are due to "blockage" of nerves. According to this system, the chief beneficial effects of chiropractic are relief of musculoskeletal pain and disability, as well as restoration of proper internal organ function. Although the first beneficial claim is intuitively understandable from the allopathic perspective, the second claim of benefit is more controversial in the allopathic viewpoint. Drawing on advances in neurophysiology, however, it is possible that chiropractic techniques may exert a physiologic response in internal organs through the somatoautonomic reflex.

For years, the American Medical Association (AMA) publicly attacked the chiropractic system, but in 1976, chiropractors won a significant lawsuit (the "Wilkes suit") against the AMA for restraint of trade. However, it was not until 1980 that the Ethics Code of the AMA was changed to reflect that each individual doctor may decide for themselves whether to accept a patient from or refer a patient to a chiropractor or other limited practitioner. In 1990, the U.S. Supreme Court upheld the decision of the lower court in its 1976 ruling.

Currently, one of the prevailing paradigms of modern chiropractic medicine is the theory of intervertebral motion and segmental dysfunction (SDF). According to this theory, it is the loss of proper spinal joint mobility, not positional misalignment, that is the key factor in the subluxation complex. Because subluxation always involves more than a single vertebra, a common finding in subluxation is restriction of a joint's range of motion, termed a fixation. The optimal therapy for fixation-subluxations is spinal manipulation therapy. SDF is said to occur when the three following signs are present: (a) point tenderness or an altered pain threshold to pressure in either the adjacent paraspinal musculature or over the spinous process, (b) abnormal contraction or tension in adjacent paraspinal musculature, and (c) loss of normal range of motion in one or more planes (26).

After evaluating the site of pain in context with the regional area and the whole body, the chiropractor must determine when and where spinal manipulative therapy would be most beneficial, as well as the type of adjustment that is most appropriate. Nonadjustment measures chiropractors may employ also include trigger point therapy, joint mobilization, and massage. It is licensed in all 50 states and most major U.S. insurance carriers, as well as Medicare, will reimburse for chiropractic treatments.

Osteopathy

Osteopathy was founded in the late 1800s in the United States by Dr. Andrew Taylor Still, who sought to develop a system of medical care that would promote the body's innate ability to heal itself. One key concept of osteopathy is that structure influences function. Hence, in this system, the structural integrity of the body mechanism is considered to be the key determinant in maintaining health and well-being. A disruption in structure in one area of the body may lead to malfunction of that area and other areas.

The other two fundamental concepts proposed by Still in the osteopathic system of practice were that the parts of the body comprised a unified whole, and the body has an innate ability to self-regulate and self-heal. The effects of any disease are felt, in varying degrees, throughout the body. Therefore, the entire body can be mobilized to help combat illness. The whole body must be treated, as treating only specific, isolated symptoms ignores the fundamental interconnectedness of the body. Preventive medicine, including good nutrition and fitness, is extremely important in maintaining healthy body systems. Appropriate therapies should stimulate and maximize the body's innate ability to heal itself.

In addition to being trained to provide standard medical care, osteopathic physicians use their hands to diagnose problems, relieve pain, restore range of motion, and balance tissues and muscles to promote the body's own innately healthy state. Osteopathy differs from chiropractic in both theory and practice. Osteopaths use arms and legs as fulcrums for bending and twisting the body (long-lever manipulation); chiropractors generally only manipulate the protruding parts of the spinal vertebrae (short-lever manipulation).

The use of manipulation in osteopathy is important but is not the sole or even primary modality of treatment. Treatment modalities are chosen based on the patient's signs and symptoms after obtaining a thorough patient history and assessing the structure and function of the musculoskeletal system to look for clues to its role in the patient's illness. Osteopathic medicine evaluates the body as an integrated unit.

Osteopathic medicine is one of two fully recognized schools of medicine in the United States with 19 osteopathic medical schools recognized by the Department of Education. Osteopathic principles and manipulative therapy are integrated into the 4-year postgraduate curriculum and include 300 to 500 hours of instruction in the study of the body's neuromusculoskeletal system.

State medical board examinations exist in all 50 states and must be passed to obtain a license to practice osteopathic medicine and prescribe medication. Specialty boards provide standards and licensing for performing surgery.

SPECIFIC CAM MODALITIES

Acupuncture

The practice of acupuncture reflects the belief that health depends on a balanced flow of qi, the vital life energy. Disturbances in qi produce illness, and by inserting needles at specific points in the body, this balance is restored, resulting in pain relief, healing, or the creation of desired physiologic changes. Moxibustion refers to the burning of powdered leaves of mugwort (*Artemis vulgairs*) to deliver warmth or focused warming either to the surface of the skin or the head of an inserted acupuncture needle.

In traditional acupuncture literature, 71 clearly defined channels or jing luo, are identified. It is along these channels that qi and blood travel. Traditional acupuncture points are located in 14 of these channels. In these 14 channels, there are 670 standard acupuncture points. Foramina, intersecting muscle sites, and spaces between tendons usually mark a significant acupuncture point. Depth of insertion, as well as the orientation and manipulation of the needle, are not arbitrary in acupuncture. Orienting the needle along the direction of channel flow is called tonifying; orienting it in the opposite direction of flow is referred to as dispersing.

Data suggest that prevalence figures in the general population range from 1% in the United States to 21% in France (27). Numerous studies have demonstrated acupuncture's relative safety, but there have been case reports of serious complications, including infections with hepatitis (28–33). For this reason, it is strongly recommended that only disposable acupuncture needles be used (34).

Research from China has found that acupuncture has a regulatory effect on the menstrual cycle, and can be used to regulate the production of luteinizing hormone (LH), follicle-stimulating hormone (FSH), and estradiol (35, 36). Acupuncture has also been used to effectively treat menorrhagia, dysmenorrhea, premenstrual syndrome (PMS), and infertility (37–40). It is believed that acupuncture exerts these, and its other gynecologic effects, in part through influencing the central effect of neuropeptides on the hypothalamic-pituitary-ovarian axis and peripherally on the uterus.

Mind–Body Therapies

Mind–body therapies (MBTs) are defined by the NIH as "interventions that use a variety of techniques designed to facilitate the mind's capacity to affect bodily function and symptoms." This would include practices such as relaxation therapy, meditation, imagery, hypnosis, biofeedback, cognitive behavioral therapy, and psychoeducational approaches. A serious limitation in most mind–body studies reviewed is the absence of any placebo or sham control condition because practitioners cannot typically be blinded to the treatment, and it is often not possible to blind patients to group assignment.

Various MBTs can improve mood, quality of life, and coping, as well as ameliorate disease and treatment-related symptoms, such as chemotherapy-induced nausea and vomiting, physical pain, and functioning (41–43). Whether MBTs can prolong cancer survival times remains an unresolved issue (44, 45).

There is strong evidence that biofeedback-assisted muscle retraining is effective in the treatment of incontinence disorders. In one randomized trial, biofeedback-assisted behavioral treatment was more effective than drug therapy in reducing incontinence episodes in elderly women (46).

MBTs have also been shown to be efficacious for the treatment of insomnia, including late-life insomnia (47, 48). Although pharmacologic treatments produce somewhat faster sleep improvements in the short term, behavioral approaches over an intermediate term (4 to 8 weeks) show comparable effects, and in the long term (6 to 24 months), behavioral approaches show more favorable outcomes than drug therapies (49).

Currently, there are no well-developed or established tools for assessing adverse events associated with MBTs. While practicing relaxation techniques, some persons report experiencing increased anxiety. Some patients might experience transitory negative effects either during or after hypnosis, including headaches, drowsiness, confusion, dizziness, or nausea, and less frequently, anxiety or panic (50).

Hypnotherapy

The use of hypnosis as a part of healing therapies goes back to ancient civilization. Modern hypnosis was developed by Franz Anton Mesmer in the 1700s; he used his techniques predominately to treat psychological disorders. Hypnosis is a technique of focused concentration. During hypnosis, the patient absorbs the words or visualization described by the hypnotherapist, dissociates from rational or internal criticisms, and responds to the hypnotherapist's suggestions. Someone may only be open to suggestions that are in accordance with their desires. Imaginative individuals are easier to hypnotize than others. During hypnosis, changes in the body occur that are similar to those that take place with other relaxation therapies. These changes can be measured in brain wave activity, oxygen and carbon dioxide metabolism, blood pressure, heart rate, and sympathetic nervous system activity. Currently, addictions and phobias are indications for hypnotherapy. Hypnotherapists should be certified by the American Board of Hypnosis or the American Council of Hypnotist Examiners.

Biofeedback

Biofeedback is a relaxation technique that allows patients to exert control over autonomic responses. Patients learn how to control physiologic responses to their own thought patterns through electrodes and monitors. The effects most frequently measured include changes in muscle tension, skin temperature and resistance, breathing patterns, and brainwaves. Usually, after eight to ten sessions, the patient no longer needs the monitoring device or electrodes to confirm the results of their efforts. It is frequently employed for the treatment of different types of chronic pain and headaches, although it has many uses. The Biofeedback Certification Institute of America certifies practitioners.

Relaxation Techniques

There are a number of different types of relaxation techniques. Autogenic training uses visual imagery and body awareness to move patients into a deep state of relaxation. While visualizing a peaceful place, the patient focuses on physical sensations in sequential order from the feet to the head, while concentrating on limbs, heartbeat, breath, and the forehead.

Progressive muscle relaxation involves the tensing and relaxing of each muscle group, beginning with the toes and ending with the head and neck.

Meditation comes in various forms and affiliations. Indian transcendental meditation is a meditative version of yoga, whereas Buddhist Vipassana is commonly referred to as mindful meditation. Prayer may be considered a form of meditation. Meditation can lower blood pressure and induce other physiologic effects as well. It may be used to relieve headaches, chronic pain, and stress.

Bodywork

Bodywork includes all healing therapies that use hands to treat the patient.

Massage

Massage is the simplest and most accessible form of bodywork. There are many varieties of massage. In most cases, massage relieves muscle tension, reduces stress, and invokes a calm feeling. Different techniques target specific parts of the body and are tailored to particular kinds of muscle stress. In addition to techniques, massage therapists are also trained in how the musculoskeletal, cardiovascular, lymphatic, and nervous systems work and interact with each other. The U.S. Department of Education's Commission on Massage Training Accreditation and Approval oversees the regulation of massage training and certification.

The most familiar form of massage in the United States is Swedish massage, a collection of techniques for muscle relaxation. Some of the specific techniques used in Swedish massage include (a) effleurage or stroking to heighten circulation, (b) pétrissage or kneading to stimulate circulation of blood and lymph, (c) tapotement or percussion to stimulate muscles, (d) friction to clear away toxins, and (e) vibration to stimulate the nervous system. Massage strokes are generally done parallel with the venous flow (i.e., toward the heart). The exception to this is when nerve strokes are used, which move outward, toward the extremities.

Lymphatic massage is intended to improve lymph flow, and involves repetitive and rapid light stroking. Lymphatic massage therapists are certified in manual lymph drainage and must have prior training as a massage therapist, physical therapist, or nurse.

Rolfing is also known as structural integration and was developed in the late 1940s. It is a massage technique based on the manipulation of the fascia. Rolfers restore proper muscle function and realign the fascia away from gravitational pull.

Myofascial release is a form of manual therapy that also focuses on the body's connective tissues and uses gentle, sustained pressure and stretching to help the patient achieve postural changes and optimal body alignment. The tissue is stretched along the direction of the muscle fibers until resistance is met, where the position is then held until the soft tissues release. This is repeated until the tissues are fully elongated.

Trigger point and myotherapy massage are techniques used to relieve muscle spasms and cramping. It is believed that by applying pressure to tender areas where muscles have been damaged (trigger points), blood flow will increase to the area and break physiologic reflex neural arcs, thus reducing the spasm or cramping.

Reflexology is a form of massage performed on the hands, feet, or ears in the belief that these locations have reflex connections throughout the body.

Postural Therapies

Postural therapies focus on the relationship between the musculoskeletal system and body movement. Each type of therapy sets its own certification guidelines. The Alexander techniques involves the use of specific movements done while sitting and standing, and is sometimes accompanied by light pressure to muscle contraction sites by the practitioner. It is taught in many acting schools as a means of reducing tension and facilitating less strained and more efficient movements.

The Feldenkrais method is used to increase awareness of bodily functions involved with movement. It is based on two principles: (a) awareness of movement can be achieved through the conscious mapping of actions involved in specific, everyday movements such as walking; and (b) the practitioner can help the patient focus on specific areas of coordination or movement and thus create an awareness of options in movement (functional integration).

Therapeutic Touch

Although therapeutic touch uses hands to treat patients, it is important to note that in this technique, the practitioner's hands may never actually touch the patient's body. The practice of therapeutic touch is based on the premise that each individual has an energy field that can be felt and manipulated therapeutically.

Intercessory Prayer and Distance or Spiritual Healing

Spiritual or distance hearing has been defined as "the intentional influence of one or more persons upon another living system without utilizing known physical means of intervention" or "a conscious, dedicated act of mentation attempting to benefit another person's physical or emotional well being at a distance" (51). Astin et al. (51) systematically reviewed the literature of distant healing, including studies that employed interventions other than prayer. They identified 23 RCTs, but as we have seen for the RCTs in other areas of CAM research, a number of technical problems were present. No formal data combination effort (meta-analysis) was attempted, however, because the amount of heterogeneity among studies was too great. Nonetheless, these systematic reviewers observed that 13 of the 23 studies reported a beneficial effect (51).

Herbs, Botanicals, and Supplements

Herbalism is the study and practice of using plant material for food, medicine, and health promotion. Herbalism not only treats disease, but it is also used to enhance quality of life, both physically and spiritually. Although a botanist defines an herb as a nonwoody, low-growing plant, herbalists will use the entire plant kingdom. Some experts prefer the term "botanical," which encompasses any plant-derived product used for a medicinal or health purpose. Herbalists may also use nonplants as healing agents, such as insects, minerals, gemstones, or animal parts. In this section, only the use of plant agents is discussed.

Traditional systems of herbal medicine do not distinguish between food and medicinal plants. The healing uses of plants and plant properties are paradigm specific. For example, in Chinese and Tibetan medicine, there are "five tastes." Each taste or flavor is associated with specific qualities and corresponding physiologic actions.

The ability to analyze the chemical composition of food and medicinal plants is viewed by many as the scientific opportunity to determine what the "active ingredients" in the plant or plant compound are, thereby allowing for the purer development of drugs and therapies. This is a rather reductionistic approach, however, and makes it extremely difficult to allow for the interaction among various plant constituents that may, as a whole, be the source of its efficacy.

The method of preparation of a plant is very important in determining its medicinal or nutritional properties. For example, the cassava root is a popular food staple in West and Central Africa. The roots and leaves of poorly processed cassava plants, however, contain cyanogens, substances that induce cyanide production. The proper processing of cassava reduces the cyanogenic content in the root. Even if the plant is properly processed, exposure to the volatile cyanide released during the processing of roots and leaves can cause health problems in workers.

Oversight and Regulation of Herbs, Botanicals, and Dietary Supplements

The Dietary Supplement Health and Education Act (DSHEA) of 1994 classified herbal preparations as dietary supplements. The DSHEA considers a substance to be a dietary supplement if it (a) is a product (other than tobacco) that is intended to supplement the diet that bears or contains one or more of the following ingredients: a vitamin, a mineral, an herb or other botanical, or an amino acid; (b) is intended for ingestion in pill, capsule, tablet, or liquid form; (c) is not used as a conventional food or as the sole item of a meal or diet; and (d) is labeled as a dietary supplement. DSHEA provides for the exemption of herbs and supplements from the safety and efficacy requirements and regulations that prescription and over-the-counter drugs must fulfill (i.e., preclinical animal studies, premarketing controlled clinical trials, and postmarketing surveillance). Manufacturers must notify the FDA within 30 days after a product is released to the public but are not required to perform any postmarketing surveillance activities.

DSHEA mandates that the following disclaimer be present on each product label, "This statement has not been evaluated by the Food and Drug Administration. This product is not intended to diagnose, treat, cure, or prevent any disease." DSHEA does allow herbal preparations to have suggested dosages on the label. Although DSHEA prevents manufacturers from making specific medical claims, it does allow descriptions of the herb's effect on "structure or function" of the body. However, it is a fine line between a medical claim and a structure or function claim.

Because of this lack of regulatory mechanisms, there is little assurance that commercial herbal preparations have predictable pharmacologic effects or that product labels provide accurate information. The potency of herbal medications has been demonstrated to vary from manufacturer to manufacturer and even from lot to lot within a manufacturer (52, 53). Although some manufacturers have tried to standardize their preparations to fixed concentrations of selected chemical constituents, the benefits of this are uncertain because many products achieve their effects through the combined or synergistic actions of different compounds (54, 55).

In the United States, the incidence and exact nature of adverse events associated with supplement use is unknown, although the empirical evidence surrounding the use of herbal medications support the claim that most of them are safe to use (56). In some instances, herbal medications (particularly those of Eastern origin) have been found to be adulterated with heavy metals, pesticides, and even conventional drugs (57–59). To remove a supplement product from the market in the United States, one of two things must happen: (a) the FDA must prove in a court of law that a product is unsafe, or (b) the Director of the Department of Health and Human Services must determine the supplement to be hazardous in an administrative hearing.

This is in stark contrast to the regulations seen in other countries (e.g., Germany). For the past 50 years, the German Commission E (equivalent to our FDA) has overseen the purity, chemical standardization, manufacture, and labeling of herbs and phytomedicines, much as with standard drugs. The commission has also fostered the full integration of herbs and phytomedicines in Germany's allopathic medical system.

The U.S. Pharmacopeia (USP), a nonprofit organization that sets the standards manufacturers must fulfill to sell their drugs in the United States, has also established standards for botanical and nonbotanical dietary supplements. The presence of the USP symbol on a product ensures the supplement fulfills USP standards for identity, strength, quality, purity, packaging, and labeling. If an herbal product carries the National Formulary designation, this signifies that it fulfills the quality standards set by the USP but does not carry FDA or USP endorsement regarding its intended use.

There are eight herbs that account for more than 50% of all single herb preparations among the 1500 to 1800 herbal medications sold in the United States (60, 61). These are echinacea, ephedra, garlic, gingko, ginseng, kava, St. John's wort, and valerian.

Herb–Drug Interactions

In 1997, 12% of the U.S. population used herbal medications—a 380% increase from 1990 (62, 63). In two studies in a preoperative patient population, between 22% and 32% of patients disclosed herbal therapy use (64, 65). Unfortunately, in one of the two studies, more than 70% of the patients failed to disclose their herbal medicine use during routine preoperative assessment (65). Failure to disclose or to ask about herb or botanical use in patients increases the risk of herb–drug interactions occurring. For example, some herbs must be discontinued at least 1 week prior to surgery because they may promote bleeding (e.g., garlic, ginkgo, ginseng). Kava and valerian have sedative effects and should be stopped 48 hours prior to surgery.

In 2001, Fugh-Berman and Ernst reviewed the medical literature for herb–drug interactions and were able to identify 108 suspected cases (66). To adequately assess the clinical data available, these authors developed a 10-point scale to evaluate the quality of a case report of an adverse interaction (Table 20.1). In their review of 108 case reports of an adverse interaction, 74 were classified as not evaluable, 20 represented possible interactions, and 14 were likely interactions. The drug most commonly involved in adverse event reports was warfarin; the herb most commonly implicated was St. John's wort.

If an adverse herb–drug interaction is suspected, it should be reported to the FDA's MedWatch program in the same manner that drug–drug interactions are reported; the number is 1-800-332-1088 or www.fda.gov/medwatch.

For an overview of the different types of herbal preparations and categories of herbal medicines, see Tables 20.2 and 20.3.

TABLE 20.1

Assessment and Evaluation of Herb–Drug Interactions

Assessment criteria

Each of the following criteria receives 1 point if it is met. The sum is totaled, and the evaluation scale is used to assess the adequacy of the case report.

- Adequate patient history is given
- Concurrently used medications are documented
- Chronology of events is complete
- Time between taking the herb and onset of adverse event is reasonable
- Adverse event is well described
- Other possible interactions are accounted for and adequately described
- Plausible, alternative explanations have been excluded
- Concurrent diseases, conditions, or medications associated with the adverse event are adequately described
- Event ceases on discontinuation of the herb
- Event recurs with reintroduction of the herb

Evaluation Scale

- 0–3 points: the possibility of an interaction is not able to be evaluated because the report contains insufficient information
- 4–7 points: a herb–drug interaction is possible, although other causes may be involved
- 8–10 points: a herb–drug interaction is likely, and the report provides reliable evidence for this asserted interaction

Adapted from Fugh-Berman A, Ernst E. Herb–drug interactions: review and assessment of report reliability. Br J Clin Pharmacol 2001;52:587–595, with permission.

Commonly Used Herbs

Echinacea

Echinacea is derived from members of the daisy family, and is used for the prevention and treatment of viral, bacterial, and fungal infections, particularly those of the upper respiratory tract (67). Preclinical studies of echinacea have shown a number of immunostimulatory effects when use is limited to less than 8 weeks (68, 69). Conversely, use for longer than 8 weeks carries the potential risk of immunosuppression (70). As a precaution, patients requiring perioperative immunosuppression should be counseled not to use echinacea compounds. Because use of echinacea has been associated with allergic reactions, it should be used cautiously in patients with asthma, allergic rhinitis, or atopy. Although definitive evidence is lacking, the potential for hepatotoxicity warrants caution in using echinacea in patients with pre-existing liver dysfunction.

Ephedra

Ephedra is referred to as ma huang in Chinese medicine, and is used to promote weight loss, increase energy, and treat respiratory tract conditions, such as asthma and bronchitis. Ephedra contains alkaloids, including ephedrine, pseudoephedrine, norephedrine, methylephedrine, and norpseudoephedrine (71). The predominant active compound is ephedrine, which is a sympathomimetic. As a result, ephedra causes dose-dependent increases in blood pressure and heart rate. Adverse effects reported with use of this drug include myocardial infarction and stroke, which are believed to result from vasoconstriction and vasospasm (72). Ephedra has been associated with hypersensitivity myocarditis, an entity characterized by cardiomyopathy with myocardial lymphocyte and eosinophil infiltration (73).

Garlic

Garlic has been extensively studied. Its potential to modify the risk of atherosclerosis effects through mediation of blood pressure, thrombus formation, and cholesterol modification is primarily attributed to the sulfur-containing compounds, particularly allicin and its transformation

TABLE 20.2

Types of Herbal Preparations

- *Powders*: These may be available as capsules, tablets, or in bulk form.
- *Infusion*: An herbal preparation that has been steeped as a tea.
- *Decoction*: A combination of bulk herbs in water that are boiled together. The mixture is then strained, and the liquid is ingested.
- *Tinctures*: The herb is soaked in a solvent (usually alcohol or water) for hours, days, or even weeks. Most tinctures are made with alcohol, although glycerin may be used to make an "alcoholfree" tincture. Glycerin tinctures usually taste more pleasant than alcohol ones, but the preparations may be weaker than alcohol-based tinctures. Tinctures are often made in a 1:5 or 1:10 concentration[a] (one part herbal material to five or ten parts [by weight] of the liquid).
- *Fluid extract*: These are more concentrated than tinctures. Although they are most often made using an alcohol or water solvent, other solvents such as glycerin, vinegar, propylene glycol, etc., may be used. Because a tincture is typically a 1:10 or 1:5 concentration, whereas a fluid extract is usually a 1:1 concentration, a fluid extract is typically at least 4 times as potent when compared with an equal amount of tincture, and a solid extract is usually 40 times as potent when compared with an equal amount of tincture.
- *Solid extracts*: The most concentrated form of an herbal preparation. This results when the solvent evaporates, leaving a solid residue. Solid extracts are most often available in powder form, although some are oil based. A typical solid extract is a 2:1 or 8:1 concentration.
- *Standardized extract*: These extracts have guaranteed levels of a certain constituent or group of constituents in the final product. The standardized component(s) are usually expressed as a percentage of the total weight of the extract.
- *Simples*: Preparations of a single herb.
- *Poultice*: May be made with either dried or fresh herbs; the poultice is made by grinding the herbal preparation, combining it with a liquid (usually water) and then spreading it on or between layers of cloth. The cloth is then placed on a body surface and is kept in place for 1 to 24 hours.
- *Aromatics*: Inhaled volatile oils or smokes.
- *Essential oil*: An herbal preparation in an oil base that has usually undergone some process of extraction.
- *Infused oil*: The "essence" of the botanical is extracted into a carrier oil; olive oil is most commonly used although other oils such as sweet almond, canola, linseed, hemp seed, and poppy seed can be used. Infused oils can be either hot or cold infused. Cold-infused oils take much longer to produce than hot-infused oils, but retain better quality.
- *Salves or ointments*: Salves are made by heating an herb with fat until the fat absorbs the plant's healing properties. A thickening and hardening agent, such as beeswax, is then added to the strained mixture to give it a thicker consistency. The key ingredient of salves is herbal oil (an oil and herb mixture that has been allowed to sit for a week or more) (herbal oils to be used in food preparation must be refrigerated during this time).

[a] Strengths of extracts: Typically, 1 g of a 4:1 solid extract is equivalent to 4 mL of a fluid extract (one-seventh of an ounce) and 40 mL of a tincture (almost 1.5 oz). Some solid extracts are concentrated as high as 100:1, meaning that it would take nearly 100 g of crude herb, or 100 mL of a fluid extract (approximately 3.5 oz), or 1000 mL of a tincture (almost 1 qt) to provide an equal amount of herbal material in 1 g of a 100:1 extract.

products (74). Commercial garlic preparations are often standardized to a fixed allicin content. Garlic inhibits platelet aggregation in a dose-dependent fashion. For this reason, discontinuation of use is recommended for at least 7 days preoperatively (75). Garlic may also adversely interact with warfarin.

Gingko Biloba

Gingko biloba has been used for a variety of ailments, including cognitive disorders, peripheral vascular disease, age-related macular degeneration, vertigo, tinnitus, erectile dysfunction, and altitude sickness.

TABLE 20.3

Categories of Herbal Medicines

- *Adaptogens*: Substances that increase the body's resistance to stress and help restore balance to the various body systems. Examples include Asian and Siberian ginseng, Astragalus, and Schizandra.
- *Antioxidants*: Substances that reduce the amount and effect of free radicals. Examples include milk thistle, ginkgo biloba, hawthorn, and bilberry.
- *Astringents*: Substances that cause protein coagulation, create a protective barrier, and help add "tone" to the tissue. These act as anti-inflammatory agents. Examples include witch hazel, tormentil, and horse chestnut.
- *Carminatives*: Herbs that help soothe and tone the digestive system. Examples include peppermint, chamomile, anise, caraway, and fennel.
- *Cholagogues*: Herbs that stimulate the production and proper flow of bile. Examples include dandelion root, turmeric, goldenseal root, Chelidonium, artichoke, and milk thistle.
- *Demulcents*: Herbs with an ability to soothe or protect irritated mucus membranes. When these are applied externally, they are referred to as emollients. Examples include marshmallow rot, slippery elm, the mucilaginous parts of aloe leaves, fenugreek seeds, and plantain leaves.
- *Digestive bitters*: Herbs that help stimulate the digestive process and increase production of digestive enzymes. Examples include gentian root and rhizome, dandelion root, barberry bark, yellow dock, and blessed thistle.
- *Immunomodulators*: Substances that promote healthy immune function. Examples include echinacea, astragalus, and Siberian ginseng.
- *Laxatives*: These may be stimulant or bulk forming. Examples include psyllium seed, senna leaves, cascara bark, and latex from the leaves of the aloe plant.

Adapted from Brown DJ. Herbal Prescriptions for Better Health. Rocklin, CA: Prima Health, 1996:28–36, with permission.

Results of randomized, double-blind, placebo-controlled clinical trials of the effect of gingko biloba on memory are mixed. The most significant negative study was conducted in 230 healthy volunteers (mean age 68.7 years) for 6 weeks. At the end of the trial, mean scores on 14 standardized neuropsychological tests of verbal and visual learning and memory, attention and concentration, and expressive language did not differ significantly between treatment and placebo groups (76).

In contrast, Mix et al. (77) found a significant difference between treatment and placebo groups in a 6-week RCT of 48 healthy adults ages 55 to 86 years. The treatment group performed significantly better on tasks assessing simple speed of processing abilities, and participants rated their overall memories as assessed by follow-up and self-report questionnaire as significantly improved compared with placebo ($p < 0.03$). No significant differences were found on any of the four objective memory tests (77).

In more recent clinical trials, there were no significant side effects reported with standardized gingko biloba extract; the most common adverse events were nausea and allergic skin reactions from either contact or ingestion of the fruit pulp of gingko.

Gingko biloba extract should not be taken with nonsteroidal anti-inflammatory drugs (NSAIDs), heparin, or Coumadin secondary to an increased risk of spontaneous bleeding (78). Because gingko has the ability to inhibit platelet-activating factor, it should be discontinued at least 36 hours prior to surgery (75, 79). Ginkgo may interact adversely with blood-thinning medications such as aspirin and warfarin.

Ginseng

The two most commonly used forms of ginseng are the Asian variety and the American variety. They are used for different purposes in Chinese medicine. Siberian ginseng is not the same genus as either Asian or American ginseng; hence, it is important to determine exactly which genus is being discussed in texts regarding herbal therapy or in instructions to use "ginseng." Asian ginseng is commonly used to protect the body against the effects of stress and to restore a feeling of equilibrium. Commercially available ginseng preparations may be standardized to ginsenoside content.

Kava

Kava comes from the root of a dried pepper plant. It is often used as an anxiolytic and sedative. Results from clinical trials suggest that kava has a therapeutic potential in the symptomatic treatment of anxiety (80). Kavalactones appear to be the active pharmacologic agents in kava and have dose-dependent effects on the central nervous system (CNS), including antiepileptic, neuroprotective, and local anesthetic properties (81, 82). Kava has been associated with 25 cases of fulminate hepatitis, 11 requiring liver transplant (83). Extensive use of kava has been associated with "kava dermopathy," a condition characterized by reversible scaly cutaneous eruptions (84). Because of its potential to synergistically act with anesthetics, its use should be discontinued at least 24 hours prior to surgery (75).

St. John's Wort

St. John's wort is the common name for *Hypericum perforatum.* Although clinical studies have demonstrated that it is as effective as sertraline and imipramine in the treatment of mild depression, it is no more effective than placebo in treating major depression (85, 86). Commercial preparations are often standardized to a fixed hypericin content of 0.3%. St. John's wort exerts its effects by inhibiting serotonin, norepinephrine, and dopamine reuptake by neurons (87, 88). There have been reports of a central serotonin excess syndrome in patients taking this drug either alone or in combination with SSRIs (89, 90). St. John's wort is known to induce the cytochrome isoform P4053A4, resulting in a doubling of its metabolic activity (91, 92). This may result in enhanced metabolism of any medications taken concurrently with St. John's wort. For example, the anticoagulant effects of warfarin may be diminished, cyclosporine may not be as effective, and the pharmakinetics of digoxin are known to be effected. In addition, the efficacy of NSAIDs may be decreased (93–95). Due to the long half-life of its metabolites, St. John's wort should be stopped at least 5 days prior to surgery (75).

Valerian

Valerian is a sedative, most commonly used in the treatment of insomnia. Commercially available preparations may be standardized to valerianic acid. Through modulation of GABA neurotransmission and receptor function, valerian produces dose-dependent sedation and hypnosis but purportedly without significant "drug hangover effects" (96–98). Patients should be told that the capsules often smell like "gym socks." There is one case report of a patient who suffered from a benzodiazepine withdrawallike symptoms after acute discontinuation of the herb (99). For patients who have become physically dependent on the drug, a slow tapering may be necessary prior to elective surgery. If this is not possible, patients are advised to continue the drug up until the day of surgery, and benzodiazepines may be used to treat any withdrawal symptoms that may develop postoperatively (75).

Chaste Tree Berry

Chaste tree berry, also known as chasteberry, monk's pepper, and Vitex, is from the fruit of the shrub *Vitex agnus castus.* Although it is not one of the "top 8" herbs in the United States, it is reviewed here because of purported effects on gynecologic conditions. Chaste tree berry has been used in Europe, particularly Germany, for many years to treat menstrual abnormalities and complaints, PMS, and breast pain associated with menses. The whole fruit extract is necessary for the medicinal activity of chaste tree berry. Chaste tree berry is believed to have anti-inflammatory properties and progesteronelike effects; it is purported to affect LH and FSH, and restore the estrogen-progesterone balance during the luteal phase of the menstrual cycle. Because chaste berry has no direct hormonal activity, it is not considered a phytoestrogen (100, 101). Two prospective trials of chaste tree berry, each lasting three menstrual cycles in women with PMS, found a significant difference in symptom improvement among women receiving chaste tree berry compared with placebo (102, 103). Side effects of chaste berry may include gastrointestinal complaints, itching or rash, headache, and increased menstrual flow (104). Use of chaste tree berry is contraindicated in pregnancy and lactation, or in patients receiving hormone therapy, haloperidol (Haldol) or thioridazine (Mellaril). For PMS or frequent or heavy menses, chaste tree berry may be used continuously for 4 to 6 months; dosage will depend on the type of preparation used.

Commonly Used Supplements

Glucosamine and Chondroitin Sulfate

Glucosamine is an aminomonosaccharide and a component of cartilage. One of the most popular supplements for the treatment of osteoarthritis is glucosamine sulfate—with or without chondroitin sulfate. Glucosamine is derived from the shells of crustaceans, and chondroitin is from cow trachea or shark cartilage. Experimental evidence in vitro suggests that glucosamine may facilitate beneficial responses in cartilage metabolism (e.g., increasing the synthesis of cartilage-specific type II collagen in human fetal chondrocytes) (105). When cultures of chondrocytes derived from cartilage afflicted with osteoarthritis are exposed to glucosamine, proteoglycan synthesis increases. Chondroitin sulfate appears to have similar effects (105).

There is evidence from a 3-year Belgian study that glucosamine slows the progression of osteoarthritis (106). In this study, patients took 1500 mg glucosamine daily, divided two or three times a day. In some cases, it took 4 to 8 weeks for effects to become apparent. A meta-analysis reviewing trials of glucosamine and chondroitin sulfate concluded that these supplements are likely to be effective for the symptomatic management of osteoarthritis, but deficiencies in study designs and conduct did not allow a definitive evaluation (107).

Coenzyme CoQ10

Coenzyme Q10 (CoQ10) is a provitamin manufactured by the body that functions as a coenzyme for mitochondrial enzymes. CoQ10 is also known as ubiquinone because it is found in almost every cell of the body. Tissue levels of CoQ10 decrease as people get older. It has also been shown to be deficient in patients with cardiovascular disease, cancer, AIDS, muscular dystrophy, spontaneous abortion, male infertility, and periodontal disease.

CoQ10 has been tested as a protective agent against the cardiac toxicity observed in cancer patients treated with the anthracycline drug doxorubicin. Studies with adults and children have confirmed the decrease in cardiac toxicity due to doxorubicin previously observed in animal studies (108–110).

Three small studies were conducted using CoQ10 as a dietary supplement in patients undergoing conventional cancer treatment (111–113). In these studies, the researchers explored the potential use of CoQ10 as an adjuvant therapy for cancer. Although some beneficial results were reported, study design flaws limited these results. These studies did not include control patients, and the participants received a variety of supplements in addition to CoQ10. Patients in the trials also received standard treatment either during or just before CoQ10 supplementation.

No serious side effects have been reported from the use of CoQ10. Doses of 100 mg/day have been reported to cause insomnia in some patients, and doses of greater than 300 mg/day for extended periods of use have been reported to elevate liver enzymes, although there have been no reports of liver toxicity (114–116). Other reported side effects have included dizziness, visual sensitivity to light, irritability, headache, heartburn, and fatigue.

Certain lipid-lowering drugs, such as the "statins" (HMG-CoA reductase inhibitors) and fibrates, as well as oral agents that lower blood sugar, such as some sulfonylureas, cause a decrease in serum levels of CoQ10 and reduce the effects of CoQ10 supplementation (117, 118). CoQ10 supplementation may interfere with warfarin and may also decrease the insulin requirements in diabetics (114).

S-adenosylmethionine

S-adenosylmethionine (SAM-e) is a physiologically essential compound that is distributed throughout all bodily tissues and fluids; it is most concentrated in the brain and liver. The human body creates SAM-e de novo from methionine and adenosine triphosphate, with the largest amounts being made in the liver. The synthesis of SAM-e is directly linked to folate and vitamin B12 metabolism. Deficiencies in these vitamins are associated with reduced concentrations of SAM-e in the CNS and with neuropsychiatric disorders (119). Lower than normal levels of SAM-e are found in cerebral spinal fluid in some patients with depression, Alzheimer's, dementia, Parkinson's disease treated with levodopa, disorders of folate metabolism, and other illnesses (120, 121).

SAM-e is promoted as a mood enhancer. It has been found to be a safe and effective treatment for depression in 16 open, uncontrolled trials (total 660 patients), 13 randomized, double-blind, placebo-controlled trials (total 535 patients), and 19 controlled, double-blind trials comparing it with other antidepressants (total 1134 patients) (122–126). SAM-e improves dopamine transmission and may have a beneficial effect on dopamine receptors.

SAM-e is also promoted for joint health because it contributes to the production of proteoglycans for cartilage repair. Natural production decreases with age, depression, or deficiencies of B vitamins or methionine (127). A meta-analysis of 11 studies showed it to be as effective as NSAIDs for arthritis pain but with fewer adverse effects (128). SAM-e should be taken with B vitamins (800 mg of folic acid and 1000 mg of B12).Currently, there are no controlled studies to determine the effects of long-term use.

The most serious adverse effect of SAM-e is the induction of mania in patients with bipolar disorder (129–131). There is no evidence that SAM-e interacts with other drugs, affects cytochrome P450 metabolism, or displaces other drugs from protein binding. The most common adverse effect reported is mild gastrointestinal distress.

The usual dosage of SAM-e for minor depression is 400 mg/day. Major depression often requires doses of 800 to 1600 mg/day. In the clinical trials of SAM-e for osteoarthritis, the usual oral dosage was 400 to 1600 mg/day. To maximize absorption, SAM-e is best taken on an empty stomach. Starting patients with 200 mg half an hour before breakfast and half an hour before lunch may help minimize the stimulation some patients report in the first few weeks of treatment. This may be switched to 400 mg before breakfast after a few weeks. The dose can be raised by 200 to 400 mg every 3 to 7 days (132).

Because of bioavailability problems, only enteric-coated formulations are recommended. Some authors recommend the butanedisulfonate form over the tosylate because they assert that it causes fewer side effects and clinically is more consistently effective (132).

SPECIFIC MEDICAL CONDITIONS AND COMMONLY USED COMPLEMENTARY AND ALTERNATIVE MEDICINE MODALITIES TO ADDRESS THEM

Weight Loss

Many weight loss supplements contain ephedra (an herb that contains ephedrine, pseudoephedrine, norephedrine, and other alkaloids), but other popular ingredients include synephrine (from bitter orange, *Citrus aurantium*), green tea (*Camellia sinensis*), chitosan, and St. John's wort (*Hypericum perforatum*). In one RCT with 48 patients completing the trial, the use of Metabolife 356 with 72 mg ephedrine and 240 mg caffeine was associated with significantly higher weight loss at the end of 8 weeks than placebo (4 kg versus 0.8 kg) (133). Despite these results, health care practitioners should discourage the use of ephedrine-containing products for weight loss, increased energy, or body building. Ephedra has been linked to many deaths, and its adverse effects include hypertension, palpitations, tachycardia, stroke, and seizures.

Interest is growing in the use of green tea and green tea extracts to promote weight loss. Because it contains polyphenols, green tea functions as an antioxidant. Traditional Chinese medicine uses green tea to help digestion, enhance mental function, and stabilize body temperature. Ayurvedic medicine uses green tea as a stimulant and diuretic. In vitro, components of green tea appear to prolong the effect of norepinephrine on thermogenesis and fat metabolism. Green tea extracts have also been shown to inhibit lipolysis—the process by which dietary fats are broken down for absorption in the small intestine. Inhibiting the breakdown of these triglycerides prevents absorption of the fat. The few studies that have been done suggest that green tea may be a safe and effective alternative to ephedra in stimulating thermogenesis for weight loss, but larger studies need to be done before this is confirmed (134, 135).

Chromium supplementation is common in many popular weight loss products. The most popular formulation is chromium picolinate, and it is available in pills, chewing gum, nutrition bars, and sports drinks. Chromium is an essential trace element and part of the insulin metabolic pathway. Deficiency of chromium leaves cells less sensitive to insulin. It is believed that chromium supplementation assists in "burning" excess fat, weight loss, and increased muscle mass through facilitating the entrance of glucose into the cells for energy production and by promoting protein synthesis. In a meta-analysis of controlled clinical trials of chromium picolinate for weight loss, the ten included trials found significantly greater weight loss in those taking chromium compared with placebo. The mean difference in weight loss between the treated and nontreated arms was only 1.1 kg over 10 to 13 weeks; a similarly small but significant difference was also found in reduction of body fat (136).

Chromium supplements are believed to be safe, with no clinical trials reporting adverse reactions. The FDA has, however, received reports of several hundred adverse events involving chromium supplements, and there have been a small number of cases of liver toxicity reported (137, 138). There are no reported adverse drug interactions, although it is known that ascorbic acid, aspirin, and indomethacin increase chromium absorption, whereas antacids lower its absorption. Complex carbohydrates also increase chromium absorption. Possible interactions may occur with drugs affecting glucose or cholesterol levels, or possibly with concurrent use of corticosteroids (139).

Caffeine is often an ingredient in weight loss agents, but its presence in the product may be hidden by listing herbs that contain caffeine instead. Herbs that contain significant amounts of caffeine include tea, kola nuts (*Cola nitida, Cola acuminate*), guarana (*Paullinia cupana*), and mate (*Ilex paraguariensis*). Despite its thermogenic effects, there is no conclusive evidence that caffeine is an effective weight loss agent.

Chitosan is another supplement growing in popularity for weight loss. The usual source of chitosan is from the shells of shrimp and crab; hence, it should not be used in patients with known shellfish allergies. It forms a positively charged gel in the stomach that can bind negatively charged fats; it can also decrease normal cholesterol emulsification. Its efficacy as a weight loss agent is believed to lie in an ability to inhibit intestinal absorption of fat from the gastrointestinal tract. In two small studies with human volunteers (total $n = 19$), one of which compared chitosan with orlistat and the other with placebo, no difference in fecal fat excretion was noted on those subjects taking the chitosan (140, 141).

In one double-blind RCT, 30 overweight volunteers completed the study in which chitosan (four capsules, each with diacetylated chitin biopolymer) was tested against placebo while maintaining a normal diet for 4 weeks. There was no difference between groups in terms of weight loss (142). In the same study, an analysis of five previous trials where chitosan use was accompanied by restricted caloric intake, there was a significant weight loss in the chitosan-treated group in comparison to placebo (142). The most common side effects seem to be mild, transient nausea and constipation, although there is one case report of possible arsenic toxicity secondary to chitosan ingestion (shellfish may contain arsenic) (143).

Adulteration is both a major concern and an ongoing problem with dietary supplements; this is also true for weight loss products. In an analysis by the Health Science Authority of Singapore, Slim 10, a Chinese herbal slimming product, was adulterated with fenfluramine and nicotinamide. A compilation of case reports has caused the FDA to warn health professionals to watch for interstitial fibrosis associated with end-stage renal disease or urologic tract tumors in patients using aristolochic acid-containing supplements (from *Aristolochia fangchi*).

Premenstrual Syndrome

Although most women experience some minor menstrual-associated physical and emotional changes (molimina) each month, the diagnosis of PMS requires that the symptoms cause considerable disruption at work, with family and friends, and in personal functioning. Surveys would suggest that 30 to 80% of women have premenstrual symptoms, but only 2 to 5% of reproductive age women suffer from severe PMS (144, 145). CAM therapies are popular with women who have PMS. In their review, Stevinson and Ernst found 27 RCTs of CAM in women with PMS published in peer-reviewed journals (146). Of these trials, 7 included the use of herbal medicine; 1 used homeopathy; and 13 relied on vitamin, mineral, and other dietary supplements; there was 1 trial each for relaxation, massage, reflexology, chiropractic, and 2 using biofeedback. This review concluded that even for modalities where more than 1 trial exists, many of the studies are methodologically quite flawed, and results are inconsistent (146).

In the Stevinson and Ernst review, none of the trials using herbal medicines had convincing evidence of their effectiveness. In one trial, chaste tree (*Vitex agnus castus*) was associated with significant improvement compared with placebo for only 1 symptom of 20 symptoms evaluated (147). The study authors did conclude that chaste tree was comparable to vitamin B6 in its efficacy, and although vitamin B6 has not been established as an efficacious treatment per se, there have been many trials evaluating its role in PMS therapy (147).

Women with PMS typically have worse dietary habits than the standard American woman. In a nutritional analysis in 1983, Abraham found that PMS patients consumed 62% more refined carbohydrates than women without PMS, 75% more refined sugar, 79% more dairy products, 78% more sodium, 53% less iron, 77% less manganese, and 52% less zinc (148). Although this reported association does not address whether poor diet is causal in PMS or an effect of PMS, encouragement of a healthier, more balanced diet is warranted for patients with PMS.

It has been postulated that PMS may reflect a deficiency of prostaglandin E_1 (PgE_1); the synthesis of PgE_1 requires magnesium, vitamin B6, and other vitamins. There have been at least two RCTs evaluating the efficacy of magnesium supplementation in PMS, and although the two independent studies reported significant effects of magnesium compared with placebo, the effects in each study were in different symptom areas (149, 150). Vitamin B6 interests PMS researchers as a possible agent for therapy because of its unique ability to increase the cerebral synthesis of several different neurotransmitters, including serotonin and dopamine. Some studies find a large effect, whereas others find none.

Linolenic acid is necessary for the synthesis of PgE_1. Hence, patients with PMS are advised to increase their consumption of vegetable oils, which are high in linolenic acid. Evening primrose oil is also a source of gamma linolenic acid and is commonly used by patients with PMS. Four small RCTs of evening primrose oil and placebo did show a significant difference in PMS symptoms, with doses of primrose oil ranging from 3 to 6 g daily (151–154). Other sources of gamma linolenic acid that may help to raise PgE_1 levels include borage oil, black currant oil, and rapeseed oil.

Another hypothesis related to the pathogenesis of PMS focuses on abnormalities in calcium regulation. In one RCT of 497 women, patients received either 1200 mg calcium carbonate or placebo for three menstrual cycles. In the luteal phase of the treated group, the symptom complex scores were significantly lower compared with the placebo group at the same cycle phase in cycles two and three. By the end of the third cycle, all four symptom factors (negative mood, water retention, food cravings, and pain) were significantly lower in the treated group in comparison to the placebo group (155).

Regular exercise has been shown to decrease the intensity and number of PMS symptoms in women. Aerobic training appears to be more effective at decreasing PMS symptomatology than strength training. The frequency of the exercise appears to be more important than the intensity (156).

Symptoms of Menopause

Phytoestrogens

One of the most popular nonprescription treatments for vasomotor symptoms is phytoestrogens. A phytoestrogen is any plant compound structurally or functionally similar to ovarian and placental estrogens and their active metabolites. Phytoestrogenic compounds may have agonistic, partial agonistic, and antagonistic interactions with estrogen receptors and other targets of estrogenic steroids involved in estrogen transport, synthesis, and metabolism. Phytoestrogens are weaker than natural estrogens, are easily broken down, and are not stored in tissue. The effects of phytoestrogens will vary with the concentration of endogenous estrogen, with the patient's gender and menopausal status, and with variability in colonic microflora.

A number of subclasses of phytoestrogens have been identified, such as lignans, isoflavones, coumestans, and resorcylic acid lactones. Isoflavones have the most potent estrogenic activity. Lignan precursors are in whole grains, seeds, fruits, and vegetables, especially flaxseed, rye, and legumes. Lignan precursors are metabolized by enteric bacteria to enterolactone and enterodiol. Isoflavone precursors are found in soybeans, clover, and alfalfa. Soy isoflavones bind with weak affinity to estrogen-receptor alpha and high affinity to estrogen-receptor beta. As a result, isoflavones in women preferentially express estrogenic activities in CNS, blood vessels, bone, and skin without causing stimulation of breast or uterus (157). Phytoestrogens are weak estrogens; the soy isoflavones, genistein and daidzein, are less than 1% as potent as estradiol in binding assays. Biological activity, however, does not correlate directly with binding assay affinity. Phytoestrogens will not be picked up by conventional testing for estrogen level measurements, although there are special assays available to measure phytoestrogen levels.

In Asia, only 10 to 20% of women experience hot flashes, whereas 70 to 80% of women in Western countries report hot flashes with menopause (158, 159). This difference is believed to be attributable to the high dietary content of soy isoflavones in the traditional Asian diet, which are believed to influence the bodily response to the changing hormone patterns of menopause (160). Consumption of legumes in Asia provides 25 to 45 mg/d total isoflavones, and in Japan, where soy consumption is very high, up to 200 mg/d of isoflavones may be consumed. In contrast, in Western countries, average isoflavone consumption is less than 5 mg/day (161, 162). There have been numerous studies of soy isoflavones, and their effects on menopausal symptoms and results have been mixed (163–166). Several found a positive effect, others a negative impact, and still other results were mixed. The longest study (24 weeks) showed no benefit for hot flashes or other symptoms at the end of the trial (163). Although none of the trials specifically asked about dyspareunia, the trial by St. Germain et al. (163) asked about vaginal dryness and found no effect of soy protein (80.4 mg isoflavones/day) on this condition. Only the study by Dalais et al. found any positive effect of soy or isoflavone supplementation on vaginal maturation index (166–168).

More recently, Secreto et al. (169) conducted a multicenter, randomized, double-blind study to determine the effectiveness of soy isoflavones and melatonin in relieving menopausal symptoms. A total of 262 women were assigned to one of four treatment groups: soy isoflavones and melatonin, soy isoflavones alone, melatonin alone, or placebo. Doses were 80 mg soy isoflavones and 3 mg pure melatonin daily for 12 weeks. The Greene Climacteric Scale was used to assess severity of menopausal symptoms. Results demonstrated similar outcomes in the four groups for somatic and vasomotor symptoms, although the combination group had slightly better improvements in psychological symptoms.

Comparisons between trials are difficult because they may use different products, types of soy proteins, and doses of isoflavones and protein. Different menopausal symptom indices may be used, and the ages of participants and menopausal status may vary significantly. Overall, however, in most of the studies, only modest effects were seen on hot flash severity, and these disappeared after 6 weeks. Studies are needed to determine whether there are important differences among whole foods, soy protein, and isoflavone extracts on menopausal symptoms and whether there is a dose-response relationship.

There are no data on the developmental effects of soy proteins in humans. The interactions between age of the individual, receptor conditioning, or effect on breast cancer prevention and soy proteins remain unknown. Some studies demonstrate that the protection offered by soy protein against breast cancer occurs only if the soy is consumed early in life or in adolescence (170, 171). Although hot flashes are the most common symptom reported in menopause, one report found that 62% of women also reported subjective changes in memory that were worse in perimenopausal women than menopausal women (172). Although the use of soy foods and products has been recommended for their effects on vasomotor symptoms, data to support the use of soy for cognitive symptom relief is not robust (173). Two more recent studies were methodologically sound and suggest the use of soy may benefit some women with significant cognitive complaints associated with menopause. In one RCT, Duffy et al. (174) tested a soy isoflavone supplement (60 mg/day) in 33 postmenopausal women. In this trial, patients were assessed not only for their cognitive function, but also for things that could confound cognitive performance such as mood, anxiety, or sleepiness. Both groups refrained from eating soy-containing foods during the trial to avoid confounding through dietary sources of soy. At the end of the study, there were significant improvements in the treated individuals. Women receiving the supplement did better in tasks requiring sustained attention, recall of pictures, and planning a task. New learning was less affected, although the manipulation of new learning was better in the treated groups. These improvements were independent of any changes in menopausal symptoms, mood, or sleepiness.

In another randomized, double-blind, placebo-controlled trial, Kritz-Silverstien et al. tested a similar population but used a higher dose of isoflavones (110 mg/day) for a 6-month period (175). Mood was assessed in trial participants, but menopausal symptoms and sleepiness were not. Compliance was good, and most women did not consume significant amounts of soy foods during the trial. Although different memory tests were used than those in the trial by Duffy et al., similar types of functions were tested. Treated patients in this trial demonstrated improved performance both in comparison to their own baselines and in comparison to the women in the placebo arm. When the results were analyzed by age categories, the older patients demonstrated a larger benefit in comparison to the younger women.

Most of the women in these two studies were fairly well educated or were of a high socioeconomic status. It is also important to note that soy products will probably not correct cognitive difficulties due to depression, dementia, or other medical conditions. Patients should be told that improvement of menopausal symptoms secondary to soy usage will probably be mild, and in the area of cognitive functions, may be fairly subtle.

Ipriflavone is a synthetic flavanoid derivative of the naturally occurring class of isoflavones and is metabolized into seven metabolites, one of which is daidzein. In humans, there is no accumulation of ipriflavone, or any of its metabolites, in any body compartments. Despite the fact that ipriflavone's structure is similar to phytoestrogens such as genistein and daidzein, ipriflavone alone has not been shown to exhibit estrogenic activity on the classic estrogen target organs. Ipriflavone has been found to improve bone density in cases of osteoporosis, and it is approved for the prevention and treatment of osteoporosis in some European and Asian countries; it is available in the United States as a supplement (176–178). The typical supplemental amount of ipriflavone is 200 mg three times a day. Taking 300 mg twice a day has been reported to be just as effective as 200 mg three times a day (179).

Many carefully controlled studies demonstrate that oral doses of 200 mg ipriflavone three times a day (often combined with 1 g oral calcium daily) can have significant effects by increasing bone mineral density, reducing bone pain, and diminishing the incidence of bone fractures—usually in postmenopausal women (180–182). Long-term trials of ipriflavone have demonstrated relative safety with prolonged use, although in one trial of ipriflavone for osteoporosis, 29 of the 132 women in the ipriflavone group completing the 3-year trial developed a clinically significant drop in lymphocytes (183). The most commonly reported side effects were mild gastrointestinal upset. Researchers recommend that patients with severe kidney disease take a lower amount of ipriflavone (200 to 400 mg daily) (184). The potential for drug–drug interactions does exist; for example, ipriflavone may increase levels of theophylline, nifedipine, and tolbutamide (a first-generation sulfonylurea).

A meta-analysis of 38 trials examining the relationship between soy products and lipid levels showed that consumption of soy protein (average intake of 47 g/day) significantly decreased serum concentrations of total cholesterol, low-density lipoprotein (LDL) cholesterol, and triglycerides (184). In the dose-response effect study by Crouse et al., a 62-mg daily intake of isoflavone aglycone reduced LDL cholesterol in 156 men and women by an average of 6% (185). The 37-mg daily aglycone dose also lowered LDL cholesterol, but by less than the higher dose. Only postmenopausal women and men demonstrated this effect. High-density lipoprotein cholesterol and triglyceride did not change significantly. Thus far, studies indicate that the lipid-lowering effect of isoflavones seems to be less than with estrogens (in humans) and is not consistent. The effects of soy intake on blood pressure have been inconsistent, although one study with sufficient power to detect a small effect did find a significant reduction in systolic, diastolic, and mean (–5.5 mm Hg) pressures with 118 mg soy isoflavone glycoside (186).

Although numerous in vitro and animal studies suggest a protective role for dietary isoflavones in the prevention of breast cancer, epidemiologic data is inconclusive (187–190). Emerging data from animal and human studies suggest it is short-term exposure to dietary isoflavones neonatally or prepubertally that decreases carcinogen-induced breast cancer by increasing the proportion of differentiated cells in the mammary gland (191, 192). This may explain why epidemiologic studies, which focus on adult intake of isoflavones, are inconclusive.

It cannot be said definitively that soy consumption exerts only protective effects on breast tissue. In one trial, the rate of DNA synthesis by breast cells taken from biopsies of normal breast tissue in premenopausal women with benign or malignant disease was increased by 14 days of soy supplementation given preoperatively (60 g/day equivalent to 45 mg isoflavones) (193). Another study has suggested that under certain circumstances, soy proteins may stimulate breast cancer growth (194).

Red Clover Isoflavones

Red clover supplements contain isoflavones (biochanin A, formononetin) not found in soy that may have additional biological activity. Soy, however, has components that red clover lacks, and it may be these components that contribute to soy's biological effectiveness. Tice et al. initiated the Isoflavone Clover Extract study to determine if two dietary supplements from red clover were more effective than placebo in diminishing hot flashes and improving quality of life for menopausal women (195). In this randomized, double-blind, placebo-controlled trial, 252 postmenopausal women were assigned to Promensil (82 mg isoflavones/day; Novogen Ltd., Sydney, Australia), Rimostil (57 mg isoflavones/day; Novogen Ltd., Sydney, Australia), or placebo and hot flush frequency and quality of life was assessed. At the end of the 12-week trial, the reductions in mean daily hot flash count were similar for all three groups, as were quality of life improvements and adverse events.

Black Cohosh

The German Botanical Regulatory Body has approved black cohosh for treating symptoms of the climacteric, and treatment is reimbursed. Use is recommended for no more than 6 months at doses of 20 to 40 mg/day; there are currently no clinical trials longer than 6 months, and most are only 2 to 3 months long. A 3-month trial is too brief to demonstrate true efficacy because hot flashes are placebo responsive, and this effect usually wanes after 3 months of therapy. Six months is adequate to evaluate efficacy but not long-term safety issues.

The primary active constituent of the black cohosh root is believed to be the terpene glycoside fraction, including acetin and cimifugoside. More recent studies show that although some constituents of the extract bind to at least one subtype of estrogen receptors, this binding produces very little, if any, estrogenic effect, and may selectively block some of these effects (196, 197). Hence, it remains unclear whether black cohosh exerts its effect via estrogen receptors or through other mechanisms. The major issue with black cohosh is the numerous preparations on the market; each one is extracted and isolated by a slightly different method. Studies of black cohosh are numerous but have poor study designs.

The best studied commercially available product containing black cohosh is Remifemin, which is manufactured in Germany by Schaper and Brummer GMBH & Co., and distributed by GlaxoSmithKline in the United States. Although the formulation of Remifemin has changed over the years, currently each tablet contains 20 mg black cohosh extract with 1 mg triterpenes, one of the major components believed to contribute to its observed clinical effects. Recommended dosages of Remifemin are one tablet in the morning and one in the evening for a total daily dose of 40 mg. Up to 12 weeks of continuous use may be needed to achieve a full therapeutic response. Remifemin Plus contains an additional product, St. John's wort.

One more recent double-blind clinical trial suggests that Remifemin does not exhibit estrogenic effects. Approximately 150 peri- and postmenopausal women were put on either a standard 39-mg dose of black cohosh extract or a dose more than three times higher (127.3 mg) for 24 weeks. Results showed no changes in vaginal cytology measures or any significant changes in serum estradiol, LH, FSH, prolactin, or sex hormone binding globulin (198). Several in vitro studies have demonstrated that black cohosh does not stimulate the growth of breast cancer cells, and no estrogen receptor binding mechanism has been demonstrated (199, 200). One RCT of

85 breast cancer survivors (59 on tamoxifen) found no benefit with Remifemin (40 mg twice a day for 2 months) for hot flashes (201).

Black cohosh has no demonstrated contraindications, mutagenicity, teratogenicity, toxicity, or known drug interactions. The two most significant adverse side effects include gastrointestinal upset and headache (which resolve with discontinuation). It is important to recognize that black cohosh is completely different from blue cohosh (*Caulophyllum thalictroides*), which has been used in the past for labor induction and augmentation, and which has considerable adverse and toxic potentialities, including coronary artery constriction, teratogenicity, and abortifacient properties.

Ginseng

Ginseng is often used as a stimulant and to impart a sense of well-being, particularly in the elderly. One RCT tested Ginsan (with 100 mg *Panax ginseng* standardized extract G115 for 14 weeks) in 384 menopausal women for symptoms of menopause and quality of life measures. No effect was seen on flushes, endometrial thickness, vaginal maturation index, or FSH (202).

Evening Primrose

Evening primrose, reviewed previously, contains the PgE_1 precursor, gamma-linolenic acid. The recommended dose is 4 to 8 g daily (203). It has been evaluated for hot flashes in one RCT of 56 menopausal women (2000 mg with 20 IU vitamin E twice a day) for 6 months, and no benefit was seen (204). Evening primrose is considered to be a benign treatment, although it is contraindicated in women taking seizure medications or antipsychotics because it lowers the seizure threshold in patients on phenothiazines.

Acupuncture

In one study evaluating the effect of acupuncture on hot flashes, 24 menopausal women were randomized to either an electroacupuncture group (electrical stimulation of acupuncture needles at standardized points) or a control group (shallow acupuncture needle insertion at the same points) (205). The women received therapy twice weekly for 2 weeks, then once weekly for 6 weeks thereafter. Hot flashes and Kupperman index scores decreased significantly for both groups, but there was no significant difference between the two groups.

Wild Yam and Progesterone Creams

Topical wild yam (*Dioscorea villosa*) and "natural" (micronized) progesterone creams have been promoted for hot flashes. Wild yam preparations contain diosgenin, a progesterone precursor. Although diosgenin can be converted to progesterone in a laboratory, human skin is incapable of duplicating this chemical process. In one double-blind, RCT 23 symptomatic menopausal women were randomized to receive either wild yam cream or placebo. At the end of 3 months, there was no significant difference between the two groups in hot flashes or night sweats (206).

Progesterone in cream form can be absorbed through the skin. Although some studies demonstrate symptom relief, serum levels of progesterone remain low and none of the studies demonstrated any improvements of other parameters, such as bone mineral density, endometrial protections, or cardiovascular lipid and lipoprotein markers (207–209). Wren et al. (208) conducted a double-blind RCT comparing the effect of a transdermal cream containing progesterone (32 mg daily) with a placebo cream in 80 postmenopausal women. The subjects were evaluated using the Greene Climacteric Scale and the Menopause Quality of Life Questionnaire, as well as blood analysis for lipids and bone markers over a period of 12 weeks. Despite a slight elevation of blood progesterone levels, the authors demonstrated no detectable change in vasomotor symptoms, mood characteristics, or sexual feelings, nor was there any change in blood lipid levels or in bone metabolic markers.

Some menopausal women believe they may use progestin creams as the progestin component of their hormone therapy. This is not true; three studies have shown that serum levels of progesterone after application of transdermal creams are insufficient to prevent estrogenic stimulation of the endometrium (207, 210, 211).

Clinical Notes

- Western or contemporary biomedicine is based on four principal tenets:
  - *Objectivism*: The observer is separated from the observed.
  - *Reductionism*: Complex phenomena are explainable by reducing or deconstructing them to their smaller component parts.
  - *Positivism*: All information can be derived from physically measurable data.
  - *Determinism*: Knowledge of scientific law and conditions allows us to make accurate predictions regarding the ensuing phenomena.
- Most forms of CAM embrace two primary principles: the body and emotions are maintained by a life force, and the body is essentially self-healing.
- Thirty-six percent of U.S. adults older than 18 years of age used some form of CAM in 2002.
- CAM use is greater among women, individuals with higher education, people who have been hospitalized within the last year, and former smokers.
- NCCAM is "dedicated to exploring complementary and alternative healing practices in the context of rigorous science, training complementary and alternative medicine (CAM) researchers, and disseminating authoritative information to the public and professionals."
- As a medical practice, Ayurveda is more than 5000 years old; it is considered by many scholars to be the oldest healing science.
- The Ayurvedic tradition believes there are basic biological energies each person manifests, known as doshas. There are three basic forms of doshas: vata, pitta, and kapha. Health is achieved by maintaining equilibrium among the three doshas.
- Fundamental concepts of Chinese medicine include yin and yang, the five phases, qi, and the essential substances of the body, essence and spirit, and zang and fu, or viscera and bowels.
- In Chinese medicine, qi pervades all things and acts as both a material substance and a force. Qi is mobile, and obstruction of blockage of qi's movement through channels in the body contributes to the formation of illness.
- In homeopathy, illness is perceived to be the organism's attempt to heal itself. Homeopathic remedies are therefore chosen to fit the illness as closely as possible and are used in the smallest possible dose.
- Naturopathy is a medical system based on the principle *Vis Medcatrix Naturae*, or the healing power of nature. This system is not associated with any particular therapy per se, but with a philosophy of life, health, and disease.
- According to the practice of chiropractic, its chief beneficial effects are relief of musculoskeletal pain and disability, as well as restoration of proper internal organ function.
- In osteopathy, the structural integrity of the body mechanism is considered to be the key determinant in maintaining health and well-being. The other two fundamental concepts of osteopathic medicine are that the parts of the body comprise a unified whole, and the body has an innate ability to self-regulate and to self-heal.
- In the practice of acupuncture, moxibustion refers to the burning of powdered leaves of mugwort (*Artemis vulgairs*) to deliver warmth or focused warming either to the surface of the skin or the head of an inserted acupuncture needle.
- Depth of insertion, as well as the orientation and manipulation of the needle, are not arbitrary in acupuncture. Orienting the needle along the direction of channel flow is called tonifying; orienting it in the opposite direction of flow is referred to as dispersing.
- Various mind–body therapies can improve mood, quality of life, and coping, as well as ameliorate disease and treatment-related symptoms, such as chemotherapy-induced nausea and vomiting, physical pain, and functioning.
- Herbalism is the study and practice of using plant material for food, medicine, and health promotion. Herbalism not only treats disease, but it is also used to enhance the quality of life, both physically and spiritually.

- The DSHEA of 1994 considers a substance to be a dietary supplement if it (a) is a product (other than tobacco) that is intended to supplement the diet that bears or contains one or more of the following ingredients: a vitamin, a mineral, an herb or other botanical, an amino acid; (b) is intended for ingestion in pill, capsule, tablet, or liquid form; (c) is not used as a conventional food or as the sole item of a meal or diet; and (d) is labeled as a dietary supplement.
- If an adverse herb–drug interaction is suspected, it should be reported to the FDA's MedWatch program in the same manner that drug–drug interactions are reported.

APPENDIX 20.1

WEBSITES

Alternative Medicine Foundation
http://amfoundation.org/info.htm
Variety of resource guides on different CAM modalities and specific health-related areas.

HealthWorld Online
Healthy Women Center
http://www.healthy.net/asp/templates/center.asp?centerid=6
Information on alternative medicine, wellness, and self-care.

InteliHealth
http://www.intelihealth.com/IH/ihtIH/WSIHW000/8513/8513.html?k=navx408x8513
From the Harvard Medical Schools and Aetna; provides a perspective on CAM from a conventional health viewpoint.

National Center for Complementary and Alternative Medicine
http://nccam.nih.gov/
NIH center specifically mandated by Congress to research CAM.

Office of Cancer Complementary and Alternative Medicine
http://www.cancer.gov/cam/
Office established to coordinate and enhance the activities of the National Cancer Institute in the arena of CAM.

Office of Dietary Supplements
http://ods.od.nih.gov/index.aspx
Provides information about the Office of Dietary Supplements, including its programs, activities, and scientific resources.

Rosenthal Center for Complementary and Alternative Medicine
Information Resources (CAM)
http://www.rosenthal.hs.columbia.edu/CAM.html
For CAM Internet resources, directory of databases, medical courses and training, legal and regulatory information, calendars, and events.

White House Commission on Complementary and Alternative Medicine Policy
http://www.whccamp.hhs.gov/finalreport.html
The commission was initiated in 2000; the Final Report is available on the site.

National Women's Health Resource Center
healthywoman.org
http://www.healthywomen.org/
A site for health professionals and consumers from the National Women's Health Resource Center. All content is reviewed by a medical advisory board.

The University of Texas MD Anderson Cancer Center
Complementary/Integrative Medicine
http://www.mdanderson.org/departments/cimer/
Short summaries of research information about CAM therapies associated with cancer treatment and side effects.

National Foundation for Alternative Medicine
http://www.nfam.org
General resources on CAM with specific information on alternative and complementary cancer therapies.

Online Databases

HerbMed
http://www.herbalgram.org/rosenthal/herbmedpro/index.asp
An evidence-based, interactive, electronic herbal database that provides hyperlinked access to the scientific data underlying the use of herbs for health.

CAM on PubMed
http://www.nlm.nih.gov/nccam/camonpubmed.html
NCCAM and the National Library of Medicine (NLM) have partnered to create CAM on PubMed, a subset of NLM's PubMed.

Peer-Reviewed Journals

- *Evidence-based Complementary and Alternative Medicine*; online journal at http://ecam.oupjournals.org
- *Journal of Alternative and Complementary Medicine*
- *Acupuncture in Medicine*
- *Alternative Medicine Alert*
- *Alternative Medicine Review*
- *Alternative Therapies in Health and Medicine*

- *American Journal of Chinese Medicine*
- *American Journal of Homeopathic Medicine*
- *BMC Complementary and Alternative Medicine*
- *Focus on Alternative and Complementary Therapies*
- *Homeopathy*
- *Journal of Manipulative and Physiological Therapies*
- *International Journal of Phytotherapy and Phytopharmacology*
- *Seminars in Integrative Medicine*

Reference Books

- *Physician's Desk Reference (PDR) for Herbal Medicine*, published by Medical Economics
- *Physician's Desk Reference (PDR) for Nonprescription Drugs and Dietary Supplements*, published by Medical Economics
- *Herb Contraindications and Drug Interactions*, 2nd ed., by Francis Brinker, Nancy Stodart, N.D. Francis, and J. Brinker, 1998, published by Eclectic Medical Publications
- *Women's Health in Complementary and Integrative Medicine: A Clinical Guide*, by Tieraona Low Dog, Marc S. Micozzi, 2004, published by Churchill Livingstone
- *Integrating Complementary Medicine into Health Systems,* by Nancy Faass, 2001, published by Jones & Bartlett Publishers

REFERENCES

1. Lopez-Jimenez F. Practicing a more scientific clinical medicine. Rev Invest Clin 2000;52(3):587–588.
2. Eisenberg D, Kessler RC, Foster C. Unconventional medicine in the United States. N Engl J Med 1993;328:246–252.
3. Kaptchuk TJ, Eisenberg DM. Varieties of healing. 1: medical pluralism in the United States. Ann Intern Med 2001;135:189–195.
4. National Center for Health Statistics, Centers for Disease Control and Prevention. The Third National Health and Nutrition Examination Survey (NHANES III), 1988–94, Series 11, No. 13A. Available at: http://www.cdc.gov/nchs/data/nhanes/nhanes3/dp-acc.pdf#search='NHANES%20III,%201988â€"1994.'. Accessed July 29, 2005.
5. Available at: www.nccam.nigh.gov/news/camsurvey.htm. Accessed month date, year.
6. Vickers A. Complementary medicine. BMJ 2000;321:683–686.
7. Cochrane Registry of Randomized Controlled Trials. Cochrane Complementary Medicine Field. Available at: http://www.compmed.ummc.umaryland.edu/Compmed/Cochrane/Cochrane.htm. Accessed month date, year.
8. Heron J. Critique of conventional research methodology. Comp Med Res 1986;1:12–22.
9. Williamson JW, Goldschmidt PG, Colton T. The quality of medical literature: an analysis of validation assessments. In: Bautar JC, Mostellar R, eds. Medical Use of Statistics. Waltham, MA: NEJM Books, 1986:370–391.
10. Sacks HS, Berrier J, Reitman D, et al. Meta-analyses of randomised controlled trials. N Engl J Med 1987;316:450–455.
11. Smith R. Where is the wisdom . . .? BMJ 1991;303:798–799.
12. Vincent CA, Furnham AF. Complementary Medicine. A Research Perspective. Chichester: Wiley, 1997.
13. Kramer MS, Shapiro SH. Scientific challenges in the application of randomised trials. JAMA 1984;252:2739–2745.
14. Pollock AV. The rise and fall of the random controlled trial in surgery. Theor Surg 1989;4:163–170.
15. Grisso JA. Making comparisons. Lancet 1993;342:157–160.
16. Bloom BS, Retbi A, Dahan S, et al. Evaluation of randomized controlled trials on complementary and alternative medicine. Int J Technol Assess Health Care 2000;16:13–21.
17. National Center for Complementary and Alternative Medicine. Available at: http://nccam.nih.gov/about/aboutnccam/index.htm. Accessed July 29, 2005.
18. Wetzel MS, Eisenberg DM, Kaptchuk TJ. Courses involving complementary and alternative medicine in U.S. medical schools. JAMA 1998;280:784–787.
19. Kligler B, Gordon A, Stuart M, et al. Suggested curriculum guidelines on complementary and alternative medicine: recommendations of the Society of Teachers of Family Medicine Group on Alternative Medicine. Fam Med 1999;31:30–33.
20. Delinick AN. A hypothesis on how homeopathic remedies work on the organism. Berl J Res Homeopath 1991;1:249–253.
21. Taylor MA, Reilly D, Llewellyn-Jones RH, et al. Randomised controlled trial of homoeopathy versus placebo in perennial allergic rhinitis with overview of four trial series. BMJ 2000;321:471–776.
22. Barnes J, Resch KL, Ernst E. Homeopathy for postoperative ileus: a meta-analysis. J Clin Gastroenterol 1997;25:628–633.
23. Ferley JP, Zmirou D, D'Adhemar D, et al. A controlled evaluation of a homeopathic preparation in the treatment of influenza-like syndromes. Br J Clin Pharmacol 1989;27:329–335.
24. Papp R, Schuback G, Beck E, et al. Oscillococcinum in patients with influenza-like syndromes: a placebo-controlled double blind evaluation. Br Homeopath J 1998;87:69–76.
25. North American Board of Naturopathic Examiners. Available at: http://www.nabne.org. Accessed July 29, 2005.
26. Leach RA. Manipulative therapy: a historical perspective from ancient times to the modern era. In: Goldstein M, ed. The Research Status of Spinal Manipulative Therapy. Washington, DC: Government Printing Office, 1994:11–17.
27. White AR, Ernst E. Introduction. In: White AR, Ernst E, eds. Acupuncture: a scientific appraisal. Oxford: Butterworth-Heinemann, 1999:1–9.
28. Ernst E, White AR. Prospective studies of the safety of acupuncture: a systematic review. Am J Med 2001;110:481–485.
29. White AR, Hayhoe S, Hart A, et al. Adverse events following acupuncture: prospective survey of 32,000 consultations with doctors and physiotherapists. BMJ 2001;323:485–486.
30. MacPherson H, Thomas K, Walters S, et al. The York acupuncture safety study. prospective survey of 34,000 treatments by traditional acupuncturists. BMJ 2001;323:486–487.
31. Ernst E, White A. Life-threatening adverse reactions after acupuncture? A systematic review. Pain 1997;71:123–126.
32. Zahger D, Moses A, Slater PE, et al. An outbreak of hepatitis B associated with acupuncture. Harefuah 1998;116:300–302.
33. Walsh B, Maguire H, Carrington D. Outbreak of hepatitis B in an acupuncture clinic. Commun Dis Public Health 1999;2:137–140.
34. Ernst E, Sherman KJ. Is acupuncture a risk factor for hepatitis? Systematic review of epidemiological studies. J Gastroenterol Hepatol 2003;18:1231–1236.

35. Aso T, Motohashi T, Murata T, Nishimura T, Kakizaki K. The influence of acupuncture stimulation on plasma levels of LH, FSH, progesterone and estradiol in normally ovulating women. Am J Chin Med 1976;4: 391–401.
36. Stener-Victorin E, Waldenstrom U, Tagnfors U, et al. effects of electro-acupuncture on anovulation in women with polycystic ovary syndrome. Acta Obstet Gynecol Scand 2000;79:180–188.
37. Zhang Y, Wang X. 50 cases of dysfunctional uterine bleeding treated puncturing the effective points—a new system of acupuncture. J Tradit Chin Med 1994;14:101–102.
38. Liu W, Zhang J, Zhang YM. Acupuncture treatment of functional uterine bleeding: a clinical observation of 30 cases. J Tradit Chin Med 1988;8:31–33.
39. Helms JM. Acupuncture for the management of primary dysmenorrhea. Obstet Gynecol 1987;69:51–56.
40. Stener-Victorin E, Wikland M, Waldenstrom U, Lundeberg T. et al. Alternative treatments in reproductive medicine: much ado about nothing. Acupuncture—a method of treatment in reproductive medicine: lack of evidence of an effect does not equal evidence of the lack of an effect. Hum Reprod 2002;17:1942–1946.
41. Classen C, Butler LD, Koopman C, et al. Supportive-expressive group therapy and distress in patients with metastatic breast cancer: a randomized clinical intervention trial. Arch Gen Psychiatry 2001;58:494–501.
42. Vasterling J, Jenkins RA, Tope DM, et al. Cognitive distraction and relaxation training for the control of side effects due to cancer chemotherapy. J Behav Med 1993;16:65–80.
43. Syrjala KL, Donaldson GW, Davis MW, et al. Relaxation and imagery and cognitive-behavioral training reduce pain during cancer treatment: a controlled clinical trial. Pain 1995;63:189–198.
44. Fawzy FI, Fawzy NW, Hyun CS, et al. Malignant melanoma. Effects of an early structured psychiatric intervention, coping, and affective state on recurrence and survival 6 years later. Arch Gen Psychiatry 1993;50:681–689.
45. Goodwin PJ, Leszcz M, Ennis M, et al. The effect of group psychosocial support on survival in metastatic breast cancer. N Engl J Med 2001;345:1719–1726.
46. Burgio KL, Locher JL, Goode PS, et al. Behavioral vs drug treatment for urge urinary incontinence in older women: a randomized controlled trial. JAMA 1998;280:1995–2000.
47. Morin CM, Hauri PJ, Espie CA, et al. Nonpharmacologic treatment of chronic insomnia. An American Academy of Sleep Medicine review. Sleep 1999;22:1134–1156.
48. Morin CM, Mimeault V, Gagne A. Nonpharmacological treatment of late-life insomnia. J Psychosom Res 1999;46:103–116.
49. Morin CM, Culbert JP, Schwartz SM. Nonpharmacological interventions for insomnia: a meta-analysis of treatment efficacy. Am J Psychiatry 1994;151:1172–1180.
50. MacHovec F. Hypnosis complications, risk factors, and prevention. Am J Clin Hypn 1988;31:40–49.
51. Astin JA, Harkness E, Ernst E. The efficacy of "distant healing": a systematic review of randomized trials. Ann Intern Med 2000;132:903–910.
52. Winslow LC, Kroll DJ. Herbs as medicines. Arch Intern Med 1998;158:2192–2199.
53. Miller LG. Herbal medicinals: selected clinical considerations focusing on known or potential drug–herb interactions. Arch Intern Med 1998;158:2200–2211.
54. Thompson CA. Herbal quality seems to be growing. Am J Health Syst Pharm 1998;55:2341–2342.
55. Wagner H. Phytomedicine research in Germany. Environ Health Perspect 1999;107:779–781.
56. Abbot NC, White AR, Ernst E. Complementary medicine. Nature 1996;381:361.
57. Ko RJ. Adulterants in Asian patent medicines. N Engl J Med 1998;339:847.
58. Vander Stricht BI, Parvais OE, Vanhaelen-Fastre RJ, et al. Safer use of traditional remedies: remedies may contain cocktail of active drugs. BMJ 1994;308:1162.
59. Espinoza EO, Bleasdell B. Arsenic and mercury in traditional Chinese herbal balls. N Engl J Med 1995;333:803–804.
60. NBJ herbal and botanical U.S. consumer sales. Nutr Business J 2000. Available at: http://www.nutritionbusiness.com. Accessed July 29, 2005.
61. Commission on Dietary Supplement Labels. Report of the Commission on Dietary Supplement Labels, Report to the President, Congress, and The Secretary of the Department of Health and Human Services. Washington, DC: U.S. Government Printing Office, 1997.
62. Eisenberg DM, Davis RB, Ettner SL, et al. Trends in alternative medicine use in the United States, 1990–1997: results of a follow-up study. JAMA 1998;280:1569–1575.
63. Eisenberg DM, Kessler RC, Foster C, et al. Unconventional medicine in the United States: prevalence, costs, and patterns of use. N Engl J Med 1993;328:246–252.
64. Tsen LC, Segal S, Pothier M, et al. Alternative medicine use in presurgical patients. Anesthesiology 2000;93:148–151.
65. Kaye AD, Clarke RC, Sabar R, et al. Herbal medications: current trends in anesthesiology practice—a hospital survey. J Clin Anesth 2000;12:468–471.
66. Fugh-Berman A, Ernst E. Herb–drug interactions: review and assessment of report reliability. Br J Clin Pharmacol 2001;52:587–595.
67. Melchart D, Linde K, Fischer P, et al. Echinacea for preventing and treating the common cold. Cochrane Database Syst Rev 2000;(2):CD000530.
68. Pepping J. Echinacea. Am J Health Syst Pharm 1999;56:121–122.
69. Rehman J, Dillow JM, Carter SM, et al. Increased production of antigen-specific immunoglobulins G and M following in vivo treatment with the medicinal plants *Echinacea angustifolia* and *Hydrastis canadensis*. Immunol Lett 1999;68:391–395.
70. Boullata JI, Nace AM. Safety issues with herbal medicine. Pharmacotherapy 2000;20:257–269.

71. Gurley BJ, Gardner SF, Hubbard MA. Content versus label claims in ephedra-containing dietary supplements. Am J Health Syst Pharm 2000;57:963–969.
72. Haller CA, Benowitz NL. Adverse cardiovascular and central nervous system events associated with dietary supplements containing ephedra alkaloids. N Engl J Med 2000;343:1833–1838.
73. Zaacks SM, Klein L, Tan CD, et al. Hypersensitivity myocarditis associated with ephedra use. J Toxicol Clin Toxicol 1999;37:485–489.
74. Stevinson C, Pittler MH, Ernst E. Garlic for treating hypercholesterolemia: a meta-analysis of randomized clinical trials. Ann Intern Med 2000;133:420–429.
75. Ang-Lee MK, Moss J, Yuan CS. Herbal medicines and perioperative care. JAMA 2001;286:208–216.
76. Solomon PR, Adams F, Silver A, et al. Ginkgo for memory enhancement. JAMA 2002;288:836–840.
77. Mix JA, Crews DW Jr. An examination of the efficacy of ginkgo extract EGb761 on the neuropsychological functioning of cognitively intact older adults. J Altern Complement Med 2000;6:219–229.
78. Miller LG. Herbal medicinals: selected clinical considerations focusing on known or potential drug–herb interactions. Arch Intern Med 1998;158:2200–2211.
79. Chung KF, Dent G, McCusker M, et al. Effect of a ginkgolide mixture (BN 52063) in antagonizing skin and platelet responses to platelet activating factor in man. Lancet 1987;1:248–251.
80. Pittler MH, Ernst E. Efficacy of kava extract for treating anxiety: systematic review and meta-analysis. J Clin Psychopharmacol 2000;20:84–89.
81. Meyer HJ. Pharmacology of kava. 1. Psychopharmacol Bull 1967;4:10–11.
82. Backhauss C, Krieglstein J. Extract of kava (*Piper methysticum*) and its methysticine constituents protect brain tissue against ischemic damage in rodents. Eur J Pharmacol 1992;215:265–269.
83. Hepatic toxicity possibly associated with kava containing products—United States, Germany and Switzerland, 1999–2002. MMWR Morb Mortal Wkly Rep 2002;51:1065–1067.
84. Norton SA, Ruze P. Kava dermopathy. J Am Acad Dermatol 1994;31:89–97.
85. Shelton RC, Keller MB, Gelenberg A. Effectiveness of St. John's wort in major depression: a randomized controlled trial. JAMA 2001;285:1978–1986.
86. Gaster B, Holroyd J. St. John's wort for depression: a systematic review. Arch Intern Med 2000;160:152–156.
87. Neary JT, Bu Y. Hypericum LI 160 inhibits uptake of serotonin and norepinephrine in astrocytes. Brain Res 1999;816:358–363.
88. Franklin M, Chi J, McGavin C, et al. Neuroendocrine evidence for dopaminergic actions of hypericum extract (LI 160) in healthy volunteers. Biol Psychiatry 1999;46:581–584.
89. Lantz MS, Buchalter E, Giambanco V. St. John's wort and antidepressant drug interactions in the elderly. J Geriatr Psychiatry Neurol 1999;12:7–10.
90. Brown TM. Acute St. John's wort toxicity. Am J Emerg Med 2000;18:231–232.
91. Obach RS. Inhibition of human cytochrome P450 enzymes by constituents of St. John's wort, an herbal preparation used in the treatment of depression. J Pharmacol Exp Ther 2000;294:88–95.
92. Ernst E. Second thoughts about safety of St. John's wort. Lancet 1999;354:2014–2016.
93. Breidenbach T, Hoffmann MW, Becker T, et al. Drug interaction of St. John's wort with cyclosporin. Lancet 2000;355:1912.
94. Yue QY, Bergquist C, Gerden B. Safety of St. John's wort. Lancet 2000;355:576–577.
95. Johne A, Brockmoller J, Bauer S, et al. Pharmacokinetic interaction of digoxin with an herbal extract from St. John's wort (*Hypericum perforatum*). Clin Pharmacol Ther 1999;66:338–345.
96. Hendriks H, Bos R, Allersma DP, et al. Pharmacological screening of valerenal and some other components of essential oil of *Valeriana officinalis*. Planta Med 1981;42:62–68.
97. Ortiz JG, Nieves-Natal J, Chavez P. Effects of *Valeriana officinalis* extracts on [^{3}H] flunitrazepam binding, synaptosomal [^{3}H]GABA uptake, and hippocampal [^{3}H]GABA release. Neurochem Res 1999;24:1373–1378.
98. Santos MS, Ferreira F, Cunha AP, et al. Synaptosomal GABA release as influenced by valerian root extract—involvement of the GABA carrier. Arch Int Pharmacodyn Ther 1994;327:220–231.
99. Garges HP, Varia I, Doraiswamy PM. Cardiac complications and delirium associated with valerian root withdrawal. JAMA 1998;280:1566–1567.
100. Blumenthal M, Goldberg A, Brinckmann J, eds. Herbal Medicine: Expanded Commission E Monographs. Newton, MA: Integrative Medicine Communications, 2000.
101. Pizzorno J, Murray M, eds. Textbook of Natural Medicine. 2nd ed. Edinburgh: Churchill Livingstone, 1999.
102. Schellenberg R. Treatment for the premenstrual syndrome with *agnus castus* fruit extract: prospective, randomized, placebo-controlled study. BMJ 2001;322:134–137.
103. Berger D, Schaffner W, Schrader E. Efficacy of *Vitex agnus castus* L. extract Ze 440 in patients with premenstrual syndrome (PMS). Arch Gynecol Obstet 2000;264:150–153.
104. Chaste Tree. In: The Review of Natural Products. St. Louis, MO: Facts and Comparisons, 1998.
105. Deal CL, Moskowitz RW. Nutraceuticals as therapeutic agents in osteoarthritis: the role of glucosamine, chondroitin sulfate, and collagen hydrolysate. Rheum Dis Clin North Am 1999;25:379–395.
106. Reginster JY, Deroisy R, Rovati LC. Long-term effects of glucosamine sulphate on osteoarthritis progression: a randomized placebo-controlled clinical trial. Lancet 2001;357:251–256.
107. McAlindon TE, Lavalley MP, Gulin JP, et al. Glucosamine and chondroitin for treatment of osteoarthritis: a systematic quality assessment and meta-analysis. JAMA 2000;283:1469–1475.
108. Iarussi D, Auricchio U, Agretto A, et al. Protective effect of coenzyme Q10 on anthracyclines cardiotoxicity: control study in children with acute lymphoblastic leukemia and non-Hodgkin lymphoma. Mol Aspects Med 1994;15(suppl):207–212.

109. Folkers K, Wolaniuk A. Research on coenzyme Q10 in clinical medicine and in immunomodulation. Drugs Exp Clin Res 1985;11:539–545.
110. Cortes EP, Gupta M, Chou C, et al. Adriamycin cardiotoxicity: early detection by systolic time interval and possible prevention by coenzyme Q10. Cancer Treat Rep 1978;62:887–891.
111. Lockwood K, Moesgaard S, Hanioka T, et al. Apparent partial remission of breast cancer in "high risk" patients supplemented with nutritional antioxidants, essential fatty acids and coenzyme Q10. Mol Aspects Med 1994;15(suppl):231–240.
112. Lockwood K, Moesgaard S, Folkers K. Partial and complete regression of breast cancer in patients in relation to dosage of coenzyme Q10. Biochem Biophys Res Commun 1994;199:1504–1508.
113. Lockwood K, Moesgaard S, Yamamoto T, et al. Progress on therapy of breast cancer with vitamin Q10 and the regression of metastases. Biochem Biophys Res Commun 1995;212:172–177.
114. Pepping J. Coenzyme Q10. Am J Health Syst Pharm 1999;56:519–521.
115. Baggio E, Gandini R, Plancher AC, et al. Italian multicenter study on the safety and efficacy of coenzyme Q10 as adjunctive therapy in heart failure. CoQ10 Drug Surveillance Investigators. Mol Aspects Med 1994;15(suppl):287–294.
116. Feigin A, Kieburtz K, Como P, et al. Assessment of coenzyme Q10 tolerability in Huntington's disease. Mov Disord 1996;11:321–323.
117. Thibault A, Samid D, Tompkins AC, et al. Phase I study of lovastatin, an inhibitor of the mevalonate pathway, in patients with cancer. Clin Cancer Res 1996;2:483–491.
118. Kaikkonen J, Nyyssönen K, Tuomainen TP, et al. Determinants of plasma coenzyme Q10 in humans. FEBS Lett 1999;443:163–166.
119. Crellin R, Bottiglieri T, Reynolds EH. Folates and psychiatric disorders. Drugs 1993;45:623–636.
120. Bottiglieri T, Godfrey P, Flynn T, et al. Cerebrospinal fluid S-adenosylmethionine in depression and dementia: effects of treatment with parenteral and oral S-adenosylmethionine. J Neurosurg Psych 1990;53:1096–1098.
121. Bottiglieri T, Hyland K, Reynolds EH. The clinical potential of ademetionine (S-adenosylmethionine) in neurological disorders. Drugs 1994;48:137–152.
122. Janicak PG, Lipinski J, Davis J, et al. S-adenosylmethionine in depression. A literature review and preliminary report. Ala J Med Sci 1988;25:306–313.
123. Bressa GM. S-adenosyl-L-methionine-(SAMe) as antidepressant: meta-analysis of clinical studies. Acta Neurol Scand 1994;89(S154):7–14.
124. Brown RP, Gerbarg PL, Bottiglieri T. S-adenosylmethionine (SAMe) in the clinical practice of psychiatry, neurology, and internal medicine. Clin Pract Altern Med 2000.
125. Brown RP, Gerbarg PL, Bottiglieri T. S-adenosylmethionine: how does SAMe work in depression, neuropsychiatric disorders, arthritis, and hepatitis? Prim Psychiatry 2001.
126. Brown RP, Gerbarg PL. Herbs and nutrients in the treatment of depression, anxiety, insomnia, migraine, and obesity. J Psychiatry Pract 2001;7:75–91.
127. Ramos L. SAMe as a supplement: can it really help treat depression and arthritis? J Am Diet Assoc 2000;100:414.
128. Soeken KL, Lee WL, Bausell RB, Agelli M. Berman BM. Safety and efficacy of S-adenosylmethionine (SAMe) for osteoarthritis. J Fam Pract 2002;51:425–430.
129. Lipinski JF, Cohen BM, Frankenburg F, et al. Open trial of S-adenosylmethionine for treatment of depression. Am J Psychiatry 1984;141:448–450.
130. Carney MWP, Chary TKN, Bottiglieri T, et al. Switch S-adenosyl methionine. Ala J Med Sci 1988;25:316–319.
131. Kagan BL, Sultzer DL, Rosenlicht N, et al. Oral S-adenosylmethionine in depression: a randomized, double-blind, placebo-controlled trial. Am J Psychiatry 1990;147:591–595.
132. Boozer CN, Nasser JA, Heymsfield SB. An herbal supplement containing Ma Huang-Guarana for weight loss: a randomized double-blind trial. Int J Obes Relat Metab Disord 2001;25:316–324.
133. Dulloo AG, Duret C, Rohrer D, et al. Efficacy of green tea extract rich in catechin polyphenols and caffeine in increasing 24-h energy expenditure and fat oxidation in humans. Am J Clin Nutr 1999;70:1040–1045.
134. Chantre P, Lairon D. Recent findings of green tea extract AR25 (Exolise) and its activity for the treatment of obesity. Phytomedicine 2002;9:3–8.
135. Pittler M, Stevinson C, Ernst E. Chromium picolinate for reducing body weight: meta-analysis of randomized trials. Int J Obes Relat Metab Disord 2003;27:522–529.
136. Porter DJ, Raymond LW, Anastasio GD. Chromium: friend or foe? Arch Fam Med 1999;8:386–390.
137. Lanca S, Alves A, Vieira AI, Barata J, de Freitas J, de Carvallo A. Chromium-induced toxic hepatitis. Eur J Intern Med 2002;13:518–520.
138. Jellin JM. Pharmacist's Letter/Prescriber's Letter: Natural Medicines Comprehensive Database. Stockton, CA: Therapeutic Research Facility, 2003.
139. Guerciolini R, Radu-Radulescu L, Boldrin M, Dallas J, Moore R. Comparative evaluation of fecal fat excretion induced by orlistat and chitosan. Obes Res 2001;9:364–367.
140. Gades MD, Stern JS. Chitosan supplementation does not affect fat absorption in health males fed a high-fat diet, a pilot study. Int J Obes Relat Metab Disord 2002;26:119–122.
141. Pittler MH, Abbott NC, Harkness EF, Ernst E. Randomized, double-blind trial of chitosan for body weight reduction. Eur J Clin Nutr 1999;53:379–381.
142. Caraccio TR, McGuigan M, Mofenson HC. Chronic arsenic (As) toxicity from chitosan supplement [Abstract 109]. Clin Toxicol 2002;40:644.

143. Singh B, Berman B, Simpson R, et al. Incidence of premenstrual syndrome and remedy usage: a national probability sample study. Altern Ther Health Med 1998;4:75–79.
144. Mortola J. Premenstrual syndrome—pathophysiologic considerations. N Engl J Med 1998;338:256–257.
145. Stevinson C, Ernst E. Complementary/alternative therapies for premenstrual syndrome: a systematic review of randomized controlled trials. Am J Obstet Gynecol 2001;185:227–235.
146. Lauritzen CH, Reuter HD, Repges R, et al. Treatment of premenstrual tension syndrome with *Vitex agnus castus*: controlled, double-blind study versus pyridoxine. Phytomedicine 1997;4:183–189.
147. Abraham G. Nutritional factors in the etiology of the premenstrual tension syndromes. J Reprod Med 1983;28:446–464.
148. Facchinetti F, Borella P, Sances G, et al. Oral magnesium successfully relieves premenstrual mood changes. Obstet Gynecol 1991;78:177–181.
149. Walker AR, De Souza MC, Vickers MF, et al. Magnesium supplementation alleviates premenstrual symptoms of fluid retention. J Womens Health 1998;7:1157–1165.
150. Puolakka J, Makarainen L, Viinikka L, et al. Biochemical and chemical effects of treating the premenstrual syndrome with prostaglandin synthesis precursors. J Reprod Med 1985;30:149–153.
151. Callender K, McGregor M, Kirk P, et al. A double-blind trial of evening primrose oil in the premenstrual syndrome: nervous symptoms subgroup. Hum Psychopharmacol 1988;3:57–61.
152. Khoo SK, Munro C, Battistutta D. Evening primrose oil and treatment of premenstrual syndrome. Med J Aust 1990;153:189–192.
153. Collins A, Cerin A, Coleman G, et al. Essential fatty acids in the treatment of premenstrual syndrome. Obstet Gynecol 1993;81:93–98.
154. Thys-Jacobs S, Starkey P, Bernstein D, et al. Calcium carbonate and the premenstrual syndrome: Effects on premenstrual and menstrual symptoms. Am J Obstet Gynecol 1988;179:444–452.
155. Aganoff J, Boyle G. Aerobic exercise, mood states and menstrual cycle symptoms. J Psychosom Res 1994;38:183.
156. Kuiper GG, Carlsson B, Grandien K, et al. Comparison of the ligand binding specificity and transcript tissue distribution of estrogen receptors alpha and beta. Endocrinology 1997;138:863–870.
157. Lock M. Contested meanings of the menopause. Lancet 1991;337:1270–1272.
158. Boulet MJ, Oddens BJ, Lehert P, et al. Climacteric and menopause in seven southeast Asian countries. Maturitas 1994;19:157–176.
159. Adlercreutz H. Western diet and Western diseases: some hormonal and biochemical mechanisms and associations. Scand J Clin Lab Invest 1990;201(suppl):3–23.
160. Adlercreutz H, Honjo H, Higashi A, et al. Urinary excretion of lignans and isoflavonoid phytoestrogens in Japanese men and women consuming a traditional Japanese diet. Am J Clin Nutr 1991;54:1093–1100.
161. Goldin BR, Adlercreutz H, Gorbach SL, et al. The relationship between estrogen levels and diets of Caucasian American and Oriental immigrant women. Am J Clin Nutr 1986;44:945–953.
162. St. Germain A, Peterson CT, Robinson JG, Alekel DL. Isoflavone-rich or isoflavone-poor soy protein does not reduce menopausal symptoms during 24 weeks of treatment. Menopause 2001;8:17–26.
163. Albertazzi P, Pansini F, Bonaccorsi G, Zanotti L, et al. The effect of dietary soy supplementation on hot flushes. Obstet Gynecol 1998;91:6–11.
164. Han KK, Soares JM Jr, Haidar MA, de Lima GR, Baracat EC. Benefits of soy isoflavone therapeutic regimen on menopausal symptoms. Obstet Gynecol 2002;99:389–394.
165. Upmalis DH, Upmalis DM, Lobo R, Bradley L, Warren M, Cone FL, Lamia CA. Vasomotor symptom relief by soy isoflavone extract tablets in postmenopausal women: a multicenter, double-blind, randomized, placebo-controlled study. Menopause 2000;7:236–242.
166. Dalais FS, Rice GE, Wahlqvist ML, et al. Effects of dietary phytoestrogens in postmenopausal women. Climacteric 1998;1:124–129.
167. Murkies AL, Lombard C, Strauss BJ, Wilcox G, Burger HG, Morton MS. Dietary flour supplementation decreases post-menopausal hot flushes: effect of soy and wheat. Maturitas 1995;21:189–195.
168. Secreto G, Chiechi LM, Amdori, et al. Soy isoflavones and melatonin for the relief of climacteric symptoms: a multicenter, double-bond randomized study. Maturitas 2004;47:11–20.
169. Peeters PH, Keinan-Boker L, van der Schouw YT, Grobbee DE. Phytoestrogens and breast cancer risk. Review of the epidemiological evidence. Breast Cancer Res Treat 2003;77:171–183.
170. Wu AH, Wan P, Hankin J, Tseng CC, Yu MC, Pike MC. Adolescent and adult soy intake and risk of breast cancer in Asian-Americans. Carcinogenesis 2002;23:1491–1496.
171. Mitchell E, Woods N. Midlife women's attributions about perceived memory changes: observations from the Seattle Midlife Women's Health study. J Womens Health Gend Based Med 2001;10:351–362.
172. Vincent A, Fitzpatrick LA. Soy isoflavones: are they useful in menopause? Mayo Clin Proc 2000;75:1174–1184.
173. Duffy R, Wiseman H, File SE. Improved cognitive function in postmenopausal women after 12 weeks of consumption of a soya extract containing isoflavones. Pharmacol Biol Behav 2003;75:721–729.
174. Kritz-Silverstein D, VonMuhlen D, Barrett-Connor E, Bressel MA. Isoflavones and cognitive function in older women: the Soy and Postmenopausal Health in Aging (SOPHIA) study. Menopause 2003;10:196–202.
175. Head KA. Ipriflavone: an important bone-building isoflavone. Altern Med Rev 1999;4:10–22.
176. Adami S, Bufalino L, Cervetti R, et al. Ipriflavone prevents radial bone loss in postmenopausal women with low bone mass over 2 years. Osteoporos Int 1997;7:119–125.
177. Gennari C, Adami S, Agnusdei D, et al. Effect of chronic treatment with ipriflavone in postmenopausal women with low bone mass. Calcif Tissue Int 1997;61:S19–S22.

178. Acerbi D, Poli G, Ventura P. Comparative bioavailability of two oral formulations of ipriflavone in healthy volunteers at steady-state. Evaluation of two different dosage schemes. Eur J Drug Metabol Pharmacokinet 1998;23:172–177.
179. Sato M, Grese TA, Dodge JA, et al. Emerging therapies for the prevention or treatment of postmenopausal osteoporosis. J Med Chem 1999;42:1–24.
180. Gennari C, Agnusdei D, Crepaldi G, et al. Effect of ipriflavone—a synthetic derivative of natural isoflavones—on bone mass loss in the early years after menopause. Menopause 1998;5:9–15.
181. Agnusedi D, Crepaldi G. Isaia G, et al. A double blind, placebo-controlled trial of ipriflavone for prevention of postmenopausal spinal bone loss. Calcif Tissue Int 1997;61:142–147.
182. Alexandersen P, Toussaint A, Christiansen C, et al. Ipriflavone in the treatment of postmenopausal osteoporosis. JAMA 2001;285:1482–1488.
183. Anderson JW, Johnstone BM, Cook-Newell ME. Meta-analysis of the effects of soy protein intake on serum lipids. N Engl J Med 1995;333:276–282.
184. Crouse JR III, Morgan T, Terry JG, et al. A randomized trial comparing the effect of casein with that of soy protein containing varying amounts of isoflavones on plasma concentrations of lipids and lipoproteins. Arch Intern Med 1999;159:2070–2076.
185. Teede H, Dalais F, Kotsopoulos D. Dietary phytoestrogens improve lipid profiles and blood pressure: a double-blind randomized placebo-controlled study in men and postmenopausal women [Abstract]. Circulation 1999;100(suppl 1):I–266.
186. Peterson TG, Coward L, Kirk M, et al. The role of metabolism in mammary epithelial cell growth inhibition by the isoflavones genistein and biochanin A. Carcinogenesis 1996;17:1861–1869.
187. Lee H, Gourley L, Duffy S, et al. Dietary effects on breast cancer risk in Singapore. Lancet 1991;337:1197–1200.
188. Wu AH, Ziegler RG, Horn-Ross PL, et al. Tofu and risk of breast cancer in Asian-Americans. Cancer Epidemiol Biomarkers Prev 1996;5:901–906.
189. Key TJ, Sharp J, Appelby PN, et al. Soya foods and breast cancer risk: a prospective study in Hiroshima and Nagasaki, Japan. Br J Cancer 1999;81:1248–1256.
190. Lamartiniere CA, Moore J, Holland M, et al. Neonatal genistein chemoprevents mammary cancer. Proc Soc Exp Biol Med 1995;208:120–123.
191. Shu X, Jin F, Wen W, et al. Soy food intake during adolescence and subsequent risk of breast cancer among Chinese women. Cancer Epidemiol Biomarkers Prev 2001;10:483–488.
192. McMichael-Phillips DF, Harding C, Morton M, et al. Effects of soy-protein supplementation on epithelial proliferation in the histologically normal human breast. Am J Clin Nutr 1998;68(suppl 6):1431–1435.
193. Kurzer MS. Phytoestrogen supplement use by women. J Nutr 2003;133:1983S–1986S.
194. Tice JA, Ettinger B, Ensrud K, et al. Phytoestrogen supplements for the treatment of hot flashes: the Isoflavone Clover Extract (ICE) study. JAMA 2003;290:207–214.
195. McKenna DJ, Jones K, Humphrey S, et al. Black cohosh: efficacy, safety, and use in clinical and preclinical applications. Altern Ther Health Med 2001;7:93–100.
196. Dog TL, Riley D, Carter T. An integrative approach to menopause. Altern Ther Health Med 2001;7:45–55.
197. Liske E, Hanggi W, Henneicke-von Zepelin HH, Boblitz N, Wustenberg P, Rahlfs VW. Physiological investigation of a unique extract of black cohosh (*Cimicifugae racemosae rhizoma*): a 6-month clinical study demonstrates no systemic estrogenic effect. J Womens Health Gend Based Med 2002;11:163.
198. Dixon-Shanies D, Shaikh N. Growth inhibition of human breast cancer cells by herbs and phytoestrogens. Oncol Rep 1999;6:1383–1387.
199. Bodinet C, Freudenstein J. Influence of *Cimicifuga racemosa* on the proliferation of estrogen receptor-positive human breast cancer cells. Breast Cancer Res Treat 2002;76:1–10.
200. Jacobsen JS, Troxel A, Evans J, et al. Randomized trial of black cohosh for the treatment of hot flashes among women with a history of breast cancer. J Clin Oncol 2001;19:2739–2745.
201. Wiklund IK, Mattsson LA, Lindgren R, Limoni C. Effects of a standardized ginseng extract on quality of life and physiological parameters in symptomatic postmenopausal women: a double-blind placebo-controlled trial. Swedish Alternative Medicine Group. Int J Clin Pharmacol Res 1999;19:89–99.
202. Seibel M. Treating hot flashes without hormone replacement therapy. J Fam Pract 2003;52:291–296.
203. Chenoy R, Hussain S, Tayob Y, O'Brien PM, Moss MY, Morse PF. Effect of oral gamolenic acid from evening primrose oil on menopausal flushing. BMJ 1994;308:501–503.
204. Wyon Y, Lindgren R, Lundeberg T, et al. Effects of acupuncture on climacteric vasomotor symptoms, quality of life, and urinary excretion of neuropeptides among postmenopausal women. Menopause 1995;2:3–12.
205. Komesaroff PA, Black CV, Cable V, et al. Effects of wild yam extract on menopausal symptoms, lipids and sex hormones in healthy menopausal women. Climacteric 2001;4:144–150.
206. Cooper A, Spencer C, Whitehead MP, et al. Systemic absorption of progesterone from Pro-Gest cream in postmenopausal women. Lancet 1998;351:1255–1256.
207. Wren BG, Champion SM, Willets K, et al. Transdermal progesterone and its effect on vasomotor symptoms, blood lipid levels, bone metabolic markers, moods, and quality of life for postmenopausal women. Menopause 2003;10:13–18.
208. Leonetti HB, Longo S, Anasti JN. Transdermal progesterone cream for vasomotor symptoms and post-menopausal bone loss. Obstet Gynecol 1999;94:225–228.
209. Wren BG, McFarland K, Edwards L. Micronised transdermal progesterone and endometrial response [Letter]. Lancet 1999;354:1447–1448.
210. Lewis JG, McGill H, Patton VM, et al. Caution on the use of saliva measurements to monitor absorption of progesterone from transdermal creams in postmenopausal women. Maturitas 2002;41:1–6.

CHAPTER 21

Intimate Partner Violence

Abbey B. Berenson

Intimate partner violence (IPV) is the primary source of violence-related injuries that affect women. Sixty-four percent of women who report being raped or physically assaulted are victimized by a current or former husband, cohabiting partner, boyfriend, or date (1). IPV cuts across all racial, ethnic, religious, educational, and socioeconomic lines (2). Until more recently, violence against women was tolerated and supported by societal and cultural norms. Harmful acts against an intimate partner were considered to be private family matters. This outlook began to change in the 1970s as opinion about violence against women shifted from a grassroots social concern to a complex medical and societal issue. By the 1990s, violence against an intimate partner was recognized as a crime in the United States.

In 1994, this issue gained further momentum when Congress passed the Violence Against Women Act and directed the National Research Council (NRC) to develop a research agenda (3). As one of its charges, the NRC reviewed all existing literature and found certain broad, consistent patterns of risk and assault. Across three different races/ethnicities (white, black, Hispanic) of women residing in urban or rural settings, a man known to the woman was the most common perpetrator of both physical and sexual assault. Their findings redirected resources and efforts away from "stranger danger" and toward the problem of violence by intimates (3).

Knowledge in this field remains limited, however, due to the relatively recent recognition of IPV as a significant problem. Furthermore, different terms have been used to describe violence that occurs between partners in a relationship, such as domestic violence, dating violence, date rape, marital rape, partner abuse, spousal abuse, and battering, and assorted descriptions have been offered for acts that may constitute relationship violence or abuse (4). These variabilities in the knowledge base create confusion and a lack of consensus for recognizing, intervening, or reporting potential cases. This problem was more recently addressed by the Centers for Disease Control and Prevention (CDC), which established standard definitions (5). According to the CDC, IPV refers to victim–perpetrator relationships among intimate partners that involve one or more types of violence including physical violence, sexual violence, threat of physical or sexual violence, and psychological or emotional abuse (Table 21.1), and may result in the victim's death by murder or suicide. Furthermore, intimate partners may be cohabiting but need not be, may be a current or former partner, may be heterosexual or same sex, and the relationship need not involve sexual activity.

Most studies on the incidence and prevalence of this crime indicate that IPV has reached epidemic proportions in the United States. However, due to the lack of consistency in defining the relationship parameters and the behaviors involved, estimates of magnitude vary depending on the data source (6). Numerous sources agree that women who reside in the United States are more likely to be injured, raped, or killed by a current or former husband, cohabiting partner, boyfriend, or date than by all other types of perpetrators combined (1, 7). Overall, approximately 2 million American women report being physically or sexually assaulted each year, and

TABLE 21.1

Categories of Intimate Partner Violence

Physical Violence: The intentional use of physical force with the potential for causing death, disability, injury, or harm.

Scratching, pushing, shoving, throwing, grabbing, biting, choking, shaking, poking, hair pulling, slapping, punching, hitting, burning, use of a weapon (gun, knife or other object); use of restraints, one's body, size, or strength against another person. Coercing other people to commit any of these acts.

Sexual Violence: The use of physical force to compel a person to engage in a sexual act against his or her will, regardless of whether the act is completed. An attempted or completed sex act involving a person who is unable to understand the nature or condition of the act, decline participation, or communicate unwillingness to engage in the sexual act. Abusive sexual contact.

Unwanted or inappropriate touching, sexual name calling, humiliating or painful acts, threatening to get another sexual partner, accusations of sleeping around, demeaning sexual ability, STDs, HIV/AIDs, refusal to use condom, sexual behaviors in public or in front of children.

Threat of Physical or Sexual Violence: The use of words, gestures, or weapons to communicate the intent to cause death, disability, injury, or physical harm, or to compel someone to engage in sex acts or abusive sexual contact when the person is unwilling or unable to consent.

"I'll kill you (beat you up) if you don't have sex with me"; brandishing a weapon; firing a gun into the air; making hand gestures; reaching toward a person's breasts or genitalia.

Psychological/Emotional Abuse (including coercive tactics): The use of techniques such as those listed here, when preceded by acts or threats of physical or sexual violence, and perceived by the victim as psychologically or emotionally abusive.

Humiliating victim; controlling victim's activities; withholding information from victim; isolating victim from friends and/or family; using victim's children to control victim's behavior; smashing/throwing objects; taking money from the victim; denying victim access to money, health care, food, and clothing.

Adapted from Saltzman LE, Fanslow JL, McMahon PM, et al. Intimate Partner Violence Surveillance: Uniform Definitions and Recommended Data Elements, Version 1.0. Atlanta: Centers for Disease Control and Prevention, National Center for Injury Prevention and Control, 1999. Available at: www.cdc.gov/ncipc/. Accessed August 1, 2005.

1.3 million of these were hurt by an intimate partner (8). Between 8% and 35% of married or cohabiting women in the United States experience IPV each year (1, 7, 9–13), whereas severe violence is experienced by 2 to 4%. The National Crime Victimization Survey estimates that in 1998, 85% (876,340 incidents) of assaults by intimate partners were against women, with an indicated rate for women about five times that of men (13). In 1998, 32% of all female homicide victims, as compared with 4% of male murder victims, were killed by an intimate partner (6). Furthermore, women abused by an intimate partner are more likely than those attacked by a stranger to be assaulted multiple times within a 12-month period (8).

As alarming as these figures are, most experts agree that data obtained by national surveys or clinical studies probably underestimate the magnitude of this crime for a variety of reasons. First, these studies have lacked a standardized definition of domestic violence or IPV, or a standard method of measurement. The lack of consistent information has limited researchers' ability to judge the magnitude of the problem, identify groups at highest risk, or monitor changes in incidence and prevalence over time (5). Second, studies have failed to include all populations. Many focused on only married and cohabiting women, and thus failed to consider abuse by boyfriends who did not live with their partner (14). National samples often have not included women who do not speak English, who are homeless, or who are incarcerated, hospitalized, or institutionalized. Third, social barriers have inhibited the collection of accurate surveillance data. Victims frequently do not report IPV even when questioned, due to shame, guilt, or fear (13). Only one-fifth of rapes and one-fourth of physical assaults against women by an intimate partner are reported to the police (8). Reporting varies with race/ethnicity, with African American (67%)

and Hispanic (65%) women reporting their victimization to the police at significantly higher rates than white women (50%) (13). Fourth, a lack of training or fear of reprisal may limit members of the criminal justice system and health care providers from reporting the violence (5). Even when victims seek medical care, their information may not be recorded in the medical record (6). Overall, the true prevalence of IPV in the United States has been estimated to be double that reported, or 4.9 million women per year (8).

Cost studies of the impact of IPV have only more recently emerged (15), growing largely out of capitation and quality components of managed care (16). The cost of IPV to the U.S. economy has been difficult to establish because of the differences in the cost components and models selected to generate the cost figures (17, 18). In the only two nationally representative studies, estimates range from more than $5.8 billion to $7.6 billion (18, 19). Gerberding et al. pointed out the conservative nature of their study, stating that their figures are not comprehensive and probably underestimate the problem of IPV in the United States (18). Miller's group used a more comprehensive model to produce tangible and intangible costs related to the victim (19). Data for 1995 indicated that two-thirds of direct costs, or $4.1 billion, related to IPV was due to medical and mental health care services alone (18).

In addition, it has been estimated by the American Association of Health Plans that IPV annually results in 100,000 days of hospitalization, almost 30,000 emergency department visits, and nearly 40,000 visits to physicians (16). Compared with a nonabused patient with the same condition, a victim of IPV who is hospitalized for any condition other than those directly resulting from IPV costs a median of $873 more, primarily due to the increased need for mental health services (20, 21). Additional costs borne by society include maintenance of shelters and programs for victims and their children, and intervention by law enforcement, judicial, and social services systems.

DYNAMICS OF INTIMATE PARTNER VIOLENCE

Two conceptual models have been used to explain the relationships, interactions, and processes of IPV. The cycle of violence model was developed in the 1970s to explain why physical violence occurs (22). In the late 1980s, the Duluth model was developed to describe coercive tactics used by the abuser to gain and maintain power and control over a partner (23, 24).

Cycle of Violence Model

The cycle of violence model proposed three distinct, escalating phases leading to an incidence of physical abuse (22).

- *Phase One*—Over a period of days, weeks, or years, the abuser reacts negatively to any stimulus. He expresses anger and hostility through abusive acts, such as name calling, use of intimidating remarks, and acts of deliberate meanness. His partner tries to relieve the tension by nurturing, appeasing, or avoiding him. As time passes, pacifying the abuser becomes more difficult as he becomes more oppressive, jealous, threatening, and possessive.
- *Phase Two*—Tension peaks and the abuser releases it in physical or sexual assault. After the assault, the abuser and victim tend to rationalize the events. The perpetrator may blame the victim for his behavior or other external forces, such as work, lack of work, bills, or family relations. If drinking or substance use accompanied the assault, the victim or abuser may blame the alcohol or drugs.
- *Phase Three*—Following the incident, the abuser becomes apologetic, promises it will not happen again, and begs for forgiveness. He is remorseful, attentive, and sincere. Initially, the victim believes the problem has passed. She assumes responsibility for the abuser's behavior, defending him to herself, family, and friends. However, the tension-building phase resumes, lasting for shorter periods of time, while the violence becomes more severe and the remorse phase diminishes. Thus, the cycle is repeated more often with escalating levels of abuse. According to this model, the accelerating abusive cycle leaves many women demoralized and lacking the self-esteem necessary to leave the situation.

This model has several limitations (25). First, experience of individual phases or a cycle of phases is not universal. Many perpetrators inflict abuse in a random fashion, with no precursors and with no remorse period. Second, this explanation of violence relieves the abuser of responsibility. It states that the violence occurs spontaneously because the abuser lacks the ability to control his anger, and thus, the behavior is beyond the abuser's control. However, this view ignores the fact that abusers usually confine their violence to their partners and the domestic context, reflecting that there is, in fact, a modicum of control they can and do exert (26). Their "lack of control" is rarely apparent to friends or coworkers. Third, the model fails to address how violence may function as a systematic coercion technique for "managing" women. Fourth, the model implicates presumed psychopathology in both victim and abuser—her low self-esteem and his emotional dependency. By focusing on psychopathology and action/reaction sequences resulting from psychopathology, the model implicates the victim as a contributor to the violence, the abuser's behavior becomes a couple's issue, and the focus shifts away from the abuser and his choice to use violence. Interventions developed from this concept strive to improve relationships and often use couple's therapy. This type of intervention, however, often results in an escalation of abuse, and now has been expressly prohibited as an intervention in batterer treatment in 20 states (27, 28).

The Duluth Model—Power and Control Tactics

Organized in 1981, the Domestic Abuse Intervention Project became a pioneer in shaping public policy to protect victims of domestic abuse. The project has contributed to major changes in judicial, social, and medical systems. These changes redirected the responsibility for dealing with violence away from the victim, and toward community agencies and the perpetrator. As a result of this work in Duluth, Minnesota institutions gained a better understanding of the complex economic, physical, and psychological conditions involved in IPV.

Of primary importance is Duluth's development of the power and control model of partner violence. This conceptual model is used currently by the National Victim Assistance Academy, a week-long training on victimology, victim's rights, and victim's services sponsored by several universities and the U.S. Department of Justice (25). The model's influence is also apparent in the CDC's efforts to standardize definitions and parameters of IPV, mentioned previously, and in information from The National Women's Health Information Center, sponsored by the U.S. Department of Health and Human Services (29). In this model, abuse is viewed as intentional and a result of individual choice. Rather than a loss of control, it is an assertion of control. Thus, partner abuse does not involve shared responsibility (27). Rather than couple's therapy, interventions are directed at the abuser through professional education, community collaboration, and abuser accountability/rehabilitation. The goal of this approach is to end the abusive behavior, not to improve the relationship.

The power and control model of partner violence (Fig. 21.1) uses a wheel with spokes as a graphic representation of its concepts. At the center or hub of the wheel are "power and control," the reasons an abuser engages in IPV. The spokes of the wheel represent the tactics used by the abuser to gain and maintain power and control, including intimidation, emotional abuse, economic abuse, isolation, minimizing, denying, blaming, or using children, male privilege, and coercion and threats. Tactics may vary slightly with culture and age of victim and abuser. The outer perimeter of the wheel is the threat or act of physical and sexual violence against the victim. Like an iron rim on a wagon wheel, the abuser's threats or acts of violence hold the system together and give strength to the tactics. These dynamics confer power on the abuser that is reflected in the actual physical, sexual, and psychological damage suffered by the victim.

This model has been the basis for rehabilitative programs for offenders and for training a diverse range of professionals who may interact with victims or abusers. With its primary focus on the abuser and its cognitive behavioral aspects, the Duluth power and control model has become the preferred conceptualization. Rehabilitative programs of this type have been shown to produce moderate effects in abusers over time (30).

FIGURE 21.1 ● The power and control model of partner violence. (Adapted from Institute for Clinical Systems Improvement, Health Care Guideline: Domestic Violence 2001, and the Domestic Abuse Intervention Project, Duluth, MN, with permission.)

BARRIERS TO LEAVING AN ABUSIVE RELATIONSHIP

Physicians and other health care workers may express frustration when encountering the victim of IPV because they cannot comprehend why an abused woman remains with an abuser (31). The frustration is verbalized as "why does she stay?" This question assumes she will be safe if she leaves and blames the woman for enduring the abuse. However, only the woman involved can judge the safest and best way to handle the situation. In addition, the belief that a woman can easily leave this environment reflects a misunderstanding of the complexity of the problem. The average victim attempts to leave the home two to five times before she is able to escape the relationship (32). Leaving an abusive partner is not a matter of simple resolution but a complex, ongoing process of decisions and changes in all aspects of daily life (33, 34). The process often includes periods of denial, self-blame, and endurance (35). The woman must give up her employment, her friends, and the normal structure of her life (36). Her children must be taken from school, their friends, and their activities. A woman demoralized by years of violence may attempt repeatedly to leave the relationship, only to return when she cannot overcome the obstacles. Thus, ambivalence, hesitance, and "relapses" in returning to the abuser may be expected as part of the process of severing the relationship (34). Consistent factors that have been demonstrated to propel women to leave include an increase in the severity of the violence, the realization and acceptance that he will not change, threats or danger to the children, and the appearance of logistical or emotional support (35). Final separation occurs when she is able to find the combination of resources that satisfy her needs and ensure her safety (25). Thus, the appropriate question from medical professionals should be "what barriers prevent her from leaving?" Knowledge of specific barriers, some of which are described in this section, will help medical personnel strengthen their abilities to intervene.

Fear

Women attempting to leave abusive relationships often report threats of harm to themselves, their children, and other family members if they act. Thus, women may believe staying in the relationship will protect other family members from violence. In many cases, the abuse does increase if they leave the home because abusers are motivated by a need to exercise power and control over the victims. The National Violence Against Women Survey found that violence

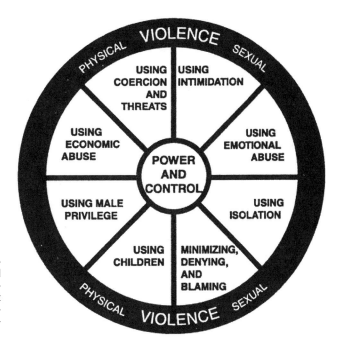

occurred more often after the termination of a relationship, with wives living apart from husbands nearly four times more likely to report that their husbands had raped, physically assaulted, or stalked them (8). The National Crime Victimization Survey demonstrated similar findings; divorced or separated persons were subjected to the highest rates of intimate partner victimization (13). Moreover, women attempting to leave an abusive environment are at increased risk for homicide (37). From 1976 to 1998, the percentage of female murder victims killed by intimate partners has remained at about 30% (10, 13).

Financial Dependence

Victims may choose to stay in an abusive environment because they fear that they could not house or feed themselves and their children. Many abused women do not have access to bank accounts, credit cards, or cash. They may not have the proper skills or experience to obtain employment. Furthermore, the need to hide from the abuser can make it difficult to obtain or continue employment. According to the U.S. General Accounting Office, up to 52% of victims lose their jobs because their abusers engage in behavior that makes it difficult to work (38). Some overcome financial obstacles, only to be tracked by their abusers through their social security numbers. To help prevent this, the Social Security Administration instituted a policy in 1998 of assigning new social security numbers to victims of harassment, abuse, or life endangerment. (For information, access the administration via the internet at www.ssa.gov or call 1-800-772-1213.)

Clinicians can assist victims by directing them to available resources, such as the National Domestic Violence Hotline (NDVH) (see Appendix 21.1 for contact information). This hotline is answered 24 hours per day, is confidential, and is staffed with both Spanish- and English-speaking operators. Other resources include state social services or human services departments, victim–witness assistance programs, and domestic or family violence coalitions. Often, a local women's shelter or United Way will assist in mortgage or rent payments. In some areas, utility companies may offer special payment plans or energy share programs. A clinician can also refer to his or her state's Internet site for regional information on resources. Go to www.__.state.us (fill in the blank with the two-letter state postal abbreviation), and search for key words "family violence," "domestic violence," or "intimate partner violence."

Social Isolation

As the abuse continues, the abuser uses tactics to enforce isolation of the victim. He may restrict her access to friends, family, telephone, care, and community support (39). He may accompany her everywhere, open her mail, go through her purse, or eavesdrop on phone conversations. The resulting isolation augments her feelings of fear. As a result, the victim loses opportunities for "reality checks" with outsiders, and becomes increasingly dependent on the abuser for social, emotional, and financial support. The only perspective available to her is that of the abuser, which may affect her judgment. This was confirmed in a study of abused women that observed that victims were unable to judge personal risk and that their assessment did not correlate with actual risk factors in their abusive relationships (34). This cognitive distortion resembles that experienced by hostages, cult members, or political prisoners (40–42). Isolation, humiliation, accusation, and unpredictable punishment are used by captors or cult leaders to create an environment controlled by fear and anticipated fear, and to instill dependency, debility, and dread (Table 21.2) (40). Exhaustion is also common among these captives (43). Such coercive stresses seriously affect a person's customary ways of thinking about themselves and dealing with their situations.

Inadequate Community or Institutional Support

Resources for victims of IPV have improved but remain inadequate. According to a Ford Foundation report, as many as 50% of all homeless women and children in the United States are fleeing domestic violence (44). The U.S. Conference of Mayors has identified domestic violence as a primary cause of homelessness (45, 46). The number of emergency shelters has increased nationwide from fewer than 10 in 1975 to 1250 in 1995, as a result of the shift from private-only

TABLE 21.2

Coercive Tactics Common to Cult Leaders, Political Captors, and Intimate Partner Violence Perpetrators

Injuries
Blunt trauma
Burns
Strangulation
Penetrating injuries
Sexual injuries

Conditions of Detention
Denial of privacy
Forced nakedness
Deprivations of physiologic needs such as sleep, food, toilet facilities, vehicle, medical care or social contacts
Humiliations: verbal abuse, performance of humiliating acts
Threats: of death, harm to family, further torture

Adapted from Physicians for Human Rights (PHR). Examining Asylum Seekers: A Health Professional's Guide to Medical and Psychological Evaluations of Torture. Washington, DC: HR, August 2001. Available at: www.phrusa.org/. Accessed August 1, 2005.

funding to combined federal-state-private funding (47). However, the need for shelter continues to exceed availability (48). Many shelters in highly populated areas are filled most of the time. For example, in New York during 1995, about 300 women and children per week were turned away due to lack of space (3). One New York City hotline reported that more than 80 requests were received each day, with an average of only four to five vacancies available (49). Even in less densely populated areas, shelters are insufficient to meet the needs of victims. For example, in Texas, shelter was provided to 27,060 victims in 1998, but 3796 adults still had to be turned away (50). In addition, some shelters are unable to accommodate women with a large number of children or those with a son older than the age of 12 (51). Victims of IPV who abuse alcohol or drugs, as well as those with mental illness or the homeless, may also be denied refuge (48, 52, 53). If a woman gains admission, her stay is usually limited to 2 to 6 weeks, which is insufficient time to locate new housing and find a job. Transitional housing is offered on a limited basis at some shelters, but most programs are unable to support second-stage housing (47). Consequently, many women return to an abusive home following a stay in a shelter because they have nowhere else to live (54).

Insurance Discrimination

Prior to the enactment of the Violence Against Women Act, abused women had difficulty obtaining health, life, or other types of insurance coverage, because several carriers deemed victims of abuse to be an excessive risk. Legislation to forbid that type of discrimination has been proposed and, in some instances, adopted. By 1998, the National Association of Insurance Commissioners, whose membership is comprised of the insurance commissioners from each state, had adopted four model acts that would protect abused women from discrimination by insurers with regard to property and casualty, health, and life and disability income. At this time, 31 states, to some degree, bar insurance discrimination against victims of domestic violence (55). However, according to the Family Violence Prevention Fund's Health Report Card, only 22 states had enacted adequate discrimination protections by 2001 (56).

Lack of Faith in the Criminal Justice System

Historically, the criminal justice system considered family violence outside their jurisdiction. Violent acts perpetrated by strangers were subject to criminal prosecution, whereas the same acts committed in the context of an intimate relationship were treated as minor transgressions or dismissed entirely. Until more recently, few laws existed to address violence occurring in the family. Consequently, women did not contact the police because they perceived the justice system as ineffective (10, 57). In addition, victims reported that they did not call police because of situational barriers, such as being physically prevented from using the telephone or being threatened with more violence (58). A previous negative experience with the police and the level of violence experienced also influenced reporting (36).

All states now have passed legislation to deter violent, abusive, or intimidating acts between intimate partners. Every jurisdiction has different policies and procedures for issuing and monitoring protection or restraining orders, devised to safeguard abused women. In most cases, the victim must file a request as soon as possible after the violence occurs. Often, financial independence and abuse of family or friends are associated with the decision to seek a protection order (59). Many women do not file for protection until an average of 4 years after the first incident, which is the average length of time abused women take to decide to end a relationship (60). Even when women do apply for a restraining order, it may not be granted; in one prospective study of 90 women, 24% who applied for a civil protective order did not qualify because of cohabitation requirements or childbearing status (61).

To obtain compliance with protection orders, there must be clear cut penalties for violations (62). Criminal sanctions are the most common mechanism used. These vary from state to state but may include charges of felony, misdemeanor, or contempt of court, with confinement from 24 hours to 30 days. Unfortunately, few data are available on the effectiveness of protection orders. An analysis of data collected from 1981 to 1991 by six police departments demonstrated that arrest is a modestly effective deterrent to subsequent aggression against a female partner (63). Two studies indicated that 86 to 92% of the women reported that after obtaining a protective order, the violence stopped (64, 65). However, two other studies demonstrated high rates (32 to 60%) of reabuse within 3 to 12 months (66, 67). These diverse findings indicate that more research is needed to predict if protection orders or arrest are effective means of providing safety for the victim (61).

PRESENTATION OF THE VICTIM OF INTIMATE PARTNER VIOLENCE

The medical community may encounter victims of IPV in primary care clinics, family planning clinics, and emergency centers. Table 21.3 lists many of the health consequences of IPV and their presenting complaints (3, 68–74).

Hospital emergency department data indicate that women represent 84% of those seeking hospital treatment for an intentional injury caused by an intimate assailant (10). Only 1 in 10 women victimized by a violent intimate seeks professional medical treatment; with 1 in 5 injured females seeking treatment (10). Among pregnant women, as many as one-third who present with trauma have an injury that was inflicted intentionally (75). However, the cause of these injuries frequently goes undetected by emergency room personnel. In one study, only 13% of victims stated that they were asked about IPV or reported its occurrence to the doctor or nurse (76). Furthermore, IPV was noted in the medical record in only 2% of those cases in which it was the reason for the emergency room visit.

Part of the problem is that there is no specific constellation of signs, symptoms, or illnesses that help health care providers recognize patients with current or past history of relationship violence (77). However, clinicians should have a high index of suspicion when women present to the emergency room or other health provider with injuries. Most perpetrators of IPV do not use a firearm, knife, or an object like a bottle or a club. Most females (81%) injured during an act of IPV face an offender with no weapon (78). Injuries are most often inflicted with the hands or fists (slapping, grabbing, punching), the teeth (biting), and legs/feet (kicking). In fact, female victims of intimate partner homicide were killed equally often by blunt objects or blows

TABLE 21.3

Health Consequences of Intimate Partner Violence

Nonfatal Outcomes

Physical Conditions

Injury, especially to head, neck, thorax, abdomen

Central injuries (chest, breasts, abdomen, pelvis, perineum)

Dental trauma

Burns, bruises in unusual locations

Human bites

Disability preventing work

Injury during pregnancy

Somatic Conditions

Headaches, migraines

Fainting

Seizures, convulsions

Back pain, neck pain, abdominal pain, stomach pain

Hypertension

Digestive problems: diarrhea, irritable bowel syndrome, nausea, constipation, stomach ulcer, gastric reflux

Insomnia, nightmares

Onset of stammering

Lack of visual acuity, even with glasses

Hearing loss

Psychological Symptoms

Depression

Anxiety/panic attacks

Posttraumatic stress disorder

Eating disorders

Suicidal ideation

Reproductive/Urogenital Symptoms

Unintended pregnancy, unsafe abortion

Pregnancy complications, miscarriage, low birth weight

Sexually transmitted diseases

Vaginal infection, discharge, itching

Vaginal bleeding, menstrual problems

Pelvic inflammatory disease

Fibroids, hysterectomy

Painful intercourse, sexual dysfunction

Chronic pelvic pain, genital area pain

Urinary tract infections

Health Risk Behaviors

Smoking

Alcohol and drug abuse

Sexual/HIV risk behaviors

Physical inactivity

Overeating

Fatal Outcomes

Homicide

Suicide

Maternal mortality

AIDS related

Adapted from Refs. 3 and 68–74.

delivered by the hands or feet (79). One reason to suspect violence is an injury to the head, face, or neck because victims of IPV are 12 times more likely to be injured in this region than those experiencing trauma from other causes. Overall, injuries that occur as a result of IPV occur on the central region of the body such as the head, face, neck, thorax, breasts, abdomen, or genitals, in contrast to accidental injuries, which tend involve the extremities (80–82). Furthermore, manual strangulation is a common method of abuse that appears to occur late in the relationship, about 3 years after physical abuse began (83). Nonlethal strangulation may cause medical complications up to 2 weeks after the strangulation incident, such as difficulty breathing, airway compromise, pneumonia, adult respiratory distress syndrome, postanoxic encephalopathy, psychosis, amnesia, cerebrovascular accident, and progressive dementia. Defensive injuries to the forearms and palms are common and always suggest violence. Fractures, dislocations, and contusions of the wrists and lower arms result from attempts to fend off blows to the chest or face (84). In addition, multiple injury sites in different stages of healing are suggestive of ongoing violence.

Time of arrival to an emergency center may also suggest the possibility of abuse because victims of IPV are more likely to present between 6:00 PM and 7:00 AM, the time frame during which most incidents occur (13, 85). Furthermore, a delay between the time of injury and arrival for care is strongly suggestive of IPV because victims often delay seeking care for their injuries (86). Dearwater et al. more recently reported that a higher proportion of women who have been battered in the past year (12 to 17%) present to emergency departments than women with acute trauma from abuse (87).

Most often, IPV victims visit clinics or private practitioners' offices, rather than a hospital urgent care facility. Commonly, the victim presents with somatic symptoms, such as a choking sensation, hyperventilation, chest pain, gastrointestinal symptoms, headaches, or chronic pain of the back, abdomen, or pelvis (68, 69, 71, 77). Complaints of insomnia, anxiety, depression, eating disorders, panic or posttraumatic stress disorder symptoms, and suicidal thoughts are also common (7, 53, 86, 88–93). The etiology for these somatic and psychological complaints may be obscured if IPV is not considered (94).

Gynecologic problems have been reported not only in sexual abuse victims, but also in those reporting physical and emotional abuse. In addition to chronic pelvic pain, abused women may present with severe dysmenorrhea or dyspareunia (95, 96). New information connects IPV with an increased risk of invasive cervical cancer (72). In this study, women with cervical cancer reported being in violent relationships longer and experiencing more frequent physical and sexual assaults than controls. Furthermore, abused women may be unable to control or negotiate correct or consistent contraceptive use, protect themselves against infection by sexually transmitted diseases (STDs), plan a pregnancy, or avoid assault during a pregnancy (97).

Abuse During Pregnancy

Studies document that between 1% and 26% of pregnant women in the United States experience IPV with most estimates falling between 4% and 8% (98–103). These percentages indicate that abuse may be more common for pregnant women than other conditions for which screening in pregnancy is routine, such as pre-eclampsia or gestational diabetes. Furthermore, the reported percentages of women experiencing violence for the *first* time while pregnant varied from 12 to 88% in three different studies (98–100). Adolescents are at especially high risk for physical abuse during pregnancy because they are vulnerable to assault from a parent and from a boyfriend or spouse. A woman whose partner is unhappy about the pregnancy or for whom the pregnancy is not planned is also more likely to experience violence than one whose partner desires the pregnancy (104). Women whose pregnancy was unintended have two to three times the risk of experiencing physical violence as compared with those with planned pregnancies (103).

Violence leads to high-risk pregnancies (35). Violence may affect pregnancy through direct mechanisms (e.g., a blow to the abdomen may cause preterm labor) or indirect mechanisms (e.g., experience of IPV leads to psychological distress or lack of access to medical care) that may cause poor outcomes (102, 105). If the mother is struck in the abdomen, the fetus may experience a direct injury. For example, Morey et al. reported a case of fetal bruising and intraventricular hemorrhage following a blow to the abdomen (106). In addition, women reporting abuse are more likely to experience complications such as infections, anemia, depression, low maternal weight gain, trauma through falls or blows to the abdomen, premature labor, and delivery by cesarean section (35, 98, 102, 107).Two controlled studies have observed that victims of IPV are more likely to deliver a low-birth-weight (less than 2500 g) infant, but other studies have not found an association between IPV and infant birth weight (98, 102, 107–112).

Unhealthy behaviors associated with IPV may also adversely affect the fetus. For example, abused women are more likely than those without a history of abuse to delay seeking prenatal care until the third trimester (108). In addition, victims of violence are more likely than nonvictims to use multiple illicit substances during pregnancy and to continue to use drugs throughout the gestation (113).

Women remain at risk for IPV during the postpartum period. Four clinically based investigations noted that the prevalence of IPV during the postpartum period ranged from 3 to 90%

(114–117). In one study of 36 women abused during pregnancy, victims reported that they were hit more frequently during the 3 months following delivery than during the pregnancy or preconception periods (114). An increase in abuse during this period may be related, in part, to the numerous stresses that accompany new parenthood, such as sleep deprivation, lack of privacy, and increased expenses. Thus, it is important to screen women for physical violence at their postpartum visit, as well as prior to and during pregnancy. The safety of all children residing in an abusive home should also be determined.

UNIVERSAL SCREENING

Primary care physicians and other health care workers (family planning, teen, and STD clinics) are in an ideal position to identify victims and refer them before they are injured or killed (118). For this reason, professional organizations such as the American Medical Association (AMA) and the American College of Obstetrics and Gynecology (ACOG) recommend that universal screening be implemented in office-based practices (2, 119). However, of physicians surveyed in 2002, only 6% reported always screening their patients, whereas 10% reported never screening for domestic violence (120). Obstetrician/gynecologists have demonstrated a strong knowledge of the prevalence and dynamics of IPV, reporting some type of training in (67%), or a familiarity with (85%), ACOG's guidelines on domestic violence, but the majority reported that they do not routinely screen for IPV (121). In comparison, they reported routinely screening for use of tobacco (95%), use of alcohol (93%), diet and exercise habits (80%), use of seat belts (73%), and symptoms of stress or depression (73%) (121). This finding would appear to indicate that training, availability of guidelines and other resources, familiarity with the topic, and willingness to screen for other health risks are not enough to change screening behaviors. This highlights the fact that there is no other health care problem that so endangers women for which routine assessments do not take place(122).

BARRIERS TO DISCLOSURE

Barriers to understanding and to disclosure exist on both sides of the clinician–patient relationship (84, 123). Social factors, psychological or personal factors, professional factors, and institutional or legal factors may all have a role (35, 84, 123–126).

Provider Factors That Hinder Disclosure

Professional and personal issues create challenges to providing adequate care for IPV victims. Providers tend to think that it is the patients, rather than the providers, who create obstacles to better care for IPV (35). However, health professionals bring personal values and biases to their clinical experiences and may make assumptions about their patients based on socioeconomic status and lifestyle choices (20). These cognitive biases may have effects on the identification of IPV victims. Various barriers to screening have been reported by providers: inadequate training, prejudices, time constraints, frustration at being unable to help the victim, fear of offending the patient, and in some cases, reticence due to a personal history of abuse. Concerns for personal safety may be an issue (127). Professional controversies over the effectiveness of universal screening and issues surrounding mandatory reporting, particularly with reference to potential legal implications, may also deter providers from screening.

Inadequate Training

Acceptance of health promotion in general, and IPV intervention specifically, as viable venues for medical involvement is still developing. Most providers who trained prior to 1985 had no formal instruction in issues related to violence or abuse. In 1988, a survey of medical schools demonstrated that 53% did not offer instruction in IPV (128). By 1994, 86% of medical school deans reported an existing adult domestic abuse curriculum (129). Although most medical schools now incorporate training in this area in their curricula, the quality of these programs varies. Most instruction occurs in the preclinical years, with only 26 schools reporting required material on

IPV in the clinical years. Required hours range from 0 to 25, with a median of only 2 hours. Curriculum on IPV may be offered during off-hours, late in the term, or close to major exams. Most often, instruction in family violence is presented as a single, stand-alone offering of less than 4 hours. It is not revisited over time, in multiple courses, or in clinical settings (122, 129). Finally, only 37% of medical texts and 63% of nursing texts published between 1990 and 1996 include some content on IPV, with only a few meeting quality criteria (medical 16%; nursing 10%) (130).

Lack of provider training has been demonstrated to correlate with failure to screen for IPV in a medical setting. In fact, a survey of ACOG fellows demonstrated that lack of training was the most common reason for failing to incorporate universal screening in their practices (131). In 1997, 57% of primary care physicians reported that they had not been trained to deal with IPV victims (132). The physicians who had received training in IPV were more likely to screen than those who had received no instruction (131). In 1998, a national sample of residents ($n = 4832$ in 632 programs) in their last year of training at U.S. academic medical centers reported on preparedness to counsel patients on several health behaviors (133). Overall, 96% were prepared to counsel patients regarding smoking, 91% about diet and exercise, 85% about substance abuse and depression, whereas less than 70% were prepared to counsel victims of IPV. Female residents, minority residents, and residents training in areas with high populations of indigent patients were more likely than Caucasian male residents to believe they were prepared to address IPV (134).

In an extensive review of IPV studies reported in the years 1992 to 1997, Waalen et al. identified 12 studies that indicated lack of provider education or experience as a barrier to screening for IPV (135). In an additional 12 studies, they found that educational programs alone increased provider knowledge but failed to increase screening. Studies that combined education with enabling strategies, such as written protocols, prompts, and written brief screening questions, were more effective in changing provider behaviors.

Mandatory Reporting Laws

An additional barrier to screening for IPV is legislation requiring mandatory reporting. Proponents of these laws point out that IPV is a crime, and as such, should be reported. Reporting is viewed as a way to improve identification of victims and provision of services to them. Mandated reporting is also viewed as a means of increasing screening for providers to avoid legal sanctions. Organizations that oppose mandated reporting, including ACOG, contend that such laws may place the woman at greater risk of retaliation, deny her the right to self-determination, threaten provider–patient confidentiality, impede her disclosure, and reduce physician's screening practices (136). The AMA acknowledges that statutory mandates create difficult dilemmas for the physician but that physicians are obligated to comply (137, 138). The AMA opposes mandatory reporting laws that would identify competent adults (139).

Mandatory reporting also receives mixed support from the general population. Overall, 52 to 80% of women stated in one study that they preferred a policy of mandatory reporting, although abused women were less likely to support it (74, 140, 141). In another study, the majority of abused patients (54%) preferred that women decide on reporting (142). Two-thirds of women in that study believed mandatory reporting policies would inhibit women from talking to their clinicians. Reasons for opposition included fear of retaliation by abuser, fear of family separation, mistrust of the legal system, and preference for confidentiality and autonomy.

The status and scope of mandatory reporting laws vary from state to state. Although 42 states require reporting of injuries resulting from firearms, knives, or other weapons to law enforcement, only seven states specifically require reporting for injuries resulting from domestic violence (143). Health care providers should be aware of reporting requirements in their state. Information may be obtained through state medical associations, the Family Violence Prevention Fund's annual Health Report Card and the Domestic Violence Statutes Database supported by the National Council of Juvenile and Family Court Judges (56, 144). In the absence of a legal requirement, the AMA advises that physicians not report IPV to authorities without the consent of a mentally competent, adult patient (137).

NATIONAL DOMESTIC VIOLENCE HOTLINE
LINEA NACIONAL SOBRE
LA VIOLENCIA DOMESTICA
1-800-799-SAFE (7233) • 1-800-787-3224 (TTY)
24 Hours • Confidential • Toll-free

FIGURE 21.2 ● A "palm card" can be handed discretely to a patient.

Time Constraints

Another reason commonly cited by physicians for not screening for IPV is lack of time (126, 131). The more recent pressure within a managed care setting to increase patient volume has exacerbated this problem. However, perception by the patient that the physician does not have enough time to talk about the cause of her injuries may result in her feeling ignored and trivialized (145). Furthermore, the perception that clinicians lack time to discuss abuse has been significantly associated with lack of disclosure (125, 146). It has been suggested that clinicians address time constraints by screening for IPV with a single question, such as "At any time has a partner ever hit you, kicked you, or otherwise physically hurt you?" An information palm card may then be offered, regardless of the response (Fig. 21.2).

Frustration at Inability to Help the Victim

Approximately one-third of gynecologists surveyed stated that they do not screen for IPV because, when abuse is detected, they are unable to help the victim. Doctors, nurses, and other medical care providers are trained to manage problems with "cure" or "fix it" as the management goal. However, management of IPV with a curative goal in mind may not be productive. Providers experienced in IPV counseling describe redefining their professional roles in helping potential victims (147). Those who understand that clinicians play a limited role in a patients' process of change focus on caring inquiry. Compassionate asking helps survivors and nonabused women by communicating that providers are concerned about this widespread problem, that women do not deserve abusive treatment, and that there are resources for those who are ready and able to make changes in their lives. Furthermore, abused women report that acknowledgment of abuse and confirmation of their worth by a health care provider "started the wheels turning" or "planted a seed" in their changing the way they perceived their situations (148). As one patient said, "Compassion is going to open the door, and when we feel safe and are able to trust, that makes a lot of difference" (149). Giving each woman a card with the NDVH number may "throw a lifeline" to the victim of IPV. She is empowered by having the information and the choice to use it. Thus, appropriate goals for management of IPV are not centered in the ability to heal or in the success in gaining direct disclosure, but in the ability to put the issue into the open, express concerns compassionately, and offer resource information.

Fear of Offending Patients

Often clinicians fear that patients will be offended by questions on abuse (150, 151). This particular fear has been expressed since the early literature of the 1980s, and the effect of time on repeated reports may perpetuate it. However, a number of studies have demonstrated that this fear is unfounded. In a more recent study on men and women seen in a primary care practice, 80% reported that they favored universal screening for assault (152). At least six additional studies confirmed that the majority of abused and nonabused women are in favor of clinical screening for violence (153). Women across the United States, representing various income levels and a mix of races/ethnicities endorse screening by their providers. A study on minority women demonstrated that this attitude is shared by Latina and Asian women (154). Abused women reported that talking about IPV could help solve the problem. The belief that patients would be uncomfortable is a serious misconception that hinders adequate access to health care.

Fear of Revisiting Personal History of Abuse

Physicians may also be reluctant to ask about IPV due to their own prior experiences. In one study, 13% of physicians cited a personal history of abuse as a barrier to screening (131). Women who have witnessed or experienced abuse in their own lives may be fearful that discussing IPV will evoke their own painful memories and make it difficult for them to maintain a professional demeanor (155).

Potential Legal Issues

Legal concerns, such as the possibility of testifying in court, having records under subpoena, or blaming an innocent partner may deter providers from screening for IPV (156). However, this apprehension may be reduced by obtaining information from the physician's state medical association and state attorney general's office or consulting with domestic violence coalition members (119). Most of these organizations or offices are available on Internet web pages. Often, a local women's shelter or a state professional organization can provide names of area lawyers experienced in working with IPV cases.

Misconceptions Based on Cultural, Socioeconomic, and Gender Prejudice

National surveys and clinical studies show that women of any age, race/ethnicity, educational level, geographic location, or socioeconomic status may be a victim of IPV. Despite this, health care providers often regard IPV as a problem limited to poor or minority patients. In one study, health care providers from five different communities stated that most cases of family violence occur in Latino, African American, Native American, or Southeast Asian communities and occur primarily in indigent families. In fact, almost 50% of obstetricians/gynecologists surveyed reported that they do not screen for IPV because they do not perceive this to be a problem among their private patients (131). When violence is detected among patients of higher socioeconomic groups, physicians are less likely to report these cases to protective services or the criminal justice agencies (157). Physicians are also less likely to recognize that abuse can occur in homosexual relationships or among the elderly.

Patient Factors That Hinder Disclosure

Patients cite many reasons for not wanting to talk with health care providers about abuse. Fear is the first barrier an abused woman must overcome in order to talk with a clinician (158). This may include fear of retaliation by the abusing partner, fear about loss of confidentiality, fear related to reporting to law enforcement and family services, and fear of judgment by the clinician (125, 145, 146, 149). Fear for themselves, their children, and their family members also acts as a barrier. Victims fear that outsiders cannot or will not help them and that they may lose whatever limited control they may have if authorities are involved.

Behaviors of the care provider may also deter disclosure (125, 146). Providers that seem uncaring, uncomfortable with the topic, inattentive, or rushed deter disclosure. Patients may feel alienated from providers of different cultural or socioeconomic background, thinking their circumstances would not be understood (84). Other problematic behaviors of providers cited by victims include accepting false explanations for injuries, treating injuries without asking the cause, minimizing the severity of the injury, implying the patient had triggered the abuse, acting angry, joking about IPV, advising patients to make up with their abusing partners, or excusing men for violence (125, 148, 159).

RECOMMENDATIONS FOR PROVIDERS

Screening: "Every Woman, Every Time"

Establish an environment that encourages providers to screen routinely, not as a result of any presenting factor or risk profile, and encourages women to disclose their victimization. This process requires an essential planning period that may include a review of current practices

Are you tired of making excuses for him?

Last week you fell. The week before it was an accident. Today you ran into a door.
Why should there be a next time?
Is someone hurting you?
Talk to your health care provider. We can help.

To find help near you, call the National Domestic Violence Hotline at:
1.800.799.7233 or 1.800.787.3224 (TTY)
TOGETHER, WE CAN STOP FAMILY VIOLENCE.

Made possible by a grant from The California Endowment. All characters depicted are models. ©2003

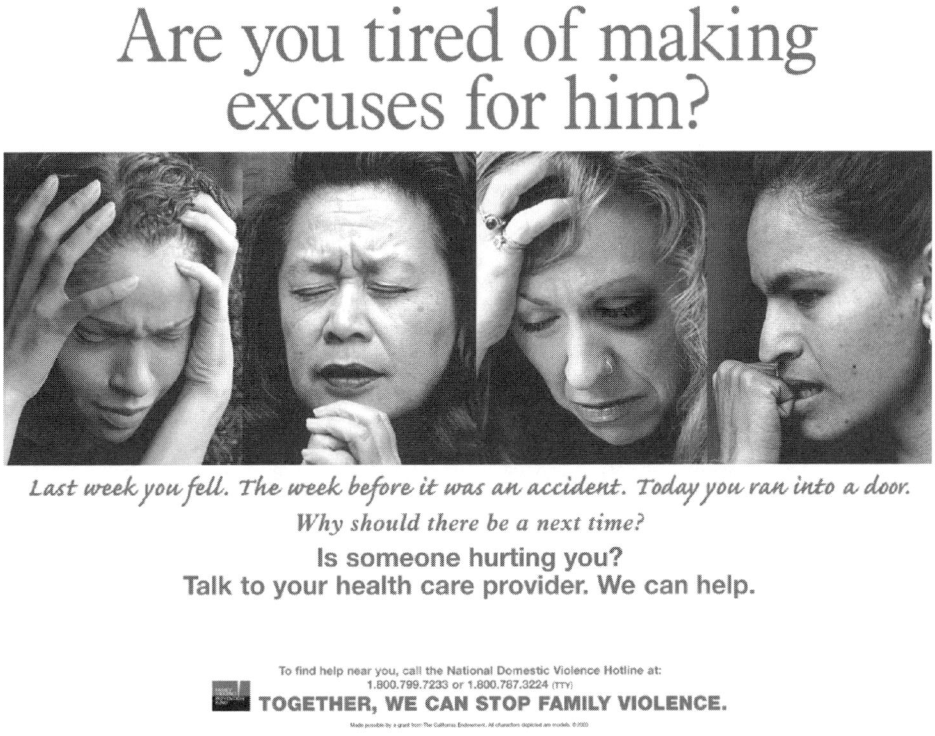

FIGURE 21.3 ● Posters placed in exam rooms and restrooms help patients trust the provider as a resource. (Reprinted with permission from the Family Violence Prevention Fund, www.endabuse.org.)

followed by developing protocols, training, modifying forms, and obtaining resource materials. Several systems approach models to accomplish this have been developed. In Texas, a systemic process-focused approach (plan change, do change, study results, act on results) was used that involved exploring what was being done elsewhere, what resources were available, and how these could work in that organization (156). Staff were trained, and when problems were discovered with physical facilities or logistics, they were dealt with as part of the continuing improvement process. Another systemic approach (the Precede/Proceed model of behavior change) described by Thompson and colleagues directed their efforts toward changing practitioner behaviors by determining factors that influenced screening practices (160). Yet another systems model approach increased clinician screening and referral by describing familiar steps for clinicians to follow if a patient disclosed IPV, providing easy and reliable referral to onsite resources, and establishing strong linkages with community services (161). These studies have promoted a number of beneficial changes and provided information for future improvements, as well as indicating that physician/staff education alone is insufficient. Systems support, including strategies such as established protocols, written questions, chart prompts, palm cards, and resource lists, are needed to increase provider's self-efficacy and performance.

Posters, such as those in Figures 21.3 and 21.4, brochures, and business-size palm cards with the NDVH on one side and local information on the other, should be placed in restrooms, exam rooms, and other locations where patient information is displayed. Such supportive information assures a victim that the provider and staff are aware and open to hearing about her issues and help establish trust that encourages women to talk about the abuse. A variety of materials is available from a number of sources (Appendix 21.1), although their use is not yet widespread. Only 5% of one group reported that such desirable support measures were available in their providers' offices (159). In addition to a supportive physical environment, the key ingredients to screening are trained providers and staff, an established IPV protocol,

Feeling alone?
Don't know who to talk to?

Is someone hurting you?
Talk to your health care provider. We can help.

To find help near you, call the National Domestic Violence Hotline at:
1.800.799.7233 or 1.800.787.3224 (TTY)
TOGETHER, WE CAN STOP FAMILY VIOLENCE.

Made possible by a grant from The California Endowment. All characters depicted are models. ©2000

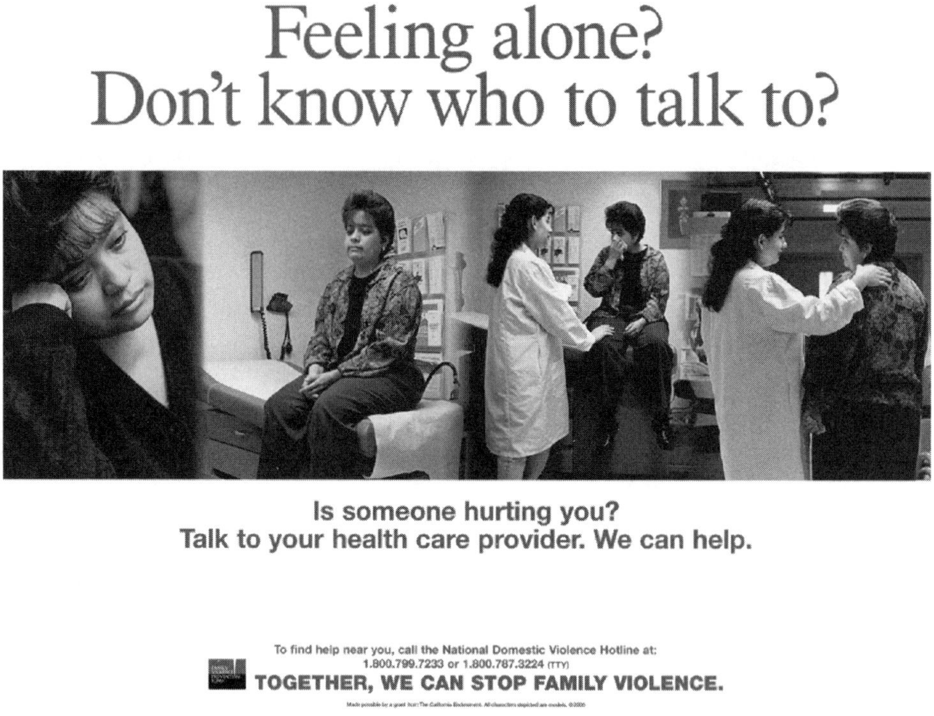

FIGURE 21.4 ● Health care providers continue to be the first and often the only professional contact made by victims of IPV. (Reprinted with permission from the Family Violence Prevention Fund, www.endabuse.org.)

a current listing of local resources, and structured, written screening questions on the patient history form (160). Furthermore, providers and staff should engage in ongoing interactive learning about IPV that includes state requirements, updates of local resources and connections, and a review of what works and does not about a particular protocol in their specific clinic setting.

The patient should be interviewed in private. In an effort to control the victim and prevent disclosure, many abusers accompany their partners to the emergency room or doctor's office. In fact, many abusers will complete medical history forms or answer medical history questions for their partners, never allowing the victim to respond (162). If this is the case, some means must be found to separate the victim from the abuser. When possible, the partner should be directed, not asked, to leave the examination room (159). An alternative strategy is to require the abuser to go to the reception area to complete forms. Another tactic is to request that the victim provide a urine sample or complete some other lab test. The nurse may accompany her to another area to complete this task and administer screening questions at this time. Once the interviewer and patient are alone, the woman must be reassured that the interview is confidential and that her answers will not be discussed with others without her permission. If confidentiality is not assured, many women will not disclose abuse because it is simply too dangerous for them to admit violence is a problem.

A patient who responds positively to direct questioning should be encouraged to elaborate. Validate her experience with assurances that she is not alone, does not deserve to be a victim of violence, and is not to blame for the abuse. Let her know resources are available to help her. Providing a woman with information and options that help her escape the abuse can give her a sense of control over her life. Avoid instructing the patient to leave her situation. If the victim declines discussing the problem during the visit, ask her at a follow-up visit if she wants to discuss it at that time.

Direct, Structured, Behavior-Specific Questions

When standard, structured questions are included as part of the health behavior inquiry, many practitioners gain confidence and easily adapt questioning about violence to their own practice style. Direct questioning is critical because 36% of all victims revealed they would divulge IPV only if asked directly (163). Following health behavior questions related to smoking, and diet and nutrition, a provider may easily introduce questions about IPV. Many physicians begin with stating, "Because violence is so common in many women's lives, I ask all my patients a few questions about it." Using specific behavioral words is more effective than asking if a patient has been physically or sexually abused because women may not identify themselves as victims of abuse. Many equate abuse with hitting or injury, not knowing that abuse may be of a sexual, psychological, or financial nature. This is also an appropriate time to mention the NDVH. Hotline information should be available to every patient and may be introduced as part of the screening process for health behaviors, much as you would introduce the availability of a smoking cessation program. Provide a palm card, such as the one in Figure 21.2, and say, "I give this card to all my patients, in case they should ever need this kind of help. The hotline can tell you how to get help in our area." The assurance that all patients are being asked these questions and provided the palm card helps prevent a woman from feeling singled out (35). To detect the verbal abuse characteristic of abuse in its earliest stage, many practitioners ask, "Does your partner threaten you, call you names, or yell at you?" (150). Various short questionnaires are also available, such as the Abuse Assessment Screen, the Woman Abuse Screening Tool (WAST), the WAST-Short, Women's Experience with Battering , the HITS Scale (hurt, insult, threat, scream), the Partner Violence Screen (PVS), and the Partner Abuse Interview (164, 165). Fogarty et al. reviewed these measures, including specific questions in 2002 (123). More recently developed measures include the Domestic Violence Survivor Assessment, which is also intended to determine the patient's current stage with regard to the change process and the Ongoing Abuse Screen (166, 167). Keep in mind that no one instrument can capture the complexity of IPV in all women's lives (166). Existing measures have been criticized for their length or impracticalities for clinical or emergency settings (167). There is some suggestion that the act of questioning itself, rather than specific sets of questions, is the heart of intervention in IPV.

Some practitioners screen patients for a history of current or past abuse using a self-reported health information questionnaire. Compared with discretionary oral inquiry, one printed question ("At any time has a partner ever hit you, kicked you, or otherwise physically hurt you?") increased identification of IPV from 0 to 11.6% (151). Although this is certainly better than not screening at all, most experts agree that direct questioning during the routine medical inquiry is a more effective way to elicit sensitive information (151). For example, in one study, identification of abuse increased from 7 to 30% when a written self-report was replaced with a nurse interview in which the same questions were asked orally (123). Use of structured interviewing questions has been demonstrated to result in higher rates of detection than a spontaneous interview that does not use a structured screen (168). However, many providers find that such measures are too long for clinical application (167, 169). The PVS, which consists of three brief questions, identified up to 71.4% of women who had experienced prior abuse (170). A fourth question is considered to be appropriate for clinical patients. Table 21.4 lists all four of these questions. In one study, a single oral question performed almost as well as the three-question PVS (169).

Most screening measures were developed in groups of White women. Specific studies on IPV and the needs of women of color are limited (73, 171, 172). No assessment tools have been developed for African American women (73). A Spanish version of WAST and WAST-Short has been validated (173).

Consent and Documentation

Providers should know their states' laws regarding informed consent and documentation. All findings should be documented clearly in the medical record. Informed consent must be obtained for the medical evaluation and treatment in all nonemergency conditions. The process includes the taking of photographs or radiographs of injuries resulting from IPV. All patients have the right to refuse such interventions. If the victim is younger than 18 years of age, parental consent

TABLE 21.4

Partner Violence Screening Questions

1. Have you been hit, kicked, punched, or otherwise hurt by someone within the past year? If so, by whom?[a]
2. Do you feel safe in your current relationship?
3. Is there a partner from a previous relationship who is making you feel unsafe now?
4. Add for clinical practice: Are you here today due to injury or illness related to partner violence?

[a] In one study, question 1 alone performed almost as well as the first three combined.

Adapted from Morrison LJ, Allan R, Grunfeld A. Improving the emergency department detection rate of domestic violence using direct questioning. J Emerg Med 2000;19:117–124; Feldhaus KM, Koziol-McLain J, Amsbury HL, et al. Accuracy of three brief screening questions for detecting partner violence in the emergency department. JAMA 1997;277:1357–1361.

is usually required. If, however, the parent is the suspected perpetrator, the physician may provide emergency treatment without parental consent. Permission to render nonemergency treatment may be obtained by court order or a court-appointed guardian. Some states also permit taking photographs and radiographs without parental consent in cases of suspected child abuse (174).

Accurate documentation in the medical record of injuries resulting from IPV will greatly assist the victim if she initiates court proceedings. The National Institute of Justice provides general recommendations for documentation (Table 21.5). Through your state medical association, you

TABLE 21.5

Documentation of Intimate Partner Violence

Do All of These	Avoid All of These
• Obtain signed informed consent form. • Take photographs of injuries known or suspected to have resulted from IPV. • Use a body map (Fig. 21.5), and mark the location, size, and age of injuries observed during the medical exam. • Write legibly or have notes transcribed and hardcopy placed in record. • Use medical terms. • Record patient's exact words, and set off patient's words with quotation marks. Use phrases such as: *patient states*. Describe the abuse by using quotation marks such as: *The patient stated, "My boyfriend kicked me."* • Describe patient's demeanor (crying, shaking, angry, calm, etc.), even if her demeanor belies evidence of abuse. • Record time of examination, and if possible, indicate how much time has elapsed since abuse occurred. Example: *Patient states that boyfriend kicked her early this morning, about 10:00 AM. Examined at 2:00 PM.*	• Avoid legal terms such as "alleged perpetrator" or "assault." • Avoid phrases such as "patient claims" or "patient alleges." • Avoid inserting your personal comments or judgments, such as "patient is a battered woman" or "a case of assault and battery." These are inadmissible in court. • Avoid making personal comments about her appearance, manner, or motive for stating abuse has occurred. • Avoid using terms such as "domestic violence," "DV," "intimate partner violence," or "IPV" in the diagnosis section of the medical record. Whether such violence has occurred is to be determined by the court.

Adapted from Refs. 175–177.

may learn your state's requirements for documentation and evidence collection. For example, some require that informed consent be signed prior to photographic documentation. Others require proof of "chain of custody" (written descriptions of sequential actions by whom and with what, with regard to clothing or other items). You must also be aware of your state's reporting requirements for injuries, IPV, human bites, and sexual assault. Your goal is to preserve evidence and to document your findings in ways that will be useful to the patient.

If a woman reports that she is not abused, but signs and symptoms seem to indicate otherwise, the provider should note that in the record. Choice of language is important. Avoid using phrases such as "alleged abuse," "abuse ruled out," or "patient denies abuse" because these could be used against the victim at a later date. These are also not permissible with external cause of injury codes. Again, states vary in their requirements.

Note in the record the date and location of the attack, and the name and relationship of the perpetrator, and the patient's description of how the injury occurred. Medical descriptions of the injury may be included but should not replace the victims' own words. For example, record "My boyfriend hit me in the lip" rather than "Patient sustained injury to lip." A patient's record may be admissible if it meets the criteria for "excited utterances" (175). The criteria require that the record demonstrate that the patient made the statement while responding to questions about the event stimulating the utterance (i.e., the abuse). Also required are documentation of the time interval between the event and the statements, and documentation of the patient's demeanor as she made the statement. Inconsistencies between the appearance of the injury and the patient's explanation of how it occurred should also be recorded.

All injuries observed should be described in the medical record and marked on a body map (Fig. 21.5). If old injuries are apparent, these should be marked on a second body map. Photographs offer visual proof of the injury but must be accompanied by written description. Color photographs of newly acquired injuries should be taken after obtaining written consent. The patient's face should be included, if possible. A card with the patient's name and hospital or patient number, as well as the date and time, should be held by a staff member and included in each photograph. If available, a camera data back will record the patient's name and identifying number directly on the photograph. The back of each photograph should be legibly marked with the photographer's name. Other physical evidence of abuse, such as torn or bloody clothing, should also be labeled and stored in paper bags or boxes, not in plastic bags. Your state may require that each item be placed in separate paper bags, labeled, and sealed. If sexual abuse has occurred, the evidence should be properly collected (after obtaining informed consent) using a forensic rape kit, labeled, and given to authorities (176).

Adult human bite marks are common, and most often are found on breasts, abdomen, or thighs of women. Adult bite marks are much larger than those of children. If compared with dog bites that feature a V-shape with deep intermittent punctures, a human bite mark is elliptical in shape, of superficial depth, and causes abrasions (177). Wear gloves when examining bite marks, and collect traces of saliva before cleaning the wound. This may help identify the abuser.

Good legible documentation often eliminates the necessity of the physician testifying in court. If the physician must testify, a carefully recorded medical chart can be useful to refresh his or her memory. Questions of confidentiality in domestic abuse cases may be affected by the Health Insurance Portability and Accountability Act of 1996 (HIPAA) (178). (See the AMA HIPAA website at www.ama-assn.org/go/hipaa.) Good documentation may also help the victim obtain a protective order, retain custody of her children, or eliminate the need for her to testify in court. The value of good documentation cannot be underestimated. If the case later comes to trial, the medical record may be the only evidence that abuse occurred besides the victim's report. The potential importance of the record underscores the provider's responsibility to know and follow state requirements for admissibility in court.

Immediate Safety Assessment

If a patient discloses abuse, assess her immediate safety by asking the victim if she is afraid to go home and if there are guns or other weapons in the house. Assess the safety of children by asking if there have been threats to them as well. If the patient is in eminent danger, help her

DOMESTIC VIOLENCE SCREENING/DOCUMENTATION FORM

DV Screen
❒ DV+ (Positive)
❒ DV? (Suspected)

Date ______________ Patient ID#____________
Patient Name ______________________________
Provider Name______________________________
Patient Pregnant? ❒ Yes ❒ No

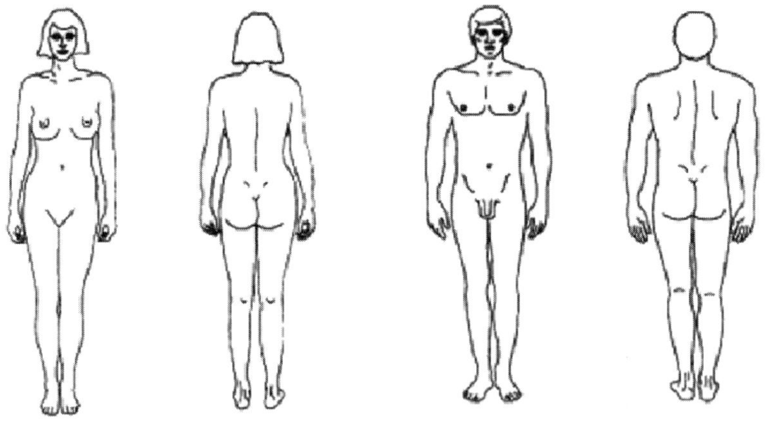

ASSESS PATIENT SAFETY

❒ Yes ❒ No Is abuser here now?
❒ Yes ❒ No Is patient afraid of their partner?
❒ Yes ❒ No Is patient afraid to go home?
❒ Yes ❒ No Has physical violence increased in severity?
❒ Yes ❒ No Has partner physically abused children?
❒ Yes ❒ No Have children witnessed violence in the home?
❒ Yes ❒ No Threats of homicide?
By whom: ______________________________
❒ Yes ❒ No Threats of suicide?
By whom: ______________________________
❒ Yes ❒ No Is there a gun in the home?
❒ Yes ❒ No Alcohol or substance abuse?
❒ Yes ❒ No Was safety plan discussed?

REFERRALS

❒ Hotline number given
❒ Legal referral made
❒ Shelter number given
❒ In-house referral made
Describe: ______________________________
❒ Other referral made
Describe: ______________________________

REPORTING

❒ Law enforcement report made
❒ Child Protective Services report made
❒ Adult Protective Services report made

PHOTOGRAPHS

❒ Yes ❒ No Consent to be photographed?
❒ Yes ❒ No Photographs taken?
Attach photograph and consent form

FIGURE 21.5 ● A standard documentation form should include a body map. (Reprinted from Clinical Guidelines on Routine Screening, from the Family Violence Prevention Fund, www.endabuse.org, with permission.)

determine if there is someone with whom she can stay. Provide her with a private space where she may make phone calls and give her a list of local shelters that includes the NDVH. Shelters often have advocates who will pick her up, if needed. They may ask to meet her at the back entrance as a safety precaution. The provider may also offer ideas for developing a safety plan for quickly leaving the abusive situation (Table 21.6). Although the physician has an obligation to counsel and refer the patient to appropriate agencies and shelters, the patient must be the one to determine when it is safe to change her life situation (179).

Intervention and Referral Options

Physicians who are knowledgeable about the resources in their community are best equipped to assist victims of IPV. Optimal care for a woman in an abusive relationship depends on the

TABLE 21.6

Establish a Safety Plan

For help in developing a personal safety plan, women may get information from the National Domestic Violence Hotline (Fig. 21.2).

Women who are ready to leave the relationship should pack a bag in advance and leave it with a neighbor or friend. Include cash, extra clothes, and perhaps bus tokens. Include a toy if there are children.

Women should hide an extra set of car and house keys outside the house in case they have to leave quickly.

Women should take important papers:

- Birth certificates for self and children
- Health insurance cards, medicine, medical records
- Deed or lease to house or apartment
- Checkbook, extra checks, bank account number, ATM cards, credit cards, bank statements, credit card statements
- Social security card or green card/work permit
- Court papers or orders, welfare papers, police reports, marriage license
- Driver's license or other photo ID
- Proof of income for self and partner, pay stubs
- Phone numbers for friends and family; cell phone, if possible

Adapted from American College of Obstetricians and Gynecologists (ACOG). Committee on Underserved Women. ACOG Educational Bulletin: Domestic Violence. No. 257. ACOG, December 1999.

provider's knowledge of community resources that can provide safety, advocacy, and support (2). Again, an excellent starting point is the NDVH. Legal assistance may be available through legal aid programs for low-income women, legal adjuncts of shelters or other agencies, bar association referral services, criminal justice advocacy units, and immigration assistance organizations (178). State coalitions on family violence or domestic violence can provide information on resources in the local area.

Assessment and intervention in these cases must respect patient's autonomy and be offered in a collaborative spirit (74). Disallowing the right to a choice may only further disempower the victim, who may feel betrayed by the abusive partner and the system that is supposed to offer protection.

Resources for Providers

During the 1990s, resources on IPV became readily available to health care providers. Professional medical associations, privately funded resource centers, and federal agencies developed instructional materials, patient education materials, computerized slide presentations, and medical education curricula on topics related to IPV (180). Videotapes, CD-ROM programs, and online training guides are also available. Help for special needs of survivors is also available through professional organizations (Appendix 21.2).

Advise patients of the 24-hour, toll-free NDVH (Fig. 21.2) (181). This is the least complicated and sometimes the most effective and immediate referral a health care provider may offer. Small announcement posters and business card-size handouts with hotline information can be generated easily on office computers. Callers receive counseling in English, Spanish, and several other languages, and can be referred directly to help in their communities, including emergency services and shelters. The number of calls to the hotline have increased by 133% since its beginning in 1996, with the millionth call in 2003. During that year, the hotline received an average of 15,000 calls per month.

Clinical Notes

INTIMATE PARTNER VIOLENCE

- IPV is no longer a private family matter. It is a crime.
- One in four women of all ages, races, educational levels, geographic locations, and socioeconomic status are affected.
- Changes in traditional services, including medical care, are needed to meet the needs of abused women.
- Safety for victims and their children is a priority.

DYNAMICS OF INTIMATE PARTNER VIOLENCE

- IPV is an ongoing, debilitating experience of physical, psychological, and/or sexual abuse in the home.
- IPV is a pattern of coercive behavior designed to exert power and control in an intimate relationship.
- Abusers use acts of and threats of physical or sexual assault to maintain control.
- Abusers use tactics such as intimidation, humiliation, blaming, or harassing behaviors. They may isolate a woman from family and friends, monitor her activities, and restrict her access to money, transportation, or medical care.

BARRIERS TO LEAVING AN ABUSIVE RELATIONSHIP

- Women may fear reprisals to themselves and to their children, friends, or family.
- Social isolation may deter women from understanding the risks in their situations. Isolation augments the effects of fear.
- Women may not know about available resources or how to access them.
- Women may leave and return to the abusive relationship several times before they are able to make a permanent change.

ROLE OF HEALTH CARE PROVIDERS

- Know state and national mandates regarding IPV, documentation, and coding.
- Recognize own attitudes about IPV.
- Provide a supportive environment with posters, brochures, and palm cards.
- Incorporate IPV screening in the preventive inquiry about smoking, alcohol use, diet/nutrition, and so on.
- Screen every woman, every time, in privacy.
- Acknowledge the widespread nature of IPV—that no woman deserves to be abused and that resources are available.
- When abuse is disclosed, (a) communicate nonjudgmentally and compassionately, (b) assess immediate safety, (c) help establish safety plan, (d) offer educational materials, (e) offer list of community and local resources, and (f) document interactions.
- Documentation should include the patient's language, photographs with consent, and a body map of injuries.

RESOURCES

- Begin with the NDVH.
- Refer to Internet web pages for the AMA, ACOG, your state government, and your particular professional organization.

APPENDIX 21.1

Selected Resources for Providers

See References for additional online resources. All URLs and telephone numbers are active as of June 2004.

American College of Obstetricians and Gynecologists (ACOG)

www.acog.org (select Women's Issues, then Violence Against Women)

- Pamphlet: The Abused Woman
- Palm cards for women and teens
- Posters
- Slide lecture presentation: Domestic Violence: The Role of the Physician in Identification, Intervention, and Prevention (English and Spanish)
- CME video and monograph: Clinical Aspects of Domestic Violence for the Ob-Gyn
- Educational Bulletin: Domestic Violence #257; Sexual Assault #242
- Committee Opinion: Mandatory Reporting of Domestic Violence #200

American Medical Association (AMA)

www.ama-assn.org

- Diagnostic and Treatment Guidelines on Domestic Violence: http://www.ama-assn.org/ama1/pub/upload/mm/386/domesticviolence.pdf
- HIPAA resource site: www.ama-assn.org/go/hipaa

American Medical Women's Association (AMWA)

- Online CME course: Domestic Violence: http://www.dvcme.org/

Minnesota Program Development, Inc.

- The Duluth Model: www.duluth-model.org
- Power Wheel Model: training programs, books, manuals, posters, online catalog and information

Family Violence Prevention Fund and National Health Resource Center

1-888-RX-ABUSE; www.endabuse.org (select Health)

- National Consensus Guidelines on Identifying and Responding to Domestic Violence Victimization in Health Care Settings 2004
- Resource and Trainer's Manual: Improving the Health Care Response to Domestic Violence
- Video: Screen to End Abuse (suggestions to health care providers) 2003
- State by State Report Card on Health Care and Domestic Violence Statutes
- Palm cards, posters, screening form with body map, practitioner reference cards, domestic violence protocols, information on privacy, coding, documentation
- Most material available online, from free CD-ROM, or at nominal cost

Institute for Clinical Systems Improvement, Bloomington, MN

952-814-7060; www.icsi.org (search keyword, "domestic violence")

- Online Health Care Guidelines: Domestic Violence (decision pathway, screening questions, etc.), updated annually (free)

National Advisory Council on Violence Against Women, Violence Against Women Office, U.S. Department of Health and Human Services

- Toolkit to End Violence Against Women: http://toolkit.ncjrs.org/

National Center for Injury Prevention and Control (NCIPC), Centers for Disease Control and Prevention (CDC)

http://www.cdc.gov/ncipc (select Intimate Partner Violence)

- Intimate Partner Violence and Sexual Assault: A Guide to Training Materials and Programs for Health Care Providers, 1998: http://www.cdc.gov/ncipc/pub-res/pdf/newguide.pdf
- Up-to-date statistics and links

National Coalition Against Domestic Violence (NCADV)

303-839-1852; http://www.ncadv.org/

- Cosmetic and Reconstructive Support Program
- Resource manual: Open Minds Open Doors: Working with Women with Disabilities
- Resource manual: Rural Task Force Resource Packet
- Resource manual: Teen Dating Violence
- Resource manual: National Directory of Domestic Violence Programs: A Guide to Community Shelter
- Video and teaching guide: Rough Love
- Online personal safety worksheet
- Posters, bumper stickers, buttons

National Domestic Violence Hotline (NDVH)

1-800-799-SAFE (7233), 1-800-787-3224 (TTY); www.ndvh.org

- Federally funded, multilingual, 24-hour advocacy and referral to local resources
- National database of emergency shelters, legal advocacy, and social service programs
- Safety planning, special programs for survivors

National Victim Assistance Academy

http://www.nvaa.org (Select Curriculum and Instruction)

- Online comprehensive text
- Annual 4-day training conducted by nationally recognized experts

National Resource Center on Domestic Violence

1-800-537-2238; www.vawnet.org

- Broad selection of online materials
- Posters, magnets, bumper stickers

APPENDIX 21.2

Resources for Survivors With Special Needs

Cosmetic and Reconstructive Support (CRS) Program

The CRS program is a direct service program of the National Coalition Against Domestic Violence (NCADV) and three medical associations to assist survivors of IPV who cannot afford cosmetic/reconstructive surgery or dentistry to repair injuries caused by a spouse or intimate partner. Facial surgeons, cosmetic dentists, and dermatologic surgeons from across the United States volunteer their services to assist survivors in removing the physical scars of abuse.

Eligibility criteria for program participation vary; however, all problems must be due to the effects of domestic violence caused by spouse or partner. If a survivor meets eligibility criteria for consideration, the appropriate program will provide a referral to a local plastic surgeon, dermatologist, or dentist. NCADV is the initial contact for eligibility screening.

Face to Face: The National Domestic Violence Project

Repair physical scars or injuries located on the head, face, and neck.

1-800-842-4546; http://www.facial-plastic-surgery.org/patient/humanitarian/pa_ffviolence.html

Partner: Educational and Research Foundation of the American Academy of Facial Plastic and Reconstructive Surgery (AAFPRS)

Give Back A Smile (GBAS) Program

Repair front teeth.

1-800-773-4227; www.givebackasmile.com

Partner: National Humanitarian Program and AACD Charitable Foundation of the American Academy of Cosmetic Dentistry (AACD)

Skin Care Outreach Empowers Survivors (S.C.O.R.E.S.) Program

Repair skin injuries (scars, burns, tattoos)

1-888-892-6702

Partner: American Society for Dermatologic Surgery (ASDS)

REFERENCES

1. Tjaden P, Thoennes N. Full Report of the Prevalence, Incidence, and Consequences of Violence Against Women. Findings from the National Violence Against Women Survey. NCJ 183781. Washington, DC: U.S. Department of Justice, Office of Justice Programs, November 2000. Available at: http://www.ncjrs.org/pdffiles1/nij/183781.pdf. Accessed August 1, 2005.
2. American Medical Association. Diagnostic and Treatment Guidelines on Domestic Violence. March 1992. Available at: http://www.ama-assn.org/ama1/pub/upload/mm/386/domesticviolence.pdf. Accessed August 1, 2005.
3. Crowell NA, Burgess AW, eds. Understanding Violence Against Women. Panel on Research on Violence Against Women, National Research Council. Washington, DC: National Academy Press, 1996.
4. Moore M. Reproductive health and intimate partner violence. Fam Plann Perspect 1999;31:304–312.
5. Saltzman LE, Fanslow JL, McMahon PM, et al. Intimate Partner Violence Surveillance: Uniform Definitions and Recommended Data Elements, Version 1.0. Atlanta: Centers for Disease Control and Prevention, National Center for Injury Prevention and Control, 1999. Available at: http://www.cdc.gov/ncipc/pub-res/udrde.pdf. Accessed August 1, 2005.
6. National Center for Injury Prevention and Control. Injury Fact Book 2001–2002. Atlanta: Centers for Disease Control and Prevention, 2001. Available at: http://www.cdc.gov/ncipc/fact_book/factbook.htm#pdf. Accessed August 1, 2005.
7. Plichta SB, Falik M. Prevalence of violence and its implications for women's health. Womens Health Issues 2001;11:244–258.
8. Tjaden P, Thoennes N. Extent, Nature, and Consequences of Intimate Partner Violence. Findings from the National Violence Against Women Survey. NCJ 181867. Washington, DC: U.S. Department of Justice, Office of Justice Programs, July 2000. Available at: http://www.ncjrs.org/pdffiles1/nij/181867.pdf. Accessed August 1, 2005.
9. Plichta SB, Weisman CS. Spouse or partner abuse, use of health services, and unmet need for medical care in U.S. women. J Womens Health 1995;4:45–54.
10. Greenfield LA, Rand MR, Craven D, et al. Bureau of Justice Statistics Factbook. Violence by Intimates. Analysis of Data on Crimes by Current or Former Spouses, Boyfriends, and Girlfriends. NCJ 167237. Washington, DC: U.S. Department of Justice, Office of Justice Programs, March 1998. Available at: http://www.ojp.usdoj.gov/bjs/pub/pdf/vi.pdf. Accessed August 1, 2005.
11. Collins KS, Schoen C, Joseph S, et al. Health Concerns Across a Woman's Lifespan: The Commonwealth Fund 1998 Survey of Women's Health. New York: The Commonwealth Fund, 1999. Available at: http://www.cmwf.org/publications/publications_show.htm?doc_id=221554. Accessed August 1, 2005.
12. Petersen R, Gazmararian J, Andersen KA. Partner violence: implications for health and community settings. Womens Health Issues 2001;11:116–125.
13. Rennison CM, Welchans S. Bureau of Justice Statistics Special Report: Intimate Partner Violence. NCJ 178247. Washington, DC: U.S. Department of Justice, May 2000. Available at: http://www.ojp.usdoj.gov/bjs/pub/pdf/ipv.pdf. Accessed August 1, 2005.
14. Wilt S, Olson S. Prevalence of domestic violence in the United States. JAMA 1996;51:77–82.
15. Laurence L, Spalter-Roth R. Measuring the Costs of Domestic Violence Against Women and the Cost-effectiveness of Interventions: An Initial Assessment and Proposals for Further Research. Washington, DC: Institute for Women's Policy Research, 1996.
16. Egger E. Capitation, quality issues make domestic violence a "medical" issue. Health Care Strateg Manage 1999;17:10–11.
17. Chalk R, King P, eds. Violence in Families: Assessing Prevention and Treatment Programs. Washington, DC: National Academy Press, 1998.
18. Gerberding JL, Binder S, Hammond WR, et al. Costs of Intimate Partner Violence Against Women in the United States. Atlanta: National Center for Injury Prevention and Control, Centers for Disease Control and Prevention, 2003. Available at: http://www.cdc.gov/ncipc/pub-res/ipv_cost/IPVBook-Final-Feb18.pdf. Accessed August 1, 2005.
19. Miller TR, Cohen MA, Wiersema B. The Extent and Costs of Crime Victimization: A New Look. National Institute of Justice Research Preview. Washington, DC: U.S. Department of Justice, Office of Justice Programs, January 1996. Available at: www.ncjrs.org/. Accessed August 1, 2005.
20. Cohn F, Salmon ME, Stobo JD, eds. Confronting Chronic Neglect: The Education and Training of Health Professionals on Family Violence. Washington, DC: National Academy Press, 2002.
21. O'Leary KD. Psychological abuse: a variable deserving critical attention in domestic violence. Violence Vict 1999;14:3–23.
22. Walker L. The Battered Woman. New York: Harper & Row, 1979.
23. Pence E, Paymar M. Education Groups for Men Who Batter: The Duluth Model. New York: Springer, 1993.
24. Minnesota Program Development, Inc. The Duluth Model. Duluth: Minnesota Program Development, Inc., 2002. Available at: www.duluth-model.org. Accessed August 1, 2005.
25. Meuer T, Seymour A, Wallace H. Domestic violence. In: Seymour A, Murray M, Sigmon J, et al., eds. National Victim Assistance Academy Textbook. Washington, DC: U.S. Department of Justice, Office of Justice Programs, June 2001. Available at: www.ojp.usdoj.gov/ovc/assist/nvaa2001. Accessed August 1, 2005.

26. Mankowski ES, Haaken J, Silvergleid CS. Collateral damage: an analysis of the achievements and unintended consequences of batterer intervention programs and discourse. J Fam Viol 2002;17:167–184.
27. Healey K, Smith C, O'Sullivan C. Batterer Intervention: Program Approaches and Criminal Justice Strategies. Washington, DC: National Institute of Justice, U.S. Department of Justice, February 1998. Available at: http://www.ncjrs.org/pdffiles/168638.pdf. Accessed August 1, 2005.
28. Bennett L, Williams O. In Brief: Controversies and Recent Studies of Batterer Intervention Program Effectiveness. Applied Research Forum. National Electronic Network on Violence Against Women (VAWnet), August 2001. Available at: http://www.vawnet.org/DomesticViolence/Research/VAWnetDocs/AR_bip.pdf. Accessed August 1, 2005.
29. National Women's Health Information Center. Violence Against Women. The Office on Women's Health, U.S. Department of Health and Human Services. Available at: http://www.4woman.gov/owh/violence.htm. Accessed August 1, 2005.
30. Taylor BG, Davis RC, Maxwell CD. The effects of a group batterer treatment program in Brooklyn. Justice Q 2001;18:170–201.
31. McGrath ME, Bettacchi A, Duffy SJ, et al. Violence against women: provider barriers to intervention in emergency departments. Acad Emerg Med 1997;4:297–300.
32. Chescheir N. Violence against women: response from clinicians. Ann Emerg Med 1996;27:766–768.
33. Landenburger K. The dynamics of leaving and recovering from an abusive relationship. JOGNN 1998;27: 700–706.
34. Martin AJ, Berenson KR, Griffing S, et al. The process of leaving an abusive relationship: the role of risk assessments and decision-certainty. J Fam Viol 2000;15:109–122.
35. Heise L, Ellsberg M, Gottemoeller M. Ending Violence Against Women. Population Reports, Series L, No. 11. Baltimore: Johns Hopkins University School of Public Health, Population Information Program, December 1999. Available at: http://www.jhuccp.org/pr/l11/violence.pdf. Accessed August 1, 2005.
36. Braude M. When should physicians report domestic violence? Hosp Pract (Off Ed) 2000;35:F12:15–16.
37. Carpenito LJ. Domestic violence: why do they stay? Nurs Forum 1996;31:3–4
38. Gemignani J. Missed opportunities in the fight against domestic violence. Bus Health 2000;18:29, 32–35.
39. Browne A. Violence against women by male partners. Am Psychol 1993;48:1077–1087.
40. Russell DEH. Rape in Marriage. Bloomington: Indiana University Press, 1990.
41. Mega LT, Mega JL, Mega BT, et al. Brainwashing and battering fatigue. Psychological abuse in domestic violence. N C Med J 2000;61:260–265.
42. Physicians for Human Rights (PHR). Examining Asylum Seekers: A Health Professional's Guide to Medical and Psychological Evaluations of Torture. Washington, DC: PHR, August 2001. Available at: http://www.phrusa.org. Accessed August 1, 2005.
43. Krishnan SP, Hilbert JC. In search of sanctuary: addressing issues of domestic violence and homelessness at shelters. Womens Health Issues 1998;8:310–316.
44. Zorza J. Woman battering: a major cause of homelessness. Clearinghouse Rev 1991;24:421–442.
45. The United States Conference of Mayors. A Status Report on Hunger and Homelessness in America's Cities: A 25-city Survey. December 2000. Available at: http://www.usmayors.org/uscm/hungersurvey/2000/hunger2000.pdf. Accessed August 1, 2005.
46. The United States Conference of Mayors. A Status Report on Hunger and Homelessness in America's Cities: A 25-city Survey. December 2001. Available at: http://www.usmayors.org/uscm/hungersurvey/2001/hungersurvey2001.pdf. Accessed August 1, 2005.
47. Roberts AR, Lewis SJ. Giving them shelter: national organizational survey of shelters for battered women and their children. J Community Psychol 2000;6:669–681.
48. Donnelly DA, Cook, KJ, Wilson LA. Provision and exclusion: the dual face of services to battered women in three deep south states. Violence Against Women 1999;5:710–741.
49. Panzer PG, Philip MB, Hayward RA. Trends in domestic violence service and leadership: implications for an integrated shelter model. Adm Policy Ment Health 2000;27:339–352.
50. Office of Attorney General. Statistics on Family Violence. State of Texas. Available at: http://www.oag.state.tx.us. Accessed August 1, 2005.
51. McKay MM. The link between domestic violence and child abuse: assessment and treatment considerations. Child Welfare 1994;73:29–39.
52. Galbraith S, Rubinstein G. Alcohol, drugs, and domestic violence: confronting barriers to changing practice and policy. J Am Med Wom Assoc 1996;51:115–117.
53. Goldberg ME. Substance-abusing women: false stereotypes and real needs. Soc Work 1995;40:189–798.
54. Correia A, Rubin J. Housing and Battered Women. Applied Research Forum, National Electronic Network on Violence Against Women (VAWnet), November 2001. Available at: http://www.vawnet.org/DomesticViolence/Research/VAWnetDocs/AR_housing.pdf. Accessed August 1, 2005.
55. The Pennsylvania Coalition Against Domestic Violence and the Women's Law Project. Insurance Discrimination Against Victims of Domestic Violence. July 1998. Available at: http://www.vawnet.org/PCADVPublications/PapersReports/PCADV_insdis.pdf. Accessed August 1, 2005.
56. Family Violence Prevention Fund. Health Report Card 2001. Available at: www.endabuse.org. Accessed August 1, 2005.
57. Easley M. Domestic violence. Ann Emerg Med 1996;27:762–763.
58. Fleury RE, Sullivan CM, Bybee DI, et al. "Why don't they just call the cops?": Reasons for differential police contact among women with abusive partners. Violence Vict 1998;13:333–346.

59. Wolf ME, Holt VL, Kernic MA, et al. Who gets protection orders for intimate partner violence? Am J Prev Med 2000;19:286–291.
60. Kernic MA, Wolf ME, Holt VL. Rates and relative risk of hospital admission among women in violent intimate partner relationships. Am J Pub Health 2000;90:1416–1420.
61. Gist JH, McFarlane J, Malecah A, et al. Women in danger: intimate partner violence experienced by women who qualify and do not qualify for a protective order. Behav Sci Law 2001;19:637–647.
62. Office for Victims of Crime. Enforcement of Protective Orders. Legal Series Bulletin #4. NCJ 189190. Washington, DC: U.S. Department of Justice, Office of Justice Programs, January 2002. Available at: http://www.ojp.usdoj.gov/ovc/publications/bulletins/legalseries/bulletin4/ncj189190.pdf. Accessed August 1, 2005.
63. Maxwell CD, Garner JH, Fagan JA. Research in Brief: The Effects of Arrest on Intimate Partner Violence: New Evidence from the Spouse Assault Replication Program. NCJ 188199. Washington, DC: U.S. Department of Justice, National Institute of Justice, July 2001. Available at: http://www.ncjrs.org/pdffiles1/nij/188199.pdf . Accessed August 1, 2005.
64. Kaci JH. Aftermath of seeking domestic violence protective orders: the victim's perspective. J Contemp Crim Just 1994;10:201–219.
65. Keilitz SL, Hannaford PL, Efkeman HS. Civil Protection Orders: The Benefits and Limitations for Victims of Domestic Violence. Williamsburg, VA: National Center for State Courts, 1997.
66. Harrell A, Smith B, Newmark L. Court Processing and the Effects of Restraining Orders for Domestic Violence Victims. Washington, DC: The Urban Institute, 1993.
67. Klein AR. Re-abuse in a population of court-restrained male batterers: why restraining orders don't work. In: Buzawa ED, Buzawa CG, eds. Do Arrests and Restraining Orders Work. Thousand Oaks, CA: Sage, 1996:192–213.
68. McCauley J, Kern DE, Kolodner K, et al. The "battering syndrome": prevalence and clinical characteristics of domestic violence in primary care internal medicine practices. Ann Intern Med 1995;123:737–746.
69. Leserman J, Li D, Drossman DA, et al. Selected symptoms associated with sexual and physical abuse among female patients with gastrointestinal disorders: the impact on subsequent health care visits. Psychol Med 1998;28:417–425.
70. Eisenstat SA, Bancroft L. Primary care: domestic violence. N Engl J Med 1999;34:886–892.
71. Coker AL, Smith PH, Bethea L, et al. Physical health consequences of physical and psychological intimate partner violence. Arch Fam Med 2000;9:451–457.
72. Coker AL, Sanderson M, Fadden MK, et al. Intimate partner violence and cervical neoplasia. J Womens Health Gend Based Med 2000;9:1015–1023.
73. Campbell DW, Sharps PW, Gary F, et al. Intimate partner violence in African American women. Online J Issues Nursing 2002;7. Available at: http://www.nursingworld.org/ojin/topic17/tpc17_4.htm. Accessed August 1, 2005.
74. Campbell JC. Health consequences of intimate partner violence. Lancet 2002;359:1331–1336.
75. Poole GV, Martin JN Jr, Perry KG Jr, et al. Trauma in pregnancy: the role of interpersonal violence. Am J Obstet Gynecol 1996;174:1873–1878.
76. Abbott J, Johnson R, Koziol-McLain J, et al. Domestic violence against women: incidence and prevalence in an emergency department population. JAMA 1995;273:1763–1767.
77. Campbell J, Snow Jones A, Dienemann J, et al. Intimate partner violence and physical health consequences. Arch Intern Med 2002;162:1157–1163.
78. Rennison CM. Bureau of Justice Statistics Special Report: Intimate Partner Violence and Age of Victim, 1993–1999. NCJ 187635. Washington, DC: U.S. Department of Justice, October 2001. Available at: http://www.ojp.usdoj.gov/bjs/pub/pdf/ipva99.pdf. Accessed August 1, 2005.
79. Paulozzi LJ, Saltzman LE, Thompson MP, et al. Surveillance for homicide among intimate partners—United States, 1981–1998. MMWR Morb Mortal Wkly Rep 2001;50(SS03):1–16.
80. McCoy M. Domestic violence: clues to victimization. Ann Emerg Med 1996;27:764–765.
81. Muellerman R, Lenaghan PA, Pakieser RA. Battered women: injury locations and types. Ann Emerg Med 1996;28:486–492.
82. Grisso JA, Schwarz DF, Hirschinger N, et al. Violent injuries among women in an urban area. N Engl J Med 1999;341:1899–1905.
83. Wilbur L, Higley M, Hatfield J, et al. Violence: recognition management, and prevention: survey results of women who have been strangled while in an abusive relationship. J Emerg Med 2001;21:297–302.
84. Guth AA, Pachter HL. Domestic violence and the trauma surgeon. Am J Surg 2000;179:134–140.
85. Olson L, Anctil C, Fullerton L, et al. Increasing emergency physician recognition of domestic violence. Ann Emerg Med 1996;27:741–745.
86. Alpert EJ. Violence in intimate relationships and the practicing internist: new "disease" or new agenda? Ann Intern Med 1995;123:774–781.
87. Dearwater SR, Coben JH, Nah G, et al. Prevalence of domestic violence in women treated at community hospital emergency department. JAMA 1998;480:433–438.
88. Richardson J, Feder G. Domestic violence: a hidden problem for general practice. Br J Gen Pract 1996;46:239–242.
89. Swett C. High rates of alcohol problems and history of physical and sexual abuse among women inpatients. Am J Drug Alcohol Abuse 1994;20:263–272.
90. Koss MP, Heslet L. Somatic consequences of violence against women. Arch Fam Med 1992;1:53–59.

91. Campbell R, Sullivan CM, Davidson WS. Women who use domestic violence shelters: changes in depression over time. Psych Women Q 1995;19:237–255.
92. Silva C, McFarlane J, Soeken K, et al. Symptoms of post-traumatic stress disorder in abused women in a primary care setting. J Womens Health 1997;6:543–552.
93. Golding JM. Intimate partner violence as a risk factor for mental disorders: a meta-analysis. J Fam Viol 1999;14:99–132.
94. McLeer SV, Anwar RAH. The role of the emergency physician in the prevention of domestic violence. Ann Emerg Med 1987;16:1155–1161.
95. Plichta SB, Abraham C. Violence and gynecologic health in women <50 years old. Am J Obstet Gynecol 1996;174:903–907.
96. Letourneau EJE, Holmes M. Gynecologic health consequences to victims of interpersonal violence. Womens Health Issues 1999;9:115–120.
97. Spitz AM, Marks JS. Violence and reproductive health. Matern Child Health J 2000;4:77–78.
98. Amaro H, Fried LE, Cabral H, et al. Violence during pregnancy and substance use. Am J Public Health 1990;80:575–579.
99. Stewart DE, Cecutti A. Physical abuse in pregnancy. CMA J 1993;149:1257–1263.
100. Helton AS, McFarlane J, Anderson ET. Battered and pregnant: a prevalence study. Am J Public Health 1987;77:1337–1339.
101. Gazmararian JA, Lazorick S, Spitz AM, et al. Prevalence of violence against pregnant women. JAMA 1996;275:1915–1920.
102. Cokkinides VE, Coker AL, Sanderson M, et al. Physical violence during pregnancy: maternal complications and birth outcomes. Obstet Gynecol 1999;93:661–666.
103. Gazmararian JA, Petersen R, Spitz AM, et al. Violence and reproductive health: current knowledge and future research directions. Matern Child Heal J 2000;4:79–84.
104. Ballard TJ, Saltzman LE, Gazmararian JA, et al. Violence during pregnancy: measurement issues. Am J Public Health 1998;88:274–276.
105. Petersen R, Gazmararian JA, Spitz AM, et al. Violence and adverse pregnancy outcomes: a review of the literature and directions for future research. Am J Prev Med 1997;13:366–373.
106. Morey MA, Begleiter ML, Harris DJ. Profile of a battered fetus. Lancet 1981;ii:1294–1295.
107. Bullock LF, McFarlane J. The birth-weight/battering connection. Am J Nurs 1989;89:1153–1155.
108. Parker B, McFarlane J, Soeken K. Abuse during pregnancy: effects on maternal complications and birth weight in adult and teenage women. Obstet Gynecol 1994;84:323–328.
109. Schei B, Samuelsen SO, Bakketeig LS. Does spousal physical abuse affect the outcome of pregnancy? Scand J Soc Med 1991;19:26–31.
110. Berenson AB, Wiemann CM, Wilkinson GS, et al. Perinatal morbidity associated with violence experienced by pregnant women. Am J Obstet Gynecol 1994;170:1760–1769.
111. O'Campo P, Gielen AC, Faden RR, et al. Verbal abuse and physical violence among a cohort of low-income pregnant women. Womens Health Issues 1994;4:29–37.
112. Grimstad H, Schei B, Backe B, et al. Physical abuse and low birthweight: a case-control study. Br J Obstet Gynaecol 1997;104:1281–1287.
113. Martin SL, English KT, Clark KA, et al. Violence and substance use among North Carolina pregnant women. Am J Public Health 1996;86:991–998.
114. Stewart DE. Incidence of postpartum abuse in women with a history of abuse during pregnancy. CMAJ 1994;151:1601–1604.
115. Gielen AC, O'Campo PJ, Faden RR, et al. Interpersonal conflict and physical violence during the childbearing year. Soc Sci Med 1994;39:781–787.
116. Hedin LW. Postpartum, also a risk period for domestic violence. Eur J Obstet Gynecol Reprod Biol 2000;89:41–45.
117. Martin SL, Mackie L, Kupper LL, et al. Physical abuse of women before, during and after pregnancy. JAMA 2001;285:1581–1584.
118. Weiss LB, Coons HL, Kripke EN, et al. Integrating a domestic violence education program into a medical school curriculum: challenges and strategies. Teach Learn Mod 2000;12:133–140.
119. American College of Obstetricians and Gynecologists (ACOG). Committee on Underserved Women. ACOG Educational Bulletin: Domestic Violence. No. 257. ACOG, December 1999.
120. Elliott L, Nerney M, Jones T, et al. Barriers to screening for domestic violence. J Gen Intern Med 2002;17:112–116.
121. Horan DL, Chapin J, Klein L, et al. Domestic violence screening practices of obstetrician-gynecologists. Obstet Gynecol 1998;92:785–789.
122. Davidson LL, Grisso JA, Garcia-Moreno C, et al. Training programs for healthcare professionals in domestic violence. J Womens Health Gend Based Med 2001;10:953–969.
123. Fogarty CT, Burge S, McCord EC. Communicating with patients about intimate partner violence: screening and interviewing approaches. Fam Med 2002;34:369–375.
124. Gremillion DH, Kanof EP. Overcoming barriers to physician involvement in identifying and referring victims of domestic violence. Ann Emerg Med 1996;27:769–773.
125. McCauley J, Yurk RA, Jenckes MW, et al. Inside "Pandora's box": abused women's experiences with clinicians and health services. J Gen Intern Med 1998;13:549–555.
126. Rodriguez MA, Bauer HM, McLoughlin E, et al. Screening and intervention for intimate partner abuse: practices and attitudes of primary care physicians. JAMA 1999;282:468–474.

127. Sugg NK, Thompson RS, Thompson DC, et al. Domestic violence and primary care: attitudes, practices, beliefs. Arch Fam Med 1999;8:301–306.
128. Centers for Disease Control and Prevention. Education About Adult Domestic Violence in 25 U.S. and Canadian Medical Schools, 1987–88. MMWR Morb Mortal Wkly Rep 1989;38(2):17–19.
129. Alpert EJ, Tonkin AE, Seeherman AM, et al. Family violence curricula in U.S. medical schools. Am J Prev Med 1998;14:273–282.
130. Parsons LH, Moore ML. Family violence issues in obstetrics and gynecology, primary care, and nursing texts. Obstet Gynecol 1997;90:596–599.
131. Parsons LH, Zaccaro D, Wells B, et al. Methods of and attitudes toward screening obstetrics and gynecology patients for domestic violence. Am J Obstet Gynecol 1995;173:381–387.
132. Reid SA, Glasser M. Primary care physicians' recognition of an attitude toward domestic violence. Acad Med 1997;72:51–53.
133. Blumenthal D, Cokhale M, Campbell EG, et al. Preparedness for clinical practice: reports of graduating residents at academic health centers. JAMA 2001;286:1027–1034.
134. Weissman JS, Campbell EG, Gokhale M, et al. Residents' preferences and preparation for caring for underserved populations. J Urban Health 2001;78:535–549.
135. Waalen J, Goodwin MM, Spitz AM, et al. Screening for intimate partner violence by health care providers: barriers and interventions. Am J Prev Med 2000;19:230–237.
136. American College of Obstetricians and Gynecologists, Committee on Health Care for Underserved Women. Committee Opinion: Mandatory Reporting of Domestic Violence. No. 200. ACOG, March 1998.
137. American Medical Association. E-2.02 Abuse of Spouses, Children, Elderly Persons, and Others at Risk. Available at: www.ama-assn.org. Accessed August 1, 2005.
138. American Medical Association. H-515.983 Physicians and Family Violence. Available at: www.ama-assn.org. Accessed August 1, 2005.
139. American Medical Association. H-515.965 Family and Intimate Partner Violence. Available at: www.ama-assn.org. Accessed August 1, 2005.
140. Koziol-McLain J, Campbell JC. Universal screening and mandatory reporting: an update on two important issues for victims/survivors of intimate partner violence. J Emerg Nurs 2001;27:602–606.
141. Rodriguez MA, McLoughlin E, Nah G, et al. Mandatory reporting of domestic violence injuries to the police: what do emergency department patients think? JAMA 2001;286:580–583.
142. Gielen AC, O'Campo PF, Campbell JC, et al. Women's opinions about domestic violence screening and mandatory reporting. J Prev Med 2000;19:279–285.
143. Houry D, Sachs CJ, Feldhaus KM, et al. Violence-inflicted injuries: reporting laws in the fifty states. Ann Emerg Med 2002;39:56–60.
144. Family Violence Department. DV Law Search: Domestic Violence Statutes Database. Available at: http://www.dvlawsearch.com/database/. Accessed August 1, 2005.
145. Gerbert B, Johnston K, Caspers N, et al. Experiences of battered women in health care settings: a qualitative study. Women Health 1996;24:1–17.
146. Rodriguez MA, Sheldon WR, Bauer HM, et al. The factors associated with disclosure of intimate partner abuse to clinicians. J Fam Pract 2001;50:338–344.
147. Gerbert B, Caspers N, Bronstone A, et al. A qualitative analysis of how physicians with expertise in domestic violence approach the identification of victims. Ann Intern Med 1999;131:578–584.
148. Gerbert B, Abercrombie P, Caspers N, et al. How health care providers help battered women: the survivor's perspective. Women Health 1999;29:115–135.
149. Rodriguez MA, Quiroga SS, Bauer HM. Breaking the silence: battered women's perspectives on medical care. Arch Fam Med 1996;5:153–158.
150. Chez RA, Jones RF III. The battered woman. Am J Obstet Gynecol 1995;173:677–679.
151. Freund KM, Bak SM, Blackhall L. Identifying domestic violence in primary care practice. J Gen Intern Med 1996;11:44–46.
152. Friedman LS, Samet JH, Roberts MS, et al. Inquiry about victimization experiences. Arch Intern Med 1992;152:1186–1190.
153. Parsons L, Goodwin MM, Petersen R. Violence against women and reproductive health: toward defining a role for reproductive health care services. Matern Child Health J 2000;4:1135–1140.
154. Rodriguez MA, Gauer HM, Flores-Ortiz Y, et al. Factors affecting patient–physician communication for abused Latina and Asian immigrant women. J Fam Pract 1998;47:309–311.
155. Warshaw C. Domestic violence: changing theory, changing practice. J Am Med Womens Assoc 1996;51:87–91.
156. Swenson-Britt E, Thornton JE, Hoppe SK, et al. A continuous improvement process for health providers of victims of domestic violence. Jt Comm J Qual Improv 2001;27:540–554.
157. Cohen S, De Vos E, Newberger E. Barriers to physician identification and treatment of family violence: lessons from five communities. Acad Med 1997;72:S19–S25.
158. Griffin MP, Koss MP. Clinical screening and intervention in cases of partner violence. Online J Issues Nurs 2002;7. Available at: http://www.nursingworld.org/ojin/topic17/tpc17_2.htm. Accessed August 1, 2005.
159. Hamberger LK, Ambuel B, Marbella A, et al. Physician interaction with battered women: the women's perspective. Arch Fam Med 1998;7:575–582.
160. Thompson RS, Rivara FP, Thompson DC, et al. Identification and management of domestic violence a randomized trial. Am J Prev Med 2000;19:253–263.

161. McCaw B, Berman WH, Syme L, et al. Beyond screening for domestic violence: a systems model approach in a managed care setting. Am J Prev Med 2001;21:170–176.
162. Shadigian E. Domestic violence: identification and management for the clinician. Compr Ther 1996;22:424–428.
163. Hayden SR, Barton ED, Hayden M. Domestic violence in the emergency department: how do women prefer to disclose and discuss the issues? J Emerg Med 1997;15:447–451.
164. Parker B, McFarlane J. Nursing assessment of the battered pregnant woman. Matern Child Nurs J 1991;16: 161–164.
165. McFarlane J, Parker B, Soeken K, et al. Assessing for abuse during pregnancy. Severity and frequency of injuries and associated entry into prenatal care. JAMA 1992;267:3176–3178.
166. Dienemann J, Campbell J, Landenburger K, et al. The domestic violence survivor assessment: a tool for counseling women in intimate partner violence relationships. Patient Educ Couns 2002;46:221–228.
167. Ernst AA, Weiss SJ, Cham E, et al. Comparison of three instruments for assessing ongoing intimate partner violence. Med Sci Monit 2002;8:CR197–201.
168. Norton LB, Peipert JF, Zierler S, et al. Battering in pregnancy: an assessment of two screening methods. Obstet Gynecol 1995;85:321–325.
169. Morrison LJ, Allan R, Grunfeld A. Improving the emergency department detection rate of domestic violence using direct questioning. J Emerg Med 2000;19:117–124.
170. Feldhaus KM, Koziol-McLain J, Amsbury HL, et al. Accuracy of three brief screening questions for detecting partner violence in the emergency department. JAMA 1997;277:1357–1361.
171. Lee RK, Thompson VL, Mechanic MB. Intimate partner violence and women of color: a call for innovations. Am J Pub Health 2002;92:530–534.
172. McNutt L, van Ryn M, Clark C, et al. Partner violence and medical encounters. African-American women's perspectives. Am J Prev Med 2000;19:264–269.
173. Fogarty CT, Brown JB. Screening for abuse in Spanish-speaking women. J Am Fam Pract 2002;15:101–111.
174. Clarke, OW. Report of the Council on Ethical and Judicial Affairs. Physicians and family violence: ethical considerations. JAMA 1992;267:3190–3193.
175. Isaac NE, Enos VP. Research in Brief: Documenting Domestic Violence: How Health Care Providers Can Help Victims. NCJ 188564. Washington, DC: National Institute of Justice, U.S. Department of Justice, September 2001. Available at: http://www.ncjrs.org/pdffiles1/nij/188564.pdf. Accessed August 1, 2005.
176. Hyman A. Domestic violence: legal issues for health care practitioners and institutions. J Am Med Womens Assoc 1996;51:101–105.
177. New York State Office for the Prevention of Domestic Violence. Domestic Violence Intervention: A Guide for Health Care Professionals. Revised, 2000 Edition. Available at: http://www.opdv.state.ny.us/health_humsvc/health/guide/contents.html. Accessed August 1, 2005.
178. Goldman J, Hudson Z, Hudson RM, et al. Health Privacy Principles for Protecting Victims of Domestic Violence. The Family Violence Prevention Fund, October 2000. Available at: http://endabuse.org/programs/display.php3?DocID=53. Accessed August 1, 2005.
179. Hyman A, Schillinger D, Lo B. Laws mandating reporting of domestic violence. JAMA 1995;273:1781–1787.
180. Albright CL. Resources for faculty development in faculty violence. Acad Med 1997;72:S93–S101.
181. National Domestic Violence Hotline. Available at: www.ndvh.org. Accessed August 1, 2005.

CHAPTER 22

Women and Sexuality

Gretchen Gross

We are, from birth to death, sexual beings. Although the expression of our sexuality, our gender identity, and, for some, sexual preference develops as our lives unfold, we crave physical contact, intimate connection, and the physical expression of our sexuality. Children of all ages experiment with their bodies in search of comfort and pleasure. At some point, we each come to understand that sexual touch, masturbation, intercourse, and other acts of physical connection and intimacy are important to our overall emotional well-being, yet many of us are woefully undereducated about our sexual selves and about the intricacies of sexual health. We understand what we should look and feel like sexually as portrayed on television and in movies, but that rarely reflects real-life sex, nor does it provide us with factual and realistic expectations of our bodies and healthy sexual functioning.

Many of us have substantial questions about our bodies, our sexual practices, and our interests. We wonder "Do I look like everyone else?" "Is my sex drive normal?" "Why can't I have an orgasm?" Therefore, it is vital for women's health care practitioners to understand that women look to them for information and answers about sexual functioning, desire, and anatomy.

To have a minimal grasp of human sexual development and functioning, doctors should have an understanding of physiology and genetics, social context, ethnic/religious/cultural responses to sex, awareness of mental health and relationship dynamics, and substance use. This asks a lot of practitioners, but they need to know that patients expect them to "be there for them" when they have questions about what is normal and abnormal and about how things can change for the better in the realm of their sexuality.

SEXUALITY: A LIFESPAN PERSPECTIVE

Practitioners should understand the range of changes that occur in women sexually across the lifespan. This is a brief overview, and surely there is much more to know and much more to tell. During early childhood, it is quite normal for young children to masturbate as soon as they find their genitals. Playing with themselves can provide both physical pleasure and comfort, and how parents react to this play will significantly impact a child's sense of their own body and of sexual touch and pleasure. Young children will explore one another, and at times, engage in mutual masturbation. They will also observe their parents' bodies. For example, watching a new mother breast-feed will likely spark questions about their own mother's breasts. Suppression of these normal behaviors is damaging to that child. Parents who take the time to talk about bodies, about privacy, and about touch as pleasurable but private are doing their children a great service in starting them off as healthy sexual beings.

Adolescence is a time of significant physical change and renowned emotional growth, which is not without its bumps and bruises. Teen girls are subject to powerful media messages, peer pressure, and their own sense of what everyone else is doing. Girls at this stage often compare themselves to other girls in body development, wondering if they are developing at the same rate as their peers. This can be the first time in a girl's life that she may wonder if she is attractive enough to warrant a partner. This is, of course, a high-risk time for the development of eating disorders, body dysmorphic disorders, and adolescent depression. Teens may be sexually active or very limited in their sexual scope. One of the current trends in middle and high school sexual practices is giving oral sex because many teens do not identify this as sex. Adolescents' levels of sexual activity are often rooted in their own level of factual knowledge about sex, in the awareness that they can masturbate to relieve increasing sexual urges, and importantly, in their own level of self-esteem and efficacy. Giving teens facts about sexual functioning and options for giving and receiving pleasure enables them to say "no" to intercourse on their own terms and for reasons that make sense to them.

WOMEN AND SEX

Many women have a huge gap in knowledge about their own bodies and about what their bodies do before, during, and after sex. Many women have no idea that, on average, it takes 15 minutes of foreplay to become fully lubricated. Many try to "keep up with" myths they believe are truths, myths that the media has portrayed regarding acceptable body size, appearance, and how they should approach and respond to sex. With the increased public popularity and acceptance of plastic surgery (e.g., among public personalities, television shows devoted to "extreme body makeovers"), it will be important to watch how this impacts women and their sense of sexuality and attractiveness as they age.

Many women have asked health care professionals questions about their libido levels, classifying themselves at the extremes of "frigid" or "oversexed." They wonder about how to communicate their needs to their partners, or if that is even acceptable. Often they do not have enough familiarity with their own anatomy to put into words what they find pleasurable. For these and more reasons, women appreciate practitioners who are ready to talk not just about their ovaries, uteruses, and menstruation, but practitioners who will also talk with them about their sexuality, which will help them find realistic answers to long-held questions. Keeping current, factual books on hand and having bibliographies readily available to women patients are signals to patients of a willingness to talk with them about their questions. It can be helpful to keep a resource library for patients that includes books such as *For Women Only* by Jennifer Berman and Laura Berman, *Female Sexual Awareness* by Emily McCarthy, and *Woman* by Natalie Angier. All are easily readable, have solid information, and speak to important aspects of healthy sexuality, as well as specifics about anatomy, desire, and functioning. In general, if a woman knows her body, knows how to please herself, and has a partner with whom she can communicate her likes and preferences easily, she will be able to have a long and healthy sexual life, with or without a partner.

Middle-age and menopausal women are increasingly healthy, active, and sexual. Although menopausal women may experience some changes in their levels of sexual functioning due to hot flash-induced sleep deprivation and lubrication changes, these symptoms are temporary and treatable. The physiologic changes in a woman's body may affect her orgasms, but sexual satisfaction can occur outside of achieving orgasm. Indeed, this seems to be the watermark of sexually satisfied elders; they have come to understand the innate value of intimacy, with or without the final result being a thunderous orgasm.

Additionally important to note when working with women of menopausal age is the consideration that the change in sexual functioning may be caused by changes in partners' functioning. In the case of erectile dysfunction (ED), sildenafil (Viagra), vardenafil (Levitra), and tadalafil (Cialis) have brought hope and pleasure back into their lives by benefiting both partners (see the Erectile Dysfunction section).

SEX COUNSELING IN THE GYNECOLOGIST'S OFFICE

Research indicates that women identify their doctor as the most likely professional they will consult for help in the areas of sexual health and functioning (1–7). The question for a women's health care provider is not whether to ask a patient about sexual health and functioning but how to approach this topic in a respectful and effective way, promoting positive discussions and information sharing.

Physicians who are open to talking with women about sexual functioning and health will find that a substantial percentage of their patients have sexually related questions or problems. Reports on the prevalence of sexual dysfunction in the general population range from 25 to 50% (1, 2). Among "normal" couples who reported that their marital and sexual relations were happy and satisfying, 40% of men reported erectile or ejaculatory dysfunction and 63% of women reported arousal or orgasmic dysfunction. Fifty percent of men and 77% of women reported difficulties such as lack of interest and inability to relax. These couples were responding to a general question regarding any sexual problems occurring in their marriage at the time of the survey (8). One survey in a family practice setting found that 56% of the patients reported having one or more sexual problems (1). Research from gynecologic practices shows that, when left entirely up to a patient, only 3% of women initiated discussions about their sexual problems. When a provider asked about sexual problems, 16% of women acknowledged problems (1).

Women have questions and concerns ranging beyond the mechanics of intercourse and orgasm, including changes in level of interest and desire, "normal" functioning, sex after childbirth, postoperative sexual functioning, and sex across the lifespan. They wonder about medication and sexual functioning, the role of anxiety and depression, the health of their relationship, their partner's functioning, and the impact of trauma, illness, and stress on their sexual lives. Health care providers should never lose sight of the roles that anxiety, stress, depression, anger, and relationship stability play in sexual functioning. Relationship issues contribute greatly to sexual functioning and satisfaction (9). When learning of a sexual dysfunction, it is important to also learn about what the woman thinks might be causing the dysfunction. Other critical questions include the following:

- When does it happen?
- Does it occur only with one specific partner?
- Does it occur with masturbation?

When practitioners view sexual functioning only from an organic or mechanical perspective, technique is usually emphasized as a remedy for the problem. This neglects the more likely scenario that the cause lies in an emotional or interpersonal realm. By the time a woman seeks advice for a sexual issue, it is likely that she and one or possibly more partners and relationships many have been troubled for months or years (1–7). The response that she receives from her health care provider sets the stage for her willingness to pursue more information, to try remedies, or to seek further treatment or counseling. A patient who feels embarrassed or ashamed when talking about her sexual health and who has these feelings reinforced by her health care provider will continue to feel isolated and "abnormal." She may not seek help again. In these cases, a problem that might otherwise have a good chance of resolution can become a deeply entrenched dysfunction.

TAKING A SEXUAL HISTORY

Physicians who routinely inquire about the sexual health of their patients identify significant concerns in at least 50% of their patients, whereas more than 75% of physicians who do not inquire estimate that less than 10% of their patients have sexual functioning issues (10).

The most effective way to integrate sexual functioning into patients' global health status is by routinely taking a sexual functioning history. At each nonemergent visit, questions such as "How has becoming a mom affected you sexually?" or "Sometimes the pressure from fibroids affects sex. Has it for you?" indicate a willingness on behalf of the provider to discuss sexual concerns.

Although the suggested scope of the sexual history remains a debated topic, one source asserts that up to 95% of sexual problems can be detected when sexual histories are routinely taken (11). In a study where physicians asked patients "Are you sexually active at this time?" and "Are you having any sexual difficulties or problems at this time?", 16% of the patients cited sexual

TABLE 22.1

Sample Questions for a Brief Sexual History

How frequently do you have intercourse or sex play (including masturbation)?
Are you sexually active with men, women, or both?
Are you satisfied with the current frequency of sexual activity?
  Is your partner satisfied with this frequency?
Do you have difficulty becoming sexually aroused?
  If so, do you have this problem with a partner and while masturbating?
  Does your partner have difficulty becoming aroused?
Do you have problems reaching orgasm?
  If so, do you have problems both with a partner and while masturbating?
Do you and your partner have similar levels of sexual interest?
Is intercourse ever painful?
  If so, when does the pain occur?

difficulties. The most common difficulties identified were dyspareunia (48%) and decreased sexual desire (21%) (1).

A brief history comprised of four salient questions has been shown to uncover sexual dysfunctions equally as effectively as a lengthier and complex questionnaire (11):

- Are you sexually active?
- Are there any problems?
- What do you think might be causing the problem?
- Do you have pain with intercourse?

These questions elicit enough information from women to allow the physician to initiate further discussion and evaluation. The physician may then continue the workup, or may refer the individual or couple to a specialist who will provide the patient with information to help resolve the dysfunction (11).

See Table 22.1 for more questions to include in a brief sexual history, with one caveat. It is becoming increasingly clear that there is a generational variation regarding what is meant by the question, "Are you sexually active?" Among college-age women and younger, anything short of vaginal/penile intercourse may not be considered "sex" or "sexual activity." It is also important to ask what gender(s) one's sexual partner(s) are. When working and talking about sexual functioning with any audience, the more specific the questions, the better.

Alternative Treatments and Internet Information

The Internet is a vast and private resource for women seeking all sorts of health and medical information. It would be valuable to ask a woman experiencing any level of sexual dysfunction if she has done any online searching for information or treatments. Anyone doing a search of treatments for female sexual dysfunction will likely be aware of multiple sexual stimulants targeted at women with dysfunction. In Chapter 20, complementary and alternative medicines are reviewed, including those purported to enhance the female libido.

Knowing what other sources and interventions your patient has tried or considered is important to a complete holistic understanding of what lengths the woman has gone to, as well as what myths she may have encountered in her research travels. Your response to her theories, searches, and considerations is important in working with her as a health care partner, as well as a provider.

SEXUAL DYSFUNCTIONS IN WOMEN

Dyspareunia and inhibited sexual desire are the most common sexual dysfunctions for which women seek help (1, 3, 11–13). Table 22.2 lists causes of these and other sexual dysfunctions. A complete history provides an understanding of the impact of the dysfunction on the woman's emotional state and their ability to fully participate in the relationship. It also includes a review of

TABLE 22.2

Sexual Dysfunctions and Their Causes in Women

Dyspareunia	
Organic Causes	
With Thrusting: Endometriosis, varices of the broad ligament, scars or adhesions, ovary adhering to cul de sac, adnexal masses, pelvic inflammatory disease, rectal problems, cystitis, orthopedic problems	*Functional Causes* Inadequate foreplay or arousal, lack of communication between partners regarding levels of arousal and excitement
At Orgasm: Endometriosis, scars, varices of broad ligament *Others:* Urinary tract infections, urethritis, hymenal strands, bacterial vaginitis, postmenopausal or postsurgical vaginal atrophy, fourchette irritation, vulvar vestibulitis, vestibular adenitis, atrophic vulvovaginitis, obstetric trauma, mediolateral episotomy, significant pelvic relaxation, leiomyomas, advanced pelvic carcinoma	*Psychological Causes* Current depressive episode, somatization or conversion disorder, phobic or panic disorder, history of chronic pelvic pain, history of sexual abuse or rape, substance abuse or chemical dependency, major anxiety-based sexual conflicts, hostility toward partner, general sexual aversion, entrenched negative sexual expectations inhibiting sexual responsiveness, fear of pregnancy or sexually transmitted diseases, lack of resolution of previous pregnancy loss or termination, low desire, nongenital chronic pain syndromes
Inhibited Sexual Desire	
Organic Causes Chronic illness (e.g., diabetes), endocrine alterations (endocrinopathy, physiologic fluctuations, panhypopituitarism, ovariectomy, adrenalectomy, use of oral contraceptives), neurologic illness or trauma (multiple sclerosis, spinal cord injury), fatigue, medications, drug and/or alcohol abuse, pregnancy	*Psychological Causes* History of sexual assault, current depressive episode, premenstrual syndrome or premenstrual dysphoric disorder
Vaginismus	
Organic Causes Vaginitis, vaginal strictures after posterior colporrhaphy, scarring from mediolateral episiotomies	*Psychological Causes* Response to past painful vaginal penetration, orthodox religious background, history of rape or sexual abuse
Anorgasmia	
Functional Causes Premature ejaculation in partner, erectile dysfunction in partner, insufficient stimulation, lack of knowledge about orgasms	*Psychological Causes* Cultural or religious restrictions, inability to relax, feelings of guilt
Vulvodynia (Also see Chapter 6)	
Organic Causes Persistent infections (especially human papilloma or *Candida*), vulvar papillomatosis, vulvar dermatoses,	cyclic vulvitis, vulvar vestibulitis, irritant contact dermatitis, steroid-induced "periorificial" dermatitis

the individual's and couple's attempts to resolve the dysfunction (13). It is important to establish the timing, situation, and duration of the disorder. The patient usually comes with her own theories of the problem, and she can provide valuable insight and information that might not otherwise be readily uncovered. A complete physical evaluation to rule out organic factors is also necessary.

Dyspareunia

There are four degrees of dyspareunia: complete, situational, primary, and secondary. The diagnosis of complete dyspareunia can be made when the patient's pain occurs with each and every attempt at vaginal penetration, both with her current partner(s) and during penetration with masturbation. It need not have occurred in all prior sexual encounters but is present with all current partners. Situational dyspareunia occurs in some situations or with some partners but not necessarily with all current partners. Primary dyspareunia involves vaginal pain that has been present from the woman's very first attempt at vaginal penetration and need not be limited to penetration with a penis. The pain persists with every penetration attempt and with each situation or partner.

Finally, secondary dyspareunia interrupts an otherwise uncomplicated history of penetration. This is often seen when there has been a change in the woman's physical or mental health status, such as in the aftermath of rape or sexual abuse, or after any number of gynecologic surgeries, illnesses, or events, including childbirth (14). A complete assessment of dyspareunia documents the history of the pain and attempts to determine the type of dyspareunia present (Table 22.3).

With the exceptions of vaginismus and problems of inadequate foreplay or lubrication, most cases of dyspareunia have an organic cause (Table 22.2). In long-standing cases of dyspareunia, organic causes are present in up to one-third of cases (13). The impact of dyspareunia is not limited solely to the presenting patient; coital pain can result in further sexual dysfunction for both partners. The fear of pain with intercourse infringes on a couple's desire for sexual intimacy. A man's erectile and ejaculatory functioning can be affected by his fear of causing his partner pain (15). Repeatedly painful sexual experiences can set up an expectation of future pain, reinforcing avoidant behaviors. The operant conditioning model explains the role that random painful or negative experiences play in the establishment of persistent and dysfunctional behaviors (13, 16).

It is important to rule out anxiety and depressive disorders in the dyspareunic patient. Untreated depressive or anxiety disorders can inhibit a woman's ability to emotionally engage in a sexual experience, resulting in inadequate lubrication and pain with intercourse. Women who have had an experience of coital pain may become focused on only their physiologic state during sex. This is called "spectatoring," which is the compulsion to judge or evaluate one's performance during sex. It is a cognitive process that virtually ensures inadequate emotional involvement and relaxation during sex.

If a patient's dyspareunia is found to be physiologic in etiology, it remains important to consider that the individual and couple may still experience some emotional sequelae, such as a negative response to intercourse, avoidance of sexual intimacy, fear of inadequacy, or a heightened level of self or partner blame. It is fairly common to see sexual dysfunctions

TABLE 22.3

Assessment of Dyspareunia

What is the chronology of the discomfort?
What is the impact of the pain on the patient?
What is the impact of the pain on the patient's relationship with her partner?
How has the patient attempted to resolve the dyspareunia before consulting her physician?

develop in the partner in response to the initial problem, frequently making medical treatment of dyspareunia itself insufficient (16). In these situations, both partners will benefit from couples' counseling to help stop the cycle of primary and secondary sexual dysfunction.

If a patient's dyspareunia is found to be physiologic in etiology, it is important to consider that the individual and couple may still experience some emotional sequelae, such as negative responses to intercourse, avoidance of sexual intimacy, fear of inadequacy, or a heightened level of self- or other blame. It is fairly common to see sexual dysfunctions develop in the partner in response to the initial problem, frequently making medical treatment of the dyspareunia itself inefficient (17). In these situations, both partners will benefit from couples' counseling to help stop the cycle of primary and secondary sexual dysfunction.

If it appears that coital pain is due to insufficient excitation and lubrication before intercourse because of insufficient foreplay, treatment options include the use of copious amounts of lubricants and encouraging the woman to determine the moment and depth of penile entry. In addition, there are some excellent books that patients and their partners can read to increase their understanding of sexual excitement and response. Barry and Emily McCarthy have authored a series of books on sexual awareness and satisfaction in men, women, and couples; these books have been well received by patients (17–19). Barbach's book, *For Yourself: The Fulfillment of Female Sexuality*, on sexual functioning and awareness in women is also well known and respected among clinicians and patients (20).

Inhibited Sexual Desire

Inhibited sexual desire is a complex dysfunction. Normally, sexual interest levels fluctuate due to any number of factors, including physical, emotional, financial, and sociologic stressors. When any couple is trying to coordinate their libidos to have mutually desired and gratifying sex, problems may arise. A couple who finds it difficult to match the timing of their desire does not meet diagnostic criteria for inhibited sexual desire (14). However, if one or both partners feel a diminished or absent ability to achieve sexual arousal or if they lack sexual interest, then a desire phase dysfunction should be considered (21).

Organic factors that can inhibit sexual desire in women include chronic physical or emotional illness, pregnancy, menopause, and use of certain medications (Table 22.4). Psychosocial factors, such as a lack of interest in the current partner, unresolved relationship issues, hostility or anger, infidelity or other breach of trust, and changes in family dynamics such as having a baby all may contribute to inhibited sexual desire. Other issues such as financial stressors, drug or alcohol abuse, and situational or chronic depression in either partner may also play an important role in the development of inhibited sexual desire.

Sexual dysfunctions often present as a symptom of a mood disorder. Depression decreases the libido, but some people attempt to improve a depressed mood by increasing sexual activity. Hypersexuality is a behavior often found in the manic state. The diagnosis of inhibited sexual desire requires symptoms specific to sexual desire rather than general symptoms of psychological functioning of the individual. If the person is describing inhibited sexual desire symptoms, but also reports changes in sleep and eating patterns, emotional liability, and lack of overall energy, it is likely that the primary diagnosis is depression rather than inhibited sexual desire. It is important to note that pharmacologic agents in the treatment of depression frequently have decreased libido as a side effect. Virtually every antidepressant currently available has some side effect that negatively affects sexual functioning and satisfaction (22–24). There is a higher incidence of sexual side effects seen with selective serotonin uptake inhibitors than was reported in initial studies of drugs in this class. Sertraline (Zoloft), fluoxetine (Prozac), and paroxetine (Paxil) have all been associated with total or partial anorgasmia, decreased libido, or delayed orgasm (25–28). Physicians play an important role in educating patients about the sexual side effects of these medications and monitoring patients for changes in sexual function. Switching medications or suggesting a drug holiday can significantly decrease the sexual dysfunction side effects and improve patient compliance.

For many women, sexual functioning and substance abuse have a complex interrelationship. Alcohol and drug abuse affects the libido, and sexual dysfunction is a commonly seen side

TABLE 22.4

Common Medications That Can Cause Sexual Dysfunction

	Decreased Desire	Increased Desire	Erectile Disorder	Ejaculatory Disorder	Orgasmic Disorder	Decreased Lubrication or Responsiveness	Gynecomastia	Priapism	Painful Clitoral Tumescence	Hormonal Alterations
Antihypertensives										
Atenolol (Tenormin)			×							
Clonidine (Catapres)	×		×	×	W					
Enalapril (Vasotec)			×							
Methyldopa (Aldomet)	×		×	×	W					
Propanolol (Inderal)	×		×							
Reserpine (Serpasil)	M		×	×						
Spironolactone (Aldactone)	×		×			×	×			
Psychotropics										
Alprazolam (Xanax)	×				×					
Barbiturates	×		×	×						
Bupropion (Wellbutrin)	×		×							
Buspirone (BuSpar)	×		×	×				×		
Clomipramine (Anafranil)	×		×	×	×					
Clonazepm (Klonopin)	×		×		×					
Diazepam (Valium)	×			×	×					
Doxepin (Adapin, Sinequan)				×						
Fluoxetine (Prozac)	×			×	×					
Imipramine (Tofranil)			×	×	W					
Lorazepam (Ativan)	×									
Nortriptyline (Pamelor)	×		×		×					
Oxazepam (Serax)	×									
Paroxetine (Paxil)			×	×	×					
Phenelzine (Nardil)				×	×					
Prochlorperazine (Compazine)	×	×	×	×		W		×		
Sertraline (Zoloft)					×					
Trazodone (Desyrel)		×						×		
Venlafaxine (Effexor)			×	×	×					
Others										
Benztropine (Cogentin)			×							
Bromocriptine (Parlodel)			×						×	

(continued)

TABLE 22.4 Continued

Common Medications That Can Cause Sexual Dysfunction

	Decreased Desire	Increased Desire	Erectile Disorder	Ejaculatory Disorder	Orgasmic Disorder	Decreased Lubrication or Responsiveness	Gynecomastia	Priapism	Painful Clitoral Tumescence	Hormonal Alterations
Carbamazepine (Tegretol)	×		×							
Cimetidine (Tagamet)			×				×			
Danazol (Danocrine)	×	×								
Disulfiram (Antabuse)			×							
Diphenhydramine (Benadryl)	×		×							
Famotidine (Pepcid)			×							
Heparin								×		
Hydroxyzine (Atarax, Vistaril)	×		×							
Isotretinoin (Acutane)				×						
Meclizine (Antivert)			×							
Medroxyprogesterone (Provera, Depo-Provera)	×		×							
Naproxen (Aleve, Anaprox, Naprosyn)	×									
Nizatidine (Axid)			×							
Phenytoin (Dilantin)	×		×							
Ranitidine (Zantac)	×		×							
Drugs of Abuse										
Alcohol, acute	×		×	×						
Alcohol, chronic	×		×							
Marijuana	×								×	

M, known effect in men; W, known effect in women; ×, effect reported in both genders or gender not specified.

effect of alcoholism in women (21, 29). Alcoholism, sexual abuse/assault history, and sexual dysfunction are now a well-recognized triumvirate. These complex issues should be carefully addressed when the patient requests treatment for any one of these three problems. Careful collaboration among the patient's physician, counselor, and other health care providers is central to the development and implementation of a sound treatment plan.

Many women will experience more emotional discomfort after they stop drinking or using the medications that previously left them emotionally numb. If the patient is not prepared for an increase in flashbacks, anxiety, and depressive symptoms during this treatment phase, she may very well relapse to avoid this dysphoric time. Therefore, it is central to the patient's recovery that she work with a professional who is well aware of the complex interrelationship between addictions, sexual dysfunction, and a history of abuse and/or assault.

Vaginismus

Vaginismus involves the involuntary spasm of the pelvic muscles that surround the vagina, specifically the perineal and levator ani muscles. These contracted muscles prevent penetration of the vagina or allow penetration only with a great deal of pain. These involuntary contractions may be strong enough to cause pain alone or may be painful only if penetration is attempted. As with other sexual dysfunctions, there are variations in severity, duration, and onset. Unfortunately, women who experience an initial episode of vaginismus often repeatedly attempt intercourse, which strengthens the psychological connection between intercourse and pain. These repeated experiences of pain and failure reinforce sexual dysfunction. Organic causes of vaginismus, including vaginitis, vaginal strictures after posterior colporrhaphy, or scarring from mediolateral episiotomies, are frequently ruled out early in the workup. More often, vaginismus is a phobic response to a painful stimulus—in this case, painful vaginal penetration. It is directly related to fear, anxiety, or guilt (13, 30). The most common etiologic factor in cases of vaginismus is an orthodox religious background (31–33), but it is not uncommon for women who have vaginismus to be victims of sexual abuse or rape. Diagnosis can help lead a woman into counseling where she can begin to resolve this response to prior trauma.

Treatment of vaginismus hinges on helping the patient break her behavioral response to negative stimuli and relearn vaginal muscle control. It is important for the woman to be in control of each phase of treatment of vaginismus. If she feels out of control or forced to proceed faster than she desires, it is likely that her behavioral response (anxiety, muscle contractions, sexual aversion) will be reinforced. She should be taught Kegel exercises for control of vaginal muscles. Vaginal dilation exercises can also be practiced in private in a relaxed and nonsexual setting; these exercises promote understanding of anatomy and being comfortable with the sensations resulting from touch. Either dilators or fingers can be used in this exercise, depending on the patient's preference and comfort level. Dilators come in four graduated sizes; the woman starts with the smallest one, covers it with lubricant, places it in her vagina, and leaves it in place for 10 to 15 minutes. The next larger size is lubricated and placed intravaginally for another 10 to 15 minutes. Gradually, the woman works up to being able to place the largest dilator intravaginally without difficulty. Steege (13) suggested that women who use their fingers rather than dilators establish a role as active participants rather than passive recipients in treatment.

The partner becomes active in the vaginal dilation exercises only when the patient is emotionally and physically ready, and after the anxiety of being touched is extinguished. At that point, specific instructions direct the experiences temporarily away from the initial goal of intercourse. Introducing the partner prematurely is counterproductive to treatment. Some women feel pressured to hurry their partner's participation as an indicator to him or her that things are moving along rapidly. It is appropriate for the health care provider to tell the patient that she is moving too rapidly and may be risking a setback in the process.

After ruling out organic causes of vaginismus, it is important to not make the only focus of treatment the patient's physiologic responses. Patients may be instructed in the use of vaginal dilators, but this is not productive if little attention is paid to the emotional sequelae of the dysfunction on both partners. It is important to understand the impact of vaginismus on both the patient and the couple. Referring them to a counselor who collaborates with their physician is a good treatment plan. If left unattended, a couple's lack of accurate sexual knowledge and/or impaired communication skills will likely cause many levels of dysfunction in their relationship.

Anorgasmia

Anorgasmia is the inability to reach orgasm. Orgasmic problems are very common, with 8 to 10% of women in the United States never achieving orgasm. A woman may have primary orgasmic problems (she has never experienced orgasm), or she may suffer secondary orgasmic problems (she previously has had orgasms but currently does not). For some women, the ability to reach orgasm is situational (e.g., some women achieve orgasm only through fantasy or with oral stimulation but not with penile stimulation).

The diagnosis of anorgasmia is based on history. Treatment depends on the type of anorgasmia and its etiology. Primary may be easier to treat than secondary, where the underlying issues must be defined and resolved. Situational anorgasmia may be resolved through the use of a bridging technique, combining an act known to allow achievement of orgasm with the technique the woman wants to use to achieve orgasm.

Orgasm is a learned response, and it can be voluntarily inhibited. Factors that may contribute to anorgasmia include cultural or religious restrictions, premature ejaculation or erectile disorders in one's partner, an inability to relax and enjoy the sexual experience without guilt, and ignorance of the basic physiology of a woman's body. A woman with primary anorgasmia may need to learn what an orgasm feels like. For some women, education on the need for sufficient clitoral stimulation, adequate communication with her partner, and "self-permission" to be sexual is necessary. Self-stimulation is also recommended as a way of learning what is arousing and what ultimately leads to orgasm. Some women may prefer to masturbate alone at first, allowing the partner to become involved later, because learning to be orgasmic alone is easier. The final step is becoming orgasmic with a partner, and the individual woman needs to learn the most effective means for her to achieve this.

SEXUAL DYSFUNCTIONS IN SPECIFIC POPULATIONS OF WOMEN

Lesbians

Lesbians often report feeling uncomfortable in heterosexually oriented clinics where there is bias and ignorance. It is discomforting to be repeatedly questioned about the need for birth control when it is not necessary or when fear of a judgment-laden response inhibits asking questions about donor insemination. Questions about sexual functioning arise throughout a woman's life cycle, and lesbian women are no exception. A lack of information and resources can lead to ongoing dysfunction that might otherwise be relatively easy to treat.

Our culture is replete with myths about lesbians. One myth suggests that because both partners are female and have matching genitalia, they will enjoy the same approaches to lovemaking, have matching levels of desire, will be expert at pleasing one another, and therefore do not need to communicate individual likes and dislikes to one another (34). As with heterosexuals, lack of communication between partners may result in sexual dysfunction. Lesbian psychosocial development includes a meshing phase, at which point the partners overidentify with one another, tending to overlook individual aspects (34). As an increased awareness of each partner's individuality grows, individual sexual appetites and preferences will also emerge.

Although most lesbians report satisfaction with their sex lives (35, 36), there is a substantial minority who report dissatisfaction or some form of sexual dysfunction. The most commonly reported dissatisfaction reported by lesbians occurs in areas of frequency and levels of sexual desire (37–39). Blumstein and Schwartz (37) found that over time lesbian couples have less frequent sex than do heterosexuals. There is conflicting data on whether lesbians in general are comfortable with this decrease in frequency (35, 37). A physician can, by sharing accurate information about patterns in lesbian couples' sexual functioning, alleviate concerns of "abnormality." A lesbian who is unaware of the trend toward decreased sexual frequency over time in long-term relationships may find this information useful because this suggests a normal pattern rather than pathology.

Breast and Gynecologic Cancer Patients

Breast and gynecologic cancer patients experience changes in their sexual functioning for several reasons. If a surgery is needed, there may be a decline in self-esteem due to the loss of reproductive organs or a change in appearance. Some women report a change in the nature of their orgasms due to the loss of their cervix or uterus, which rhythmically contracts during orgasm (40). Surgical scars may result in coital pain. Treatment may result in disfigurement, physical and emotional fatigue, and a profoundly lowered self-esteem.

It is not uncommon for women who have undergone treatment for breast and gynecologic cancers to present in counseling offices with many issues, including questions about their femininity, body image, and sexual desirability. If a patient has had surgery or radiation treatment, she may have problems with vaginal lubrication or stenosis leading to dyspareunia. If dyspareunia develops, one should consider a concomitant sexual dysfunction in her partner. Partners can develop a sexual dysfunction or aversion secondary to their fear of causing physical pain or in response to anatomic or emotional changes in their partners. Partners of women who experience coital pain frequently develop erectile difficulties (15).

The woman's age at the time of diagnosis and treatment has an impact on her emotional experience and functioning. A 32-year-old patient who must have a hysterectomy to prevent the spread of cancer will face issues of infertility, self-image, and sexual attractiveness differently than will a 68-year-old woman undergoing the same treatment. Although the issues of sexual attractiveness, desirability, and functioning are universal, in the case of the younger woman, the additional experience of surgical infertility complicates an already traumatic diagnosis and treatment plan.

Both partners usually have questions beyond the scope of the immediate diagnosis and treatment plan but hesitate to ask the physician. A woman who wants to ask her physician about possible changes in orgasmic functioning, physical sensations, and desire level, yet feels that her physician is only concerned with the cancer, may not ask these relevant questions. Partners may feel a need to alter their sexual patterns, fearing they might hurt their partner. Physicians can help a patient and her partner by simply leaving time for ancillary questions. Open-ended question are useful, such as "At some point, many people have important questions about how the disease (or surgery, radiation, chemotherapy) will affect their sexual functioning. What are your concerns at this point?" Asking these questions at various stages of treatment, regardless of the woman's age, is important. The woman who initially had no questions may find that she has questions 4 months postoperatively. Encouraging direct and open communication between the physician, the patient, and her partner decreases misunderstandings about the immediate and long-term impact of cancer and its treatment on their lives.

Cancer patients may be hesitant to express anger or sadness about changes in sexual function or relationships. The patient may report "I'm alive. I beat cancer. So I feel petty to be angry that I have pain when my husband and I try to make love. But our sex life has been so important to us that I feel such a loss now that it's changed." The physician should hear her concerns and offer appropriate treatment. The dyspareunia can be addressed by telling the patient about over-the-counter lubrication gel, as well as the relationship between adhesions and discomfort. Discussing the woman's need to experience sexual intimacy as a celebration of her life and her marriage, both of which outlasted the cancer, conveys empathy and helps the woman with feelings of guilt she may be experiencing over her anger.

Many women report that a return to their precancer level of sexual desirability and functioning is an integral part of their recovery process. Despite a good recovery and a positive prognosis, women are still vulnerable to developing reactive depression secondary to the profound impact of cancer on their lives, changes in their sexual self-image and functioning, their perceived desirability, or their surgically or medically induced infertility. Physician awareness of these concerns and potential responses to cancer diagnosis and treatment will support the patient's need to deal with many facets of a cancer diagnosis.

Infertility Patients

By the time a couple is seen in an infertility clinic, they have usually endured at least 12 months of trying, and failing, to become pregnant. Each unsuccessful month leaves them with a greater sense of concern, anxiety, guilt, blame, or anger at not becoming pregnant. After establishing a relationship with a specialist, it is possible that there will be several more months of evaluations and pharmacologic or surgical interventions. In the course of this process, the couple might learn more about the nature of their infertility, and their diagnosis may lessen their hopes of pregnancy.

Because of the invasive nature of an infertility workup and treatment regimen, intimate sexual behavior comes under the scrutiny and direction of strangers. Couples are told when to have sex and when to abstain. Men are asked to produce semen samples for analysis, and postcoital mucus may be examined. As conception becomes more strongly linked to attendance at the infertility clinic than to lovemaking, many couples experience diminished sexual desire and increased problems with arousal and orgasmic functioning (40, 41). The emphasis on timed intercourse can eventually result in decreased sexual activity during nonfertile periods (42–44). Patients report that the changes in their sexual relationships that become established during infertility treatment linger long after the treatment itself has ended, irrespective of the outcome (40, 45).

Furthermore, there is a population of patients who are infertile because of their sexual dysfunctions, such as an anejaculation. It is possible for some men to ejaculate with masturbation but not while having intercourse with their partners. Although these couples may become pregnant as a result of insemination, the problem itself has not been addressed and may actually be aggravated by treatment. Artificial insemination in this population may make it easier for the couple to resist psychotherapy, which would direct treatment at the root of the dysfunction (46). Because infertility due to sexual dysfunctions can be successfully treated in one-half to two-thirds of cases by brief therapy with the couple, this offers an opportunity for the couple to experience full sexual functioning and, possibly, pregnancy without clinical intervention (47).

Infertility patients are a population particularly vulnerable to sexual dysfunction, both iatrogenic and pre-existing. Taking an accurate sexual history before, during, and after treatment, and educating the couple on the impact of treatment on their sexual functioning, may prompt a couple to seek help relatively rapidly if symptoms of dysfunction develop.

Sexual Abuse and Rape Victims

Physicians encounter sexual assault victims in many different settings in the course of their practice. They will meet them in the emergency room soon after an assault when the injuries and experience are raw, in well-woman clinics, during routine obstetric care, and in delivery rooms. The women may be forthcoming and fully aware of the extent of the abuse, or they may only be aware of strong visceral responses to internal or breast examinations. They may present with panic disorder, depression, or substance abuse. They may be hypersexual or, conversely, avoidant of sex altogether. This might appear as conscious or subconscious avoidance behaviors, as in the case of vaginismus. The most frequently cited symptom of childhood sexual abuse in adult women is depression (48–51). Adults abused in childhood generally experience chronic sexual problems in adulthood, including fear and avoidance of intimate emotional or sexual relationships, aversion to sexual contact, dysfunctions of desire and arousal, and primary or secondary anorgasmia (50). These patients are equally likely to appear as sexually promiscuous women needing repeated treatment for sexually transmitted diseases and unwanted pregnancies as they are to be avoidant of gynecologic care and sexual behavior altogether.

Incest survivors and rape victims often experience “flashback” memories triggered by seemingly benign situations and individuals. Because of the nature of the gynecologic or obstetric visit, the medical setting is ripe for intrusive memory flooding. Triggers can be as minute as words used, being in an unfamiliar place, body position reminiscent of the abuse position, being physically moved or touched by someone, feeling sexually aroused, or feeling similar physical responses to touch, hair color, facial features, or caring gestures (52).

Sexual abuse and assault survivors still struggle with the stigma placed on them in our society. For this reason, women may not be initially forthcoming about their trauma, fearing judgmental responses by physicians and others. They may continue to carry their own sense of guilt and blame for the assault. This often prevents them from telling their stories to helping professionals. Adults who were molested as young children may have taken the blame for the abuse; this defense fits a child's developmental vulnerability to assume responsibility for events out of his or her control. Many predators also instruct their child victims that the child wanted the abuse or liked the special attention. Thus, when a woman tells a physician who is a relative stranger about her abuse history, the physician should be aware that his or her response to this information is integral to the patient's recovery process. This woman may not have told anyone else about her history, or she may be quite comfortable telling her story; compassion and respect are always warranted.

Alcohol and drug abuse is frequently seen in this patient population. Women use medications and alcohol to numb their emotional pain, as well as to suppress conscious memories and flashbacks. Some medicate themselves in an attempt to help themselves be sexually active without being emotionally present. Whether the substance abuse predated the assault or was adopted as a dysfunctional coping mechanism in the wake of the trauma, treatment must include the complex relationship between the assault, the patient's sexual dysfunction, and her abuse of or dependence on medications or alcohol.

Maintaining boundaries with these patients is essential; lack of boundaries and role clarity makes victims feel vulnerable. Ongoing communication between physician and patient before and during exams is frequently welcomed by the patient. It decreases the likelihood of intrusive memory flooding by keeping the woman in the present.

Abused women may access counseling at various stages in their lives. Each developmental phase may raise more issues relating back to the trauma. If the physician recognizes symptoms such as sexual dysfunctions of various degrees, avoidance of health care visits, or drug-seeking behaviors, he or she should not hesitate to support the patient by referring her to counseling.

SEXUAL DYSFUNCTIONS IN MEN

Sexual dysfunction is certainly not limited to women. Men experience a variety of dysfunctions (Table 22.5), and, like women, some of these have organic causes, physiologic causes, or may result from specific medications (Table 22.4).

TABLE 22.5

Sexual Dysfunctions and Their Causes in Men

Erectile Dysfunction (Impotence)	
Organic Causes	*Psychological Causes*
Peyronie's disease of the penis, prostatic surgical procedures, testicular failure, seminal vesiculities, hypospadias, endocrine alterations (Addison's disease, acromegaly, pituitary insufficiency, low androgen level), chronic illnesses/conditions (diabetes, liver disease, adrenal neoplasms, obesity, fatigue), use/abuse of substances (alcohol, narcotics, estrogenic, or parasympatholytic medications), neurologic diseases (multiple sclerosis, amyotrophic lateral sclerosis, transection of the spinal cord, parkinsonism, peripheral neuropathies, lesions of the hypothalamus/ limbic system/spinal cord, spina bifida)	Depression, marital discord, guilt associated with sexuality, sexual phobias, performance anxiety (fear of failure, pressure of sexual demands, inability to abandon self to sexual feelings)
Premature Ejaculation	
Organic Causes	*Psychological Causes*
(should be ruled out in men with prior history of good ejaculatory control) Prostatitis, neurologic disorders	Repetition of acquired patterns of rapid ejaculation, anxiety, low sensitivity threshold
Retarded Ejaculation (Including Anejaculation)	
Organic Causes	*Psychological Causes*
Neurologic injury or illness, use/abuse of alcohol	History of traumatic sexual events (sexual abuse, partner's infidelity, being discovered while mastur-bating as a youth), sexual guilt, suppressed anger, ambivalence toward partner, anxiety

Premature Ejaculation

Premature ejaculation occurs when men pass rapidly from the excitement phase of the sexual response to the orgasmic phase with little (if any) time spent in the plateau state. It is as disconcerting for men as it is for their partners. Men cite limited gratification and feelings of frustration and anxiety, and may develop performance anxiety that can, if left untreated, result in ED.

To effectively treat this disorder, it is helpful to understand the physiology of ejaculation, which occurs in two phases. In the first phase, the terminal vas deferens, seminal vesicles, and prostate contract while the bladder sphincter closes. The bolus of semen is forced into the prostatic urethra at this time. The second phase is manifested in the rhythmic contractions of the perineal muscles, forcing the semen out of the urethra in spurts. Once the first phase of ejaculation has begun, ejaculation cannot be consciously stopped.

There are two avenues for effective treatment of this dysfunction. The first is behavioral, often referred to as the "squeeze technique." This is used as a means of interrupting the response cycle at the excitement phase, allowing the man to better experience his body's response and enabling him to create a plateau state. The squeeze technique consists of the partner placing their thumbs over the frenulum of the penis, index fingers on top of the glans penis, and middle fingers just behind (proximal to) the corona, applying pressure for 10 to 15 seconds. This is done at the point when the man feels that he is very close to orgasm. Ordinarily, this prevents the man from ejaculating and causes him to lose some of his erection. The pressure does not hurt the erect penis. Stimulation of the penis then starts again, and the squeeze technique is used for a second time. The third time the man is allowed to ejaculate (53).

An alternate treatment focuses on the theory that premature ejaculation is a response to a lack of sexual stimulation over time, which leads to a "hungry kid in the candy store" response. In this case, the couple is encouraged to have frequent and "nonevaluated" sex. If the man experiences premature ejaculation during any of these encounters, there is no negative response, no stopping of lovemaking, but rather just a switch in focus to the not yet orgasmic partner to ensure her pleasure as well. Men who use this approach are not focused on their orgasm, feel competent in being able to satisfy their partners, and in time decrease their premature ejaculation (54).

Erectile Dysfunction

ED is the inability to obtain an erection sufficient to penetrate or to maintain an erection until ejaculation. Although it is tempting to classify ED into either psychogenic or organic etiologies, there is enormous overlay between the two. A man may have had erectile difficulties initially because of an organic cause and later develop a psychogenic component as a response. The presence of one cause does not preclude the presence of another, especially if ED has been present for some time.

It is common for EDs associated with psychogenic causes to appear with a sudden onset and to occur intermittently. Erectile disorders with an organic basis often present with gradual onset and are persistent or progressive. One commonly used test to distinguish psychogenic from organic ED is nocturnal penile tumescence monitoring. Nocturnal erections occur in healthy boys and men ages 3 to 79 years approximately every 90 to 100 minutes during sleep. These last an average of 20 to 40 minutes per episode, commonly accompanying rapid eye movement states of sleep, and decrease in quantity and quality as men age (55). One commonly used clinical technique to prove the absence of nocturnal erections is to place an intact ring of postage stamps around the flaccid penis, using the adhesive on the back of the last stamp to secure the circle. During sleep, the pressure of even a partial erection is sufficient to cause visible breakage in the perforations between the stamps. Nocturnal penile tumescence can be measured during a study in a formal sleep lab or with a RigiScan instrument (Bard Instruments).

If a man is not depressed and has normal nocturnal penile tumescence for his age, his ED is considered to be largely psychogenic, and the treatment of choice is individual or couples' counseling. If there are no nocturnal erections, only partial nocturnal erections, or if sufficient rigidity is not achieved, the cause is more likely organic.

The primary organic causes of ED include vascular disorders, neurologic disorders, use of medications or substances, endocrinologic disorders, and surgical complications (Table 22.5). For patients with vascular, neurologic, or surgical causes, penile implants or the use of vasoactive agents injected into the cavernosa are treatment options. Medications that are commonly associated with the onset of erectile disorders include antihypertensives, antidepressants, central nervous system sedatives or anxiolytics, H_2-blockers, alcohol, and antipsychotics (Table 22.4). Changing the medication, altering the dose or dosing schedule, or taking a drug holiday may provide relief from sexual side effects.

Pharmacologic interventions are popular. Sildenafil (Viagra), vardenafil (Levitra), and tadalafil (Cialis) have all emerged as treatment options. These medications work to increase blood flow to the penis, enabling a man to achieve and/or maintain erection. However, it is clear that they do not increase essential desire and will not help a man with decreased desire or an arousal disorder. Pfizer (manufacturer of Viagra) points out in their patient literature that more than 30 million men in the United States have ED to some degree, meaning there are also 30 million partners affected by ED who will also reap the benefits of the use of medication.

It is often the woman who requests information about such medical treatments on her partner's behalf. Her partner should be encouraged to see his own physician for evaluation for reversible organic causes and a decision as to whether this medication would be safe for his use.

SUMMARY

There are many opportunities to recognize sexual dysfunction in a medical practice specializing in women's reproductive health. Prevalence rates of sexual dysfunction in a general population range from 25 to 50%. The challenge for most physicians lies in establishing a comfort level with the subject matter and gaining the necessary sensitivity and interpersonal communication skills needed when discussing sexual functioning. Approaching sexual health as an integral part of a patient's overall health helps practitioners decrease their own hesitancy and embarrassment when talking about sex with patients. This increases awareness, diagnosis, and treatment, enabling the patient to return to an optimal level of sexual function.

Managed care has ensured the role of family practitioners and gynecologists as gatekeepers and primary providers for women's health care. To do justice to their patients, physicians must consider the emotional and physical well-being of their patients. However, the physician cannot be expected to provide counseling or ongoing therapy in areas in which they have no specific training. The physician's duty to his or her patients is to inquire, listen, and integrate care for her physical and emotional well-being, referring to a counselor when appropriate.

Clinical Notes

TAKING A SEXUAL HISTORY

- Women want to be able to discuss sexual questions and problems with their primary care physicians and obstetricians/gynecologists.
- Sexual dysfunction diagnoses are often missed because key questions are not asked.

SEXUAL DYSFUNCTIONS IN WOMEN

- Dyspareunia may be complete, situational, primary, or secondary; it has many organic, functional, and psychological causes.
- Inhibited sexual desire has many causes, but it is important to rule out depression or other mood disorders as the primary problem.

- Vaginismus can often be overcome with Kegel and vaginal dilation exercises in addition to counseling.
- Anorgasmia may be primary, secondary, or situational. Behavioral treatment techniques are available.

SEXUAL DYSFUNCTIONS IN SPECIFIC POPULATIONS OF WOMEN

- Lesbians are just as susceptible to sexual dysfunctions as heterosexuals but may be even more hesitant to ask their physicians questions.
- Breast and gynecologic cancer patients and their partners have sexual dysfunction sequelae from their diseases and their treatments.
- Infertility patients have a tendency to develop new sexual dysfunctions because of the regimentation of intercourse that is part of their treatment.
- Sexual abuse and assault victims may be sexually promiscuous or sexually avoidant; remember, the gynecologist may be the first person who has asked them about their prior traumas.

SEXUAL DYSFUNCTIONS IN MEN

- Premature ejaculation can be treated with behavioral techniques.
- ED may be differentiated into organic or psychogenic (or both) etiologies based on nocturnal penile tumescence testing.
- Medications for ED have revolutionized treatment of this disorder, but they should only be prescribed after appropriate evaluation of the man.

REFERENCES

1. Bachmann GA, Leiblum SR, Grill J. Brief sexual inquiry in gynecologic practice. Obstet Gynecol 1989;73: 425–427.
2. Ende J, Rockwell S, Glasgow M. The sexual history in general medical practice. Arch Intern Med 1984;144: 558–561.
3. Frenken J, Van Tol P. Sexual problems in gynaecological practice. J Psychosom Obstet Gynaecol 1987;6:143–155.
4. Ketting E. Gynaecology—duty or service? J Psychosom Obstet Gynaecol 1984;3:107–114.
5. Lewis CE. Sexual practices: are physicians addressing the issues? J Gen Intern Med 1990;5(suppl):78–81.
6. Nease DE, Liese BS. Perceptions and treatment of sexual problems. Fam Med 1987;19(6):468–470.
7. Hansen JP, Bobula J, Meyer D, et al. Treat or refer: patients' interest in family physician involvement in their psychosocial problems. J Fam Pract 1987;24(5):499–503.
8. Frank E, Anderson C, Rubinstein D. Frequency of sexual dysfunction in "normal" couples. N Engl J Med 1978;299:111–115.
9. Baker M. A GP's view of sexual dysfunction and its treatment. Med J Aust 1991;155:612–614.
10. Burnap DW, Golden JS. Sexual problems in medical practice. Med Educ 1967;42:673–680.
11. Plouffe L. Screening for sexual problems through a simple questionnaire. Am J Obstet Gynecol 1985;151: 166–169.
12. Hammond DC. Screening for sexual dysfunction. Clin Obstet Gynecol 1984;27:232–237.
13. Steege JF. Dyspareunia and vaginismus. Clin Obstet Gynecol 1984;27:750–759.
14. American Psychiatric Association. Diagnostic and Statistical Manual of Mental Disorders, Fourth Edition, Text Revision. Washington, DC: American Psychiatric Press, 2000.
15. Sarrel PM. Sex problems after menopause: a study of fifty married couples in a sex counseling programme. Maturitas 1981;4:231–237.
16. Fink P. Dyspareunia: current concepts. Med Aspects Human Sex 1972;6:28–47.
17. McCarthy B, McCarthy E. Male Sexual Awareness. New York: Carroll & Graf, 1989.
18. McCarthy B, McCarthy E. Female Sexual Awareness. New York: Carroll & Graf, 1989.
19. McCarthy B, McCarthy E. Couple Sexual Awareness. New York: Carroll & Graf, 1990.
20. Barbach LG. For Yourself: The Fulfillment of Female Sexuality. New York: Doubleday, 1975.
21. LaFerla JJ. Inhibited sexual desire and orgasmic dysfunction in women. Clin Obstet Gynecol 1984;27:738–749.
22. Finger WW, Lund M, Slagle MA. Medications that may contribute to sexual disorders: a guide to assessment and treatment in family practice. J Fam Pract 1997;44:33–43.
23. Segraves RT. Antidepressant-induced orgasm disorder. J Sex Marital Ther 1995;2:192–201.
24. Margolese HC, Assalian P. Sexual side effects of antidepressants: a review. J Sex Marital Ther 1996;22:209–217.

25. Shen WW, Hsu JH. Female sexual side effects associated with selective serotonin reuptake inhibitors: a descriptive clinical study of 33 patients. Int J Psychiatry Med 1995;25:239–248.
26. Rothschild AJ. Selective serotonin reuptake inhibitors—induced sexual dysfunction: efficacy of a drug holiday. Am J Psychiatry 1995;152:1514–1516.
27. Ayd FJ Jr. Pertinent medical intelligence: fluoxetine's impact on sexual function. Md Med J 1995;44:526–527.
28. Dorevitch A, Davis H. Fluvoxamine-associated sexual dysfunction. Ann Pharmacother 1994;28:872–874.
29. Murphy WD, Coleman E, Hoon E, et al. Sexual dysfunctions and treatment in alcoholics. Sex Disabil 1980;3:240–245.
30. LoPiccolo J, Lobitz WC. The role of masturbation in the treatment of orgasmic dysfunction. In: LoPiccolo J, LoPiccolo L, eds. Handbook of Sex Therapy. New York: Plenum Press, 1978.
31. Schover LR, Montaugue DK, Youngs DD. Multidisciplinary treatment of an unconsummated marriage with organic factors in both spouses. Cleve Clin J Med 1993;60:72–74.
32. Branley HM, Brown J, Draper KC, et al. Non-consummation of marriage treated by members of the Institute of Psychosexual Medicine: a prospective study. Br J Obstet Gynaecol 1983;90:908–913.
33. Scholl GM. Prognostic variables in treating vaginismus. Obstet Gynecol 1988;72:231–235.
34. Falco KL. Psychotherapy With Lesbian Clients: Theory Into Practice. New York: Brunner/Mazel, 1991.
35. Loulan J. Preliminary Report on Survey of Lesbian Sex Practices. Unpublished manuscript, 1986.
36. Loulan J. Lesbian Passion: Loving Ourselves and Each Other. San Francisco: Spinsters/Aunt Lute, 1987.
37. Blumstein P, Schwartz P. American Couples. New York: William Morrow, 1983.
38. Nichols M. The treatment of inhibited sexual desire (ISD) in lesbian couples. Women Ther 1982;1:49–66.
39. Hall M. Sex therapy with lesbian couples: a four stage approach. J Homosex 1987;14:137–156.
40. Keye WR. Psychosexual responses to infertility. Clin Obstet Gynecol 1984;27:760–766.
41. Gervaise PA. The psychosexual impact of infertility and its treatment. Can J Human Sex 1993;2:141–149.
42. Burns LH. Infertility as boundary ambiguity: one theoretical perspective. Fam Process 1987;26:359–372.
43. Reading A. Sexual aspects of infertility. Infertil Reprod Clin North Am 1993;2:559–564.
44. Bain J. Sexuality and infertility in the male. Can J Human Sex 1993;2:157–160.
45. Baram D, Tourtelot T, Muechler E, et al. Psychological adjustment following unsuccessful in vitro fertilization. J Psychosom Obstet Gynaecol 1988;9:181–190.
46. Barwin NB. Sexual problems resulting in the need for homologous artificial insemination (AIH) as a treatment for infertility: psychotherapeutic considerations. Can J Human Sex 1993;2:179–182.
47. Delafontaine D. Artificial insemination: definition, indications, technique and results. Contracept Fertil Sex 1993;21:511–516.
48. Bachmann GA, Moeller TP, Bennett J. Childhood sexual abuse and the consequences in adult women. Obstet Gynecol 1988;71:631–642.
49. Tsai M, Feldman-Summers S, Edgar M. Childhood molestation: variables related to differential impacts on psychosexual functioning in adult women. J Abnorm Psychol 1979;88:407–417.
50. Becker JV, Skinner, LJ, Abel GG, et al. Incidence and types of sexual dysfunction in rape and incest victims. J Sex Marital Ther 1982;8:65–74.
51. Finklehor D, Browne A. The traumatic impact of child sexual abuse. Am J Orthopsychiatry 1985;55:530–541.
52. Maltz W, Holman B. Incest and Sexuality. Lexington, MA: Lexington Books, 1987.
53. Lowe JC, Mikulas WL. Use of written material in learning self control of premature ejaculation. In: LoPiccolo J, LoPiccolo L, eds. Handbook of Sex Therapy. New York: Plenum Press, 1978.
54. Schnarch DM. Constructing the Sexual Crucible: An Integration of Sexual and Marital Therapy. New York: WW Norton, 1991.
55. Karacan I. Advances in the psychophysiological evaluation of male erectile impotence. In: LoPiccolo J, LoPiccolo L, eds. Handbook of Sex Therapy. New York: Plenum Press, 1978.

CHAPTER 23

Psychiatric Disorders

James M. Martinez and Lauren B. Marangell

INTRODUCTION

Many major psychiatric illnesses occur more frequently in women than in men and may be exacerbated at various phases of the female reproductive cycle. Not surprisingly, these disorders are frequently encountered in obstetric and gynecologic practices. This chapter briefly reviews some of the major psychiatric diagnoses and their management, with an emphasis on disorders and treatments that are most relevant to the gynecologist. The psychiatric diagnoses discussed in this chapter and their initial management are listed in Table 23.1.

DEPRESSION DISORDERS

Psychiatric disorders with predominant depressive symptoms are commonly seen in the gynecologist's office. Although it may seem easier to diagnose "depression not otherwise specified (NOS)," attempting to clarify the type of mood disorder a patient has will lead to a more focused treatment approach. The following section first reviews the diagnosis and treatment of major depressive disorder (MDD) because the clinical approach to other forms of depression builds on this foundation.

Patients with depressive symptoms should also be assessed for a history of mania or hypomania, which would indicate the presence of bipolar disorder (discussed later in this chapter) and require a different treatment approach.

Major Depressive Disorder

MDD is one of the most common psychiatric illnesses worldwide and is associated with as much disability as several other chronic illnesses, including arthritis and coronary artery disease. Relapse rates are estimated at more than 50% after a single depressive episode, and 80 to 90% after a second depressive episode (1). MDD is projected to be the second leading cause of disability by the year 2020 (2).

Evidence suggests a genetic component in the etiology of MDD and other major affective disorders. Life's major stressors also predispose to the development of MDD. However, although individuals under great stress (e.g., trauma, bereavement, terminal cancer) have higher rates of MDD in comparison to the general population, most individuals do not develop MDD as a response to a major life stressor. Thus, the presence or absence of an identifiable "trigger" event is irrelevant to the diagnosis of MDD.

Several gender differences exist in the epidemiology, presentation, and course of an episode of major depression. Major depression is nearly twice as common in women compared with men; the lifetime prevalence of depression among women is 10 to 25%, whereas it is only 5 to

TABLE 23.1

Summary of Common Psychiatric Disorders and Initial Treatment Options

Psychiatric Disorder	Initial Treatment Options
Mood Disorders	
Major and minor depressive disorders, dysthymia	Antidepressants and psychotherapy (alone or in combination)
Premenstrual dysphoric disorder	SSRI, daily or only during the symptomatic days in the late luteal phase (see Chapter 7)
Bipolar Disorder	Psychiatric referral
Anxiety Disorders	
Generalized anxiety disorder	SSRI, venlafaxine (Effexor), buspirone (BuSpar), or benzodiazepine; consider referral for psychotherapy
Panic disorder	SSRI (start at one-half the usual starting dose for depression); high-potency benzodiazepine if needed for the short-term treatment of acute anxiety; strongly consider referral for psychotherapy
Social phobia	SSRI; beta-blocker (short-term use for performance anxiety); consider referral for psychotherapy
PTSD, OCD	SSRI plus psychotherapy
Psychotic Disorders	Psychiatric referral
Anorexia nervosa, bulimia nervosa	Management of medical complications; restoration of nutrition and normal weight; psychotherapy; support groups; SSRI for the treatment of bulimic symptoms and comorbid depression and anxiety; family interventions; psychiatric referral
Personality disorders	Psychiatric referral
Delirium	Full medical workup, often in hospitalized setting; high-potency antipsychotics for severe agitation; benzodiazepines for alcohol or sedative-hypnotic withdrawal only; avoid anticholinergics; psychiatric consultation

OCD, obsessive-compulsive disorder; PTSD, post-traumatic stress disorder; SSRI, selective serotonin reuptake inhibitor.

12% among men (3, 4). Depressive episodes may be more chronic in women, and recurrence rates are higher among women than men (5, 6).

Major depression in women often begins during the childbearing years and follows a chronic, recurrent course. Women have a greater likelihood of having comorbid anxiety disorders (7) and eating disorders (8). Several events during the female reproductive cycle may precipitate or exacerbate depressive episodes, and these are discussed here and in Chapter 7.

Diagnosis

MDD is characterized by a history of one or more major depressive episodes in which patients experience a predominantly depressed mood or anhedonia (a loss of interest in pleasurable activities) over a period of at least 2 weeks, with associated physical disturbances in sleep, appetite, energy level, libido, and concentration, and changes in psychomotor activity (9). Affected individuals may report feelings of guilt, hopelessness, helplessness, irritability, anxiety, somatic complaints, and thoughts of death. Difficulty falling asleep is nonspecific, but waking up too early

TABLE 23.2

The Harvard Department of Psychiatry/National Depression Screening Day Scale (HANDS™)

Over the Past 2 Weeks, How Often Have You:	None/Little of the Time (0 Points)	Some of the Time (1 Point)	Most of the Time (2 Points)	All the Time (3 Points)
1. been feeling low in energy, slowed down?				
2. been blaming yourself for things?				
3. had poor appetite?				
4. had difficulty falling asleep, staying asleep?				
5. been feeling hopeless about the future?				
6. been feeling blue?				
7. been feeling no interest in things?				
8. had feelings of worthlessness?				
9. thought about or wanted to commit suicide?				
10. had difficulty concentrating or making decisions?				

MDE, major depressive episode.

Score of 0–8, MDE is unlikely. Unless item 9 elicited a positive response, a complete evaluation is not recommended. Score of 9–16, MDE is likely, complete evaluation is recommended. Score of 17–30, MDE is very likely, complete evaluation is strongly recommended, immediate attention may be required.

Adapted from Baer L, Jacobs DG, Meszler-Reizes J, et al. Development of a brief screening instrument: the HANDS. Psychother Psychosom 2000;69:35–41, with permission of Screening for Mental Health, Inc.

(Obstetricians, gynecologists, and other primary care clinicians are invited to screen patients for mood disorders by participating free of charge in National Depression Screening Day. Clinicians can participate by screening on one day in October or November and/or throughout the year. CEUs are provided. To register, e-mail info@mentalhealthscreening.org or call 781-239-0071.)

in the morning and being unable to go back to sleep, or alternatively, consistent hypersomnia are quite characteristic of major depression.

Despite the global nature of the symptoms of depression, only about 50% of depressed patients are recognized as such by clinicians. Patients with depression often do not complain specifically of depression. They may seek medical attention for a variety of somatic symptoms, including chronic aches and pains with anatomic bases but out of proportion to what the patient usually encounters; alternatively, the patient may express nonspecific nervous complaints. It is important to incorporate routine screening for MDD at annual exams and when vague symptoms raise suspicion.

Screening instruments for depression such as the Zung scale or Beck Inventory of Depression may be used to rate the severity of symptoms. More recently, Baer et al. developed a shorter scale, which they found performed at least as well as Zung and Beck (10). Table 23.2 reproduces their depression screening questionnaire, which has been used for National Depression Screening Day, included in 2003. A score of 9 or higher indicates that the patient should be more thoroughly evaluated for MDD. However, the *diagnosis* of MDD should made using *DSM-IV-TR* criteria (Table 23.3).

Although making the diagnosis of MDD requires ruling out nonpsychiatric causes of the symptoms (Table 23.4), a true diagnosis of MDD does not preclude the concurrent presence of other medical, or even psychiatric, diagnoses. Lab studies to rule out an underlying medical condition may include a complete blood count, urinalysis, urine drug screen, chemistry profile, or thyroid panel.

TABLE 23.3

DSM-IV-TR Criteria for Major Depressive Episode

$\geq$ of the following symptoms present during the same 2-week period and representing a change from previous functioning. Either (1) or (2) *must* be present.

(1) Depressed mood most of the day, nearly every day, as indicated by either subjective report or observation by others
(2) Markedly diminished interest or pleasure in all, or almost all, activities most of the day, nearly every day (subjective or observational)
(3) Significant weight loss when not dieting or weight gain ($>$5% body weight in 1 month) or decrease or increase in appetite nearly every day
(4) Insomnia or hypersomnia nearly every day
(5) Psychomotor agitation or retardation nearly every day
(6) Fatigue or loss of energy nearly every day
(7) Feelings of worthlessness or excessive or inappropriate guilt nearly every day (not merely self-reproach about being sick)
(8) Diminished ability to think or concentrate, or indecisiveness, nearly every day (subjective or observational)
(9) Recurrent thoughts of death (not fear of dying), recurrent suicidal ideation with or without a specific plan, or a suicide attempt

Modified from American Psychiatric Association. Diagnostic and Statistical Manual of Mental Disorders, Fourth Edition, Text Revision. Washington, DC: American Psychiatric Press, 2000.

TABLE 23.4

Common Medical Causes of Psychiatric Symptoms

Symptoms of	Common Medical Causes
Depression	Hypothyroidism and other endocrine disorders; CVA; vitamin B12 deficiency; infection; medication side effects; drug intoxication or withdrawal states
Mania	CVA; substance intoxication (e.g., stimulants, alcohol, hallucinogens); hyperthyroidism; Cushing's disease; CNS infections; temporal lobe epilepsy; Wilson's disease
Anxiety	Endocrine disorders (e.g., adrenal or thyroid dysfunction, hypoglycemia, pheochromocytoma); anemia; cardiovascular disorders (e.g., myocardial infarction, arrhythmias, mitral valve prolapse); pulmonary disorders (e.g., pulmonary embolus, asthma); alcohol or drug intoxication or withdrawal states; infection; medication side effects or interactions
Psychosis	Endocrine disorders; heavy metal poisoning; neurologic disorders (e.g., Wilson's disease, dementia, epilepsy); nutritional deficiencies; alcohol or drug intoxication or withdrawal states; medication side effects or interactions; CNS infections
Delirium	Metabolic disorders; systemic illnesses/infections; postoperative states; severe trauma; postictal states; CNS disorders; medication side effects or interactions; toxins/poisonings

CNS, central nervous system; CVA, cerebral vascular accident.

Patients with severe depression may experience psychotic symptoms (e.g., hallucinations, delusions, catatonia) and/or suicidal thoughts. The presence of either is a red flag for referral. Direct questions about the presence of suicidal thoughts, plans, and the availability of the means to carry out the plan must be openly discussed with the patient. Asking about suicide will not increase a patient's risk for committing suicide. Inquiries about it may actually reassure the patient, and allow the patient and clinician to make plans to prevent it.

Treatment

Treatment of major depression should be aimed at complete symptom remission and functional recovery, and is effective in more than 90% of patients. After other causes have been ruled out or effectively treated, treatment options for MDD include antidepressant medications, psychotherapy alone or in combination with medications, and electroconvulsive therapy (ECT). ECT, though effective, is reserved for pharmacology-refractory patients and other special circumstances that are beyond the scope of this chapter.

Prior to the initiation of psychoactive medication for MDD, and for all psychiatric disorders that may respond to psychoactive agents, a clear diagnosis of a psychiatric illness must be made. In addition, a clear treatment plan, including the length of time the medication will be used should be developed. The absence of a diagnosis and plan increases the likelihood the patient will overuse, misuse, or become psychologically dependent on the psychoactive medication. Numerous antidepressant medications are available (Table 23.5). Elderly patients should typically be started at dosages half that of usual initial dose because they often achieve treatment goals at lower doses.

All antidepressants are believed to be equally effective in treating major depression, although individual patients may preferentially respond to a particular agent. The choice of agent is generally based on the side effect profile, convenience of use, and price. Response typically occurs 4 to 6 weeks after initiation of antidepressant treatment, although therapeutic effects may be seen after 10 to 14 days in some patients. If no response is seen, the dose should be titrated upward, as tolerated, to the upper dose range. If an adequate response is still not achieved, switching to a different antidepressant is indicated. Patients with MDD often suffer from other comorbid psychiatric illnesses, which may contribute to inadequate treatment response, treatment nonadherence, and a poorer overall prognosis. Such patients should be referred to a psychiatrist for further evaluation and management.

For the first 6 to 8 weeks after the diagnosis is made, the patient with MDD should be seen frequently (every 1 to 3 weeks, depending on symptom severity) to adjust medications as necessary and for brief supportive psychotherapy. Major life decisions should be delayed if possible during this time. Frank discussions about suicidal plans, thoughts, and intentions need to be assessed with each visit. Patients need to be asked routinely about medication side effects. The more depressed a patient is, the less tolerant they will be of even minor adverse effects, and they may self-discontinue their medication without discussing it with their provider.

When response and remission are achieved, patients should continue the antidepressant medication at the same dose for maintenance treatment to prevent recurrences of major depression (11). Lowering the dose for maintenance therapy is not recommended. The duration of maintenance treatment depends on numerous factors, including number of prior depressive episodes. In general, patients with one major depressive episode should be treated for at least 6 to 12 months after achieving remission before considering treatment discontinuation. Patients with a history of three or more depressive episodes should consider indefinite maintenance treatment due to the high risk of recurrent depressive episodes.

Psychotherapy

Current office-based psychotherapies for MDD are very oriented toward the present and often use the techniques of cognitive therapy and interpersonal therapy in counseling sessions. The patient with MDD often experiences cognitive distortions, and cognitive therapy works to address and negate these distortions. Interpersonal therapy focuses on the social contexts and consequences of MDD, and helps patients develop skills in three key areas: identifying and dealing with stressful situations, recognizing the assets they possess to deal effectively with those situations, and becoming aware of alternative choices. However, in most acute depressive states, pharmacotherapy is still required because psychotherapy requires that the patient be able to concentrate, then later recall and effectively begin to use new coping mechanisms.

Pharmacotherapy

The selective serotonin reuptake inhibitors (SSRIs) are commonly used as first-line medications for the treatment of major depression and most major anxiety disorders. The available SSRIs include citalopram (Celexa), escitalopram (Lexapro), fluoxetine (Prozac, Sarafem, Prozac Weekly), fluvoxamine (Luvox), paroxetine (Paxil, Paxil CR), and sertraline (Zoloft). The advantages of SSRIs include improved tolerability as compared with older antidepressants, relative safety in the elderly and medically ill patients, relative safety in overdose situations (when taken alone), ease of use, and, for some agents, anticompulsive and antianxiety effects. Individual SSRIs differ from one another with respect to dosage guidelines, half-life, metabolism to active or inactive metabolites, drug interaction potential, and risk for discontinuation symptoms on abrupt cessation of treatment. The starting dose of an SSRI may be the effective treatment dose (Table 23.5).

Common side effects of SSRIs include insomnia, sedation, gastrointestinal upset, nausea, vomiting, diarrhea, sweating, headaches, restlessness, and dose-related sexual dysfunction. Weight gain is not common with SSRIs. Most side effects are transient, with the exception of sexual dysfunction, which typically persists but is reversible on medication discontinuation. Approximately 20% of patients on SSRIs will report sexual dysfunction as a side effect of the therapy. Although the most common complaint is a delay to orgasm or anorgasmia, problems such as loss of interest and erectile dysfunction may also occur. Sildenafil (Viagra) has been used in women with antidepressant-induced sexual dysfunction with moderate success in open trials (12). Antidepressants with fewer propensities for sexual dysfunction include bupropion (Wellbutrin, Wellbutrin SR, Wellbutrin XR, Zyban), nefazodone (Serzone), and mirtazapine (Remeron).

An uncomfortable discontinuation syndrome is associated with the abrupt cessation of SSRIs and venlafaxine (Effexor) after 2 or more months of use; this is particularly true for all but fluoxetine, which has a very long half-life. Symptoms of the withdrawal syndrome include irritability, insomnia, restlessness, headaches, and mild paresthesias. These symptoms can be avoided or alleviated by slowly tapering the SSRI over a period of about 10 to 14 days. For discontinuation of fluoxetine, tapering can be done first by lengthening the dosing interval to every other day and eventually to once or twice a week before its discontinuation.

SSRIs can elevate levels of other medications, including heterocyclic antidepressants, anticonvulsants, warfarin (Coumadin), quinidine (Quinidex, Quinora), benzodiazepines, digoxin (Lanoxin, Digitek), and flecainide (Tambocor).

Venlafaxine, a dual norepinephrine and serotonin reuptake inhibitor, is also considered a first-line option in the treatment of major depression. An extended-release preparation is available (Effexor XR) and is preferred due to once-daily dosing and improved tolerability as compared with the immediate-release formulation. Doses above 300 mg daily can cause diastolic hypertension (13).

Bupropion, a norepinephrine and dopamine reuptake inhibitor, is recognized as a first-line agent for the treatment of major depression. It is also U.S. Food and Drug Administration (FDA) approved for the indication of smoking cessation. Common side effects include anxiety, insomnia, and headaches, although it is relatively devoid of sexual side effects or weight gain. In 2003, a once-daily preparation became available, Wellbutrin XR. A disadvantage to the use of bupropion is a dose-dependent risk of seizures. Patients with a history of a seizure disorder or eating disorder are at particularly increased risk for seizures when using bupropion, so its use in these patient populations is contraindicated.

Other antidepressants are relatively safe and commonly prescribed as second-line or adjunct therapy. Nefazodone and trazodone (Desyrel) block presynaptic serotonin reuptake and postsynaptic serotonin-2 receptors. Common side effects of nefazodone include sedation, dizziness, and visual disturbances, but it is not typically associated with weight gain or sexual dysfunction. There are rare reports of liver failure in patients taking nefazodone. Coadministration of antihistaminics should be avoided. Trazodone side effects include excessive sedation, orthostatic hypotension, and risk of priapism. Many clinicians prescribe trazodone at low doses (25 to 100 mg) at night for the short-term treatment of insomnia, although this is not an FDA-approved

TABLE 23.5

Commonly Prescribed Antidepressants, FDA-Approved Uses, Dosages, and Key Side Effects

Medication	FDA-Approved Uses	Antidepressant Dose		Key Side Effects
		Initial Dose[a]	Dose Range	
Selective Serotonin Reuptake Inhibitors (SSRIs)				
Citalopram (Celexa)	Depression	20 mg daily	20–40 mg daily	Nausea, dry mouth, somnolence, insomnia, sweating, sexual dysfunction
Escitalopram (Lexapro)		10 mg daily	10–20 mg daily	
Fluoxetine (Prozac, Sarafem)	Depression; OCD; bulimia nervosa; PMDD	20 mg qAM	20–80 mg qAM	Nausea, headaches, insomnia, nervousness, somnolence, sexual dysfunction
Fluvoxamine (Luvox)	OCD	50 mg qhs	50–150 mg twice a day	Nausea, headaches, somnolence, insomnia, dry mouth, asthenia, nervousness, sexual dysfunction
Paroxetine (Paxil, Paxil-CR)	Depression; OCD; panic disorder; social phobia; GAD	20 mg daily, _ mg daily for CR	20–50 mg daily, _ mg daily for CR	Nausea, somnolence, headaches, dry mouth, asthenia, constipation, sexual dysfunction
Sertraline (Zoloft)	Depression; OCD; panic disorder; PTSD	50 mg daily	50–200 mg daily	Nausea, diarrhea, insomnia, dry mouth, somnolence, sweating, sexual dysfunction
Other Antidepressants				
Bupropion extended release (Wellbutrin XR)	Depression; aid in smoking cessation (see Chapter 19)	150 mg qAM	150–300 mg qAM	Agitation, headaches, dizziness, anorexia, constipation, sweating, insomnia, sedation, dose-dependent seizure risk
Mirtazapine (Remeron)	Depression	15 mg qhs	15–45 mg qhs	Somnolence, weight gain
Nefazodone (Serzone)	Depression	50 mg twice a day	150–300 mg twice a day	Headaches, nausea, sedation, visual changes, hepatic failure (rare)
Venlafaxine extended-release (Effexor XR)	Depression; GAD	37.5–75 mg daily	75–225 mg daily	Similar to SSRIs; dose-dependent risk of increase in blood pressure, especially above 300 mg/day

FDA, U.S. Food and Drug Administration; GAD, generalized anxiety disorder; OCD, obsessive-compulsive disorder; PMDD, premenstrual dysphoric disorder; PTSD, post-traumatic stress disorder.

[a]Starting doses for SSRIs in the treatment of anxiety disorders may be lower than those listed in this table.

indication. Mirtazapine is an antidepressant medication with multiple neuroreceptor interactions. Although it has a low risk for sexual dysfunction and cytochrome P-450 enzyme-related drug interactions, common side effects include sedation and weight gain.

Heterocyclic antidepressants, a category that includes the tricyclic antidepressants (TCAs), are older antidepressants that are still used. Because the newer antidepressants described previously have fewer severe (including cardiac) side effects and are safer in overdose, the heterocyclics/tricyclics should not be considered first-line therapy for depression. Monoamine oxidase inhibitors (MAOIs) are also an older class of antidepressants. Because of multiple side effects and drug–drug interactions (including common foods and over-the-counter medications), these drugs should be avoided in the primary care setting.

Major Depressive Disorder and Pregnancy

Available data suggest that rates of major depression are similar in pregnant and nonpregnant women. However, numerous factors may increase the risk for depression in pregnancy, including a prior history of depression, young maternal age, greater number of children, poor social support, ambivalence regarding the pregnancy, and marital problems (14–17). For individuals with a history of major depression, discontinuation of antidepressant medications during pregnancy may precipitate a relapse of depression (18, 19). Women with depression during pregnancy are at risk for poor mother–infant interactions during the postpartum period (20).

There are several issues regarding the pharmacologic treatment of depression during pregnancy. The risk of potential harmful effects of early fetal exposure to antidepressants must be considered against the risk of untreated maternal depression with its negative health and safety consequences for both mother and fetus.

Bupropion (Wellbutrin) is a Category B drug in pregnancy. Available data suggest that SSRIs are probably safe for use during pregnancy (18, 21–23), even though all SSRIs and venlafaxine are Category C in pregnancy. Although a prospective study reported minor malformations and perinatal complications in infants exposed to fluoxetine in utero during late pregnancy (24), the methodology of this study has been criticized. Women choosing to take antidepressants preconceptually or during pregnancy should be informed of the known and unknown risks of fetal exposure to antidepressants. These issues have been reviewed at length elsewhere (23, 25).

Pregnancy loss and miscarriage may increase the risk of major depression (26). Patients with a recent history of pregnancy loss, particularly those with a prior history of major depression, should be monitored for the emergence of depressive symptoms.

Major Depressive Disorder and the Postpartum Period

The postpartum period can be associated with a range of affective symptoms, from the mild and self-limited "postpartum blues" to the more severe syndromes of postpartum depression and postpartum psychosis. The "postpartum blues" typically arise within days after delivery and remit spontaneously within 2 weeks. Treatment involves reassurance and social support, although close monitoring may be indicated because some women with the postpartum blues will develop postpartum depression (27, 28).

Postpartum depression affects approximately 10% of postpartum women. The *DSM-IV-TR* diagnosis of "major depressive disorder with postpartum onset" requires the onset of symptoms within 1 month after delivery (9, 14), although the obstetric literature indicates women may be at an increased risk for depression for several months after delivery. Symptoms are similar to those of nonpostpartum depression and may include marked anxiety, sleep problems, and feelings of doubt regarding parental abilities. Affected individuals may also have thoughts of harming themselves or their infants. Postpartum depression can interfere with a woman's functioning as a new mother and negatively impact the infant's development (29–33).

Risk factors for the development of postpartum affective disorders include a prior history of postpartum affective disorders, a history of nonpostpartum affective disorders, a family history of depression, inadequate social support, marital discord, and adverse life events during pregnancy (34–38). Treatment usually consists of a combination of pharmacotherapy (SSRIs and TCAs are usually effective) and supportive psychotherapy.

Prophylactic administration of antidepressant treatment to asymptomatic women (with a prior history of postpartum depression) during the postpartum period may prevent the onset of a new depressive episode (39). Women should be educated about the signs and symptoms of postpartum depression as part of routine prenatal care.

Postpartum psychosis, a severe form of postpartum depression, occurs in 1 to 2 women per 1000 deliveries, or approximately 0.1% of postpartum women (40). There is always a symptom-free interval between delivery and the onset of symptoms. Symptoms of irritability and sleep changes may arise within days after delivery, rapidly followed by hallucinations, delusions, disorganized behavior, and mood lability (41). When symptoms present within days of delivery, the most common presentation is affective psychosis, which may include intense feelings of guilt and worthlessness, uncontrollable crying, and death wishes. A late onset of postpartum psychosis (i.e., greater than 3 weeks after delivery) often presents with a schizophreniform syndrome and tends to occur in older women with a history of pre-existing psychopathology. Suicide and infanticide are possible consequences. Risk factors for postpartum psychosis include a past history of postpartum psychosis or bipolar disorder (42). Recurrence rates are high (43).

Postpartum psychosis is a psychiatric emergency and mandates immediate psychiatric involvement. Treatment includes antipsychotic medications and mood stabilizers (particularly in those individuals with an underlying bipolar disorder). Hospitalization, with separation of mother and newborn, is almost always necessary.

Major Depressive Disorder Therapies and Lactation

Breast-feeding women should be informed that antidepressants are secreted into breast milk, and detectable levels of antidepressants and their metabolites may be found in the plasma of some infants (44). The effects of such neonatal antidepressant exposure on infant development are unknown, and the physician and patient should weigh the potential benefits of treatment with antidepressants against the unknown risks of neonatal exposure to medication through the breast milk. For women who choose to take or continue antidepressant medications, sertraline is considered safest among the SSRIs. Bupropion, although Category B in pregnancy, is generally not considered safe in breast-feeding.

For individuals who choose not to take antidepressant medications while breast-feeding, there are limited data supporting the use of psychotherapy, including interpersonal therapy (45) and cognitive behavioral therapy (46).

Major Depressive Disorder and the Perimenopause

The perimenopausal period may be associated with an increased risk of a recurrence or exacerbation of depression in women with a prior history of major depression (47). Women without a prior history of major depression may experience depressive symptoms but are not at an increased risk for new-onset major depression (48, 49). Various factors may contribute to the increased risk of depression during this period, including declining ovarian function (50) and numerous age-related psychosocial stressors (51).

Antidepressants are first-line treatment for perimenopausal MDD. Some studies have suggested a role for hormone replacement therapy in reducing depressive symptoms (52, 53), though available data regarding estrogen therapy as either monotherapy or adjunctive therapy to antidepressants for the treatment of perimenopausal depression are conflicting.

Minor Depressive Disorder

Many patients may not meet *DSM-IV-TR* criteria for MDD but suffer from depressive symptoms nonetheless. The diagnosis requires at least two, but less than five, of the criteria used to diagnose MDD (Table 23.3), with the additional stipulations that there has never been an MDD, criteria are not met for dysthymic disorder (discussed later), and the patient has never had manic or psychotic symptoms.

The prevalence of minor depression is twice that of MDD. Its classification as "minor" is misleading because it is associated with significant functional impairments and with adverse clinical outcomes (54). Approximately 8% of patients suffering minor depression will have persistent symptoms, whereas 10 to 18% will develop MDD within 1 year (55). Because trial data are limited, there are no definitive treatment options for this disorder. One commonly accepted approach is to use supportive office visits coupled with educational efforts for 4 to 6 weeks, and if this is not successful, a trial of antidepressants and/or referral for cognitive behavioral therapy may be initiated.

Premenstrual Syndrome and Premenstrual Dysphoric Disorder

Premenstrual syndrome (PMS) is a term often used to describe a syndrome that occurs during the luteal phase of the menstrual cycle and peaks prior to menstrual bleeding. Characteristic symptoms include somatic complaints such as bloating, breast tenderness, and nonspecific aches, as well as impairments in concentration, appetite, sleep, and mood. The public often uses the term "PMS" to describe mild symptoms that do not impair functioning and in fact occur in the majority of women. Premenstrual dysphoric disorder (PMDD) refers to a more severe syndrome that occurs regularly and exclusively during the late luteal phase of the menstrual cycle and affects 3 to 8% of fertile women. For a more complete discussion of PMS and PMDD, see Chapter 8.

Adjustment Disorder With Depressed Mood

Adjustment disorder with depressed mood is a psychiatric condition resulting from an identifiable stressor in which the accompanying level of emotional and mental impairment is greater than what would be expected for most individuals. An example of this diagnosis might be the patient who on experiencing a loss, and instead of an uncomplicated bereavement, experiences excessive depressed mood, tearfulness, and hopelessness. This must also be distinguished from posttraumatic stress disorder (PTSD), discussed in the Anxiety Disorders section. The diagnosis is applicable only within the first 6 months after the stressor occurs. If the impairment lasts longer than 6 months, a diagnosis of another form of depression should be sought. Treatment is generally psychotherapy and/or crisis intervention. Judicious and time-limited use of antidepressants may also be helpful.

Dysthymia

Dysthymia is a milder form of depression (compared with major depression and minor depression) marked by considerable chronicity. It is a depressed state that lasts for 2 or more years. Because the depressed mood is so persistent in dysthymia, many of the patient's family and friends may attribute the lowered mood and functional impairments and difficulties as being "just the way she is."

Patients with dysthymia may present with a multiplicity of medical complaints and excessive use of medical services; marital, family, or job difficulties that are ongoing; or suicide attempts. Symptoms commonly seen include hypersomnia, loss of energy and libido, increased appetite, and weight gain.

There is a high rate of MDD among patients with dysthymia, so it is important to remember the two may coexist. SSRIs and heterocyclic antidepressants have been shown to be effective, and brief episodes of psychotherapy may also be helpful.

Depression Secondary to a Medical Condition, Medication, or Substance of Abuse

Prior to making a diagnosis of depressive disorder, the clinician must rule out nonpsychiatric causes of depressive symptoms, including medical conditions, medications, and substances of abuse. Common nonpsychiatric causes of depressive symptoms are shown in Table 23.4. Almost any medical condition may cause depression, either through the psychological trauma of being ill or through a combined psychobiological effect. The treatment of a secondary depression focuses on the resolution of the medical condition and/or withdrawal of the substance. Psychiatric therapy is also often needed and recommended, depending on the etiology.

BIPOLAR DISORDER

Bipolar disorder is a mood disorder with a cyclical course of illness in which affected patients experience major depressive episodes and manic (bipolar I disorder) or hypomanic (bipolar II disorder) episodes (9). Manic episodes are periods of elevated, euphoric, or irritable mood accompanied by several characteristic symptoms. These include a lack of insight, significant increase in energy, decreased need for sleep, impulsivity, racing thoughts, pressured speech, distractibility, increased libido, psychomotor restlessness, and involvement in activities that have potentially harmful consequences, such as spending sprees or sexual indiscretions (9). Patients may be delusionally grandiose, believing they have a special significance in the world or developing expansive projects or plans. Similarly, patients with hyperreligiosity may feel a special connection with a higher power or pray excessively. Alternatively, patients' delusions may be of a persecutory and paranoid nature.

In most instances, manic patients are referred for psychiatric evaluation and treatment. The *DSM-IV-TR* diagnostic criteria for mania require that patients presenting with psychosis or other symptoms lasting for at least 1 week that impair functioning warrant psychiatric hospitalization (9). This may be very difficult because most acutely manic patients do not believe their behavior is disturbed. Although voluntary hospitalization is optimal, civil commitment may be necessary to initiate therapy. Less severe episodes that do not significantly impair functioning are referred to as hypomania.

The lifetime prevalence of bipolar I disorder, based on cross-national epidemiologic data, is approximately 0.3 to 1.5% (56). First-degree relatives of persons affected by bipolar depression are at increased risk of developing mood disorders. Approximately 10% of children with one affected parent will develop the illness themselves. Bipolar disorder typically begins during young adulthood and follows a chronic and episodic, though variable, course. It is highly comorbid with other psychiatric disorders and is associated with an increased risk of suicide.

Treatment includes mood-stabilizing medications, such as lithium (Eskalith, Lithobid, Lithonate), valproic acid (Depakene, Depakote, Depacon), and olanzapine (Zyprexa), as well as other antipsychotic medications. Patients with bipolar disorder that are being treated with antidepressants must be monitored closely because one of the side effects for the antidepressant therapy may be a shift in mood toward mania. Patients with known or suspected bipolar disorder should be referred to a psychiatrist for further evaluation and management.

ANXIETY DISORDERS

Anxiety disorders are the most common psychiatric disorders in the United States, with a lifetime prevalence of nearly 25% (3). They tend to develop at an early age. The etiology of anxiety disorders appears to be multifactorial, and there is some evidence of a genetic contribution for some of the specific anxiety disorders.

Women are three times more likely to suffer an anxiety disorder than men (57). Certain conditions associated with secondary anxiety are more common in women than men, including hyperthyroidism, mitral valve prolapse, stimulant use for weight loss, and certain collagen diseases. For other conditions associated with secondary anxiety, see Table 23.4.

The various anxiety disorders can be more difficult to diagnose than depression or psychosis. This is due in part to vague symptoms, or alternatively, symptoms suggestive of a serious underlying medical condition. In addition, patients with anxiety disorder may report numerous physical symptoms, and other emotional problems may coexist with the anxiety disorder.

Generalized Anxiety Disorder

Generalized anxiety disorder (GAD) involves excessive, uncontrollable anxiety and worry about numerous aspects of daily life. Symptoms of GAD overlap considerably with symptoms of major depression and include restlessness, fatigue, impaired concentration and sleep, irritability, and muscle tension. *DSM-IV-TR* diagnostic criteria (Table 23.6) require that at least three symptoms be present for most days during a 6-month period or longer, be severe enough to impair normal

TABLE 23.6

DSM-IV-TR Criteria for Generalized Anxiety Disorder

A. Excessive anxiety and worry (apprehensive expectation), occurring more days than not for ≥6 months, about a number of events or activities
B. The person finds it difficult to control the worry
C. The anxiety and worry are associated with ≥3 of the following 6 symptoms (with at least some symptoms present for more days than not for the past 6 months)
   (1) Restlessness or feeling keyed up or on edge
   (2) Being easily fatigued
   (3) Difficulty concentrating or mind going blank
   (4) Irritability
   (5) Muscle tension
   (6) Sleep disturbance
D. The focus of the anxiety and worry is not confined to features of an Axis I (psychiatric) disorder, e.g., the anxiety or worry is not about having a panic attack (as in panic disorder), being embarrassed in public (as in social phobia), being contaminated (as in obsessive-compulsive disorder), being away from home or close relatives (as in separation anxiety disorder), gaining weight (as in anorexia nervosa), having multiple physical complaints (as in somatization disorder), or having a serious illness (as in hypochondriasis), and the anxiety and worry do not occur exclusively during post-traumatic stress disorder
E. The anxiety, worry, or physical symptoms cause clinically significant distress or impairment in social, occupational, or other important areas of functioning
F. The disturbance is not due to the direct physiologic effects of a substance (drug of abuse or prescribed medication) or a general medical condition and does not occur exclusively during a mood disorder, psychotic disorder, or a pervasive developmental disorder

Modified from American Psychiatric Association. Diagnostic and Statistical Manual of Mental Disorders, Fourth Edition, Text Revision. Washington, DC: American Psychiatric Press, 2000.

functioning, and are not caused by another psychiatric disorder, medication or substance of abuse, or me dical condition (9).

The lifetime prevalence of GAD is approximately 5%, with women being affected nearly twice as often as men (3). GAD is a chronic illness that tends to develop insidiously, often in the teens or early twenties during times of stress (the mean age of onset is 21 years), and fluctuates in severity throughout its course (58). Comorbidity with other psychiatric disorders is common (59), particularly other mood disorders, alcoholism, and other anxiety disorders, and when this occurs the prognosis for recovery is poorer (58). There is little evidence for a genetic basis for GAD, but traumatic early life experiences may serve as predisposing factors.

The clinical dilemma in patients with GAD symptoms revolves around the question of how much examination and testing needs to be done to rule out medical conditions that may present with symptoms of anxiety (e.g., heart disease in a patient presenting with chest pain and palpitations). Patients should have a complete medical and focused physical examination to rule out underlying medical conditions. Patients should be counseled about moderating or eliminating alcohol, caffeine, and other drugs, such as weight loss pills, that may cause worsening of their symptoms. Inquires about life stressors and attempts made by the patient to engage in relaxation techniques or efforts should be made.

Psychotherapy, particularly cognitive behavioral therapy, may be effective alone or in combination with pharmacologic agents in the treatment of GAD (60).

Pharmacotherapy

Benzodiazepines are effective anxiolytic agents (61) with a rapid onset of symptomatic relief and are the most commonly prescribed drugs for anxiety. The available benzodiazepines differ mainly in their pharmacokinetic properties and metabolism to active or inactive metabolites.

Most benzodiazepines are metabolized in the liver through oxidative degeneration, except for lorazepam (Ativan) and oxazepam (Serax), which are metabolized through conjugation with glucuronic acid only. This is significant because glucuronic conjugation occurs even in the presence of impaired liver function due to illness or age. For this reason, in elderly patients or in patients with impaired liver function, lorazepam (Ativan) or oxazepam (Serax) are the preferred benzodiazepines of use.

Common side effects of benzodiazepines include sedation, anterograde amnesia, dizziness, and psychomotor impairment. They are relatively safe when taken in overdose. There is, however, a high potential for both physiologic dependence and abuse with benzodiazepines. Tolerance to the euphoric effects in abusers often develops, leading to progressively increased doses. Conversely, tolerance to the anxiolytic effects is uncommon. A dangerous withdrawal syndrome is associated with abrupt benzodiazepine discontinuation; thus, a slow taper is recommended when discontinuing benzodiazepines.

SSRIs and venlafaxine are also effective in the treatment of GAD, and because of their relative safety and lack of potential for addiction, are considered by many to be preferred (over benzodiazepines) as first-line therapy (62–65). These may be particularly useful in patients with comorbid depression.

Buspirone (BuSpar), an anxiolytic agent that modulates serotonin activity, is FDA approved for the treatment of GAD. The effective dose range is 20 to 60 mg/day divided twice a day (66). The onset of action may be delayed for several weeks, and some patients may require higher doses. Buspirone does not share the anticonvulsant, sedating, or muscle relaxant properties associated with benzodiazepines, but it also does not carry their risk for dependence or withdrawal syndrome (67, 68). Though effective in treating GAD, it is not effective in treating other comorbid anxiety disorders or comorbid major depression.

Panic Disorder

Panic attacks are discrete episodes of sudden, intense anxiety and fear with associated affective, somatic, and cognitive symptoms. Panic disorder includes recurrent panic attacks with anticipatory anxiety about future attacks (9). The frequency and intensity of attacks vary widely. The object of the fear may, or may not, be defined. Panic disorder is diagnosed when the patient experiences panic attacks four times or more in 1 month, and when the symptoms produce persistent fear and significant disruption of the patient's normal functioning.

Panic attacks begin abruptly, increase rapidly in a crescendolike manner to peak within minutes of onset, and typically resolve within 30 minutes. Symptoms may awaken patients from sleep. Common symptoms include heart palpitations, chest pain, sweating, trembling, a choking or smothering sensation, dyspnea, chills or hot flushes, paresthesias, feelings of unreality or detachment, and fear of losing control or impending danger (9). The intensity of physical symptoms, such as heart palpitations and shortness of breath, coupled with feelings of impending danger, often lead to multiple emergency room visits. The severity of the symptoms and the fear of their recurrence is quite significant; it is very common for patients with panic disorder to develop agoraphobia within 6 months of the first attack.

The lifetime prevalence of panic disorder is approximately 3.5% (3), with a higher prevalence in women. Panic disorder typically begins in late adolescence or early adulthood and follows a chronic waxing and waning course. Women with panic disorder may be prone to developing avoidance behaviors or agoraphobia. Comorbid psychiatric conditions such as GAD, simple phobia, somatization disorder, MDD, and alcohol dependence may exist with panic disorder (69–71).

Patients with panic disorder are a differential diagnostic challenge to primary care physicians and cardiologists. Because the panic symptoms may be difficult to distinguish from angina or other cardiac conditions, unnecessary cardiac catheterization may be ordered. Patients with panic disorder do have an increased mortality incidence from cardiovascular disease, however, possibly from coronary vasospasm induced by hyperventilation (72).

Panic disorder is increasingly viewed as a primary biological disorder. There is a strong genetic component. Among first-degree relatives of patients with panic disorder, there is a tenfold increase in risk of also developing the disorder.

Pharmacologic therapies for the treatment of panic disorder are available; nonpharmacologic treatment such as cognitive behavioral therapy is also effective.

SSRIs offer several advantages over other pharmacologic treatments for panic disorder, such as tolerability, ease of dosing, safety, and efficacy in major depression and other anxiety disorders, and should be considered first-line agents. SSRIs should be started at low doses and titrated to doses similar to those used in the treatment of depression (Table 23.5).

Compared with benzodiazepines, antidepressants are as effective in treating anxiety and agoraphobic avoidance, and more effective in treating depressive symptoms in panic disorder. However, starting antidepressants at full doses will make most patients with panic disorder acutely worse, often leading to treatment discontinuation.

Because of their potential for addiction and abuse, and with the availability of other effective agents, benzodiazepines are generally not preferred as first-line therapy in panic disorder. One treatment strategy is to start therapy with both a daily SSRI and an as-needed, short-acting benzodiazepine, and then taper the benzodiazepine after several weeks as the antidepressant takes effect.

The TCAs clomipramine (Anafranil) and imipramine (Tofranil, Impril), as well as the MAOI phenelzine (Nardil), are also effective treatments but are limited by safety and tolerability issues.

Social Phobia

Excessive anxiety and fear of embarrassment characterize social phobia (also known as social anxiety disorder) while under the potential scrutiny of others. Performance situations, such as public speaking or using the public restroom, are commonly feared, although interactional situations such as going to social gatherings or dealing with authority figures may also invoke symptoms of anxiety and fear. The condition is common and the lifetime prevalence is estimated to range from 2 to 13%. Rates of occurrence are similar for men and women, and the prevalence decreases with age (9). The disorder can be disabling because individuals may develop phobic avoidance of the feared situations, such as the workplace or school. Physical symptoms such as abdominal pain, sweating, diarrhea, tremors and palpitations, or flushing may occur and tend to be worse right before the feared event. Social phobia differs from panic disorder because the symptoms of social phobia are anticipated and occur in a predictable situation.

The anxiety invoked by the phobia may interfere with an individual's ability to maintain friendships and intimate relationships. Social anxiety typically begins in adolescence and has a chronic course (73). Patients with social phobia may become addicted to alcohol or other substances in an attempt to decrease their social anxiety. Patients suffering from phobias and phobic anxiety may be at increased risk for cardiovascular disease and events, possibly secondary to coronary vasospasm, cardiac ischemia, or anxiety-induced arrhythmias.

Social anxiety disorder goes unrecognized in both clinical and mental health settings. Patients with other psychiatric disorders may have undiagnosed comorbid social anxiety disorder, making the use of screening questions an important component of the clinical encounter. Strong positive responses to the three following questions were found to have a sensitivity of 89% and a specificity of 90% for social anxiety disorder (74): Is being embarrassed or looking stupid among your worst fears? Does fear of embarrassment cause you to avoid doing things or speaking to people? Do you avoid activities in which you are the center of attention?

Cognitive behavioral therapies, such as exposure therapy, cognitive restructuring, and social skills training, are effective in the treatment of phobic disorders, including social phobia. Heimberg reviewed the literature on this topic (75). Cognitive therapy teaches patients to recognize, analyze, and refute irrational fears, whereas behavioral therapy exposes patients to graded exposures and simulations of anxiety-provoking situations to lead to desensitization. Cognitive behavioral therapy for social phobia is usually done in a group setting, appears to be as effective as pharmacotherapy, and is associated with a relatively durable response. Cognitive behavioral therapy may be used as a primary treatment for social phobia or in conjunction with pharmacotherapy.

A number of pharmacologic options are effective in the treatment of social phobia. SSRIs, particularly paroxetine (Paxil), have been well studied in the treatment of social phobia and are reasonable first-line agents for individuals who prefer medications to psychotherapy (76–78).

Although higher doses of the SSRIs may ultimately be required for effective therapy, patients with anxiety disorders may be unusually sensitive to medication side effects, so it is recommended the medication be started at one-half of the usual starting dose. As the rate of improvement may be slow, the medication should be continued for at least 12 weeks once the target dose is reached before concluding the medication trial is a success or a failure. If one SSRI is not effective or not tolerated, switching to another SSRI might be effective, just as in depression. Only about 50% of patients taking SSRIs for social phobia will see a substantial improvement in their symptoms.

High-potency benzodiazepines, such as alprazolam (Xanax), clonazepam (Klonopin), and lorazepam (Ativan), are also effective for social phobia. Average doses in clinical trials have been 2.5 mg/day of clonazepam or its equivalent (79).

For performance anxiety or "stage fright," beta-blockers taken 1 to 2 hours before the feared situation may prevent anxiety-related autonomic symptoms (Pollack 2001). Propranolol (Inderal) 20 to 40 mg or atenolol (Tenormin) 50 to 100 mg would be acceptable dosing regimens.

Buspirone, although effective in GAD, has not been found effective in the treatment of social phobia (80).

Adjustment Disorder With Anxiety

This diagnosis is made when patients have excessive and maladaptive symptoms of anxiety for less than 6 months and are experiencing, or have experienced, a major life stressor but do not meet the criteria for another anxiety disorder. The anxiety resolves when either the stressor is alleviated or the patient achieves a new level of adjustment or adaptation to the stressor. Treatment for this may include moderation or avoidance of caffeine or other stimulants, short-term counseling, instruction in techniques of relaxation or other forms of self-regulation, and a short course of anxiolytic therapy.

Post-traumatic Stress Disorder

PTSD is an anxiety disorder that results from experiencing or witnessing a severe traumatic event, where the initial response is horror and hopelessness. Events that typically are associated with PTSD involve interpersonal violence, exposure to life-threatening accidents, or disasters. Incidents of interpersonal violence give rise to PTSD more often than other types of events. The *DSM-IV-TR* diagnostic criteria include distressing or impairing symptoms of re-experiencing the trauma, avoidance of reminders of the trauma, numbing of responsiveness, and hyperarousal (9). PTSD symptomatology is complex, with some symptoms that are obviously directly associated with the traumatic event (e.g., nightmares of the event, avoidance of stimuli that symbolize or trigger memories of the event) and other symptoms that are not (e.g., insomnia, detachment from others, labile mood, exaggerated startle response). PTSD is associated with a high risk of suicide.

In the general population, the lifetime prevalence of PTSD for men is 5 to 6%, and 10 to 14% for women (81–83). Women have a higher risk for developing PTSD than men, despite less frequent exposure to typical triggering traumatic events (81). In women, PTSD often results from an assault episode or episodes (82), particularly sexual assault (84).

When symptoms develop immediately after an event and subside within a month, the diagnosis of acute stress disorder is made. When symptoms continue for more than 1 month, however, the diagnosis of PTSD is warranted. Although most people exposed to trauma do not develop PTSD, those that do will usually develop symptoms shortly after the traumatic event and recover within months.

Initial treatment of PTSD in the early days and weeks after the trauma includes psychosocial support. An example would be referral of a rape victim to a rape counseling team. Using specialized techniques, patients are encouraged to discuss the trauma to help deal with their distress, without becoming overwhelmed. Effective treatments include techniques such as exposure therapy, cognitive therapy, anxiety management, and interpersonal therapies.

Antidepressants are also effective in treating core symptoms of PTSD. Specifically, the SSRIs are considered first-line drug therapy for PTSD and are started at low doses with gradual titration to doses similar to or higher than those used in the treatment of major depression (85). The only drugs with FDA approval specifically for the treatment of PTSD are sertraline (Zoloft) and paroxetine (Paxil). Failure to respond would be an indicator for psychiatric referral because atypical antidepressants or mood stabilizers may be needed.

Obsessive-Compulsive Disorder

Obsessive-compulsive disorder (OCD) is characterized by the presence of obsessive thoughts and/or compulsive behaviors that cause distress and impairment and are not due to a medical condition or the effects of medication or substances of abuse (9). Obsessions are intrusive, repetitive thoughts that are associated with marked anxiety. Compulsions are repetitive physical or mental acts that are usually done in response to compulsions and are intended to relieve anxiety or prevent some dreadful, although seemingly unrelated, event. Examples of common compulsions include excessive handwashing, counting, ordering or arranging, checking (e.g., checking stoves, locks, alarm clocks), and hoarding. Patients can become severely impaired, spending hours each day in their obsessions and compulsions. Patients are often aware that their obsessions and/or compulsions are excessive and irrational, yet are unable to resist them.

The estimated lifetime prevalence of OCD is approximately 3% (86). The onset of OCD often occurs in adolescence or early adulthood but can begin as early as 2 years old. It is much less common to begin after age 35 years. The course is chronic and fluctuating, and stress often precipitates an acute exacerbation of the disorder.

Other psychiatric disorders such as MDD, simple phobia, and panic disorder may coexist with OCD. Evidence supports the idea of a biological origin for OCD as brain imaging studies have seen an increase in site-specific brain changes among patients with OCD, and there are clinical studies linking OCD with head trauma and other neurologic disorders (87–89).

Effective treatments for OCD include cognitive behavioral therapy, SSRIs, and some TCAs. Effective SSRI dosages may be similar to or higher than those used in the treatment of depression. Response to medication may take 8 to 12 weeks, although obsessions are less responsive to medications than compulsions. The combination of cognitive behavioral therapy, plus antidepressant medication, is preferred in moderate to severe OCD.

EATING DISORDERS

The most common eating disorders are anorexia nervosa and bulimia nervosa, both of which have specific diagnostic criteria (Tables 23.7 and 23.8). These disorders typically begin in adolescence or young adulthood, and more than 90% of affected patients are female. Bulimia is more common

TABLE 23.7

DSM-IV-TR Criteria for Anorexia Nervosa

A. Refusal to maintain body weight at or above a minimally normal weight for age and height (e.g., weight loss leading to maintenance of body weight less than 85% of that expected; or failure to make expected weight gain during period of growth, leading to body weight less than 85% of that expected).
B. Intense fear of gaining weight or becoming fat, even though underweight.
C. Disturbance in the way in which ones body weight or shape is experienced, undue influence of body weight or shape on self-evaluation, or denial of the seriousness of the current low body weight.
D. In postmenarcheal girls and women, amenorrhea (i.e., the absence of at least three consecutive menstrual cycles; a woman is also considered amenorrheic if her periods only occur following hormone administration).

Specify *Binge Eating/Purging Type*, where during the current episode patient has regularly engaged in self-induced vomiting or the misuse of laxatives, diuretics, or enemas; or *Restricting Type*, where she has not engaged in binge eating/purging behaviors during the current episode.

Adapted from American Psychiatric Association. Diagnostic and Statistical Manual of Mental Disorders, Fourth Edition, Text Revision. Washington, DC: American Psychiatric Press, 2000, with permission.

TABLE 23.8

DSM-IV-TR Criteria for Bulimia Nervosa

A. Recurrent episodes of binge eating. An episode is characterized by both (1) and (2).
   (1) eating, in a discrete time period (e.g., within any 2-hour period), an amount of food that is definitely larger than most people would eat during a similar time/under similar circumstances.
   (2) a sense of lack of control over eating during the episode.
B. Recurrent inappropriate compensatory behavior in order to prevent weight gain, such as self-induced vomiting misuse of laxatives, diuretics, enemas, other medications; fasting; or excessive exercise.
C. The binge eating and inappropriate compensatory behaviors both occur, on average, at least twice a week for 3 months.
D. Self-evaluation is unduly influenced by body shape and weight.
E. The disturbance does not occur exclusively during episodes of anorexia nervosa (Table 23.7).

Specify *Purging Type*, where during the current episode, patient has regularly engaged in self-induced vomiting or the misuse of laxatives, diuretics, or enemas; or *Nonpurging Type*, where she has not engaged in purging behaviors during the current episode but has used other inappropriate compensatory behaviors, such as fasting or excessive exercise.

Adapted from American Psychiatric Association. Diagnostic and Statistical Manual of Mental Disorders, Fourth Edition, Text Revision. Washington, DC: American Psychiatric Press, 2000, with permission.

than anorexia, affecting up to 2 to 3% of adult women (90). The prevalence of anorexia is 1 to 2% (91).

Anorexic and bulimic behaviors may result in gastroesophageal irritation or Mallory-Weiss tears from vomiting, melanosis coli (an abnormal pigmentation of the colon lining), and colon dysfunction due to laxative abuse. Dental erosion, salivary gland enlargement, and scarring of the hand (Russell's sign) due to self-induced vomiting may also be present. Patients may complain of sore throats or chronic hoarseness. Both bulimic and anorectic patients may engage in excessive amounts of exercise, and this behavior often precedes the development of the formal eating disorder (92).

Both disorders are associated with substantial psychiatric comorbidity, including mood disorders, anxiety disorders (particularly OCD and social phobia), substance abuse, and personality disorders (93–96).

Patients are often brought, under protest, to the clinician by friends or family. The management of eating disorders is complex, involving various treatment modalities that aim to restore nutritional state and weight, manage medical complications, treat comorbid psychiatric disorders, target maladaptive thoughts related to the eating disorder, provide education, and prevent relapse (97). Hospitalization and close monitoring may be necessary for patients with significant medical sequelae. For the treatment of comorbid depression and anxiety, the SSRIs are the preferred antidepressants due to their safety and tolerability relative to other antidepressants.

Anorexia Nervosa

Although the common image of anorexia nervosa is that of a white, middle-class teenager or young woman, this disorder occurs in men, the elderly, and all ethnic groups. The mean age of onset is 14, with another peak in incidence at age 18. The exact etiology is unknown but is believed to be multifactorial. Anorexia nervosa is characterized by an intense fear of gaining weight, maintenance of a weight that is 85% or less than expected for age and height, and excessive or distorted self-evaluation of weight or body shape. Patients with anorexia nervosa attempt to control their weight by excessive dieting or starvation (restricting type, which is the more common type), or by compensatory measures after binge eating episodes (binge eating/purging type). Despite their food-deprived state, patients with anorexia nervosa often have a high energy level.

As a result of excessive weight loss or low weight maintenance, amenorrhea may result and is considered one of the diagnostic symptoms of anorexia nervosa if it is of 3 months duration or more, or if the female patient fails to menstruate without hormonal usage (Table 23.7) (9). Other common physical complications of anorexia nervosa include malnutrition, osteopenia, or osteoporosis (98, 99), dehydration, hypothermia, muscle wasting, cardiac arrhythmias, disrupted gastrointestinal motility, lanugo, and infertility (97, 100). It is important to examine these patients without clothing, and to document both their height and weight.

Despite excessive weight loss, laboratory tests in most patients with anorexia are often normal. In some cases, lab studies may reveal macrocytic anemia and leukopenia. These resolve with weight gain and are not clinically significant (101). Hypoglycemia, when present, indicates a poor prognosis (102). Hypokalemia or a metabolic alkalosis should raise suspicions that the patient is inducing vomiting or may be abusing diuretics (103). The amount of weight loss, symptomatology, and duration of illness do not necessarily correlate with the severity of any laboratory abnormalities.

Treatment for this disorder is individualized, multifaceted, and requires an interdisciplinary team approach. A mental health expert with experience in treating eating disorders should manage the psychiatric component of the treatment plan, which often includes individual and group psychotherapy. The initial therapy is geared toward restoration of a weight compatible with survival, and this may require hospitalization.

The long-term prognosis for patients with anorexia nervosa is variable. Several studies have found a less favorable outcome for anorexia nervosa in comparison to bulimia (104, 105). There is a high association of comorbid affective disorders in patients with anorexia nervosa. Anorexia nervosa is associated with a mortality rate between 5% and 18%, with the main causes of death being starvation, arrhythmias, and suicide. The degree of social integration achieved during therapy is a strong predictor of a favorable outcome.

Bulimia Nervosa

Bulimia nervosa is an eating disorder characterized by recurrent episodes of binge eating and subsequent efforts to prevent weight gain, such as purging (e.g., vomiting or laxative use), fasting, or excessive exercise (9). As with anorexia nervosa, patients with bulimia are pathologically concerned with weight and body shape. However, patients with bulimia are typically not grossly underweight.

The etiology of bulimia is not known but is most likely multifactorial. Patients suffering from bulimia are at increased risk of developing affective disorders, and there is an increased rate of alcoholism seen among patients with a history of bulimia. The diagnosis of bulimia nervosa is primarily a clinical one, although *DSM-IV-TR* criteria have been established (Table 23.8).

Patients with bulimia may note the development of secondary amenorrhea, despite being an appropriate weight for their height. Physical examination of the patient with bulimia is often benign and laboratory evaluation is commonly normal. The most common electrolyte abnormality seen in bulimia is an increase in serum bicarbonate, which is indicative of a metabolic alkalosis, although decreases in chloride, potassium, or magnesium, or an increase in serum amylase secondary to increased salivary isoenzymes, may also be seen.

Several antidepressants have shown efficacy in bulimia nervosa, and fluoxetine (Prozac) is FDA approved for the treatment of bulimia nervosa. Behavioral approaches to address the symptoms of binging and purging must be included in the nonpharmacologic treatment plan.

DELIRIUM

Delirium is a syndrome characterized by global cognitive impairment that develops rapidly and fluctuates over the course of hours or days (9). Patients may exhibit confusion, disorientation, inattentiveness, labile mood, and perceptual disturbances, such as hallucinations or illusions. These symptoms typically wax and wane, with intermittent periods of clear sensorium. Early diagnosis and management is critical because delirium is associated with substantial morbidity and mortality. These patients usually require a more immediate and extensive workup than is available in a gynecology office.

PSYCHOSIS

Psychosis is a term generally used to describe a loss of contact with reality. Examples of psychotic symptoms include hallucinations; delusions (fixed, false beliefs that are held tightly by an individual and are not concordant with the individual's culture); gross disorganization in speech, thought, or behavior; and catatonia. Psychotic symptoms can be seen in a variety of psychiatric illnesses, including primary psychotic disorders, such as schizophrenia, and severe mood disorders. In addition, acute psychotic symptoms may be associated with the effects of a medication or substance of abuse, an underlying medical problem, or a delirium. Treatment of psychotic symptoms typically involves the use of antipsychotic medications. Patients with psychotic symptoms should be referred for psychiatric evaluation and management.

PERSONALITY DISORDERS

Personality disorders are a group of disorders characterized by enduring patterns of rigid, maladaptive thinking and behavior that are pervasive across numerous situations and cause distress and functional impairment. The *DSM-IV-TR* personality disorders include paranoid, schizoid, schizotypal, antisocial, borderline, histrionic, narcissistic, avoidant, dependent, and obsessive-compulsive personality disorders (9).

Although a complete review of each personality disorder is beyond the scope of this chapter, several points warrant discussion. First, patients with personality disorders rarely present specifically for evaluation and treatment of the personality disorder because they often have little or no insight into their maladaptive patterns of thinking and behavior. Second, personality disorders are often comorbid with other psychiatric disorders, and may adversely affect treatment adherence and outcomes if not recognized and referred for appropriate treatment. Furthermore, certain behaviors may arouse negative feelings in the treating physician or treatment team toward that patient and adversely affect their treatment.

Borderline personality disorder (BPD) is a fairly common entity, and 75% of BPD patients are women. BPD is manifested by inflexible, maladaptive patterns of behavior, including impulsive and unpredictable actions, mood instability, and unstable interpersonal relationships. Some patients with BPD use a defense mechanism in which they view themselves and others as "all good" or "all bad" without being able to appreciate contradictory attributes simultaneously. The term splitting is often used to describe a situation in which the patient develops alliances with "good" health care team members, who may then argue with other members of the health care team about the appropriate care of the patient. This dynamic should be considered when office staff members are in conflict about a particular patient. Psychiatric referral can be helpful in this situation.

Clinical Notes

PSYCHIATRIC EMERGENCIES WARRANTING PSYCHIATRIC REFERRAL

- Suicide threats, intent, or plan
- Command-type hallucinations (e.g., voices telling patient to kill self or others)
- Psychosis during pregnancy or the postpartum period

SITUATIONS WHEREIN PSYCHIATRIC REFERRAL IS RECOMMENDED

- Patients with past history of psychiatric illness who are planning pregnancy or are pregnant
- Patients on psychiatric medications who are planning pregnancy or are pregnant
- Patients with psychiatric illness during pregnancy
- Patients with postpartum depression

- Patients with bipolar disorder
- Patients with a psychotic disorder (e.g., schizophrenia)
- Patients with complex psychiatric or medical comorbidity
- Patients who have failed an initial treatment trial for a psychiatric illness
- Children or adolescents with psychiatric symptoms

REFERENCES

1. Kupfer DJ. Long-term treatment of depression. J Clin Psychiatry 1991;52(suppl):28–34.
2. Murray CJ, Lopez AD. Alternative projections of mortality and disability by cause 1990–2020: Global Burden of Disease Study. Lancet 1997;349:1498–1504.
3. Kessler RC, McGonagle KA, Zhao S, et al. Lifetime and 12-month prevalence of DSM-III-R psychiatric disorders in the United States: results from the National Comorbidity Survey. Arch Gen Psychiatry 1994;51: 8–19.
4. Maier W, Gansicke M, Gater R, et al. Gender differences in the prevalence of depression: a survey in primary care. J Affect Disord 1999;53:241–252.
5. Sargeant JK, Bruce ML, Florio LP, et al. Factors associated with 1-year outcome of major depression in the community. Arch Gen Psychiatry 1990;47:519–526.
6. Winokur G, Coryell W, Keller M, et al. A prospective follow-up of patients with bipolar and primary unipolar affective disorder. Arch Gen Psychiatry 1993;50:457–465.
7. Rapaport MH, Thompson PM, Kelsoe JR Jr, et al. Gender differences in outpatient research subjects with affective disorders: a comparison of descriptive variables. J Clin Psychiatry 1995;56:67–72.
8. Kendler KS, Maclean C, Neale M, et al. The genetic epidemiology of bulimia nervosa. Am J Psychiatry 1991;148:1627–1637.
9. American Psychiatric Association. Diagnostic and Statistical Manual of Mental Disorders, Fourth Edition, Text Revision. Washington, DC: American Psychiatric Press, 2000.
10. Baer L, Jacobs DG, Meszler-Reizes J, et al. Development of a brief screening instrument: the HANDS. Psychother Psychosom 2000;69:35–41.
11. American Psychiatric Association. Practice guideline for the treatment of patients with major depressive disorder (revision). Am J Psychiatry 2000;157(suppl):1–45.
12. Nurnberg HG, Hensley PL, Lauriello J, et al. Sildenafil for women patients with antidepressant-induced sexual dysfunction. Psychiatr Serv 1999;50:1076–1078.
13. Thase ME. Effects of venlafaxine of blood pressure: a meta-analysis of original data from 3744 depressed patients. J Clin Psychiatry 1998;59:502–508.
14. O'Hara MW, Zekoski EM, Philipps LH, et al. Controlled prospective study of postpartum mood disorders: comparison of childbearing and nonchildbearing women. J Abnorm Psychol 1990;99:3–15.
15. Frank E, Kupfer DJ, Perel JM, et al. Three-year outcomes for maintenance therapies in recurrent depression. Arch Gen Psychiatry 1990;47:1093–1099.
16. Murray D, Cox JL, Chapman G, et al. Childbirth: life event or start of a long-term difficulty? Further data from the Stoke-on-Trent controlled study of postnatal depression. Br J Psychiatry 1995;166:595–600.
17. Kumar R, Robson KM. A prospective study of emotional disorders in childbearing women. Br J Psychiatry 1984;144:35–47.
18. Cohen LS, Rosenbaum JF. Psychotropic drug use during pregnancy: weighing the risks. J Clin Psychiatry 1998;59(suppl):18–28.
19. Prien RF, Kupfer DJ. Continuation drug therapies for major depressive episodes: how long should it be maintained? Am J Psychiatry 1986;143:18–23.
20. Zuckerman B, Bauchner H, Parker S, et al. Maternal depressive symptoms during pregnancy, and newborn irritability. J Dev Behav Pediatr 1990;11:190–194.
21. Ericson A, Kallen B, Wiholm B. Delivery outcome after the use of antidepressants in early pregnancy. Eur J Clin Pharmacol 1999;55:503–508.
22. Kulin NA, Pastuszak A, Sage SR, et al. Pregnancy outcome following maternal use of the new selective serotonin reuptake inhibitors: a prospective controlled multicenter study. JAMA 1998;279:609–610.
23. Wisner KL, Gelenberg AJ, Leonard H, et al. Pharmacologic treatment of depression during pregnancy. JAMA 1999;282:1264–1269.
24. Chambers CD, Johnson KA, Dick LM, et al. Birth outcomes in pregnant women taking fluoxetine. N Engl J Med 1996;335:1010–1015.
25. Altshuler LL, Cohen L, Szuba MP, et al. Pharmacologic management of psychiatric illness during pregnancy: dilemmas and guidelines. Am J Psychiatry 1996;153:592–606.
26. Janssen HJ, Cuisinier MC, Hoogduin KA, et al. Controlled prospective study on the mental health of women following pregnancy loss. Am J Psychiatry 1996;153:226–230.
27. Cox JL, Connor Y, Kendell RE. Prospective study of the psychiatric disorders of childbirth. Br J Psychiatry 1982;140:111–117.
28. Hannah P, Adams D, Lee A, et al. Links between early post-partum mood and post-natal depression. Br J Psychiatry 1992;160:777–780.

29. Breznitz Z, Friedman SL. Toddlers' concentration: does maternal depression make a difference? J Child Psychol Psychiatry 1988;29:267–279.
30. Cogill SR, Caplan HL, Alexandra H, et al. Impact of maternal depression on cognitive development of young children. BMJ 1986;292:1165–1167.
31. Cummings EM, Davies PT. Maternal depression and child development. J Child Psychol Psychiatry 1994;35: 73–112.
32. Murray L. The impact of postnatal depression on infant development. J Child Psychol Psychiatry 1992;33: 543–561.
33. Whiffen VE, Gotlib IH. Infants of postpartum depressed mothers: temperament and cognitive status. J Abnorm Psychol 1989;98:274–279.
34. Cooper PJ, Murray L. Course and recurrence of postnatal depression: evidence for the specificity of the diagnostic concept. Br J Psychiatry 1995;166:191–195.
35. Davidson J, Robertson E. A follow-up study of post partum illness, 1946–1978. Acta Psychiatr Scand 1985;71:451–457.
36. O'Hara MW, Schlechte JA, Lewis DA, et al. Prospective study of postpartum blues: biologic and psychosocial factors. Arch Gen Psychiatry 1991;48:801–806.
37. O'Hara MW. Social support, life events, and depression during pregnancy and the puerperium. Arch Gen Psychiatry 1986;43:569–573.
38. Warner R, Appleby L, Whitton A, et al. Demographic and obstetric risk factors for postnatal psychiatric morbidity. Br J Psychiatry 1996;168:607–611.
39. Wisner KL, Wheeler SB. Prevention of recurrent postpartum major depression. Hosp Community Psychiatry 1994;45:1191–1196.
40. Stowe ZN, Nemeroff CB. Women at risk for postpartum-onset major depression. Am J Obstet Gynecol 1995;173:639–645.
41. Brockington IF, Cernik KF, Schofield EM, et al. Puerperal psychosis: phenomena and diagnosis. Arch Gen Psychiatry 1981;38:829–833.
42. Suri R, Burt VK. The assessment and treatment of postpartum psychiatric disorders. J Pract Psychiatry Behav Health 1997;3:67–77.
43. Robling SA, Paykel ES, Dunn VJ, et al. Long-term outcome of severe puerperal psychiatric illness. Psychol Med 2000;30:1263–1271.
44. Wisner KL, Perel JM, Findling RL. Antidepressant treatment during breast-feeding. Am J Psychiatry 1996;153:1132–1137.
45. Stuart S, O'Hara MW. Interpersonal psychotherapy for postpartum depression: a treatment program. J Psychother Pract Res 1995;4:18–29.
46. Appleby L, Warner R, Whitton A, et al. A controlled study of fluoxetine and cognitive-behavioural counselling in the treatment of postnatal depression. BMJ 1997;314:932–936.
47. Kessler RC, McGonagle KA, Nelson CB, et al. Sex and depression in the National Comorbidity Survey. II: cohort effects. J Affect Disord 1994;30:15–26.
48. Schmidt PJ, Roca CA, Bloch M, et al. The perimenopause and affective disorders. Semin Reprod Endocrinol 1997;15:91–100.
49. Burt VK, Altshuler LL, Rasgon N. Depressive symptoms in the perimenopause: prevalence, assessment, and guidelines for treatment. Harv Rev Psychiatry 1998;6:121–132.
50. Schmidt PJ, Rubinow DR. Menopause-related affective disorders: a justification for further study. Am J Psychiatry 1991;148:844–852.
51. Avis NE, McKinlay SM. The Massachusetts Women's Health Study: an epidemiologic investigation of the menopause. J Am Med Womens Assoc 1995;50:45–49, 63.
52. Schmidt PJ, Nieman L, Danaceau MA, et al. Estrogen replacement in perimenopause-related depression: a preliminary report. Am J Obstet Gynecol 2000;183:414–420.
53. Soares CN, Almeida OP, Joffe H, et al. Efficacy of estradiol for the treatment of depressive disorders in perimenopausal women: a double-blind, randomized, placebo-controlled trial. Arch Gen Psychiatry 2001;58:529–534.
54. Beck DA, Loenig HG. Minor depression: a review of the literature. Int J Psychiatry Med 1996;26: 177–209.
55. Maier W, Gansicke M, Weiffenbach O. Relationship between major and subthreshold variants of unipolar depression. J Affect Disord 1997;45:41–51.
56. Weissman MM, Bland RC, Canino GJ, et al. Cross-national epidemiology of major depression and bipolar disorder. JAMA 1996;276:293–299.
57. Pigott TA. Gender differences in the epidemiology and treatment of anxiety disorders. J Clin Psychiatry 1999;60(suppl):4–15.
58. Yonkers KA, Warshaw MG, Massion AO, et al. Phenomenology and course of generalised anxiety disorder. Br J Psychiatry 1996;168:308–313.
59. Brawman-Mintzer O, Lydiard RB, Emmanuel N, et al. Psychiatric comorbidity in patients with generalized anxiety disorder. Am J Psychiatry 1993;150:1216–1218.
60. Gorman JM. Treatment of generalized anxiety disorder. J Clin Psychiatry 2002;63(suppl):17–23.
61. Hoehn-Saric R, McLeod DR, Zimmerli WD. Differential effects of alprazolam and imipramine in generalized anxiety disorder: somatic versus psychic symptoms. J Clin Psychiatry 1988;49:293–301.
62. Rocca P, Fonzo V, Scotta M, et al. Paroxetine efficacy in the treatment of generalized anxiety disorder. Acta Psychiatry Scand 1997;95:444–450.

63. Davidson JR, Dupont RL, Hedges D, et al. Efficacy, safety, and tolerability of venlafaxine extended release and buspirone in outpatients with generalized anxiety disorder. J Clin Psychiatry 1999;60:528–535.
64. Gelenberg AJ, Lydiard RB, Rudolph RL, et al. Efficacy of venlafaxine extended-release capsules in non-depressed outpatients with generalized anxiety disorder: a 6-month randomized controlled trial. JAMA 2000;283:3082–3088.
65. Rickels K, Pollack MH, Sheehan DV, et al. Efficacy of extended-release venlafaxine in nondepressed outpatients with generalized anxiety disorder. Am J Psychiatry 2000;157:968–974.
66. Ballenger JC. Current treatments of the anxiety disorders in adults. Biol Psychiatry 1999;46:1579–1594.
67. Ninan PT. The functional anatomy, neurochemistry, and pharmacology of anxiety. J Clin Psychiatry 1999;60(suppl):12–17.
68. Rakel RE. Long-term buspirone therapy for chronic anxiety: a multicenter international study to determine safety. South Med J 1990;83:194–198.
69. Andrade L, Eaton WW, Chilcoat HD. Lifetime co-morbidity of panic attacks and major depression in a population-based study: age of onset. Psychol Med 1996;26:991–996.
70. Battaglia M, Bernardeschi L, Politi E, et al. Comorbidity of panic and somatization disorder: a genetic-epidemiological approach. Compr Psychiatry 1995;36:411–420.
71. Yonkers KA, Zlotnick C, Allsworth J, et al. Is the course of panic disorder the same in women and men? Am J Psychiatry 1998;155:596–602.
72. Coryell W, Noyes R, Clancy J. Excess mortality in panic disorder: a comparison with primary unipolar depression. Arch Gen Psychiatry 1982;39:701–703.
73. Ost LG. Age of onset in different phobias. J Abnorm Psychol 1987;96:223–229.
74. Kobak KA, Schaettle SC, Greist JH, et al. Computer-administered rating scales for social anxiety in a clinical drug trial. Depress Anxiety 1998;7:97–104.
75. Heimberg RG. Current status of psychotherapeutic interventions for social phobia. J Clin Psychiatry 2001;62(suppl):36–42.
76. Baldwin D, Bobes J, Stein DJ, et al. Paroxetine in social phobia/social anxiety disorder: randomised, double-blind, placebo-controlled study. Br J Psychiatry 1999;175:120–126.
77. Katzelnick DJ, Kobak KA, Greist JH, et al. Sertraline for social phobia: a double-blind, placebo-controlled crossover study. Am J Psychiatry 1995;152:1368–1371.
78. Stein MB, Fyer AJ, Davidson JR, et al. Fluvoxamine treatment of social phobia (social anxiety disorder): a double-blind, placebo-controlled study. Am J Psychiatry 1999;156:756–760.
79. Davidson JR, Ford SM, Smith RD, et al. Long-term treatment of social phobia with clonazepam. J Clin Psychiatry 1991;52(suppl):16–20.
80. van Vliet IM, den Boer JA, Westenberg HG, et al. Clinical effects of buspirone in social phobia: a double-blind placebo-controlled study. J Clin Psychiatry 1997;58:164–168.
81. Kessler RC, Sonnega A, Bromet E, et al. Posttraumatic stress disorder in the National Comorbidity Survey. Arch Gen Psychiatry 1995;52:1048–1060.
82. Resnick HS, Kilpatrick DG, Dansky BS, et al. Prevalence of civilian trauma and posttraumatic stress disorder in a representative national sample of women. J Consult Clin Psychol 1993;61:984–991.
83. Breslau N, Davis GC, Peterson EL, et al. Psychiatric sequelae of posttraumatic stress disorder in women. Arch Gen Psychiatry 1997;54:81–87.
84. Foa EB. Trauma and women: course, predictors, and treatment. J Clin Psychiatry 1997;58(suppl):25–28.
85. Ballenger JC, Davidson JR, Lecrubier Y, et al. Consensus statement on posttraumatic stress disorder from the International Consensus Group on Depression and Anxiety. J Clin Psychiatry 2000;61(suppl):60–66.
86. Weissman MM, Bland RC, Canino GJ, et al. The cross-national epidemiology of obsessive-compulsive disorder: the Cross-National Collaborative Group. J Clin Psychiatry 1994;55(suppl):5–10.
87. Baxter LR, Phelps ME, Mazziotta JC, et al. Local cerebral glucose metabolic rates in obsessive-compulsive disorder. Arch Gen Psychiatry 1987;44:211–218.
88. Luxenberg JS, Swedo SE, Flament MF, et al. Neuroanatomical abnormalities in OCD detected with quantitative x-ray computed tomography. Am J Psychiatry 1988;145:1089–1093.
89. McKeon J, McGuffin P, Robinson P. Obsessive compulsive neurosis following head injury: a report of 4 cases. Br J Psychiatry 1984;144:190–192.
90. Becker AE, Grinspoon SK, Klibanski A, et al. Eating disorders. N Engl J Med 1999;340:1092–1098.
91. Shisslak CM, Crago M, Estes LS. The spectrum of eating disturbances. Int J Eat Disord 1995;18:209–219.
92. Taub DE, Blinde EM. Eating disorders among adolescent female athletes: influence of athletic participation and sport team membership. Adolescence 1992;23:267–275.
93. Halmi KA, Eckert E, Marchi P, et al. Comorbidity of psychiatric diagnoses in anorexia nervosa. Arch Gen Psychiatry 1991;48:712–718.
94. Braun DL, Sunday SR, Halmi KA. Psychiatric comorbidity in patients with eating disorders. Psychol Med 1994;24:859–867.
95. Herzog DB, Keller MB, Sachs NR, et al. Psychiatric comorbidity in treatment-seeking anorexics and bulimics. J Am Acad Child Adolesc Psychiatry 1992;31:810–818.
96. Skodol AE, Oldham JM, Hyler SE, et al. Comorbidity of DSM-III-R eating disorders and personality disorders. Int J Eat Disord 1993;14:403–416.
97. American Psychiatric Association. Practice guideline for the treatment of patients with eating disorders [Revised]. Am J Psychiatry 2000;157(suppl):1–39.
98. Bachrach LK, Guido D, Katzman D, et al. Decreased bone density in adolescent girls with anorexia nervosa. Pediatrics 1990;86:440–447.

99. Rigotti NA, Neer RM, Skates SJ, et al. The clinical course of osteoporosis in anorexia nervosa: a longitudinal study of cortical bone mass. JAMA 1991;265:1133–1138.
100. Stewart DE, Robinson E, Goldbloom DS, et al. Infertility and eating disorders. Am J Obstet Gynecol 1990;163:1196–1199.
101. Devuyst O, Lambert M, Rodhain J, et al. Haematological changes and infectious complications in anorexia nervosa: a case-control study. QJM 1993;86:791–799.
102. Rich LM, Caine MR, Findling JW, et al. Hypoglycemic coma in anorexia nervosa: case report and review of the literature. Arch Intern Med 1990;150:894–895.
103. Mehler PS. Electrolyte disorders in bulimia. Eating Disorders: The Journal of Treatment and Prevention 1998;6:65–68.
104. Strober M, Freeman JR, Morrel W. The long-term course of severe anorexia nervosa in adolescents: survival analysis of recovery, relapse, and outcome predictors over 10–15 years in a prospective study. Int J Eat Disord 1997;22:339–360.
105. Fichter MM, Quadflieg N. Six-year course and outcome of anorexia nervosa. Int J Eat Disorder 1999;26: 359–385.

CHAPTER 24

Management of the HIV-Positive Woman

Nancy L. Eriksen

INTRODUCTION

Despite the dramatic advances in the treatment of HIV and AIDS, the epidemic continues to soar, particularly among women. The growing number of women of reproductive age living with HIV/AIDS is a dominant feature of this disease. Because most women with HIV/AIDS are asymptomatic, they tend to be diagnosed later in the disease process then men and have poorer access to HIV specialists and medications (1). They are also more vulnerable than men by virtue of the fact that they tend to have a unique set of social needs. Some of these include poverty, domestic violence, depression, and children, some of whom may be HIV positive (2).

Because most women of reproductive age are healthy, the only time they may visit a physician is for routine gynecologic care. Thus, it is important for the health care provider to be able to recognize the signs and symptoms that might suggest HIV infection so they can be diagnosed early in the disease. This allows for early intervention prior to the onset of opportunistic infections (OIs) in order to delay the progression to AIDS. In addition, the management of common gynecologic problems may need to be altered due to their HIV/AIDS status.

This chapter provides an overview of the diagnosis and primary care of patients with HIV/AIDS, along with issues unique to HIV-infected women that are related to the transmission of the virus, contraception, reproductive options, and gynecologic manifestations of the disease.

Epidemiology

From 1999 through 2003, the estimated number of AIDS cases increased 15% among females and estimated rates of AIDS cases in 2003 were 9.2 per 100,000 among females (3). The proportion of women infected with HIV is estimated to be much higher, but accurate figures are not known because not all states have mandatory reporting of HIV cases.

In the United States, the HIV epidemic initially centered on women who were injection drug users in the Northeast. Although the Northeast still has the largest number of women living with AIDS, the fastest rate of growth of new cases has now shifted to women living in the South. This region traditionally has the highest rates of sexually transmitted diseases (STDs), which are a known risk factor for acquiring HIV infection. Among women, the leading HIV exposure category has shifted from intravenous drug use to heterosexual contact. In 2003, 63% of newly reported HIV infections among women were attributed to heterosexual transmission (3). In addition, younger women are disproportionately at risk because nearly 50% of all heterosexually transmitted cases occur when they are either teenagers or in their early twenties (3).

Minority women have also been disproportionately affected. African American and Hispanic women together represent less than one-fourth of all U.S. women, yet they account for 33% of newly reported AIDS cases in 2000 (3). Furthermore, in 1998, AIDS was the third leading cause of death in African American and Hispanic women ages 25 to 44, reflecting the devastating effect this infection has taken on women of color (5). Overall, these figures underscore the need for effective prevention strategies starting at a young age, along with early diagnosis and treatment of women with HIV.

Screening

Since 1995, major advances in the treatment of HIV has led to the prolonged survival and improved quality of life for those living with HIV (6). Prophylactic therapy during pregnancy has also led to a substantial reduction in the perinatal transmission of HIV (7). These advances increase the benefit of early identification of one's HIV status. Currently, HIV testing is recommended as a routine part of prenatal care with targeted screening of nonpregnant women in low prevalence (less than 1%) areas based on behavioral and clinical risk factors (8).

Providers of reproductive health care can potentially play an important role in identifying women at risk for, or infected with, HIV. These providers are particularly well suited to screen for HIV because the same issues that bring women to them, both sexual and reproductive health, provide a convenient opportunity for discussion of sexual risks. Early diagnosis of HIV infection may have a tremendous impact on the health and survival of these women, and would afford an opportunity to counsel these women about reducing the risk of transmission to their partner and future offspring. A more recent survey of women infected with HIV determined that in the year prior to their diagnosis, 73% had at least one reproductive or gynecologic health concern for which they sought treatment, yet were not offered HIV testing (9). Furthermore, private obstetricians/gynecologists were less likely to offer the test compared with internists, nurse practitioners, and obstetricians/gynecologists in an inner-city clinic. These results underscore the need to extend voluntary HIV screening with informed consent to all gynecologic health encounters to allow women the opportunity for earlier diagnosis.

Studies that examine the routine offering of HIV testing to all pregnant patients can serve as a model for offering testing outside pregnancy. When offered, 75 to 95% of pregnant women accept HIV testing (10). In the prenatal setting, HIV testing is readily accepted by patients because it is offered to everyone, which significantly reduces stigma and provider bias (11, 12). The routine offering of HIV testing is most successful if the health care provider emphasizes the advantages of HIV testing. These include (a) discussing the interaction of HIV infection in pregnancy before conception; (b) educating patients on the risk of HIV infection and the steps that can be taken to avoid it; (c) discussing contraceptive options so patients understand that birth control methods, other than condoms, are not protective against HIV; and (d) discussing the importance of detecting HIV infection early in order to receive treatment, which has been shown to improve survival.

Trying to assess a patient's risk for HIV infection can be difficult for both the woman and the provider. Even when a provider can accurately assess a woman's potential risk of HIV infection, risk factors will only detect 57% of women infected (13). Because most newly diagnosed cases of HIV are in asymptomatic women and are the result of unrecognized heterosexual transmission, it is no longer acceptable to offer testing only to individuals with "high-risk" behaviors. In a study by Landesman et al. (14), 40% of infected women did not realize they had been involved in high-risk behavior. Women who are in what they believe to be a mutually monogamous relationship may not see themselves at risk for HIV infection. Yet an increasing number of women who acquired the virus via heterosexual transmission reported being in a monogamous relationship (15). Thus, a woman's current risk cannot be determined unless her partner's risk factors are also assessed. The provider should remind the patient that due to the latency period of the virus, they or their partner may have been infected as long as 15 years ago. Most patients do not realize that HIV infection can be clinically dormant, but transmissible, for long periods of time.

In the case where a woman may decline HIV testing initially, additional opportunities may occur to offer testing based on the history, clinical findings, or laboratory test results. These risk factors for HIV infection are listed in Table 24.1. These risk factors include high-risk sexual behavior of the patient or partner, country of origin in an HIV-endemic area, prior or current STD or OI, and cytologic atypia. Once identified, the patient should be informed that he or she is at higher risk of having HIV and be asked to reconsider HIV screening.

TABLE 24.1

Risk Factors for HIV Infection

Social/Sexual History
- Substance abuse
- Partner is intravenous drug user
- Sex partners of bisexual men
- Sex partner is HIV positive
- History of rape or sexual abuse
- History of anal intercourse
- Multiple sexual partners
- Country of origin from an endemic area (Sub-Saharan Africa, Caribbean, Central Asia)
- Prior STD
- Prior cervical dysplasia or cervical cancer

Clinical Findings
← STD/PID
← Recurrent vulvovaginal candidiasis
← Cervical dysplasia or cervical cancer
← Unexplained persistent constitutional symptoms
← Opportunistic infection
← Genital ulcers
← Oral thrush
← Herpes zoster
← Recurrent bacterial pneumonia

Laboratory Tests
← Abnormal PAP smear
← Positive RPR or VDRL test
← Positive PPD
← Hepatitis B or C antibody
← Thrombocytopenia

STD, sexually transmitted disease; PID, pelvic inflammatory disease; RPR, rapid plasma reagent; VDRL, Venereal Disease Research Laboratory; PPD, purified protein derivative.
Adapted from Centers for Disease Control and Prevention. 1993 Revised classification system for HIV infection and expanded surveillance case definition for AIDS among adolescents and adults. MMWR Morb Mortal Wkly Rep 1993;41:1–47, Stein MD, Rosene KA. Clues to enhancing the identification of human immunodeficiency virus-infected women. Obstet Gynecol 1992;80: 317–320, World Health Organization. The current global situation of the HIV/AIDS pandemic. Wkly Epidemiol Rec 1995;27:193–196.

Diagnostic Testing

HIV infection is usually diagnosed by serologic tests that detect antibody to the virus. Infection may also be detected by nucleic acid-based assays that measure the number of copies of the virus in plasma (RNA polymerase chain reaction [PCR] or viral load [VL] test) or by detecting the virus in cells (DNA PCR testing). Other less common means of diagnosing HIV include detection of viral antigens or direct viral culture.

The most common method of HIV detection is with an enzyme-linked immunosorbent assay (ELISA) test for screening, also referred to as an enzyme immunosorbent assay. If the ELISA is reactive, the test is repeated in duplicate. If both tests are reactive, the sample is considered positive. This is followed by a confirmatory test such as a Western blot (WB) or immunofluorescent assay. The sensitivity and the specificity of the ELISA are both greater than 99%. False-negative ELISA results usually occur in the first 1 to 2 weeks of HIV infection known as the "window"

TABLE 24.2

Potential Causes of Indeterminate Western Blot

- Serologic tests in the process of seroconversion (low levels of antibody)
- End-stage AIDS with loss of core antibody
- Technical or clerical error
- Infection with HIV-2
- Cross-reacting nonspecific antibodies, as seen with collagen-vascular disease, autoimmune diseases, injection drug use, multiple sclerosis, and parity or recent immunization

period or late in the disease when antibody production is low (16, 17). ELISA screening fails to detect up to one-third of patients with HIV-2 (18).

False-positive ELISA results have been reported in patients with autoantibodies, such as autoimmune diseases, liver disease, hemodialysis, multiparity, transfusion, renal disease, or vaccinations, including those enrolled in HIV vaccine trials (19, 20).

The WB assay detects antibodies to specific HIV proteins, including core (gag) (p17, p24, p55), polymerase (pol) (p31, p51, p66), and envelope (env) (gp41, gp120, gp160) proteins (21). The absence of all bands is a negative test. A WB is positive if reactivity is detected to gp41 and gp120/160 *or* p24 and gp120/160 (21). The presence of any bands that do not meet these criteria for a positive result is considered an indeterminate Western blot (IWB) result. The WB has a reported specificity of 97.8% (22). Indeterminate WB results account for 4 to 20% of WB assays with positive bands for HIV proteins (20). Potential causes of an IWB are listed in Table 24.2. The most important factor in evaluating indeterminate results is risk assessment. Patients at low risk (i.e., a stable mutually monogamous relationship) with IWB tests are almost never infected with either HIV-1 or HIV-2. Repeat testing usually continues to show IWB results, and the cause of this pattern is infrequently established. In a study that followed 89 patients with prior repeated IWB results, the authors recommended that patients at low risk for HIV should not undergo further follow-up, whereas those at high risk should be observed serologically for at least 6 months (23). A suggested algorithm for follow-up of indeterminate tests is shown in Figure 24.1. Patients at low risk should be retested after 30 days to quickly diagnose those who may be in the "window" period before seroconversion. If the results are still indeterminate, the WB should be repeated in 6 months because antibodies are detected in 95% of HIV-positive patients by 6 months (24). Using this protocol for the diagnosis of HIV-1 has been more than 99% accurate (22).

Patients who have flulike symptoms suggestive of acute HIV infection or who are at high risk for HIV (Table 24.1) should have a plasma VL test performed. During the initial 3 to 4 weeks of HIV infection, the HIV viral replication is very high, although host antibody responses may be very low. Thus, a plasma VL test may be positive when the WB is indeterminate. The most common VL test is the reverse transcriptase PCR (RT-PCR). Two other VL tests available are the branched chain DNA and the nucleic acid sequence-based amplification. These tests report the number of copies of virus per millimeter of plasma. The lower limit of detection for standard tests is 400 copies/mL, but ultrasensitive assays can detect as few as 20 to 50 copies/mL. False-positive rates are 2 to 3%, usually with low HIV titers (less than 15,000 copies/mL) (25, 26). If the VL is negative, then the patient is considered negative. Repeat HIV screening should be continued every 6 to 12 months for women with high-risk behavior. However, repeat HIV screening is not needed in low-risk women with an IWB after 6 months, unless they develop a risk factor.

Women for whom HIV-1 WB exhibits the unusual indeterminate test band pattern of gag (p55, p24, or p17) plus pol (p66, p51, or p31) in the absence of env (gp120/160 or gp41) should be tested for HIV-2 (27). Additional risk factors for HIV-2 include origin from a country where

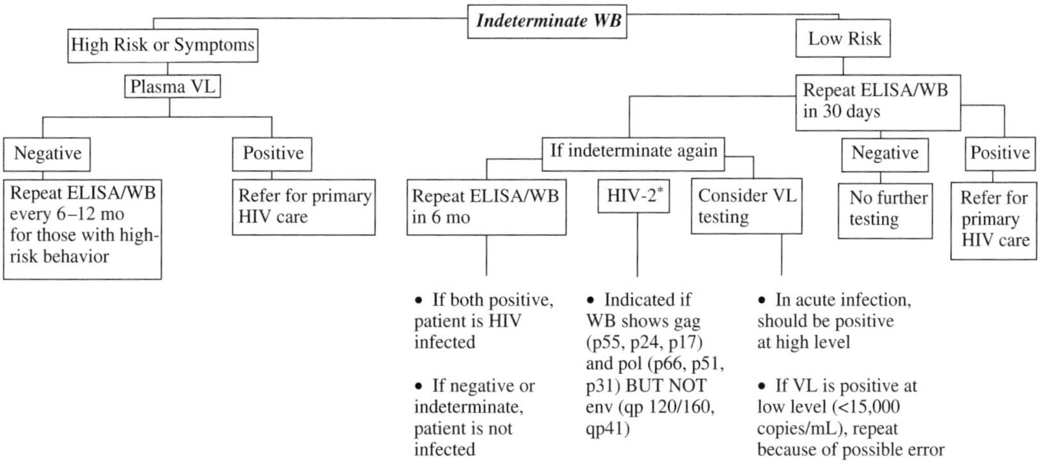

FIGURE 24.1 • Suggested algorithm for an indeterminate Western blot (WB). ELISA, enzyme-linked immunosorbent assay; VL, viral load (plasma).*HIV-2 testing is also indicated for persons from endemic areas, such as the west coast of Africa, or if their sex or intravenous drug abuse partner has HIV-2 or is from West Africa.

infection is endemic, especially West Africa; unprotected sex with a person know to be infected with HIV-2 or if the person is from West Africa; and sharing needles with a person from a country in which HIV-2 is endemic or receiving a transfusion from a country in which HIV-2 is endemic.

Patients who have a confirmatory positive test for HIV or fall outside the recommendations outlined in this section should be referred to an infectious disease specialist.

PRIMARY HIV CARE

For the majority of women of reproductive age, a visit for a routine annual exam or gynecologic problem may be the only opportunity for HIV testing and assessment of the potential gynecologic manifestations of HIV. Thus, reproductive health care providers are in a unique position to both diagnose and manage these complications.

The special needs of women with HIV require a multidisciplinary approach to care because they frequently have medical, gynecologic, and psychosocial needs. The primary care provider is often best suited to perform the initial evaluation of the HIV-infected women and coordinate referrals to specialty providers. The prompt assessment of immunologic and virologic status of the patient allows for the identification of those women needing OI prophylaxis, as well as those who would most benefit from treatment with highly active antiretroviral therapy (HAART). (OIs are listed in Table 24.4 under CDC classification.) Women with a CD4 count of less than 350 cells/mm^3 merit special attention because they are at greater risk for progression to AIDS without HAART when matched for RNA copy number (28).

A comprehensive evaluation of the HIV-infected patient includes a thorough history and physical examination, including pelvic exam, laboratory tests, and psychological and social service assessment. Beginning with the history, the provider should inquire about the possible mode of infection, number of current and past sexual partners, and the possible date of infection. A patient with a documented seroconversion of HIV within the last 6 months may still be in the acute phase of infection and benefit from immediate referral to an HIV specialist for treatment with HAART (29). The patient should also be questioned regarding prior STDs, history of hospitalizations, or other treatments of OIs. A list of current medications and prior immunizations is also needed. The review of systems should target the early symptoms of HIV (fevers, night sweats, lymphadenopathy, fatigue) and symptoms suggestive of an undiagnosed symptomatic HIV-related condition (weight loss, diarrhea, dysphagia, skin changes, cervical dysplasia, pelvic inflammatory disease [PID], recurrent yeast infections, mental status changes, severe headaches, shortness of breath, cough, neurologic changes, oral/genital sores). A psychosocial history should include current living conditions, as well as the number and ages of children who may be at risk for HIV infection. Questions should be asked that pertain to symptoms of depression and current or past substance abuse, including smoking and alcohol, sexual abuse, and domestic violence. These questions may identify urgent social needs that would prompt referral to a social worker.

The physical exam should begin with the patient's general appearance and vital signs. Cachexia and alopecia are associated with advanced disease and may indicate the development of wasting syndrome. Lymphadenopathy or fever in a patient with AIDS may also suggest an infectious complication. The oropharynx should be examined closely because 40% of seropositive women on initial exam have oral pathology. The most common findings are oral candidiasis, oral hairy leukoplakia, gingivitis, and aphthous ulcers (30). A funduscopic exam that reveals retinal hemorrhage or yellow-white infiltrates is suggestive of either cytomegalovirus (CMV) or toxoplasmosis retinitis. The abdominal exam should note any organomegaly that may suggest hepatitis, lymphoma, or fungal infection. A breast and pelvic exam are essential, and special attention should be given to genital or perirectal ulcers, condyloma, and vaginal infection. A Papanicolaou (Pap) smear should be obtained, along with cervical cultures for gonorrhea and chlamydia. If symptoms warrant, a wet mount with both sodium chloride and potassium hydroxide should be performed to identify bacterial vaginosis, trichomonas, and candidiasis. Other less common manifestations include Kaposi's sarcoma and bacillary angiomatosis, which mimics the lesions of Kaposi's sarcoma. Both have been reported as vulvar and cervical lesions (31–33). A neurologic assessment that reveals either sensory or motor deficits could suggest AIDS-related neuropathy or a central nervous system infectious complication such as toxoplasmosis. Finally, skin manifestations are common, particularly bacterial folliculitis, seborrheic dermatitis, herpes zoster, and molluscum contagiosum (34).

A baseline laboratory evaluation is needed to establish the stage of disease, risk for OIs, need for HAART or immunizations, and the exposure to other infectious diseases. A list of these laboratory tests is presented in Table 24.3 (35). The CD4 count and VL (quantitative HIV PCR) are of vital importance in assessing the degree of immunosuppression and risk of progression to AIDS. Recommendations for OI prophylaxis and HAART are based on these values. A hepatitis panel is used to screen for past infection and identify women who are candidates for immunization. Serologic evidence of previous exposure to toxoplasmosis may be relevant for decisions on prophylaxis, evaluation of neurologic symptoms in patients with advanced immunosuppression, and avoidance of exposure in those who have not been previously infected. CMV antibody status can guide the provider to use CMV-negative blood products, if necessary, or in the presence of severe immunosuppression, to refer the patient to an ophthalmologist for CMV retinitis screening. A positive cryptococcal antigen would also alert the clinician to a patient who needs prophylaxis. Serum chemistry and lipid panel are also important in assessing any underlying problems that might complicate the clinical course, particularly if HAART is initiated. A Pap smear and cervical cultures for gonorrhea and chlamydia should be performed at the initial exam and annually thereafter.

At the conclusion of the exam, patient education should be provided that focuses on five areas. First, the provider should emphasize the importance of close medical follow-up, particularly with an HIV specialist. In general, a patient has a VL and CD4 count performed every 3 to 6 months, regardless of the decision to initiate or delay HAART. The importance of continuing gynecologic follow-up should also be emphasized because a large number of women still do not receive gynecologic care from their HIV specialist (36). Second, counseling regarding the modes of transmission, as well as the means to reduce transmission through safer sex practices, should be provided. Third, every effort should be made to encourage the woman to disclose her status to her current and former partners so they can be tested. However, many women may fear being harmed by disclosing their status, particularly if they have been involved in a physically violent relationship. The provider must use caution in these cases not to force a woman to disclose her status. A multidisciplinary approach enlisting the assistance of social workers may be helpful. Fourth, prepregnancy counseling should be provided to all women of reproductive age, regardless of whether they indicate a desire to have children in the future. Decisions regarding the choice of HAART may be influenced by the information given. A detailed description of prepregnancy counseling is provided later in the chapter. Finally, the patient should be encouraged to find resources that will help her cope with this disease. Most

TABLE 24.3

Initial Evaluation of the HIV-Infected Woman

Complete History and Physical Baseline Laboratory Evaluation
- Complete blood count with platelets
- Serum chemistry panel (electrolytes, liver and renal function)
- Fasting lipid profile
- Syphilis serology
- Hepatitis panel (A, B, and C)
- Quantitative PCR HIV RNA (VL)
- CD4 subsets
- Toxoplasmosis serology (IgG)
- Cytomegalovirus serology (IgG)
- Cryptococcal antigen
- PPD skin testing
- Pap smear
- Chlamydia and gonorrhea cultures
- Wet mount

Patient Education Referrals
- HIV specialist
- Social services
- Mental health
- Ophthalmologist (CD4 $<$ 100, CMV IgG+)
- Dental

PCR, polymerase chain reaction; VL, viral load; PPD, purified protein derivative; CMV, cytomegalovirus.
From Kaplan JE, Masur H, Holmes KK, et al. USPHS/IDSA guidelines for the prevention of opportunistic infections in persons infected with human immunodeficiency virus: an overview. Clin Infect Dis 1995;21(suppl 1):S12–S31, with permission.

urban areas have AIDS service organizations that can help with education, support groups, social work referrals, transportation, and child care.

Once the patient has been assessed, she may require referrals to a variety of health care professionals (Table 24.3). It is of utmost importance that all patients be referred to an HIV specialist. HIV-infected patients have been shown to have a significant decrease in mortality when treated by physicians who are HIV experienced (37). This is because patients who go to physicians who are not HIV specialists are less likely to receive OI prophylaxis or HAART, which significantly reduces their survival (38). An ophthalmology consult by a physician experienced in manifestations of HIV is also indicated for the patient with antibody to CMV and/or a CD4 less than 100 cells/mm^3. These patients are at greatest risk of acquiring CMV retinitis, regardless of whether they have visual field changes. A complete dental exam is also needed. Children younger than the age of 4 should be referred to a pediatrician for HIV testing if not already done. Chronic depression has been linked to a more rapid decline in CD4 count and a two-fold greater risk of dying compared with those with no depressive symptoms (39). Depression may also have an impact on adherence to medication or whether one even decides to initiate HAART. Therefore, referral to a therapist or psychiatrist is critical to ensure that, when present, present depression is actively treated. In most cases, it is prudent to delay starting HAART until depression is addressed. Socioeconomic issues must also be addressed in HIV-positive women to provide optimal care. Women with HIV often lack adequate familial or social support. For example, only 14% of HIV-infected women of reproductive age are married compared with 50% of all women in the same age group (40). Many feel isolated due to the stigma of the disease, which causes many of them not to divulge their HIV status or seek care for their HIV infection. If the partner or her children are infected, it increases the emotional burden she must endure.

TABLE 24.4

Classification System of HIV Disease

CD4 Count	A	B	C
>500	A1	B1	C1
200–500	A2	B2	C2
<200	A3	B3	C3

Category A

Asymptomatic HIV infection
Persistent generalized lymphadenopathy
Acute retroviral syndrome

Category B (Formerly "ARC")

Bacillary angiomatosis
Candidiasis (oral or recurrent vaginal)
Cervical dysplasia
Constitutional symptoms (e.g., fever or diarrhea) for >1 mo
Hairy leukoplakia (oral)
Herpes zoster
Idiopathic thrombocytopenic purpura
Listeriosis
Pelvic inflammatory disease
Peripheral neuropathy

Category C (Aids-Defining Conditions)

CD4 count < 200 cells/mm^3
Candidiasis (pulmonary or esophageal)
Cervical cancer
Coccidioidomycosis
Cryptococcosis (extrapulmonary)
Cryptosporidiosis
Cytomegalovirus
Encephalopathy (HIV)
Herpes simplex (chronic or esophageal)
Histoplasmosis
Isosporiasis
Kaposi's sarcoma
Lymphoma
Mycobacterium avium
Mycobacterium kansasii
Mycobacterium tuberculosis
Pneumocystis carinii
Pneumonia (recurrent)
Progressive multifocal leukemia
Salmonellosis

From Centers for Disease Control and Prevention. 1993 Revised classification systems for HIV infection and expanded surveillance case definitions for AIDS among adolescents and adults. MMWR Morb Mortal Wkly Rep 1993;41(RR-17):1–19.

In addition, the majority of these women are unemployed, have less years of formal education, and live in households with incomes of less than $10,000 per year (40). Nearly 50% of HIV-infected women have been sexually abused as children, and 41% have been in physically violent relationships (41). A history of substance abuse is also common, particularly in women with a history of sexual abuse. Lack of housing and the need for transportation and child care are other common problems seen in HIV-positive patients. These disturbing facts re-emphasize the need to consider referral to a social worker for assessment and assistance in dealing with these and other barriers to consistent and specialized health care.

Once the patient has been assessed and the laboratory tests results are available, the patient should be counseled regarding her immunologic status, classification, and need for prophylaxis or immunizations. The CD4 count can be used to classify the patient into asymptomatic or symptomatic HIV/AIDS (42). Table 24.4 shows the detailed 1993 classification system. Any patient with a CD4 less than 200 cells/mm^3 or in Category C is considered to have AIDS. Any patient with a CD4 less than 200 cells/mm^3 should also be assessed for primary OI prophylaxis according to guidelines given in Table 24.5. The patient's prior immunization record, as well as pertinent laboratory test, such as the toxoplasmosis IgG , CMV IgG, and hepatitis panel, should be reviewed with the patient. Immunizations should also be given according to

TABLE 24.5

Recommended Primary Opportunistic Infection Prophylaxis

Pathogen	Regimen
Pneumocystis pneumonia (PCP) (CD4 <200 mm^3 *or* oropharyngeal candidiasis)	TMP-SMX 1 DS or 1 SS q day -OR- TMP-SMX 1 DS three times weekly
Toxoplasmosis (CD4 <100 mm^3 *and* positive Toxo IgG)	TMP-SMX 1 DS q day
Mycobacterium avium complex (CD4 <50 mm^3	Azithromycin 1200 mg every week -OR- Clarithromycin 500 mg bid
Mycobacterium tuberculosis-Isoniazid sensitive (TST reaction >5 mm *or* prior positive TST result without treatment *or* contact with case of active tuberculosis regardless of TST result *or* high probability of exposure to isoniazid resistant tuberculosis)	Isoniazid, 300 mg po *plus* pyridoxine, 50 mg po q.d. × 9 months -OR- isoniaztd 900 mg po plus pyridoxine 100 mg po twice a week × 9 months
Mycobacterium tuberculosis-Isoniazid resistant (TST reaction >5 mm *or* prior positive TST result without treatment *or* contact with case of active tuberculosis regardless of TST result *or* high probability of exposure to isoniazid resistant tuberculosis)	Rifampin 600 mg po -OR- rifabutin 300 mg po q day × 4 mo
Mycobacterium tuberculosis-Multidurg- (isoniazid and rifampin) resistant (TST reaction >5 mm *or* prior positive TST result without treatment *or* contant with case of active tuberculosis regardless of TST result *or* high probability of exposure to multidrug resistant tuberculosis)	Choice of drugs requires consultation with public health authorities. Depends on susceptibility of isolate from source patient.

TMP-SMX, trimethoprim-sulfamethoxazole; DS, double strength; SS, single strength.

the guidelines in Table 24.6. Recommendations for the initiation of antiretroviral therapy are beyond the scope of this chapter, and patients should be referred to an HIV specialist for consideration of HAART and long-term virologic follow-up. More information on OI prophylaxis or initiation of HAART can be obtained by reviewing the most recent recommendations available at http://www.aidsinfo.nih.gov.

TABLE 24.6

Recommended Immunizations

S. pneumoniae (CD4 >200 mm^3)
Hepatitis B series for susceptible (anti-HBc-negative) patients
Hepatitis A for susceptible (anti-HAV-negative) patients
Influenza—annually
Tetanus—repeat every 10 years

Anti-HBc, antibody to hepatitis B core antigen; HAV, hepatitis A virus.
From 2001 USPHS/IDSA Guidelines for the Prevention of Opportunistic Infections in Persons Infected With Human Immunodeficiency Virus. November 28, 2001. Available at: http://www.aidsinfo.nih.gov. Accessed August 2, 2005.

TABLE 24.7

Risk Factors for Transmission of HIV

- Bacterial vaginosis
- Sexually transmitted diseases
- Genital ulcers
- Cervical ectopy
- Sex during menses
- Multiple sexual partners
- Anal sex
- Traumatic sex
- High-risk partner
- Elevated plasma viral load
- Acute primary HIV infection
- Lack of condom use
- Uncircumcised male

From DeVincenzi I, the European Study Group. A longitudinal study of human immunodeficiency virus transmission by heterosexual partners. N Engl J Med 1994;331:341–346, Royce RA, Sena A, Cates W, et al. Sexual transmission of HIV. N Engl J Med 1997;336:1072–1078, Plummer FA, Simonsen JN, Cameron DW, et al. Cofactors in male–female sexual transmission of human immunodeficiency virus type 1. J Infect Dis 1991;163:233–239.

Prevention of Transmission

Once a patient has been diagnosed with HIV, counseling should be given regarding the various modes of transmission. Transmission of HIV can occur via exposure to blood, blood products, or body fluids, including breast milk or sexual contact. To date, there are no confirmed cases of female-to-female HIV transmission, but barrier precautions should be considered in these cases. Vertical transmission can also occur and is dealt with specifically later in this chapter.

HIV-positive patients should be counseled that they may not donate blood or body organs and to avoid exposure of their blood or body fluids to others. Practices that should be avoided include, but are not limited to, sharing needles, toothbrushes, or razors that may be contaminated with occult blood. Ordinary household exposure does not cause the transmission of HIV, and no special precautions need to be taken for cleaning dishes or laundry.

Transmission of HIV through sexual contact accounts for the vast majority of HIV cases in the United States and worldwide. Information regarding this mode of transmission is vital not only to those women already infected, but also to those women testing negative for HIV who engage in high-risk behavior. Many factors influence the susceptibility of HIV transmission through sexual contact and are listed in Table 24.7. Women and their partners should be counseled regarding these potential risk factors for transmission and be educated as to how to reduce sexual transmission. The risk of HIV infection per sexual contact is estimated to range between 0.001% and 0.3% (43, 44). Nevertheless, some partners become infected after even a single exposure or a few sexual exposures (45), whereas others remain uninfected despite hundreds of exposures. In addition, the rate of male-to-female and female-to-male sexual transmission of HIV is similar (43, 46).

The primary strategies for reducing the sexual transmission of HIV infection focus on four main areas: encouraging the use of condoms, treating STDs, treatment with HAART, and reducing the amount of unsafe sexual behavior by promoting abstinence, by delaying sexual intercourse, or by decreasing the number of sexual partners. In one of the largest longitudinal studies of the heterosexual transmission of HIV, deVincenzi et al. followed 304 serodiscordant couples for an average of 20 months (43). Of the 124 couples who used condoms consistently for vaginal and anal intercourse, no seroconversions occurred in HIV-negative partners despite 15,000 episodes of sexual contact. In contrast, the seroconversion rate was 12.7% at the end of

2 years for couples who used condoms inconsistently. The incidence of seroconversions did not differ significantly between the female and male index partners (11.4% and 13.4%, respectively). A more recent meta-analysis of 12 cohort studies of serodiscordant couples revealed a seroconversion rate of 0.9% for couples who always used condoms compared with a 6% seroconversion rate in couples who never used condoms over a 2-year period (47).

DeVincenzi et al. (43) also noted that having an STD enhanced the risk of seroconversions (33% for nonulcerative and 40% for ulcerative STDs) even more than the practice of anal intercourse (28%). Vaginal infections, including candidiasis, trichomoniasis, and bacterial vaginosis, have been associated with up to a three-fold increase in the risk for HIV seroconversions (48, 49). Studies demonstrate that aggressive treatment of STDs results in a 40% reduction in HIV seroconversions (50, 51). In light of this evidence, patients should be encouraged to use condoms not only to prevent the transmission of HIV, but also to prevent the transmission of STDs, which enhance the risk of HIV transmission. In addition, condoms should be used even if both partners are infected because of the potential risk of transmission of drug-resistant variants, which may lead to treatment failure (52).

Antiretroviral therapy taken to decrease a patient's VL can also reduce the quantity of virus present in the male and female genital tract (53–55). However, there is not always a direct correlation between plasma VL and that found in the genital tract because up to one-third of women with an undetectable VL still have virus present in cervicovaginal fluids (55). Despite this finding, antiretroviral therapy is critical for reducing the quantity of virus found in the female genital tract. Overall, the odds of detecting HIV RNA virus in the female genital tract triples for each ten-fold increase in plasma HIV RNA VL (54). In a study designed to determine the influence of VL for the heterosexual transmission of HIV, Quinn et al. prospectively followed 415 serodiscordant couples for 2 years (46). There were no instances of transmission among couples in which the HIV-infected partners' HIV RNA level was less than 1500 copies/mL. There was a significant dose response of increased transmission with increasing VL. In multivariate analysis, it was determined that for each log increase in plasma HIV RNA levels there is an associated increase in transmission with a rate ratio of 2.5 for seroconversion. Thus, it appears that VL is the chief predictor of the risk of heterosexual transmission of HIV-1 and that transmission is very low in persons with a VL less than 1500 copies/mL.

With the advent of antiretroviral chemotherapy for postexposure prophylaxis (PEP), reproductive health care providers may encounter situations in which counseling is sought following a rape, unprotected intercourse with a partner who is suspected of having HIV, or serodiscordant couples that have experienced condom breakage. Although there are no data yet that demonstrate a reduction in the transmission of HIV in this situation, PEP is recommended after unprotected receptive anal and vaginal intercourse with a partner who is, or is likely to be, HIV infected. Prophylaxis should also be offered for receptive fellatio with ejaculation, although the lack of per-contact estimate for this behavior makes it more difficult to weigh the benefits against the risks (56). Prophylaxis is not recommended after cunnilingus or receptive fellatio without ejaculation, unless factors are present that increase the likelihood of transmission, such as exposure to menstrual blood. Prophylaxis should only be given to individuals with isolated exposures or exposures in a patient who is likely to practice safer behaviors in the future. Treatment should be modeled after that used for occupational exposures (57). Ideally, treatment should be given immediately, but no later than 72 hours, after exposure (58). Two-drug therapy, such as zidovudine and lamivudine for 4 weeks, is an effective regimen and has proven efficacy in needlestick exposures. A protease inhibitor, such as nelfinavir or indinavir, may be added if the patient is known to have HIV. Consultation with an HIV specialist is recommended in these situations for recommendations and for follow-up of potential side effects.

GYNECOLOGIC ISSUES

Contraception

Knowledge of contraceptive methods for family planning and prevention of STDs is of paramount importance to health care providers giving care to HIV-infected women and women at risk for HIV infection. Unfortunately, methods that prevent conception may not necessarily prevent HIV transmission, and the most effective means of preventing HIV infection is not necessarily the ideal contraceptive method. Any discussion of contraception with patients must address two issues: prevention of unintended pregnancy, and the prevention of HIV and other STDs. In evaluating and prescribing a contraceptive method, the provider must consider its effectiveness, side effects, contraindications, convenience of use, and cost. With the HIV-infected woman, potential for preventing HIV transmission and drug–drug interactions must also be considered.

Barrier methods such as condoms have become the mainstay in preventing transmission of HIV and other STDs. Condoms do not cover all exposed areas and are most effective in preventing infections transmitted by fluids from mucosal surfaces (e.g., HIV, gonorrhea, chlamydia, trichomoniasis) than in preventing those transmitted by skin-to-skin contact (e.g., herpes simplex virus [HSV], human papilloma virus [HPV], syphilis) (59). Women should be encouraged to use condoms in addition to any other form of contraceptive method they use. This recommendation is also extended to couples in whom both partners are HIV infected because of the potential risk of transmitting drug-resistant strains of the virus to each other, which may eventually result in treatment failure (52).

Because the use of male condoms requires the cooperation of the male partner, it is important to solicit their help, as well as empower the patient to negotiate their use. Women who receive partner support for contraceptive use, as well as behavioral intervention to teach negotiating skills in the use of contraceptives, are more likely to consistently use condoms (60, 61). Women and their sexual partners should be instructed on the proper use of condoms. Latex condoms are impermeable to HIV but not natural membrane (skin) condoms are not. Using oil-based lubricants (e.g., petroleum jelly, baby or cooking oils, lotions) weakens latex and should be avoided. Condoms need to be stored in a cool, dry place to prevent deterioration. Exposure to direct sunlight, excessive heat (e.g., wallet), and excessive humidity (e.g., bathroom) should be avoided.

Barrier methods other than condoms, including the diaphragm, vaginal contraceptive sponge, and female condom, have also been recommended for women. Both the contraceptive sponge and diaphragm are effective in providing contraception and decreasing the risk of STDs. Unfortunately, both devices do not completely cover the lower vagina, which is exposed to semen and other secretions. Seroconversion after only vaginal exposure to infectious secretions has been demonstrated in both animals and humans. Thus, ascension of the virus into the endometrium is not essential for HIV transmission (63). The female condom has been shown to prevent the transmission of HIV in vitro, but its ability to prevent transmission in vivo has not been well studied (64). Because of these issues, the female condom, diaphragm, and contraceptive sponge should not be used alone for the prevention of HIV transmission.

For the past two decades, spermicides, including nonoxynol-9 (N-9), have been recommended for the prevention of STDs, including HIV. However, more recent studies indicate that N-9 causes an increase in genital ulcers and vaginal inflammation (65, 66), which raised concerns regarding the possibility of increasing the risk of HIV transmission. As a result, several randomized trials have been performed to evaluate the effectiveness of N-9 in prevention of STDs. Three different preparations of N-9 have been examined, including film, gel, and vaginal sponge. These investigators concluded that N-9 is not effective in preventing gonorrhea, chlamydia, trichomoniasis, syphilis, or HIV infection (65, 67, 68). In addition, in one study using vaginal sponges with N-9, there was nearly a 50% increase in the transmission of HIV compared with the placebo group (67). As a result of these findings, the Centers for Disease Control and Prevention (CDC) no longer recommends the use of spermicides containing N-9 for vaginal or anal intercourse (59). This recommendation also extends to condoms lubricated with N-9.

The intrauterine device (IUD) has been associated with an increase in infectious complications in patients with high-risk sexual behavior. Currently, the World Health Organization and the International Planned Parenthood Federation do not recommend the use of the IUD in HIV-infected women, based on theoretical concerns about the increased risk of pelvic infection and female-to-male transmission. (It is believed that if the IUD causes a pelvic infection, this will further increase the risk of female-to-male HIV transmission [69, 70].) Despite these recommendations, the IUD has been studied for use as a contraceptive method, primarily for use in developing countries. Available evidence shows there is no increase in the cervical shedding of HIV in women using the IUD (71). Furthermore, the only study measuring the impact of female-to-male transmission of HIV found no association in more than 500 serodiscordant couples (72).

Likewise, the only longitudinal study examining the use of the IUD and acquisition of HIV by women from their infected partners also found no association (73). The incidence of infectious complications, including PID, is also not increased in HIV-infected women (74). These studies did not control for the use of condoms; thus, the role condom use played in preventing the transmission of HIV cannot be assessed.

Oral contraceptive pills (OCPs) are known to be effective for preventing pregnancy, but several issues need to be considered when prescribing them to the HIV-infected woman. These include the impact of OCPs on the immune system and their effect on HIV transmission, as well as potential drug–drug interactions, particularly for patients on HAART.

There is evidence that both estrogen and progesterone can alter both systemic and mucosal immunity. Progesterone has been shown to have an inhibitory effect on the immune system, and estrogen can inhibit cell-mediated responses to various stimuli (75). Animal studies also show that the local absorption of antigens through the vagina is influenced by the serum concentrations of estrogen and progesterone, which can manifest as a decrease in cell-mediated immunity (76). These data suggest that women who are HIV positive and using oral contraceptives may be at risk for progression of their disease because of decreased cell-mediated immunity. Unfortunately, there are no clinical studies to reliably answer this question.

Another significant issue is whether OCPs increase the risk of HIV transmission. Several clinical studies have generated mixed results, with nearly half concluding that OCPs increase the risk of HIV transmission, whereas the remainder concluded the opposite (77). The major criticism of these studies lies in their inability to control for confounding variables, such as risk-taking behavior, which may account for the transmission of HIV rather than the OCPs themselves. A separate but related question is whether OCPs affect the infectiousness of HIV-infected women. OCPs are known to cause cervical ectopy, which theoretically increases the risk for viral shedding. Studies that have addressed the amount of viral shedding in HIV-infected women on OCPs are also inconclusive primarily because many did not control for the presence of other STDs, which also affect the amount of viral shedding (77).

Perhaps the most significant concern about the use of OCPs in HIV-infected women is the potential for drug–drug interactions. In addition to anticonvulsant medications and some antibiotics, there are antiretroviral drugs that have been shown to decrease the effectiveness of OCPs. Several of the protease inhibitors, including nelfinavir, lopinavir, and ritonavir, along with the nonnucleoside reverse transcriptase inhibitor nevirapine, have been shown to decrease the levels of ethinyl estradiol in OCPs, which decrease their effectiveness (78). Rifampin, which is used to treat tuberculosis, also significantly decreases the levels of ethinyl estradiol. The potential clinical impact of these medications on the effectiveness of the OCPs is great, and it is generally not recommended to use OCPs in patients taking these medications because of the risk of contraceptive failure leading to pregnancy. Women using OCPs should also be instructed to use condoms to decrease the risk of sexual transmission of HIV.

The use of progestational agents has also raised concern regarding its effect on increasing the risk of HIV transmission to women using these agents. In animal studies by Marx et al. (79), monkeys treated with high doses of progesterone and then inoculated vaginally with simian immunodeficiency virus demonstrated a marked increase in HIV transmission. This was believed to be due to the thinning of the vaginal epithelium, making the macaques treated with progesterone more susceptible to HIV transmission. Since this study was published, two longitudinal studies have been performed to address the question of the risk of HIV transmission in women using medroxyprogesterone acetate (DMPA) (80, 81). Both studies found a clinically and statistically significant positive association between DMPA and HIV seroconversion. Given these findings, women using progestational agents should be advised to use condoms to decrease their risk of HIV transmission.

Menstrual Irregularities

Menstrual abnormalities reported in women with HIV, particularly amenorrhea in AIDS patients with wasting syndrome (82), have led investigators to postulate that HIV may cause abnormalities of the hypothalamic-pituitary axis. Most studies reporting on menstrual cycle data have used retrospective data and thus have yielded conflicting results (83–85). A more recent prospective study with HIV-negative controls examined this issue further by controlling for confounding variables such as age, body mass index, and substance abuse. The study demonstrated that women with HIV are at slightly more risk for very short cycles (less than 18 days), but in general, HIV infection did not affect cycle length (86). In addition, women with AIDS (who are at higher risk for AIDS wasting and weight loss) were 50% more likely to have a menstrual cycle greater than 40 days than HIV-negative controls, and those with a high VL had more variable cycles. Overall, the present data suggest that HIV serostatus appears to have little effect on menstrual cycle length, at least until immunodeficiency is advanced.

Women who have abnormal uterine bleeding (AUB) and who are HIV infected are two times more likely to have chronic plasma cell endometritis of a higher severity than HIV-negative controls (87). For this reason, diagnosis and treatment of chronic endometritis should be strongly considered in HIV-positive women with AUB and/or uterine tenderness. Once endometritis is excluded, however, management of AUB or amenorrhea in women with HIV should be similar to that received by women without HIV infection.

Abnormal Cervical Cytology/Human Papilloma Virus

Women infected with HIV are known to have a higher incidence of cervical intraepithelial neoplasia (CIN) than uninfected women. As a result, moderate cervical dysplasia and severe cervical dysplasia have been added to Category B of the 1993 CDC classification revision (42).

The prevalence of abnormal cervical cytology, such as squamous intraepithelial lesion (SIL), at study entry ranges from 19 to 41% of HIV-positive women compared with 10% in HIV-negative women (88–91). However, the cumulative incidence of abnormal cervical cytology in the HIV-positive population is much higher. In a longitudinal study of HIV-infected women, the Women's Interagency HIV Study Group demonstrated that 73% of HIV-infected women had an abnormal Pap smear over a 5-year period as compared with 42% in controls (92). In addition, HIV-positive women were four times more likely to develop low-grade SIL after a normal Pap smear at baseline than HIV-uninfected women.

Studies have shown that HIV is an independent risk factor for SIL and HPV (89, 90, 92–94). Approximately two-thirds of HIV-infected women will have any type of HPV as compared with one-third of uninfected women (90, 93). In addition, the risk of identifying an oncogenic type of HPV (16/18) in the HIV-positive women in one study was 24%, nearly three times higher than controls (93). Women with AIDS causing severe immunosuppression (CD4 less than 200 cell/mm^3) are more likely to have HPV infection, abnormal cervical cytology, and/or CIN, along with persistence of HPV (88, 90, 92–95). In addition, a high VL (more than 30,000 copies/mL) was also shown to increase a patient's risk for HPV infection and viral shedding, but not for SIL, in the HIV Epidemiology Research Study (HERS) (90, 94). The presence of HPV is a predictor of a higher likelihood of progression and lower regression of CIN in those who are HIV positive, suggesting that severe immunodeficiency plays a role in the natural history of HPV (92).

Screening for cervical cancer and preinvasive lesions is of vital importance to HIV-infected women. Based on their findings of a higher prevalence of dysplasia in HIV-infected women, some investigators advocate screening with colposcopy instead of Pap smears (96). However, most controlled studies show the sensitivity and specificity of Pap smears in HIV-positive women to be similar to those reported in HIV-negative women (97–100). Furthermore, colposcopy has not been shown to be cost effective as a screening tool in this population (101). Published guidelines for screening HIV-infected women currently recommend a Pap smear twice in the first year after diagnosis, and if the results are normal, annually thereafter (59). Routine colposcopy is not recommended.

Pap smears must be interpreted somewhat differently among seropositive women. Wright et al., in a prospective study, showed that 38% of HIV-positive women with mild cervical atypia, including atypical squamous cells of undetermined significance (ASCUS) and atypical glandular cells of undetermined significance, had CIN on colposcopic biopsy compared with 14% in the control group (102). Furthermore, 12% of seropositive women with severe inflammation with reparative atypia also had CIN. Based on these findings, Wright et al. recommended colposcopic examination after a single Pap smear showing cytologic atypia, including severe inflammation (102). In the latter case, an alternative method would be to examine the patient for infection and perform colposcopy only if the inflammation does not resolve after disease-specific treatment. (If there is no disease-specific entity to treat, the practitioner should proceed directly to colposcopy.) These patients should not be treated for a presumed diagnosis of cervicitis. All HIV-positive women with ASCUS and SIL should have a colposcopic exam.

Treatment of SIL is similar in HIV-infected patients, yet despite the method of treatment, recurrences are more common. Persistence of CIN after treatment occurs in up to 62% of patients after 3 years of follow-up, compared with 18% of HIV-uninfected women (103). The factors most predictive of recurrence are the severity of immunosuppression and residual CIN but not the type of treatment modality (103). HIV-infected women are also more likely to have excessive bleeding and cervicovaginal infections after a cone biopsy or laser ablation (104).

Because women with HIV are more likely to have higher recurrence rates after treatment, they should be educated about the necessity for close follow-up with Pap smears. A Pap test should be performed every 4 to 6 months the first 2 years following treatment because 90% of recurrences occur in this time (105, 106). Closer surveillance (e.g., Pap smears performed every 3 months) may be necessary for high-grade lesions. After three consecutive negative Pap smears, the patient can return to having an annual evaluation. If repeated Pap smears show abnormalities, repeat colposcopy and directed biopsies are indicated.

Treatment failures can occur even if the margins of the cervical specimen are clear, as exemplified by the fact that patients often require a second or third therapeutic procedure. Hysterectomy has been associated with a 50% recurrence rate of intraepithelial neoplasia at the vaginal cuff of the same grade and is therefore not indicated for the treatment of cervical dysplasia in HIV-infected women (107). Adjuvant therapy such as 5-fluorouracil after treatment for high-grade cervical dysplasia has been shown to reduce the frequency of recurrence, as well as the proportion of recurrences that were high grade (108). Another finding of this same study by Maimen et al. was that women receiving HAART had lower recurrence rates, whereas those with low CD4 cell counts had higher recurrence rates (108). Other adjuvant therapies currently under investigation include isotretinoin and 5% imiquimod cream.

Vulvar, vaginal, and perianal intraepithelial neoplasia are common among HIV-seropositive women. In the largest, well-controlled prospective cohort study to date, Conley et al. found vulvovaginal and perianal condyloma acuminata or intraepithelial neoplasia in 6% of HIV-positive women and 1% of controls (109). The incidence of condyloma acuminata or vulvar intraepithelial neoplasia (VIN) occurring over the 3-year study period was 16 times higher in women infected with HIV. Moreover, VIN lesions were significantly associated with immunosuppression, particularly with a CD4 less than 200 cells/mm^3. Overall, 2% of HIV-infected women without VIN at study entry developed high-grade VIN or invasive cancer of the vulva during the study. Treatment of VIN is difficult because of the higher likelihood of recurrence after excisional or ablative therapy (110). Close follow-up of these lesions is recommended in consultation with a gynecologic oncologist.

All HIV-positive women should undergo careful inspection of the vulva and perianal region for evidence of condyloma or VIN. It may be possible to enhance the detection of VIN by applying 5% acetic acid solution to a 4 × 4 sponge and applying it to the vulva for 5 minutes, as well as using low-power magnification (magnifying glass) to perform the exam (111). Women with any degree of abnormality, except typical exophytic condylomata acuminata, should be referred for colposcopy and biopsy so VIN or invasive disease can be ruled out (109).

The prevalence of invasive cervical cancer (ICC) has been reported to occur nearly twice as often in HIV-infected patients as noninfected patients, leading to it becoming an AIDS-defining illness (42, 112, 113). Despite these findings, the CDC has not seen an increase of ICC between 1992 and 1997 in their surveillance of AIDS-defining illnesses. Many factors could account for this discrepancy, including lack of cervical cancer screening and poor follow-up among HIV-infected patients as compared with uninfected patients.

Vaginal and Cervical Infections

Considerable interest has been shown regarding the relationship of HIV-1 and lower genital tract infections. Initial studies reported an increase in the frequency of most lower genital tract infections, but these studies either did not have control groups or involved select populations such as prostitutes or pregnant women (114–116). More recently, a prospective study by the HERS group looked at the prevalence of lower genital tract infections in HIV-positive women and compared them to high-risk HIV-seronegative women. This study showed no significant difference in the prevalence of chlamydia trachomatis, *Neisseria gonorrhea*, bacterial vaginosis (BV), or trichomoniasis between the two groups (117). Of these infections, BV was the most common, occurring in approximately 35% of all women participating in the study, regardless of HIV status. In a subsequent study by the same group, it was shown that although HIV-infected women were not more likely to have incident infections of BV, they were more likely to have persistence of their infections (118). Similarly, HIV-positive women with a CD4 count of less than 200 mm^3 were more likely to have persistence of any type of lower genital tract infection than women with higher CD4 counts.

STDs have been associated with increased shedding of HIV in cervical-vaginal secretions (119–121). Because heterosexual and most cases of perinatal transmission occur through direct contact with virus in the genital tract, the presence of these infections has significant clinical implications. It has been hypothesized that lower genital tract infections cause mucosal inflammation, resulting in the disruption of the normal epithelium leading to increased amounts of HIV shedding. Treatment of cervicitis, as well as vaginal infections, has been shown to decrease the shedding of HIV in cervical-vaginal secretions by three- to six-fold (119, 121). However, no studies have directly examined the role of vaginal STDs on female-to-male transmission of HIV.

Women with HIV infection should be encouraged to use condoms to decrease their risk of other STDs. Treatment of vaginal and cervical infections is the same as for uninfected women.

Considerable controversy has surrounded the role of vulvovaginal candidiasis in HIV-infected women. Early in the HIV epidemic, reports suggested that vulvovaginal candidiasis was more frequent and more recurrent in HIV-infected women (122, 123). In response to these findings, the CDC in 1993 added vulvovaginal candidiasis that is defined as persistent or poorly responsive to therapy, as a symptomatic condition (Category B) of HIV infection. Since then, however, two prospective cohort studies using at-risk, HIV-negative controls have not demonstrated an increase in the incidence of vulvovaginal candidiasis, except in severely immunocompromised women with a CD4 less than 200 cells/mm^3 (30, 124).

Presently, there are no data to suggest that refractory vulvovaginal candidiasis does not respond to conventional antifungal therapy. Reports are conflicting as to whether HIV-positive women have a higher frequency of non-albicans *Candida* species, in particular, *Candida glabrata* (30, 125). So far, the clinical and microbiological spectrum of vulvovaginal candidiasis appears to be similar in HIV-positive and HIV-negative women. Treatment principles should be identical to those in HIV-negative women. Schuman et al. showed that use of suppressive prophylactic therapy with fluconazole 200 mg once weekly effectively decreased the recurrence of symptomatic vulvovaginal candidiasis in HIV-positive women (126). This study also observed that there was a tendency for *C. glabrata* to replace *Candida albicans* as a colonizing organism. Fortunately, azole resistance of *C. albicans* vaginal isolates has been rare, in contrast to resistance of *C. albicans* oropharyngeal isolates. Presently, primary prophylaxis of vulvovaginal candidiasis is not recommended because it is expensive and deemed unnecessary (127). In the event recurrent vulvovaginal candidiasis occurs, topical antifungal therapy should be extended to 10 to 14 days to achieve clinical remission. For those with candidiasis recalcitrant to topical therapy, an initial regimen of oral fluconazole 200 mg daily for 14 days should be administered. Once clinical remission and a negative culture have been achieved, a suppressive regimen is indicated. Several possible regimens are clotrimazole 500-mg vaginal suppository administered once weekly, ketoconazole 100 mg daily for 6 months, or fluconazole 100 mg weekly for 6 months (128). Women who have azole-resistant infections should be treated with nystatin, boric acid, or flucytosine. Boric acid suppositories prescribed as 600-mg gelatin capsules inserted into the vagina daily for 14 days are particularly useful for *C. glabrata* vaginitis (129).

Syphilis

The seroprevalence of HIV among women with syphilis in the United States is high, ranging from 8.3 to 20.5% (130). All patients with syphilis should have HIV testing, with a retest after 3 months if the initial test is negative for those who continue to exhibit high-risk behavior.

Syphilis is more commonly seen at the time of initial diagnosis of HIV than many other STDs (131). Thus, serologic tests for syphilis should be part of the initial workup of the HIV-infected patient.

Unusual serologic responses have been observed among HIV-infected patients who have syphilis. Most reports involve serologic titers that were higher than normal, but false-negative serologic results have also been seen (59). Nevertheless, both treponemal and nontreponemal serologic tests for syphilis can be interpreted in the usual manner for diagnosing syphilis in the HIV-infected patient. However, the microhemagglutination assay to *Treponema pallidum* (MHA-TP) is somewhat less likely (88.6%) than the fluorescent treponemal antibody absorbent (FTA-ABS) test (99.2%) to be reactive in cases of primary syphilis (132). For the most part, the clinical manifestations of syphilis are similar in HIV and uninfected patients. However, HIV-infected patients with primary syphilis are more likely to have multiple chancres at initial presentation and to have genital ulcers with secondary syphilis than HIV-uninfected patients (133, 134). HIV-positive women are also more likely to present with secondary syphilis than HIV-infected men (134). HIV-infected patients frequently have cerebrospinal fluid abnormalities in early syphilis, but the majority of patients are asymptomatic. This finding, along with initial retrospective reports suggesting HIV-infected patients were more likely to have neurosyphilis than uninfected patients, prompted investigators to question the adequacy of the CDC-recommended treatment for HIV-infected patients with early syphilis (135). In an effort to answer this question of whether outcomes of treatment for syphilis in HIV-infected patients differ from outcomes in uninfected patients, Rolfs et al. (133) designed a randomized trial of enhanced therapy for early syphilis. Patients diagnosed with early syphilis received the CDC-recommended treatment of 2.4 million units of intramuscular penicillin G benzathine, and were then randomized to enhanced therapy with 2 g amoxicillin and 500 mg probenecid three times daily for 10 days or placebo. Results were then stratified based on HIV status. The rate of detection of *T. pallidum* in the cerebrospinal fluid (CSF) did not differ according to HIV status prior to treatment, nor were HIV-infected patients more likely to have *T. pallidum* in their CSF than uninfected patients after receiving standard therapy with penicillin alone compared with the enhanced therapy (133). In addition, the response to treatment was similar for patients with AIDS compared with HIV-infected patients with less immunosuppression.

Overall, the clinical response rate of HIV-infected patients with syphilis is similar to those without HIV infection. Serologically, a less than four-fold decrease in titer at 6 to 12 months is considered a treatment failure. Among patients with primary or secondary syphilis, HIV-infected patients are more likely to have serologically defined treatment failure at 6 to 12 months (133). The explanation for this finding is currently unknown. Posttreatment serologic evaluation should be more frequent in HIV-infected patients. The CDC guidelines currently recommend serologic tests at 3, 6, 9, 12, and 24 months after therapy for HIV-positive patients (59). HIV-infected patients who meet the criteria for treatment failure should be managed the same as those without HIV infection. This includes a CSF examination and treatment for neurosyphilis if *T. pallidum* is detected.Most experts would retreat patients with 7.2 million units of benzathine penicillin G (administered as three weekly doses of 2.4 million units each), even if the CSF examination is negative (59). Seroreversion of treponemal-specific tests occurs in 5 to 10% of HIV-infected patients and is similar to HIV-uninfected patients 1 year following treatment (132). Seroreversion of nontreponemal tests typically occurs after 1 year in HIV-negative patients with syphilis (136). This is frequently not the case in HIV-infected patients who may continue to have persistently elevated titers to nontreponemal tests (135).

Pelvic Inflammatory Disease

PID is a common STD and is frequently seen in the HIV-positive patient. This finding eventually led to the addition of PID to the 1993 revised classification system for HIV infection. It is currently listed as a symptomatic, but not AIDS-defining, illness under Category B (42). Thus, HIV testing should be offered to all women with a diagnosis of PID. The seroprevalence of HIV in patients with PID is high and ranges between 4.2% and 16.7% (137, 138). The rate of seroprevalence is even higher in women with tubo-ovarian abscesses (TOAs) (23.5%) or with a low white blood cell count (WBC) (less than 10,000/mm^3) (47.4%) (139).

HIV appears to alter the clinical course of PID. Several retrospective studies have shown that HIV-positive women with PID are more likely to have a higher temperature, lower WBC count (less than 10,000 cells/mm^3), and decreased abdominal tenderness on admission as compared with HIV-negative controls (139–142). However, patients with lower CD4 counts (less than 200 cells/mm^3) were more likely to have a temperature less than 38°C on admission in one study (142). Some of these studies have shown that HIV-positive women are more likely to have a TOA and require surgical intervention than uninfected women (139, 141, 142). In a more recent prospective study, Cohen et al. (143) performed laparoscopy on women admitted with PID in Kenya. TOAs were found in 33% of HIV-infected women as compared with only 15% of HIV uninfected women. Among HIV-positive women, a TOA was found in 55% of those with AIDS (as defined by a CD4 count of less than 200 cell/mm^3) versus 14% of those without AIDS. A prospective study on American women with PID also confirmed a lower WBC count on admission, along with a higher rate of TOAs in HIV-infected women (144). These same investigators showed that the microbiology of PID did not differ between groups, with the exception that the HIV-infected women had a higher percentage of *Streptococcus* and *Mycoplasma* species. The presence of these bacteria also correlated with a significantly higher rate of plasma cell endometritis, a condition commonly associated with these two organisms.

Despite the clinical differences in how HIV-positive patients present with PID, they generally respond well to both intravenous and oral regimens recommended by the CDC STD treatment guidelines (59, 143–145). HIV-infected women do however take a longer period of time to defervesce, resulting in a significantly longer hospital stay compared with HIV-uninfected women (140, 143, 144). This is particularly true in women with TOAs or AIDS (143–145). The CDC currently recommends parenteral regimens to treat HIV-positive women with PID (59). This may not be warranted in patients who do not meet criteria for hospitalization as outlined in the CDC treatment guidelines, particularly because there are studies that have more recently substantiated the outpatient treatment guidelines by the CDC (144, 145).

Herpes

Herpes simplex virus 2 (HSV-2) is the most common cause of genital ulcers in the United States and occurs more commonly in HIV-infected patients (146). The higher occurence in HIV-infected patient is a result of increased viral shedding of HSV-2, which is four times higher in HIV-infected patients than in HIV-uninfected patients (147). HSV-2 shedding is even greater in AIDS patients who have more severe immunosuppression than those with HIV alone (148). Other factors that increase HSV-2 shedding in HIV patients are the use of oral contraceptives or DMPA, as well as pregnancy (149).

Herpetic lesions are more likely to be atypical in appearance or location. They frequently do not look vesicular or have a base of erythema around the ulcer as in the classic presentation of herpes simplex. Instead they may appear flat with evidence of secondary bacterial infection (Fig. 24.2). Immunocompromised patients (CD4 less than 200 cells/mm^3) are 16 times more likely to have recurrent episodes of herpes than those whose CD4 counts are greater than 500 cells/mm^3(114). In fact, HSV-2 lasting longer than 1 month suggests immunodeficiency and is an AIDS-defining illness (59).

HSV can activate latent HIV or enhance the replication of HIV, particularly during an acute attack of herpes (150, 151). This explains why herpes ulcers have such a strong association with the sexual transmission of HIV. In a recent meta-analysis of 17 studies that addressed the effect of HSV-2 on HIV, Wald et al. determined that 52% of sexually transmitted HIV infections can be facilitated by HSV-2 infection (146). This finding underscores the need to counsel HIV-infected persons to use latex condoms during every act of intercourse, even if they do not have a history of herpes, to decrease the rate of sexual transmission of HIV and other STDs such as HSV-2.

Treatment of herpes is similar to uninfected patients; however, longer treatment courses are often required, particularly when the patient is severely immunocompromised (59). Treatment should continue until all lesions are healed, and close outpatient follow-up is necessary. An important component of HSV treatment in these patients is ensuring the patient is on HAART in order to decrease the VL so the patient's immune system can reconstitute itself, which will raise the CD4 count. This in turn decreases the frequency of recurrent herpetic outbreaks.

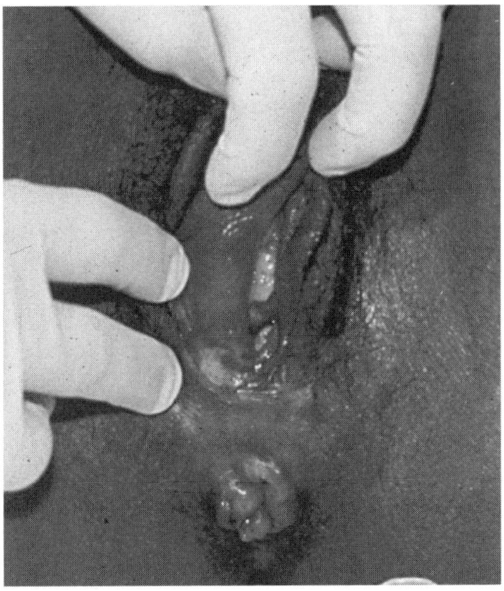

FIGURE 24.2 • A 1-cm lesion on lower right labia minora.

If lesions persist in a patient receiving acyclovir or valacyclovir, resistance testing should be performed. Acyclovir resistance has been reported in 11 to 17% of patients with HSV who are also HIV positive (152). All acyclovir-resistant strains are resistant to valacyclovir, and most are resistant to famciclovir, leaving few desirable options for treatment. Foscarnet, 40 mg/kg intravenously every 8 hours for 3 weeks, or until the lesions are gone, is an effective alternative treatment. Unfortunately, the requirement for parenteral infusion, as well as the potential renal and metabolic toxicities of foscarnet, are major limitations to this therapy and require that these patients be managed in consultation with an infectious disease specialist. Topical cidofovir gel 1% applied to the lesions once daily for 5 days has also been demonstrated to be effective (153).

Prophylaxis for recurrent herpes is similar to regimen used in the uninfected patient, although many HIV specialists have a lower threshold for initiating prophylaxis than what current guidelines suggest (six or more recurrences per year) (59). Ideally, these woman should be initiated on HAART or have their HAART regimen optimized to prevent severe immunosuppression. Daily suppressive therapy in a woman with AIDS can potentially risk acyclovir resistance. Therefore, long-term suppressive therapy is a less desirable option than optimizing the patient's HAART regimen to restore her CD4 count, which in and of itself lowers the risk for recurrent herpes.

Genital Ulcer Disease

Genital ulcers are often seen in HIV-infected women and may be difficult to diagnose. Often, these lesions appear large and necrotic, are painful (Fig. 24.3), and may persist or enlarge in size if untreated (Fig. 24.4) (154). These lesions typically appear in women who are severely immunosuppressed with accompanying high VLs because they are either not on treatment for their HIV or are failing treatment (154, 155). Approximately half of the genital lesions in HIV-infected women are idiopathic (termed aphthous ulcers), with the remainder having an infectious etiology (155–157). In the largest series of HIV-positive women with genital ulcer disease (GUD), LaGuardia et al. found no etiology for the ulcers in 60% of the women. Of those with an infectious etiology, 28% had HSV, 10% mixed bacteria, and 2% CMV (155). Women with idiopathic GUD should also have a careful examination of the oral cavity because nearly 40% will also have oral aphthous ulcers (154).

The diagnostic approach to the patient with GUD is outlined in Table 24.8. Vaginal discharge on the perineum can cause local irritation and be the source of secondary bacterial infection that is often seen in these cases. Thus, any vaginal infection should be identified and treated to decrease the risk of further tissue breakdown. In addition, aerobic, anaerobic, viral, and fungal cultures

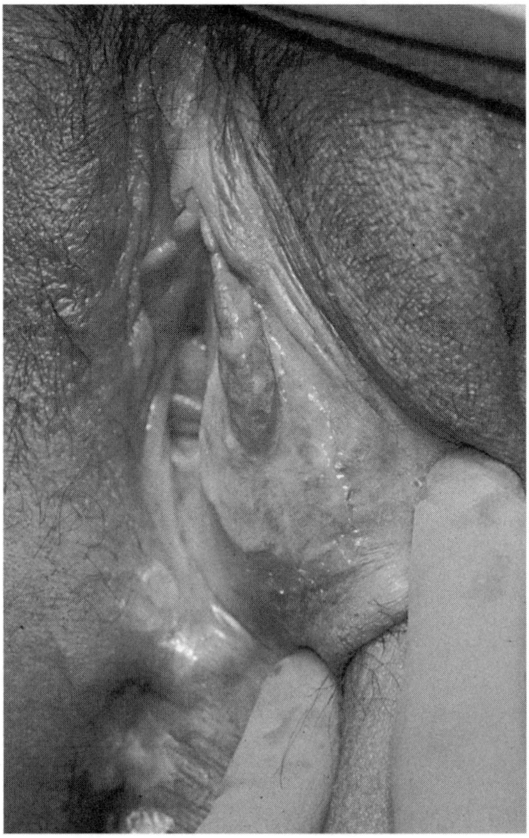

FIGURE 24.3 ● A 2 × 3 cm genital ulcer disease lesion on left vulva.

should be obtained along with a serologic test for syphilis to search for an infectious etiology. Although the most common infectious cause of genital ulcers is HSV, other causes to be considered include syphilis, cytomegalovirus, *H. ducreyi*, and mycobacteria. A comprehensive investigation of a woman with GUD should include a biopsy of the lesion. Because these lesions are often exquisitely painful, regional anesthesia is often necessary. Because part of the biopsy is sent for cultures, the lesion(s) should not be cleansed with an antiseptic until *after* the biopsy is completed. An elliptical biopsy encompassing a normal edge of tissue should be obtained and then bisected horizontally. Excision of the lesion is not necessary and does not prevent recurrence. Once bisected, the specimens should be placed in two separate containers with normal saline. One is marked for cultures, and the other is for histology and immunohistochemical staining. It is beneficial to describe in detail all potential bacteria, viruses, and fungal organisms for which to evaluate in the culture and histologic examination. If acyclovir resistance is suspected, send a portion of the specimen for sensitivity testing. Once the biopsy has been obtained, cleanse the lesions with a dilute (i.e., approximately one part chlorhexidine to two parts water) chlorhexidine solution. Betadine should be avoided if possible because it inhibits fibroblast formation. It is also not necessary to debride these lesions. A monofilament such as 3-0 Prolene should be used to close the wound. Interrupted sutures are best, and subcutaneous closure should be avoided. Chromic or cat gut suture should be avoided because it cause more inflammation. Sutures can be removed 7 to 10 days after the biopsy. Antibiotics are generally not useful and should not be used empirically; their use should be reserved for cases where a specific vaginal infection is being treated.

The treatment of GUD requires individualization based on the etiology of the disease and is outlined in Table 24.9. However, the cornerstone of treatment in all patients is HAART. Treatment needs to be started or optimized in consultation with an HIV specialist. Failure of the patient to either receive or adhere to HAART can result in the lesions not healing or healing very slowly. Aerobic cultures may yield mixed bacteria from the perineum but does not require treatment as a general rule because it is most likely contamination from vaginal discharge. If the patient

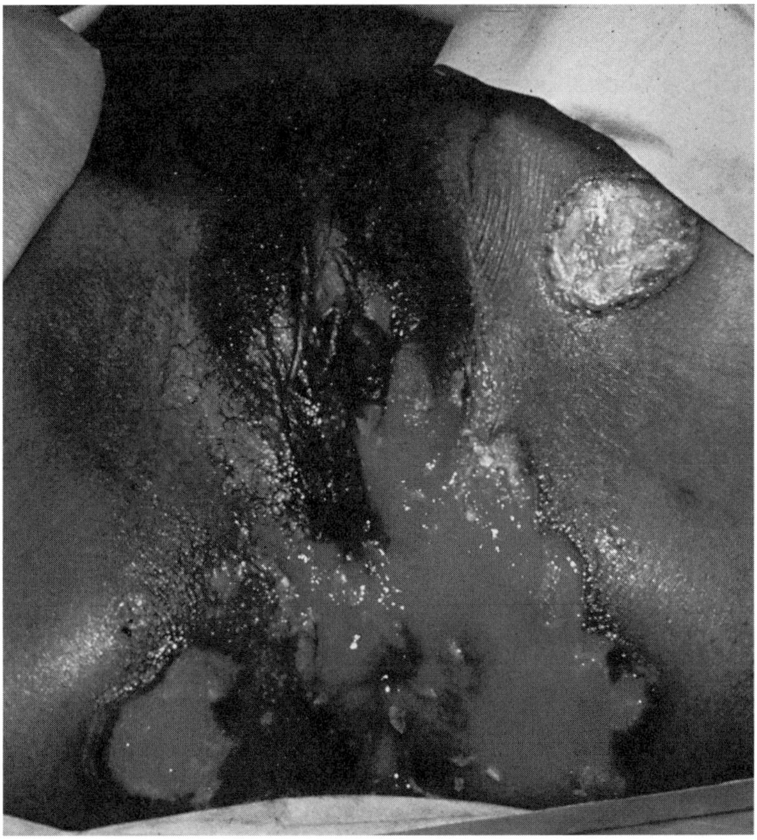

FIGURE 24.4 ● Advanced genital ulcer disease.

TABLE 24.8

Diagnostic Approach to the Patient With Genital Ulcer Disease

- Wet prep of vaginal discharge
- Serologic test for syphilis
- Aerobic and anaerobic culture
- Herpes simplex virus culture
- Cytomegalovirus culture
- AFB smear and mycobacterial cultures
- Tissue biopsy (include normal tissue margins)

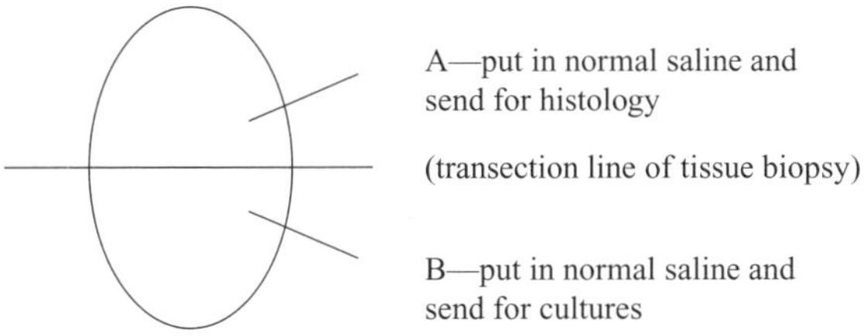

- Acyclovir sensitivity testing of tissue, if needed

TABLE 24.9

Treatment for Genital Ulcer Disease

General
- Treat underlying HIV/AIDS with HAART
- Sitz baths twice a day
- Treat any vaginal infection
- Adequate analgesia for pain relief

Infectious Etiology
- Herpes simplex virus—valacyclovir 1 g three times a day
- Cytomegalovirus—valganciclovir 900 mg twice a day
- If the initial treatment fails or the patient is acyclovir resistant, use foscarnet cream (2.5%) twice daily for 20 min or intravenously (40 mg/kg every 8 hr for 3 weeks)

Idiopathic
- Many lesions respond empirically to HAART
- Steroids
- Thalidomide 200 mg every day for 14 days

HAART, highly active antiretroviral therapy.

becomes febrile, a systemic bacterial or fungal infection should be suspected, and consultation with an infectious disease specialist is advised. Ideally, treatment other than HAART should await culture and biopsy results, but presumptive treatment with valacyclovir can be initiated while these results are pending. Anti-HSV agents should be given until the lesion is completely gone with weekly outpatient follow-up to monitor the progress of treatment (Fig. 24.5). Once the lesion has been completely healed, and if the HSV culture is positive, a suppressive dose should

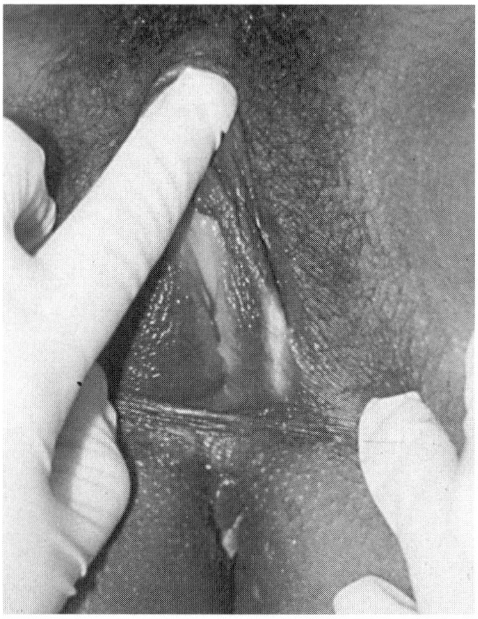

FIGURE 24.5 ● Lesion (same as in Fig. 24.2) 2 weeks after acyclovir treatment.

be initiated until the CD4 count goes above 200 cell/mm^3. Long-term suppressive therapy can result in acyclovir resistance and should be avoided if possible, especially if the CD4 cells have reconstituted. If acyclovir resistance is present, there will also be resistance to valacyclovir and famciclovir, leaving foscarnet as the only treatment option. A dilemma arises when no etiologic agent is found. In these cases, many respond to HAART with or without valacyclovir. Mixed results have been seen with the use of topical and systemic steroids (154). In cases of aphthous ulcers that are unresponsive to all therapies mentioned, consideration can be given to the use of thalidomide, which has been found to be a very effective treatment for oral aphthous ulcers (158). Because thalidomide is known to cause phocomelia, it should be used with caution in women who are not using an effective means of birth control. One way to administer treatment would be to do an initial pregnancy test, give 1 week of thalidomide at a time, and monitor with weekly pregnancy tests. If a positive test result occurs, the thalidomide should be discontinued immediately. Any exposure of the drug within 31 days from the last menstrual period during the "all or none" period would not increase the risk of anomalies.

Once treatment is underway, a weekly follow-up is necessary to monitor the course of therapy. Once the GUD is completely healed, suppressive therapy can be considered based on the underlying cause. Patients should be informed that GUD may recur, and close follow-up is warranted.

Reproductive Options in Women With HIV

More recent advances in HAART have produced a significant increase in the life expectancy of HIV-infected adults. Because the majority of men and women infected with HIV are of reproductive age, they are likely to consider becoming parents. Most of the attention has been focused on preventing vertical transmission of HIV to the infants of women infected with HIV. However, with serodiscordant couples there is the added concern about the possibility of transmission of HIV to the uninfected partner through unprotected intercourse. Having an undetectable VL does not eliminate the possibility of transmission because the level of HIV between plasma and semen or vaginal secretions is poorly correlated (55). The risk per act of unprotected intercourse is estimated to be between 1 in 500 and 1 in 1000 (159, 160). Nevertheless, a single act of unprotected intercourse is sufficient to infect one's partner. Careful preconceptual counseling of the risks involved and advice on how to time intercourse accurately are necessary for couples prepared to risk unprotected intercourse to have a child. Couples may try to minimize the risk of exposure by accurately timing intercourse using ovulation detection methods. The CDC does not recommend postexposure prophylaxis in cases of repeated unprotected intercourse between discordant couples (58).

For the woman who is HIV positive, another option to consider is washed intrauterine insemination (IUI). This would eliminate any risk of transmission of HIV to the uninfected male partner through unprotected intercourse. The pregnancy rate per cycle of IUI is 10 to 12% and is relatively inexpensive compared with other artificial reproductive technologies (ARTs).

There are several options available to couples in whom the male is HIV positive and the woman is negative. Conception through unprotected intercourse is not recommended because of the high concentration of HIV in the lymphocytes of semen. Insemination using donor sperm eliminates the risk of transmitting the virus to the woman and subsequently to her infant. However, removing the possibility of genetic parenthood from one partner, particularly the one whose life is threatened with disease, has tremendous moral and ethical implications, and requires thorough counseling beforehand. Although a perfectly safe method, this is not the option of choice for most serodiscordant couples.

Semprini et al. (161) pioneered a technique to enable HIV-negative women to undergo IUI with sperm washed free of HIV. By using PCR technology to eliminate the cell-associated and free virus from the semen, one can significantly reduce the risk of transmitting HIV. However, false-negative results may occur if the number of infected cells or virions is below the sensitivity limit of the techniques used. To date, more than 2000 IUIs using this sperm washing technique have been performed without any reported seroconversions (162). Although this technique is widely used in Europe, especially in Spain and Italy, the CDC recommended against using washed IUI of women with semen from men infected with HIV in 1990, following a single case report in the United States of HIV transmission to a woman who underwent IUI from her HIV-positive husband (163). This case report led to the American Society of Reproductive Medicine to advise against the provision of ART services to HIV-infected individuals (164). To date, this is the only documented case in the world literature of HIV seroconversion following IUI and is presumed to be the result of inadequate washing. In Europe, washed IUI is usually tested for HIV using PCR technology, but this is not routinely done in the United States.

Another option that is more commonly performed in the United States is in vitro fertilization (IVF). This should be considered when IUI is either not feasible or successful. HIV has been isolated from spermatogonia (less than 1%) but has not been detected from mature spermatozoa (165, 166). Spermatozoa are not considered to be a major target because they do not express significant levels of CD4, CCR5, or CXCR4 receptors, which are critical for HIV entry into cells (167). A technique known as intracytoplasmic sperm injection (ICSI) is used to minimize the number of spermatozoa exposed to oocytes. After undergoing ovulation induction, a woman's oocytes are harvested, and each oocyte is fertilized with one spermatozoa. (This is in contrast to the millions of spermatozoa an oocyte is exposed to using IUI.) The fertilized ova are then transferred back into the uterus and the woman is monitored to determine if a pregnancy has occurred. In the largest single series of IVF-ICSI cases reported in HIV-1 discordant couples, Sauer et al. at Columbia University did not have any seroconversions in 34 women or their offspring (168). The clinical pregnancy rate and the delivery rate per embryo transfer was 45% and 31%, respectively (168). Although this technique yields a higher pregnancy rate per cycle than IUI, it is also considerably more expensive. Serodiscordant couples interested in ICSI should contact the Center for Reproductive Care at Columbia University at 646-756-8282 and inform them they are interested in the HIV serodiscordant program.

Adoption is the final option for those couples that do not want to risk HIV transmission from unprotected intercourse or who fail or choose not to undergo ART. In practice, however, the presence of HIV infection in one or both partners may make adoption a difficult process.

PRECONCEPTION COUNSELING

The American College of Obstetrics and Gynecology advocates that all women of reproductive age receive preconceptual counseling as part of routine primary care. Unintended pregnancy accounts for almost half the pregnancies that occur annually in the United States, and the diagnosis of pregnancy frequently occurs either when or after organogenesis is nearly completed. The purpose of preconceptual counseling is to identify risk factors for adverse maternal or fetal outcome, provide appropriate patient education, and treat or stabilize conditions prior to conception to optimize maternal–fetal outcome (169).

The recommended components of preconceptual counseling for HIV-infected women are listed in Table 24.10 (170). Discussion of these issues are necessary for the patient to make informed decisions regarding the desire to become pregnant and how her treatment will affect both her and her unborn fetus. In addition, it allows for the medical care of HIV-infected women to be coordinated between the HIV specialist and the patient's reproductive health care provider prior to conception, which may have significant advantages over waiting to treat after the woman has conceived.

Most perinatal transmission (75 to 80%) occurs during childbirth, with the remainder occurring in utero (171). HIV is also present in breast milk so patients should be counseled to refrain from breast-feeding (8). Patients should also be educated that treatment with antiretroviral agents significantly reduces the vertical transmission of HIV.

In February 1994, the Pediatric AIDS Clinical Trials Group (PACTG) 076 protocol demonstrated that the three-part zidovudine regimen significantly reduced the transmission of HIV from 25 to 8.3%. This amounted to a nearly 70% reduction in the transmission of HIV (172). Since then, advances in the understanding of HIV have shown that the treatment of HIV by potent antiretroviral drugs significantly reduces the VL, which further lowers the risk of vertical transmission of HIV. Currently, triple combination therapy, including the PACTG 076 protocol, is the standard of care during pregnancy (170). Women receiving triple combination antiretroviral therapy who achieve an undetectable VL have a less than 1% risk of vertical transmission (7, 173).

TABLE 24.10

Recommended Components of Preconceptual Counseling for HIV-Infected Women

- Selection of appropriate contraception to reduce likelihood of unintended pregnancy
- Education about risks of perinatal transmission and strategies to lower vertical transmission
- Initiation or modification of HAART prior to conception to
  - Avoid teratogenic drugs
  - Maximally suppress maternal viral load
  - Evaluate and control potential side effects that may adversely impact maternal–fetal outcome
- Evaluation and prophylaxis of opportunistic infection and administration of immunizations
- Screening for psychological and substance abuse disorders
- Assessment of reproductive and familial genetic history, screening for STDs, initiation of folic acid supplementation
- Planning for perinatal consultation, if indicated

HAART, highly active antiretroviral therapy; STD, sexually transmitted disease.
From Public Health Service Task Force. Recommendations for the Use of Antiretroviral Drugs in Pregnant HIV-1 Infected Women for Maternal Health and Interventions to Reduce Perinatal Transmission in the United States. February 4, 2002. Available at: http://www.aidsinfo.nih.gov. Accessed August 2, 2005.

More than half of all women currently entering the first trimester with a known HIV diagnosis are not currently on any HAART. In addition, nearly 40% of those on antiretroviral therapy may require adjustment of their regimen (170). Treatment of eligible patients with HAART should be initiated or optimized prior to conception in accordance to the adult treatment guidelines, with the goal of achieving an undetectable VL (78). This will theoretically eliminate both in utero and perinatal transmission of HIV, assuming an undetectable VL is maintained during the pregnancy. In some cases, women who are not pregnant may not be a candidate for HAART according to the Guidelines for the Use of Antiretroviral Agents in HIV-Infected Adults and Adolescents (78). If so, these women should be encouraged to contact their HIV specialist if they are contemplating pregnancy to determine if treatment with HAART is indicated. If so, it can be started in order to achieve an undetectable VL prior to conception. Women whose VL and CD4 count do not currently meet the guidelines for therapy can delay HAART until 10 to 12 weeks' gestation to avoid any teratogenic risk. Women who are already on HAART, but who do not have an undetectable VL, should also consult their HIV specialist preconceptually to maximally suppress their VL prior to conception.

The reproductive health provider should also counsel HIV-infected women regarding the potential adverse effects of antiretroviral medications during pregnancy. The vast majority of these medications are either FDA Pregnancy Category B or C. Although some drugs are teratogenic in animal studies, the benefit of taking HAART outweighs the risk of congenital anomalies in most cases. The exception is the nonnucleoside drug efavirenz, which has caused neural tube defects in animal studies and recently in a neonate (170, 174). Because these types of defects occur in the first 4 weeks after conception, a woman conceiving on this drug has the greatest risk for this anomaly. Women who desire to conceive should reconsider either starting or continuing on this drug. Those who are currently on efavirenz should use an effective method of contraception to avoid pregnancy. Women on this drug who want to conceive should ideally switch from efavirenz to another nonnucleoside analog drug prior to conception. For women in whom changing to another drug is impossible due to adverse side effects or prior failed combinations, 1 mg folic acid daily should be taken preconceptually because this has been shown to reduce the risk of neural tube defect by 70% (175, 176). If a patient inadvertently conceives on efavirenz, they should be referred to a maternal–fetal specialist for a targeted ultrasound and genetic counseling.

Another adverse side effect of HAART that clinicians should be aware of is mitochondrial toxicity from nucleoside analogs. Among the disorders associated with mitochondrial dysfunction are symptomatic lactic acidosis and hepatic steatosis, which may have a female preponderance. Lactic acidosis has been reported in pregnant women and can mimic acute fatty liver of pregnancy. This syndrome has resulted in three maternal deaths and fetal demise in two women who were on stavudine and didanosine, along with another antiretroviral agent (170). Clinicians should advise their patients to avoid this combination of drugs during pregnancy unless other combinations have failed or cause unacceptable side effects.

Finally, due to the evolving and complex nature of the management of HIV-1 infection, a specialist with experience in the treatment of pregnant women with HIV infection should be involved in the care of these patients. Detailed recommendations for the management of HIV infection are available on the HIV/AIDS Treatment Information Service website at http://www.aidsinfo.nih.gov.

Clinical Notes

SCREENING

- Reproductive health care providers play an important role in identifying women at risk for HIV.
- Most women with HIV are asymptomatic and have acquired it through sexual transmission.
- A woman is often unaware of her risk for HIV. Her partner's risk must also be assessed.
- Women who have been sexually active within the past 10 to 15 years, as well as women with risk factors, should be offered HIV testing (Table 24.1).

PRIMARY CARE

- The special needs of women require a multidisciplinary approach to care.
- A comprehensive evaluation includes a complete history and physical, along with baseline laboratory evaluation (Table 24.3).
- Depression, domestic violence, and a history of sexual abuse are common in women with HIV.
- Patients should be counseled on how to reduce the risk of HIV transmission.
- The patient should be referred to an HIV specialist for HAART.

GYNECOLOGIC HEALTH ISSUES

- All patients should be encouraged to use condoms to reduce the risk of sexual transmission of HIV.
- N-9 is no longer recommended by the CDC for reducing the transmission of HIV.
- Abnormal cervical cytology requires colposcopy and aggressive treatment. The recurrence risk of cervical dysplasia is high (60%), regardless of the treatment used.
- PID is common in women with HIV, and they respond well to intravenous antibiotics.
- HSV infection may have an atypical presentation, especially in immunocompromised patients.
- Genital ulcer disease is difficult to diagnose. Approximately 60% of cases are idiopathic, with the remainder having an infectious etiology. Bacterial, viral, fungal cultures, and biopsy are needed to thoroughly investigate the cause of GUD (Table 24.8). Treatment must be individualized (Table 24.9), but all patients should be given HAART.

- Artificial reproductive techniques can assist serodiscordant couples to become pregnant without risking the transmission of HIV to the uninfected partner.
- Prepregnancy counseling should be offered to all women of reproductive age with HIV to counsel them as to the means of reducing the vertical transmission of HIV.

REFERENCES

1. Bozzette SA, Berry SH, Duan N, et al. The care of HIV-infected adults in the United States. N Engl J Med 1998;339:1897–1904.
2. Hader SL, Smith DK, Moore JS, et al. HIV infection in the United States: status at the millennium. JAMA 2001;285:1186–1192.
3. Centers for Disease Control and Prevention. HIV/AIDS Surveillance Report, 2003 (vol 15) Atlanta. US Dept Health & Human Services Centers for Disease Control & Prevention 2004: p6 Also at http://www.cdc.gov/hiv/stats/hasrlink.htm. Available at: http://www.cdc.gov/hiv/graphics/women.htm. Accessed August 2, 2005.
4. Centers for Disease Control and Prevention. Mortality L285 slide series (through 2002). Available at: http://www.cdc.gov/hiv/graphics/mortalit.htm. Accessed August 2, 2005.
5. Moore RD, Chaisson RE. Natural history of HIV infection in an era of combination antiretroviral therapy. AIDS 1999;13:1933–1942.
6. Ioannidis JP, Abrams EJ, Ammann A, et al. Perinatal transmission of human immunodeficiency virus type 1 by pregnant women with RNA virus loads <1000 copies/ml. J Infect Dis 2001;183:539–545.
7. Centers for Disease Control and Prevention. Revised recommendations for HIV screening of pregnant women. MMWR Morb Mortal Wkly Rep 2001;50(RR20):1–20.
8. MacDonald SR, Skor A, Socol ML, et al. Human immunodeficiency virus infection and women: a survey of missed opportunities for testing and diagnosis. Am J Obstet Gynecol 1998;178:1264–1271.
9. Fernandez MI, Wilson TE, Ethier KA, et al. Acceptance of HIV testing during prenatal care. Public Health Rep 2000;15:460–468.
10. Stringer EM, Stringer JA, Cliver SP, et al. Evaluation of a new testing policy for human immunodeficiency virus to improve screening rates. Obstet Gynecol 2001;98:1104–1108.
11. Carusi D. Human immunodeficiency virus test refusal in pregnancy: a challenge to voluntary testing. Obstet Gynecol 1998;91:540–545.
12. Barabacci M, Repke JT, Chaisson RE. Routine prenatal screening for HIV infection. Lancet 1991;337:709–711.
13. Landesman S, Minkoff H, Holman S, et al. Serosurvey of human immunodeficiency virus infection in parturients: implications for human immunodeficiency virus testing programs of pregnant women. JAMA 1987;258:2701–2703.
14. Castro KG, Lifson AR, White CR, et al. Investigations of AIDS patients with no previously identified risk factors. JAMA 1987;257:2039.
15. Morens SM. Serological screening tests for antibody to human immunodeficiency virus—the search for perfection in an imperfect world. Clin Infect Dis 1997;25:101–103.
16. Farzadegan H, Polis MA, Wolinsky SM, et al. Loss of human immunodeficiency virus type 1 (HIV-1) antibodies with evidence of viral infection in asymptomatic homosexual men. A report from the Multicenter AIDS Cohort Study. Ann Intern Med 1988;108:785–790.
17. Centers for Disease Control and Prevention. Identification of HIV-1 group O infection—Los Angeles County, California, 1996. MMWR Morb Mortal Wkly Rep 1996;45:561–564.
18. Proffitt MR, Yen-Lieberman B. Laboratory diagnosis of human immunodeficiency virus infection. Infect Dis Clin North Am 1993;7:203–219.
19. Mylonakis E, Paliou M, Lally M, et al. Laboratory testing for infection with the human immunodeficiency virus: established and novel approaches. Am J Med 2000;109:568–576.
20. Centers for Disease Control and Prevention. Interpretation and use of the Western blot assay for serodiagnosis of human immunodeficiency virus type 1 infections. MMWR Morb Mortal Wkly Rep 1989;38:1–7.
21. Centers for Disease Control and Prevention. Update: serologic testing for HIV-1 antibody—United States, 1988 and 1989. MMWR Morb Mortal Wkly Rep 1990;39:380–383.
22. Celum CL, Coombs RW, Lafferty W, et al. Indeterminate human immunodeficiency virus type 1 Western blots: seroconversion risk, specificity of supplemental tests, and an algorithm for evaluation. J Infect Dis 1991;164:656–664.
23. Busch MP, el Amad Z, McHugh TM, et al. Reliable confirmation and quantification of human immunodeficiency virus type 1 antibody using a recombinant-antigen immunoblot assay. Transfusion 1991;31:129–137.
24. Rich JD, Merriman NA, Mylonakis E, et al. Misdiagnosis of HIV infection by HIV-1 plasma viral load testing: a case series. Ann Intern Med 1999;130:37–39.
25. Havlicheck DH Jr, Hage-Korban E. False-positive HIV diagnosis by HIV-1 plasma viral load testing. Ann Intern Med 1999;131:794.
26. Centers for Disease Control and Prevention. Human Immunodeficiency Virus Type 2. Available at: http://www.cdc.gov/hiv/pubs/facts/hiv2.htm. Accessed August 2, 2005.
27. Sterling TR, Lyles CM, Vlahov D, et al. Sex differences in longitudinal human immunodeficiency type 1 RNA levels among seroconverters. J Infect Dis 1999;180:666–672.

28. Hoen B, Dumon B, Harzic M, et al. Highly active antiretroviral treatment initiated early in the course of symptomatic primary HIV-1 infection: results of the AWRS 053 trial. J Infect Dis 1999;180:1342–1346.
29. Schuman P, Sobel JD, Ohmit SE, et al. Mucosal candidal colonization and candidiasis in women with or at risk for human immunodeficiency virus infection. Clin Infect Dis 1998;27:1161–1167.
30. Long SR, Whitfield MJ, Eades C, et al. Bacillary angiomatosis of the cervix and vulva in a patient with AIDS. Obstet Gynecol 1996;88:709–711.
31. Macasaet MA, Duerr A, Thelmo W, et al. Kaposi sarcoma presenting as a vulvar mass. Obstet Gynecol 1995;86:685–697.
32. Darai E, Vlastos G, Madelenat P. Acquired immunodeficiency syndrome-related Kaposi's sarcoma: two cervical cases. Am J Obstet Gynecol 1995;173:979.
33. Mirmirani P, Hessol NA, Maurer TA, et al. Prevalence and predictors of skin disease in the Women's Interagency HIV Study (WIHS). J Am Acad Dermatol 2001;44:785–788.
34. Kaplan JE, Masur H, Holmes KK, et al. USPHS/IDSA guidelines for the prevention of opportunistic infections in persons infected with human immunodeficiency virus: an overview. Clin Infect Dis 1995;21(suppl 1):S12–S31.
35. Solomon L, Stein M, Flynn C, et al. Health services use by urban women with or at risk for HIV-1 infection: the HIV Epidemiology Research Study (HERS). J Acquir Immune Defic Syndr 1998;17:252–261.
36. Kitihata MM, Koepsell TD, Deyo RD, et al. Physicians' experience with the acquired immunodeficiency syndrome as a factor in patient's survival. N Engl J Med 1996;334:701–706.
37. Gardner LI, Holmberg SD, Moore J, et al. Use of highly active antiretroviral therapy in HIV-infected women: impact of HIV specialist care. J Acquir Immune Defic Syndr 2002;29:69–75.
38. Ickovics JR, Hamburger ME, Vlahov D, et al. Mortality, CD4 cell count decline, and depressive symptoms among HIV-seropositive women: Longitudinal analysis from the HIV epidemiology research study. JAMA 2001;285:1466–1474.
39. Ellerbrock TV, Bush TJ, Chamberland ME, et al. Epidemiology of women with AIDS in the United States 1981–1990: a comparison with heterosexual men with AIDS. JAMA 1991;265:2971–2975.
40. Wyatt GE, Myers HF, Williams JK, et al. Does a history of trauma contribute to HIV risk for women of color? Implications for prevention and policy. Am J Public Health 2002;92:660–665.
41. Centers for Disease Control and Prevention. 1993 Revised classification system for HIV infection and expanded surveillance case definition for AIDS among adolescents and adults. MMWR Morb Mortal Wkly Rep 1993;41:1–47.
42. DeVincenzi I, the European Study Group. A longitudinal study of human immunodeficiency virus transmission by heterosexual partners. N Engl J Med 1994;331:341–346.
43. Peterman TA, Stoneburner RL, Allen JR, et al. Risk of human immunodeficiency virus transmission from heterosexual adults with transfusion-associated infection. JAMA 1988;259:55–58.
44. Henry K. Documented male-to-female transmission of HIV-1 after minimal vaginal exposure in the absence of other cofactors for infection. Minn Med 1991;74:32–34.
45. Quinn TC, Wawer MJ, Sewankambo N, et al. Viral load and heterosexual transmission of human immunodeficiency virus type 1. N Engl J Med 2000;342:921–929.
46. Davis K, Weller SC. The effectiveness of condoms in reducing heterosexual transmission of HIV. Fam Plan Perspec 1999;31:272–279.
47. Laga M, Manoka A, Kivuvu M, et al. Non-ulcerative sexually transmitted diseases as risk factors for HIV-1 transmission in women: results from a cohort study. AIDS 1993;7:95–102.
48. Taha TE, Hoover DR, Dallabeta GA, et al. Bacterial vaginosis and disturbances of vaginal flora: association with increased acquisition of HIV. AIDS 1998;12:1699–1706.
49. Hayes R, Mosha F, Nicoll A, et al. A community trial of the impact of improved sexually transmitted disease treatment on the HIV epidemic in rural Tanzania. AIDS 1995;9:919–926.
50. Mayaud P, Mosha F, Todd J, et al. Improved treatment services significantly reduce the prevalence of sexually transmitted diseases in rural Tanzania: results of a randomized controlled trial. AIDS 1997;11:1873–1880.
51. Yerly S, Vors S, Rizzardi P, et al. Acute HIV infection: impact on the spread of HIV and transmission of drug resistance. AIDS 2001;15:2287–2292.
52. Liuzzi G, Chirianni A, Clementi M, et al. Analysis of HIV-1 load in blood, semen and saliva: evidence for different viral compartments in a cross-sectional and longitudinal study. AIDS 1996;10:F51–F56.
53. Coombs RW, Wright DJ, Reichelderfer PS, et al. Variation of human immunodeficiency virus type 1 viral RNA levels in the female genital tract: implications for applying measurements to individual women. J Infect Dis 2001;184:1187–1191.
54. Kovacs A, Wasserman SS, Burns D, et al. Determinants of HIV-1 shedding in the genital tract of women. Lancet 2001;358:1593–1601.
55. Katz MH, Gerberding JL. The care of persons with recent sexual exposure to HIV. Ann Intern Med 1998;128:306–312.
56. Centers for Disease Control and Prevention. Updated U.S. public health service guidelines for the management of health-care worker exposures to HBV, HCV, and HIV and recommendations for postexposure prophylaxis. MMWR Morb Mortal Wkly Rep 2001;50(RR-11):1–42.
57. Centers for Disease Control and Prevention. Management of possible sexual, injecting-drug-use, or other nonoccupational exposure to HIV, including considerations related to antiretroviral therapy. MMWR Morb Mortal Wkly Rep 1998;47(RR-17):1–14.
58. Centers for Disease Control and Prevention. Sexually transmitted diseases treatment guidelines 2002. MMWR Morb Mortal Wkly Rep 2002;51(RR-6):1–78.

59. Cabral RJ, Galavotti C, Armstrong K, et al. Reproductive and contraceptive attitudes as predictors of condom use among women in an HIV prevention intervention. Women and Health 2001;33:117–132.
60. DiClemente RJ, Wingood GM. A randomized controlled trial of an HIV sexual risk reduction intervention for young African-American women. JAMA 1995;274:1271–1276.
61. Centers for Disease Control and Prevention. Update: barrier protection against HIV infection and other sexually transmitted diseases. MMWR Morb Mortal Wkly Rep 1993;42:589–597.
62. Kell PD, Barton SE. Unrevealing the mysteries of vulval ulceration in human immunodeficiency virus-seropositive women. Am J Obstet Gynecol 1991;164:935–936.
63. Drew WL, Blair M, Miner RC, et al. Evaluation of the virus permeability of a new condom for women. Sex Transm Dis 1990;17:110–112.
64. Roddy RE, Zekeng L, Ryan K, et al. A controlled trial of nonoxynol-9 film to reduce male-to-female transmission of sexually transmitted diseases. N Engl J Med 1998;339:504–510.
65. Stafford MK, Ward H, Flanagan A, et al. Safety study of nonoxynol-9 as a vaginal microbicide: Evidence of adverse effects. J Aquir Immune Defic Syndr Hum Retrovirol 1998;17:327–331.
66. Kreiss J, Ngugi E, Holmes, et al. Efficacy of nonoxynol-9 contraceptive sponge use in preventing heterosexual acquisition of HIV in Nairobi prostitutes. JAMA 1992;268:447–482.
67. Richardson BA, Lavreys, Martin HL, et al. Evaluation of a low-dose nonoxynol-9 gel for the prevention of sexually transmitted diseases. Sex Transm Dis 2001;28:394–400.
68. World Health Organization (WHO) Scientific Working Group on Improving Access to Quality Care in Family Planning. Medical Eligibility Criteria for Initiating and Continuing Use of Contraceptive Methods. Geneva: WHO, 1996.
69. IPPF International Medical Advisory Panel. Statement on contraception for clients who are HIV positive. IPPF Med Bull 1991;25:1–2.
70. Richardson BA, Morrison CS, Sekadde-Kigondu C, et al. Effect of intrauterine device use on cervical shedding of HIV-1 DNA. AIDS 1999;13:2091–2097.
71. European Study Group on Heterosexual Transmission of HIV-1. Comparison of female to male and male to female transmission of HIV-1 in 563 stable couples. BMJ 1992;304:809–813.
72. Kapiga SH, Lyamuya EF, Lwihula GK, et al. The incidence of HIV infection among women using family planning methods in Dar-es-Salaam, Tanzania. AIDS 1998;12;75–84.
73. Morrison CS, Sekadde-Kigondu C, Sinei SK, et al. Is the intrauterine device appropriate contraception for HIV-1 infected women? Br J Obstet Gynaecol 2001;108:784–790.
74. Grossman CJ. Interactions between the gonadal steroids and the immune system. Science 1985;227:257–261.
75. Apr MB, Apr EL. Antigen recognition in the female reproductive tract. I. Update of intraluminal protein traces in the mouse vagina. In: MacDonald TC, Challacombe SJ, Bland PW, et al., eds. Advances in Mucosal Immunology. Norwell, MA: Kluwer Academic, 1990:608–609.
76. Stephenson JM. Systematic review of hormonal contraception and risk of HIV transmission: when to resist meta-analysis. AIDS 1998;12:545–553.
77. Department of Health and Human Services. Guidelines for the Use of Antiretroviral Agents in HIV-infected Adults and Adolescents. February 4, 2002. Available at: http://www.aidsinfo.nih.org. Accessed August 2, 2005.
78. Marx PA, Gettie A, Dailey P, et al. Progesterone implants enhance SIV vaginal transmission and early virus load. Nature Med 1996;2:1084–1089.
79. Martin HL, Nyange PM, Richardson BA, et al. Hormonal contraception, sexually transmitted diseases, and the risk of heterosexual transmission of human immunodeficiency virus type 1. J Infect Dis 1998;178:1053–1059.
80. Ungchusak K, Rehle T, Thammapornpilap P, et al. Determinants of HIV infection among female commercial sex workers in northeastern Thailand: results from a longitudinal study. J Acquir Immune Defic Syndr Hum Retrovirol 1996;12:500–507.
81. Grinspoon S, Corcoran C, Miller K, et al. Body composition and endocrine function in women with AIDS wasting. J Clin Endocrin Metab 1997;82:1332–1337.
82. Shah PN, Smith JR, Wells C, et al. Menstrual symptoms in women infected by the human immunodeficiency virus. Obstet Gynecol 1994;83:397–400.
83. Ellerbrock TV, Wright TC, Bush TJ, et al. Characteristics of menstruation in women infected with human immunodeficiency virus. Obstet Gynecol 1996;87:1030–1034.
84. Chirgwin KD, Feldman J, Muneyyirci-Delale O, et al. Menstrual function in human immunodeficiency virus-infected women without acquired immunodeficiency syndrome. J Acquir Immune Defic Syndr 1996;12:489–494.
85. Harlow SD, Schuman P, Cohen M, et al. Effect of HIV infection on menstrual cycle length. J Acquir Immune Defic Syndr 2000;24:68–75.
86. Kerr-Layton JA, Stamm CA, Peterson LS, et al. Chronic plasma cell endometritis in hysterectomy specimens of HIV-infected women: a retrospective analysis. Infect Dis Obstet Gynecol 1998;6:186–190.
87. Schafer A, Freidmann W, Mielke M, et al. The increased frequency of cervical dysplasia-neoplasia in women infected with the human immunodeficiency virus is related to the degree of immunosuppression. Am J Obstet Gynecol 1991;164:593–599.
88. Ellerbrock TV, Chiasson MA, Bush TJ, et al. Incidence of cervical squamous intraepithelial lesions in HIV-infected women. JAMA 2000;283:1031–1037.
89. Jamieson DJ, Duerr A, Burk R, et al. Characterization of genital human papillomavirus infection in women who have or who are at high risk of having HIV infection. Am J Obstet Gynecol 2002;186:21–27.

90. Mitchell MF, Tortolero-Luna G, Wright T, et al. Cervical human papillomavirus infection and intraepithelial neoplasia: a review. Monogr Natl Cancer Inst 1996;21:17–25.
91. Massad LS, Ahdieh L, Benning L, et al. Evolution of cervical abnormalities among women with HIV-1: evidence from surveillance cytology in the Women's Interagency HIV Study. J Acquir Immune Defic Syndr 2001;27:432–442.
92. Sun XW, Ellerbrock TV, Lungu O, et al. Human papillomavirus infection in human immunodeficiency virus-seropositive women. Obstet Gynecol 1995;85:680–686.
93. Duerr A, Kieke B, Warren D, et al. Human papillomavirus-associated cervical cytologic abnormalities among women with or at risk of infection with human immunodeficiency virus. Obstet Gynecol 2001;184: 584–590.
94. Ahdieh L, Klein RS, Burk R, et al. Prevalence, incidence, and type-specific persistence of human papillomavirus in human immunodeficiency virus (HIV)-positive and HIV-negative women. J Infect Dis 2001;184:682–690.
95. Maiman M, Fruchter RG, Sedis A, et al. Prevalence, risk factors, and accuracy of cytologic screening for cervical intraepithelial neoplasia in women with the human immunodeficiency virus. Gynecol Oncol 1998;68:233–239.
96. Wright TC, Ellerbrock TV, Chiasson MA, et al. Cervical intraepithelial neoplasia in women infected with human immunodeficiency virus: prevalence, risk factors, and validity of Papanicolaou smears. Obstet Gynecol 1994;84:591–597.
97. Korn AP, Autry M, DeRemer PA, et al. Sensitivity of the Papanicolaou smear in human immunodeficiency virus-infected women. Obstet Gynecol 1994;83:401–404.
98. Boardman LA, Peipert JF, Cooper AS, et al. Cytologic-histologic discrepancy in human immunodeficiency virus-positive women referred to a colposcopy clinic. Obstet Gynecol 1994;84:1016–1020.
99. Fahey MI, Irwig L, Macaskill P. Meta-analysis of PAP test accuracy. Am J Epidemiol 1995;141:680–689.
100. Goldie SJ, Weinstein MC, Kuntz KM, et al. The costs, clinical benefits, and cost effectiveness of screening for cervical cancer in HIV-infected women. Ann Intern Med 1999;130:97–107.
101. Wright TC, Moscarelli RD, Dole P, et al. Significance of mild cytologic atypia in women infected with human immunodeficiency virus. Obstet Gynecol 1996;87:515–519.
102. Fruchter RG, Maiman M, Sedlis A, et al. Multiple recurrences of cervical intraepithelial neoplasia in women with the human immunodeficiency virus. Obstet Gynecol 1996;338–344.
103. Cuthill S, Maiman M, Fruchter RG, et al. Complications after treatment of cervical intraepithelial neoplasia in women infected with the human immunodeficiency virus. J Reprod Med 1995;40:823–828.
104. Kurman RJ, Henson DE, Herbst AL, et al. Interim guidelines for management of abnormal cervical cytology. JAMA 1994;271:1866–1869.
105. Balduaf JJ, Dreyfus M, Ritter J, et al. Cytology and colposcopy after loop electrosurgical excision: implications for follow-up. Obstet Gynecol 1998;92:124–130.
106. Tate DR, Anderson RJ. Recrudescence of cervical dysplasia among women who are infected with the human immunodeficiency virus: a case-control analysis. Am J Obstet Gynecol 2002;186:880–882.
107. Maiman M, Watts DH, Anderson J, et al. Vaginal 5-flurouracil for high-grade cervical dysplasia in human immunodeficiency virus infection: a randomized trial. Obstet Gynecol 1999; 94:954–961.
108. Conley LJ, Ellerbrock TV, Bush TJ, et al. HIV-1 infection and risk of vulvovaginal and perianal condylomata and intraepithelial neoplasia: a prospective cohort study. Lancet 2002;359:108–113.
109. Korn AP, Abercrombie PD, Foster A. Vulvar intraepithelial neoplasia in women infected with human immunodeficiency virus. J Reprod Med 1996;61:384–386.
110. Korn AP. Gynecologic care of women infected with HIV. Clin Obstet Gynecol 2001;44:226–242.
111. Chin KM, Sidhu JS, Janssen RS, et al. Invasive cervical cancer in human immunodeficiency virus-infected and uninfected hospital patients. Obstet Gynecol 1998;92:83–87.
112. Cooksley CD, Hwang LY, Waller DK, et al. HIV-related malignancies: community-based study using linkage of cancer registry and HIV registry data. Int J STD AIDS 1999;10:795–802.
113. Fennema J S, van Ameijden EJ, Coutinho RA, et al. HIV, sexually transmitted diseases and gynecologic disorders in women: Increased risk for genital herpes and warts among HIV-infected prostitutes in Amsterdam. AIDS 1995;9:1071–1078.
114. Lindsay MK, Adefris W, Willis S, et al. The risk of sexually transmitted diseases in HIV infected parturients. Am J Obstet Gynecol 1993;169:1031–1035.
115. Clark RA, Brandon W, Dumestre J, et al. Clinical manifestations of infection with human immunodeficiency virus in women in Louisiana. Clin Infect Dis 1993;17:165–172.
116. Cu-Uvin S, Hogan JW, Warren D, et al. Prevalence of lower genital tract infections among human immunodeficiency virus (HIV) seropositive and high-risk HIV seronegative women. Clin Infect Dis 1999;29:1145–1150.
117. Jamieson DJ, Duerr A, Klein RS, et al. Longitudinal analysis of bacterial vaginosis: Findings from the HIV Epidemiology Research Study. Obstet Gynecol 2001; 98:656-663.
118. Wang CC, McClelland RS, Reilly M, et al. The effect of treatment of vaginal infections on shedding of human immunodeficiency virus type 1. J Infect Dis 2001;183:1017–1022.
119. Mostad SB, Overbaugh J, DeVange DM, et al. Hormonal contraception, vitamin A deficiency, and other risk factors for shedding of HIV-1-infected cells from the cervix and vagina. Lancet 1997;350:922–927.
120. McClelland RS, Wang CC, Mandaliya K, et al. Treatment of cervicitis is associated with decreased cervical shedding of HIV-1. AIDS 2001;15:105–110.
121. Carpenter CJ, Mayer KH, Fisher A, et al. Natural history of acquired immunodeficiency syndrome in women in Rhode Island. Am J Med 1989;86:771–775.

122. Rhoads JL, Wright DC, Redfield RR, et al. Chronic vaginal candidiasis in women with human immunodeficiency virus infection. JAMA 1987;257:3105–3107.
123. Duerr A, Sierra MF, Feldman J, et al. Immune compromise and prevalence of *Candida vulvovaginitis* in human immunodeficiency virus-infected women. Obstet Gynecol 1997;90:252–256.
124. Spinillo A, Michelone G, Cavann C, et al. Clinical and microbiological characteristics of symptomatic vulvovaginal candidiasis in HIV seropositive women. Genitourin Med 1994;70:268–272.
125. Schuman P, Capps L, Peng G, et al. Weekly fluconazole for the prevention of mucosal candidiasis in women with HIV infection. Ann Intern Med 1997;126:689–696.
126. Sobel JD. Gynecologic infections in human immunodeficiency virus-infected women. Clin Infect Dis 2000;31:1225–1233.
127. Sobel JD, Faro S, Force RW, et al. Vulvovaginal candidiasis: epidemiologic, diagnostic, and therapeutic considerations. Am J Obstet Gynecol 1998;178:203–211.
128. Prutting SM, Cerveny JD. Boric acid vaginal suppositories: a brief review. Infect Dis Obstet Gynecol 1998;6:191–194.
129. Blocker ME, Levine WC, St. Louis ME. HIV prevalence in patients with syphilis, in the United States. Sex Transm Dis 2000;27:53–59.
130. Greenblatt RM, Bacchetti P, Barken S, et al. Lower genital tract infections among HIV-infected and high risk uninfected women: findings of the Women's Interagency HIV Study (WIHS). Sex Transm Dis 1999;26:143–151.
131. Augenbraun M, Rolfs R, Johnson R, et al. Treponemal specific tests for the serodiagnosis of syphilis. Sex Transm Dis 1998;25:549–552.
132. Rolfs RT, Joesoef MR, Hendershot EF, et al. A randomized trial of enhanced therapy for early syphilis in patients with and without human immunodeficiency virus infection. N Engl J Med 1997;337:307–314.
133. Rompalo AM, Joesoef MR, O'Donnell JA, et al. Clinical manifestations of early syphilis by HIV status and gender: Results of the syphilis and HIV study. Sex Transm Dis 2001;28:158–165.
134. Musher DM, Hamill RJ, Baughn RE. Effect of human immunodeficiency virus (HIV) infection on the course of syphilis and on the response to treatment. Ann Intern Med 1990;113:872–881.
135. Fiumara N. Treatment of primary and secondary syphilis. JAMA 1980;243:2500–2502.
136. Safrin S, Dattel BJ, Hauer L, et al. Seroprevalence and epidemiologic correlates of human immunodeficiency virus infection in women with acute pelvic inflammatory disease. Obstset Gynecol 1990;75:666–670.
137. Sperling RS, Friedman F, Joyner M, et al. Seroprevalence of human immunodeficiency virus in women admitted to the hospital with pelvic inflammatory disease. J Reprod Med 1991;36:122–124.
138. Hoegsberg B, Abulafia O, Sedlis A, et al. Sexually transmitted disease and human immunodeficiency virus infection among women with pelvic inflammatory disease. Am J Obstet Gynecol 1990;163:1135–1139.
139. Barbosa C, Macasaet M, Brockmann S, et al. Pelvic inflammatory disease and human immunodeficiency virus infection. Obstet Gynecol 1997;89:65–70.
140. Korn AP, Landers DV, Green JR, et al. Pelvic inflammatory disease in human immunodeficiency virus-infected women. Obstet Gynecol 1993;82:756–758.
141. Kamenga MC, DeCock KM, St. Louis ME, et al. The impact of human immunodeficiency virus infection on pelvic inflammatory disease: a case-control study in Abidjan, Ivory Coast. Am J Obstet Gynecol 1995;172:919–925.
142. Cohen CR, Sinei S, Reilly M, et al. Effect of immunodeficiency virus type 1 infection upon acute salpingitis: a laparoscopic study. J Infect Dis 1998;178:1352–1358.
143. Irwin KL, Moorman AC, O'Sullivan MJ, et al. Influence of human immunodeficiency virus infection on pelvic inflammatory disease. Obstet Gynecol 2000;95:525–534.
144. Bukusi EA, Cohen CR, Stevens CE, et al. Effects of human immunodeficiency virus 1 infection on microbial origins of pelvic inflammatory disease and on efficacy of ambulatory oral therapy. Am J Obstet Gynecol 1999;181:1374–1381.
145. Wald A, Link K. Risk of human immunodeficiency virus infection in herpes simplex virus type 2-seropositive persons: a meta-analysis. J Infect Dis 2002;185:45–52.
146. Augenbraun M, Feldman J, Chirgwin K, et al. Increased genital shedding of herpes simplex virus type 2 in HIV-seropositive women. Ann Intern Med 1995;123:845–847.
147. Mostad SB, Kreiss JK, Ryncarz AJ, et al. Cervical shedding of herpes simplex virus and cytomegalovirus throughout the menstrual cycle in women infected with human immunodeficiency virus type 1. Am J Obstet Gynecol 2000;183:948–955.
148. Mostad SB, Kreiss JK, Ryncarz AJ, et al. Cervical shedding of herpes simplex virus in human immunodeficiency virus-infected women: effects of hormonal contraception, pregnancy, and vitamin A deficiency. J Infect Dis 2000;181:58–63.
149. Golden MP, Sunyoung K, Hammer HM, et al. Activation of human immunodeficiency virus by herpes simplex virus. J Infect Dis 1992;166:494–499.
150. Mole L, Ripich S, Margolis D, et al. The impact of active herpes simplex virus infection on human immunodeficiency virus load. J Infect Dis 1997;176:766–770.
151. Stewart JA, Reef SE, Pellett PE et al. Herpesvirus infections in persons infected with human immunodeficiency virus. Clin Infect Dis 1995;21(suppl 1):S114–S120.
152. Lalezari J, Schacker T, Feinberg J, et al. A randomized, double blind, placebo-controlled trial of cidofovir gel for the treatment of acyclovir-unresponsive mucocutaneous herpes simplex virus infection in patients with AIDS. J Infect Dis 1997;176:892–898.

153. Anderson J, Clark RA, Watts DH, et al. Idiopathic genital ulcers in women infected with human immunodeficiency virus. J Aquir Immune Defic Syndr Hum Retrovirol 1996;13:343–347.
154. LaGuardia KD, White MH, Saigo PE, et al. Genital ulcer disease in women infected with human immunodeficiency virus. Am J Obstet Gynecol 1995;172:553–562.
155. Schuman P, Christensen C, Sobel J. Aphthous vaginal ulceration in two women with acquired immunodeficiency syndrome. Am J Obstet Gynecol 1996;174:1660–1663.
156. Covino JM, McCormack WM. Vulvar ulceration of unknown etiology in a human immunodeficiency virus-infected woman: response to treatment with zidovudine. Am J Obstet Gynecol 1990;163:116–118.
157. Jacobson JM, Greenspan JS, Spritzer J, et al. Thalidomide for the treatment of oral aphthous ulcers in patients with human immunodeficiency virus infection. N Engl J Med 1997;336:1487–1493.
158. Saracco A, Musicco M, Nicolosi A, et al. Man to woman sexual transmission of HIV: a longitudinal study of 343 steady partners of infected men. J Acquir Immune Defic Syndr 1993;6:497–502.
159. Mastro TD, DeVincenzi I. Probabilities of sexual HIV transmission. AIDS 1996;10(suppl A):575–582.
160. Semprini AE, Levi-Setti P, Bozzo M, et al. Insemination of HIV-negative women with processed semen of HIV-positive partners. Lancet 1992;340:1317–1319.
161. Semprini AE. Viral transmission in ART: risks for patients and healthcare providers. Hum Reprod 2000;15:69.
162. Centers for Disease Control and Prevention. HIV-1 infection and artificial insemination with processed semen. MMWR Morb Mortal Wkly Rep 1990;39:249–256.
163. American Society for Reproductive Medicine. Guidelines for therapeutic insemination of sperm. Fertil Steril 1993;59(suppl 1):1S–4S.
164. Nuovo GJ, Becker J, Simsir A, et al. HIV nucleic acid localize to the spermatogonia and their progeny. A study by polymerase chain reaction in situ hybridization. Am J Pathol 1994;144:1142–1148.
165. Quale AJ, Xu C, Mayer KH, et al. T lymphocytes and macrophages, but not motile spermatozoa are a significant source of human immunodeficiency virus in semen. J Infect Dis 1997;176:960–968.
166. Kim LU, Johnson MR, Barton S, et al. Evaluation of sperm washing as a potential method of reducing HIV transmission in HIV-discordant couples wishing to have children. AIDS 1999;13:645–651.
167. Sauer M, Chang P. Establishing a clinical program for human immunodeficiency virus 1-seropositive men to father seronegative children by means of in vitro fertilization with intracytoplasmic sperm injection. Am J Obstet Gynecol 2002;186:627–633.
168. American College of Obstetricians and Gynecologist Technical Bulletin. Preconceptual Care. No. 205. May 1995.
169. Public Health Service Task Force. Recommendations for the Use of Antiretroviral Drugs in Pregnant HIV-1 Infected Women for Maternal Health and Interventions to Reduce Perinatal Transmission in the United States. February 4, 2002. Available at: http://www.aidsinfo.nih.gov. Accessed August 2, 2005.
170. Mofenson L. Epidemiology and determinants of vertical transmission. Semin Pediatr Infect Dis 1994;5:252–265.
171. Conner EM, Sperling RS, Gelber R, et al. Reduction of maternal-infant transmission of human immunodeficiency virus type 1 with zidovudine treatment. N Engl J Med 1994;331:1173–1180.
172. Van Dyke RB, Korber BT, Popek E, et al. The Ariel Project: a prospective cohort study of maternal-child transmission of human immunodeficiency virus type 1 in the era of maternal antiretroviral therapy. J Infect Dis 1999;179:319–328.
173. Fundaro C, Genovese O, Rendeli C, et al. Myelomeningocele in a child with intrauterine exposure to efavirenz. AIDS 2002;16:299–301.
174. Milunsky A, Jick H, Jick SS, et al. Multivitamin/folic acid supplementation in early pregnancy reduces the prevalence of neural tube defects. JAMA 1989;262:2847–2852.
175. Czeizel AE, Dudas I. Prevention of the first occurrence of neural tube defects by preconceptual vitamin supplementation. N Engl J Med 1992;327:1832–1835.
176. Stein MD, Rosene KA. Clues to enhancing the identification of human immunodeficiency virus-infected women. Obstet Gynecol 1992;80:317–320.
177. World Health Organization. The current global situation of the HIV/AIDS pandemic. Wkly Epidemiol Rec 1995;27:193–196.
178. 2001 USPHS/IDSA Guidelines for the Prevention of Opportunistic Infections in Persons Infected With Human Immunodeficiency Virus. November 28, 2001. Available at: http://www.aidsinfo.nih.gov. Accessed August 2, 2005.
179. Royce RA, Sena A, Cates W, et al. Sexual transmission of HIV. N Engl J Med 1997;336:1072–1078.
180. Plummer FA, Simonsen JN, Cameron DW, et al. Cofactors in male–female sexual transmission of human immunodeficiency virus type 1. J Infect Dis 1991;163:233–239.

CHAPTER 25

Diagnosis and Management of Hereditary Cancer

Monique A. Spillman and Andrew Berchuck

Most cancers arise due to accumulation of genetic alterations in critical genes over the course of a lifetime. In contrast to "sporadic" cancers, in which all mutations are acquired, hereditary cancers arise in individuals who have inherited a mutation in a cancer-causing gene. These individuals generally develop cancer at a younger age than sporadic cases and often develop multiple primary cancers. Several hereditary cancer syndromes have been identified and are characterized by clustering of specific types of cancers within families. Since the mid-1990s, many of the genes responsible for hereditary cancer syndromes have been identified, and this has facilitated genetic testing and clinical interventions aimed at decreasing cancer mortality. This chapter summarizes progress to date in the diagnosis and management of hereditary cancer syndromes.

It was previously understood that cancer arises due to genetic alterations, and some families were described as being "full of cancer." For example, a grandmother might have had breast cancer, a mother had ovarian cancer, and two sisters had breast cancer. In other families, every generation was observed to have had at least one case of colon cancer that arose at surprisingly young ages. Individuals in these families believed they were predestined to get cancer. The first description in the medical literature of such a "cancer family" was by Warthin in 1913, when he described "family G" in which there were many cases of gastrointestinal and uterine cancer (1). He followed this family for many years and found that 17 of the 48 descendants died of cancer or had been operated on for cancer (2).

Subsequently, numerous other large families in which cancer is extremely common have been reported (3). For many years, we were unable to explain this phenomenon. It was believed that perhaps some dietary or environmental carcinogen might be at fault. Although substances in the environment, hormones, and individual behaviors play a role in the genesis of many cancers, in the past decade a hereditary basis has been found for most familial cancers. Malignancies of the colon, breast, and ovary are the most common hereditary cancers in women, and approximately 10% of these cancers have a hereditary basis (4–8). The identification of autosomal dominant cancer susceptibility genes represents a milestone in the management of hereditary cancer syndromes. With the availability of genetic testing, cancer prevention and early detection efforts can be focused on mutation carriers, whereas noncarriers in these families can be reassured they are not at greater risk than the general population. The ability to reassure families with negative tests is limited somewhat by the possible existence of other as yet undiscovered genes.

BASIC CANCER GENETICS

Cancer is a disease in which there is loss of growth regulatory control. Normal cellular proliferation is regulated by complex molecular pathways that contain numerous checks and balances. The proteins that comprise these pathways are encoded by genes within the cellular DNA. Oncogenes encode proteins that stimulate proliferation, whereas tumor suppressor genes encode proteins that inhibit proliferation. In each organ, there is a carefully programmed balance between these opposing classes of gene products. In some organs, such as the bone marrow, the genetic program allows for constant proliferation, whereas in others, such as the brain, proliferation rarely occurs. In addition, these same genes are involved in regulating differentiation and apoptosis (programmed cell death), which are processes that also serve to control the population of cells within an organ.

Alterations in the genes that control cellular growth can cause malignant transformation. Oncogenes can be activated by several mechanisms. In some types of cancers, activation occurs by amplification of oncogenes (e.g., c-*myc,* HER-2/*neu*). Instead of 2 copies of one of these growth stimulatory genes, there may be as many as 40 copies. Some oncogenes may become overactive if affected by point mutations (e.g., K-*ras*). Finally, oncogenes may be translocated from one chromosomal location to another, and they may come under the influence of promoter sequences that cause overexpression of the gene (e.g., *abl).*

Loss of tumor suppressor gene function can also result in overactive proliferation and outgrowth of a tumor. This usually involves a two-step process in which both copies of a given tumor suppressor gene are inactivated. In most cases, mutation of one copy of a tumor suppressor gene occurs, along with complete loss of the other copy of the gene due to deletion of a large segment of the chromosome where the gene resides.

DNA repair genes play an important role in preventing the development of human cancers. Each time a cell divides, the DNA is copied so both cells will receive a complete set of the

TABLE 25.1

Hereditary Cancer Syndromes

Syndrome	Gene	Chromosome	Predominant Cancers
Familial breast/ovarian cancer	BRCA1	17q21	Breast, ovary
	BRCA2	13q12	Breast, ovary
	CHEK2	22q12.1	Breast
Ataxia-telangiectasia	AT	11q22	Breast
Hereditary nonpolyposis colon cancer	MSH2	2p16	Colon, endometrium, ovary and others
	MLH1	3p21	
	PMS1	2q31	
	PMS2	7p22	
	MSH6	2p16	
Familial adenomatous polyposis coli	APC	5q21	Colonic polyps, cancer
Li-Fraumeni syndrome	p53	17p13	Sarcomas, leukemias, breast, brain, and others
Wilms' tumor	WT1	11p13	Kidney
von Hippel-Lindau	VHL	3p25	Kidney and others
Neurofibromatosis	NF1	17q11	Neurofibromas
	NF2	22q12	Neurofibromas
Retinoblastoma	Rb	13q14	Retinoblastoma sarcomas
Familial melanoma	MLM	1p36	Melanoma
	CDKN2 (p16)	9p21	
Multiple-endocrine neoplasia			
Type 1	MEN1	11q13	Thyroid, adrenal, pancreas, pituitary, parathyroid
Type 2	ret	10q11	Thyroid, adrenal, parathyroid
Hereditary papillary renal carcinoma	met	7q31	Papillary kidney

genetic code. Although DNA synthesis occurs with high fidelity, it is estimated that spontaneous errors (mutations) occur about once every million bases. In nondividing cells, mutations may arise due to endogenous processes such as DNA methylation and deamination. The cellular DNA repair systems are able to fix much of this genetic damage, but some mutations elude this surveillance system. In general, cancer occurs only after damage to several growth regulatory oncogenes and tumor suppressor genes. The rate at which critical mutations occur in cells may be accelerated if the DNA repair genes themselves have undergone inactivating mutations.

Hereditary cancers arise due to inherited mutations in tumor suppressor genes, DNA repair genes, and oncogenes (Table 25.1). Persons who inherit a mutation in a cancer gene have a strikingly increased lifetime risk of developing one or more cancers. These cancers often develop at a younger age than would be expected. Cancers in young children, such as retinoblastoma and Wilms' tumor, often result from inherited mutations in tumor suppressor genes. Although carriers have the mutation in every cell of their body, most cells do not undergo malignant transformation.

PRINCIPLES OF CANCER GENETIC COUNSELING

Obtaining a thorough cancer history from the patient and/or the family is a vital first step in caring for families with hereditary cancer. The seemingly simple act of gathering information forms the foundation on which the rest of the process is based. The importance of careful documentation of family history, including review of clinical materials from other cancer cases in the family, has been stressed for many years by Dr. Henry T. Lynch, one of the pioneers of hereditary cancer genetics. His own compulsively assembled pedigrees allowed him to define two familial cancer syndromes: Lynch I (colon cancer), and Lynch II (colon cancer and other cancers).

A complete family cancer history should begin by ascertaining cancer information of all first-degree relatives, including mother, father, siblings, and children. Data on second-degree relatives, including grandparents, aunts, and uncles, should also be obtained from *both* maternal and paternal sides. Family members without cancer should be included because their unaffected status can provide clues to the inheritance pattern. A family cancer history should ideally be obtained from more than one individual in families where there is a suspicion of a hereditary syndrome (9). This information can be depicted diagrammatically in a pedigree (Fig. 25.1). To

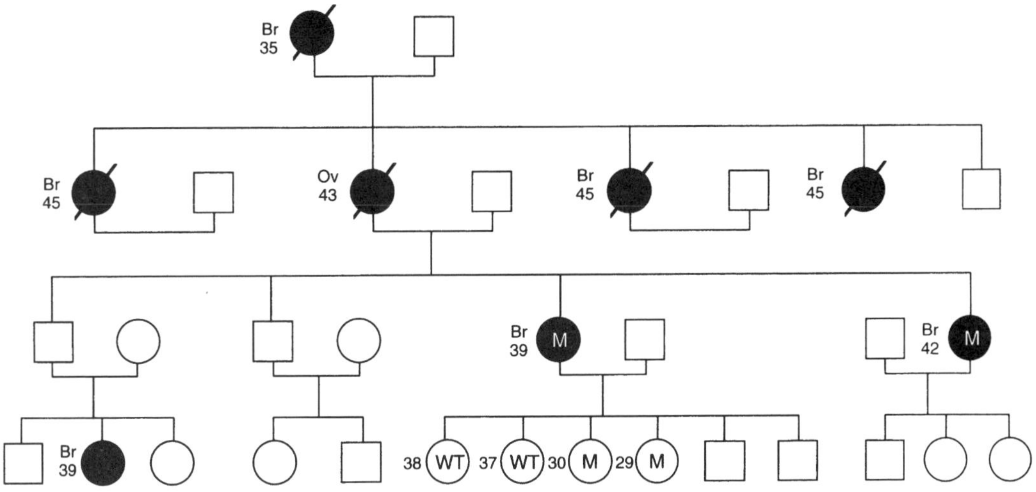

FIGURE 25.1 ● Familial ovarian cancer pedigree with BRCA1 mutation. The ages of family members and types of cancer are noted. Slashes denote individuals who have died of cancer. Individuals denoted M have the 5382insC mutation in BRCA1, whereas individuals denoted WT have normal BRCA1. □, males; ○, females; ■, affected males; ●, affected females.

TABLE 25.2

Ashkenazi Jewish Cancer Susceptibility Mutations

Breast/Ovarian Cancer	
BRCA1 185delAG	1.0%
BRCA1 5382insC	0.1%
BRCA2 6174delT	1.4%
Total	**2.5%**
Colorectal Cancer	
APC 1307 T>A	6.1%

make a pedigree as accurate as possible, cancer diagnoses should be confirmed when possible by review of pathologic specimens or medical records.

Pedigrees concisely convey a large amount of information, including the presenting cancer case (proband), others with cancer, cancer decedents, and potential mutation carriers. Important additional information recorded includes the age of onset of cancers, second cancers, bilaterally of a cancer, stage of the cancer, and metastatic location. In addition, cancer histology, age of unaffected individuals, exposure to carcinogenic agents, suspected extended family history of cancers, and the pattern of cancer occurrence among generations is recorded (10). Male breast cancer cases are likely to harbor an inherited BRCA2 mutation and should be specifically included in the assembled pedigree (11, 12). The ratio of female-to-male births in an affected family may also provide important information about the hereditary gene (13).

A known genetic disorder in the family should be prominently noted because some syndromes also predispose individuals to cancers (e.g., Fanconi's anemia, xeroderma pigmentosa, Bloom's syndrome, ataxia-telangiectasia). An ethnic history should also be elucidated, especially for patients of Ashkenazi (Eastern European) Jewish heritage. Specific mutations, called founder mutations, can segregate in closely related members of ethnic groups (14). The most common founder mutations described thus far are the BRCA1 185delAG and BRCA2 6174delT mutations, which occur in about 1.0% and 1.4% of Ashkenazi Jews, respectively (15, 16). A third less common founder mutation (BRCA1 5382insC) has been noted in Ashkenazi populations (Table 25.2). One Israeli study found that about half of women with ovarian cancer and one-third of women with breast cancer had one of the three Ashkenazi founder mutations (17).

Finally, a complete history of potential modifying factors should be obtained, including hormone use, birth control pill use, menopausal status, diet, parity, breast-feeding history, and concomitant medical conditions (Table 25.3).

TABLE 25.3

Assessment of Hereditary Cancer Risk

Obtain personal and family history of cancer
Confirm precise cancer diagnosis in affected individuals
Estimate risk of hereditary cancer syndrome
Education and informed consent
Genetic testing
Posttest counseling and follow-up

Once a family is suspected of having a hereditary cancer syndrome, genetic counselors who are specially trained in patient education should be involved in all phases of the genetic testing process (18). Extensive nondirective counseling and education is essential prior to genetic testing. Individuals should understand the risk of testing positive, potential benefits of the test, and the social and psychological implications of testing. Testing should be offered to both women and men in a high-risk family (19, 20). Approximately three-fourths of candidates who seek genetic counseling elect to undergo cancer genetic testing. If possible, a family member who has already had cancer should be tested first. If a mutation is found in an affected individual, this greatly facilitates testing of other family members for this specific mutation.

Test results should be conveyed in a setting that includes multidisciplinary input from genetic counselors, oncologists, and others. Additional psychological support and encouragement is also offered at this juncture. Negative test results can produce survivor guilt. The lifetime cancer risk for mutation carriers, as well as the options for prevention, should be reviewed.

Some families with a strong cancer history do not carry a mutation in a known susceptibility gene. Referral of these families to institutions with expertise in cancer genetics will assist in the identification of other cancer-causing genes. In the meantime, clinical decisions in such families are made on a case-by-case basis. In some cases, preventive strategies, including surgical prophylaxis, may be warranted even when genetic testing does not reveal an alteration in a known cancer susceptibility gene.

HEREDITARY OVARIAN AND BREAST CANCER GENETICS

Autosomal dominant hereditary syndromes account for 5–7% of breast cancers and 10% of ovarian cancers. Germline mutations in BRCA1 and BRCA2 account for the vast majority of hereditary ovarian cancer cases and at least half of hereditary breast cancers. Population-based studies have demonstrated that BRCA mutations are rare in the non-Ashkenazi general population, affecting approximately 1 in 300 to 1 in 800 individuals (14). In the Ashkenazi Jewish population, it is estimated at 2%.

BRCA1

The BRCA1 gene on chromosome 17q21 encodes a protein of 1863 amino acids that plays a role in repair of double-stranded DNA breaks. Loss of BRCA1 function initiates the development of other genetic alterations that eventually lead to clinically recognizable cancer. Mutations in BRCA1 are 1.5 to 2 times more common than BRCA2 mutations, except in Iceland where BRCA2 mutations predominate. Initial lifetime risk estimates of breast cancer were approximately 80 to 90% in large BRCA1 pedigrees, whereas the estimated risk of ovarian cancer was 30 to 60% (21). Initial estimates of the fraction of BRCA1-associated cancers and the cumulative lifetime risks may have been too high due to ascertainment bias in large extended cancer families (22–25). The lifetime risk of ovarian cancer in BRCA1 carriers is now believed to be 20 to 30% (6, 7, 26, 27). The lifetime risk of breast cancer by age 70 is now believed to be 65% (27).

Increased breast cancer risk begins earlier than risk for ovarian cancer (28). Carriers have an increased breast cancer risk in their twenties, whereas their ovarian cancer risk does not rise appreciably until the mid-thirties. In addition to a primary breast cancer, BRCA1 mutation carriers are at 40.5% risk of developing a second primary breast cancer by the age of 70 (11).

Various BRCA1 mutations may differ in the extent to which they predispose to breast or ovarian cancer. Mutations in the carboxy terminus of the gene may result in a higher frequency of breast cancer relative to ovarian cancer (29, 30). Conversely, ovarian cancer seems to be associated with mutations in the proximal amino terminus. However, not all studies have confirmed these findings. Differences in penetrance have also been noted among families with identical BRCA1 mutations. Two hypotheses, both of which may be relevant, have been proposed to explain variable penetrance. First, other genes may modify the penetrance of BRCA1. Alternatively, it is possible that gene–environment interactions may modify risk. For example, pregnancy and oral contraceptive pill use decrease the risk of ovarian cancer in the general population. Reproductive risk factors that affect breast and ovarian cancer incidence in the general population may also modify risk in BRCA1 carriers. For example, oral contraceptives may reduce ovarian cancer risk by at least 50% in women with hereditary ovarian cancer syndromes (31).

BRCA1 mutation carriers face a three- to four-fold higher risk of prostate, colon, pancreatic, and stomach cancers (11, 28). A more recent study of Ashkenazi Jewish carriers confirmed the increased risk of prostate cancer, but colon cancer risk was not increased (11, 26). BRCA1 mutation carriers face a significantly increased risk of fallopian tube cancer and primary peritoneal cancer (11, 32–35).

BRCA1-associated breast cancers have been characterized by higher-grade, medullary features, aneuploidy, and high proliferation index relative to sporadic breast cancers (36–38). Rare basal epithelial breast cancers are likely to occur in BRCA mutation carriers (39). Despite these poor prognostic features, BRCA1-associated breast cancers presented at lower stage and had relatively favorable outcome in one study (38). Chemotherapy in addition to conservative surgery for breast cancer increased the survival of Ashkenazi women with BRCA mutations (40).

The histologic features of ovarian cancers in BRCA1 carriers do not differ strikingly from sporadic cancers. Most cases are advanced stage, moderate to poorly differentiated serous cancers, but survival of BRCA1 carriers with ovarian cancer was longer than sporadic cases matched for age, stage, and other prognostic factors (41–44). The improved survival in BRCA1-associated ovarian cancer may be due to a better response to platinum-based chemotherapy (45).

BRCA2

A significant fraction of breast cancer families that do not have BRCA1 mutations were found to be linked to chromosome 13q12 in 1994 (46). In 1995, this second breast cancer susceptibility gene (BRCA2) was identified (47). Notable attributes of BRCA2 families include early age of onset and the occurrence of male breast cancer (48, 49). Ovarian cancer is a less prominent feature of these families, and there are about ten female breast cancer cases and one male breast cancer case for each ovarian cancer case in BRCA2 families. Fallopian tube cancer risk is also increased (32, 34).

BRCA2 is considered to be responsible for a similar proportion of hereditary breast cancer as BRCA1 (4 to 5%), and studies indicate that mutations in BRCA2 confer a similar lifetime risk of female breast cancer as for BRCA1. As noted for BRCA1, earlier initial penetrance estimates that were much higher may have been artifactually high due to ascertainment bias (24, 25). The current estimated BRCA2 lifetime risk of ovarian cancer is between 10 and 20% (6, 7, 26, 34). Ovarian cancer is most often observed in families with mutations in the large exon 11 (50).

Similar to BRCA1, the BRCA2 gene appears to play a role in DNA repair (51). BRCA2 is now known to be identical with a gene for Fanconi's anemia (52). The clinicopathologic characteristics of BRCA2-associated breast cancers appear similar to sporadic cases, but BRCA2-associated cases are less often tubular and are of higher grade (36). Carriers of the BRCA2 mutations are also at increased risk of other cancers, including prostate, laryngeal, and pancreatic cancer.

Genetic Testing for Hereditary Ovarian and Breast Cancer

Mutations have been observed throughout the large BRCA1 and 2 genes, and approximately 80 to 90% of the mutations predict truncated protein products (53–55). Missense mutations alter a single amino acid in a full-length protein product and occur in about 10 to 15% of hereditary cases (54, 55). Alteration of a single amino acid may create a disease-causing mutation or may not affect gene function (56). Segregation of a missense mutation with breast and ovarian cancer in a family suggests, but does not prove, its significance. Because mutations in BRCA1 and BRCA 2 occur throughout these large genes, the most reliable method of detecting mutations is to sequence the entire coding region, including intronic splice sites. The sensitivity of DNA sequencing for detecting mutations is excellent and the false-negative rate is estimated to be very low. Reliance on methods other than DNA sequencing probably lowers sensitivity for detecting mutations to about 70 to 90%. Although automated DNA sequencing is labor intensive and expensive, it remains the gold standard for mutational testing.

Although mutations in BRCA1 and BRCA2 have been noted in some women in the absence of a family history of breast or ovarian cancer, the incidence is low and cost considerations

TABLE 25.4

Clinical Characteristics of BRCA1 and BRCA2 Carriers

Primary Risk Factors
Two or more first-degree relatives with breast or ovarian cancer
Early onset of breast cancer (20–40 years old)
Early onset of ovarian cancer (30–50 years old)
Male breast cancer (BRCA2 only)
Ashkenazi Jewish heritage
Associated Cancers
Prostate cancer (BRCA1 only)
Colon cancer (BRCA1 only)
Pancreatic cancer (BRCA2 only)

prohibit BRCA mutational screening in the general population. A postmenopausal woman with breast or ovarian cancer who does not have a family history of ovarian or breast cancer has a 3% risk of carrying a mutation. At the other extreme, in families with two cases of breast cancer and two cases of ovarian cancer, the probability of finding a mutation may be as high as 80 to 90% (30). Those who believe it is reasonable to test "high-risk" individuals generally advocate testing when the family history suggests at least a 5 to 10% probability of finding a mutation. In practical terms, this translates into two first-degree relatives with either ovarian cancer at any age, breast cancer prior to age 50, and those in a high-risk ethnic group, such as the Ashkenazi Jewish population (Table 25.4). Within the Ashkenazi population, 1 in 40 individuals carry one of three germline BRCA1 or BRCA2 mutations (6–8, 14, 57).

It is preferable to test affected individuals in a "high-risk" family first because a negative test in an unaffected individual may reflect failure to inherit the mutant allele, even though others in the family carry a mutation. Another option is to retrieve tissue blocks from deceased individuals from which DNA can be extracted and analyzed for a mutation. Once a specific mutation is identified in an affected individual, other family members can be tested faster and less inexpensively because the analysis is focused on one mutation.

Confidentiality remains a critical issue in cancer susceptibility testing. Misuse of genetic information potentially could have devastating consequences, including difficulty in securing employment and life, health, or disability insurance (58). Most individuals ask their insurance company to pay for BRCA1/2 testing and are willing to have this information recorded in their medical records. Strong state and federal statutes have been enacted to protect the confidentiality of genetic testing information and enact penalties for genetic discrimination. In view of this, results of pedigree analysis and genetic testing should be entered into the medical record.

Hereditary Ovarian Cancer Surveillance and Treatment

With the discovery of BRCA1 and BRCA2, only a minority of cases of familial ovarian cancer should have to be managed as we have in the past by simply recommending prophylactic oophorectomy on the basis of a strong family history (59–61). Although the penetrance of various mutations is still somewhat uncertain, it is clear that carriers have a strikingly increased risk of ovarian cancer relative to the general population (29, 50, 62).

Patients who desired continued fertility may be offered surveillance options such as annual screening with CA 125 and/or ultrasound (Table 25.5). Such a conservative approach is reasonable, but lacks proven efficacy in women during the reproductive years. The National Cancer

TABLE 25.5

Management Options for BRCA1/BRCA2 Carriers

Ovaries
Oral contraceptive pill until childbearing complete
Breast-feeding
Prophylactic oophorectomy after childbearing
Annual transvaginal ultrasound, CA-125 level, and physical/pelvic examination in individuals choosing not to have oophorectomy or in untested high-risk individuals
Breasts
Prophylactic bilateral total mastectomy, including tissue under the nipple
Biannual mammography, clinical examination and monthly self-breast exam in individuals choosing not to undergo mastectomy or untested high-risk individuals beginning at age 25

Institute (NCI) Cancer Genetics Network is currently sponsoring a pilot study of these screening modalities in high-risk women.

Another ovarian cancer risk reducing strategy for BRCA mutation carriers may be the use of oral contraceptives, which decrease the risk of ovarian cancer in the general population by as much as 80%. Oral contraceptives might be a particularly attractive alternative for young women who have not yet completed childbearing, and limited data indicate that BRCA mutation carriers may benefit from oral contraceptive use (31, 63). However, another study found no benefit of oral contraceptive use for reducing ovarian cancer risk (64).

Prophylactic Bilateral Oophorectomy

Fortunately, the incidence of ovarian cancer in carriers does not begin to rise appreciably until the late thirties when many women have completed their family (28). Prophylactic oophorectomy after completion of childbearing represents a rational approach to decreasing ovarian cancer mortality in mutation carriers. Surveys show that 75% of high-risk women undergoing BRCA testing would consider prophylactic oophorectomy (65).

Prophylactic oophorectomy is an attractive option in mutation carriers for several reasons (Table 25.6). First, this procedure can now be performed laparoscopically in an outpatient setting, and the costs will generally be covered by medical insurance for BRCA mutation carriers (66). Prophylactic oophorectomy causes only modest changes in body image and self-esteem, and is not viewed as cosmetically mutilating by most women. In addition, there is now strong evidence that prophylactic bilateral salpingo-oophorectomy (BSO) provides strong protection against both ovarian cancer and breast cancer. In one more recent study, the risk of breast and ovarian cancer was decreased 75% (67). Another large multicenter study followed women for a mean of 8.8 years after prophylactic BSO and concluded that the procedure reduced the risk of epithelial ovarian cancer by 96% compared with nonovariectomized controls (68). Prophylactic BSO reduced the risk of ovarian, primary peritoneal, and fallopian tube cancers by 98% in a study of 248 cases and 245 controls, all of whom were BRCA mutation carriers (69).

Four areas require particular attention when performing a prophylactic BSO in a known BRCA carrier. First, all ovarian tissue must be removed. This is particularly important in cases where scar tissue or endometriosis has encapsulated the ovary. Dense adhesions may require a conversion to a laparotomy to ensure complete removal of both ovaries.

Second, it is critical that the surgical pathologist be notified that a prophylactic oophorectomy specimen is from a BRCA mutation carrier. The specimen should be serially sectioned through *both* the ovaries and the fallopian tubes. In one series of prophylactic BSO samples, 12% contained occult cancers (70, 71). The emphasis should be on the identification of cancerous

TABLE 25.6

Pros and Cons of Prophylactic Salpingo-Oophorectomy

Pros
Decreases ovarian and fallopian tube cancer incidence and mortality
Can be delayed to allow completion of childbearing
Laparoscopic approach possible in most cases
Impact on body image generally acceptable
Estrogen replacement can prevent consequences of surgical menopause
Decreases breast cancer risk
Cons
Cost
Potential morbidity and mortality
Small but residual potential for subsequent primary peritoneal carcinoma
Surgical menopause in premenopausal patients who elect not to take hormone replacement

tissue within the specimen because no significant premalignant features have been identified consistently in normal ovaries from BRCA mutation carriers (72, 73).

Third, malignant cells have also been found in pelvic washings performed at the time of prophylactic BSO (74). In one study, pelvic washings were positive for malignant cells in women with occult fallopian tube cancers (75). Based on these findings, obtaining pelvic washings during the initial laparoscopic survey of the pelvis is a critical addition to prophylactic laparoscopic BSO.

Finally, due to the increased risk of fallopian tube cancers in BRCA mutation carriers, it is important for as much of the fallopian tube as possible to be removed (11, 32, 33, 68). A concomitant hysterectomy ensures resection of the cornual portion of the tube, but may not be desired by the patient or feasible by a completely laparoscopic approach (75).

Postoophorectomy Treatment and Surveillance

In premenopausal women without a personal history of breast cancer, the risk and benefits of estrogen replacement should be discussed with the patient as a method to avoid the deleterious side effects of surgical premature menopause (76). The observation that oophorectomy alone reduces the subsequent risk of breast cancer has now been demonstrated in BRCA carriers (67, 68, 77). Although there is some concern that estrogen replacement might increase the risk of breast cancer in these women, the limited available data do not demonstrate an increased risk (78).

One concern regarding prophylactic oophorectomy is the observation that a small fraction of women subsequently have developed intraperitoneal carcinomatosis that was indistinguishable from ovarian cancer (79, 80). This rarely occurs, however, and it is believed oophorectomy should be greater than 90% protective, and statistical outcomes modeling suggests that a prophylactic oophorectomy results in an average of 2.6 life-year increase (77).

Hereditary Breast Cancer Surveillance and Treatment

Prevention of breast cancer mortality in BRCA1 and BRCA2 carriers presents different issues because these cancers are much more readily detected at an early stage than ovarian cancers. As a result, overall breast cancer 5-year survival in the United States is approximately 70% compared with only 30% for ovarian cancer. Furthermore, unlike oophorectomy, mastectomy causes marked alterations in self-esteem and body image, even when breast reconstruction is performed. A recent trial in women with BRCA1 and BRCA2 mutations showed a significant decrease in breast cancer after mastectomy (81).

Previous surgical practice for prophylactic mastectomies included subcutaneous mastectomies in which most of the breast tissue was removed, but the nipple was preserved. Advocates of prophylactic mastectomy today generally recommend total mastectomy, including the tissue under the nipple, because malignancy can potentially form in the nipple. Even if a total mastectomy is performed, there is no guarantee that all breast tissue will be successfully excised.

Although some women will continue to choose mastectomy, close surveillance with mammography and breast self-exam may prove equally effective in reducing mortality in view of the good prognosis for women with early breast cancer. In this regard, Lynch found that although 76% of BRCA1 mutation carriers accepted prophylactic oophorectomy, only 35% considered mastectomy a reasonable option (82). In a large BRCA1 kindred in Utah, 82% of female BRCA1 mutation carriers obtained a mammogram in the year after their genetic diagnosis, but only 11% were considering a mastectomy (19). Beginning in the 20s, biannual mammography and clinical breast exams are recommended for individuals choosing intensive screening (83). Mammography should be initiated at least 5 years before the youngest case of breast cancer in the family. Tumors in BRCA1 and BRCA2 mutations differ in estrogen receptor status; BRCA1 tumors are more likely to lack estrogen and progesterone receptors. Tamoxifen, when started at age 35, reduced breast cancer incidence by 62% among healthy BRCA2 carriers but not in healthy BRCA1 carriers (84).

HEREDITARY COLON CANCER

Colon cancer represents the third most common cause of cancer mortality in American women after breast and lung cancer. Colon cancer develops in a stepwise progression from normal mucosa, to hyperplasia and polyp, and finally, to dysplasia, cancer in situ, and invasive cancer (9). Because this disease has a well-defined clinically recognizable precancerous phase, colon cancer mortality can be decreased by screening programs (85). Effective screening methods include fecal occult blood testing and sigmoidoscopy and/or colonoscopy. When a positive screening result is obtained, colonoscopy and/or barium enema is performed to search for polyps and cancers. Unfortunately, available screening tests are underused; therefore, half of all patients with colon cancer die of their disease.

Most colon cancers are believed to arise due to sporadic mutations that accumulate over a lifetime, but some cases are the result of a hereditary predisposition. Among the 70,000 women diagnosed with a colorectal cancer this year in the United States, about 15% will have a first-degree relative with colon cancer. Individuals who have a first-degree relative with colon cancer are twice as likely to develop colon cancer compared with the general population (86). The risk is substantially greater if the relative was younger than 45 years of age at diagnosis.

Familial Adenomatous Polyposis

The familial adenomatous polyposis coli (APC or FAP) syndrome is inherited as an autosomal dominant trait with almost complete penetrance (87, 88). FAP affects 1 in 7000 persons, accounting for about 1% of all colon cancers. Virtually all individuals who inherit this syndrome develop hundreds of polyps throughout the colon and invasive colon cancer at a young age (89). Each polyp is believed to have the same chance of malignant transformation as a sporadic polyp. The sheer number of polyps in the inherited syndrome makes the combined risk for malignant transformation at multiple sites substantial. Patients with this syndrome may also develop gastric, periampullary, and duodenal precancerous polyps.

In 1991, Bodmer et al. localized the gene-causing familial polyposis to chromosome 5q21 (90). Most mutations in the FAP gene are frameshift or nonsense changes that cause early termination of the protein product. The exact function of the FAP protein remains unclear but is believed to act as a tumor suppressor. The FAP protein may also be involved in signal transduction, cellular adhesion, and microtubule function (91, 92).

Unlike most tumor suppressor genes in which inactivation of both copies of the gene is necessary, mutation of only one copy of the FAP gene is required for polyp formation (93).

Progression from polyp to a fully invasive cancer is accompanied by alterations in other genes such as p53, DCC (deleted in colon cancer), and K-*ras* (94). In addition to being responsible for familial polyposis syndrome, the FAP gene is frequently mutated in the course of sporadic colon cancer development (92).

A founder mutation of the FAP gene has been identified in 6% of Ashkenazi Jews (T to A in codon 1307) (Table 25.2). Although the polymorphism does not affect the function of the APC protein, it creates a stretch of eight adenine bases that is highly susceptible to inactivating mutations. Affected individuals appear to have about a 20% lifetime risk of colorectal cancer. Although the penetrance of this APC polymorphism is lower than that of clearly deleterious APC mutations, because the polymorphism is much more frequent, it is estimated to be responsible for about 28% of familial colorectal cancer in the Ashkenazi population (95, 96).

Hereditary Nonpolyposis Colorectal Cancer

The most common form of hereditary colon cancer is a hereditary nonpolyposis colorectal cancer (HNPCC) which accounts for about 5 to 10% of colorectal cancers. HNPCC was originally described as the Lynch syndromes type I and II. The Lynch type I syndrome described families with predominantly large bowel cancers, whereas the Lynch type II syndrome included large bowel cancers and cancers in other abdominal organs.

Clinically, HNPCC syndrome is characterized by early age of onset (average age: 44 years), proximal colon cancers (70%), and a high rate of metachronous cancers (97). Patients with HNPCC generally form premalignant widely based sessile colonic adenomas rather than polyps. Colonic cancers in individuals with HNPCC are usually proximal to the splenic flexure, diploid, and have a more favorable prognosis than sporadic colon cancers. Patients treated with subtotal colectomy have a 45% chance of developing another colon cancer in the remaining colon (98).

Lynch type II syndrome patients have an increased risk of other organ site cancers. Endometrial cancer is the second most common malignancy in women with HNPCC, with a cumulative risk of 20 to 60% (99–101). The average age of onset of HNPCC-associated endometrial cancers is in premenopausal women in their forties (101–103). HNPCC-associated endometrial cancers have the good prognostic features of other early stage, well-differentiated, endometrioid histologic types, and a resultant 90% survival (103, 104).

In addition, HNPCC carriers have an increased risk of ovarian, small bowel, stomach, pancreatic, ureteral, and renal cancers (Table 25.7). HNPCC-associated ovarian cancer cases represent

TABLE 25.7

Clinical Characteristics of Hereditary Nonpolyposis Colorectal Cancer Families

Patient Characteristics
Early onset of colorectal cancer
Proximal tumor localization
Multiple primary colorectal cancers
Extracolonic cancers (endometrium, stomach, small intestine, upper urologic tract, and ovary; skin) (Muir-Torre syndrome)
Family Characteristics
Histologically confirmed colorectal cancer in at least three relatives, one of whom is a first-degree relative of the other two
Occurrence of disease in at least two successive generations
At least one family member with colon cancer before age 50
Autosomal dominant inheritance
High penetrance (90%)

approximately 1% of all ovarian cancers (5). The risk of a HNPCC carrier developing ovarian cancer is increased to 5 to 12% (99–101). The age of onset of HNPCC-associated ovarian cancers is in the early forties, and the clinical features of the ovarian cancers are generally more favorable than sporadic cases (105). About 20% of HNPCC-associated ovarian cancers occur concurrently with endometrial cancer in the same patient.

In 1991, the International Collaborative Group on Hereditary Non-Polyposis Colorectal Cancer met and established the Amsterdam criteria for the diagnosis of the syndrome (Table 25.7) (106). These criteria include (a) histologically verified colorectal cancer in three or more relatives, one of whom is a first-degree relative of the other two, with exclusion of familial adenomatous polyposis syndrome; (b) colorectal cancer involving at least two successive generations; and (c) at least one family member who has developed colorectal cancer by age 50. The updated Amsterdam Criteria II account for the presence of noncolorectal inherited cancers in the pedigree evaluation (97).

HNPCC syndrome occurs due to inherited mutations in one of a family of genes involved in DNA mismatch repair. The first of the HNPCC genes to be identified was MSH2 on chromosome 2p (107, 108). Subsequently, the MLH1 gene on chromosome 3p was noted to be responsible for other HNPCC familial mutations. Mutations in these two genes appear to account for the majority of HNPCC families in which mutations can be identified, and for 3 to 5% of all colorectal cancers (109). Other DNA repair genes, including PMS1, PMS2, and MSH6, have been implicated in some cases. The function of the DNA repair genes is well known from studies in yeast and bacteria. Mutation in DNA repair genes leads to the accumulation of mutations, particularly in areas of the DNA that have repetitive sequences (e.g., CACACA). These repetitive sequences, called microsatellites, are dispersed throughout all chromosomes and are a frequent site of mutations in humans who inherit mutations in one of the DNA repair genes. Although some microsatellites are within the coding sequence of genes, most reside in the intervening noncoding regions. Microsatellite mutations within growth regulatory genes may contribute to malignant transformation, but it is unclear whether microsatellite instability outside genes is important in carcinogenesis or merely a symptom of the underlying problem.

Genetic Testing for Hereditary Colon Cancer

With the identification of genes responsible for hereditary colon cancer, families suspected of having familial colon cancer can now undergo genetic testing. Many of the issues that were discussed with regard to BRCA1 and BRCA2 testing in families with breast and ovarian cancer apply to genetic testing for hereditary colon cancer. Pedigrees should be thoroughly documented, and the other critical steps in the genetic counseling process must occur. The previously described Amsterdam criteria requiring at least one family member with a diagnosis of colon cancer at an early age and at least three affected individuals in two contiguous generations serves as a reasonable guideline for selecting candidates for genetic testing. A consensus conference of the NCI in Bethesda developed guidelines for screening of cancer patients with suspected inherited colorectal cancers.

The NCI screening strategy uses microsatellite instability in tumor DNA because microsatellite instability is present in most colon cancers that arise in individuals who inherit mutations in the DNA repair genes. If microsatellite instability is found, the specific DNA repair genes are then screened for mutations (Table 25.1). There is no apparent correlation between the spectrum of HNPCC-associated cancers and involvement of a specific DNA repair gene.

Once a mutation is detected, testing can be offered to all family members. In view of the high penetrance of these mutations (approximately 90%), every effort should be made to identify all of the carriers within a family. Identification of HNPCC mutations and genetic testing reduces the number of colon carcinomas and resulting mortality (91).

Hereditary Colon Cancer Surveillance and Treatment

Current recommendations for colon cancer surveillance in HNPCC patients begin with genetic counseling at age 20. A full colonoscopy should be performed starting at age 25, or at least 5 years earlier than the youngest affected family member (110). The International Collaborative Group

TABLE 25.8

Surveillance Recommendations for Hereditary Nonpolyposis Colorectal Cancer Carriers

Test	Age at Initiation (yr)	Frequency
Colonoscopy[a]	20–25	Every 2 years until age 35; annually thereafter
Endometrial sampling	25–35	1–2 years
Transvaginal ultrasound, CA125 level	25–35	1–2 years
Gastroscopy	30–35	1–2 years
Urinary bladder ultrasound Urine cytology	30–35	1–2 years

[a] Subtotal colectomy is indicated when a polyp or cancer is found.

on HNPCC currently recommends colonoscopy screening every 1 to 3 years. The American Society of Colon and Rectal Surgeons recommends colonoscopy every 2 years from age 21 to 40, then annually (110). Colonoscopy rather than sigmoidoscopy is appropriate because most of the colon cancers in this syndrome are right sided (91). If cancer is found, at least a subtotal colectomy is indicated. Patients found to have an adenoma on colonoscopic screening are advised to undergo surgery because colonoscopic polyp resection is often inadequate with these broad-based lesions. In addition, patients who develop adenomas have a substantial risk of recurrent polyps and cancer formation (Table 25.8). Patients with HNPCC can develop invasive lesions from adenomas in as little as 2 years, in contrast to the general population where this transition is believed to require 8 to 10 years. For this reason, screening and surveillance must be performed frequently.

Patients in FAP families should undergo genetic testing between ages 10 to 12, if possible. If genetic testing is not possible, current recommendations suggest yearly sigmoidoscopy from age 12 (97). Frequent endoscopic screening of the upper gastrointestinal tract, including the stomach, duodenum, and periampullary region, is recommended (97).

Surgical prophylaxis for hereditary colon cancer varies by the syndrome type. APC mutation carriers generally should undergo prophylactic total colectomy (97). Half of APC patients will develop colon cancer by age 40, and all develop cancer by age 70 (98). Prophylactic colectomy with ileorectal anastomosis is a reasonable option for asymptomatic HNPCC mutation carriers (97, 110). The choice between close surveillance and prophylactic surgery is one that each carrier must decide for themselves after nondirective counseling.

A low-fat and high-fiber diet with lots of fruits and vegetables is associated with a decreased incidence of colorectal cancer in the general population. However, it is not known whether dietary interventions would decrease the incidence of cancer in HNPCC families. There is some evidence that chemoprevention with sulindac (a nonselective COX-1 inhibitor) reduces adenoma development in some APC carriers (111). In addition, data have linked aspirin intake to a reduction in colon cancer risk, but it is not known if this affects the incidence of hereditary colon cancers (112). New COX-2 inhibitors, such as celecoxib, are currently being evaluated for HNPCC patients in clinical trials (110).

HNPCC Families and the Risk of Endometrial and Ovarian Cancer

Due to the increased risk of endometrial cancer in HNPCC families, yearly endometrial sampling is suggested beginning at age 30 (113, 114). However, the efficacy of this approach remains unproven because most HNPCC-associated endometrial cancers are curable when diagnosed due to the presence of abnormal uterine bleeding.

Although pelvic ultrasound and serum CA 125 levels have been advocated for ovarian cancer screening in HNPCC families, the utility of these techniques for diagnosing ovarian cancer while it is still confined to the ovaries is unproven. Prophylactic hysterectomy and adnexectomy should be considered in patients undergoing colectomy if childbearing has been completed. Ideally, concurrent hysterectomy, salpingo-oophorectomy, and any necessary surgical staging will have been planned in advance with both the general surgery team and the gynecologic team. Intraoperative opening and examination of the uterus is important, especially if a preoperative endometrial biopsy has not been obtained. Some HNPCC mutation carriers will decline colectomy in favor of periodic colorectal cancer screening due to quality of life issues after colectomy. In that case, a prophylactic hysterectomy with oophorectomy can be performed by either the abdominal or vaginal route.

HNPCC mutation carriers may be eligible for estrogen replacement therapy after prophylactic oophorectomy. Although no data specifically related to HNPCC carriers have been published, estrogen replacement therapy is believed to decrease the risk of colon cancer in the general population (76). The risk and benefits of hormone replacement therapy must be discussed and individualized for each patient.

In summary, gynecologists have an important role in the identification of high-risk patients through the assembly of family history and pedigrees, as well as referral for appropriate genetic testing. Increasingly, prophylactic surgery and chemoprophylaxis are part of the gynecologists' arsenal in these families as we strive to reduce mortality from the hereditary breast, ovarian, colon, and endometrial cancer syndromes.

Clinical Notes

- Up to 10% of certain cancer types can be traced through family lines.
- Cancer of the colon, breast, and ovary are the most common hereditary cancers in women; it is believed that 5 to 10% of these cancers have a hereditary basis.
- Cancer results from loss of growth regulatory controls. Oncogenes encode proteins that stimulate proliferation, whereas tumor suppressor genes encode for proteins that inhibit proliferation.
- In caring for a patient or family with hereditary cancer, a thorough cancer history is absolutely essential. Data on all first- and second-degree relatives must be obtained. Other extended family history should be recorded, if available.
- Ten percent of breast and ovarian cancers are due to autosomal dominant hereditary syndromes. Most hereditary ovarian cancer cases are due to germ-line mutations in BRCA1 and BRCA2. At least half of hereditary breast cancers are due to germ-line mutations in BRCA1 and BRCA2.
- In families with BRCA1 mutations, the lifetime risk of breast cancer by age 70 is 65%, and the lifetime risk of ovarian cancer is 20 to 30%. The incidence of prostate, colon, pancreatic, and stomach cancers is also increased.
- In families with BRCA2 mutations, the elevated lifetime risk of breast cancer approximates the risk seen in families with BRCA2 mutations, but the lifetime risk of ovarian cancer is 10 to 20%.
- The probability of finding a BRCA1 or BRCA2 mutation in a woman older than age 50 who is the only individual in her family with ovarian or breast cancer is 3%.
- Prior to genetic testing, all women must receive adequate educational materials and counseling explaining the postulated risks and benefits before deciding to undergo testing. Confidentiality remains a critical issue in cancer susceptibility testing.
- Prophylactic oophorectomy for carriers of BRCA1 or BRCA2 mutations is an attractive option because it can be done laparoscopically, usually only causes modest changes in body image or self-esteem, and costs are generally covered by medical insurance for BRCA mutation

carriers. It does not guarantee that malignancy such as intraperitoneal carcinomatosis will not develop, although this rarely occurs.

- Prevention of breast cancer in BRCA1 and BRCA2 carriers is more complex. Mastectomy causes marked alterations in body image and self-esteem, even with breast reconstruction. Total mastectomy is recommended because cancer may form in the nipple if it is not removed. There is still no guarantee with total mastectomy that all breast tissue will be excised.
- Close surveillance with frequent mammography and breast examinations are recommended to begin between ages 25 and 35 for those affected individuals.
- Colon cancer is the third most common cause of cancer mortality in American women.
- Familial APC syndrome is an autosomal dominant trait and accounts for about 1% of all colon cancers. Individuals with APC mutations should undergo prophylactic total colectomy because half of these patients will develop colon cancer by age 40, and all develop cancer by age 70.
- A polymorphism in the gene associated with FAP affects approximately 6% of all Ashkenazi Jews. Affected individuals have a 20% lifetime risk of colon cancer.
- The most common form of hereditary colon cancer is HNPCC, which accounts for about 5 to 10% of colorectal cancers. There are three criteria for this diagnosis: colorectal cancer in three or more relatives with one being a first-degree relative of the other two, colorectal cancer in two successive generations or more, and one family member who developed colorectal cancer by age 50.
- Patients with mutations in MLH1 or MSH2 genes are at risk for HNPCC. They should undergo genetic counseling at age 20, and a full colonoscopy should be done every 2 years until age 35 and then annually thereafter.

REFERENCES

1. Warthin AS. Heredity with reference to carcinoma. Arch Intern Med 1913;12:546–555.
2. Warthin AS. A further study of a cancer family. J Cancer Res 1925;9:279–286.
3. Lynch HT, Albano WA, Lynch JF, et al. Recognition of the cancer family syndrome. Gastroenterology 1983;84:672–673.
4. Hardcastle JD. Colorectal cancer. CA Cancer J Clin 1997;47:66–69.
5. Rubin SC, Blackwood MA, Bandera C, et al. BRCA1, BRCA2, and hereditary nonpolyposis colorectal cancer gene mutations in an unselected ovarian cancer population: relationship to family history and implications for genetic testing. Am J Obstet Gynecol 1998;178(4):670–677.
6. Reedy M, Gallion H, Fowler JM, et al. Contribution of BRCA1 and BRCA2 to familial ovarian cancer: a gynecologic oncology group study. Cancer Res 2002;85:255–259.
7. Risch HA, McLaughlin JR, Cole D, et al. Prevalence and penetrance of germline BRCA1 and BRCA2 mutations in a population series of 649 women with ovarian cancer. Am J Hum Genet 2001;68(3):700–710.
8. Whittemore AS, Gong G, Itnyre J. Prevalence and contribution of BRCA1 mutations in breast cancer and ovarian cancer: results from three U.S. population-based case-control studies of ovarian cancer. Am J Hum Genet 1997;60(3):496–504.
9. Muto T, Bussey HJR, Morson BC. The evolution of cancer of the colon and rectum. Cancer 1975;36:2251–2270.
10. Lynch HT, Lynch JF. Breast cancer genetics: family history, heterogeneity, molecular genetic diagnosis and genetic counseling. Curr Probl Cancer 1996;20:329–365.
11. Brose MS, Rebbeck TR, Calzone KA, et al. Cancer risk estimates for BRCA1 mutation carriers identified in a risk evaluation program. J Natl Cancer Inst 2002;94(18):1365–1372.
12. Frank TS, Deffenbaugh AM, Reid JE, et al. Clinical characteristics of individuals with germline mutations in BRCA1 and BRCA2: analysis of 10,000 individuals. J Clin Oncol 2002;20:1480–1490.
13. de la Hoya M, Fernandez JM, Tosar A, et al. Association between BRCA1 mutations and ratio of female to male births in offspring of families with breast cancer, ovarian cancer or both. JAMA 2003;290(7):929–931.
14. Ford D, Easton DF, Peto J. Estimate of the gene frequency of BRCA1 and its contribution to breast and ovarian cancer incidence. Am J Hum Genet 1995;57:1457–1462.
15. Oddoux C, Struewing JP, Clayton CM, et al. The carrier frequency of the BRCA2 6174delT mutation among Ashkenazi Jewish individuals is approximately 1%. Nat Genet 1996;14:188–190.
16. Struewing JP, Abeliovich D, Collins FS, et al. The carrier frequency of the BRCA1 185delAG mutation is approximately 1 percent in Ashkenazi Jewish individuals. Nat Genet 1995;11:198–200.
17. Abeliovich D, Kaduri L, Lerer I, et al. The founder mutations 185delAG and 5382insC in BRCA1 and 6174delT in BRCA2 appear in 60% of ovarian cancer and 30% of early-onset breast cancer patients among Ashkenazi women. Am J Hum Genet 1997;60:505–514.

18. Lynch HT, Fusaro RM, Lemon SJ, et al. Survey of cancer genetics: genetic testing implications. Cancer 1997;80:523–532.
19. Botkin JR, Smith KR, Croyle RT, et al. Genetic testing for a BRCA1 mutation: prophylactic surgery and screening behavior in women 2 years post testing. Am J Med Genet 2003;118A:201–209.
20. American Society of Clinical Oncology. American Society of Clinical Oncology policy statement update: genetic testing for cancer susceptibility. J Clin Oncol 2003;21(12):2397–2406.
21. Easton DF, Ford D, Bishop DT. Breast and ovarian cancer incidence in BRCA1-mutation carriers. Breast Cancer Linkage Consortium. Am J Hum Genet 1995;56(1):265–271.
22. Couch FJ, DeShano ML, Blackwood MA, et al. BRCA1 mutations in women attending clinics that evaluate the risk of breast cancer. N Engl J Med 1997;336(20):1409–1415.
23. Langston AA, Malone KE, Thompson JD, et al. BRCA1 mutations in a population-based sample of young women with breast cancer. N Engl J Med 1996;334:137–142.
24. Rebbeck TR, Couch FJ, Calzone K, et al. Genetic heterogeneity in hereditary breast cancer: role of BRCA1 and BRCA2. Am J Hum Genet 1996;59:547–553.
25. Serova OM, Mazoyer S, Puget N, et al. Mutations in BRCA1 and BRCA2 in breast cancer families: are there more breast cancer—susceptibility genes? Am J Hum Genet 1997;60:486–495.
26. Struewing JP, Hartge P, Wacholder S, et al. The risk of cancer associated with specific mutations of BRCA1 and BRCA2 among Ashkenazi Jews. N Engl J Med 1997;336:1401–1408.
27. Antoniou A, Pharaoh PD, Narod S, et al. Average risks of breast and ovarian cancer associated with BRCA1 or BRCA2 mutations detected in case series unselected for family history: a combined analysis of 22 studies. Am J Hum Genet 2003;72:1117–1130.
28. Ford D, Easton DF, Bishop DT, et al. Risks of cancer in BRCA1-mutation carriers. Breast Cancer Linkage Consortium. Lancet 1994;343:692–695.
29. Gayther SA, Warren W, Mazoyer S, et al. Germline mutations of the BRCA1 gene in breast and ovarian cancer families provide evidence for genotype-phenotype correlation. Nat Genet 1995;11:428–433.
30. Shattuck-Eidens D, McClure M, Simard J, et al. A collaborative survey of 80 mutations in the BRCA1 breast and ovarian cancer susceptibility gene. Implications for presymptomatic testing and screening. JAMA 1995;273:535–541.
31. Narod SA, Risch H, Moslehi R, et al. Oral contraceptives and the risk of hereditary ovarian cancer: Hereditary Ovarian Cancer Clinical Study Group. N Eng J Med 1998;339:424–428.
32. Aziz S, Kuperstein G, Rosen B, et al. A genetic epidemiological study of carcinoma of the fallopian tube. Gynecol Oncol 2001;80(3):341–345.
33. Zweemer RP, van Diest PJ, Verheijen RH, et al. Molecular evidence linking primary cancer of the fallopian tube to BRCA1 germline mutations. Cancer Res 2000;76:45–50.
34. Levine DA, Argenta PA, Yee CJ, et al. Fallopian tube and primary peritoneal carcinomas associated with BRCA mutations. J Clin Oncol 2003;21(22):4222–4227.
35. Menczer J, Chetrit A, Barda G, et al. Frequency of BRCA mutations in primary peritoneal carcinoma in Israeli Jewish women. Gynecol Oncol 2003;88:58–61.
36. Breast Cancer Linkage Consortium. Pathology of familial breast cancer: differences between breast cancers in carriers of BRCA1 or BRCA2 mutations and sporadic cases. Lancet 1997;359:1505–1510.
37. Eisinger F, Stoppa-Lyonnet D, Longy M, et al. Germ line mutation at BRCA1 affects the histoprognostic grade in hereditary breast cancer. Cancer Res 1996;56(3):471–474.
38. Marcus JN, Watson P, Page DL, et al. Hereditary breast cancer: pathobiology, prognosis, and BRCA1 and BRCA2 gene linkage. Cancer 1996;77(4):697–709.
39. Foulkes WD, Stefansson IM, Chappuis PO, et al. Germline BRCA1 mutations and a basal epithelial phenotype in breast cancer. J Natl Cancer Inst 2003;95(19):1482–1485.
40. Robson ME, Chappuis PO, Statgopan J, et al. A combined analysis of outcome following breast cancer: differences in survival based on BRCA1/BRCA2 mutation status and administration of adjuvant treatment. Breast Cancer Res 2003;6(1):R8–R17.
41. Rubin SC, Benjamin I, Behbakht K, et al. Clinical and pathological features of ovarian cancer in women with germ-line mutations of BRCA1. N Engl J Med 1996;335:1413–1416.
42. Stratton JF, Gayther SA, Russell P, et al. Contribution of BRCA1 mutations to ovarian cancer. N Engl J Med 1997;336:1125–1130.
43. Berchuck A, Heron KA, Carney ME, et al. Frequency of germline and somatic BRCA1 mutations in ovarian cancer. Clin Cancer Res 1998;4(10):2433–2437.
44. Boyd J, Sonada Y, Federici M. Clinicopathologic features of BRCA-linked and sporadic cancer. JAMA 2000;283:2260–2265.
45. Cass I, Baldwin RL, Varkey T, et al. Improved survival in women with BRCA-associated ovarian carcinoma. Cancer 2003;97:2187–2195.
46. Wooster R, Neuhausen SL, Mangion J, et al. Localization of a breast cancer susceptibility gene, BRCA2, to chromosome 13q12–13. Science 1994;265:2088–2090.
47. Wooster R, Bignell G, Lancaster J, et al. Identification of the breast cancer susceptibility gene BRCA2. Nature 1995;378:789–791.
48. Lancaster JM, Wooster R, Mangion J, et al. BRCA2 mutations in primary breast and ovarian cancers. Nat Genet 1996;13(2):238–240.
49. Phelan CM, Lancaster JM, Cumbs C, et al. Mutation analysis of the BRCA2 gene in 49 site-specific breast cancer families. Nat Genet 1996;13:120–122.

50. Gayther SA, Mangion J, Russell P, et al. Variation of risks of breast and ovarian cancer associated with different germline mutations of the BRCA2 gene. Nat Genet 1997;15:103–105.
51. Vaughn JP, Cirisano FD, Huper G, et al. Cell cycle control of BRCA2. Cancer Res 1996;56:4590–4594.
52. D'Andrea AD, Grompe M. The Fanconi anaemia/BRCA pathway. Nat Rev 2003;3:23–34.
53. Couch FJ, Weber BL, Breast Cancer Information Core. Mutations and polymorphisms in the familial early-onset breast cancer (BRCA1) gene. Hum Mutat 1996;8:8–18.
54. Deffenbaugh AM, Frank TS, Hoffman M, et al. Characterization of common BRCA1 and BRCA2 variants. Genet Test 2002;6(2):119–121.
55. Frank TS, Manley SA, Olopade OI, et al. Sequence analysis of BRCA1 and BRCA2: correlation of mutations with family history and ovarian cancer risk. J Clin Oncol 1998;16(7):2417–2425.
56. Miki Y, Swensen J, Shattuck-Eidens D, et al. A strong candidate for the breast ovarian cancer susceptibility gene BRCA1. Science 1994;266:66–71.
57. King M-C, Marks J, Mandell J, et al. Breast and ovarian cancer risks due to inherited mutations in BRCA1 and BRCA2. Science 2003;302:643–646.
58. The ad hoc committee on genetic testing/insurance issues. Genetic testing and insurance. Am J Hum Genet 1995;56:327–331.
59. Castilla LH, Couch FJ, Erdos MR, et al. Mutations in the BRCA1 gene in families with early-onset breast and ovarian cancer. Nat Genet 1994;8:387–391.
60. Friedman LS, Ostermeyer EA, Szabo CI, et al. Confirmation of BRCA1 by analysis of germline mutations linked to breast and ovarian cancer in ten families. Nat Genet 1994;8(4):399–404.
61. Wilson CA, Payton MN, Elliott GS et al. Differential subcellular localization, expression and biological toxicity of BRCA1 and the splice variant BRCA1-11b. Oncogene 1997;14:1–16.
62. Shattuck-Eidens D, Oliphant A, McClure M, et al. BRCA1 sequence analysis in women at high risk for susceptibility mutations. Risk factor analysis and implications for genetic testing. JAMA 1997;278(15): 1242–1250.
63. Narod SA, Risch H, Moslehi R, et al. Oral contraceptives and the risk of hereditary ovarian cancer. Hereditary Ovarian Cancer Clinical Study Group. N Engl J Med 1998;339(7):424–428.
64. Modan B, Hartge P, Hirsh-Yechezkel G, et al. Parity, oral contraceptives, and the risk of ovarian cancer among carriers and noncarriers of a BRCA1 or BRCA2 mutation. N Engl J Med 2001;345(4):235–240.
65. Lynch HT, Lemon SJ, Durham C, et al. A descriptive study of BRCA1 testing and reactions to disclosure of test results. Cancer 1997;79(11):2219–2228.
66. Kauff ND, Scheuer L, Robson ME, et al. Insurance reimbursement for risk-reducing mastectomy and oophorectomy in women with BRCA1 or BRCA2 mutations. Genet Med 2001;3:422–425.
67. Kauff ND, Satagopan JM, Robson ME, et al. Risk-reducing salpingo-oophorectomy in women with a BRCA1 or BRCA2 mutation. N Engl J Med 2002;346(21):1609–1615.
68. Rebbeck TR. Prophylactic oophorectomy in BRCA1 and BRCA2 mutation carriers. J Clin Oncol 2000;18(21 suppl):100S–103S.
69. Weber BL, Punzalan C, Eisen A, et al. Ovarian cancer risk reduction after bilateral prophylactic oophorectomy (BPO) in BRCA1 and BRCA2 mutation carriers. Am J Hum Genet 2000;67(suppl 2):58.
70. Colgan TJ, Murphy J, Cole DE, et al. Occult carcinoma in prophylactic oophorectomy specimens: prevalence and association with BRCA germline mutation status. Am J Surg Pathol 2001;25(10):1283–1289.
71. Lu KH, Garber JE, Cramer DW, et al. Occult ovarian tumors in women with BRCA1 or BRCA2 mutations undergoing prophylactic oophorectomy. J Clin Oncol 2000;18:2728–2732.
72. Barakat RR, Federici MG, Saigo PE, et al. Absence of premalignant histologic, molecular, or cell biologic alterations in prophylactic oophorectomy specimens from BRCA1 heterozygotes. Cancer 2000;89:383–390.
73. Stratton JF, Buckley CH, Lowe D, et al. Comparison of prophylactic oophorectomy specimens from carriers and noncarriers of a BRCA1 or BRCA2 gene mutation. United Kingdom Coordinating Committee on Cancer Research (UKCCCR) Familial Ovarian Cancer Study Group. J Natl Cancer Inst 1999;91:626–628.
74. Colgan TJ, Boerner SL, Murphy J, et al. Peritoneal lavage cytology: an assessment of its value during prophylactic oophorectomy. Cancer Res 2002;85:397–403.
75. Paley PJ, Swisher EM, Garcia RL, et al. Occult cancer of the fallopian tube in BRCA-1 germline mutation carriers at prophylactic oophorectomy: a case for recommending hysterectomy at surgical prophylaxis. Cancer Res 2001;80:176–180.
76. Rossouw JE, Anderson GL, Prentice RL, et al. Risks and benefits of estrogen plus progestin in healthy postmenopausal women: principal results from the Women's Health Initiative randomized controlled clinical trial. JAMA 2002;288(3):321–333.
77. Grann VR, Jacobson JS, Thomason D, et al. Effect of prevention strategies on survival and quality-adjusted survival of women with BRCA1/2 mutations: an updated decision analysis. J Clin Oncol 2002;20(10):2520–2529.
78. DiSaia PJ, Grosen EA, Kurosaki T, et al. Hormone replacement therapy in breast cancer survivors: a cohort study. Am J Obstet Gynecol 1996;174(5):1494–1498.
79. Piver MS, Jishi MF, Tsukada Y, et al. Primary peritoneal carcinoma after prophylactic oophorectomy in women with a family history of ovarian cancer. A report of the Gilda Radner Familial Ovarian Cancer Registry. Cancer 1993;71:2751–2755.
80. Struewing JP, Watson P, Easton DF, et al. Prophylactic oophorectomy in inherited breast/ovarian cancer families. Monogr Natl Cancer Inst 1995;(17):33–35.

81. Meijers-Heijboer H, Van Gecl B, Van Putten WL J, et al. Breast cancer after prophylactic bilateral mastectomy in women with a BRCA1 or BRCA2 mutation. N Engl J Med 2001;345:159–164.
82. Lynch HT. Many at risk consider prophylactic oophorectomy. Ob/Gyn News July 1, 1997.
83. Hoskins KF, Stopfer JE, Calzone KA, et al. Assessment and counseling for women with a family history of breast cancer. A guide for clinicians. JAMA 1995;273:577–585.
84. King MC, Wieand S, Hale K, et al. Tamoxifen and breast cancer incidence among women with inherited mutations in BRCA1 and BRCA2: National Surgical Adjuvant Breast and Bowel Project (NSABP-1) Breast Cancer Prevention Trial. JAMA 2001;286(18):2251–2256.
85. Winawer SJ, Zauber AG, Ho MN, et al. Prevention of colorectal cancer by colonoscopic polypectomy. N Engl J Med 1993;329:1977–1981.
86. St.John DJ, McDermott FT, Hopper JL, et al. Cancer risk in relatives of patients with common colorectal cancer. Ann Intern Med 1993;118:785–790.
87. Bussey HJR. Gastrointestinal polyposis. Gut 1970;11:970–978.
88. Bussey HJR. Familial polyposis coli. Pathol Annu 1979;14:61–81.
89. Lipkin M, Sherlock P, DeCosse JJ. Risk factors and preventative measures in the control of cancer of the large intestine. Curr Probl Cancer 1980;4(10):1–57.
90. Bodmer WF, Bailey CJ, Bodmer J, et al. Localization of the gene for familial adenomatous polyposis on chromosome 5. Nature 1987;328:614–616.
91. Parsons R. Molecular genetics and hereditary cancer: hereditary nonpolyposis colorectal carcinoma as a model. Cancer 1997;80:533–536.
92. Solomon E, Voss R, Hall V, et al. Chromosome 5 allele loss in human colorectal carcinoma. Nature 1987;328:616–619.
93. Fearon ER. Molecular abnormalities in colon and rectal cancer. In: Mendelsohn J, Howley PM, Israel MA, et al., eds. The Molecular Basis of Cancer. Philadelphia: WB Saunders, 1995:340.
94. Fearon ER, Vogelstein B. A genetic model for colorectal tumorigenesis. Cell 1990;61:759–767.
95. Laken SJ, Peterson GM, Gruber SB, et al. Familial colorectal cancer in Ashkenazim due to a hypermutable tract in APC. Nat Genet 1997;17:79–83.
96. Gryfe R, Di Nicola N, Geeta L, et al. Inherited colorectal polyposis and cancer risk of the APC I1307K polymorphism. Am J Hum Genet 1999;64:378–384.
97. American Gastroenterological Association (AGA). AGA technical review on hereditary colorectal cancer and genetic testing. Gastroenterology 2001;121:198–213.
98. Lynch HT, Lynch J. Genetic counseling for hereditary cancer. Oncology 1996;10:27–32.
99. Aarnio M, Mecklin JP, Aaltonen LA, et al. Life-time risk of different cancers in hereditary non-polyposis colorectal cancer (HNPCC) syndrome. Int J Cancer 1995;64(6):430–433.
100. Dunlop MG, Farrington SM, Carothers AD, et al. Cancer risk associated with germline DNA mismatch repair gene mutations. Hum Mol Genet 1997;6(1):105–110.
101. Watson P, Vasen HF, Mecklin JP, et al. The risk of endometrial cancer in hereditary nonpolyposis colorectal cancer. Am J Med 1994;96(6):516–520.
102. Brown GJ, St. John DJ, Macrae FA, et al. Cancer risk in young women at risk of hereditary nonpolyposis colorectal cancer: implications for gynecologic surveillance. Cancer Res 2001;80(3):346–349.
103. Vasen HF, Watson P, Mecklin JP, et al. The epidemiology of endometrial cancer in hereditary nonpolyposis colorectal cancer. Anticancer Res 1994;14(4B):1675–1678.
104. Boks DE, Trujillo AP, Voogd AC, et al. Survival analysis of endometrial carcinoma associated with hereditary nonpolyposis colorectal cancer. Int J Cancer 2002;102(2):198–200.
105. Watson P, Butzow R, Lynch HT, et al. The clinical features of ovarian cancer in hereditary nonpolyposis colorectal cancer. Cancer Res 2001;82(2):223–228.
106. Vasen HF, Mecklin J-P, Khan M, et al. The International Collaborative Group on hereditary nonpolyposis colorectal cancer. Discuss Colon Rectum 1991;34:424–425.
107. Leach FS, Nicolaides NC, Papadopoulos N, et al. Mutations of a mutS homolog in hereditary nonpolyposis colorectal cancer. Cell 1993;75:1215–1225.
108. Fishel R, Rao MRS, Copeland NG, et al. The human mutator gene homolog MSH2 and its association with hereditary nonpolyposis colorectal cancer. Cell 1993;75:1027–1038.
109. Salovaara R, Loukola A, Kristo P, et al. Population-based molecular detection of hereditary nonpolyposis colorectal cancer. J Clin Oncol 2000;18(11):2193–2200.
110. Yu H-J, Lin K, Ota D, et al. Hereditary nonpolyposis colorectal cancer: preventive management. Cancer Treat Rev 2003;29:461–470.
111. Giardiello FM, Hamilton SR, Krush AJ, et al. Treatment of colonic and rectal adenomas with sulindac in familial adenomatous polyposis. N Engl J Med 1993;328:1313–1316.
112. Thun MJ, Namboodiri MM, Heath CW Jr. Aspirin use and reduced risk of fatal colon cancer. N Engl J Med 1991;325:1593–1596.
113. Burke W, Peterson G, Lynch P, et al. Recommendations for follow-up care of individuals with an inherited predisposition to cancer. JAMA 1997;227:915–919.
114. Menko FH, Wijnen JT, Vasen HFA, et al. Genetic counseling in hereditary nonpolyposis colorectal cancer. Oncology 1996;10:71–76.

CHAPTER 26

Occupational and Environmental Exposures

Linda M. Frazier and David A. Grainger

There are some well-established links between gynecologic disorders and environmental exposures. Environmental exposures can occur in the course of employment or outside the workplace. Exposures include chemicals, physical agents such as radiation, biological agents such as infectious organisms or biological products, and others such as shift work. Most of the gynecologic pathology caused by occupational and environmental exposures are due to chemicals and job physical demands. In this chapter, we summarize the evidence for occupational and environmental contributions to gynecologic disorders, and then outline a clinical approach to the patient. To help estimate the risk in a given woman, an approach to assessing and interpreting the types and magnitude of her exposures is described.

EXPOSURES AND REGULATIONS

Despite occupational and environmental laws and regulations, exposures to hazardous agents continue to occur. Regulatory protections in Westernized countries significantly reduced certain toxic exposures during the 20th century. Blood lead levels in the United States dropped, and air, water, and food quality improved. Occupational exposure limits were developed, repeatedly revised downward, and enforced. However, these approaches remain imperfect for four reasons: (a) protections available in Westernized countries are not available to many people in developing countries; (b) exposures over recommended limits continue to occur, even in Westernized countries; (c) new exposure agents are constantly being developed, especially new chemical entities; and (d) occupational and environmental exposure limits are only as good as the data on which they are based. The research database is incomplete. There are many thousands of chemicals in current use, but few of them have been fully tested for human health effects.

Unlike the U.S. Food and Drug Administration (FDA), which requires extensive testing in humans before pharmaceutical products can be marketed, the Occupational Safety and Health Administration (OSHA) does not require toxicity testing before a chemical can be used in the workplace. The U.S. Environmental Protection Agency (EPA) does require premarket testing of some agents, primarily pesticides. Testing relies on rodent models, which approximate human outcomes relatively well for acute toxicity, fertility, teratogenesis, and induction of cancer. Because rodent toxicology protocols used for regulatory purposes are less robust for predicting effects on the endocrine system, puberty, and endometriosis, new screening tests are being investigated (1). Menstrual dysfunction, spontaneous abortion, cervical cancer, and certain neurobehavioral end points, however, have no direct equivalent in rodents.

Environmental exposures are ubiquitous. Low levels of metals such as lead, mercury, and arsenic are commonly found in drinking water or food, in household dust samples, or in human serum, urine, or hair specimens. Almost all homes (97%) contain pesticide products, with an average of six products per household (2). More than 90% of serum and adipose samples from women contain polychlorinated biphenyls (PCBs) and other organochlorine chemicals at levels of about 4 parts per billion (3). PCBs are persistent pollutants with a widespread geographic distribution and may be consumed at high levels in foods such as fatty sport fish taken from contaminated waters. Dozens of pharmaceuticals and their metabolites have been detected downstream from municipal sewage treatment plants, and a few have been measured at trace concentrations in drinking water (4). Polycarbonate resins from consumer products and packaging can leach bisphenol A into food, although the estimated dietary exposure is 0.25 parts per billion (5). Do these low levels of exposure cause disease? Evidence for and against harmful effects from occupational and environmental exposures is discussed in this chapter for common problems seen in office gynecology.

MECHANISMS OF ACTION

A great deal of the environmental health research has been conducted on agents such as diethylstilbestrol (DES), PCBs, the insecticide dichlorodiphenyl trichloroethane (DDT), and dioxins such as 2,3,7,8-tetrachlorodibenzo-p-dioxin (TCDD). Dioxins are pollutants produced from certain chemical manufacturing processes or from combustion. DES, PCBs, DDT, and TCDD are no longer being actively used in the United States to treat obstetric conditions, to manufacture products, or to control insect infestations. Exposure to PCBs, dioxins, and DDT metabolites still occurs today because the compounds are highly persistent in the environment, and they are still used in other countries. The mechanisms of action of these agents have been elucidated through ongoing studies, and results of research may be generalizable to other exposures that act by similar mechanisms. Research on tobacco, an agent still in use, is also pertinent because of its cytotoxic, mutagenic, and other effects.

Known mechanisms of action for many environmental exposures include inhibition of enzymes such as estrogen sulfotransferase, suppression of the hypothalamic-pituitary axis,

TABLE 26.1

Selected Endocrinologically Active Agents

Synthetic Chemicals
PCBs, DDT and its metabolites, TCDD, certain insecticides (chlordecone, endosulfan, methoxychlor), components of plastics (bisphenol A), components of detergents and their biodegradation products (4-octylphenonol, nonylphenol)
Phytoestrogens
Flavonoids
Genistein, daidzein, formononetin, biochanin, apigenin, chrysin, diadnaringenin, kaempferol, quercetin, narnigenin, phloretin, ipriflavone, flavone
Coumestans
Coumestrol
Lignans
Enterodiol, enterolactone
Mycoestrogens
Zearalenone or derivatives

DDT, dichlorodiphenyl trichloroethane; PCBs, polychlorinated biphenyls; TCDD, 2,3,7,8-tetrachlorodibenzo-p-dioxin.

interference with genes or chromosomes, and cumulative destruction of oocytes. Studies of prenatal exposures suggest that fetal programming may play a role in disorders that do not become apparent until adulthood (the Barker hypothesis). These disorders may include immune dysfunction and cardiovascular disease, as well as pregnancy-induced hypertension and low birth weight.

Disruption of endocrine activity at receptors in target organs is another mechanism through which environmental agents can cause health problems in women. Certain chemicals have endocrinologic activity (6, 7). These include industrial chemicals, phytoestrogens produced by plants, and mycoestrogens produced by fungi (Table 26.1). Mechanisms of action of endocrinologically active compounds include antiestrogenic effects, androgenic effects, and effects on other endocrine pathways.

Because research on breast and endometrial cancer has elucidated the mechanisms of action for selective estrogen receptor modulators such as tamoxifen and raloxifene, a parallel field of inquiry is determining specific mechanisms by which endocrinologically active environmental exposures operate at the molecular and cellular levels. Many agents have agonistic interaction with alpha and beta estrogen receptors. Although a few phytoestrogens such as genistein (found in soy) are relatively close in potency to estradiol, most synthetic chemicals with estrogenic properties are at least 1000 times less potent than estradiol (6).

GYNECOLOGIC DISORDERS

Environmental exposures that have been associated with gynecologic disorders in women are shown in Table 26.2. When evaluating the potential impact of an exposure in the workplace or at home, the patient's health history must also be considered. Factors such as maternal age, family history, and others may outweigh the risks of low-level exposure to chemicals or other environmental hazards.

Gynecologic Congenital Anomalies

Uterine malformations are relatively common among women with subfecundity. In a study of 3181 women who underwent hysterosalpingography, 3 to 6% had a uterine anomaly, most commonly a uterine septum (8). Whether environmental chemicals make a major contribution to gynecologic malformations in humans is unknown.

Prenatal exposure to DES causes structural anomalies of the uterus, including hypoplasia of the uterine cavity, uterine corpus, and cervix (9). Because approval for use of DES in pregnancy was withdrawn by the FDA in 1972, DES should not account for uterine anomalies in younger women. Inadvertent in utero exposure of girls to oral contraceptives does not appear to cause congenital malformations.

The amount of research on environmental exposures and human female urogenital abnormalities is limited. Environmental exposures have been associated with congenital anomalies of the urogenital system in animal models in males, although there is no direct evidence that similar exposures cause gynecologic anomalies in females. Phthalates are used to create cellulose plastics and the polymers in certain adhesives, inks, and cosmetics. Hypospadias in male offspring can be induced after in utero exposure to di (n-butyl) phthalate (10). Fungicides are used in agriculture to protect grain seeds and crops such as flowers and berries. The fungicides vinclozolin or procymidone can cause hypospadias or undescended testes in rats (11–13). Reduced penis size in male animal models can be caused by a single gestational dose of the dioxin, 2,3,7,8-tetrachlorodibenzo-p-dioxin (14). Time trend studies have suggested that male genital defect rates may be rising in some Westernized countries, although it is unclear whether this is related to environmental chemicals.

Disorders of Puberty

Concerns about environmental chemicals and puberty are based on a few clusters of premature puberty in girls and on circumstantial evidence from animal studies. Time trend studies in the United States suggest that puberty occurs somewhat earlier among today's children

TABLE 26.2

Selected Gynecologic Effects Associated With Environmental Exposures Among Women

Gynecologic Disorders	Examples of Exposures
Uterine anomalies	DES
Altered puberty	Cranial radiation therapy; possibly phthalate esters
Menstrual disorders	DES, tobacco, 2-bromopropane, intensive exercise, significant psychological stress
	Exposures among oncology nurses, hairdressers
Subfecundity	DES, tobacco, xylene, toluene, formaldehyde, 2-bromopropane, ethylene glycol ethers and other solvents, pesticides, nitrous oxide, mercury, PCBs, intensive job physical demands, shift work
	Exposures among dental hygienists, laboratory technicians, agricultural workers or women employed in semiconductor or electronics manufacturing
Spontaneous abortion	Tobacco, organic solvents (e.g., chloroform, xylene, toluene, methylene chloride), ethylene glycol ethers, formaldehyde, lead and other heavy metals, certain pesticides, antineoplastic or antiviral drugs, waste anesthetic gases, intensive job physical demands, shift work, tap water with high levels of trihalomethanes
	Exposures among laboratory technicians, hairdressers, agricultural workers, certain health care workers, semiconductor manufacturing employees
Ovarian dysfunction	Tobacco, cytotoxic drugs, radiation therapy, 2-bromopropane; possibly metabolic products of DDT, and some of the agents listed previously for subfecundity
Tubal disorders	Tobacco; possibly PCBs, phytoestrogens
Endometriosis	Possibly TCDD
Leiomyoma	Possibly organochlorine pesticides and phytoestrogens
Birth defects	Certain organic solvents, heavy metals, fungicides, herbicides, insecticides, PCBs, ionizing radiation and others
Menopausal disorders	Tobacco; possibly some of the agents listed previously for ovarian dysfunction and subfecundity
Osteoporosis	Tobacco; Possibly lead
Ovarian cancer	Possibly exposures among women in health care, cosmetology, and occupations using polycyclic aromatic hydrocarbons
Breast cancer	Radiation therapy, especially during adolescence; inconsistent findings for PCBs, DDT metabolites, and occupations with pesticide exposure
Endometrial cancer	None
Cervical cancer	Tobacco; possibly exposures in certain industrial and cleaning occupations
Vaginal cancer	DES

DDT, dichlorodiphenyl trichloroethane; DES, diethylstilbestrol; PCB, polychlorinated biphenyl; TCDD, 2,3,7,8-tetrachlorodibenzo-p-dioxin.

than among children in the past. More detailed records from the Netherlands demonstrate that during the past 42 years, the age at menarche decreased by 6 months (15). Improvements in child health and an increasing incidence of childhood obesity are probably related to this trend.

There are relatively few epidemiologic studies that assess the effects of environmental exposures on puberty. One study showed that girls who had modest PCB exposures in the perinatal period (greater than or equal to 4 ppm in maternal fat samples) underwent puberty at the same age as girls with negligible exposure levels (16). In a cluster of girls with premature thelarche in Puerto Rico, phthalate esters were found in the serum of 68% of the cases but only 3% of the controls (17). Animal research shows that accelerated puberty occurs among females after exposure to the phytoestrogen genistein or to the synthetic chemical 4-nonylphenol (18, 19). Cranial radiation for cancer accelerates puberty in girls, although there are no studies assessing whether chemical neurotoxicants accelerate puberty in humans.

Menstrual Disorders

Exposures can result in menstrual disorders through interference with the hypothalamic-pituitary-ovarian axis, destruction of oocytes, or reversible ovarian toxicity. An example of an ovarian toxicant is cigarette smoke, which increases the risk for menstrual disorders in epidemiologic studies (20). In another study, occupational exposure to a solvent containing 2-bromopropane caused ovarian failure and secondary amenorrhea in a group of female workers (21).

Studies of women exposed to solvents such as toluene, dry cleaning agents, and styrene have not found increased rates of menstrual dysfunction, although menstrual disorders have been noted in nurses who handle cytotoxic antineoplastic drugs (22).

Hairdressers who work with disinfectants such as formaldehyde have an increased risk of menstrual disorders in some studies (23). Hairdressers who work only with modern hair dyes are not believed to be at increased risk. Menstrual disorders can also be caused by exposure to substances such as DES in the prenatal period (24). Phytoestrogens in soy products have been associated with increased menstrual cycle length in some studies but not others (25, 26).

Intense physical activity or substantial psychological stress can lead to menstrual disorders and hence can theoretically confound studies of occupational chemical exposures.

Subfecundity

Environmental exposures among women are associated with reductions in overall fecundity rates and with increased rates of common diagnoses related to subfecundity, such as spontaneous abortion and ovarian dysfunction. Male factors contribute to subfecundity in 40% of couples. Table 26.3 lists environmental toxicants related to male fertility problems, spontaneous abortions in female partners of exposed men, and birth defects or preterm birth among the man's children (27–32).

TABLE 26.3

Selected Agents Associated With Male-Mediated Adverse Reproductive Outcomes

Metals
Alkyl mercury, boron, lead (inorganic or tetraethyl), manganese, welding fumes
Solvents
Carbon disulfide, ethylene glycol ethers, solvents involved in painting occupations, styrene and acetone (combined exposure)
Pesticides
Carbaryl, chlordecone, dibromochloropropane
Others
Anesthetic gases, chloroprene, ethylene dibromide

Epidemiologic studies show that women who work with organic solvents (e.g., in biomedical laboratories, in woodworking industries, and in the manufacture of electronics and semiconductors) are at increased risk for subfecundity (33–36). Potentially hazardous solvents and other chemicals include xylene, toluene, formaldehyde, 2-bromopropane, and ethylene glycol ethers. Dental hygienists are at increased risk for fertility problems if they have uncontrolled exposures to mercury or the anesthetic gas nitrous oxide (37, 38). Female agricultural workers have reduced fertility if they have significant exposure to pesticides through spraying and nonuse of gloves (39, 40).

Intensive job physical demands increase the risk for subfecundity and for spontaneous abortions that can lead to subfecundity (41–43). The related ergonomic factors include standing more than 7 hours per shift, rotating shifts, and a high overall score for intensive physical demands.

Some studies of nonworkplace exposures have noted associations with difficulty becoming pregnant. A woman's fecundity is clearly reduced by cigarette smoking (44). Ovarian toxicity can be caused by drugs or radiation exposure when women are treated for autoimmune disorders or cancer. Frequently consuming fish contaminated with PCBs from Lake Ontario was associated with reduced fertility among women in one study (45). Prenatal DES exposure among girls is associated later with a 16% prevalence of primary infertility, compared with a 6% chance in controls (24). Because prenatal DES exposure is no longer occurring, these findings are principally used today to generate hypotheses about whether endocrine-disrupting chemicals could be causing reduced fertility.

Spontaneous Abortion

There is excellent evidence that environmental exposures of particular types and magnitudes cause spontaneous abortion. In the preconception period, occupational studies among men suggest that some miscarriages could be mediated by an exposure-related effect on germ cells, especially if the father works with organic solvents, lead, mercury, welding fumes, or certain pesticides (27, 29, 31). Animal studies show that paternal exposures can reduce litter size, even when the mother is not exposed (27).

Karyotyping of fetal material from miscarriages shows an increased incidence of chromosomal abnormalities that were not present in the parents. Although this is commonly interpreted as a random mistake during cell division, germ cell DNA from the man or woman may also have been affected by an exposure in the distant past or near the time of conception. Tobacco-related chemical additions to DNA remain in lung tissue after cessation of smoking (46). In mice, exposure to butadiene produces concentration-related heritable translocations in germ cells (47). Alcohol exposure to the ovaries in the immediate preconception period can interfere with spindle formation, and this can lead to aneuploidy (48).

Many types of hazardous exposures to pregnant female rodents cause early fetal loss as manifested by fetal resorptions and decreased litter size (27). Women working with organic solvents have an increased risk for miscarriage, especially if exposure levels are high enough to cause mucous membrane irritation or headaches (49, 50). Some of these solvents are commonly used, including xylene, toluene, methylene chloride, perchloroethylene, chloroform, and others (27, 29, 49, 51). Women with solvent-intensive semiconductor manufacturing jobs who also have exposures to ethylene glycol ethers are at increased risk for spontaneous abortions (36). Formaldehyde, used in manufacturing and as a disinfectant by health care workers and hairdressers, also increases the risk of miscarriage if exposure levels are uncontrolled (23, 34).

Maternal lead exposure increases the risk of spontaneous abortions, as do other heavy metals. Women agricultural workers who use certain pesticides are at increased risk (52). Personnel working in operating rooms that are not properly ventilated, and nurses or pharmacists who handle cytotoxic and antiviral medications without using proper safety procedures are at increased risk (53, 54).

Ionizing radiation shortly after conception was embryo-toxic among atomic bomb survivors, presumably causing subclinical miscarriages. In animal studies, the dose required to cause early fetal loss exceeds the occupational exposure limit by a large margin. Electromagnetic fields from personal computers do not increase the risk for spontaneous abortion (55).

Intensive physical job demands such as standing for more than 7 hours per shift increase the risk for spontaneous abortion, especially among women who have a history of previous spontaneous abortions (43). Shift work is also an independent risk factor in most studies (41, 42).

Lower-level environmental exposures outside the workplace have also been associated with increased rates of spontaneous abortion, although few of these studies have been conducted, and the results have been contradictory. Chlorinated drinking water obtained from surface sources (e.g., lakes) contains trihalomethanes; high levels of these contaminants were associated with increased risk for miscarriage in some studies (56). Maximum allowable concentrations of trihalomethanes in municipal drinking water have now been lowered to a level below the apparent threshold for miscarriage. In a small study from China, increased maternal serum levels of metabolites of DDT were found in women who had a miscarriage compared with full-term controls (57).

Ovarian Dysfunction

In animal models, ovarian toxicity occurs after exposure of adult females to many compounds. TCDD appears to cause ovarian dysfunction through depletion of androstenedione and induction of apoptotic cell death (7). Women who suffered ovarian failure from workplace exposure to 2-bromopropane had reduced ovarian follicle numbers and developmental arrest of the follicles (21). Low levels of persistent pollutants such as DDE (a metabolite of DDT) have been found in samples of follicular fluid and may reduce fertilization rates among women undergoing in vitro fertilization (58).

Cigarette smoking induces ovarian dysfunction that is not entirely reversible (44). Radiation exposure at high doses can cause toxic effects to the ovary not only during adult life, but also during fetal life. In one study, pregnant female rats were exposed to 1.5 Gy of gamma irradiation (59). The female offspring that were exposed in utero had a substantial reduction in the number of oocytes. These offspring had normal puberty and fertility at the beginning of reproductive life but had decreased fertility due to premature ovarian failure later in life. Some chemicals (e.g., dioxins) given to rats can also reduce the number of antral follicles in female offspring exposed in utero (60). Due to the length of required follow-up, there are almost no studies like this in humans. The cohort studies of women exposed to DES in utero suggest that most of their fertility problems are related to uterine anomalies rather than ovarian dysfunction.

Tubal Disorders

There is thus some suggestion that environmental exposures could contribute to tubal infertility, although research on exposures other than tobacco is limited. Tobacco smoke slows embryo transport in the oviducts of hamsters and alters the oviduct epithelium in mice. Also, smoking is a risk factor for ectopic pregnancy in women.

PCBs alter fallopian tube structure in rats. Phytoestrogens such as genistein stimulate leukemia inhibitory factor in human oviduct cells, which could adversely affect embryo implantation (61).

Endometriosis

Endometriosis is induced in a dose-dependent manner among monkeys exposed to TCDD, although the exposure levels are higher than those typically found among women (62). Human studies, however, are inconsistent. Two studies show that infertile women with endometriosis have higher serum TCDD levels than women with tubal infertility (statistically significant in only one of the studies), whereas another study found similar plasma TCDD levels in women with endometriosis compared with a variety of control women (63–65). The amount of TCDD in tampons is six orders of magnitude lower than exposures from food (66).

Smoking appears to reduce the risk for endometriosis, probably through effects on estrogen metabolism (44).

Leiomyoma

Kepone and endosulfan, two endocrinologically active organochlorine pesticides, promote the growth of leiomyoma cell lines derived from Eker rats (67). Endosulfan also displays agonist activity in uterine myometrium, as do the phytoestrogens coumestrol, genistein, and naringin (68).

No epidemiologic studies are available for these exposures, although smokers are less likely to have uterine fibroids (44).

Birth Defects

A huge number of agents have been tested for teratogenicity, and many of these have been positive in at least one animal species. A number of these relationships have been confirmed in human studies. A complete review of chemical teratogenicity is beyond the scope of this chapter. Among the agents of concern, significant human exposures are most common for the organic solvents, heavy metals, and pesticides (27, 49, 50, 69).

Organic solvents are used during manufacturing processes, industrial cleaning applications, health care, and a wide variety of other occupational settings or hobby activities. Examples of teratogens include acetaldehyde, formamide, glycol ethers (e.g., ethylene glycol monomethyl ether), methanol, methyl pyrrolidone, tetrachloroacetone, toluene and others. Metals demonstrating teratogenicity in animal studies include lead acetate and lead nitrate, organic mercury compounds (e.g., methylmercury), cadmium chloride, chromium trioxide, nickel carbonyl, and others. Pesticides demonstrating teratogenicity in animal studies include the fungicides, benomyl and thiram, the herbicides 2.4-D and dinoseb, and the insecticides aldrin, chlorfenvinphos, dieldrin, methyl parathion, phosmet, toxaphene, and trichlorfon. Examples of other teratogenic exposures include ionizing radiation at relatively high doses, and PCBs. Prenatal exposure to PCBs is associated with mild neurodevelopmental effects in children (70).

Menopausal Disorders

Environmental exposures that cause ovarian dysfunction can lead to premature ovarian failure and early menopause. Thus far, the only well-established toxicants that cause this problem are anticancer drugs and cigarette smoke, although few studies have investigated this issue (71).

Osteoporosis

Environmental exposure to toxicants that interfere with bone calcium or vitamin D metabolism could theoretically increase a woman's risk for osteoporosis later in life. Lead affects vitamin D metabolism in humans; lead also affects the function of both osteoblasts and osteoclasts in experimental systems. Calcium homeostasis in bone can be disrupted by hexachlorobenzene, aluminum, and cadmium. There is no research available to indicate whether these exposures are clinically important in the development of osteoporosis. Higher serum DDT levels were correlated with bone lower mineral density in some studies (72) but not in others (73). Smoking is a risk factor for osteoporosis.

Cancer

Ovarian Cancer

Ovarian cancer rates are increased in several occupations that entail intensive exposure to disinfectants, antineoplastic drugs, polycyclic aromatic hydrocarbon solvents, and other chemicals that affect ovarian reproductive function. These occupations include health care and cosmetology (74–76). Maternal use of hormone therapy during pregnancy was associated with a 3.6-fold increase in the risk of ovarian germ cell cancer in their daughters in one case-control study (77). The hormonal therapy included treatment of the mothers with DES or other supportive hormones and inadvertent use of oral contraceptives. This hypothesized relationship has not been assessed in other populations, and no studies of ovarian cancer rates after exposure to synthetic or plant-derived endocrinologically active agents were located.

Breast Cancer

Breast cancer risk increases with earlier age at menarche and estrogen receptor status is intimately related to prognosis, highlighting the potential role of endogenous estrogens in this disease. Data are inconsistent on whether breast cancer risk is affected by exposure to exogenous estrogenic compounds. Phytoestrogens may exert a protective effect (78). Some studies have suggested that women in occupations with pesticide contact are at increased risk for breast cancer, although other studies do not confirm this. A group of investigators found that PCB and DDE levels in breast adipose tissue were associated with estrogen receptor-negative breast cancer (79). A number of well-controlled research investigations have found no increase in organochlorine levels among women with breast cancer compared with women without breast cancer (3, 80).

Future studies may evaluate environmental exposures during adolescence, a critical period for breast development. Radiation treatment at 10 to 14 years of age creates a greater risk for breast cancer than receiving this treatment at later ages (81).

Tobacco, a weak risk factor for premenopausal breast cancer, appears to convey higher risk for those who began smoking at a young age (82).

Endometrial Cancer

Prenatal DES exposure induces uterine adenocarcinomas in mice. Although unopposed estrogen therapy increases risk for endometrial cancer, endocrinologically active PCBs and chlorinated pesticides appear to have no effect. In case-control studies, women with endometrial cancer do not have higher serum concentrations of these organochlorine chemicals (83, 84). Endometrial cancer rates are lower in smokers, consistent with an antiestrogen effect of tobacco smoke (44).

Cervical Cancer

Cervical cancer risk is increased among smokers, suggesting that smoke-related toxicants entering the body can act as cocarcinogens with human papilloma virus. Rates of cervical cancer are also increased among printers, typesetters, manufacturing workers, maids, and cleaners (74, 85). Organic solvents that may be used in some of these occupations are carcinogens (e.g., benzene, carbon tetrachloride, formaldehyde). The cervical cancer studies were not able to measure specific occupational exposures to ascertain whether organic solvents could have functioned as cocarcinogens.

Vaginal Cancer

Vaginal clear cell adenocarcinoma is a well-known sequela of prenatal DES exposure. In utero exposure to bisphenol A causes nonmalignant morphologic changes in the vagina of rats (86). No other in utero exposure studies of endocrinologically active compounds were located.

PATIENT MANAGEMENT

Our goal should be to help the patient (and her partner in preconception and infertility counseling) to make an informed decision about risks in the setting of limited information and to achieve as low an exposure level as possible. Accomplishing this while not placing undue burdens on patients or causing unnecessary alarm is challenging but achievable.

Estimating Exposure Levels

"The dose makes the poison," so it is crucial to determine if exposure levels are high, low, or negligible. Workplace exposure levels can be estimated through the occupational and environmental history. This process can be expedited by having the patient record potential exposures and work procedures and bring them to the office visit. Examples of such forms have been published, and a patient questionnaire as shown in Figure 26.1 can be used to supplement the clinician's history (27). Clues that workplace exposure levels are high include frequent use of large quantities of a chemical, inhalation (of vapors, aerosols, or dust), skin contact, lack of protective equipment,

Occupational and Environmental History

Please help us by finding out the following information.
Fill out this form and bring it to your clinic visit.

Name:	Date:	Clinic ID #:
Job Title:	Work Area:	Employer:

A. Are you worried that your job or home is unsafe? NO YES
If yes, please describe:

B. Chemicals

Chemical Names List chemicals to which you may be exposed. Obtain chemical names from labels or Material Safety Data Sheets. Don't list abbreviations or brand names. Attach extra pages to this form, if needed.	**How Often** Do you come in contact with the chemical—daily, weekly, monthly, rarely?	**How Much** Are you around a large or small amount of the chemical?	**Protective Equipment** When you are around the chemical, do you use gloves, special clothing, or a mask?

Do you ever get chemicals on your skin?	NO	YES
Have there been any chemical spills lately?	NO	YES
Has a safety professional inspected your work area?	NO	YES
Can you wash up before eating or going home?	NO	YES
Was your home built before 1946?	NO	YES
Is your home under construction?	NO	YES

C. Are you exposed to infections or radiation? NO YES
If yes, please describe:

D. Physical demands of your work:
Standing: ___ hours per shift
Lifting: ___ lb How often?
Shift length: ___ hours
Shift rotations (day/night, etc.): NO/YES

E. Your partner's occupation: ______________________
Is he exposed to chemicals or radiation? NO YES
If yes, please complete a form for him.
Does he smoke? NO YES Do you smoke? NO YES

F. Is there anything else you want to discuss?

FIGURE 26.1 ● Patient questionnaire for identifying and recording potential occupational and environmental exposures.

and lack of access to washing facilities. Latex gloves are good for handling blood and body fluids but are a poor barrier against organic solvents and many other chemicals.

The contrast between a negligible exposure level and a moderate to high exposure level is suggested by the following examples:

- Wearing clothing that has been dry cleaned versus unloading clothing from machines 8 hours a day in a dry cleaning plant
- Living in a home built in the 1960s versus sanding or using a heat gun to remove paint while renovating a home built in the 1940s
- Inhaling solvent vapors while using a small amount of rubber cement versus degreasing parts for 8 hours a day in an open vat at a manufacturing facility
- Occasionally using a permethrin mosquito repellent versus spraying fungicides on greenhouse plants all day while wearing street clothing and latex gloves
- Mixing cytotoxic drugs in a properly functioning biological safety cabinet while wearing impervious gloves versus mixing these drugs in a clinic without protective equipment

In each case, the exposure level in the second scenario would be substantially higher.

Exposure levels in workplace air, food, or water samples, or in household dust, can be measured precisely, although physicians often do not have access to this information. Lead was banned from interior paints in 1978, so the older the home, the more likely that lead exposure could occur. The local health department may be able to assess a patient's home for serious contamination with lead. Commonly available laboratory tests can be used to measure recent exposures to lead or other heavy metals; they can also measure inhibition of cholinesterase by organophosphate or carbamate pesticides. Biological fluids and tissues can also be tested for other types of exposures, although the patient may need to be sent to an occupational health clinic that is experienced in collecting these specimens. Many compounds are rapidly metabolized, so the test must be done while exposure is still occurring.

Finding Data From the Literature

Chemical components of products used in the workplace can be identified from labels and material safety data sheets. Although material safety data sheets have a section on health effects, this information is often incomplete and outdated. Data on reproductive effects may be omitted. Textbooks devoted to reproductive hazards, teratogens, or occupational and environmental medicine are useful to scan for information on compounds to which the patient or her partner may be exposed. When data in textbooks are missing or equivocal, a literature search can ascertain if there are new data since the books went to press.

Websites of the EPA (www.epa.gov), the National Institute for Occupational Safety and Health (www.cdc.gov/niosh), and the Agency for Toxic Substances and Disease Registry (ATSDR) (www.atsdr.cdc.gov) provide information on hazardous effects of environmental exposures. On the ATSDR website, the "Frequently Asked Questions" and "Case Studies" sections are particularly useful.

Poison control centers have a number of computerized databases on hand and are glad to assist clinicians in evaluating the literature on a patient's exposures. As of 2003, there is a nationwide number for access to the 62 U.S. poison control centers. The number, 1-800-222-1222, is functional in all 50 states, the District of Columbia, the U.S. Virgin Islands, and Puerto Rico, and routes the caller to their local poison center.

Counseling the Patient

After talking with the patient and searching the literature for additional information, the clinician will need to make a decision. Often, there will be significant limitations in health effects data. Because the stakes are high for each patient, we should be cautious about reassuring her that an exposure is probably safe just because there are no studies proving it otherwise. Animal research does not approximate human responses 100% of the time, and epidemiologic population-based studies may not be entirely generalizable to an individual patient's situation. Also, her estimates of exposure levels may be imprecise.

History also confirms the need to be cautious. Regulatory limits on occupational and environmental exposures have been repeatedly lowered as new evidence became available. For example, the occupational exposure limit for ethylene glycol monomethyl ether was 100 ppm in 1946, which is now considered much too high; today, the limit is as low as 1 ppm in some countries. It is reasonable to conclude that many of today's occupational and environmental exposure limits will be further lowered in the future as new evidence becomes available.

If a patient already has a gynecologic disorder and she wants to know if an exposure caused it, placing her environmental exposures in the context of her medical risk factors is warranted. The patient should be informed of the main strengths and limitations of available information about her exposures. Evaluation of a woman with subfecundity or spontaneous abortions should include a review of exposures in her partner. It can be misleading to think of a chemical as either good or bad because the exposure dose and interactions with other risk factors determines the risk for health effects.

When the goal of counseling is to prevent a future health problem such as subfecundity, spontaneous abortion, or an adverse fetal effect, counseling should begin at a young age—during a woman's late teens and early twenties. The clinical assessment should include a history of workplace or environmental exposures, such as those shown in Table 26.2, that may increase the risk of subfecundity and spontaneous abortion. Preconception counseling should also emphasize the rapid pace of embryonic development in the first few weeks of pregnancy. Exposure to occupational or environmental hazards that have been linked to birth defects should be stopped in the preconception period because birth defects can occur before the woman confirms that she is pregnant.

Genetic predisposition, parental age, certain infections, poorly controlled diabetes mellitus, nutritional deficiency, and substance abuse are risk factors for birth defects that often outweigh risks from low-level chemical exposures. A number of pharmaceuticals are known or suspected teratogens, or may cause fetal health problems later in pregnancy (see Appendix 26.1). Risk from these agents varies depending on the dose or the gestational timing of exposure. Agents classified as pregnancy Categories B or C that are not listed in Appendix 26.1 may also convey fetal risk. To make a clinical decision about a drug, risks must be weighed against benefits, and more detailed information from the manufacturer and other sources should be reviewed (69, 87). The large number of drugs ranked as pregnancy Category D or X illustrates the importance of reviewing the patient's medications as part of the process of placing occupational or environmental exposures into context.

Occupational or environmental exposures may also increase risk for problems later in pregnancy, such as pre-eclampsia and preterm birth. Some of these exposures are the same ones that can lead to subfecundity, spontaneous abortion, or birth defects.

If a patient has potential exposures in the workplace, she can be more scrupulous about her work practices and take advantage of information and safety training that is offered. She can find out information about her benefits and the availability of transfers within the company. If the workplace is hostile to these efforts and the exposures are significant, she may need to postpone a pregnancy or look for another job.

If she lives in a city, the municipal water supplier is required to provide her with information on any contaminants in her tap water that are subject to regulations. She can use the student sections of the EPA website listed previously to find out about topics, including pollutants in food. A varied and balanced diet is good not only because it provides an array of nutrients, but also because it limits intake of particular foods that may contain pollutants. Both the EPA and the FDA advise pregnant women to limit their consumption of cooked fish to an average of 12 oz per week because of contamination with mercury and chlorinated compounds (a typical serving is 3 to 6 oz). Because fish that are high in the food chain accumulate higher levels of pollutants, pregnant women should avoid consumption of these fish entirely: shark, swordfish, king mackerel, and tile fish. Although the advisory does not discuss preconception health, it seems reasonable to take the same precautions when planning a pregnancy.

Clinical Notes

- Environmental exposures can cause subfecundity, spontaneous abortions, and birth defects.
- Chemicals that can cause these problems include substantial exposures to solvents, some disinfectants, heavy metals such as lead, certain pesticides, cytotoxic drugs, waste anesthetic gases, mercury, and other contaminants in fish, trihalomethanes in tap water, and others.
- Exposures must be at a sufficient dose to cause a problem.
- Intensive job physical demands and shift work also increase risk for subfecundity and spontaneous abortion.
- Higher-risk occupations include certain health care workers, hairdressers or cosmetologists, dental hygienists, laboratory technicians, agricultural workers, manufacturing workers, and others. If exposures are well controlled, however, women in these jobs are not at risk.
- Mechanisms of action include disruption of endocrine activity at target organs, suppression of the hypothalamic-pituitary axis, interference with genes or chromosomes, and cumulative destruction of oocytes. Fetal programming may play a role.
- Ovarian toxicity can cause early menopause.
- Environmental exposures are suspected as etiologic agents in premature puberty, endometriosis, breast cancer, and other gynecologic disorders, but data are not certain.
- Most synthetic chemicals with estrogenic properties are at least 1000 times less potent than estradiol.
- Assessment of occupational and environmental exposures is an essential component of preconception counseling.
- Male environmental exposures should be considered when evaluating infertile couples or counseling women about preconception health.
- Exposure dose is very important, and can be estimated through the occupational and environmental history.
- Regulatory exposure limits are not always protective.
- Clues that workplace exposure levels are high include use of large quantities of a chemical, inhalation (of vapors, aerosols, or dust), skin contact, lack of protective equipment, and lack of access to washing facilities.
- Laboratory tests can be used to measure recent exposures to certain agents such as heavy metals and cholinesterase-inhibiting pesticides.
- Tests for other types of exposures are available through an occupational medicine specialty clinic or research laboratory.
- Because the stakes are high for the patient and the research database is limited, be cautious about reassuring women that an exposure is probably safe.

APPENDIX 26.1

Potential Fetal Risks From Pharmaceuticals: Selected Drugs Ranked as Pregnancy Category D or X

Anti-Infectives:

Amebicides
Carbarsone (D)

Aminogylcosides
Amikacin (C; D per manufacturer)
Kanamycin (D)
Tobramycin (C; D per manufacturer)

Antimalarials
Quinine (D; X per manufacturer)

Iodine
Iodine (D)
Ovidone-Iodine (D)

Sulfonamides
Sulfasalazine (B; D near term)
Sulfonamides (B; D near term)

Tetracyclines
Chlortetracycline (D)
Clomocycline (D)
Demeclocycline (D)
Doxycycline (D)
Methacycline (D)
Minocycline (D)
Oxytetracycline (D)
Tetracycline (D)

Urinary Germicides
Methylene Blue (D)

Antilipemic Agents
Fluvastatin (X)
Lovastatin (X)
Pravastatin (X)
Simvastatin (X)

Antineoplastics
Aminopterin (X)
Azathioprine (D)
Bleomycin (D)
Busulfan (D)
Cisplatin (D)
Chlorambucil (D)
Cyclophosphamide (D)
Cytarabine (D)
Daunorubicin (D)
Doxorubicin (D)
Etoposide (D)
Fluorouracil (D)
Hydroxyurea (D)
Idarubicin (D)
Leuprolide (X)
Mechlorethamine (D)
Melphalan (D)
Mercaptopurine (D)
Methotrexate (D)
Mitoxantrone (D)
Plicamycin or Mithramycin (D)
Procarbazine (D)
Tamoxifen (D)
Teniposide (D)
Thioguanine (D)
Thiotepa (D)
Tretinoin (Systemic) (D)
Vinblastine (D)
Vincristine (D)

Autonomics

Sympatholytics
Acebutolol (B; D second and third trimesters)
Atenolol (D)
Betaxolol (C; D second and third trimesters)
Bisoprolol (C; D second and third trimesters)
Carteolol (C; D second and third trimesters)
Ergotamine (D)
Labetalol (C; D second and third trimesters)
Mepindolol (C; D second and third trimesters)
Metoprolol (C; D second and third trimesters)
Nadolol (C; D second and third trimesters)
Oxprenolol (C; D second and third trimesters)
Penbutolol (C; D second and third trimesters)
Pindolol (B; D second and third trimesters)
Propranolol (C; D second and third trimesters)
Sotalol (B; D second and third trimesters)
Timolol (C; D second and third trimesters)

Sympathomimetics (adrenergic)
Cocaine (X)
Levarterenol (D)
Metaraminol (D)

Cardiovascular drugs

Antihypertensives

1. Angiotensin-Converting Enzyme Inhibitors
Benazepril (C first trimester; D second and third trimesters)
Captopril (C first trimester; D second and third trimesters)

Enalapril (C first trimester; D second and third trimesters)
Fosinopril (C first trimester; D second and third trimesters)
Lisinopril (C first trimester; D second and third trimesters)
Quinapril (C first trimester; D second and third trimesters)
Ramipril (C first trimester; D second and third trimesters)

2. Other antihypertensives

Acebutolol (B; D second and third trimesters)
Atenolol (D)
Betaxolol (C; D second and third trimesters)
Bisoprolol (C; D second and third trimesters)
Carteolol (C; D second and third trimesters)
Celiprolol (B; D second and third trimesters)
Irbesartan (C first trimester; D second and third trimesters)
Labetalol (C first trimester; D second and third trimesters)
Losartin (C first trimester; D second and third trimesters)
Mepindolol (C; D second and third trimesters)
Metoprolol (C; D second and third trimesters)
Nadolol (C; D second and third trimesters)
Oxprenolol (C; D second and third trimesters)
Penbutolol (C; D second and third trimesters)
Pindolol (B; D second and third trimesters)
Propranolol (C; D second and third trimesters)
Sotalol (B; D second and third trimesters)
Timolol (C; D second and third trimesters)

Antiarrythmic agents

Amiodarone (D)

Central Nervous System Drugs

Analgesics and antipyretics

Aspirin (C in low dose (< 150 mg/day; D in standard dose)
Propoxyphene (C; D if used for prolonged periods)

Anticonvulsants

Aminoglutethimide (D)
Bromides (D)
Carbamazepine (D)
Clonazepam (D)
Divalproex (D)
Ethotoin (D)
Mephobarbital (D)
Paramethadione (D)
Phenobarbital (D)
Phensuximide (D)
Phenytoin (D)
Primidone (D)
Trimethadione (D)
Valproic acid (D)

Antidepressants

Amitriptyline (D)
Butriptyline (D)
Dibenzepin (D)
Dothiepin (D)
Imipramine (D)
Iprindole (D)
Nortriptyline (D)
Opipramol (D)

Antimigraine agents

Ergotamine (D)

Hallucinogens

Phencyclidine (X)

Narcotic Analgesics (*all narcotics may produce withdrawal syndrome in neonates with prolonged use)

Alfentanil (D)
Alphaprodine (D)
Anileridine (D)
Butorphanol (D)
Codeine (D)
Dihydrocodeine Bitartrate (D)
Fentanyl (D)
Heroin (D)
Hydrocodone (D)
Hydromorphone (D)
Levorphanol (D)
Meperidine (D)
Methadone (D)
Morphine (D)
Nalbuphine (D)
Opium (D)
Oxcodone (D)
Oxymorphone (D)
Pentazocine (D)
Phenazocine (D)

Narcotic antagonists

Cyclazocine (D)
Levallorphan (D)
Nalorphine (D)

Nonsteroidal anti-inflammatory drugs

Diclofenac (D in third trimester or near delivery)
Diflunisal (D in third trimester or near delivery)
Etodolac (D in third trimester or near delivery)
Fenoprofen (D in third trimester or near delivery)
Flurbiprofen (D in third trimester or near delivery)
Ibuprofen (D in third trimester or near delivery)
Indomethacin (D in third trimester or near delivery)
Ketoprofen (D in third trimester or near delivery)
Ketorolac (D in third trimester or near delivery)
Meclofenamate (D in third trimester or near delivery)
Mefanamic acid (D in third trimester or near delivery)
Nabumetone (D in third trimester or near delivery)
Naproxen (D in third trimester or near delivery)
Oxaprozin (D in third trimester or near delivery)

Phenylbutazone (D in third trimester or near delivery)
Piroxicam (D in third trimester or near delivery)
Sulindac (D in third trimester or near delivery)
Tolmetin (D in third trimester or near delivery)

Sedatives and Hypnotics

Alprazolam (D)
Amobarbital (D)
Bromides (D)
Butalbital (D)
Chlordiazepoxide (D)
Clorazepate (D)
Diazepam (D)
Ethanol (D/X)
Flunitrazepam (D)
Flurazepam (X)
Lorazepam (D)
Mephobarbital (D)
Meprobamate (D)
Methaqualone (D)
Metharbital (D)
Middazolam (D)
Oxazepam (D)
Pentobarbital (D)
Phenobarbital (D)
Quazepam (X)
Secobarbital (D)
Temazepam (X)
Triazolam (X)

Tranquilizers

Lithium (D)

Chelating agents

Pencillamine (D)

Coagulants and anticoagulants

Anticoagulants

Anisindione (D)
Coumarin derivatives (D/X)
Dicumarol (D)
Diphenadione (D)
Ethyl biscoumacetate (D)
Nicoumalone (D)
Phenidione (D)
Phenprocoumon (D)
Warfarin (D)

Diagnostic agents

Diatrozoate (D)
Ethiodized oil (D)
Gallium-69 (X)
Iocetamic acid (D)
Iodamide (D)
Iodipamide (D)
Iodoxamate (D)
Iopanoic acid (D)
Iothalamate (D)
Ipodate (D)
Methylene blue (D)
Metrizamide (D)
Metrizoate (D)
Technetium-99m (X)
Tyropanoate (D)

Diuretics

Bendroflumethiazide (D)
Benzthiazide (D)
Bumetanide (D)
Chlorothiazide (D)
Chlorthalidone (D)
Cyclopenthiazide (D)
Cyclothiazide (D)
Ethacrynic acid (D)
Hydrochlorothiazide (D)
Hydroflumethiazide (D)
Indapamide (D)
Methyclothiazide (D)
Metolazone (D)
Polythiazide (D)
Quinethazone (D)
Sprionolactone (D)
Triamterene (D)
Trichlormethiazide (D)

Gastrointestinal agents

Antidiarrheals

Opium (D)
Paregoric (D)

Anti-inflammatory bowel disease agents

Sulfasalizine (D)

Gallstone solubilizing agents

Chenodiol (X)

Hormones

Adrenal

Cortisone (D)

Androgen

Danazol (D)

Antiestrogen

Tamoxifen (D)

Antiprogestogen

Mifepristone (X)

Antithyroid

Carbimazole (D)
Methimazole (D)
Propylthiouracil (D)
Sodium Iodide I^{131} or I^{125} (X)

Estrogens

Chlorotrianisene (X)
Clomiphene (X)
Dienestrol (X)
Diethylsti8lbestrol (X)
Estradiol (X)
Esttrogens, conjugated (X)
Estrone (X)
Ethinyl estradiol (X)
Mestranol (X)
Oral contraceptives (X)

Pituitary

Leuprolide (X)

Progestogens

Ethisterone (X)
Ethynodiol (X)
Hydroxyprogesterone (X)
Lynestrenol (X)
Medroxyprogesterone (X)
Norethindrone (X)
Norethynodrel (X)
Norgestrel (X)
Oral contraceptives (X)

Immunosuppressant agents

Azathioprine (D)

Radiopharmaceuticals

Sodium Iodide I^{125} (X)
Sodium Iodide I^{131} (X)

Respiratory drugs

Antitussives

Codeine (C; but D if used for prolonged periods or in high doses at term)
Hydrocodone (C; but D if used for prolonged periods or in high doses at term)

Expectorants

Hydriodic acid (D)
Iodinated glycerol (X)
Potassium iodide (D)
Sodium iodide (D)
Terpin hydrate (D)

Vaccines

Measles (X)
Rubella (X)
Smallpox (X)
TC-83 Venezuelan equine encephalitis (X)
Yellow fever (D)

Toxin

Ciguatoxin (X)

Vitamins

Calcifediol (D in high doses)
Calcitirol (D in high doses)
Cholecalciferol (D in high doses)
Dihydrotachysterol (D in high doses)
Ergocalciferol (D in high doses)
Etretinate (X)
Isotretinoin (X)
Menadione (X)
Tretinoin (systemic) (D)
Vitamin A (X in high doses)
Vitamin D (D in high doses)

Miscellaneous

Colchicine (D)
Electricity (D)

REFERENCES

1. Melnick R, Lucier G, Wolfe M, et al. Summary of the National Toxicology Program's report of the endocrine disruptors low-dose peer review. Environ Health Perspect 2002;110:427–431.
2. Adgate JL, Kukowski A,. Stroebel C, et al. Pesticide storage and use patterns in Minnesota households with children. J Expo Anal Environ Epidemiol 2000;10:159–167.
3. Laden F, Hankinson SE, Wolf MS, et al. Plasma organochlorine levels and the risk of breast cancer: an extended follow-up in the Nurse's Health Study. Int J Cancer 2001;91:568–574.
4. Heberer T. Occurrence, fate, and removal of pharmaceutical residues in the aquatic environment: a review of recent research data. Toxicol Lett 2002;131:5–17.
5. Howe SR, Borodinsky L. Potential exposure to bisphenol A from food-contact use of polycarbonate resins. Food Addit Contam 1998;15:370–375.
6. Kuiper GG, Lemmen JG, Carlsson G, et al. Interaction of estrogenic chemicals and phytoestrogens with estrogen receptor beta. Endocrinology 1998;139:4252–4263.
7. Heimler I, Rawlins RG, Owen H, et al. Dioxin perturbs, in dose- and time-dependent fashion, steroid secretion, and induces apoptosis of human luteinized granulosa cells. Endocrinology 1998;139:4373–4379.
8. Raga F, Bauset C, Remohi J, et al. Reproductive impact of congenital Müllerian anomalies. Hum Reprod 1997;12:2277–2281.
9. Van Gils AP, Tham RT, Falke TH, et al. Abnormalities of the uterus and cervix after diethylstilbestrol exposure: correlation of findings on MR and hysterosalpingography. AJR Am J Roentgenol 1989;153:1235–1238.
10. Mylchreest E, Wallace DG, Cattley RC, et al. Dose-dependent alterations in androgen-regulated male reproductive development in rats exposed to di (n-butyl) phthalate during late gestation. Toxicol Sci 2000;55:143–151.
11. Gray LE JR, Ostby J, Monosson E, et al. Environmental antiandrogens: low doses of the fungicide vinclozolin alter sexual differentiation of the male rat. Toxicol Ind Health 1999;15:48–64.
12. Ostby J, Kelce WR, Lambright C, et al. The fungicide procymidone alters sexual differentiation in the male rat by acting as an androgen-receptor antagonist in vivo and in vitro. Toxicol Ind Health 1999;15:80–93.
13. Wolf CJ, LeBlanc GA, Ostby JS, et al. Characterization of the period of sensitivity of fetal male sexual development to vinclozolin. Toxicol Sci 2000;55:152–161.
14. Gray LE, Ostby JS, Kelce WR. A dose-response analysis of the reproductive effects of a single gestational dose of 2, 3, 7, 8-tetrachlorodibenzo-p-dioxin in male Long Evans hooded rat offspring. Toxicol Appl Pharmacol 1997;146:11–20.
15. Fredriks AM, van Buuren S, Burgmeijer RJ, et al. Continuing positive secular growth change in the Netherlands, 1955–1997. Pediatr Res 2000;47:316–323.
16. Gladen BC, Ragan NB, Rogan WJ. Pubertal growth and development and prenatal and lactational exposure to polychlorinated biphenyls and dichlorodiphenyl dichloroethane. J Pediatr 2000;136:490–496.
17. Colon I, Caro D, Bourdony CJ, et al. Identification of phthalate esters in the serum of young Puerto Rican girls with premature breast development. Environ Health Perspect 2000;198:895–900.
18. Casanova M, You L, Gaido KW, et al. Developmental effects of dietary phytoestrogens in Sprague-Dawley rats and interactions of genistein and daidzein with rat estrogen receptors alpha and beta in vitro. Toxicol Sci 1999;51:236–244.
19. Chapin RE, Delaney J, Wang Y, et al. The effects of 4-nonylphenol in rats: a multigeneration reproduction study. Toxicol Sci 1999;52:80–91.
20. Windham GC, Elkin EP, Swan SH, et al. Cigarette smoking and effects on menstrual function. Obstet Gynecol 1999;93:59–65.
21. Koh JM, Kim CH, Hong SK, et al. Primary ovarian failure caused by a solvent containing 2-bromopropane. Eur J Endocrinol 1998;138:554–6.
22. Shortridge LA, Lemasters GK, Valanis B et al. Menstrual cycles in nurses handling antineoplastic drugs. Cancer Nurs 1995;18:439–444.
23. Kersemaekers WM, Roeleveld N, Zeilhuis GA. Reproductive disorders due to chemical exposures among hairdressers. Scand J Work Environ Health 1995;21:325–334.
24. Herbst AL, Hubby MM, Azizi F, et al. Reproductive and gynecologic surgical experience in diethylstilbestrol-exposed daughters. Am J Obstet Gynecol 1981;141:1019–1028.
25. Watanbe S, Terashima K, Sato Y, et al. Effects of isoflavone supplement on healthy women. Biofactors 2000;12:133–141.
26. Strom BL, Shcinnar R, Ziegler EE, et al. Exposure to soy-based formula in infancy and endocrinologic and reproductive outcomes in young adulthood. JAMA 2001;286:807–814.
27. Frazier LM, Hage ML. Reproductive hazards of the workplace. New York: Wiley, 1998.
28. Baranski B. Effects of the workplace on fertility and related reproductive outcomes. Environ Health Perspect 1993;101(suppl 2):81–90.
29. Lindbohm ML, Hemminki K, Bonhomme MG, et al. Effects of paternal occupational exposure on spontaneous abortions. Am J Public Health 1991;81:1029–1033
30. Kristensen P, Irgens LM, Daltveit AK, et al. Perinatal outcome among children of men exposed to lead and organic solvents in the printing industry. Am J Epidemiol 1993;137:134–144.
31. Blatter BM, Hermens R, Bakker M, et al. Paternal occupational exposure around conception and spina bifida in offspring. Am J Ind Med 1997;32:283–291.
32. Lindbohm ML. Effects of parental exposure to solvents on pregnancy outcome. J Occup Environ Med 1995;37:908–914.

33. Wennborg H, Bodin L, Vainio H, et al. Solvent use and time to pregnancy among female personnel in biomedical laboratories in Sweden. Occup Environ Med 2001;58:225–231.
34. Taskinen HK, Kyyronen P, Sallmen M, et al. Reduced fertility among female wood workers exposed to formaldehyde. Am J Ind Med 1999;36:206–212.
35. Chen PC, Hsieh GY, Wang JD, et al. Prolonged time to pregnancy in female workers exposed to ethylene glycol ethers in semiconductor manufacturing. Epidemiology 2002;13:191–196.
36. Correa A, Gray RH, Cohen R, et al. Ethylene glycol ethers and risk of spontaneous abortion and subfertility. Am J Epidemiol 1996;143:707–717.
37. Rowland AS, Baird DD, Weinberg CR, et al. Reduced fertility among women employed as dental assistants exposed to high levels of nitrous oxide. N Engl J Med 1992;327:993–997.
38. Rowland AS, Baird DD, Weinberg CR, et al. The effect of occupational exposure to mercury vapor on the fertility of female dental assistants. Occup Environ Med 1994;51:28–34.
39. Abell A, Juul S, Bonde JP. Time to pregnancy among female greenhouse workers. Scand J Work Environ Health 2000;26:131–136.
40. Curtis KM, Savitz DA, Weinberg CR, et al. The effect of pesticide exposure on time to pregnancy. Epidemiology 1999;10:112–117.
41. Bisanti L, Olsen J, Basso O, et al. Shift work and fecundity: a European multicenter study. European Group on Infertility and Subfecundity. J Occup Environ Med 1996;38:352–358.
42. Nurminen T. Shift work and reproductive health. Scand J Work Environ Health 1998;24(suppl 1):28–34.
43. Fenster L, Hubbard AE, Windham GC, et al. A prospective study of work-related physical exertion and spontaneous abortion. Epidemiology 1997;8:66–74.
44. Shiverick KT, Salafia C. Cigarette smoking and pregnancy I: ovarian, uterine and placental effects. Placenta 1999;20:265–272.
45. Buck GM, Vena JE, Schisterman EF, et al. Parental consumption of contaminated sport fish from Lake Ontario and predicted fecundability. Epidemiology 2000;11:388–393.
46. Wiencke JK, Thurston SW, Kelsey KT, et al. Early age at smoking initiation and tobacco carcinogen DNA damage in the lung. J Natl Cancer Inst 1999;91:614–619.
47. Anderson D. Genetic and reproductive toxicity of butadiene and isoprene. Chem Biol Interact 2001;135–136:65–80.
48. Kaufman MH. The teratogenic effects of alcohol following exposure during pregnancy, and its influence on the chromosome constitution of the pre-ovulatory egg. Alcohol Alcohol 1997;32:113–128.
49. Khattak S, K-Moghtader G, McMartin K, et al. Pregnancy outcome following gestational exposure to organic solvents: a prospective controlled study. JAMA 1999;281:1106–1109.
50. McMartin KI, Chu M, Kopecky E, et al. Pregnancy outcome following maternal organic solvent exposure: a meta-analysis of epidemiologic studies. Am J Indus Med 1998;34:288–292.
51. Doyle P, Roman E, Beral V, et al. Spontaneous abortion in dry cleaning workers potentially exposed to perchloroethylene. Occup Environ Med 1997;848–853.
52. Arbuckle TE, Sever LE. Pesticide exposures and fetal death: a review of the epidemiologic literature. Crit Rev Toxicol 1998;28:229–270.
53. Valanis G, Vollmer WM, Steele P. Occupational exposure to antineoplastic agents: self-reported miscarriages and stillbirths among nurses and pharmacists. J Occup Environ Med 1999;41:632–638.
54. Occupational Safety and Health Administration (OSHA). Controlling occupational exposure to hazardous drugs. In: OSHA Technical Manual. OSHA Instruction CPL 2-2.20B CH-4. Washington, DC: U.S. Department of Labor, 1995:1–34.
55. Schnorr TM, Grajewski BA, Hornung RW, et al. Video display terminals and the risk of spontaneous abortion. N Engl J Med 1991;324:727–733.
56. Bove F, Shim Y, Zeitz P. Drinking water contaminants and adverse pregnancy outcomes. Environ Health Perspect 2002;110(suppl 1):61–74.
57. Korrick SA, Chen C, Damokosh AI, et al. Association of DDT with spontaneous abortion: a case-control study. Ann Epidemiol 2001;11:491–496.
58. Younglai EV, Foster WG, Hughes EG, et al. Levels of environmental contaminants in the follicular fluid, serum, and seminal plasma of couples undergoing in vitro fertilization. Arch Environ Contam Toxicol 2002;43:121–126.
59. Mazaud S, Guigon CJ, Lozach A, et al. Establishment of the reproductive function and transient fertility of female rats lacking primordial follicle stock after fetal gamma-irradiation. Endocrinology 2002;143:4775–4787.
60. Heimler I, Trewin AL, Chaffin CL, et al. Modulation of ovarian follicle maturation and effects on apoptotic cell death in Holtzman rats exposed to 2,3,7,8-tetrachlorodibenzo-o-dioxin (TCDD). Reprod Toxicol 1998;12:69–73.
61. Reinhart KC, Dubey RK, Keller PJ, et al. Xeno-oestrogens and phyto-oestrogens induce the synthesis of leukaemia inhibitory factor by human and bovine oviduct cells. Mol Hum Reprod 1999;5:899–907.
62. Rier SW. The potential role of exposure to environmental toxicants in the pathophysiology of endometriosis. Ann N Y Acad Sci 2002;955:201–212.
63. Mahyani A, Barel S, Soback S, et al. Dioxin concentrations in women with endometriosis. Hum Reprod 1997;12:373–375.
64. Pauwels A, Schepens PJ, D'Hooghe T, et al. The risk of endometriosis and exposure to dioxins and polychlorinated biphenyls: a case-control study of infertile women. Hum Reprod 2001;16:2050–2055.

65. Lebel G, Dodin S, Ayotte P, et al. Organochlorine exposure and the risk of endometriosis. Fertil Steril 1998;69:221–228.
66. Scialli AR. Tampons, dioxins, and endometriosis. Reprod Toxicol 2001;15:231–238.
67. Walker CL. Role of hormonal and reproductive factors in the etiology and treatment of uterine leiomyoma. Recent Prog Horm Res 2002;57:277–294.
68. Hunter DS, Hodges LC, Vonier PM, et al. Estrogen receptor activation via activation function 2 predicts agonism of xenoestrogens in normal and neoplastic cells of the uterine myometrium. Cancer Res 1999;59:3090–3099.
69. Schardein JL. Chemically Induced Birth Defects. 3rd ed. New York: Marcel Dekker, 2000.
70. Jacobson JL, Jacobson SW. Evidence for PCBs as neurodevelopmental toxicants in humans. Neurotoxicology 1997;18:415–424.
71. Cramer DW, Xu H. Predicting age at menopause. Maturitas 1996;23:319–326.
72. Beard J, Marshall S, Jong K, et al. 1,1,1-Tricholoro-2,2-bis (p-chlorophenyl)-ethane (DDT) and reduced bone mineral density. Arch Environ Health 2000;55:177–180.
73. Bohannon AD, Cooper GS, Wolff MS, et al. Exposure to 1,1,1-tricholoro-2,2-bis (p-chlorophenyl)-ethane (DDT) in relation to bone mineral density and rate of bone loss in menopausal women. Arch Environ Health 2000;55:386–391.
74. Sala M, Dosemeci M, Zahm SH. A death certificate-based study of occupation and mortality from reproductive cancers among women in 24 US states. J Occup Environ Med 1998;40:632–639.
75. Hartge P, Stewart P. Occupation and ovarian cancer: a case-control study in the Washington, DC, metropolitan area, 1978–1981. J Occup Med 1994;36:924–927.
76. Spinelli JJ, Gallagher RP, Band PR, et al. Multiple myeloma, leukemia and cancer of the ovary in cosmetologists and hairdressers. Am J Ind Med 1984;6:97–102.
77. Walker AH, Ross RK, Haile RW, et al. Hormonal factors and risk of ovarian germ cell cancer in young women. Br J Cancer 1988;57:418–422.
78. Ingram D, Sanders K, Kolybaba M, et al. Case-control study of phyto-oestrogens and breast cancer. Lancet 1997;350:990–994.
79. Woolcott CG, Aronson KJ, Hanna WM, et al. Organochlorines and breast cancer risk by receptor status, tumor size and grade (Canada). Cancer Causes Control 2001;12:395–404.
80. Laden F, Collman G, Iwamoto K, et al. 1,10dichloro-2,2-bis (p-chlorophenyl) ethylene and polychlorinated biphenyls and breast cancer: combined analysis of five US studies. J Natl Cancer Inst 2001;93:768–776.
81. Miller AB, Howe GR, Sherman GJ, et al. Mortality from breast cancer after irradiation during fluoroscopic examinations in patients being treated for tuberculosis. N Engl J Med 1989;321:1285–1289.
82. Khuder SA, Mutgi AB, Nugent S. Smoking and breast cancer: a meta-analysis. Rev Environ Health 2001;16: 253–261.
83. Weiderpass E, Adami HO, Baron JA, et al. Organochlorines and endometrial cancer risk. Cancer Epidemiol Biomarkers Prev 2000;9:487–493.
84. Sturgeon SR, Brock JW, Potischman N, et al. Serum concentrations of organochlorine compounds and endometrial cancer risk (United States). Cancer Causes Control 1998;9:417–424.
85. Savitz DA, Andrews KW, Brinton LA. Occupation and cervical cancer. J Occup Environ Med 1995;37:357–361.
86. Schonfelder G, Flick G, Mayr E, et al. In utero exposure to low doses of bisphenol A lead to long-term deleterious effects in the vagina. Neoplasia 2002;4:98–102.
87. Briggs GG, Freeman RK, Yaffe SJ. Drugs in Pregnancy and Lactation: A Reference Guide to Fetal and Neonatal Risk. 6th ed. Philadelphia: Lippincott Williams & Wilkins, 2002:1528–1539.

Index

Page numbers in *italic* represent figures; page numbers followed by a "t" represent tables.